Fundamentals of Periodontics

Second Edition

Fundamentals of PERIODONTICS

Second Edition

Edited by

Thomas G. Wilson, Jr, DDS
Private Practice in Periodontics and Dental Implants
Dallas, Texas

Clinical Associate Professor
Department of Periodontics
Baylor College of Dentistry
Dallas, Texas

Clinical Associate Professor
Department of Periodontics
University of Texas Health Science Center
San Antonio, Texas

Kenneth S. Kornman, DDS, PhD
Chief Scientific Officer
Interleukin Genetics
Waltham, Massachusetts

Lecturer
Harvard School of Dental Medicine
Boston, Massachusetts

Quintessence Publishing Co, Inc

Chicago, Berlin, Tokyo, Copenhagen, London, Paris, Milan, Barcelona, Istanbul, São Paulo, New Delhi, Moscow, Prague, and Warsaw

Dedications

To my wonderful sons, Trey and John. May you find your true path.
—TGW

To the incredibly dedicated teachers from whom I have received so much throughout all phases of my career: Jane Eldridge, my high school debating coach; Steve Kreitzman, my research mentor at Emory School of Dentistry; Sig Ramfjord, Harald Löe, Walter Loesche, Raul Caffesse, Klaus Lang, and Thorkild Karring, who were both periodontal teachers and colleagues; and Gordon Duff, my research colleague in inflammation genetics.
—KSK

Library of Congress Cataloging-in-Publication Data

Fundamentals of periodontics / [edited by] Thomas G. Wilson, Jr.,
Kenneth S. Kornman.—2nd ed.
      p. ; cm.
Includes bibliographical references and index.
  ISBN 0-86715-405-5 (hardcover)
  1. Periodontics. I. Wilson, Thomas G. II. Kornman, Kenneth S. [DNLM:
1. Periodontal Diseases. 2. Periodontium. WU 242 F981 2003]
RK361 .F86 2003
617.6'32—dc21

                        2002013762

quintessence
books

© 2003 Quintessence Publishing Co, Inc

Quintessence Publishing Co, Inc
551 Kimberly Drive
Carol Stream, IL 60188
www.quintpub.com

A caveat: Dentistry is a constantly changing science; our knowledge is ever expanding. This particularly applies to the procedures, instruments, and therapeutic drugs described in this book. Although the authors, editors, and publisher have made every attempt possible to ensure that the information is current and correct, it falls to the reader to verify from independent sources the information found here. This is especially true of drugs and their dosages.

Disclosure: Both of the editors have been actively involved in developing and transferring new technology into periodontics for many years. They currently have financial interests that involve subjects detailed in this text. Dr Wilson holds stock in Interleukin Genetics and receives research funding from Biora, DentalView, Interleukin Genetics, and Straumann. Dr Kornman is a shareholder, employee, and member of the Board of Directors for Interleukin Genetics.

Editor: Arinne Dickson
Production: Susan Robinson
Printed in Hong Kong

Table of Contents

Preface

This book is designed as an introduction to the science and art of periodontics for students new to the subject and for clinicians who wish to expand their knowledge. The material is organized as a guide to what must be seen and what must be done to successfully diagnose and treat periodontal diseases.

Experts in any clinical area interpret the findings from a clinical examination by means of preformed mental patterns based on published knowledge and practical experience with patients. The expert clinician therefore quickly limits the mental "search space" to focus on the important issues for each individual patient. Students have no preformed mental patterns on which to draw for guidance. They must search exhaustively through all the pieces of information they have remembered to determine which pieces apply to the specific patient.

This book has been organized to bring the experts' thought process to the student. Seeing the same flexible process applied to a variety of conditions, the student will gain not only information but a lens through which to view information. This is the beginning of the quick selectivity and judgment that is the essence of expertise.

This second edition has been extensively updated to incorporate substantial new biologic and practical knowledge of periodontal and implant dentistry that has become available since the first edition was published. In addition, the text has been clarified and many new figures have been added to make the information especially accessible to those who are new to the study of dentistry.

This book is written to be as user-friendly as possible given the complexity of the subjects covered. Part I details the knowledge needed to understand periodontal diseases and their treatment, providing essential information on the examination process and how to interpret clinical findings. Part II explains the clinical management of periodontal diseases. As in the first edition, this section first explains how to determine an initial diagnosis and uses case reports to illustrate the different disease categories and suggested therapies. Special emphasis is given to various treatment outcomes. Part III deals with restorative and esthetic dentistry as they relate to periodontal therapy. New to this edition, Part IV is designed to lead the clinician through diagnosis, placement, restoration, and maintenance of cases involving implant reconstructions.

As always, we very much appreciate the tremendous contributions made by many to our understanding of the diagnosis, prevention, and treatment of periodontal diseases. We are grateful to the outstanding scholars who synthesized these contributions into the chapters of this second edition.

Contributors

Terry B. Adams, DDS, MSD
Private Practice in Orthodontics;
Clinical Assistant Professor
Department of Graduate Orthodontics
Baylor College of Dentistry
Texas A&M University System Health Science Center
Dallas, Texas

Olav F. Alvares, BDS, MS, PhD
Associate Professor
Department of Periodontics
University of Texas Health Science Center
San Antonio, Texas

William F. Ammons, Jr, BA, DDS, MSD
Professor Emeritus
Department of Periodontics
School of Dentistry
University of Washington;
Part-Time Private Practice in Periodontics
Seattle, Washington

Gary C. Armitage, DDS, MS
R. Earl Robinson Distinguished Professor
Division of Periodontology
Department of Stomatology
School of Dentistry
University of California
San Francisco, California

Oded Bahat, BDS, MSD
Private Practice in Periodontics
Beverly Hills, California

Erwin P. Barrington, DDS, PhD
Professor of Periodontics
University of Illinois;
Private Practice in Periodontics
Chicago, Illinois

P. Mark Bartold, DDSc, PhD
Professor and Director
Colgate Australian Clinical Dental Research Center
University of Adelaide
Adelaide, Australia

James D. Beck, PhD
Professor of Dental Ecology
Center for Oral and Systemic Diseases
University of North Carolina at Chapel Hill
Chapel Hill, North Carolina

Barbara D. Boyan, PhD
Price Gilbert, Jr, Chair in Tissue Engineering
Professor
Department of Biomedical Engineering
Georgia Institute of Technology
Atlanta, Georgia;
Professor
Departments of Cell Biology and Orthopaedics
School of Medicine
Emory University
Atlanta, Georgia

Michael A. Brunsvold, DDS, MS
Associate Professor
Department of Periodontics
University of Texas Health Science Center
San Antonio, Texas

Richard F. Caudill, DMD
Private Practice in Periodontics
Tequesta, Florida

Catherine C.M.E. Champagne, PhD
Research Assistant Professor
Center for Oral and Systemic Diseases
University of North Carolina at Chapel Hill
Chapel Hill, North Carolina

David L. Cochran, DDS, PhD
Professor and Chair
Department of Periodontics
University of Texas Health Science Center
San Antonio, Texas

Jason B. Cope, DDS, PhD
Private Practice in Orthodontics;
Clinical Assistant Professor
Department of Graduate Orthodontics
Baylor College of Dentistry
Texas A&M University System Health Science Center
Dallas, Texas

David D. Dean, PhD
Professor
Department of Orthopaedics
University of Texas Health Science Center
San Antonio, Texas

Chester W. Douglass, DMD, PhD
Professor of Oral Health Policy
School of Dental Medicine;
Professor of Epidemiology
School of Public Health
Harvard University
Boston, Massachusetts

Jeffrey L. Ebersole, PhD
Alvin L. Morris Professor of Oral Health Research
Director, Center for Oral Health Research
College of Dentistry
University of Kentucky
Lexington, Kentucky

Gülnur Emingil, DDS, PhD
Associate Professor
Department of Periodontology
School of Dentistry
Ege University
Izmir, Turkey

Steven P. Engebretson, DMD, MS
Assistant Professor
Division of Periodontics
School of Dental and Oral Surgery
Columbia University
New York, New York

Neil L. Frederiksen, DDS, PhD
Professor and Director, Oral and Maxillofacial
    Radiology
Diagnostic Sciences
Baylor College of Dentistry
Texas A&M University System Health Science Center
Dallas, Texas

Tommy W. Gage
Professor and Vice Chairman
Department of Oral Surgery/Pharmacology
Baylor College of Dentistry
Texas A&M University System Health Science Center
Dallas, Texas

Michael Glick, DMD
Professor and Acting Chair
Department of Diagnostic Sciences
University of Medicine and Dentistry of New Jersey
New Jersey Dental School
Newark, New Jersey

Mark E. Glover, DDS, MSD
Private Practice in Periodontics
Dallas, Texas

Janet M. Guthmiller, DDS, PhD
Associate Professor
Department of Periodontics
College of Dentistry
University of Iowa
Iowa City, Iowa

William W. Hallmon, DMD, MS
Director, Graduate Training
Department of Periodontics
Baylor College of Dentistry
Texas A&M University System Health Science Center
Dallas, Texas

Mark Handelsman, DDS
Private Practice in Periodontics
Beverly Hills, California;
Clinical Assistant Professor
Departments of Periodontics and Implant Dentistry
School of Dentistry
University of Southern California
Los Angeles, California

Stephen K. Harrel, DDS
Clinical Associate Professor
Department of Periodontics
Baylor College of Dentistry
Texas A&M University System Health Science Center;
Private Practice in Periodontics
Dallas, Texas

Joachim S. Hermann, Dr med dent, FICOI
Assistant Professor, Head, and Postgraduate
    Program Director
Division of Periodontics
Dental School
University of Zürich
Zürich, Switzerland;
Clinical Assistant Professor
Department of Periodontics
University of Texas Health Science Center
San Antonio, Texas

Frank L. Higginbottom, DDS
Private Practice in Restorative and Implant Dentistry;
Clinical Associate Professor
Department of Restorative Dentistry and Graduate
    Prosthodontics
Baylor College of Dentistry
Texas A&M University System Health Science Center
Dallas, Texas

Palle Holmstrup, DDS, PhD, Dr Odont
Associate Director and Professor
Department of Periodontology
School of Dentistry, Health Science Faculty
University of Copenhagen
Copenhagen, Denmark

Marjorie Jeffcoat, DMD
James R. Rosen Professor of Dental Research and
    Chairman
Department of Periodontology
School of Dentistry
University of Alabama at Birmingham
Birmingham, Alabama

Bradley D. Johnson, DDS, MSD
Private Practice in Periodontics
Seattle, Washington

Kenneth L. Kalkwarf, DDS, MS
Professor of Periodontics and Dean
Dental School
University of Texas Health Science Center
San Antonio, Texas

Ira B. Lamster, DDS, MMSc
Dean
School of Dental and Oral Surgery
Columbia University
New York, New York

**Niklaus P. Lang, DMD, Prof Dr med dent,
  MS, Dr odont hc, FRCPS (Glasg)**
Professor and Chairman
Department of Periodontology and Fixed Prosthodontics
School of Dental Medicine
University of Berne
Berne, Switzerland

Burton Langer, DMD, MSD
Private Practice Limited to Periodontics and
    Oral Diagnosis
New York, New York

Laureen Langer, DDS
Private Practice Limited to Periodontics and
    Oral Diagnosis;
Associate Clinical Professor
School of Dental and Oral Surgery
Columbia University
New York, New York

Christoph H. Lohmann, MD
Assistant Professor
Department of Orthopaedics
University of Texas Health Science Center
San Antonio, Texas;
Department of Orthopaedics
University of Eppendorf
Hamburg, Germany

Dan M. Loughlin, DDS, MS
Private Practice in Periodontics
Arlington, Texas

Robert M. Loughlin, DDS
Resident
Department of Prosthodontics
University of Texas Health Science Center
San Antonio, Texas

Ingvar Magnusson, Odont Dr, DDS
Professor
Department of Oral Biology
College of Dentistry
University of Florida
Gainesville, Florida

William C. Martin, DMD, MS
Clinical Assistant Professor
Department of Prosthodontics
Center for Implant Dentistry
College of Dentistry
University of Florida
Gainesville, Florida

Michael K. McGuire, DDS
Private Practice in Periodontics;
Clinical Associate Professor
University of Texas at Houston Dental Branch
Houston, Texas;
Clinical Associate Professor
University of Texas Health Science Center
San Antonio, Texas

James T. Mellonig, DDS, MS
Professor and Director of the Specialist Division
Department of Periodontics
University of Texas Health Science Center
San Antonio, Texas

John A. Molinari, PhD
Chair
Department of Biomedical Sciences
School of Dentistry
University of Detroit Mercy
Detroit, Michigan

A. Sampath Narayanan, PhD
Research Professor
Department of Pathology
School of Medicine
University of Washington
Seattle, Washington

Steven Offenbacher
Professor and Director
Center for Oral and Systemic Diseases
University of North Carolina at Chapel Hill
Chapel Hill, North Carolina

Richard J. Oringer, DDS, DMSc
Assistant Professor
Director, Predoctoral Periodontics
Department of Periodontics
School of Dental Medicine
Stony Brook University
Stony Brook, New York

Thomas J. Pallasch, DDS, MS
Professor of Dentistry (Pharmacology and
    Periodontics)
School of Dentistry
University of Southern California
Los Angeles, California

Mark R. Patters, DDS, PhD
Professor and Chair
Department of Periodontology
College of Dentistry
University of Tennessee
Memphis, Tennessee

Terry D. Rees, DDS, MSD
Professor
Department of Periodontics
Director, Stomatology Center
Baylor College of Dentistry
Texas A&M University System Health Science Center
Dallas, Texas

Bengt G. Rosling, DDS, Dr Odont
Associate Professor
Department of Periodontology
University of Göteborg
Göteborg, Sweden;
Research Associate
Periodontal Disease Clinical Research Center
Department of Oral Biology
New York State University
Buffalo, New York

Mark I. Ryder, DMD
Division of Periodontology
Department of Stomatology
School of Dentistry
University of California
San Francisco, California

Zvi Schwartz, DMD, PhD
Professor
Department of Periodontics
Hadassah Faculty of Dental Medicine
Hebrew University
Jerusalem, Israel;
Professor
Department of Biomedical Engineering
Georgia Institute of Technology
Atlanta, Georgia

Jørgen Slots, DDS, DMD, PhD, MS, MBA
Professor
Department of Periodontology
School of Dentistry
University of Southern California
Los Angeles, California

John S. Sottosanti, DDS
Associate Professor
Department of Continuing Education
University of Southern California
Los Angeles, California;
Private Practice in Periodontics
San Diego, California

Bjorn Steffensen, DDS, MS
Associate Professor
Department of Periodontics
University of Texas Health Science Center
San Antonio, Texas

Ray C. Williams, DMD
Chair
Department of Periodontology
School of Dentistry
University of North Carolina at Chapel Hill
Chapel Hill, North Carolina

Richard D. Wilson, DDS, FACD, FICD
Private Practice in General Dentistry;
Clinical Professor
Department of Periodontics
School of Dentistry
Virginia Commonwealth University
Richmond, Virginia

John M. Wright, DDS, MS
Professor and Director of Pathology
Baylor College of Dentistry
Texas A&M University System Health Science Center
Dallas, Texas

Samuel J. Zeichner, DMD, MA, MS(Hyg)
Director of Oral and Maxillofacial Radiology
The Maxillofacial Radiology Center
New York, New York;
Associate Professor
Department of Oral Pathology, Biology, and
    Diagnostic Science
University of Medicine and Dentistry of New Jersey
Newark, New Jersey

Basic Terms and Classification of Diseases

As we learn more about the nature and pathogenesis of periodontal diseases, changes in nomenclature become necessary. Such changes often lead to confusion and misunderstanding. To minimize these problems, definitions of key terms used in this book, along with other relevant terminology, are provided below. The most recent classification of periodontal diseases is provided as well.

Gingivitis

Plaque-induced gingivitis (also called *chronic gingivitis*): That form of the disease that is *primarily* plaque associated and will resolve completely when plaque is removed on a regular basis.

Other forms of gingivitis (those forms other than chronic, known by various names): Although plaque is often an aggravating factor in these conditions, the inflammation is not completely resolved by plaque removal.

Periodontitis

Chronic periodontitis

- *Chronic periodontitis with early attachment loss:* These patients have 4- to 6-mm probing depths, with the free gingival margin at or slightly coronal to the cementoenamel junction and no furcation invasion.
- *Chronic periodontitis with moderate attachment loss:* Patients with 4- to 6-mm probing depths, with the free gingival margin at or slightly coronal to the cementoenamel junction and frequently Class 1 or 2 furcation invasion.
- *Recurrent periodontitis* (also called *relapsing periodontitis*): Chronic periodontitis that was never in remission due to inadequate removal of local factors by either the patient or the therapist.

Aggressive forms of periodontitis

- *Localized aggressive periodontitis in a juvenile:* May begin around puberty; severe disease localized to molars and incisors with minimal periodontitis in other sites; minimal plaque and inflammation may be evident clinically.
- *Generalized aggressive periodontitis in a juvenile:* May begin around puberty; generally involves severe disease around molars, incisors, and premolars; thought to follow localized aggressive periodontitis; if seen in the primary dentition, it is likely that there are systemic diseases that have compromised host defenses.
- *Generalized aggressive periodontitis in an adult/Chronic periodontitis with severe generalized attachment loss:* Severe generalized bone loss and attachment loss; 7-mm or greater probing depths are evident in many sites; there may be evidence of rapid bone loss with periods of exacerbation or remission.
- *Refractory periodontitis:* Periodontitis in which further loss of attachment continues or recurs following thorough removal of local factors by the therapist and the patient.
- *Periodontitis associated with systemic disease* (such as HIV and diabetes; usually seen in adults)

All of these conditions can be additionally classified as treated or untreated, arrested or active, and may be seen alone or in various combinations.

CLASSIFICATION OF PERIODONTAL DISEASES AND CONDITIONS*

I. Gingival Diseases

A. Dental plaque–induced gingival diseases
  1. Gingivitis associated with dental plaque only
    a. without other local contributing factors
    b. with local contributing factors
  2. Gingival diseases modified by systemic factors
    a. associated with the endocrine system
      1) puberty-associated gingivitis
      2) menstrual cycle–associated gingivitis
      3) pregnancy-associated
        a) gingivitis
        b) pyogenic granuloma
      4) diabetes mellitus–associated gingivitis
    b. associated with blood dyscrasias
      1) leukemia-associated gingivitis
      2) other
  3. Gingival diseases modified by medications
    a. drug-influenced gingival diseases
      1) drug-influenced gingival enlargements
      2) drug-influenced gingivitis
        a) oral contraceptive–associated gingivitis
        b) other
  4. Gingival diseases modified by malnutrition
    a. ascorbic acid–deficiency gingivitis
    b. other

B. Non–plaque-induced gingival lesions
  1. Gingival diseases of specific bacterial origin
    a. *Neisseria gonorrhea*–associated lesions
    b. *Treponema pallidum*–associated lesions
    c. streptococcal species–associated lesions
    d. other
  2. Gingival diseases of viral origin
    a. herpesvirus infections
      1) primary herpetic gingivostomatitis
      2) recurrent oral herpes
      3) varicella-zoster infections
    b. other

3. Gingival diseases of fungal origin
  a. *Candida* species infections
    1) generalized gingival candidosis
  b. linear gingival erythema
  c. histoplasmosis
  d. other
4. Gingival lesions of genetic origin
  a. hereditary gingival fibromatosis
  b. other
5. Gingival manifestations of systemic conditions
  a. mucocutaneous disorders
    1) lichen planus
    2) pemphigoid
    3) pemphigus vulgaris
    4) erythema multiforme
    5) lupus erythematosus
    6) drug-induced
    7) other
  b. allergic reactions
    1) dental restorative materials
      a) mercury
      b) nickel
      c) acrylic
      d) other
    2) reactions attributable to
      a) toothpastes/dentifrices
      b) mouthrinses/mouthwashes
      c) chewing gum additives
      d) foods and additives
    3) other
6. Traumatic lesions (factitious, iatrogenic, accidental)
  a. chemical injury
  b. physical injury
  c. thermal injury
7. Foreign body reactions
8. Not otherwise specified (NOS)

continued

*From the American Academy of Periodontology. See *Annals of Periodontology*, volume 4, 1999.

II. Chronic Periodontitis
A. Localized
B. Generalized

III. Aggressive Periodontitis
A. Localized
B. Generalized

IV. Periodontitis as a Manifestation of Systemic Diseases
A. Associated with hematological disorders
  1. Acquired neutropenia
  2. Leukemias
  3. Other
B. Associated with genetic disorders
  1. Familial and cyclic neutropenia
  2. Down syndrome
  3. Leukocyte adhesion deficiency syndromes
  4. Papillon-Lefèvre syndrome
  5. Chediak-Higashi syndrome
  6. Histiocytosis syndromes
  7. Glycogen storage disease
  8. Infantile genetic agranulocytosis
  9. Cohen syndrome
  10. Ehlers-Danlos syndrome (Types IV and VII)
  11. Hypophosphatasia
  12. Other
C. Not otherwise specified (NOS)

V. Necrotizing Periodontal Diseases
A. Necrotizing ulcerative gingivitis (NUG)
B. Necrotizing ulcerative periodontitis (NUP)

VI. Abscesses of the Periodontium
A. Gingival abscess
B. Periodontal abscess
C. Pericoronal abscess

VII. Periodontitis Associated with Endodontic Lesions
A. Combined periodontic-endodontic lesions

VIII. Developmental or Acquired Deformities and Conditions
A. Localized tooth-related factors that modify or predispose to plaque-induced gingival diseases/periodontitis
  1. Tooth anatomic factors
  2. Dental restoration/appliances
  3. Root fractures
  4. Cervical root resorption and cemental tears
B. Mucogingival deformities and conditions around teeth
  1. Gingival/soft tissue recession
    a. facial or lingual surfaces
    b. interproximal (papillary)
  2. Lack of keratinized gingiva
  3. Decreased vestibular depth
  4. Aberrant frenum/muscle position
  5. Gingival excess
    a. pseudopocket
    b. inconsistent gingival margin
    c. excessive gingival display
    d. gingival enlargement
  6. Abnormal color
C. Mucogingival deformities and conditions on edentulous ridges
  1. Vertical and/or horizontal ridge deficiency
  2. Lack of gingiva/keratinized tissue
  3. Gingival/soft tissue enlargement
  4. Aberrant frenum/muscle position
  5. Decreased vestibular depth
  6. Abnormal color
D. Occlusal trauma
  1. Primary occlusal trauma
  2. Secondary occlusal trauma

Part I

Essential Information for Clinical Decision Making

The Pathogenesis of Periodontitis

Kenneth S. Kornman
- General Patterns
- Details of Pathogenesis
- Are All Patients the Same?
- Interrelationships of Pathogenic Mechanisms
- Biochemical and Cellular Steps in Pathogenesis
- Disease Progression Versus Disease Control

Periodontitis is a bacterially induced chronic inflammatory disease. This simple definition describes the complexity of the elements that must be considered to understand the clinical management of periodontitis. Bacteria "cause" the disease, yet the biochemical destruction that leads to clinical signs of disease is the result of the chronic inflammatory processes in the periodontal tissues. This chapter describes the general elements in the pathogenesis of periodontal disease, and subsequent chapters contain detailed discussions of the biology of specific elements.

Pathogenesis is the sequence of events leading to a clinically detectable disease. We know that at the clinically observable level of periodontitis, bacterial accumulations lead to inflammatory changes in the periodontal tissues (Fig 1-1). The inflammation, if uncontrolled, leads to clinically detectable loss of connective tissue attachment and bone.

To understand the pathogenesis of periodontitis, we must explore how bacterial accumulations on the teeth lead to clinical signs of disease. The study of this process proceeds by adding successive levels of detail to Fig 1-1.

The pathogenesis of all chronic diseases is complex because the time frame allows for many varied individual patient responses. On the clinical level, it is usually possible to describe the pathogenic events of most chronic diseases. In addition, histologic analyses of the tissues involved provide a description of cellular and tissue differences for different clinical states of the disease. Investigators then use these histologic observations as landmarks to speculate on the biochemical and cellular pathways involved in the development and progression of disease.

This chapter provides an overview of the pathogenic events involved in periodontal disease. The description of the integrated sequence of events in periodontitis, although mostly hypothetical, is based on strong data for specific elements in periodontal disease and other related diseases. The pathogenesis of periodontal disease has been reviewed in detail in the literature.[1] Specific mechanisms that contribute to it are described in detail in chapters on the microbiology (chapter 5), inflammatory response (chapter 9), immune response (chapter 8), connective tissue metabolism (chapter 6), and bone metabolism (chapter 7) associated with periodontal diseases.

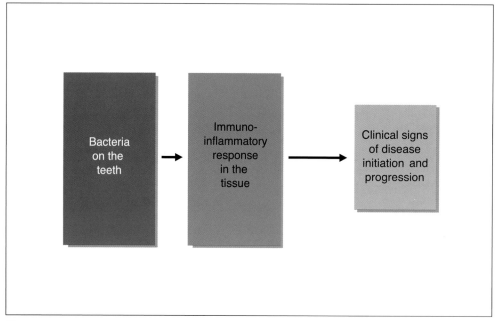

Fig 1-1 In periodontal disease, the biologic conditions in the tissues of each host are activated by the bacterial challenge to produce the pathology and clinical signs of disease.

General Patterns

Describing Periodontitis to the Patient

We must be able to describe to the patient what we know about how periodontitis develops. This is obviously not a discussion of either biochemistry or molecular biology but rather a description of basic principles.

Start by defining the clinical outcome of periodontitis (Fig 1-1), and then explain that periodontitis is the destruction of gingival tissue and bone that support the teeth. If untreated, this destruction leads to loose teeth, and ultimately the teeth will be lost. Next, briefly describe the central process involved in periodontal disease (Fig 1-2). Bacterial accumulation on the teeth causes inflammation in the gingival tissues. The inflammation destroys the gingival tissue and bone. This is similar to how arthritis, another inflammatory disease, causes destruction of the tissue and bone of the joints.

Finally, explain that when bacteria accumulate on the teeth, the amount of inflammation in the tissues and the amount of destruction of bone and gingival tissue differs widely among patients. We know that both genetic factors and acquired factors (such as smoking) modify the body's responses to the bacteria (Fig 1-3). Therefore, the severity of disease in an individual patient is the combined effect of the bacterial accumulations and the body's responses to the bacteria.

Describing Periodontal Disease to a Physician or Researcher in Another Field

The next level of detail, shown in Fig 1-4, may be useful in discussing periodontal disease with individuals who are more knowledgeable about biology and medicine than the typical patient. At this level we can describe the primary biologic mechanisms of the disease and explain how poor oral hygiene leads to bacterial accumulation and periodontal disease:

1. Certain products from the bacteria that accumulate on the teeth enter the gingival tissues and initiate immuno-inflammatory processes. Small-molecular-weight bacterial products enter the tissues first and increase tissue permeability to allow larger-molecular-weight bacterial antigens and lipopolysaccharides (LPS) to enter the tissue.
2. The tissue responds by recruiting white blood cells to the local area to fight the bacterial challenge. One key cell involved in the local fight is the polymorphonuclear leukocyte (PMN). Large numbers of PMNs rush through the gingiva into the gingival sulcus, where the bacteria are located. Other lymphocytes recruited to the area produce antibodies to help with the bacterial fight.

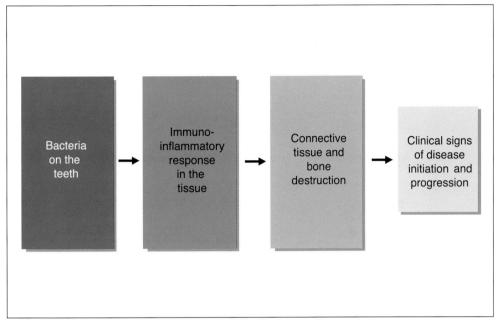

Fig 1-2 Bacteria on the teeth cause inflammation in the gingival tissues. Some of the chemicals involved in inflammation destroy gingival tissue and bone.

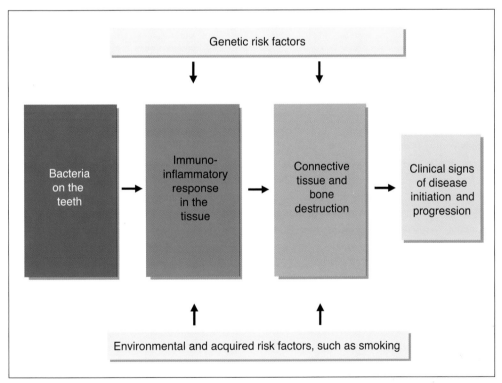

Fig 1-3 When bacteria activate inflammation in the tissues, the amount of inflammation and the severity of destruction of connective tissue and bone differs widely among patients. This variability in disease expression is the result of genetic and acquired (eg, smoking) factors that modify the body's response to bacteria.

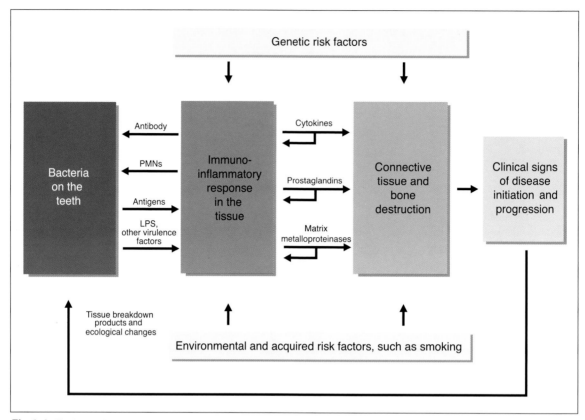

Fig 1-4 The bacteria activate the immunoinflammatory responses by means of antigens, LPS, and other products. The host attempts to control the bacteria by means of PMNs and antibodies. Many chemicals are produced in the tissues as part of the immunoinflammatory response. Three groups of those chemicals—cytokines, prostaglandins, and matrix metallopro- teinases—are involved in the protection against bacteria but also lead to destruction of connective tissues and bone, which support the teeth.

3. When the lymphocytes enter the gingiva and are acti- vated to fight the bacteria, they produce several chem- icals to coordinate the battle. The most important chemicals in periodontal disease are cytokines, prosta- glandins, and matrix metalloproteinases (MMPs). All these products are critical to inducing inflammation in the tissues. The same chemicals activate destruction of bone and connective tissues that support the teeth.

Details of Pathogenesis

The pathogenesis of plaque-induced gingivitis is relatively well defined. Bacterial accumulations initiate vascular changes typical of acute inflammatory reactions. This re- sults in a vascular leakage of fluid and active migration of PMNs, or neutrophils, out of the vessels into the tissues and into the gingival sulcus. There are also early losses of collagen just apical to the junctional epithelium. These changes are initiated within hours of plaque accumula- tion. Within days, lymphocytes accumulate adjacent to the junctional epithelium, and fibroblasts in the area begin to show morphologic changes. Some proliferation of epi-

thelial cells is evident at this time, and collagen destruc- tion becomes more noticeable. The chronic gingivitis state is limited to the tissues closely adjacent to the sulcular and junctional epithelium. By definition, gingivitis does not in- clude activation of osteoclastic activity beyond that ob- served with normal bone remodeling, nor does it include apical migration of the junctional epithelium. Details of the histologic findings in gingivitis have been described by Page and Schroeder.[2]

The pathogenesis of periodontitis is reasonably clear at a clinical and microscopic level, but the details of spe- cific mechanisms are still being defined. The pathogene- sis of periodontitis, as currently understood, will be de- scribed in terms of the distinct categories of mechanisms depicted in Fig 1-3. Although it is valuable for discussion purposes to divide the mechanisms into discrete cate- gories, it is important to recognize that most of the factors are interrelated.

At each stage of disease progression (Fig 1-4) many cells are producing various chemicals. The details of each stage are described in subsequent chapters. Only the key elements of the pathogenesis are described in this chapter.

Plaque Bacteria Needed in Initiation and Progression of Periodontitis

Clinical studies have proven that bacterial accumulations on the teeth are necessary to initiate the processes that lead to periodontitis. If bacteria are removed on a regular basis, the tissue-destructive mechanisms are not activated. If periodontitis has already developed, bacterial removal and regular cleaning are necessary to halt the disease and allow the tissue to heal. It is clear that some bacteria attaching to the teeth are associated with gingival health. After dental cleaning, the bacteria that are early colonizers on the teeth are compatible with health. As the plaque ecosystem matures, due to incomplete and inconsistent cleaning, gram-negative anaerobic bacteria become more prominent. Extensive data implicate the following bacteria in the initiation and progression of periodontitis: *Porphyromonas gingivalis*, *Bacteroides forsythus*, and *Actinobacillus actinomycetemcomitans*.

Bacteria Activate Host Immunoinflammatory Responses

Bacteria and their products interact with the junctional epithelium, and the bacterial products penetrate into the underlying connective tissue. As the bacteria accumulate, low-molecular-weight soluble products, such as amines and hydrogen sulfide, easily pass through the intact epithelium and initiate early inflammatory changes in the tissues. Larger chemotactic products from the bacteria enter the tissue and activate adhesion molecules on the small blood vessels just beneath the junctional epithelium and on the inflammatory and immune cells circulating in the blood. This process results in a staged and sequential influx of different cell populations, beginning with PMNs and followed by macrophages and lymphocytes.

There is a very large increase in the number of leukocytes, especially neutrophils, migrating through the junctional epithelium, through the connective tissue, and into the sulcus or pocket. The collagen and other components of the extracellular matrix around the small blood vessels in the area are destroyed. If the bacterial challenge remains, the junctional epithelium proliferates, extends apically along the root surface, and subsequently is converted into an ulcerated pocket epithelium.

T cells, macrophages, and neutrophils are all present and activated, although the histologic lesion becomes dominated by B cells. The activated B cells differentiate into antibody-producing plasma cells. The full expression of the inflammatory and immune responses in the periodontal tissues appears to be controlled locally, because local antibody patterns in the gingival tissue of periodontitis patients are distinctly different from systemic patterns.

With chronic, prolonged inflammation and exposure to endotoxins, some immune mechanisms start to shut down or malfunction.

Potential for Destruction

As in any chronic inflammation, in periodontitis a wide variety of host-destructive mechanisms assist in both the inflammatory and wound-healing processes. Because the inflammation is allowed to persist chronically, it has the potential to be very destructive. In the periodontium, connective tissue is destroyed by enzymes such as collagenases from PMNs and fibroblasts. Bone destruction is activated by cytokines and inflammatory mediators such as interleukin 1β (IL-1β) and prostaglandin E_2 (PGE_2). As these processes occur, the epithelial cells in the junctional epithelium are migrating in an apical direction, as a result of cell proliferation activated by the inflammatory process and loss of collagen fibers that inhibit epithelial migration. The destructive changes are most likely the result of products from a specific subset of bacteria with great potential to activate many of the body's destructive mechanisms (see chapter 5).

Different Bacteria Produce Different Products

Although bacteria produce low-molecular-weight compounds, such as hydrogen sulfide and butyrate, that are capable of inducing some of the early signs of inflammation, the chronic signs of periodontitis, including inflammation, loss of collagen, and loss of bone, are primarily the result of bacterial products entering the tissues and activating inflammatory and immune processes that result in bone and connective tissue destruction. Although some bacteria found in the subgingival plaque are capable of producing enzymes that destroy collagen, the primary collagenase activity in the periodontium appears to be due to the MMPs, enzymes released from PMNs, macrophages, and fibroblasts. In addition, although LPS from subgingival bacteria is capable of directly activating bone resorption in tissue culture systems, the same LPS activates many other host mechanisms that appear to be primarily responsible for the bone destruction seen in periodontitis.

Very little is known about the processes that initiate a shift from chronic gingivitis to progressing periodontitis. One may speculate on mechanisms that may alter either the bacterial challenge or the host defenses. For example, substantial microbial shifts may occur even in very stable complex ecosystems. Subtle changes in bacterial populations may lead to sufficient drift in the surface characteristics of a particular species, causing a temporary disadvantage for the host. Because some specific protective mechanisms—for example, antibodies—may be less efficient against changes on the bacterial surfaces, there may be short-term changes in the body's ability to control certain bacterial populations. Likewise, several factors are known to dramatically influence host defenses on a transient or prolonged basis. For example, transient viral infections, psychologic stress, and chemical stresses such as smoking have been shown to produce significant alterations in the immune response.

Several potential bacterial pathogens are routinely found in a chronically balanced state. These include *Porphyromonas gingivalis,* certain types of *Prevotella intermedia, Bacteroides forsythus, Actinobacillus actinomycetemcomitans, Fusobacterium nucleatum,* and several others. These bacteria produce factors that activate processes destructive to host tissue, as well as factors that interfere with host defense mechanisms.

Are All Patients the Same?

Although the above processes describe the pathogenesis of chronic periodontitis in many patients, modifications in one or more of these steps appear to be involved in shifting a patient to a disease that is more aggressive and less predictable in its response to therapy. Approximately 7% to 13% of the adult population in industrialized countries have generalized severe periodontitis. For example, in patients with diabetes, periodontitis may take on an aggressive nature that is most likely the result of altered immune response, wound healing, and connective tissue metabolism. More subtle changes are likely to be the basis for many of the severe cases seen in practice.

The clinical condition at any time is a function of the destructive and repair processes in the tissues; therefore, relatively minor differences in some biochemical pathways may produce substantial differences in clinical disease over time. Certain medical conditions, such as diabetes, and lifestyle factors, such as smoking, influence the function of multiple biochemical pathways. Within the range of "normal" biology, there are also substantial and common genetic differences in certain key biochemical pathways.

Interrelationships of Pathogenic Mechanisms

The bacteria in the subgingival area form a complex ecosystem. In turn, that ecosystem is influenced by the adjacent tissues. The bacteria secrete products that enter the tissue and initiate inflammation, including vascular leakage, and tissue destruction. Tissue factors that were activated by the bacteria then leak out into the sulcus area, where the bacteria reside, and many of these tissue factors become nutrients or cell modifiers for the bacteria. For example, it has long been known that in shigella bacterial infections, the gut epithelial cells become activated when shigella cells attach to them. The activated epithelial cells release cytokines as part of the host response. It has been determined recently that the shigella cells actually use the epithelial cytokines as the signaling mechanism to convert into microbial cells with the ability to invade the tissue.[3] This demonstrates that it is not possible to think of the biology of the bacterial mass on mucous membranes without considering integration with the host.

Biochemical and Cellular Steps in Pathogenesis

Early Steps

Bacteria that are early colonizers of the tooth surface are usually found adjacent to the healthy gingival margin. These bacteria include gram-positive facultative streptococci and *Actinomyces* sp, gram-negative capnophilic *Capnocytophaga* sp, and the gram-negative anaerobes *Fusobacterium nucleatum* and *Prevotella intermedia.*[4]

The microbial mass releases large quantities of metabolites, which may diffuse through the junctional epithelium. These metabolites may include fatty acids, such as butyric acid and propionic acid, that are toxic to the tissues; peptides of the N-formyl-1-methionyl-1-leucyl-1-phenylalanine (FMLP) type, which are potent chemoattractants for leukocytes; and the LPSs of gram-negative bacteria. Several other products of periodontal bacteria have been shown to activate various host mechanisms, but their relative importance in the disease process is unknown.[5] These chemicals cross the junctional epithelium and enter the tissues. At the same time, they activate the junctional epithelial cells to produce proinflammatory mediators, including IL-1, IL-8, PGE_2, and MMPs, as further signals to connective tissue; these substances can traverse the junctional epithelium and enter the connective tissues.[6] It is via this mechanism that gingival vessels become inflamed and leukocytes are guided to the location of the microbial plaque. As serum begins to leak out of the superficial blood vessels, LPS can also activate the complement cascade via the indirect pathway, as well as induce the production of kinins, all of which can act on the blood vessels and their endothelial cells.

Biochemical and Cellular Steps in Pathogenesis

Epithelium: An Early Signaling Mechanism and Barrier

In addition to providing a protective barrier and a rapid cell turnover, which leads to constant shedding of the mucosal surface exposed to bacterial colonization, mucosal epithelia also play a crucial role in intraepithelial recruitment of phagocytes and specific lymphocyte subsets and thus in the control of bacterial penetration through the mucosal integuments.[7] Keratinocytes may play an active role in this process. This finding is not unexpected, because keratinocytes represent the interface between the body and the external environment exposed to bacterial challenges. Substantial evidence indicates that keratinocytes can respond to a variety of bacterial stimuli via the production of a wide array of proinflammatory mediators, and of cytokines in particular.[8,9] Such ability to "sense" the external environment and to respond with the generation of specific autocrine and paracrine messages has been confirmed in a series of in vitro investigations on mucosal and cutaneous keratinocyte cultures. Emerging evidence indicates that interaction between periodontal bacteria and keratinocytes leads to keratinocyte activation to express a variety of inflammatory mediators.[10] These stimuli may act locally to transmit the inflammatory message in a centripetal direction toward the subepithelial microvessels, and therefore induce an inflammatory reaction.

IL-8 messenger RNA was found to be present in gingival tissue and was localized primarily to the junctional epithelium.[11–13] This localization may play a role in directing neutrophils to the gingival sulcus area. In addition, epithelial cells in general are known to produce a broad range of cytokines, including IL-1α, IL-1β, granulocyte-macrophage colony-stimulating factor (GM-CSF), interferon β (IFN-β), tumor necrosis factor α (TNF-α), transforming growth factor β (TGF-β), IL-3, IL-6, IL-7, IL-8, IL-10, IL-11, and IL-12.[7,9,14–20] The cytokines produced by the responding epithelial cells are also known to activate adhesion molecules on endothelial cells and cytokine production by endothelial cells.

Selective Accumulation of Inflammatory Cells in Gingival Tissues

Although most PMNs recruited into the gingival tissues emigrate out into the gingival sulcus, the majority of the mononuclear cells persist in the perivascular connective tissue and form the local inflammatory infiltrate. Specific mononuclear cell phenotypes are selectively recruited to the local site. Specific chemokines produced within the inflammatory infiltrate, such as the monocyte chemotactic protein-1 (MCP-1), have been suggested as partly responsible for the spatial demarcation of the area of leukocyte in-

filtration.[21] Initial evidence seems to indicate that specific lymphocyte clones may selectively home into the gingiva.[22] The molecular basis of this selectivity is largely unknown; locally processed antigens presented with class II molecules on the endoluminal aspect of endothelial cells may be a mechanism able to selectively enrich cells committed to periodontal bacteria.

Activation of Local Tissue Mononuclear Cells That Shape Local Immune Response

Soon after the initiation of the acute inflammatory response, small lymphocytes consisting of both T cells and B cells predominate in the tissue infiltrate. The B cells are driven to differentiate into clones of antibody-producing plasma cells.

With a bacterial challenge, the macrophage is activated through surface receptors that influence the antigen-specific immune response that will directly target the pathogen. Macrophages exposed to LPS produce several cytokines,[23] including IFN-γ,[24] TNF-α,[25] TGF-β,[26] IL-1α, IL-β,[15,27] IL-6,[28,29] IL-10,[30,31] IL-12,[32,33] and IL-15[34]; the chemokines MCP, macrophage inflammatory protein, and RANTES; MMPs; and PGE$_2$. Some of the factors from monocytes (in particular, IL-1β, TNF-α, and PGE$_2$) are prominent components of the periodontitis lesion and have been strongly implicated in the pathogenesis of periodontal diseases (for review, see Offenbacher[35]).

The macrophage products substantially alter the local environment in several ways:

1. The macrophages in the gingival area produce chemokines[36] that recruit additional monocytes and lymphocytes into the local area.
2. The factors produced by activated macrophages, such as PGE$_2$, MMPs, and various cytokines, alter the environment to favor collagen degradation.
3. Antigen-specific T lymphocytes are activated by interactions with the macrophages and differentiate to cytokine-producing T cells that provide help for B-cell differentiation and antibody production.

Inflammatory Mediators Prominent in Gingival Tissues

The events that make up the pathogenesis of periodontitis are initiated, driven, and regulated by mediators of the inflammatory process. They are known to be major participants in acute and chronic inflammation, regardless of its location, and there is strong evidence for participation of these mediators in periodontitis. They are produced by activated resident gingival cells and infiltrating leukocytes, as well as by the complement cascade and kinin system in blood plasma. Monocytes from individuals who are susceptible to or who have severe periodontitis produce elevated amounts of mediators,[37] and elevated concentrations of mediators are present in inflamed gingiva and gingival crevicular fluid from diseased sites.[38] Concentrations decrease following successful therapy.

IL-1 is a major mediator in periodontitis.[39–41] IL-1β comes mostly from activated macrophages and PMNs and IL-1α, from keratinocytes of the junctional or pocket epithelium. Production is induced by LPS and other bacterial components and by IL-1, which is autostimulatory. Production is suppressed by bacterial metabolites such as butyric acid and propionic acid, as well as by IL-1 receptor antagonist, which is also produced by macrophages.

IL-1 upregulates complement and Fc receptors on neutrophils and monocytic cells, along with adhesion molecules on fibroblasts and leukocytes. It induces homing receptors for lymphoid cells in the extracellular matrix and induces osteoclast formation and bone resorption. It enhances production of itself, MMPs, and prostaglandins by macrophages, fibroblasts, and neutrophils. IL-1 upregulates major histocompatibility complex expression by B cells and T cells to facilitate their activation, clonal expansion, and immunoglobulin (Ig) production. In conjunction with TNF-α and IL-6, IL-1 induces the production of acute-phase proteins by the liver.

IL-2, IL-3, IL-4, and IL-5 are involved in lymphocyte clonal expansion and the differentiation of B cells into antibody-producing plasma cells. IL-2 is produced by T cells and antigen-presenting cells and, in the presence of antigen, induces expression of clones of specific T cells and secretion of IL-3 and IL-4. IL-4 regulates IgG1 and IgE production and suppresses activated macrophages and causes their apoptosis. IL-6 is produced by macrophages, fibroblasts, lymphocytes, and endothelial cells. Production is induced by IL-1 and LPS.

The major sources of prostaglandins and leukotrienes in inflamed periodontal tissues are the activated macrophage and PMN, although they can also be produced by other cells, such as fibroblasts. Prostaglandins, especially PGE_2, make up the primary pathway of alveolar bone destruction in periodontitis. Leukotrienes, especially LTB-4, are potent chemoattractants for neutrophils. Endothelial cells activated by cytokines or LPS secrete another bioactive lipid known as platelet-activating factor, which induces vasodilation and platelet aggregation and degranulation.

The MMPs make up a large family of zinc ($Zn++$) dependent enzymes produced by macrophages, fibroblasts, and keratinocytes activated by LPS or cytokines. MMPs collectively can digest all the components of the extracellular matrix. Production of these enzymes is tightly controlled, complex, and not well understood. Transcription

is upregulated by IL-1, TGF-α, epidermal growth factor, and TGF-β. With some exceptions, transcription is downregulated by TGF-β and IFN-γ. MMP activity is suppressed by tissue inhibitors of metalloproteinases (TIMPs), which are also produced by macrophages.

Activation of Local Antibody Response

As the bacterial challenge increases, protection of the host tissues is achieved by PMN activity in the sulcus, facilitated by a specific antibody that is produced systemically and in the local tissues. Circulating antibody may be more abundant and important than locally produced antibody. Most, although not all, patients with aggressive or chronic periodontitis mount a systemic humoral immune response to antigens of the infecting bacteria.[42] This response probably results from the access of subgingival plaque bacteria and bacteria cell wall components to local lymph nodes and, through the circulation, to the spleen. Antibody titers can be remarkably high, although biologic activity is often low, as measured by antibody avidity and capacity to opsonize and enhance phagocytosis and killing. Specific antibody from the blood makes up a major portion of the specific antibody in gingival crevicular fluid.[43,44] The local antibody response is directed by the cytokine profile within the tissues and the presentation of antigens by professional antigen-presenting cells, such as the macrophage.

Studies of the antibody response in subjects without periodontitis found that individuals with low antibody titers tended to have high antibody avidity and opsonic ability, suggesting that the antibody response is capable of providing protective functions in healthy subjects with gingivitis.[45] This is also consistent with the finding that antibody from gingivitis subjects recognized fewer specific *P gingivalis* epitopes than antibody from periodontitis subjects.[46]

Disease Progression Versus Disease Control

The local cellular and humoral responses described above appear to be sufficiently competent in most individuals to control a limited bacterial challenge. In at least two conditions, it appears that the routine host response becomes more destructive at the local level. The first condition appears to involve a specific bacterial biomass that directly inhibits key components of the host defense mechanism. Some subgingival biomasses and the specific bacteria that accumulate in those ecosystems are capable of interfering with PMN function in multiple ways. There is also reason to believe that certain bacterial challenges are capable of shifting the T-cell and B-cell responses to result in less effective antibody. Selected periodontal bacteria produce proteases that cleave the Fc regions of IgG or degrade the C3 component of the complement, thereby interfering with phagocytosis and killing.[47–49]

The second factor that may result in a more destructive response to the bacterial challenge is host response modifiers, such as smoking, systemic disease, and genetic variations. In general, these appear to predispose the individual to a more destructive response.

With a chronic bacterial challenge, the periodontal tissues are continuously exposed to specific bacterial components that have the ability to alter many local cell functions. The tissues are populated with T lymphocytes and macrophages that are producing selective subsets of cytokines and prostanoids that favor net loss of collagen and bone, as well as less effective antibody production. The efficiency of PMN migration is reduced, and it is likely that more PMNs are activated within the tissue. The total impact of the above changes is to subtly shift the scene from one in which the host is controlling the bacterial challenge to one in which the challenge is less well controlled and the tissue-destructive phase dominates. Factors such as smoking and genetic influences on cytokine expression, which are capable of modifying critical aspects of the PMN-antibody protection and/or fibroblast function, alter the protective-destructive balance of the systems.

References

1. Page RC, Kornman KS (eds). The pathogenesis of human periodontitis. Periodontol 2000 1997;14:1–248.
2. Page RC, Schroeder HE. Pathogenesis of inflammatory periodontal disease: A summary of current work. Lab Invest 1976; 34:235.
3. Sansonetti PJ. Rupture, invasion and inflammatory destruction of the intestinal barrier by Shigella, making sense of prokaryote-eukaryote cross-talks. FEMS Microbiol Rev 2001;25:3–14.
4. Listgarten MA. The structure of dental plaque. Periodontol 2000 1994;5:52–65.
5. Watanabe K, Hagen KL, Andersen BR. CD11b expression on neutrophils in human crevicular fluid collected from clinically healthy gingivae. J Periodontal Res 1991;26:91–96.
6. Abe T, Hara Y, Aono M. Penetration, clearance and retention of antigen en route from the gingival sulcus to the draining lymph node of rats. J Periodontal Res 1991;26:429–439.
7. Sundqvist GK, Carlsson J, Herrmann BF, et al. Degradation in vivo of the C3 protein of guinea-pig complement by a pathogenic strain of *Bacteroides gingivalis*. Scand J Dent Res 1984; 92:14–24.
8. Kupper TS. The activated keratinocyte: A model for inducible cytokine production by non-bone marrow-derived cells in cutaneous inflammatory and immune responses [review]. J Invest Dermatol 1990;94(suppl 6):146S–150S.
9. Spertini O, Kansas GS, Munro JM, et al. Regulation of leukocyte migration by activation of the leukocyte adhesion molecule-1 (LAM-1) selectin. Nature 1991;349:691–694.
10. Fiero D, Langkamp H, Piesco N, et al. Characterization of human oral epithelial cell immune response [abstract 1116]. J Dent Res 1995;74:540.
11. Fitzgerald JE, Kreutzer DL. Localization of interleukin-8 in human gingival tissues. Oral Microbiol Immunol 1995;10: 297–303.
12. Temeles DS, McGrath HE, Kittler EL, et al. Cytokine expression from bone marrow derived macrophages. Exp Hematol 1993; 21:388–393.
13. Tonetti MS, Gerber L, Lang NP. Vascular adhesion molecules and initial development of inflammation in clinically healthy human keratinized mucosa around teeth and osseointegrated implants. J Periodontal Res 1994;29:386–392.
14. Campochiaro PA. Cytokine production by retinal pigmented epithelial cells. Int Rev Cytol 1993;146:75–82.
15. Durum SK, Schmidt JA, Oppenheim JJ. IL-1: An immunological perspective. Annu Rev Immunol 1985;3:263.
16. Elias JA, Zheng T, Einarsson O, et al. Epithelial interleukin-11: Regulation by cytokines, respiratory syncytial virus, and retinoic acid. J Biol Chem 1994;269:22261–22268.
17. Friedman RM. Interferons. In: Oppenheim JJ, Shevach EM (eds). Textbook of Immunophysiology. New York: Oxford, 1988:194.
18. Hedges S, Agace W, Svensson M, et al. Uroepithelial cells are part of a mucosal cytokine network. Infect Immun 1994;62: 3215–3221.
19. Kirnbauer R, Koch A, Schwartz T, et al. IFN-beta 2, B cell differentiation factor 2, or hybridoma growth factor (IL-6) is expressed and released by human epidermal cells and epidermoid carcinoma cell lines. J Immunol 1989;142:1922–1928.
20. Payne JB, Reinhardt RA, Masada MP, et al. Gingival crevicular fluid IL-8: Correlation with local IL-1α levels and patient estrogen status. J Periodontal Res 1993;28:451–453.
21. Wilson M, Reddi K, Henderson B. Cytokine-inducing components of periodonto-pathogenic bacteria. J Periodontal Res 1996;31:393–407.
22. Eastcott JW, Yamashita K, Taubman MA, et al. Adoptive transfer of cloned T helper cells ameliorates periodontal disease in nude rats. Oral Microbiol Immunol 1994;9:284–289.
23. Manthey C, Vogel SN. Interactions of lipopolysaccharide with macrophages. In: Zwilling BS, Eisenstein TK (eds). Macrophage-Pathogen Interactions. New York: Marcel Dekker, 1994:63–81.
24. Fultz MJ, Barber BA, Dieffenbach CW, Voegel SN. Induction of IFN-gamma in macrophages by lipopolysaccharide. Int Immunol 1993;5:1383–1392.
25. Carswell EA, Old LJ, Kassel RL, et al. An endotoxin-induced serum factor that causes necrosis of tumors. Proc Natl Acad Sci USA 1975;72:3666–3670.
26. Khalil N, Whitman C, Zuo L, et al. Regulation of alveolar macrophage transforming growth factor-beta secretion by corticosteroids in bleomycin-induced pulmonary inflammation in the rat. J Clin Invest 1993;92:1812–1818.
27. Beuscher HU, Rausch UP, Otterness IG, Tollinghoff M. Transition from interleukin 1 beta (IL1 beta) to IL1 alpha production during maturation of inflammatory macrophages in vivo. J Exp Med 1992;175:1793–1797.
28. Tajima Y, Yokose S, Kashimata M, et al. Epidermal growth factor expression in JE of rat gingiva. J Periodontal Res 1992;27: 299–300.

29. Tsai C-C, McArthur WP, Baehni PC, et al. Serum neutralizing activity against *Actinobacillus actinomycetemcomitans* leukotoxin in juvenile periodontitis. J Clin Periodontol 1981;8:338–348.

30. Benjamin D, Park CD, Sharma V. Human B cell interleukin 10. Leuk Lymphoma 1994;12:205–210.

31. Moore KW, O'Garra A, De Waal MR, et al. Interleukin-10. Annu Rev Immunol 1993;11:165–190.

32. Heinzel FP, Rerko RM, Ling P, et al. Interleukin 12 is produced in vivo during endotoxemia and stimulates synthesis of gamma interferon. Infect Immun 1994;62:4244–4249.

33. Whitney C, Ant J, Moncla B, et al. Serum immunoglobulin G antibody to *Porphyromonas gingivalis* in rapidly progressive periodontitis: Titer, avidity, and subclass distribution. Infect Immun 1992;60:2194–2200.

34. Grabstein KH, Eisenman J, Shanebeck K, et al. Cloning of a T cell growth factor that interacts with the beta chain of the interleukin-2 receptor. Science 1994;264:965–968.

35. Offenbacher S. Periodontal diseases: Pathogenesis. Ann Periodontol 1996;1:821–878.

36. Xiaohui Y, Antoniades H, Graves D. Expression of monocyte chemoattractant protein 1 in human inflamed gingival tissues. Infect Immun 1993;61:4622–4628.

37. Garrison SW, Nichols FC. LPS elicited secretory response in monocytes: Altered release of PGE_2 but not IL-1 beta in patients with adult periodontitis. J Periodontal Res 1989;24:88–95.

38. Offenbacher S, Heasman PA, Collins JG. Modulation of host PGE2 secretion as a determinant of periodontal disease expression. J Periodontol 1993;64:432–444.

39. Page RC. The role of inflammatory mediators in the pathogenesis of periodontal disease. J Periodontal Res 1991;26:230–242.

40. Springer TA. Adhesion receptors of the immune system [review]. Nature 1990;346:425–434.

41. Stadnyk AW. Cytokine production by epithelial cells. FASEB J 1994;8:1041–1047.

42. Ishikawa I, Nakashima K, Koseki T, et al. Induction of the immune response to periodontopathic bacteria and its role in the pathogenesis of periodontitis. Periodontol 2000 1997;14:79–111.

43. Kinane D, Mooney J, MacFarlane T, McDonald M. Local and systemic antibody response to putative periodontopathogens in patients with chronic periodontitis: Correlation with clinical indices. Oral Micriobiol Immunol 1993;8:65–68.

44. Stashenko P, Jandinski JJ, Fujiyoshi P, et al. Tissue levels of bone resorptive cytokines in periodontal disease. J Periodontol 1991; 62:504–509.

45. Walters JD, Miller TJ, Cario AC, et al. Polyamines found in gingival fluid inhibit chemotaxis by human polymorphonuclear leukocytes in vitro. J Periodontol 1995;66:274–278.

46. Picker L, Kishimoto T, Smith C, et al. ELAM-1 is an adhesion molecule for skin homing T-cells. Nature 1991;349:796–799.

47. Gregory RL, Kim DE, Kindle JC, et al. Immunoglobulin-degrading enzymes in localized juvenile periodontitis. J Periodontal Res 1992;27:176–183.

48. Prabhu A, Michalowicz BS, Mathur A. Detection of local and systemic cytokines in adult periodontitis. J Periodontol 1996; 67:515–522.

49. Stashenko P, Fujiyoshi P, Obernesser MS, et al. Levels of interleukin-1α in tissue from sites of active periodontal disease. J Clin Periodontol 1991;18:548–554.

CHAPTER 2

The Epidemiology of Periodontal Diseases

Chester W. Douglass

- Definitions
- Epidemiology of Periodontal Diseases
- Trends in Prevalence and Severity
- Risk Factors
- Forecasting the Future

Definitions

Epidemiology

Epidemiology, from *epi* (upon) + *demos* (people), is the study of the distribution of disease within a population. Knowledge of the basic epidemiology of periodontal diseases is important for clinicians as they attempt to understand risk factors for periodontal disease and how these risk factors are related to their clinical observations.

Because the frequently cited disease estimates of the 1985–1986 National Institute of Dental Research (NIDR)[1] survey of employed adults and senior citizens' centers are at noticeably lower levels than the estimates of previous or more recent surveys, these differences are thoroughly discussed.

Prevalence

Prevalence is the frequency or number of cases of a disease that can be identified within a specified population at a given point in time. It is the proportion of the population that has the disease. Prevalence relates to clinical questions such as, How many patients of every 1,000 patients are likely to have periodontal disease? Knowing the frequency of occurrence raises or lowers the clinician's suspicion of a disease when conducting examinations.

Incidence

Incidence is the number of new cases of disease that occur during a specific time. By convention, incidence is usually expressed as new cases per 100,000 persons per year. For chronic diseases such as periodontal disease, incidence is usually referred to as the incidence of progression (eg, of attachment loss) during a given time.

Because as many as 32 teeth in each adult patient are at risk for periodontal disease, and the number of sites around each tooth at which bacteria can attack the periodontium is literally infinite, the epidemiology of periodontal disease commonly uses three terms: *prevalence*, the presence of disease; *extent*, the number of teeth or sites at which disease has been identified; and *severity*, the depth, in millimeters, to which pocket depth or attachment loss has progressed.

Table 2-1 Relative Risk: Elements

Exposure	Disease present	Disease absent	Total
Exposed	a	b	a + b
Unexposed	c	d	c + d
Total	a + c	b + d	

Table 2-2 Smoking and Periodontal Disease: A Case-Control Study

| Smoking status | Periodontal disease | | |
	Present	Absent	Odds ratio
Heavy smokers	210	243	4.41
Never smoked	20	102	1.00

Risk Factors

Risk factors are variables such as behaviors, agents, or conditions that can be associated with increased prevalence, extent, or severity of periodontal disease. Examples of risk factors for periodontal disease include poor oral hygiene, systemic diseases, local irritants, oral pathogens, and cultural values. The term *risk indicator* is sometimes used for factors that are associated with disease but are not etiologically involved, such as age, race, gender, or socioeconomic status. There is no way for the clinician or patient to change these factors.

Hazard Rate

The *hazard rate* is the instantaneous risk of disease incidence. In periodontics, for example, it is the extent or rate at which chronic repetitive occurrences of gingivitis, local irritants, or bacterial attacks progress suddenly into periodontitis. This concept is consistent with the so-called burst theory of periodontal destruction.[2,3]

Relative Risk

Relative risk (RR) is a measure of the association between exposure to a particular factor and the risk (or chance) of developing periodontal disease. It is expressed as a ratio of the incidence of disease among those who are exposed to a particular risk factor to the incidence of disease among those who are not exposed. The population under study may be divided into four groups, based on the presence or absence of periodontal disease among those who are either exposed to the factor under question or not exposed (Table 2-1).

The relative risk (RR) can be computed as:

$$RR = \frac{\text{(disease rate in exposed group)}}{\text{(disease rate in unexposed group)}} = \frac{\dfrac{a}{a + b}}{\dfrac{c}{c + d}} = \frac{a(c + d)}{c(a + b)}$$

A practitioner can observe patients in a systematic way and compare patients who have advanced periodontal disease (cases) with similar patients who do not (controls). In such a case-control study, the row totals (a + b or c + d) are not meaningful population estimates of patients who are exposed and not exposed to whatever exposure factor is being studied, and therefore they cannot be used to calculate relative risk. Thus, when analyzing data from a case-control study, we are estimating the relative risk and use the term *relative odds*, or *odds ratio*.

Because the percentage of the population in which the disease develops to severe levels is usually small in comparison with the total population, (c + d) is approximately equal to d and (a + b) is approximately equal to b. The formula in Table 2-1 then becomes an estimate of the relative risk or relative odds, which is most commonly referred to as the *odds ratio (OR)*:

$$OR = \frac{ad}{bc}$$

The concept of odds ratio can be seen in an epidemiological study of smoking and advanced periodontal disease (Table 2-2). Using the odds ratio formula, which estimates relative risk, the risk of developing advanced periodontal disease in smokers compared with nonsmokers can be calculated as follows:

$$OR = ad/bc = (210 \times 102) \div (243 \times 20) = 4.41$$

Odds ratios are expressed relative to a risk of 1.0 for the control patients who are not exposed. Therefore, these data show that this group of heavy smokers has a 4.41 times greater chance (risk) of developing advanced periodontal disease than does a group of patients who have never smoked.

Epidemiology of Periodontal Diseases

Our ability to apply valid and reliable measures to representative samples of the population gives us our present understanding of periodontal diseases. A number of the diagnostic tests described in Part II of this text describe new ways to detect disease activity either directly, from local antibody reactions, or indirectly, from crevicular fluid, temperature, and enzyme levels. Unfortunately, these measures have not been used in large-scale epidemiological studies of periodontal disease, and we are left with measures of what are essentially observable morphologic changes: pocket depth (PD) and loss of attachment (LOA). Two direct clinical observations, gingival bleeding and the presence of calculus, are also commonly used in epidemiological studies. The severity of periodontal disease is thought to be moderate when patients have up to 4 to 5 mm of attachment loss or pocket depth; it is considered advanced or serious at 6 mm or greater. Periodontal disease measures below these levels—for example, at 2 mm or less—tend to be normally distributed throughout the population. Early detection of risk factors should be targeted at patients who have shallow pockets to prevent the progression of disease past this initial 2-mm level.

Gingivitis

Gingivitis is an inflammation of the marginal gingiva. Early epidemiological measures of gingivitis consisted of a visual assessment of redness and edema of the free gingival margin. More recently, a probing assessment has been used, defining gingivitis as present when a light probing of the free gingival margin causes bleeding from within the gingival sulcus. Gingivitis apparently declined from the 1960s to the mid-1970s, with half of adults aged 18 to 79 showing no disease and only about 25% exhibiting gingivitis by 1974[4] (Table 2-3). This estimate, however, is obtained from a cross-sectional survey, which means that at

Table 2-3 Adults Aged 18–79 with Gingivitis and No Disease

	1960–1962	1971–1974
No disease	26.1%	51.4%
Gingivitis	48.5%	25.2%

Data from National Center for Health Statistics.[5,6]

any one point in time, 25% of the population exhibits visual signs of gingivitis. The percentage of the population that experiences some transient gingivitis, a low-level chronic inflammation, over a period of a year would be much higher. The most likely explanation for decreases in gingivitis is improved general oral hygiene levels across the general population. The more recent studies[1,2,7] continue to show that gingivitis is highly prevalent within the United States.

Periodontitis

Because of the need to measure observable clinical changes, the epidemiological definition of *periodontitis* is "disease with pocket formation and/or loss of periodontal attachment." Four national cross-sectional studies[2,5,6] that provide a picture of the prevalence, extent, and severity of periodontal destruction since 1960 and associations with risk factors are summarized in Tables 2-4 and 2-5. One regional study is also discussed because it is directly comparable to the same region of the country in the most recently reported national survey. Table 2-4 summarizes the population, general sampling strategy, and periodontal measures of the four national studies conducted since 1960. Although these studies have been conducted on different populations using different measurement methods, a general picture begins to emerge. The periodontal measures used in these national studies were the Russell Periodontal Index (PI)[11] full mouth in the two early National Center for Health Statistics (NCHS) studies, a modified Russell PI with probing of the mesial site conducted full mouth in the 1981 Research Triangle Institute (RTI) study, and periodontal probing for direct pocket depth and attachment loss measures in millimeters conducted half mouth on the midbuccal and mesiobuccal line angle sites. The prevalence estimates shown in Table 2-5 are the percentage of the population with at least one tooth with a PI of 6, which defined "periodontitis with pockets" in the two NCHS studies, and with periodontal pocket measurements of at least 4 mm in the RTI and NIDR studies. Because the distribution of disease at less than 2 or 3 mm of

Table 2-4 National Surveys: Study Population, Sampling Strategy, and Measures Used*

	1960–1962 NCHS HES[5,8]	1971–1974 NCHS NHANES-I[6,9]	1981 RTI[2]	1985–1986 NIDR[1]
Population	General	General	Dental patients	Employed adults
General sampling strategy	Stratified area probability sample	Stratified area probability sample	Stratified sample of dentists Probability sample of insured dental patients familiar	Dunn & Bradstreet business sample
Periodontal measures collected	Russell PI full mouth	Russell PI full mouth	Russell PI with probe, mesial site full mouth	Pocket depth and attachment loss, half mouth mesial and buccal sites
Periodontal measures compared	No disease Disease without pockets Disease with pockets	No disease Disease without pockets Disease with pockets	< 4 mm 4–6 mm > 6 mm	Pocket depth in mm 4 mm

*HES = Health Examination Survey; NHANES = National Health and Nutrition Examination Survey.
Reprinted from Douglass and Fox[10] with permission.

Table 2-5 Prevalence of Periodontal Disease with Pockets by Year, Age, and Gender (%)

Age group	Disease with pockets 1960–1962[5]		Disease with pockets 1971–1974[6]		Pocket depth ≥ 4 mm 1981 RTI[2]	Pocket depth ≥ 4 mm 1985–1986 NIDR[1]	
	Male	Female	Male	Female	Male and female	Male	Female
35–39	39.7	20.5	30.5	22.2	28.8 (ages 19–44)	18.9	15.7
40–44						20.5	12.4
45–49	36.9	29.6	37.7	29.7	47.6 (ages 45–64)	25.5	14.2
50–54						19.6	14.2
55–59	45.6	35.5	46.9	35.8		23.3	14.9
60–64						24.3	17.9

Reprinted from Douglass and Fox[10] with permission.

pocket depth is so common, the 4-mm level becomes the first cutoff point that begins to define a smaller subpopulation of higher-risk persons who exhibit moderate levels of periodontal destruction. Table 2-5 shows data that suggest that age and gender should be considered risk factors for advancing periodontal destruction. Males show a higher prevalence of periodontal disease pockets than do females, and the percentage of persons with pocket depths greater than 4 mm increases with age. The 1985–1986 NIDR study reports a lower proportion of the population with periodontal pockets than was reported 20 to 30 years earlier by the NCHS studies, implying a decline in the prevalence of periodontal disease. An alternative explanation is that the population on which the study was conducted and the periodontal disease measurement methods are in fact responsible for these lower numbers.

Trends in Prevalence and Severity

Capilouto and Douglass[12] examined data on the trend in periodontal disease and found equivocal evidence for confirming a decline in the prevalence of periodontitis. They summarize by stating, "It appears that approximately 20% of adults in the United States continue to experience a level of periodontal disease severity that requires professional treatment." Other reports seem to support this conclusion. Brown et al,[2] analyzing the 1981 RTI study, found a 33% prevalence of periodontitis. The NIDR employed-adult survey (see Table 2-4) was conducted just 5 years after the RTI study. It seems that the differences in these two surveys can be explained not by a true decline in the

Table 2-6 Comparison of NEEDS to the National and Region 1 Senior Survey

| | NIDR Senior | | | |
	National (1986)	Region 1*[15]	NEEDS (1990) Region 1[16]	NEEDS 95% confidence interval
Gingival bleeding	47%	40%	85%	(82–88)
Calculus	66%	53%	89%	(86–91)
Probing depth 4 mm	22%	19%	87%	(85–90)
Attachment loss 4 mm	68%	70%	95%	(93–97)
Probing depth 6 mm	4%	3%	21%	(18–25)
Attachment loss 6 mm	34%	36%	56%	(51–60)

*USPHS Region 1 represents the six New England states.[7]

prevalence of pocketing in the adult population over such a short period of time but rather by the sampling methods employed. By observing only employed adults from larger businesses, the NIDR study excluded the majority of the population. Not included in this study were small-business owners, the self-employed, miners, agricultural workers, people in the military, women who did not work outside the home, and the unemployed, most of whom would seem more likely to have more untreated periodontal disease than would employed workers, many of whom receive dental insurance as part of their employee benefits plans.

Another possible explanation of the NIDR results is that the methods used to measure the prevalence, extent, and severity of periodontal disease were themselves too conservative and so resulted in false-negative findings in a consistent and pervasive way. The reliability of the probing method is not in question, but rather the validity of the sites selected as truly representative. The midbuccal aspect of each tooth avoids the furcation in multirooted teeth, and the mesiobuccal line angle, with the probe held parallel to the long axis of the tooth, avoids the deep interproximal area. Fox and Douglass[13] and Kingman et al[14] both explored this problem and found that measuring the mesial sites, alone or with the midbuccal site, underestimated the prevalence of attachment loss greater than 4 mm by 10% to 52%, depending on the population surveyed.

Table 2-6 presents a direct comparison for the six New England states (Region 1) of the 1985–1986 NIDR senior survey and the New England Elders Dental Study (NEEDS) conducted between 1990 and 1992. The data show substantial differences on all six periodontal disease measures collected by these two studies. The prevalence of gingival bleeding, calculus, probing depth greater than 4 mm, and attachment loss greater than 4 mm were found on 85%, 89%, 87%, and 95% of New England elders, respectively, as opposed to 40%, 53%, 19%, and 70% of those attend-

ing senior centers surveyed by the NIDR in the same region of the country. Probing depth and attachment loss greater than 6 mm in the NIDR study are also far lower than in the New England Elders Dental Study.

The examination method was substantially different in these two studies. The NEEDS project examined all teeth present, while the NIDR examined only half the mouth[17] and excluded third molars. NEEDS examined three sites per tooth, including the distal lingual sites, and also searched for the deepest site per tooth (similar to the Community Periodontal Index of Treatment Needs [CPITN]). The NIDR examination included only the buccal and mesiobuccal sites, which are sites at which severe periodontal disease is less likely to occur. In addition to greater prevalence, Table 2-7 shows that gingival pocketing and loss of attachment are both extensive (affecting five to seven teeth per person) and severe, with 21% of the senior population having pockets greater than 6 mm and 56% showing loss of attachment greater than 6 mm. With the data from the more complete periodontal examination, it can be concluded that periodontitis continues to be widespread throughout middle-aged and older adults.

Risk Factors

Many studies have shown that the risk factors most directly associated with increases in prevalence and severity of periodontal disease are *(1)* gender, with men experiencing greater levels than women; *(2)* socioeconomic status, with higher education and income associated with lower levels; *(3)* number of teeth, with more teeth per person associated with greater severity; *(4)* smoking, with heavy smoking associated with greater severity; and *(5)* age, with older adults exhibiting more loss of attachment than younger adults. Diabetes mellitus and a number of bacterial pathogens are also risk factors for periodontal disease.

Table 2-7 Periodontal Disease in 554 Dentate New England Elderly Subjects Eligible for Periodontal Examination

| Sex | Age | Total n | Bleeding | | Gingival pocketing | | | | | | | |
| | | | | | Mild (0–3 mm) | | Moderate (4–6 mm) | | | Severe (> 6 mm) | | |
			n	%	n	%	n	%	Affected teeth*	n	%	Affected teeth*
Female	70–74	108	89	82	15	14	78	72	5.3 ± 3.6	15	14	2.5 ± 2.3
	75–79	95	79	83	9	9	69	73	4.6 ± 3.6	17	18	1.7 ± 0.9
	80–84	62	57	92	10	16	41	66	4.9 ± 2.7	11	18	2.5 ± 1.4
	85+	48	44	92	12	25	29	60	6.1 ± 4.0	7	15	1.7 ± 1.9
	Total	313	269	86	46	15	217	69	5.1 ± 3.5	50	16	2.1 ± 1.7
Male	70–74	108	92	82	10	6	65	54	5.9 ± 4.4	33	31	2.8 ± 2.4
	75–79	76	65	87	7	3	43	41	4.7 ± 3.7	26	34	1.7 ± 1.0
	80–84	40	31	84	4	5	28	40	4.9 ± 3.7	8	20	1.8 ± 1.1
	85+	17	14	92	3	6	12	31	8.1 ± 3.9	2	12	1.0 ± 0.0
	Total	241	202	86	24	5	148	44	5.6 ± 4.1	69	29	2.2 ± 1.9
Total		554	471	85	70	13	365	66	5.3 ± 3.8	119	21	2.2 ± 1.8

| Sex | Age | Total n | Calculus | | Loss of attachment | | | | | | | |
| | | | | | Mild (0–3 mm) | | Moderate (4–6 mm) | | | Severe (> 6 mm) | | |
			n	%	n	%	n	%	Affected teeth*	n	%	Affected teeth*
Female	70–74	108	89	82	6	6	57	54	6.6 ± 4.2	43	41	2.4 ± 2.2
	75–79	95	83	87	3	3	39	41	6.8 ± 4.1	52	55	2.3 ± 1.6
	80–84	62	52	84	3	5	25	40	6.7 ± 3.9	34	55	2.4 ± 1.5
	85+	48	44	92	3	6	15	31	6.7 ± 4.4	30	63	2.6 ± 2.1
	Total	313	268	86	15	5	136	44	6.7 ± 4.1	159	51	2.4 ± 1.8
Male	70–74	108	98	91	3	3	40	38	7.5 ± 5.1	63	59	3.3 ± 2.6
	75–79	76	71	93	2	3	20	27	5.8 ± 4.2	53	71	2.9 ± 2.2
	80–84	40	38	95	1	3	15	39	6.3 ± 3.5	22	58	2.7 ± 2.2
	85+	17	16	94	0	0	6	35	6.3 ± 4.4	11	65	3.9 ± 3.3
	Total	241	223	93	6	3	81	34	6.7 ± 4.5	149	63	3.1 ± 2.4
Total		554	491	89	21	4	217	39	6.7 ± 4.3	308	56	2.7 ± 2.2

*Mean ± SD, restricted to subjects with at least one affected tooth.
Reprinted from Douglass et al[18] with permission.

The third factor may seem paradoxical, but is really just a matter of arithmetic: the greater the number of teeth, the more chances for disease. Data from the New England Elders Study,[19] which involved a more complete examination than most epidemiology studies (Tables 2-8 and 2-9), show that a representative sample of elders throughout the six New England states who have 25 to 32 teeth have four times as many PD sites of at least 4 mm and twice as many sites with LOA at least 4 mm than do elders with 1 to 10 teeth. In the group of elders with 1 to 10 teeth, the rate (or risk) of a 4-mm pocket may be higher per tooth than in the group with 25 to 32 teeth. However, the number of instances of periodontal disease that need to be professionally managed is greater in the elders with 25 to 32 teeth. This group, who successfully retained their natural dentition, has on average 10 PD and 16 LOA sites of at least 4 mm. The elders with fewer teeth may have a higher rate of

disease per tooth, but they have fewer teeth (a lower denominator) and on average have only 2.5 PD and 8 LOA sites of at least 4 mm. Hence, older adults with more teeth need more periodontal services.

Should age per se be considered a risk factor for periodontal disease? This question needs further examination. At present, opinions differ on whether older adults are at higher risk for periodontal disease or not. One view is that adults who survive to old age are the "survivors" and that teeth still present in this group are less susceptible to periodontitis.[18] That is, the risk or likelihood of exhibiting periodontitis is less because susceptible persons and susceptible teeth had experienced the disease when they were younger.[20]

Further, what has previously been thought of as an age effect may be more correctly understood as a cohort effect. That is, the differences observed between age groups

Table 2-8 Number of Sites* with Pocket Depth ≥ 4 mm[†] in Subjects ≥ 70 Years Old [‡]

No. of teeth (tooth group)	Pocket depth (≥ 4 mm)		Group comparison	P value
	Mean	SE		
01–10 (1)	2.48	0.61	1 vs 2	.001
11–24 (2)	6.96	0.47	1 vs 3	.001
25–32 (3)	10.50	0.84	2 vs 3	.001

* Mean scores.
† Adjusted for age and gender.
‡ F statistic = 32.41 (*P* < .001). Analysis of variance model with number of sites with pocket depth ≥ 4 mm as dependent variable, and age, gender, and tooth group as main effects and possible interaction effects, Reprinted from Joshi et al[19] with permission.

Table 2-9 Number of Sites* with Loss Attachment ≥ 4 mm[†] in Subjects ≥ 70 Years Old [‡]

No. of teeth (tooth group)	Pocket depth (≥ 4 mm)		Group comparison	P value
	Mean	SE		
01–10 (1)	8.04	0.91	1 vs 2	.001
11–24 (2)	16.79	0.70	1 vs 3	.001
25–32 (3)	16.37	1.25	2 vs 3	.77

* Mean scores.
† Adjusted for age and gender.
‡ F statistic = 31.09 (*P* < .001). Analysis of variance model with number of sites with loss of attachment ≥ 4 mm as dependent variable, and age, gender, and tooth group as main effects and possible interaction effects. Reprinted from Joshi et al[19] with permission.

in studies probably result from the fact that each successive generation of adults is paying better attention to dental care and so is experiencing better oral health than the previous generation. Thus, greater use of dental care, improved oral hygiene habits, and the significant increases in retention of teeth are the factors that predict greater or lesser experience with periodontal disease. Each succeeding generation of elders has improved on all of these predictive factors, so previous cross-sectional studies have been misleading.

The greatest difference in cohorts has been the increase in the number of teeth. Older adults had 7.2 teeth per person in 1962, but by 1993 they had 17.2 teeth per person.[18] Hence, the number of teeth at risk for periodontal disease is increasing as the number of teeth per person increases. Because of the large increase in the numbers of elders living into their seventh, eighth, and ninth decades of life,[21] this trend should be expected to continue for some time. Clinicians, therefore, should expect to see more moderate to severe periodontal disease in older adults not because age is a risk factor but rather because there are so many more older adults with more teeth liable to the encroachments of periodontal disease in the long term. In addition, these older adults are taking more medications and have more chronic systemic conditions, both of which are factors associated with higher risk of periodontal disease.

Forecasting the Future

The substantial prevalence, severity, and extent of periodontal disease documented in this chapter suggests that while our understanding of the pathophysiology of peri-

odontal diseases has improved greatly over the last two decades, there is still a substantial and unmet need for periodontal services within the population. Looking over the long term, a number of conclusions seem warranted:

1. Periodontal diseases are still prevalent in a significant minority of the population.[1,16]
2. Periodontal disease is severe for many millions of high-risk subgroups within the population.[1,2,12]
3. The data show that older adults who retain their teeth are at high risk.[10,21]
4. There will be a large increase in the number of older adults in the next few decades.[22,23]
5. There is a shortage of dental hygienists, and the dentist-to-population ratio has already begun to decline.[24]
6. There is evidence of an underdemand for periodontal services by the public.[25,26]
7. There is evidence of underdocumentation of periodontal disease by dentists.[27]
8. The epidemiological data probably underestimate the true distribution and severity of periodontal disease.[10,28,29]
9. Substantial numbers of fixed partial dentures currently being provided may not be in the best long-term interests of periodontium.

Substantial efforts are required by periodontists, general practitioners, and dental hygienists to meet the need for periodontal care in the 20% of the US adult population (40 million people) who have advanced periodontal disease, as well as to treat the large and growing amount of moderate periodontal disease within the large, growing, and aging population of the nation.[6]

References

1. Löe H. Oral Health of United States Adults: National Findings. US Dept Health and Human Services, NIDR, 1987.

2. Brown LJ, Oliver RC, Löe H. Periodontal diseases in the U.S. in 1981: Prevalence, severity, extent, and role in tooth mortality. J Periodontol 1989;60:363.

3. Douglass CW, Gillings D, Sollecito W, Gammon MD. National trends in the prevalence and severity of the periodontal diseases. J Am Dent Assoc 1983;107:403–412.

4. Douglass CW, Gillings D, Sollecito W, Gammon MD. The potential for increase in the periodontal diseases of the aged population. J Periodontol 1983;54:721–730.

5. Kelly JE, Van Kirk LE. Periodontal Disease in Adults, United States, 1960–62. National Center for Health Statistics. Government Printing Office, 1965.

6. Kelly JE, Harvey CR. Basic Data on Dental Examination Findings of Persons 1–74 Years, United States, 1971–74. National Center for Health Statistics. Government Printing Office, 1979.

7. Miller AJ, Brunelle JA, Carlos JP, et al. Oral Health of United States Adults: The National Survey of Oral Health in U.S. Employed Adults and Seniors: 1985–86, Regional Findings. Bethesda: National Institutes of Health, 1987.

8. Johnson ES, Kelly JE, Van Kirk LE. Selected Dental Findings in Adults by Age, Race and Sex, United States, 1960–62. National Center for Health Statistics. Government Printing Office, 1965.

9. Harvey CR, Kelly JE. Decayed, Missing, and Filled Teeth Among Persons 1–74 Years, United States, 1971–74. Government Printing Office, Aug 1981.

10. Douglass C, Fox C. Cross-sectional studies in periodontal disease: Current status and implications for dental practice. Adv Dent Res 1993;7(1):25–31.

11. Russell A. A system of classification and scoring for prevalence surveys of periodontal disease. J Dent Res 1956;35:350–359.

12. Capilouto ML, Douglass CW. Trends in the prevalence and severity of periodontal diseases in the U.S.: A public health problem? J Public Health Dent 1988;48:245–251.

13. Fox CH, Douglass CW. Periodontal destruction assessed by two sites per tooth vs. six sites. J Dent Res 1989;68:954.

14. Kingman A, Morrison E, Löe H, Smith J. Systematic errors in estimating prevalence and severity of periodontal disease. J Periodontol 1988;59:707.

15. Miller AJ, Brunelle JA, Carlos JP, et al. Oral Health of United States Adults: The National Survey of Oral Health in U.S. Employed Adults and Seniors: 1985–86, National Findings. Bethesda: National Institutes of Health, 1987.

16. Fox CH, Jette AM, McGuire SM, et al. Periodontal disease among New England elders. J Periodontol 1994;65:676–684.

17. Hunt R. The efficiency of half-mouth examinations in estimating the prevalence of periodontal disease. J Dent Res 1987;66:1044–1048.

18. Douglass CW, Jette AM, Fox CH, et al. Oral health status of the elderly in New England. J Gerontol 1993;48(2):M39–M46.

19. Joshi A, Douglass CW, Jette AM, et al. Consequences of success: Do more teeth translate into more disease and utilization? J Public Health Dent 1996;56:190–197.

20. Burt BA, Eklund SA. Dentistry, Dental Practice, and the Community, ed 4. Philadelphia: Saunders, 1992:339.

21. Reinhardt JW, Douglass CW. The need for operative dentistry services: Projecting the effects of changing disease patterns. Oper Dent 1989;14:114–120.

22. Douglass CW. Implications of demographic and dental disease changes for the financing of geriatric dental services. Health Matrix 1988;6(3):13.

23. Rice DP, Douglass CW, Gillings DB, Yordy KD. Public policy options for better dental health. J Dent Educ 1981;45:746.

24. Solomon ES. Dentists and dentist-to-population ratios 1985–2020. Manpower Project. Washington, DC: American Association of Dental Schools, 1988.

25. Bailit H, Manning W. The need and demand for periodontal services: Implications for dental practice and education. J Dent Educ 1988;52:458.

26. Gillings D, Sollecito W, Douglass CW. A need-based model to project national dental expenditures. J Public Health Dent 1983;43:8.

27. McFall WT, Bader JD, Rozier RG, Ramsey D. Presence of periodontal data in patient records of general practitioners. J Periodontol 1988;59:445.

28. Oliver RC. Patient evaluation. Int Dent J 1977;27:103.

29. Fox CH. Validity, Reliability, and Comparability of Cross-sectional Surveys of Periodontal Status [thesis]. Cambridge, MA: Harvard Univ, 1991.

CHAPTER 3

Anatomy of the Periodontium

> **Palle Holmstrup**
> • Macroanatomy
> • Microanatomy

Knowledge of the architecture and biology of normal tissue is a prerequisite for understanding diseased tissue. Diagnosis of disease involves distinguishing deviations from normal characteristics, and knowledge of the normal state is essential to defining the goals of therapy.

The periodontium is a dynamic structure composed of the tissues supporting and investing the teeth. These tissues include the gingiva, the periodontal ligament, the cementum, and the alveolar bone. The vascular and nerve supplies of the involved periodontal tissues are also vital to their normal functioning.

The structure and function of the tissue components of the periodontium are interdependent. Their dynamic biologic adaptation and renewal processes maintain a harmonious relationship under normal conditions.

Macroanatomy

Gingiva

The gingiva covers the alveolar process, and it is the only one of the periodontal tissues that under healthy conditions is directly visible upon inspection. The healthy gingiva (Figs 3-1a and 3-1b) is pale pink (salmon or coral pink), but variations are common, depending on epithelial thickness and keratinization, vascularity, and pigmentation. Accumulations of melanin pigmentation are normal (Figs 3-2a and 3-2b); they are more frequently observed in Africans and Asians than in Caucasians, and more frequently in Caucasians with dark skin than in those with light skin. The pigmentation may vary and range in color from light brown to black. It may be regularly or irregularly deposited.[1]

The coronal border with its scalloped outline is the free gingival margin (Fig 3-3), a thin, rounded edge formed by a coronal slope of the tissue. After teeth penetrate the mucosa during eruption, the gingival margin is located between the occlusal surface and the terminal position slightly coronal to the cementoenamel junction. The shape of the gingival margin usually gives rise to a small sulcus between the gingival tissue and the tooth. The attached gingiva extends apically from the free gingiva to the mucogingival line or junction, where the gingiva fuses with the alveolar mucosa (Fig 3-4). This demarcation is most obvious on the vestibular aspects of the jaws but may also occur on the lingual aspect of the mandible. There is, however, no demarcation in the palate, because the palatal mucosa, like gingiva, is keratinized and firmly attached to the underlying periosteum continuous with the attached gingiva.

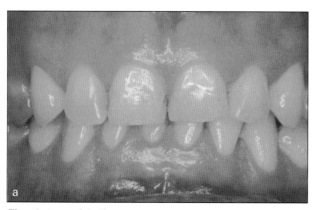
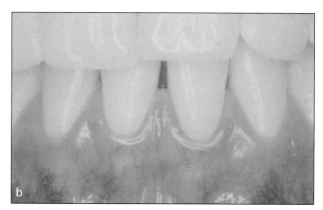

Figs 3-1a and 3-1b Nonpigmented gingiva: *(a)* broad zone of attached gingiva with surface stippling; *(b)* narrow zone of attached gingiva with visible vessels almost to the gingival margin.

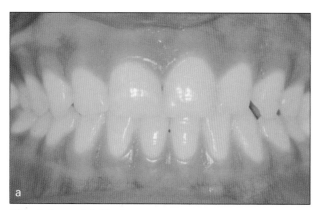
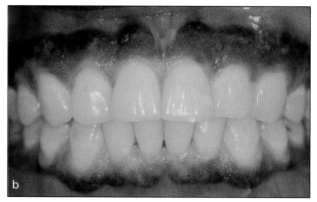

Figs 3-2a and 3-2b Gingival pigmentation: *(a)* slight and *(b)* heavy. Surface stippling is particularly evident in *(b)*.

The free gingiva (Fig 3-4) comprises the gingival tissue extending from the gingival margin in an apical direction to the free gingival groove, which is a furrow situated according to the most coronally inserting periodontal ligament fibers at the level of the cementoenamel junction. The free gingival groove is not present in relation to all teeth and is not present in all individuals.

The free gingiva includes the interdental papillae, and part of its internal surface forms the lateral aspect of the small gingival sulcus. When no disease is present, there is little or no free gingiva, and the free and attached gingiva together are sometimes referred to merely as the gingiva.

The apicocoronal width of the attached gingiva shows regional and individual variations and in health tends to increase with age due to vertical growth of the alveolar process. However, the level of the mucogingival line is relatively stable with increasing age,[2] and an inadequate

width of attached gingiva in childhood will correct itself from 6 to 12 years of age without surgical intervention.[3] The vestibular attached gingiva is widest in the incisor and molar regions, whereas it is narrowest in the canine and premolar regions. In areas of inserting ligaments, the width usually is reduced. The lingual attached gingiva of the mandible is widest in the molar regions and narrowest in the incisor area. The texture of healthy attached gingiva is firm, with a tight anchoring to the teeth and the periosteum. Surface stippling resembling orange peel is present to varying degrees on vestibular surfaces.

In young individuals, the interdental papillae fill the interproximal spaces, with the coronal height of the papillae being immediately apical to the contact area of adjacent teeth. In the most coronal part, the interdental papilla frequently shows a concavity, or col (Fig 3-5), as determined by the shape of the contact areas of the neighboring teeth

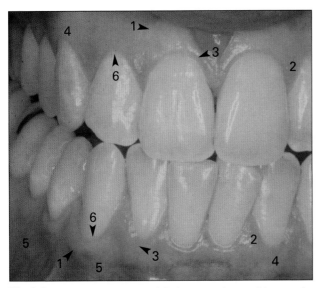

Fig 3-3 Gingival structures and their nomenclature: (1) mucogingival junction, (2) interdental papilla, (3) free gingiva, (4) attached gingiva, (5) alveolar mucosa, and (6) gingival margin.

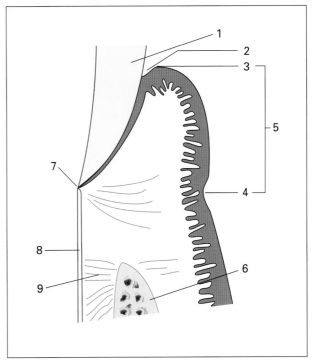

Fig 3-4 Free gingiva and surrounding structures: (1) Enamel, (2) small gingival sulcus, (3) gingival margin, (4) free gingival groove, (5) free gingiva, (6) alveolar bone, (7) cementoenamel junction, (8) cementum, and (9) periodontal ligament.

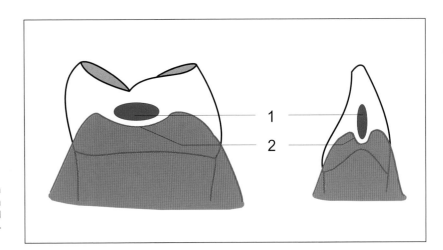

Fig 3-5 Shape of interdental papilla between molars and incisors. The interdental papilla shows a concavity, or col (2), as determined by the shape of the contact areas (1) of neighboring teeth.

between which the papilla is situated. This is most prominent in the premolar and molar regions. In the incisor regions, the papillae are more pyramidal.

There are major variations in gingival architecture as determined by the degree of eruption, position of teeth, missing teeth or diastemata, and underlying bone morphology. With increasing age, gingival recession becomes more common as the result of inflammatory processes, trauma from toothbrushing, and other oral hy-

giene procedures. The alveolar mucosa, in contrast to the gingiva, is nonkeratinized and loosely connected to the underlying tissues, and it is movable. It is darker red than the gingiva, and the surface is smooth. The difference in color results from differences in keratinization pattern and proximity to the surface of underlying blood vessels. Indeed, small blood vessels are visible beneath the alveolar mucosa.

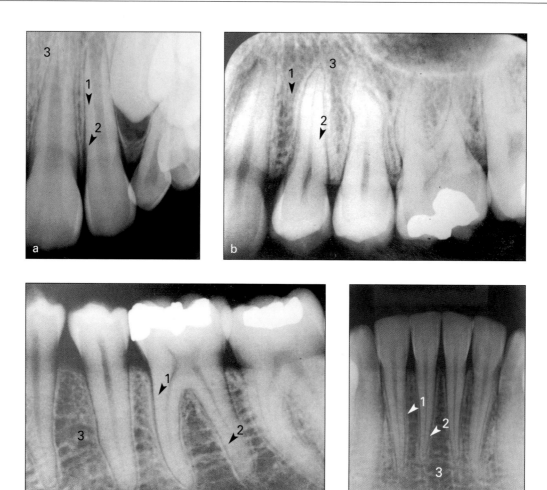

Figs 3-6a to 3-6d Radiographic demonstration of periodontal structures: *(a)* maxillary right canine and incisor region, *(b)* maxillary left premolar and molar region, *(c)* mandibular right molar region, and *(d)* mandibular incisor region. In each illustration, the following elements are identified: (1) periodontal ligament space, (2) lamina dura of dental alveolus, and (3) trabecular bone.

Periodontal Ligament

The periodontal ligament connects the tooth with the surrounding alveolar bone, and it is consequently situated in the narrow space between these two (see Fig 3-4). The periodontal ligament space, which is normally between 0.1 and 0.25 mm in width,[4] is visible on radiographs as a radiolucent line surrounding the root (Figs 3-6a to 3-6d). The ligament is widest near the cementoenamel junction and near the apex, whereas it is narrowest near the middle of the root. The width depends on the age and functionality of the tooth, with a maximum width for teeth in heavy function as opposed to unerupted teeth and teeth without antagonists. Tooth mobility may occur if the width is increased, if the ligament is partly lost, or if it is altered due to inflammation.

Cementum

The cementum covers the root surface. The fibers of the periodontal ligament are attached to this layer. The thickness of the cementum at the cementoenamel junction is about 50 µm in the age group 11 to 20 years, while at the age of 70 years it has increased to about 130 µm. The deposition of new cementum continues periodically throughout life, which is how root fractures may be repaired. Apically, the thickness of the cementum is about 200 µm in the age group 11 to 20 years, while at the age of 70 years it may exceed 500 µm.[5] The cementum is indistinguishable on radiographs.

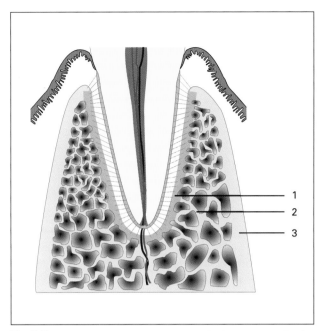

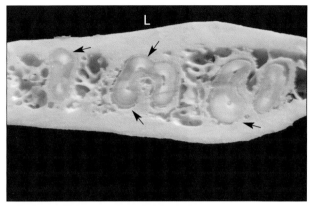

Fig 3-7 Alveolar bone structure: (1) alveolar bone proper (lamina dura in radiographs), (2) trabecular bone, and (3) compact bone.

Fig 3-8 Horizontal cross section of left mandibular alveolar process of the molar region at the midroot level. *Arrows* indicate areas of fusion of alveolar walls (lamina dura) and compact cortical bone. (L) lingual aspect.

Alveolar Bone

The alveolar processes are the parts of the maxilla and the mandible that provide the housing for the roots of the teeth. These processes are dependent on the presence of teeth; they develop in accordance with tooth formation and eruption, and they are subjected to atrophy if the teeth are lost. The coronal margin of the alveolar processes shows a wavy configuration that corresponds to the course of the cementoenamel junctions of the teeth, and it is situated 1 to 1.5 mm from these junctions. The alveolar processes are covered by compact bone (Fig 3-7), which overlies a trabecular bone structure. Within the trabecular bone structure, the alveoli are situated with their 0.1- to 0.4-mm-thick compact-bone plate; this is the alveolar bone proper, which is seen on radiographs as the lamina dura (see Fig 3-6). The alveolar walls, in which the periodontal ligament fibers anchor, are perforated with numerous small canals allowing vessels and nerves to enter the periodontal ligament space.[6] This is why the alveolar walls are sometimes referred to as the *cribriform plates*. The walls of the alveoli are often situated in and continuous with the compact cortical bone of the buccal and lingual or palatal aspects of the alveolar processes (Fig 3-8).

The thickness of the compact cortical bone on the superficial/outer aspects of the alveolar processes varies. In the incisor, canine, and premolar regions, the buccal cortical bone is thin and sometimes missing at the coronal part of the roots.[7] The morphology of the alveolar processes is closely tooth dependent. When there is vestibular tipping of a tooth, the vestibular cortical bone frequently becomes thin, whereas the lingual cortical bone becomes massive. Tipping is often associated with fenestrations and dehiscences of the cortical bone plates (Figs 3-9a and 3-9b). The outer cortical bone is covered by a periosteum.

The shape of the alveoli follows that of the roots of the teeth. The root morphology of the teeth has been extensively described by Carlsen.[8] The interdental septa are the parts of bone separating adjacent alveoli. The shape of the interdental septa follows the alignment of the adjacent cementoenamel junctions. When neighboring teeth are in close approximation, the interdental septum is narrow or even nonexistent. Progression of periodontal disease in such areas may give rise to rapid destruction of the tooth-bearing structures. In the anterior region, the coronal parts of the septa form peaks, and because of a fusion of the inner and outer cortical bone, trabecular bone in this area is often minute. The septa of posterior teeth are relatively wide and contain more trabecular bone.

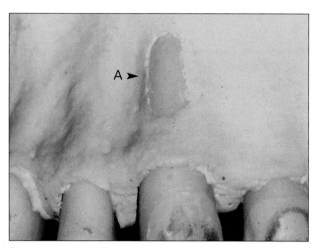

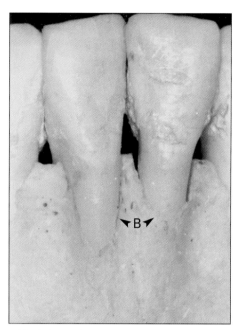

Figs 3-9a and 3-9b Fenestration (A) of the maxillary, and dehiscences (B) of the cortical bone of the mandibular alveolar process.

Vascular Supply of the Periodontium

The most important arterial supply for the maxillary alveolar bone, periodontal ligament, and gingiva is provided by the anterior and posterior superior alveolar arteries, the infraorbital artery, and the greater palatine artery. The mandible is supplied chiefly by the inferior alveolar artery and its branches, including the mental artery and the sublingual, buccal, and facial arteries.

The dental artery (Fig 3-10) is a branch of the superior or inferior alveolar artery, and it dismisses intraseptal arteries, which again have branches penetrating the bone and entering the alveolus. These branches are the rami perforantes, which form a dense anastomosing network in the periodontal ligament. The maxillary gingiva is mainly supplied from terminal supraperiosteal branches of the posterior alveolar arteries, the infraorbital artery, and the greater palatine artery (Fig 3-11). Accordingly, the mandibular gingiva receives its main supply from terminal branches of the buccal, facial, mental, and sublingual arteries.

It is important to note that there are numerous anastomoses between the arteries mentioned. Consequently, rather than single arteries supplying only certain regions, the blood vessels form an extended network that supplies the soft and hard tissues.[9,10] The network ensures a sufficient blood supply, even when single vessels are blocked or surgically cut. The network includes bone-penetrating

anastomoses between arteries of the bone, those of the periodontal ligament, and those of the gingiva. The free gingiva receives its blood supply from vessels originating in all three tissues. Adjacent to the junctional epithelium, the vessels form a plexus with sufficient supply for immediate defense mechanisms (see Fig 3-10).

From the venous and lymphatic capillaries, the venous blood and lymph accordingly pass into larger vessels. The course of the venous and the lymphatic vessels extensively parallels that of the arterial supply.

The lymph from the periodontal tissues passes through lymph nodes before re-entering the bloodstream. The submandibular lymph nodes (Fig 3-12) drain all the periodontal tissues except the following: *(1)* the palatal gingiva, which is drained by the deep cervical lymph nodes; *(2)* the periodontal tissues of the third molars, which are drained by the jugulodigastric lymph nodes; and *(3)* the periodontal tissues of the mandibular incisors, which are drained by the submental lymph nodes.[10]

Nerve Supply of the Periodontium

All nerve branches supplying the periodontium are ramifications from the trigeminal nerve, and the nerves of the periodontal tissues follow a course that resembles that of the blood vessels. The nerves register pressure, touch, temperature, and pain. In addition, the periodontal liga-

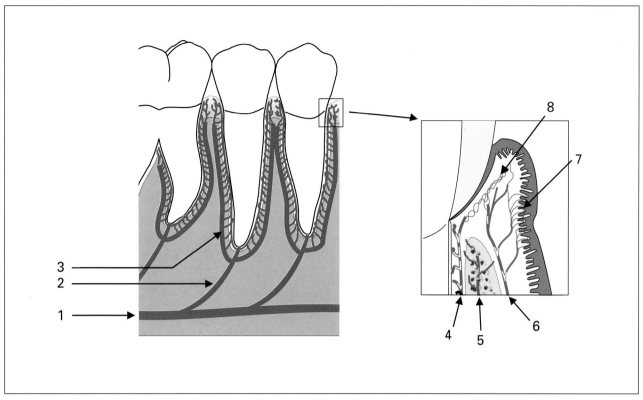

Fig 3-10 Blood supply of the periodontium: (1) superior or inferior alveolar artery, (2) dental artery, (3) intraseptal artery, (4) periodontal ligament vessels, (5) terminal branches of intraseptal artery with rami perforantes, (6) supraperiosteal vessels, (7) subepithelial plexus with capillary loops in connective tissue between epithelial ridges of oral epithelium, and (8) dentogingival (junctional) plexus of vessels.

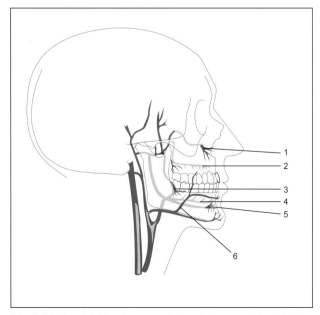

Fig 3-11 Arterial blood supply of the gingiva: (1) infraorbital artery, (2) greater palatine artery, (3) buccal artery, (4) sublingual artery, (5) mental artery, and (6) facial artery.

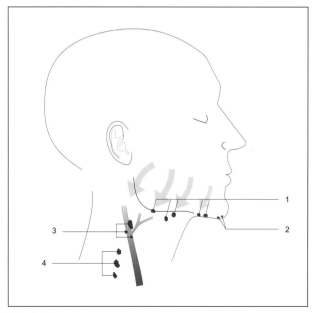

Fig 3-12 Lymph nodes draining the periodontium: (1) submandibular lymph nodes; (2) submental lymph nodes; (3) upper deep cervical lymph nodes, the largest being the jugulodigastric lymph node; and (4) lower deep cervical lymph nodes.

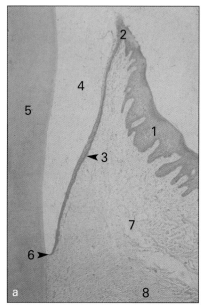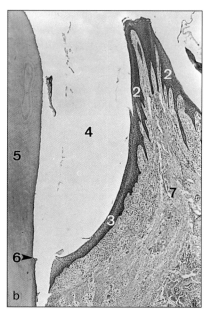

Figs 3-13a and 3-13b Histologic features of clinically normal human gingival tissue: *(a)* facial gingiva and *(b)* interproximal gingiva. Both illustrations identify (1) gingival oral epithelium, (2) gingival sulcular epithelium, (3) gingival junctional epithelium, (4) enamel, (5) dentin, (6) cementoenamel junction, (7) gingival connective tissue, and (8) alveolar bone.

ment also harbors proprioceptors recording position and movement, which is very important for the regulation of chewing forces. The receptors of the periodontal ligament are able to identify objects a few micrometers thick between teeth in occlusion.

The periodontal ligaments in the mandible are all supplied by the inferior alveolar nerve, while those of the maxilla are supplied by branches of the posterior, middle, and anterior superior alveolar nerves. The maxillary gingiva is also supplied by branches from these latter nerves and from the infraorbital, greater palatine, and nasopalatine nerves. The vestibular mandibular gingiva is supplied by the mental and buccal nerves, whereas the lingual aspect of the mandibular gingiva is supplied by the lingual nerve.

In addition to the above-mentioned sensory nerves of the periodontium, autonomic nerves control the smooth muscles associated with the periodontal vasculature.[11,12] The autonomic nerves originate from the superior cervical ganglion.

Microanatomy

Gingiva

Epithelium

The gingiva is covered by stratified squamous epithelium with architectural characteristics specific for the areas related to the teeth. Based on these characteristics, the gin-

gival epithelium can be divided into the following (Figs 3-13a and 3-13b):

1. The oral epithelium
2. The sulcular epithelium
3. The junctional epithelium

Oral epithelium. The gingival oral epithelium faces the oral cavity and extends from the gingival margin to the mucogingival junction. It thereby covers the clinically visible part of the free gingiva and the attached gingiva. The vast majority of cells in the epithelium are keratinocytes characterized by their ability to produce cytoplasmic keratin filaments (tonofilaments). Keratin polypeptides, the cytoskeleton molecules, form a complex family in humans, with molecular weights from 40 to 68 kd; their function is to give mechanical strength to the epithelial sheet.[13]

Surface epithelia are constantly renewed tissues characterized by surface sloughing of mature keratinocytes and cell renewal obtained by mitotic division of keratinocytes in the basal cell layer. There is an equilibrium between cell renewal and desquamation from the surface. About 10 days are required for a new cell to traverse the epithelium and reach the stratum corneum.[14] This interval is called the *epithelial turnover time.* The newly formed keratinocytes change their appearance as they move toward the epithelial surface. During this process, the synthesis of keratin polypeptides is altered, and when the keratinocytes get closer to the surface, other characteristic proteins are synthesized.

The genetically determined sequence of events during the movement of the keratinocytes from the basal cell layer toward the surface is referred to as *terminal differentiation*. Furthermore, the production of the various keratins shows topographic specificity, including variation between different gingival epithelia.[15,16] The epithelial keratinization processes appear to be prompted by the underlying connective tissue.[17,18] The events of continuous differentiation occurring in the epithelial cell from its birth to its final sloughing from the surface have been summarized as follows:[19]

1. Cells lose the ability to multiply by mitotic division.
2. Cells produce increased amounts of protein and accumulate keratohyalin granules, keratin filaments, and macromolecular matrix material in their cytoplasm.
3. Cells lose the cytoplasmic organelles responsible for protein synthesis and energy production.
4. Cells eventually degenerate into a cornified layer due to the process of intracellular keratinization, but without loss of cell-to-cell attachment.
5. Cells are ultimately sloughed away from the epithelial surface and into the oral cavity as the cell-to-cell attachment mechanisms (ie, desmosome and gap junctions) finally disintegrate.

If cell nuclei are lacking in the cornified layer of keratinized cells (stratum corneum), the epithelium, as well as the stratum corneum itself, is called *orthokeratinized*; it is *parakeratinized* if the cells of this layer contain nuclei. The epithelium consists of several cell layers making up the classic epithelial strata of a keratinized epithelium: stratum basale, stratum spinosum, and stratum corneum (keratin layer) (Fig 3-14). If the epithelium is orthokeratinized, it also comprises a stratum granulosum (granular layer) between the stratum spinosum and the stratum corneum. The granular layer contains keratohyalin granules.

Keratinocytes have a characteristic shape, depending on their position in the epithelium (see Fig 3-14). The stratum basale is the germinative layer, and the basal cells, which are attached to the basement membrane, are cuboidal or columnar. The spinous cells in the middle of the epithelium are the largest cells. They are polygonal, whereas the cells of the granular layer and the superficial layer are flattened, with their long axes parallel to the epithelial surface.

The oral epithelium under normal conditions also contains cells with functions and morphology different from the keratinocytes. These cells are melanocytes, which are dendritic cells producing melanin, a pigment that protects

against actinic radiation.[20] Another intraepithelial dendritic cell that does not produce keratin is the Langerhans cell, which is a macrophage-like cell that probably plays an important role in the early host response to microbial antigens at the gingival margin.[21,22]

The epithelial–connective tissue interface is wavy, with prominent epithelial ridges and with connective tissue papillae projecting into the epithelium.[23,24] Intersections between the epithelial ridges at the epithelial subsurface correspond to depressions on the surface, which can be seen clinically in the stippled appearance.[25–27]

The folded and digitating junction between the epithelium and the underlying connective tissue ensures a sufficient adhesion of the epithelium to the connective tissue, with a high resistance to mechanical influences on the gingival surface during masticatory function. The extensive area of the interface also provides the epithelial cells sufficient nutrition and disposal of metabolic byproducts, which depend solely on diffusion between the epithelial layer and the capillary loops within the connective tissue projections.[28]

At the ultrastructural level, the epithelial–connective tissue junction demonstrates a complicated architecture (Fig 3-15). As in other mammalian squamous epithelia, the basal epithelial cells are separated from, and attached to, the connective tissue by the basal lamina, which comprises components produced by the epithelial cells. Visible by electron microscopy are the lamina lucida and the lamina densa. The lamina lucida is a 40-nm-wide electron-lucent zone immediately beneath the basal cell membrane. This zone contains the proteoglycan laminin.[29] The epithelial cell membrane has numerous electron-dense, thick zones dispersed along the cell membrane at intervals. These zones are called *hemidesmosomes*, and groups of tonofilaments in the epithelial cell cytoplasm anchor in these zones.

Underneath the lamina lucida is an electron-dense zone, called *lamina densa*, of approximately the same thickness as the lamina lucida. Lamina densa contains type IV collagen.[29] Anchoring fibrils formed of type VII collagen and secreted primarily by the keratinocyte are associated with type IV collagen in the lamina densa and bind the basal lamina to the underlying connective tissue.[30] The structural composition of the epithelial–connective tissue interface is also influenced by interactions between the two tissues.[31,32] Between the epithelial cells, intercellular attachment structures are similar to those found in other squamous epithelia, including gap junctions and desmosomes, which are pairs of hemidesmosomes (Figs 3-16a and 3-16b). Desmosomes are most prominent in the spinous layer.

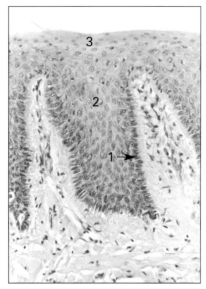

Fig 3-14 Parakeratinized gingival oral epithelium and its stratification: (1) basal cell layer (stratum basale), (2) spinous cell layers (stratum spinosum), and (3) parakeratinized cell layer (stratum corneum).

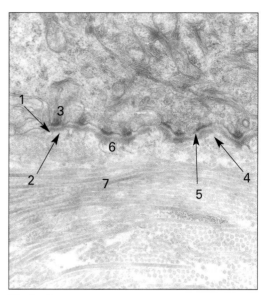

Fig 3-15 Ultrastructure of basal lamina area of gingival oral epithelium: (1) cell membrane of epithelial basal cell, (2) hemidesmosome, (3) tonofilaments inserting in hemidesmosome, (4) lamina lucida, (5) lamina densa, (6) anchoring fibrils, and (7) collagen fibrils.

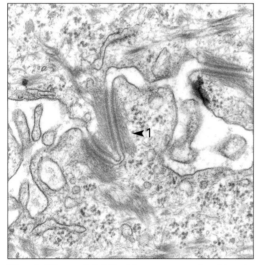

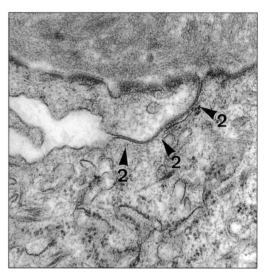

Figs 3-16a and 3-16b Ultrastructure of cell junctions of gingival oral epithelial cells: (1) desmosome and (2) gap junction.

Sulcular epithelium. The gingival sulcular epithelium, which is of very restricted distribution in healthy individuals, extends from the oral epithelium into the gingival sulcus facing the tooth. This epithelium thus forms the external wall of the 0.5-mm-deep gingival sulcus (see Fig 3-13), the internal border of which is the tooth. Apically, the border of the sulcular epithelium is the surface of the junctional epithelium. The sulcular epithelium is similar to the oral epithelium except for its lack of a stratum corneum. This lack of keratinization has given rise to

speculations that the gingival sulcus is particularly susceptible to influences from microorganisms.[28]

Junctional epithelium. The gingival junctional epithelium is part of the attachment between tooth and gingiva and thereby plays an extremely important role in periodontal health and disease. Because it is adapted for adherence to the tooth surface, this epithelium differs from the sulcular and oral epithelia in several aspects. In a healthy condition it is thinner, demonstrates a specific cytokeratin profile, and has an even interface with the connective tissue (see Fig 3-13). The junctional epithelium is thickest in its coronal part—15 to 30 cell layers—but toward the cementoenamel junction (which is the level of the most apical part of the epithelium in a patient without attachment loss), it thins to a few cell layers.

The suprabasal cells of the junctional epithelium are flattened, with their long axes parallel to the tooth surface. There are relatively few intercellular junctions and distensible intercellular spaces, and the adhesion between the epithelial cells thereby is reduced as compared with the other gingival epithelia. The spaces also enable diffusion of tissue fluids from the connective tissue through epithelium into the gingival sulcus. However, the unkeratinized surface, the orientation of cells with their long axes parallel to the tooth, and the intercellular spaces also permit the passage of some bacterial products from the gingival sulcus to the connective tissue.[33]

The junctional epithelium has two basal laminas, one being attached to the connective tissue (the external basal lamina) and another being attached to the tooth surface (the internal basal lamina).[34] The junctional epithelium is specialized to adhere organically by the basal lamina to the calcified dental tissues and to some extent protects the underlying periodontal ligament from invasion by noxious substances. The internal as well as the external basal lamina seem to include the same ultrastructural components as described for the basal lamina of the oral epithelium. However, it has not been possible to demonstrate the presence of type IV collagen in the internal basal lamina, whereas laminin was found in both areas.[35]

The junctional epithelium is constantly renewed by mitotic division of basal cells, coronal migration, and sloughing from the small surface at the base of the gingival sulcus, the turnover rate being only 4 to 6 days. The number of desquamated cells per surface area unit is many times higher than elsewhere in the oral mucosa. These flattened, elongated suprabasal cells do not resemble the cells of the suprabasal strata of the sulcular and oral epithelia, and their specificity suits the junctional epithelium to a situation in which the tooth penetrates and merges with the soft tissue.

Like the sulcular and the oral epithelia, the junctional epithelium contains Langerhans cells.[15] Even in clinical health, the junctional epithelium contains neutrophils migrating toward the bottom of the gingival sulcus. These cells therefore appear important in preserving the integrity of the healthy periodontium. The processes involved in breakdown of periodontal attachment originate in the gingival sulcus, which thereby constitutes an area of particular importance in diagnosing, treating, and researching the pathogenesis of periodontitis.

The primary junctional epithelium derives from the reduced enamel epithelium.[34] However, a junctional epithelium can also be regenerated after surgery from the basal cells of the gingival oral epithelium.[36]

Gingival Connective Tissue

The major portion of the connective tissue (lamina propria) of the free and attached gingiva consists of dense networks of collagen fibers, which interdependently fulfill numerous functions and provide firmness to the gingiva and to the attachment of the gingiva to the underlying cementum and alveolar bone. The collagen fibers course in various directions, and although they are intimately blended, they are classified into groups with presumed functions based on their location and insertion[28,37] (Figs 3-17a and 3-17b):

1. *Circular*—maintain contour and position of free marginal gingiva
2. *Dentogingival*—provide gingival support
3. *Alveologingival*—attach gingiva to bone
4. *Periostogingival*—attach gingiva to bone
5. *Transseptal*—maintain relationships of adjacent teeth and protect interproximal bone
6. *Transgingival*—secure alignment of teeth in arch
7. *Interpapillary*—provide support for interdental gingiva
8. *Intercircular*—stabilize teeth in arch
9. *Intergingival*—provide support and contour of attached gingiva

Collagen accounts for about 60% of gingival protein. The most common of the various collagen types in mucosa, as in skin, bone, dentin, and cementum, is type I collagen. Its molecules are aggregated into fibrils, which again are grouped into collagen fiber bundles, as seen with the light microscope.[38] Type I collagen of gingiva, however, is somewhat different biochemically from the collagen found in other parts of the body, including the skin.[39] The collagen turnover in normal gingiva is not as rapid as in the periodontal ligament but is significantly greater than in other tissues, such as skin, tendon, and palate tissues.[40]

Reticular or argyrophilic fibers are thin, loosely packed collagen fibers that take up silver stain. They are present at the interfaces between the surface epithelium and underlying connective tissue, and between endothelium and connective tissue surrounding the vessels.[41] The elastic fiber system, responsible for elastic properties of the gingiva, accounts for about 6% of total gingival protein. Mature elastic fibers are found adjacent to alveolar bone, whereas immature stages (represented by oxytalan) are found in the subepithelial connective tissue.[30]

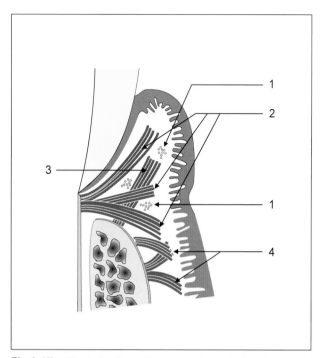

Fig 3-17a Gingival collagen fiber groups in vertical section: (1) circular fibers, (2) dentogingival fibers, (3) alveologingival fibers, and (4) periostogingival fibers.

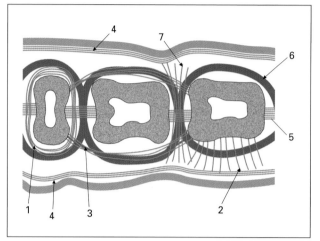

Fig 3-17b Gingival collagen fiber groups in horizontal section: (1) circular fibers, (2) dentogingival fibers, (3) intercircular fibers, (4) intergingival fibers, (5) transseptal fibers, (6) transgingival fibers, and (7) interpapillary fibers.

The ground substance in which cells and fibers of the connective tissue are embedded is composed of glycosaminoglycans, the most common being dermatan sulfate (accounting for 60% of total glycosaminoglycans), followed by chondroitin-4-sulfate (28%).[30]

Several cell types can be identified within the gingival connective tissue, where they constitute approximately 8% by volume. Fibroblasts, which account for 65% of connective tissue cells, are by far the predominating cells of the healthy gingival lamina propria.[42] They are most likely responsible for the constant functional adaptation of the tissues, since they possess abilities for synthesis, resorption, and enzymatic degradation of collagen and ground substance. Recent evidence suggests that these cells may also be involved in inflammation-mediated destruction of periodontal tissues.[43–46]

Red and white blood cells are present in the gingival connective tissue, the vast majority residing inside the vessels. However, even in connective tissue from sites devoid of clinical signs of inflammation, histologic examination commonly reveals neutrophils, macrophages, lymphocytes, mast cells, and few plasma cells.[47–49] Such accumulations are most prominent in the subsulcular region, which often exhibits local lysis of connective tissue fibers. Smaller numbers of cells may be found scattered between the gingival fibers elsewhere in the gingival connective tissue.[50] It is therefore plausible that the inflammatory cells contribute to the constant maintenance of the periodontal tissue integrity even in the healthy condition. That these cells can both protect the tissue from destruction and promote tissue breakdown is no longer surprising. It is the particular balance achieved among the wide spectrum of cellular activities taking place in the tissue that accounts for a final outcome of either protection or destruction. The cellular activities are widely mediated by growth factors and cytokines released from the cells in the periodontal environment. Other mediating functions rely on extracellular matrix components. The cells may be triggered to release mediators, which results in either catabolic or anabolic processes.[30,51] An intimate understanding of how these various signals are coordinated is necessary for deeper insight into the destructive processes.

Periodontal Ligament

The periodontal ligament serves a number of functions, the main one being anchorage of the tooth. This is achieved by collagen fibers attaching the cementum of the root to the alveolar bone proper (Fig 3-18). In addition, the periodontal ligament contains vessels, nerves, epithelial islands, ground substance, and cells. The periodontal ligament, which covers the entire root from the apex to the

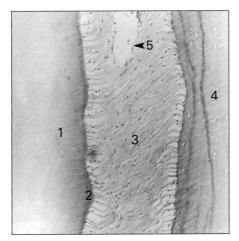

Fig 3-18 Photomicrograph of principal periodontal ligament fibers and their insertion: (1) dentin, (2) cementum, (3) principal periodontal ligament fibers, (4) alveolar bone, and (5) vessel.

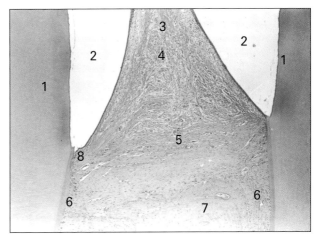

Fig 3-19 Interproximal periodontal tissues: (1) dentin, (2) enamel, (3) interdental papilla, (4) interpapillary fibers, (5) transseptal fibers, (6) periodontal ligament, (7) alveolar bone, and (8) dentogingival fibers.

cementoenamel junction of the healthy tooth, occupies the space between the root surface and alveolar bone, and in the coronal part the ligament is continuous with the subepithelial connective tissue of the gingiva (Fig 3-19; see Fig 3-13). The fibers and the ground substance of the periodontal ligament have a relatively high turnover rate, but the cellular turnover is rather slow.[52–54]

Type I collagen accounts for about 80% of periodontal ligament collagen; type III is second most common.[55] As in the gingiva, most of the collagen of the periodontal ligament is arranged into bundles called *principal fiber groups*. Among these is the loose connective tissue, in which periodontal ligament cells, secondary fibers, vessels (including lymphatic vessels), and nerves are all embedded. The fiber bundles of the periodontal ligament are inserted as Sharpey fibers into the cementum at one end and into the compact bone plate of the alveolus at the other end (Fig 3-20).

The principal fibers are wavy in their course, traversing the space between root and alveolar wall. Thus, sufficient elasticity is achieved to compensate minute movements of the tooth resulting from chewing. The principal fibers of the periodontal ligament can be divided into six groups, with presumed functions based on location and insertion[28] (Fig 3-21):

1. *Alveolar crest*—retain the tooth in the alveolus, oppose lateral forces, and protect deeper periodontal ligament structures
2. *Oblique*—oppose axially directed forces
3. *Transseptal*—prevent teeth from losing contact
4. *Horizontal*—oppose lateral forces
5. *Interradicular*—prevent tooth tipping and extrusion
6. *Apical*—prevent tooth tipping and extrusion, protect vessel and nerve supply to the tooth

There are secondary collagen fibers, as well as oxytalan and reticulin or argyrophilic fibers, with random orientation between the principal fiber groups. Such fibers are often associated with vessels and nerves, and they do not attach to bone and cementum. It has been hypothesized that oxytalan fibers function in a supportive, developmental, and/or sensory role in the periodontal ligament.[30] The periodontal ligament also contains a few elastic fibers, which are incorporated in the walls of arterial blood vessels.

The periodontal ligament, the cementum, and the alveolar bone are dynamic tissues that constantly adapt to altered functional states and to attrition of the teeth. The major cellular component of the periodontal ligament is fibroblasts. They are spindle shaped, their long axes being parallel to the principal fibers. The potential function of the fibroblasts includes both synthesis and degradation of collagen, as mentioned. These cells therefore play a key role in maintenance, re-formation, and degradation of the periodontal ligament. Periodontal ligament fibroblasts are capable of producing various types of collagen and ground substance components, depending on their origins.[56] Consequently, the distribution of various types of fibroblasts, with capabilities to produce the different connective tissue elements currently needed for adaptation and repair, is necessary for preserving optimal tissue health.

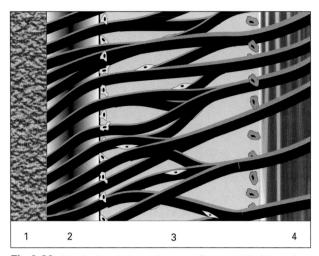

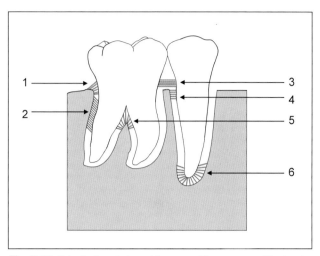

Fig 3-20 Principal periodontal ligament fibers and their insertion: (1) dentin; (2) cementum with Sharpey fibers, surface covered by cementoblasts; (3) periodontal ligament space with principal collagen fibers and scattered fibroblasts; and (4) alveolar bone with Sharpey fibers, surface covered by osteoblasts.

Fig 3-21 Principal periodontal ligament fiber groups: (1) alveolar crest fibers, (2) oblique fibers, (3) transseptal fibers, (4) horizontal fibers, (5) interradicular fibers, and (6) apical fibers.

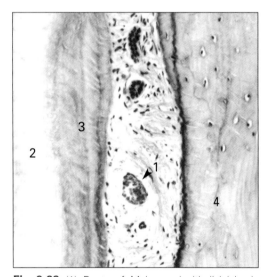

Fig 3-22 (1) Rests of Malassez (epithelial islands within the periodontal ligament), (2) dentin, (3) cementum, and (4) alveolar bone.

Remnants of the Hertwig epithelial root sheath, known as the *cell rests of Malassez*, are always present in the periodontal ligament[58] (Fig 3-22). The function of these cells is unknown, but their proliferative capability is preserved.[59] Inflammatory stimulation of their proliferation may result in the formation of cysts.

In the clinically noninflamed periodontium, inflammatory cells within the periodontal ligament are few. Where they do exist, they may include any type.

Cementum

The major function of the cementum, which covers the dentin of the tooth roots, is to attach periodontal ligament fibers to the root surface. Occasionally cementum covers small portions of the enamel of the crown. In composition and structure, cementum has several similarities to bone. One is the laminated structure, presumably reflecting a rhythmic deposition. The resting lines, in particular, are bonelike, having a higher content of ground substance and minerals, and a lower content of collagen, than adjacent cementum layers. Cementum differs from bone in the absence of vascularization and innervation. Bone, in contrast, has constant remodeling processes; in cementum, deposition is continuous. Cementum is not resorbed as a result of moderate compression forces, whereas bone is. This is an important characteristic of cementum, protecting the roots, for instance, from resorption during orthodontic movement of teeth. The calcified tissue is needed for the Sharpey fiber attachment to the roots to occur. The development of regenerative therapeutic procedures for

The periodontal ligament may also be the source of other cells, including cementoblasts and osteoblasts, with the various cell populations exhibiting specific bioavailability-signaling molecules. Presumably, future treatment strategies will be based on further elucidation of intercellular signaling and the possible application of molecular replacement where needed.[57]

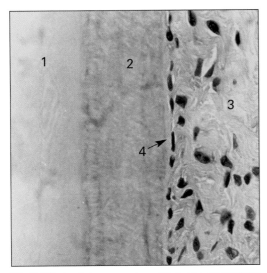

Fig 3-23 Acellular cementum: (1) dentin, (2) acellular cementum covered by a single layer of cementoblasts, (3) periodontal ligament with fibroblasts, and (4) cementoblast.

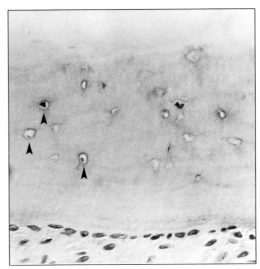

Fig 3-24 Cellular cementum. *Arrows* indicate cementocytes within lacunae of the cementum.

restoring lost periodontal attachment therefore has emphasized the need for more information about cementum and its deposition.

About 50% of mature cementum contains organic materials, including collagens, glycoproteins, and proteoglycans, with collagens accounting for the vast majority. Type I collagen makes up 90%, and type III collagen about 5%, of the organic matrix.[60] Cementum may be acellular, characterized by lack of embedded cells (Fig 3-23), or cellular, containing cementocytes in lacunae within the mineralized tissue[61] (Fig 3-24). Fibrillar cementum contains densely packed collagen fibrils, whereas afibrillar cementum has few, if any, fibrils in its matrix.[34] The bulk of the mineral portion of cementum is made up of calcium and phosphate, which is present in the form of hydroxyapatite.

The primary cementum formed before the tooth reaches occlusion is acellular, with few collagen fibrils. After occlusion is accomplished, additional secondary cementum deposition overlies the primary cementum. The secondary cementum is either acellular or cellular and contains more collagen fibrils.[62] Cellular cementum is often deposited on the apical third of the roots and in furcation areas. All cementum is formed by cementoblasts, which in cellular cementum are sometimes incorporated in the mineralized matrix to become cementocytes. Cementoblasts are relatively scarce; they reside within the periodontal ligament, at the surface of the cementum, and they resemble periodontal fibroblasts[63] (see Figs 3-23 and 3-24). During the

formation of cementum, the principal periodontal ligament fibers become embedded in the cementum, continuing there as the Sharpey fibers. Multinucleated giant cells, cementoclasts, may also be seen at the surface of the cementum, these cells being responsible for the resorption of the roots.

Alveolar Bone

Unlike cementum, alveolar bone is a vascular and innervated mineralized tissue. Although mineralized, it is constantly undergoing remodeling as a result of its adaptation to functional needs, such as those raised by attrition and migration of teeth. To maintain these processes, the alveolar bone comprises a population of bone-forming cells, osteoblasts, which secrete an extracellular organic matrix, osteoid; the main constituents of osteoid are collagen, glycoprotein, and proteoglycans. Bone collagen is composed predominantly of type I collagen, with only small amounts of type III and type IV collagen.[64] Once secreted, osteoid mineralizes as the result of mineral deposition and transformation to hydroxyapatite, and it gradually becomes mature bone (Fig 3-25). During the initial secretion phase, the osteoblasts and the small vessels are situated on the outer surface of bone trabeculae and cortical bone and on the inside of cortical bone plates, but with time they become engulfed by the osteoid produced. The osteoblasts are thereby transformed into osteocytes (see Fig 3-25) located in lacunae surrounded first

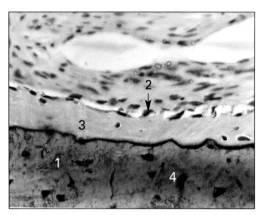

Fig 3-25 Osteoblasts secreting osteoid: (1) bone, (2) osteoblasts, (3) osteoid, and (4) osteocytes surrounded by bone.

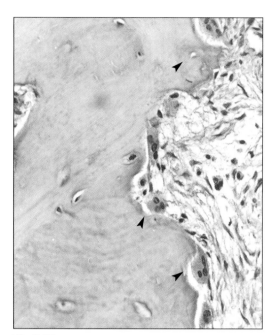

Fig 3-26 Howship lacunae (osteoclasts in resorption) on surface of interdental bone septum indicated by *arrows.*

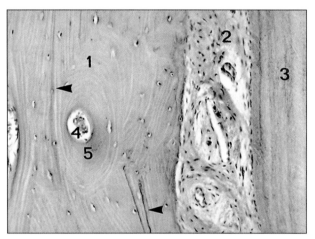

Fig 3-27 Haversian canal and osteon in lamellated alveolar bone with resting lines: (1) alveolar bone with lamellated bone structure, (2) periodontal ligament, (3) root, (4) haversian canal, and (5) osteon. *Arrows* indicate resting lines.

by osteoid and subsequently by bone. Osteocytes and osteoblasts are connected to each other by a network of cytoplasmic projections located in canaliculi.

The resorption of bone is carried out by multinucleated osteoclasts, but monocytes and osteoblasts may also participate. The osteoclasts are usually situated in lacunae of the bone surface (Howship lacunae) (Fig 3-26). The outer

surfaces of bone are lined by the periosteum containing collagen fibers, vessels, nerves, bone-forming cells, and bone-resorbing cells. The inner surfaces of bone, the marrow spaces, are similarly lined by the endosteum. The nutrition of bone is further provided by blood vessels inside the bone, frequently situated in canals (haversian canals) in the center of osteons (Fig 3-27).

The compact-bone lining of the tooth-bearing alveolus, apart from numerous canals allowing vessels and nerves to penetrate, exhibits a special architecture because the principal fibers of the periodontal ligament insert here as Sharpey fibers, the peripheries of which are mineralized.

Periods of bone formation frequently alternate with periods of bone resorption. New bone deposited on previously formed bone is separated from the old bone by reversal lines, whereas periodic bone apposition alternating with periods of quiescence give rise to resting lines resulting in a lamella structure of the bone (see Fig 3-27). Bone formation and resorption are mediated by numerous signal molecules, cytokines, and growth hormones, the activities of which are influenced by inflammation. The bone-forming cells, the bone-resorptive cells, and inflammatory cells communicate by producing and releasing these signal molecules, which bind to receptors on the surface of the target cells, altering cellular function. As an example of such a process, synthesis and release of the cytokine interleukin 1, the main source of which is the macrophage, may result in activation of bone resorption by osteoclasts and downregulation of bone formation by osteoblasts. Also, interleukin 1 stimulates the synthesis of metalloproteinases with abilities to degrade connective tissue components.[40,65]

Induction of interleukin 1 synthesis can be due to stimulation by antigens or other cytokines. Downregulation of interleukin 1 expression is mediated by a number of cytokines and by corticosteroids. Tissue homeostasis, for bone as for connective tissues, involves a perfect coordination of anabolic and catabolic processes and is obtained as the result of a balance in complex interactions of synergistic and antagonistic molecules. In addition to these processes, evidence has accumulated to support the idea of an integrated system whereby the organization of a tissue matrix couples with interactive mechanisms to produce selected cellular responses.[30] Consequently, the dynamics of the periodontium also reflect a complicated interaction whereby the architecture and function of the periodontium depend on the extracellular matrix.

Acknowledgments

Photographs prepared by Leise Elgaard, Department of Oral Medicine and Oral Surgery, University Hospital of Copenhagen. Radiographs courtesy of Dr Ib Sewerin, Department of Radiology, School of Dentistry, University of Copenhagen. Schematic illustrations prepared by Dr Finn Holm-Petersen, Copenhagen, Denmark. Histologic sections courtesy of Dr Jesper Reibel and Dr Finn Praetorius, Department of Oral Pathology, and Dr Søren Schou, Department of Oral and Maxillofacial Surgery, School of Dentistry, University of Copenhagen. Ultrastructural illustrations courtesy of Dr Lis Andersen, Department of Oral Pathology, School of Dentistry, University of Copenhagen.

References

1. Dummett CO, Barens G. Oromucosal pigmentation: An updated literary review. J Periodontol 1971;42:726–736.
2. Ainamo A, Ainamo J, Poikkeus R. Continuous widening of the band of attached gingiva from 23 to 65 years of age. J Periodontal Res 1981;16:595–599.
3. Saario M, Ainamo A, Mattila K, Ainamo J. The width of radiologically-defined attached gingiva over permanent teeth in children. J Clin Periodontol 1994;21:666–669.
4. Coolidge ED. The thickness of the human periodontal membrane. J Am Dent Assoc 1937;24:1260.
5. Zander HA, Hurzeler B. Continuous cementum apposition. J Dent Res 1958;37:1035.
6. Birn H. The vascular supply of the periodontal membrane: An investigation of the number and size of perforations in the alveolar wall. J Periodontal Res 1966;1:51–68.
7. Elliot JR, Bowers GM. Alveolar dehiscence and fenestrations. Periodontics 1963;1:245.
8. Carlsen O. Dental Morphology. Copenhagen: Munksgaard, 1987.
9. Mormann W, Meier C, Firestone A. Gingival blood circulation after experimental wounds in man. J Clin Periodontol 1979;6:417–424.
10. Lindhe J, Karring T. The anatomy of the periodontium. In: Lindhe J (ed). Textbook of Clinical Periodontology. Copenhagen: Munksgaard, 1989:19.
11. van Steenberghe D. The structure and function of periodontal innervation: A review of the literature. J Periodontal Res 1979; 14:185–203.
12. Linden RWA, Millar BJ, Scott BJJ. The innervation of the periodontal ligament. In: Berkowith BKB, Moxham BT, Newman HN (eds). The Periodontal Ligament in Health and Disease. New York: Mosby-Wolfe, 1995:133–159.
13. Moll R, Franke WW, Schiller DL, et al. The catalog of human cytokeratins: Patterns of expression in normal epithelia, tumors and cultured cells. Cell 1982;31:11–24.
14. Skougaard MR. Cell renewal with special reference to the gingival epithelium. In: Stable PH (ed). Advances in Oral Biology, vol 4. New York: Academic Press, 1970:261–288.
15. Juhl M, Reibel J, Stoltze K. Immunohistochemical distribution of keratin proteins in clinically healthy human gingival epithelia. Scand J Dent Res 1989;97:159–170.
16. Feghali-Assaly M, Sawaf MH, Serres G, et al. Cytokeratin profile of the junctional epithelium in partially erupted teeth. J Periodontal Res 1994;29:185–195.
17. Karring T, Lang NP, Löe H. The role of gingival connective tissue in determining epithelial differentiation. J Periodontal Res 1975;10:1–11.
18. Holmstrup P. Epithelial-mesenchymal interaction in human oral mucosa: Studies on heterotransplants in nude mice [thesis]. Copenhagen: Royal Dental College, 1985.
19. Schroeder HE, Page R. The normal periodontium. In: Schluger S, Yuodelis R, Page R, Johnson R (eds). Periodontal Diseases, ed 2. Philadelphia: Lea & Febiger, 1990:3–52.
20. Schroeder HE. Melanin containing organelles in cells of the human gingiva, II. Epithelial melanocytes. J Periodontal Res 1969;4:1–18.
21. Newcomb G, Seymour GJ, Powell RN. Association between plaque accumulation and Langerhans cell numbers in the oral epithelium of attached gingiva. J Clin Periodontol 1982;9:297–304.
22. Juhl M, Stoltze K, Reibel J. Distribution of Langerhans cells in clinically healthy human gingival epithelium with special emphasis on junctional epithelium. Scand J Dent Res 1988;96:199–208.
23. Karring T, Löe H. The three-dimensional concept of the epithelium-connective tissue boundary of gingiva. Acta Odontol Scand 1970;28:917–933.
24. Klein-Szanto AJ, Schroeder HE. Architecture and density of the connective tissue papillae of the human oral mucosa. J Anat 1977;123:93–109.
25. Soni NN, Silberkweit M, Hayes RL. Histological characteristics of stippling in children. J Periodontol 1963;34:427.
26. Rosenberg HM, Massler M. Gingival stippling in young adult males. J Periodontol 1967;38:473–480.
27. Owings JR Jr. A clinical investigation of the relationship between stippling and surface keratinization of the attached gingiva. J Periodontol 1969;40:588–592.
28. Hassell TM. Tissues and cells of the periodontium. Periodontol 2000 1993;3:9–38.
29. Salonen J, Pelliniemi LJ, Foidart JM, et al. Immunohistochemical characterization of the basement membranes of the human oral mucosa. Arch Oral Biol 1984;29:363–368.

30. Mariotti A. The extracellular matrix of the periodontium: Dynamic and interactive tissues. Periodontol 2000 1993;3:39–63.

31. Holmstrup P, Andersen L, Harder F. The junction zone of human epithelium and foreign stroma: Ultrastructural observations in human oral mucosal transplants in nude mice. Acta Pathol Microbiol Immunol Scand [A] 1984;92:211–218.

32. Holmstrup P. Studies on the deposition of laminin and type IV collagen in human oral mucosa transplanted to nude mice. Acta Pathol Microbiol Immunol Scand [A] 1985;93:1–8.

33. Listgarten MA. Pathogenesis of periodontitis. J Clin Periodontol 1986;13:418–430.

34. Schroeder HE, Listgarten MA. Fine Structure of the Developing Epithelial Attachment of Human Teeth, Monographs in Developmental Biology. Basel: Karger, 1977.

35. Salonen J, Santti R. Ultrastructural and immunohistochemical similarities in the attachment of human oral epithelium to the tooth in vivo and to an inert substrate in an explant culture. J Periodontal Res 1985;20:176–184.

36. Frank R, Fiore-Danno G, Cimasoni G, Ogilvie A. Gingival reattachment after surgery in man: An electron microscopic study. J Periodontol 1972;43:597–605.

37. Rateitschak KH, Rateitschak EM, Wolf HF, Hassell TM. Color Atlas of Dental Medicine. Vol 1: Periodontology, ed 2. Stuttgart:Thieme, 1989.

38. Chavrier C, Couble ML, Magloire H, Grimaud JA. Connective tissue organization of healthy human gingiva: Ultra-structural localization of collagen types I-III-IV. J Periodontal Res 1984;19: 221–229.

39. Narayanan AS, Page RC. Connective tissues of the periodontium: A summary of current work. Coll Relat Res 1983;3:33–64.

40. Page RC, Ammons WF. Collagen turnover in the gingiva and other mature connective tissues of the marmoset *Sanguinus oedipus*. Arch Oral Biol 1974;19:651–658.

41. Melcher AH. Gingival reticulin: Identification and role in histogenesis of collagen fibers. J Dent Res 1966;45:426.

42. Schroeder H, Münzel-Pedrazzoli S, Page R. Correlated morphometric and biochemical analysis of gingival tissue in early chronic gingivitis in man. Arch Oral Biol 1973;18:899–923.

43. Eley BM, Harrison JD. Intracellular collagen fibrils in the periodontal ligament of man. J Periodontal Res 1975;10:168–170.

44. Birkedal-Hansen H. From tadpole collagenase to a family of matrix metalloproteinases. J Oral Pathol 1988;17:445–451.

45. Page RC. The role of inflammatory mediators in the pathogenesis of periodontal disease. J Periodontal Res 1991;26:230–242.

46. Sodek J, Overall CM. Matrix metalloproteinases in periodontal tissue remodelling. In: Birkedal-Hansen H, Werb Z, Welgus H, Van Wart H (eds). Matrix Metalloproteinases and Inhibitors. Stuttgart: Gustav Fischer, 1992:352.

47. Seymour GJ, Powell RN, Aithen J. Experimental gingivitis in humans: A clinical and histologic investigation. J Periodontol 1983;54:522–528.

48. Seymour GJ, Powell RN, Cole KL, et al. Experimental gingivitis in humans: A histochemical and immunological characterization of the lymphoid cell subpopulations. J Periodontal Res 1983;18:375–385.

49. Laurell L, Rylander H, Sundin K. Histologic characteristics of clinically healthy gingiva in adolescents. Scand J Dent Res 1987;95:456–462.

50. Moskow BS, Polson AM. Histologic studies on the extension of the inflammatory infiltrate in human periodontitis. J Clin Periodontol 1991;18:534–542.

51. Hefti AF. Aspects of cell biology of the normal periodontium. Periodontol 2000 1993;3:64–75.

52. Crumley P. Collagen formation in the normal and stressed periodontium. Periodontics 1964;2:53.

53. Minkoff R, Engström TG. A long-term comparison of protein turnover in subcrestal vs supracrestal fibre tracts in the mouse periodontium. Arch Oral Biol 1979;24:817–824.

54. McCulloch CA, Melcher AH. Continuous labelling of the periodontal ligament of mice. J Periodontal Res 1983;18:231–241.

55. Butler WT, Birkedal-Hansen H, Beegle WF, et al. Proteins of the periodontium: Identification of collagens with the [alpha1(I)] 2alpha2 and [alpha1(III)]3 structures in bovine periodontal ligament. J Biol Chem 1975;250:8907–8912.

56. Limeback H, Sodek J, Aubin JE. Variation in collagen expression by cloned periodontal ligament cells. J Periodontal Res 1983; 18:242–248.

57. Pitaru S, McCulloch CAG, Narayanan SA. Cellular origins and differentiation control mechanisms during periodontal development and wound healing. J Periodontal Res 1994;29:81–94.

58. Reeve CM, Wentz FJ. The prevalence, morphology and distribution of the epithelial cell rests in the human periodontal ligament. Oral Surg 1962;15:785.

59. Johansen JR. Incorporation of tritiated thymidine by the epithelial rests of Malassez after attempted extraction of rat molars. Acta Odontol Scand 1970;28:463–470.

60. Birkedal-Hansen H, Butler WT, Taylor RE. Proteins of the periodontium: Characterization of the insoluble collagens of bovine dental cementum. Calcif Tissue Res 1977;23:39–44.

61. Gottlieb B. Biology of the cementum. J Periodontol 1942;13:13.

62. Stern I. An electron microscopic study of the cementum: Sharpey's fibers and periodontal ligament in the rat incisor. Am J Anat 1964;115:377.

63. Furseth R. The fine structure of the cellular cementum of young human teeth. Arch Oral Biol 1969;14:1147–1158.

64. Hauschka PV, Wians FH. Osteocalcin-hydroxyapatite interaction in the extracellular organic matrix of bone. Anat Rec 1989; 224:180–188.

65. Kjeldsen M, Holmstrup P, Bendtzen K. Marginal periodontitis and cytokines: A review of the literature. J Periodontol 1993;64: 1013–1022.

CHAPTER 4

Histopathology of Periodontal Diseases

Palle Holmstrup
- Gingivitis
- Periodontitis

Gingivitis

Usually, gingivitis is a chronic disease. However, there is no sharp border that histologically distinguishes healthy gingiva from gingivitis. Even the clinically healthy gingiva exhibits accumulations of inflammatory cells. Based on findings in experimental animal studies, a sequential development of histologic changes in the gingival tissues from healthy gingiva to periodontitis has been posited: the initial lesion, the early lesion, the established lesion, and the advanced lesion.[1] However, not all these stages have been proven histologically in human subjects. The character of the cellular infiltrate in neither gingivitis nor periodontitis seems to follow a logical, consistent progression, so the concept of sequential development remains questionable.[2,3]

The tissue changes seen microscopically vary, with the mildest of changes not being related to clinically visible pathology. These subclinical findings are early stages of inflammation as revealed by the presence of few neutrophils, macrophages, lymphocytes, and very few plasma cells in the subsulcular connective tissue[4–6.] (Figs 4-1a and 4-1b).

Even the subclinical inflammatory reactions are accompanied by localized areas of lysis of connective tissue fibers, particularly in the region beneath the sulcular epithelium.[3,7]

Plaque-induced clinical gingivitis is characterized by reddening, swelling, and bleeding on probing. The condition is reversible and may persist without further progression into periodontitis with loss of connective tissue attachment.

Epithelial Changes

Histologically, the gingival tissues demonstrate a response to bacterial plaque accumulation in the gingival sulcus area. Low-molecular-weight products from the bacteria penetrate the epithelium and initiate a number of changes in both the epithelium and the connective tissue. Gingivitis is characterized by the formation of a small gingival pocket or pseudopocket resulting from loss of junctional epithelial attachment, as well as by edema of gingival tissue (Figs 4-2a and 4-2b). There is no apical migration of the junctional epithelium, but the junctional epithelium has widened intercellular spaces, and it has proliferated into the underlying connective tissue with the formation of

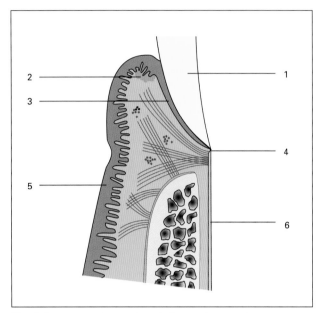

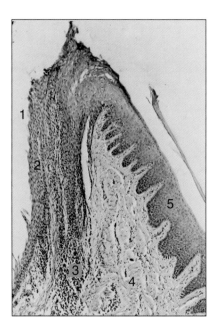

Fig 4-1a Tissue changes in subclinical gingivitis: (1) enamel, (2) limited loss of subsulcular connective tissue in slightly inflamed area—inflammatory infiltrate dominated by neutrophils, (3) gingival sulcular epithelium, (4) cementoenamel junction, (5) gingival oral epithelium, and (6) cementum.

Fig 4-1b Subclinical gingivitis with slight inflammation: (1) enamel; (2) gingival junctional epithelium with migration of few neutrophils into the gingival sulcus; (3) limited inflammatory infiltrate, dominated by neutrophils; (4) gingival connective tissue; and (5) gingival oral epithelium.

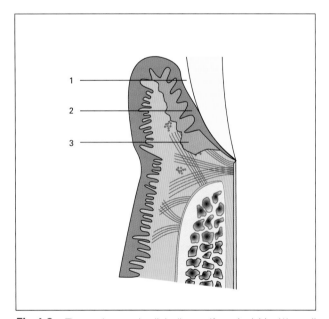

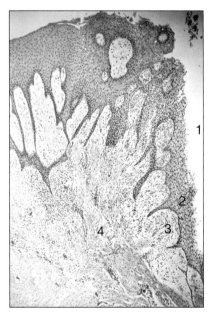

Fig 4-2a Tissue changes in clinically manifest gingivitis: (1) small gingival pocket due to loss of junctional epithelial attachment and edema of the tissue; (2) gingival junctional epithelium with proliferations into underlying connective tissue and with neutrophils migrating into the gingival sulcus; and (3) area infiltrated with inflammatory cells, mainly neutrophils and lymphocytes, with loss of collagen.

Fig 4-2b Gingivitis with more intensive inflammation and visible loss of collagen: (1) enamel; (2) gingival junctional epithelium with proliferations into underlying connective tissue—neutrophils migrate through the epithelium; (3) area infiltrated with inflammatory cells, predominantly neutrophils and lymphocytes, with loss of collagen; and (4) gingival connective tissue.

extensive rete pegs. Usually, there is a substantial migration of inflammatory cells, particularly neutrophils, through the junctional epithelium into the gingival sulcus. These cells protect the periodontal tissues against microbial attack, and neutrophils often form a wall between the microbial plaque and the sulcular and junctional epithelia. Thus, neutrophils in the gingival crevice form the first barrier of defense against the accumulating bacteria. The neutrophils in the sulcus phagocytose bacteria by engulfing the microorganisms in vacuoles.[8]

Although the bacteria in the gingival sulcus are in a close relationship to the sulcular and junctional epithelia, the bacteria in general do not penetrate the epithelium in chronic gingivitis. Bacterial aggregations, however, may be seen in contact with the epithelial surface, and sometimes they are found in the intercellular spaces.

The basal lamina separating the connective tissue from the sulcular and junctional epithelia in the inflamed area shows changes commonly seen in inflammation, which are observable with electron microscopy (Fig 4-3). These changes include duplications, interruptions, and altered width. Detached basal lamina fragments may also be seen in the subjacent connective tissue.[9]

The oral epithelium shows an altered expression of cytokeratins, particularly where the oral epithelium merges with the sulcular epithelium.[10] It is unknown whether these changes are due to altered epithelial differentiation control, but they might be a result of the release of inflammatory mediators. The number of Langerhans cells, the intraepithelial dendritic macrophage-like cells, increases numerically in early gingival inflammation,[11] probably because foreign antigen processing and stimulation of T-cell responses at this stage of the disease are particularly important.

Connective Tissue Changes

The subsulcular connective tissue is characterized by inflammation with dilation of blood vessels and exudation of serum, including serum antibodies.[12,13] The exudation is the background of increased crevicular fluid, characteristic of gingivitis and periodontitis. Histologically, the inflammatory process usually has both acute and chronic characteristics, as manifested by the presence of neutrophils, lymphocytes, macrophages, mast cells, and plasma cells in the infiltrate. The intensity and extension of the infiltrate vary with the challenges presented by the local microflora, the individual inflammatory reactions to the microflora, and the durations of these reactions.

The mildest forms of inflammation are dominated by neutrophils and T lymphocytes,[4,5] whereas the gingivitis lesions with subsequent progression into periodontitis appear to be dominated by B lymphocytes, which transform

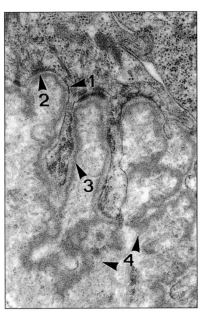

Fig 4-3 Ultrastructure of epithelial basal lamina area in gingivitis: (1) cell membrane of junctional epithelial basal cell, (2) hemidesmosome, (3) lamina densa, and (4) duplications of lamina densa.

into plasma cells.[1,14–16] In advanced lesions, widespread distribution of inflammatory cells involving larger segments of the gingiva is seen.[3]

The inflammatory effector cells migrate from the peripheral circulation to accumulate in the periodontal tissues, as seen by microscopic examination. The mechanism behind this is first triggered by adhesion of the inflammatory effector cells to the vessel walls of the target tissue. The adhesion is mediated by adhesion molecules expressed on the surface of the endothelial cells and on the surface of the leukocytes. After adhesion to the endothelium, the leukocytes penetrate the vessel wall and migrate into the tissue. As an example, the migration of neutrophils is known as a chemotactic response to bacteria. The chemotaxis is a directed movement of the cells in response to a chemoattractant. After chemotactic migration, the neutrophil recognizes the microorganism in the gingival sulcus, binds to it, and phagocytoses it.[17]

Tissue Damage

It appears that many processes are involved in a successful first defense. If one or more of these processes are inadequate because of either genetic or acquired host deficiencies, the defense mechanisms suffer, and further microbial colonization and tissue damage may succeed. Such deficiencies have been described for certain patient categories of periodontitis. Depressed chemotaxis and phagocytosis have been reported in patients with localized aggressive periodontitis.[17] However, some periodontal bacteria, such as *Actinobacillus actinomycetemcomitans*, *Porphyromonas gingivalis*, and *Fusobacterium nucleatum*, may jeopardize the protective functions of neutrophils by the inhibition of phagocytosis, production of superoxide dismutase, and direct leukocytotoxicity.[18]

There is no evidence of alveolar bone resorption in gingivitis lesions. The connective tissue in the subsulcular area is subjected to lysis of collagen, which in 4 days of experimentally induced gingivitis in dogs may amount to as much as 70% of the collagen fraction.[7,19] The number of fibroblasts within the area of inflammation is reduced, and those fibroblasts still residing in the area are altered, presumably with reduced capacity for collagen synthesis.[20,21] Vascular proliferation and edema also appear.

The collagen loss, which can be total in the heavily inflamed area of a chronic gingivitis lesion, may be mediated by inflammatory signal molecules produced by the cells participating in the inflammatory process and by proteases released from neutrophils, macrophages, and fibroblasts in the area. There are, however, several pathways by which collagen degradation can be processed in the periodontal tissues. Phagocytosis and intracellular digestion of enzymatically degraded collagen fragments may be accomplished by macrophages,[22] but gingival fibroblasts have been shown to possess the capability of total denaturation of collagen. Furthermore, the constant turnover through degradation and synthesis of periodontal connective tissue achieves a fine balance on which the tissue integrity depends. Alterations with downregulation or decreased capacity of collagen synthesis of some fibroblasts may also result in loss of connective tissue.

It has been demonstrated that the gingival collagen loss due to inflammation is characterized not only by constant proportions of type I and type III collagens but also by marked increases in the relative content of type V collagen.[23] This may reflect a differentiated response in gingival fibroblasts during inflammation.

Tissue Formation

Extensive formation of new collagen fibers is sometimes the predominant histologic reaction to inflammation, especially in its border zones.[3] This is one characteristic response of fibroblasts. The microscopically observable changes in the gingival connective tissue presumably reflect the variability in inflammatory cell activities, the most important of which are mediated by cytokines and

growth factors. These are released by the involved cells as the result of inflammatory exacerbation alternating with periods of quiescence.

Periodontitis

Pocket Formation

The most characteristic feature distinguishing periodontitis from gingivitis is loss of connective tissue attachment and bone in conjunction with the formation of a pocket due to the apical migration of the junctional epithelium. As a consequence of this apical migration, the junctional epithelium becomes attached to the root cementum, and the external wall of the pocket is covered by an epithelium, the so-called pocket epithelium (Figs 4-4a and 4-4b). The initial stages of periodontitis are easily detectable microscopically but very difficult to reveal clinically. Loss of attachment can be measured with the periodontal probe, but probing is crude compared with microscopy.

The formation of a pocket between the epithelium and the root surface enables further retention of bacteria,[24] and the low reduction-oxidation (redox) potential favors colonization by periodontal pathogens, most of which are anaerobic.[2] The pocket epithelium, which is invaded by neutrophils, is characterized by thickening with irregular proliferations of rete pegs, and the epithelium becomes microulcerated.[25–27] This facilitates the entry of bacteria and their products into the connective tissue, whereby the host's local defense mechanisms may be further challenged. The possible initiation of a burst of destructive activity is obvious. However, it should be emphasized that even in the absence of ulceration, the junctional epithelium is permeable. Therefore, the junctional epithelium itself can offer a route for noxious stimuli, and the importance of ulceration as a prerequisite in the pathogenesis of a burst of disease activity is debatable.[2]

Loss of Attachment

The pathologic connective tissue changes characteristic of gingivitis spread apically in periodontitis. The process involves first the dentogingival and dentoperiosteal collagen fibers and later the periodontal ligament fibers. The loss of connective tissue attachment in the root surface is irreversible, because the pocket epithelium between cementum and connective tissue prevents reinsertion of collagen fibers in the root surface.[28]

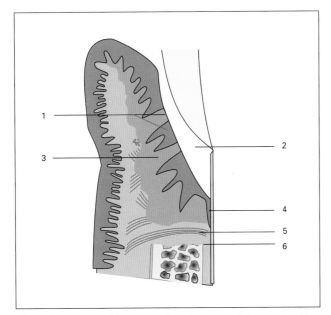

Fig 4-4a Periodontitis in periodontal tissues: (1) pocket epithelium with scattered ulceration and with migrating neutrophils; (2) gingival pocket due to apical migration of junctional epithelium and loss of periodontal ligament fibers; (3) area infiltrated with inflammatory cells, including increased numbers of plasma cells—the loss of connective tissue is expanded apically; (4) junctional epithelium attached to root cementum; (5) intact transseptal fibers; and (6) resorption of alveolar bone that has resulted in a more apical position of the bone margin.

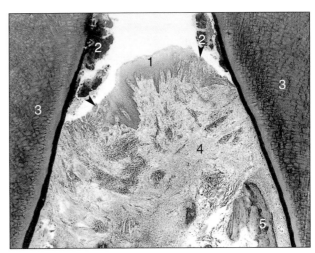

Fig 4-4b Periodontitis in interproximal tissues with apical migration of pocket epithelium, loss of connective tissue attachment, and loss of bone in interproximal papilla: (1) gingival oral epithelium, (2) calculus, (3) dentin, (4) gingival connective tissue with inflammation, and (5) alveolar bone. Arrows indicate ulcerated pocket epithelium.

Inflammatory Reaction

Beneath the pocket epithelium, the connective tissue shows mixed populations of neutrophils, macrophages, lymphocytes, and plasma cells infiltrating the area.[3,29,30] The infiltrate generally extends from the pocket epithelium to the underlying crest of the alveolar bone, which is undergoing osteoclastic resorption. Frequently, small lymphocytes are closest to the sulcular epithelium, and underlying these cells are accumulations of plasma cells and macrophages. Neutrophils are predominantly seen in the pocket and pocket epithelium. Perivascular plasma-cell infiltration is common. According to most studies, the irreversible changes in attachment level appear to be associated with increased numbers of plasma cells in the gingival connective tissue.

Disease activity, however, may be reflected not in a shift of inflammatory cell populations visible in the light microscope but rather in a switching on and off of activities of cells present in the tissues.[15] Even small numbers of certain T-lymphocyte and monocyte/macrophage subsets[31] may exert profound modulatory effects on other cell types by release of cytokines.[15] Some of these cytokines, including interleukin 1, tumor necrosis factor, and interleukin 6, have

at this point been identified in periodontitis-affected tissue, or they have been produced by pathogen-stimulated inflammatory and noninflammatory cells isolated from periodontal tissues.[32] Data now suggest that disease progression is not linear, as previously described.[33,34] It is obvious from the array of potentials of the cells present in the gingival tissues that disease progression may occur as a rapid response consisting of activation of processes with a catabolic outcome. Likewise, processes with an anabolic dominance may occur intermittently.

Changes of the Alveolar Bone

The collagen of the gingival connective tissue is reduced in the area subjacent to the pocket epithelium, but areas with formation of new collagen are commonly seen in the periphery of this region as well. Most frequently, intact transseptal fibers over the crestal bone are present independently of the severity of alveolar destruction.[3,35] The inflammatory infiltrate may spread beyond the gingival collagen fibers. Lymphocytes and plasma cells have been revealed not only between transseptal fibers but also in marrow spaces of crestal alveolar bone and within the periodontal ligament. Bone resorption by osteoclast activity is common. Remodeling and simultaneous deposition of new bone with progressive thickening of marginal alveolar bone and endosteal resorption of crestal bone also occur as the result of inflammation. Fibrosis of the fatty bone marrow is commonly found associated with the spread of periodontal inflammation.[3]

Along the root surface, the inflammatory process results in the complete breakdown of collagen fibers from 0.5 to 1.0 mm apical to the base of the pocket epithelium.[36,37]

In periodontal inflammation, the cementum at the root surface is more resistant to resorption than is bone. This is probably due to the reduced metabolic processes characteristic of nonvascularized cementum as compared with vascularized bone. Cementum also has a higher fluoride content than bone, which gives it a greater resistance to the dissolving acids produced by the resorbing cells.[38]

Following destruction of the periodontal attachment, the root cementum becomes exposed to the pocket or, if gingival recession occurs, to the oral cavity. Inorganic and organic substances may thereby gain access to the surface cementum. Inorganic substances—including fluoride, calcium, and phosphate—may, depending on the environment, increase the mineral content of the surface cementum. This results in increased resistance to caries. However, adsorption of organic substances (including bacterial toxins such as lipopolysaccharide and leukotoxin) to the exposed root cementum is a complicating phenomenon that may necessitate therapeutic intervention such as removal of root cementum.

Categories of Periodontitis

There are no major histologic differences in the various categories of periodontitis (except for acute necrotizing periodontitis). However, local exacerbation may result in acute lesions with abscess formation. Such abscesses show accumulations of neutrophils, bacteria, and necrotic lesions.

Aggressive Periodontitis

Bacterial tissue invasion has been demonstrated in aggressive periodontitis, where bacteria have been found in the epithelium, between collagen fibers, and inside phagocytotic cells. The invading species has been identified as *Actinobacillus actinomycetemcomitans*, an organism commonly associated with aggressive periodontitis.[39–41] The significance of the tissue invasion by pathogenic bacteria is that such bacteria may remain unaffected by scaling and root planing, thereby giving rise to continuous infection of the tissues and persistence of disease. In aggressive periodontitis lesions, the destruction of the supporting tissues is more extensive than in chronic periodontitis. Extracellular structures occupy only 20% of the volume, compared with 50% in chronic periodontitis.

Also, the plasma-cell infiltration appears to be more massive in aggressive periodontitis than in chronic periodontitis,[42] and there is a greater number of degenerating plasma cells as well.[43]

Acute Necrotizing Gingivitis and Periodontitis

The histologic findings in acute necrotizing forms of gingivitis and periodontitis differ from those in the more common forms of gingivitis and periodontitis. The acute necrotizing forms are characterized by ulceration, with a surface necrosis involving epithelium and superficial connective tissue. Clinically, this necrosis can appear light yellow to gray. At the ultrastructural level, the necrotic lesions exhibit four layers.[44] The superficial bacterial zone typically contains bacteria of varying form and size, including spirochetes. Apical to this zone a neutrophil-rich zone is characteristic, with leukocytes dominated by neutrophils, as well as bacteria, including spirochetes. Further apical is a necrotic zone, with necrotic cells intermingled with bacteria, including spirochetes and fusobacteria. In the most apical zone of the necrotic lesion, the intact tissue is invaded by spirochetes. The connective tissue shows proliferation of vessels and vasodilation, as well as acute inflammation with dense neutrophilic infiltrates containing macrophages. Deeper in the tissues, the inflammatory process exhibits plasma cells.

Acknowledgments

Photographs prepared by Leise Elgaard, Department of Oral Medicine and Oral Surgery, University Hospital of Copenhagen. Histologic sections courtesy of Dr Jesper Reibel and Dr Finn Praetorius, Department of Oral Pathology, and Dr Søren Schou, Department of Oral and Maxillofacial Surgery, School of Dentistry, University of Copenhagen. Ultrastructural illustrations courtesy of Dr Lis Andersen, Department of Oral Pathology, School of Dentistry, University of Copenhagen. Schematic illustrations by Dr Finn Holm-Petersen, Copenhagen, Denmark.

References

1. Page RC, Schroeder HE. Pathogenesis of inflammatory periodontal disease: A summary of current work. Lab Invest 1976; 34:235–249.

2. Gillett IR, Johnson NW, Curtis MA, et al. The role of histopathology in the diagnosis and prognosis of periodontal diseases. J Clin Periodontol 1990;17:673–684.

3. Moskow BS, Polson AM. Histologic studies on the extension of the inflammatory infiltrate in human periodontitis. J Clin Periodontol 1991;18:534–542.

4. Seymour GJ, Powell RN, Aithen J. Experimental gingivitis in humans: A clinical and histologic investigation. J Periodontol 1983;54:522–528.

5. Seymour GJ, Powell RN, Cole KL, et al. Experimental gingivitis in humans: A histochemical and immunological characterization of the lymphoid cell subpopulations. J Periodontal Res 1983;18:375–385.

6. Laurell L, Rylander H, Sundin Y. Histologic characteristics of clinically healthy gingiva in adolescents. Scand J Dent Res 1987;95:456–462.

7. Payne WA, Page RC, Ogilvie AL, Hall WB. Histopathologic features of the initial and early stages of experimental gingivitis in man. J Periodontal Res 1975;10:51–64.

8. Brecx M, Patters MR. Morphology of polymorphonuclear neutrophils during periodontal disease in the cynomolgus monkey. J Clin Periodontol 1985;12:591–606.

9. Selvig KA. Ultrastructural changes in periodontal diseases. In: Genco RJ, Goldman HM, Cohen DW (eds). Contemporary Periodontics. St Louis: Mosby, 1990.

10. Bosch FX, Ouhayoun JP, Bader BL, et al. Extensive changes in cytokeratin expression patterns in pathologically affected human gingiva. Virchows Arch B Cell Pathol Incl Mol Pathol 1989;58:59–77.

11. Hitzig C, Monteil RA, Charbit Y, Teboul M. Quantification of T6+ and HLA/DR+ Langerhans cells in normal and inflamed gingiva. J Biol Buccale 1989;17:103–108.

12. Platt D, Crosby RG, Dalbow MH. Evidence for the presence of immunoglobulins and antibodies in inflamed periodontal tissues. J Periodontol 1970;41:215–222.

13. van Swol RL, Gross A, Setterstrom JA, D'Alessandro SM. Immunoglobulins in periodontal tissues, II. Concentrations of immunoglobulins in granulation tissue from pockets of periodontosis and periodontitis patients. J Periodontol 1980;51:20–24.

14. Mackler BF, Frostad KB, Robertson PB, Levy BM. Immunoglobulin bearing lymphocytes and plasma cells in human periodontal disease. J Periodontal Res 1977;12:37–45.

15. Gillett R, Cruchley A, Johnson NW. The nature of the inflammatory infiltrates in childhood gingivitis, juvenile periodontitis and adult periodontitis: Immunocytochemical studies using a monoclonal antibody to HLADR. J Clin Periodontol 1986;13:281–288.

16. Schroeder HE, Munzel-Pedrazzoli S, Page RC. Correlated morphometric and biochemical analysis of gingival tissue in early chronic gingivitis in man. Arch Oral Biol 1973;18:899–923.

17. Van Dyke TE, Vaikuntam J. Neutrophil function and dysfunction in periodontal disease. Curr Opin Periodontol 1994;(2):19–27.

18. Slots J, Genco RJ. Black-pigmented *Bacteroides* species, *Capnocytophaga* species, and *Actinobacillus actinomycetemcomitans* in human periodontal disease: Virulence factors in colonization, survival, and tissue destruction. J Dent Res 1984;63:412–421.

19. Schroeder HE, Graf-de Beer M, Attström R. Initial gingivitis in dogs. J Periodontal Res 1975;10:128–142.

20. Simpson DM, Avery BE. Pathologically altered fibroblasts within lymphoid cell infiltrates in early gingivitis. J Dent Res 1973;52:1156.

21. Simpson DM, Avery BE. Histopathologic and ultrastructural features of inflamed gingiva in the baboon. J Periodontol 1974;45:500–510.

22. Perez-Tamayo R. Collagen degradation and resorption: Physiology and pathology. In: Perez-Tamayo R, Rojkind M (eds). Molecular Pathology of Connective Tissues. New York: Marcel Dekker, 1973.

23. Narayanan AS, Clagett JA, Page RC. Effect of inflammation on the distribution of collagen types I, III, IV and V and type I trimer and fibronectin in human gingivae. J Dent Res 1985;64:1111–1116.

24. Muller-Glauser W, Schroeder HE. The pocket epithelium: A light- and electronmicroscopic study. J Periodontol 1982;53:133–144.

25. Schroeder HE. Histopathology of the gingival sulcus. In: Lehner T (ed). Borderland Between Caries and Periodontal Disease. London: Academic Press, 1977:43–78.

26. Kaplan GB, Ruben MP, Pameijer CH. Scanning electron microscopy of the epithelium of the periodontal pocket, II. J Periodontol 1977;48:634–638.

27. Saglie R, Carranza FA Jr, Newman MG, Pattison GA. Scanning electron microscopy of the gingival wall of deep periodontal pockets in humans. J Periodontal Res 1982;17:284–293.

28. Nyman S, Gottlow J, Lindhe J, et al. New attachment formation by guided tissue regeneration. J Periodontal Res 1987;22:252–254.

29. Seymour GJ, Greenspan JS. The phenotypic characterization of lymphocyte subpopulations in established human periodontal disease. J Periodontal Res 1979;14:39–46.

30. Okada H, Kida T, Yamagami H. Identification and distribution of immunocompetent cells in inflamed gingiva of human chronic periodontitis. Infect Immun 1983;41:365–374.

31. Topoll HH, Zwadlo G, Lange DE, Sorg G. Phenotypic dynamics of macrophage subpopulations during human experimental gingivitis. J Periodontal Res 1989;24:106–112.

32. Kjeldsen M, Holmstrup P, Bendtzen K. Marginal periodontitis and cytokines: A review of the literature. J Periodontol 1993;64:1013–1022.

33. Lindhe J, Haffajee AD, Socransky SS. Progression of periodontal disease in adult subjects in the absence of periodontal therapy. J Clin Periodontol 1983;10:433–442.

34. Socransky SS, Haffajee AD, Goodson JM, Lindhe J. New concepts of destructive periodontal disease. J Clin Periodontol 1984;11:21–32.

35. Goldman HM. The behavior of transseptal fibers in periodontal disease. J Dent Res 1957;36:249.

36. Selvig KA. Ultrastructural changes in cementum and adjacent connective tissue in periodontal disease. Acta Odontol Scand 1966;24:459.

37. Deporter DA, Brown DY. Fine structural observations on the mechanism of loss of attachment during experimental periodontal disease in the rat. J Periodontal Res 1980;15:304–313.

38. Yoon SH, Brudevold F, Smith FA, et al. Distribution of fluorine in teeth and alveolar bone. J Am Dent Assoc 1960;61:565.

39. Gillett R, Johnson NW. Bacterial invasion of the periodontium in a case of juvenile periodontitis. J Clin Periodontol 1982;9:93–100.

40. Carranza FA Jr, Saglie R, Newman MG, Valentine PL. Scanning and transmission electron microscopic study of tissue-invading microorganisms in localized juvenile periodontitis. J Periodontol 1983;54:598–617.

41. Christersson LA, Albini B, Zambon JJ, et al. Tissue localization of *Actinobacillus actinomycetemcomitans* in human periodontitis, I. Light, immunofluorescence and electron microscopic studies. J Periodontol 1987;58:529–539.

42. Liljenberg B, Lindhe J. Juvenile periodontitis: Some microbiological, histopathological and clinical characteristics. J Clin Periodontol 1980;7:48–61.

43. Joachim F, Barber P, Newman HN, Osborn J. The plasma cell at the advancing front of the lesion in chronic periodontitis. J Periodontal Res 1990;25:49–59.

44. Listgarten MA. Electron microscopic observations on the bacterial flora of acute necrotizing ulcerative gingivitis. J Periodontal Res 1965;36:328.

Microbiology and Etiology of Periodontal Diseases

Kenneth S. Kornman
- Ecology: Bacteria and Host on Mucous Membranes
- Plaque Biofilms: A Teeming Community
- Bacterial Complexes
- Calculus: What Is It and Why Remove It?
- Bacterial Associations with Health and Disease
- Therapeutic Goals and Bacterial Outcomes of Therapy

Jørgen Slots
- Herpesvirus in Human Periodontal Disease

Infectious diseases have influenced many aspects of human history. In fact, until the 1940s a great part of human evolution appears to have been driven by the challenge of surviving in a microbe-dominated environment. Because of our efforts to protect ourselves from microbial pathogens and the science of host-parasite interactions, we have traditionally thought of bacteria and viruses as outside invaders to be eliminated, or at least controlled. Microorganisms have been considered different from humans, and life has been a constant battle between "them" and "us." But of course, the bacteria that cover most of our body surfaces are not just benign but actually essential to our life on earth. Although we have known about the beneficial roles of bacteria for many years, only in the past few years have we better understood the extent of integration that exists between the bacteria and the host.

The human mouth contains more than 300 bacterial species.[1] Although some of these species are transients, found infrequently in samples taken from the mouth, most are common inhabitants of the oral cavity of adults. Out of all these species, very few have been shown to have any potential to damage the host. This is characteristic of a relationship that has evolved carefully over many, many years. Within certain conditions, such as in a well-nourished, systemically healthy individual with reasonable oral hygiene practices, a health-associated balance is achieved. The bacteria benefit from tissue products that provide es-

sential nutrients, and the host benefits from having a primed systemic defense system that is alert to microbial challenges that are potentially destructive to the host. In addition, many of the host systems that evolved to manage bacterial challenges are now known to be involved in the pathogenesis of chronic diseases of middle and later life. For example, the body's reaction to lipopolysaccharide, the very toxic cell-wall constituent of gram-negative bacteria, is greatly controlled by lipoproteins in the serum, which are components of the lipids that are involved in the risk for cardiovascular disease.

There is therefore a complex and continual adjustment of the host mechanisms to manage the challenge of the bacteria that colonize the mucous membranes and adjacent teeth. It is easy to understand how, in some individuals, the host systems either are less capable of maintaining this balance for a prolonged period or are actually innately destructive. For example, some degree of local inflammation in the gingiva is probably valuable to maintain the flow of protective cells into and through the tissue. However, if that chronic inflammation is either excessive or qualitatively different—for example, in overexpression of prostaglandins or matrix metalloproteinases—there may be adverse local or systemic implications.

Simple and well-documented relationships exist between the accumulation of supragingival plaque and the existence of periodontal inflammation and destruction of periodontal tissues. Although these general patterns are very clear statistically and on a population-wide basis, many patients do not fit them. For example, some patients have plaque and calculus accumulations for years, but although they have gingival inflammation, they have minimal to no loss of attachment or loss of bone. Other individuals with minimal accumulations of supragingival plaque show extensive destruction of both bone and connective tissue. And some patients exhibit a severity of disease consistent with plaque and calculus accumulations, yet they do not show the expected healing response when these accumulations are removed.

The diagnosis and treatment of periodontal diseases therefore must be based on an understanding of dental plaque and its formation, as well as an understanding of the complex bacterial host defense interactions that appear to explain periodontal diseases and their treatment outcomes. The host responses to bacterial challenges are discussed in chapters 8 and 9. This chapter will present and discuss information that can be summarized in the following conclusions about the role of bacteria in the initiation, progression, and treatment of periodontal diseases:

1. Bacteria accumulate as plaques on the teeth in a predictable pattern dictated by ecological factors, which include host responses.
2. Because of host and ecological factors, some bacterial plaques develop microbial complexes that cause periodontal diseases.
3. Regular disruption of bacterial plaque prevents most periodontal disease and halts most existing disease.
4. Clinical periodontitis occurs only when the body responds in certain ways to the bacterial challenge.
5. The goal of treatment is to disrupt the bacterial plaque and prevent the development of the microbial complexes that have the potential to cause tissue destruction.

Ecology: Bacteria and Host on Mucous Membranes

Two simple concepts appear to explain much of our new understanding of bacteria-host interactions. These concepts clarify both the cause and the treatment of periodontal disease:

1. Bacterial plaques on the teeth behave as a multicellular organ that is often called a *biofilm.*
2. The bacteria and host continuously interact in a dynamic equilibrium that is mostly protective, but selective changes on either side of the equation may lead to periodontal destruction.

The Pattern of Bacterial Ecology

The oral cavity has multiple ecological niches that represent very different bacterial ecosystems. There are five major bacterial ecosystems in the oral cavity: *(1)* tongue, *(2)* buccal mucosa, *(3)* tooth-adherent bacteria that are coronal to the gingival margin (supragingival plaque), *(4)* bacteria that reside apical to the gingival margins (subgingival plaque), and *(5)* saliva. Most of the bacteria found in the saliva are organisms from the tongue and buccal mucosa. In an individual with moderate to heavy plaque accumulations, the saliva will also reflect the bacteria found in the dental plaque. Therefore, the saliva represents primarily a collection of bacteria shed from other ecosystems on their way to being swallowed.

After a tooth is cleaned, specific bacteria accumulate in a predictable and reproducible pattern. Immediately after cleaning, salivary proteins selectively attach to the tooth surface and form an acquired pellicle.[2–4] When further tooth cleaning is not allowed, the bacterial succession can be monitored.[5–8]

Within the first 2 days after cleaning, the tooth surface is colonized primarily by gram-positive facultative cocci, which are primarily *Streptococcus* species. Over the next 7-day period, other early colonizers enter the plaque (Figs 5-1 and 5-2), including *Veillonella* species, a gram-negative anaerobic cocci; gram-positive rods that are primarily *Actinomyces* species; and *Capnocytophaga* species, a gram-negative rod. At this time more strictly anaerobic species become prominent, in particular *Fusobacterium* species and *Prevotella intermedia.* The morphology of the plaque at this time is primarily filamentous instead of coccoid and reflects the dominance of *Actinomyces* and *Fusobacterium* species. This ecological structure remains relatively stable if undisturbed physically and represents the layer of plaque attached to the tooth surface. Late colonizers appear at different times on the surface of this bacterial mat. *Porphyromonas gingivalis,* motile rods, and spirochetes are major components of the late colonizers.

Clinical signs of gingivitis may be detectable in many sites after 4 to 5 days of undisturbed plaque accumulation and maturation. If the teeth are cleaned professionally every 2 days with no other cleaning in between these times, clinical signs of gingivitis do not appear.[10] Gingivitis is a predictable consequence of plaque ecological succession and maturation. Most forms of periodontitis are associated with microorganisms that are found in the later stages of bacterial succession in plaque. Early plaque col-

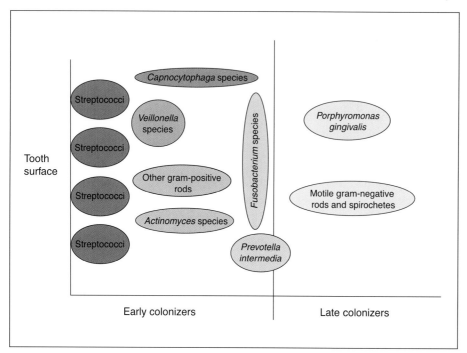

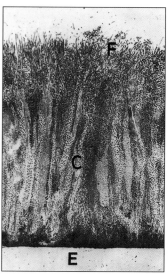

Fig 5-1 The successive appearance of different bacterial types on a tooth surface after cleaning. The different bacterial species colonize at different times and depend on attachment to either the tooth surface or to bacteria that have attached previously.

Fig 5-2 One-week-old supragingival plaque on an epoxy resin crown. The epoxy crown (E) is shown at the bottom of the photograph. The majority of the plaque bulk at 1 week consists of columns of coccoid bacteria (C). Some filamentous bacteria (F) have colonized the surface of the plaque. Original magnification ×1,200. (Reprinted from Listgarten MA,[9] with permission of Munksgaard International Publishers.)

onizers do not appear to be capable of producing periodontitis in dogs, monkeys, or humans.

These principles may be summarized as follows:

1. Supragingival plaque accumulation involves a predictable ecological maturation.
2. Gingivitis and most forms of periodontitis are the result of bacterial plaque maturation.
3. Prevention of bacterial plaque maturation by regular cleaning is a predictable way to prevent periodontal diseases.
4. Physical disruption of the plaque by cleaning the teeth influences the type of bacteria that are found on the tooth surface.

Supragingival Maturation, Subgingival Formation

The inflammatory changes that result from supragingival plaque maturation produce a swelling of the gingival margin and an increase in fluid flow from the gingival crevice (gingival crevicular fluid). The supragingival plaque that is covered by the swollen gingival margin and bathed by gingival crevicular fluid undergoes ecological changes that result in the bacterial composition characteristic of subgingival plaque. The structure of the subgingival plaque is very

different than that seen in supragingival areas. The tooth-adherent subgingival plaque is dominated by gram-positive filamentous bacteria and therefore may be very similar to supragingival plaque. In addition, some *Capnocytophaga* species may bind directly to cementum and provide a different basis for ecological succession. Some bacteria also bind directly to the epithelial surface of the gingiva and allow the formation of a loose adherent mat on the epithelial side of the subgingival area. The bottom or apical portion of the sulcus or pocket usually has loosely adherent and somewhat unorganized filamentous gram-negative rods and spirochetes separated from the epithelium by a layer of leukocytes. The subgingival plaque therefore has three zones: the tooth-adherent bacteria, epithelial-associated bacteria, and apical bacteria.

Determinants of Bacterial Load and Bacterial Composition

Although the interactions that lead to a specific bacterial ecology and the subsequent ecological succession involve many complex, redundant processes, the plaque mass and bacterial composition at a particular site appear to be determined primarily by three factors: bacterial attachment, bacterial metabolism and nutrition, and mechanical cleaning (Fig 5-3).

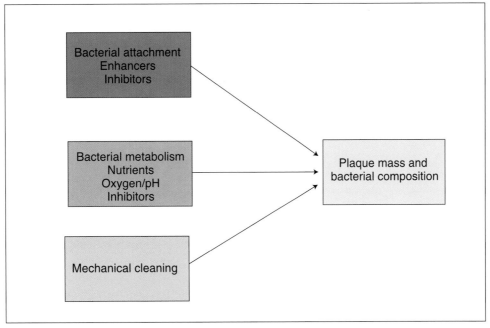

Fig 5-3 Factors that influence plaque mass and the bacterial species that will be present in the plaque.

Bacterial Attachment

The first factor that influences whether a specific bacterial species is present at a site is bacterial attachment. Bacteria may attach directly to the salivary pellicle on the tooth surface as described, or it may adhere to the plaque by interbacterial aggregation processes. These attachments are modified by enhancers such as adhesins contained in the saliva and specific inhibitors such as secretory immunoglobulin A (IgA). This important influence on bacterial ecology may be altered in situations in which there are aberrations in the content of saliva or in the production of IgA.

Bacterial Metabolism and Nutrition

Most of the growth and structural change in plaque after the first few days occurs as the result of bacterial proliferation. Once a bacterial cell attaches, it will divide and continue to proliferate if it is metabolically favored in that particular environment. If the environment is not favorable, the cell must expend a great deal of energy protecting itself and capturing nutrients. Although bacteria are very well adapted to withstand stress conditions, the gene regulation that favors the stress response is not conducive to cell division. The metabolic environment is determined by the nature and availability of nutrients, the pH and oxidation-reduction potential, and metabolic inhibitors.

Supragingival bacteria acquire most of their nutrient needs from food passing through the oral cavity. Most of the supragingival bacteria prefer carbohydrates as a nutrient source and are amply supplied with these nutrients

through the host's diet. The availability of dietary nutrients for bacterial metabolism depends on the chemical composition of the diet and the bacterial cell's access to it. Large molecules such as starches and proteins are not available for use until they are broken down into much smaller compounds. Although some degradation occurs in the oral cavity, it is thought to be too little to provide substantial nutrients for the plaque or bacteria. Low-molecular-weight carbohydrates such as sucrose and lactose are readily available for metabolism.

Other factors, such as the stickiness of foods and the frequency of intake, influence the availability of certain substrates to the plaque bacteria. For example, if starches are retained in the oral cavity, sufficient enzymatic degradation may occur to make the breakdown products of these large compounds available for metabolism. Nutrients may also be provided by interbacterial feeding mechanisms. For example, *Veillonella alkalescens* is not capable of metabolizing glucose but readily metabolizes lactic acid produced by streptococci in the environment. The use of lactic acid by *V alkalescens* also benefits the streptococci by helping to raise the pH of the environment, thereby facilitating additional carbohydrate metabolism by the streptococci.

It is thus easy to see how dietary patterns, including types of food consumed and frequency of consumption, may greatly influence the supragingival plaque composition. Dietary effects on *Streptococcus mutans* and dental caries are very well established.

The subgingival bacteria do not utilize dietary nutrients for their metabolism. Many of the subgingival bacterial species may use glucose but actually preferentially metabolize peptides and amino acids. Most of the nutrients for the subgingival bacteria come from tissue breakdown products, gingival crevicular fluid, and interbacterial feeding. Because inflammation produces an increase in both gingival crevicular fluid flow and tissue breakdown, the subgingival bacteria are greatly favored when the adjacent tissues are inflamed.

Because the metabolic process depends on the transfer of electrons, bacterial composition is greatly influenced by the pH and oxidation-reduction potential in the environment. Some enzymes, and hence the metabolic processes of some bacteria, are more sensitive than others. Some bacteria actually function very well in a low-pH (acidic) environment and are referred to as *acidophilic bacteria*. *Lactobacillus* species are acidophilic and are frequently found associated with dental caries where the environment is highly acidic. Although most mammalian biochemistry, as well as that of many bacterial species, is based on transferring electrons to oxygen to produce water, some bacterial species do not have this type of metabolism and are actually killed in the presence of oxygen. They are referred to as *anaerobic bacteria*. Different bacterial species utilize and react to oxygen in subtly different ways.

Although the mouth is constantly exposed to oxygen, the subgingival bacteria are mostly anaerobic. In addition, although the supragingival plaque bacteria are facultative—that is, they can metabolize in either an aerobic or anaerobic environment—they usually live in the oral cavity as anaerobes. As supragingival plaque matures, its oxidation-reduction potential is poised toward anaerobic growth, meaning that anaerobic bacteria can more easily metabolize and proliferate. Therefore, mature supragingival plaque and undisturbed subgingival plaque should provide the most predictable anaerobic environment, which should favor the growth of anaerobic bacteria.

Finally, the bacterial metabolism may be negatively influenced by a variety of inhibitors produced by certain bacteria to inhibit the growth and metabolism of other species. For example, certain *Streptococcus* species produce compounds that inhibit the growth of *Actinobacillus actinomycetemcomitans*, a pathogen associated with localized aggressive periodontitis.

Mechanical Cleaning

Perhaps the dominant influence on plaque mass and composition is mechanical cleaning. The mature bacterial ecosystem found in dental plaque is complex, and mechanical disruption forces the ecological succession to start over. In areas that are cleaned regularly, a mature ecology will not be able to develop. The cleaner the tooth surface, the more immature the ecological system, and the longer the system will take to reach full maturity. Although most patients clean their teeth regularly, many do not routinely clean interproximal areas or do not clean them well.

Supragingival plaque formation follows a very predictable pattern and sets the stage for subgingival plaque formation. As supragingival plaque matures, inflammation develops in the adjacent gingival tissues. The mature supragingival plaque therefore provides nutrients directly to the subgingival bacteria, and also induces inflammation in the tissue, thereby providing additional nutrients indirectly to the subgingival bacteria. It also provides attachment mechanisms and reduces the oxygen tension in the area. Although supragingival plaque appears to be required for the initial establishment of the subgingival flora, once the subgingival plaque is established, supragingival plaque is no longer essential. Once the environment has been established, the subgingival bacteria have sufficient nutrients, attachment opportunities, and an established oxidation-reduction environment for their metabolism and proliferation. The supragingival plaque may be removed with only minimal impact on an already established subgingival ecology. It is therefore essential that professional cleanings include attention to both supragingival and subgingival environments.

Periodontal Pocket Depth

Periodontal pocket depth integrates many of the determinants of bacterial plaque mass and composition. The bacterial species that are commonly found in mature dental plaques—that is, the plaques that have been relatively undisturbed for many weeks—are the same species that are frequently associated with initiating periodontitis. These species include *P gingivalis* and *Bacteroides forsythus*. The frequency of detection (ie, prevalence) and the level of these bacterial species are strongly correlated with the periodontal pocket depth; that is, *P gingivalis* and *B forsythus* are more commonly detected and are in higher numbers in periodontal pockets deeper than 6 mm as compared with sites that probe to less than 4 mm. It is likely that deeper pockets provide many of the ecological features listed above that are conducive to plaque maturation and growth of the anaerobic bacteria that are more pathogenic.

For example, the subgingival bacteria in deep pockets are protected from toothbrush cleaning, so the ecosystem is more mature than in shallow pockets. Also, there is a constant flow of gingival crevicular fluid in deep pockets, thereby providing the host-derived nutrients that are essential for growth of certain bacterial species. Finally, the deep pockets are likely to be more protected from the aerobic environment of the oral cavity, thereby facilitating an anaerobic environment that is conducive to expansion of the populations of certain species.

Smoking and Bacterial Ecology

Although bacteria are essential for the initiation of peri-odontitis, smoking is one of the strongest risk factors for severe disease. This means that if a group of young adults have low to moderate levels of bacterial plaque, the smokers are highly likely to develop clinical signs of peri-odontitis earlier than the nonsmokers, and the smokers are also more likely to develop generalized severe disease.

Smoking is known to have a negative influence on con-nective tissue metabolism and wound healing. In addi-tion, smoking inhibits multiple host immunological re-sponses that should help to control the bacterial challenges. It is not surprising, therefore, that smoking produces a substantial risk of earlier and more severe pe-riodontitis.

Several studies[11–13] have examined the relationship of smoking to the bacterial populations in the plaque, but until recently the story was confusing. Socransky and Haf-fajee[14] have now clarified this important relationship by showing that current smokers do not have higher levels of bacterial pathogens such as *B forsythus* or *P gingivalis*, but that the pathogens are found in more subgingival sites than in subjects who never smoked or who stopped smok-ing. Smokers generally had periodontal pathogens present at 10% to 25% more sites than nonsmokers. Of interest is that the greatest difference between the distribution of pathogens in smokers and nonsmokers was in sites less than 4 mm in probing depth. This finding may have im-portant implications for the more generalized nature of periodontitis in smokers.

All of these pathogenic factors interconnect (see Fig 1-4). Although smoke products may have a direct effect on the bacteria, smoking most likely alters the tissue re-sponses to the bacterial challenge, which may change the tissue defense mechanisms involving polymorphonuclear leukocytes and antibody, thus allowing easier spread or proliferation of certain bacteria.

Plaque Biofilms: A Teeming Community

The ecological interactions described above are reflected in the complex physical structure of dental plaque that is generally referred to as a *biofilm*. Biofilms are defined as "matrix-enclosed bacterial populations adherent to each other and/or to surfaces or interfaces."[15]

Although biofilms have been described for many years relative to adherent bacterial masses in water pipes, beer-brewing tanks, and other structures, recent observations have clarified the sophistication and complexity of their organization, properties, and growth characteristics.[16,17] Subgingival and supragingival dental plaques exhibit all the primary characteristics of biofilms,[18–20] including a primitive circulatory system and a mixed microbial com-munity that is highly integrated in terms of nutritional needs and outputs. Understanding the characteristics of biofilms and that dental plaque is a biofilm is critical to the clinical practice of periodontics, because special efforts are required to control bacteria that live in biofilms. Most im-portant, bacteria living in biofilms are not easily eradicated by antimicrobial agents,[17] and antimicrobial agents have been shown to have reduced efficacy against oral bacteria living in biofilms.[21,22] This means that control of the bacte-ria living in dental plaque biofilms must start with physical disruption of the plaque. Most studies of antimicrobial agents have confirmed the principle that such agents work best when used in conjunction with mechanical cleaning procedures that disrupt the plaque. The corollary of this finding is that once dental plaque has formed, the bacteria cannot be treated effectively by antimicrobial agents alone.

Streptococcus species are the most predominant early tooth colonizers and provide an abundant array of adhe-sions after attachment. *Fusobacterium* species congregate with all other oral bacteria examined to date and bind readily to dental pellicle. Both *Streptococcus* and *Fuso-bacterium* species therefore appear to play a major role in biofilm formation and structure.

Bacterial Complexes

Specific bacteria in dental plaque reach a level that is de-pendent on the nutrients and environment provided by the other bacteria in the biofilm and the host products that flow into the gingival sulcus area. For this reason it is not surprising that the toxic products produced by bacterial plaque at a specific site in the mouth are the summation of the products produced by the total biofilm at that site. Therefore, the biologic activity of bacterial plaque at a specific site is the result of the complex of bacterial types that have formed the ecosystem at that time. The charac-ter of the plaque is thus best described by the complex of multiple bacterial species that dominate at that site, rather than by a single microbial type. Only in recent years have the statistical and microbial techniques been available to provide an understanding of microbial complexes and their relationship to disease.

Socransky and colleagues[23] at the Forsyth Institute used DNA probe technology to study the bacterial composition of large numbers of sites in many subjects. When they an-alyzed the bacterial composition of dental plaques from different clinical situations, it was clear that groups of bac-terial species were consistently found together in clusters

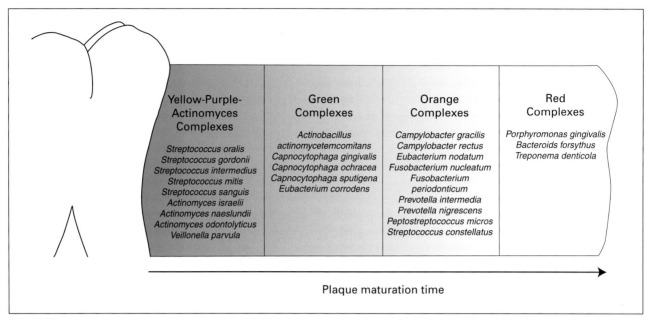

Fig 5-4 The specific microorganisms in dental plaque are found in predictable ecological complexes—ie, the bacterial species in a "complex" are most commonly found together. The complexes, as defined by Socransky and coworkers,[23] were color coded, as shown. The complexes tend to form ecological layers out from the tooth surface that represent maturation of the plaque ecology. (Based on Socransky et al.[23])

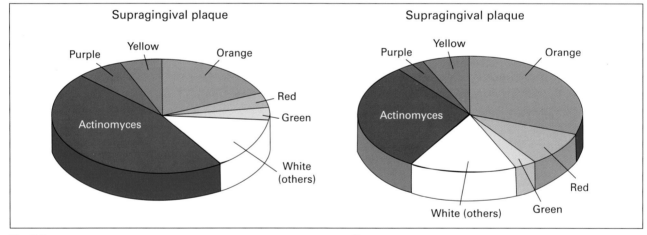

Fig 5-5 The microbial complexes, as defined by Socransky and coworkers[23] and shown in Fig 5-4, are in different proportions in supragingival and subgingival plaque. These differences most likely reflect the different ecological determinants that are found in the two environments. (Based on Ximenez-Fyvie et al.[24,25])

that were characteristic of the bacterial ecosystem in a specific clinical situation (Figs 5-4 and 5-5). The bacterial species that were associated with clinical disease most frequently fit into the red or orange complexes.

Why are specific bacteria frequently found together? As discussed above, the bacteria that are localized to a specific site at a specific time are the direct result of the ecology at that local site. The ecological determinants therefore define *groups* of bacteria that are selected by the environment. Such bacterial complexes reinforce the sta-

bility of the ecology, support the growth of other members of the complex, and also change the environment to allow development of another complex.

"Biochemical Soup"

Although it is important to understand the individual characteristics of each bacterial species as they relate to periodontal health or disease, at any point in time the gingival tissues are exposed to all of the products released by the bacterial complexes at that site. The tissue changes are therefore the result of the total ecosystem and bacterial complexes at a specific site. Before bacterial populations could be studied in great detail, most investigators focused on a few bacterial species that were consistently associated with disease. Most of these species are now known to be components of the red and orange complexes.

Therapeutic Disruption of Ecosystems Alters Entire Bacterial Complexes

Mechanical therapies such as scaling and root planing remove much of the bacterial biofilm and disrupt the bacterial complexes at a specific site. The result of such disruption is that the bacterial ecology must start to re-form in the sequential manner that over time will allow redevelopment of the well-defined complexes. If the patient regularly disrupts the bacterial deposits, the plaque maturation must again start at the beginning. The red and orange complexes, with the bacteria that cause periodontal destruction, cannot form at a site unless the ecosystem is first prepared by the establishment of other complexes, as shown in Fig 5-4. Thus, one of the effects of mechanical cleaning is to force the ecological maturation of the bacterial complexes to re-start. If patients do not clean interproximal sites regularly, specific ecosystems there can mature and develop the bacterial complexes that lead to tissue destruction.

Calculus: What Is It and Why Remove It?

Composition

Calculus is primarily mineralized bacterial plaque. Calculus deposits have been reported in germ-free animals in the absence of any bacteria and may be the result of calcification of salivary proteins on the tooth surface. Supragingival calculus is clinically visible coronal to the gingival margin. The presence and amount of supragingival calculus are the result of the level of bacterial deposits on the teeth but are also influenced by salivary gland secretion. As a result, the greatest quantity of supragingival plaque is usually seen on the buccal surfaces of the maxillary molars adjacent to the duct from the parotid gland and on the lingual surfaces of the mandibular anterior teeth, which are exposed to the duct of the submandibular glands. Supragingival calculus may range in color from white to dark brown, depending on stain from food.

Subgingival calculus forms apical to the gingival margin and is usually not visible. It may be detected by tactile ex-

ploration with a periodontal probe or a fine explorer and is usually evident as a roughened surface. If the gingival margin is retracted by a blast of air or a dental instrument, subgingival calculus may be evident at and just apical to the cementoenamel junction. Subgingival calculus frequently appears brown or black, which reflects the presence of bacterial and blood products.

Supragingival calculus consists of 70% to 90% inorganic salts, which are mainly in the form of calcium phosphate ($Ca_3[PO_4]_2$). Calculus also contains varying amounts of calcium carbonate and magnesium phosphate. The inorganic portion of calculus is chemically similar to the inorganic portion of bone, dentin, and cementum. The organic component of calculus involves protein and polysaccharide complexes derived from dental plaque and desquamated epithelial cells and white blood cells.

The mixture of inorganic crystals changes in relative composition as the calculus ages. Brushite ($Ca[HPO_4] \cdot 2H_2O$) is the first crystal form to appear and is followed by octocalcium phosphate ($Ca_8[HPO_4]_4$). In mature deposits that have accumulated for over 6 months, the major crystalline form is hydroxyapatite ($Ca_{10}[PO4]_6 \cdot OH_2$), with minor components of octocalcium phosphate and whitlockite, a magnesium-containing tricalcium phosphate ($Ca_3[PO_4]_2$).

Dental calculus has been associated with periodontal diseases by both ancient and modern writers. Although calculus does not have a direct traumatic effect on the gingival tissues, as previously believed, it may well be a factor that contributes to disease by amplifying the impact of primary factors.

Clinical Significance of Calculus

Epidemiological studies show strong associations between calculus and periodontitis, but there is no evidence to implicate calculus as a primary cause of periodontitis. This conclusion is the result of the following observations:

1. The mineralized surface of calculus is always covered by unmineralized bacterial plaque, and therefore the calculus itself does not contact the gingival tissues.
2. In animals treated with antimicrobial agents, bacterial plaque is eliminated from the calculus surface, and the junctional epithelium may actually attach directly to the calculus. In such artificially induced situations, the presence of calculus without bacterial plaque is associated with gingival health, not disease.

Calculus may amplify the effects of bacterial plaque, however. For example, calculus growth keeps the bacterial plaque in close contact with the tissue surface and also limits the patient's ability to remove the plaque. In addition, since calculus has the potential to concentrate both nutrients and toxins,[26] one might reasonably expect it to influence both the bacterial ecology and tissue inflammation. But this is currently speculative.

Although it may be possible to use chemical agents to remove plaque from the calculus surface without removing the calculus itself, this is not currently an accepted approach to therapy. Well-controlled studies have clearly demonstrated that the removal of both subgingival calculus and subgingival bacterial deposits allows one to maintain a state of periodontal health for long periods. No long-term studies have assessed the results of removing plaque without removing calculus.

Bacterial Associations with Health and Disease

The bacteria associated with gingival health and various forms of periodontal disease have been studied in great detail over the past 30 years. Due to the availability of research funding and exciting speculations about the role of specific bacteria in periodontal disease, most of these data were generated during the 1980s. The techniques available at that time did not allow the detailed characterization of different genotypes of bacteria that may be distinctly different in terms of pathogenic potential but that look very similar when grown in the laboratory. For example, the association between *P intermedia* and periodontitis has been confusing. What were previously identified as *P intermedia* are now known to make up at least two different genotypes. These different genotypes appear to have different associations with disease, which may explain past confusion. As a result, much of the information available today on the microbiology of periodontal diseases should be viewed as ecological patterns. The impact of this fact on demonstrating specific bacterial etiologies in periodontal disease is discussed below.

Gingival Health

At gingival sites that are clinically or relatively healthy, the bacterial pattern is consistent with that described for relatively immature supragingival plaque. *Streptococci*, *Actinomyces* species (especially *A viscosus* and *A naeslundii*), and *Veillonella* species account for the majority of the bacteria that can be grown in gingival health.[5,6,27–29] If a plaque sample taken from healthy gingiva is examined in a wet mount using phase-contrast or dark-field microscopy, the bacteria are found to be primarily nonmotile, with a ratio of motile to nonmotile forms of about

1:40.[30] Although many other bacterial species may be isolated from subgingival plaque samples of individuals with healthy gingiva,[6] these bacteria are primarily minor or transient components of a maturing dental plaque. Some bacterial species believed to be periodontal pathogens may be found in association with gingival health. In addition, the subgingival microflora of sites that have been recently scaled and root planed is similar to that observed in gingival health.[30] The bacteria associated with gingival health are found primarily in the actinomyces, purple, and yellow complexes (see Fig 5-4).

Microflora Associated with Gingivitis

Early studies of the microbiology of gingivitis used stained plaque smears. The investigators[31] reported that the microflora shifted from a gram-positive dominance to a more complex flora that included large numbers of gram-negative and spiral forms. Later studies that cultured the bacteria associated with experimental gingivitis reported a shift from a *Streptococcus*-dominated plaque to one in which *Actinomyces* species predominated.[6,29] Although *Actinomyces* species increase every time plaque mass increases, gingival bleeding is specifically associated with an increase in *A viscosus* and pigmented *Bacteroides* species that would most likely be identified today as *P intermedia* and *P gingivalis*.[6,29] Other investigators looking at plaque-induced gingivitis[32] and pregnancy-associated gingivitis[33] observed increased gram-negative anaerobic rods and increased pigmented *Bacteroides* (now *Prevotella* and *Porphyromonas* species) as compared with healthy sites.

Other, more extensive studies[34] found that levels of gram-negative rods, including *Eikenella corrodens*, *Fusobacterium nucleatum*, and *Capnocytophaga* species, were increased in plaque samples taken from gingivitis sites. These observations were put into perspective by Moore and coworkers[5] (for review, see Moore and Moore[1]). These investigators noted that the bacterial composition of the developing plaque showed a very predictable ecological succession for the first 4 days of plaque accumulation. The composition of the plaque then became more diverse, with the bacterial patterns reflecting the level of inflammation at the sample site. In sites with gingivitis, increases were observed in *F nucleatum*, *Eubacterium timidum*, and specific *Treponema* and *Bacteroides* species. The bacteria associated with gingivitis are found primarily in the actinomyces, purple, and yellow complexes, with representation also from the orange complex (see Fig 5-4).

The above studies are consistent with the earlier observations that plaque accumulation involves a sequential ecological progression of bacterial changes. As a certain level of bacterial complexity is achieved, an increase in gram-negative anaerobic species is observed together with a clinical increase in inflammation. These conditions set the stage for colonization by the bacteria that have been associated with chronic periodontitis.

Microflora Associated with Chronic Periodontitis

The subgingival microflora associated with chronic periodontitis has been studied extensively. The intent of these studies has been diverse and has ranged from extensive taxonomic assessments to describe the predominant bacterial species associated with periodontitis to highly selective studies focusing on the potential role of an individual species in the disease process. Although bacteria are clearly the initiating agents in periodontitis, the complexity of the microflora and the critical role of the host in determining the outcome of the bacterial challenge have greatly complicated attempts to implicate specific microorganisms in the disease. The evidence to support the etiologic role of specific microorganisms in periodontal diseases has been reviewed by Haffajee and Socransky.[35]

Chronic periodontitis appears to involve bacterial maturation in a susceptible host. Adult patients with periodontitis and no previous periodontal therapy have a predictable microbial pattern in the subgingival plaque. Although the pattern may vary somewhat, depending on how the ecosystem has been disrupted by cleaning and on the techniques used for sampling and identifying the bacteria, in general most patients with chronic periodontitis will have the bacterial species that are consistent with a complex mature ecosystem.

As a result of the changing ecology as plaque matures and inflammation develops, the bacteria associated with chronic periodontitis are different from those found in periodontal health. Because of the ecological influence on the presence of these microorganisms, the microbiology of chronic plaque-induced gingivitis lies between that of periodontal health and chronic periodontitis. Although plaque from periodontitis sites includes bacteria found in the actinomyces, purple, yellow, and green complexes, certain bacterial species from the orange and red complexes (see Fig 5-4) are now strongly associated with chronic periodontitis as well.

Microbial Pathogens in Chronic Periodontitis

Many bacteria—as many as 500 different bacterial taxa—have been isolated from subgingival plaque samples. Many of these bacterial species have not actually been grown but have been identified as new species based on nucleic acid composition. It is likely that some of these new, but as yet uncultured, bacterial species will be found to participate in the initiation and progression of periodontitis. It should be emphasized that the new species are also found in complexes that are determined by the ecology of that specific site. It remains to be seen whether these new species will define subclusters (eg, red complex 1.1 or 1.2) that discriminate risk for disease more effectively than the current complexes. The species discussed below have been studied for many years relative to their ecology and disease association.

Porphyromonas gingivalis

P gingivalis is an anaerobic nonmotile rod that has been associated with chronic periodontitis for many years. On gram stains this microorganism appears as a gram-negative short rod or slightly elongated coccus. On blood agar plates it forms brownish black colonies and belongs to a group of species once referred to as *black-pigmenting bacteroides*. These bacteria were originally classified as *Bacteroides melaninogenicus* and over the years have been reclassified and subdivided into *Porphyromonas* and *Prevotella genera*.

P gingivalis populations have been shown to be increased in sites with periodontitis and lower or nondetectable in sites with gingival health or plaque-induced gingivitis.[24,25,28,32,36–50] In addition, the elimination of *P gingivalis* has been associated with successful clinical outcomes, whereas persistence of the microorganism has been associated with disease recurrence.[37,40,51–59] This microorganism has been shown to have extensive virulence factors, including a true collagenase, endotoxin, IgA (and other) proteases, and low-molecular-weight compounds including hydrogen sulfide and ammonia. The net result of these virulence factors is that *P gingivalis* has the ability to induce bone resorption, destroy connective tissue, induce a variety of cytokines, and inhibit host protective mechanisms. *P gingivalis* may also enter the junctional epithelium and multiply in that location.[60] The addition of *P gingivalis* to a complex microbial ecosystem in monkeys has been shown to initiate progressive bone loss and clinical signs of periodontitis.[61]

Bacteroides forsythus

B forsythus has gained increasing attention in recent years as the availability of specific DNA probes and new culture techniques have allowed the study of this difficult-to-grow microorganism. *B forsythus* is found most commonly in subgingival plaque samples and is usually associated with deep pockets.[62–64] This microorganism is frequently detected in aggressive periodontitis subjects as well.[65]

B forsythus is a gram-negative anaerobic rod that is usually elongated with pointed ends but may be very pleomorphic, depending on the growth conditions. This species has unusual growth requirements and is not usually isolated on standard anaerobic growth media.

Actinobacillus actinomycetemcomitans

A actinomycetemcomitans has been strongly associated with aggressive periodontitis, such as localized aggressive periodontitis and other aggressive forms.[49,66–82] Although this microorganism is not routinely found in chronic periodontitis cases, it has previously been observed in 25% to 30% of such cases.[45,46,83–86] *A actinomycetemcomitans* may be associated with progressive destructive disease[62] and may be especially difficult to eradicate with mechanical treatment.[28,46,87–89] Therefore, the role of *A actinomycetemcomitans* in chronic periodontitis is now viewed as significant. In addition, recent observations[90] indicate that in family units in which one of the parents has periodontitis and *A actinomycetemcomitans*, the children are highly likely to acquire the same microorganism from that parent.

A actinomycetemcomitans has an extensive collection of virulence factors comparable to those of *P gingivalis*. These include a true collagenase, endotoxin, IgA proteases, and toxins, all of which alter leukocyte function and epithelial cell function. The net result of these virulence factors is that *A actinomycetemcomitans* is capable of evading normal host responses and destroying both connective tissue and bone.

Fusobacterium nucleatum

F nucleatum is found in early stages of plaque-induced gingivitis and increases proportionately as periodontitis is initiated and becomes more severe.[1] This microorganism produces high concentrations of butyric acid and is capable of initiating early inflammatory changes. *F nucleatum* is a well-established pathogen in other body sites and may represent an important component of periodontitis initiation in adults. It is a prominent component of the subgingival plaque in periodontitis with severe attachment loss.[62]

F nucleatum is a gram-negative anaerobic rod that is elongated and has pointed ends. Its potential importance in the initiation and progression of periodontitis is complicated by the fact that several variations of this species—including *F vincentii*, *F nucleatum*, and *F polymorphum*—were previously placed into one microbial group. At present there are no data to indicate pathogenic differences among the species, but such findings would not be unusual.

Prevotella intermedia

P intermedia is another species that was previously characterized as a black-pigmented bacteroides. As a result of this characterization, much of the early data inadvertently combined *Prevotella* species, including *P intermedia*, with multiple black-pigmented *Bacteroides* species that are now known to be distinct, such as *P gingivalis*. Although *P intermedia* has been isolated in association with both aggressive periodontitis[66,67] and advancing periodontitis,[28] it is found prominently in gingivitis and rapidly returns after therapy.[41,51,57] In general, the association between *P intermedia* and disease progression or disease resolution has not been strong.[51,57]

P intermedia does have many of the virulence factors that are found in *P gingivalis* and does produce extensive tissue damage when injected subcutaneously. *P intermedia* has recently been subdivided into two species, *P intermedia* and *Prevotella nigrescens*.[91] Recent studies[92] indicate that in plaque samples from patients with periodontitis, *P intermedia* was detected more frequently than *P nigrescens*, whereas samples from healthy gingival sites were dominated by *P nigrescens*. No studies have evaluated the relative pathogenic potential of the two species, but it is hoped that separate monitoring of them will clarify the role of *P intermedia* in periodontitis.

Several other microorganisms have been strongly associated with chronic periodontitis (for review, see Haffajee and Socransky[35]).

Microflora of Aggressive Periodontitis

Aggressive forms of periodontitis, including localized aggressive periodontitis and disease in children, have been studied extensively. *A actinomycetemcomitans* has been repeatedly implicated in localized aggressive periodontitis. This microorganism is routinely isolated from patient lesions and is often found in very high numbers. It is rarely seen in healthy subjects, those with plaque-induced gingivitis, or edentulous subjects.[34,49,69,85,93–95] Perhaps most important, good clinical outcomes have been associated with the elimination or suppression of *A actinomycetemcomitans* in patients with aggressive periodontitis, and residual or recurrent disease has been associated with failure to eliminate or reduce this microorganism.[51,66,96–103] Other microorganisms, such as *Capnocytophaga* species and *P intermedia*, are routinely isolated from aggressive periodontitis lesions. *P gingivalis* is rarely seen at such sites, but it may appear in adults with aggressive periodontitis since chronic periodontitis may be superimposed on the localized aggressive periodontitis lesions.

The infection with *A actinomycetemcomitans* is not substantially reduced by mechanical cleaning procedures[56,66] but may be reduced by systemic antibiotics or surgical therapy.[66,95,96,103] These findings appear to be related to the observation that *A actinomycetemcomitans* is routinely found within the tissues of subjects with aggressive periodontitis.[104,105] The inability to reduce this microorganism by routine mechanical means and the lack of responsiveness of localized aggressive periodontitis to plaque-focused therapy further emphasize the probable role of *A actinomycetemcomitans* in the initiation and progression of aggressive periodontitis. Some studies[66] have suggested that the outcomes of therapy are different for individuals harboring both *A actinomycetemcomitans* and *P intermedia* as compared with individuals without *P intermedia*.

Some aggressive forms of periodontitis affect the primary dentition and frequently progress to produce disease in the permanent dentition. Patients with this type of disease may have a localized form affecting only a few teeth, or the disease may be generalized throughout the mouth. In general, individuals with a generalized form of the disease have a more overt host defect than those individuals with only localized disease. The microbial patterns of this type of periodontitis are more diverse than those reported for aggressive periodontitis affecting the permanent dentition, but *A actinomycetemcomitans*, *Capnocytophaga sputigena*, and *P intermedia* appear to be the most prominent members of the microflora.[71,106]

Microflora Associated with Refractory Chronic Periodontitis

Refractory periodontitis lesions have been studied extensively and appear to show the same microflora as deep pockets from chronic periodontitis.[37,40,52,53,55,65,86,107,108] In general, these studies show three patterns for the microflora[86]:

1. The plaque microflora resembles the complex ecosystem found in patients with chronic periodontitis and includes high levels of *F nucleatum*, *P gingivalis*, and *P intermedia*. *E corrodens*, *Campylobacter rectus*, and *B forsythus* are also found.
2. Minimal to no *P gingivalis*, *P intermedia*, or *B forsythus* are found. These samples are usually dominated by surface translocating bacteria, such as *Capnocytophaga* species, *E corrodens*, and *C rectus*.
3. *A actinomycetemcomitans* is a prominent component of the microflora, together with either of the two patterns listed above.

Microflora Associated with Necrotizing Ulcerative Gingivitis

Acute necrotizing ulcerative gingivitis was originally thought to be unique among the periodontal diseases in that bacteria are found within the tissue, as discovered by microscopic analysis. As indicated above, in recent years, it has been shown that *A actinomycetemcomitans* and

Table 5-1 Longitudinal Studies of Bacterial Prediction of Disease Progression

Bacteria	Positive samples	Negative samples
A actinomycetemcomitans[53]	46.2%*	NA†
P gingivalis[96] *C ochracea*	66.7%	NA
P micros and *C rectus*	100.0%	NA
A actinomycetemcomitans[97]	25.0%	NA
P gingivalis	0.0%	NA
P intermedia	28.6%	NA
A actinomycetemcomitans, *P gingivalis*, and *P intermedia*	NA	0%‡
A actinomycetemcomitans,[98] *P gingivalis*, and *P intermedia*	51.4%	42.3%
P gingivalis (>10⁶)§[21]	Relative risk = 4.1‖	NA
A actinomycetemcomitans (>10⁶)	Relative risk = 4.3	NA

* 46.2% of the sites that were positive for the indicated bacteria showed disease progression during the study.
† Not available.
‡ None of the sites that were negative for the indicated bacteria showed disease progression during the study.
§ *P gingivalis* was detected at a level of > 10⁶ cells per sample.
‖ Disease progression was 4.1 times more likely in sites that were positive for the indicated bacteria than in sites that were negative.

sometimes *P gingivalis* may invade the tissue and proliferate within the epithelium and, in some cases, within connective tissue. The microbial proliferation and extension within the tissues in acute necrotizing ulcerative gingivitis is still dramatic and is certainly the most extensive of that observed for any periodontal disease. The microbiology of this condition appears to involve predominantly *P intermedia*, *F nucleatum*, and spirochetes (primarily *Treponema* species).[109]

Bacterial Prediction of Disease

The chronic nature of most periodontitis lesions and the complexity of the subgingival microflora do not allow the simple identification of classic bacterial pathogens. However, there are convincing data to implicate certain bacteria as at least markers or indicators of disease initiation and progression. The identification and elimination of certain bacteria appear to make up an important part of therapy, because the failure to eliminate these specific microorganisms substantially increases the risk of future disease progression.

Although cross-sectional studies showing an association between specific bacteria and disease states are of great importance, they do not definitively show the role of selected microorganisms in disease initiation or progression. For that reason, it is very important to look at the few longitudinal studies that have assessed how specific microbial findings affect the future disease pattern (Table 5-1).[110-112]

Therapeutic Goals and Bacterial Outcomes of Therapy

Why not just treat periodontal disease with systemic antibiotics? One of the characteristics of biofilms is that many of the bacteria are not accessible to the antibiotic, and therefore only relatively small components of the bacterial populations are altered by antibiotic therapy. With established bacterial complexes in the dental plaque biofilm, antibiotics by themselves will have limited benefit in reducing bacteria and in improving the clinical characteristics of periodontal disease.

It should be emphasized that scaling and root planing by a highly skilled clinician, combined with diligent and regular home care, will produce outstanding and predictable clinical benefits in most cases. There are, however, both local tooth site and systemic limitations to how cases respond to this regimen. Even the most experienced clinicians are unable to remove most subgingival bacterial deposits in sites with probing depths of more than 6 mm or in furcations, unless surgical access is used to accomplish scaling and root planing. In addition, some patients have different host responses, and their clinical improvement after scaling and root planing may not be as predictable as it is in other patients.

When antibiotics are combined with mechanical therapy, such as scaling and root planing, to disrupt the bacterial biofilm, they may provide significant benefits in certain clinical situations. The greatest benefit of systemic antibiotics is generally seen in patients with deep periodontal pockets—where scaling and root planing alone produces incomplete bacterial reduction—and in patients with generalized severe disease, which is often an indication of a compromised host defense system.

The benefits of systemic antibiotics appear to result from more complete elimination of selective bacterial populations. For example, metronidazole plus amoxicillin, in conjunction with scaling and root planing, is effective in reducing the red-complex bacteria for up to 1 year after therapy.[113] Members of the orange complex are reduced for shorter periods, and the other complexes are minimally altered.

For many individuals, conventional therapy including scaling, root planing, and plaque control effectively reduces or eliminates key pathogens. These bacteria persist, however, in some individuals. It is in treating this group of patients that knowledge about specific bacteria is most valuable.

Herpesvirus in Human Periodontal Disease

Most viruses known to cause oral diseases in human beings are DNA viruses that are contracted in childhood or early adulthood through contact with saliva, blood, or genital secretions. Herpesviruses are the most important DNA viruses in oral pathology. The hallmark of herpesvirus infections is immune impairment. Figure 5-6 describes the infectious process of herpesviruses.

Herpesviruses share at least four characteristics[114]:

1. The typical particle consists of an icosahedral capsid assembly of 162 capsomers enclosed in a viral envelope.
2. The genome is a single double-stranded DNA molecule ranging in size from 120 to 250 kilobase pairs.
3. Viral infection exhibits a tendency to tissue tropism; that is, the herpesvirus is highly selective in regard to the surfaces or organs it infects or invades.
4. The viral productive phase is followed by a latent phase in host cells, which ensures survival of the viral genome throughout the lifetime of the infected individual. Latent herpesviruses can undergo sporadic reactivation and reenter the productive phase.

Eight human herpesvirus species have been identified so far (Table 5-2). In the latent phase of infection, herpesviruses reside in the following cells:

1. Herpes simplex virus type 1 and type 2 (HSV-1 and HSV-2) in sensory nerve ganglia and monocytes
2. Varicella-zoster virus (VZV) in sensory nerve ganglia and monocytes
3. Epstein-Barr virus (EBV) in B lymphocytes and salivary gland tissue
4. Human cytomegalovirus (HCMV) in monocytes, macrophages, lymphocytes, and salivary gland tissue
5. Human herpesvirus 6 (HHV-6) in lymphocytes and ductal epithelium of salivary gland tissue
6. Human herpesvirus 7 (HHV-7) in lymphocytes and salivary gland tissue
7. Human herpesvirus 8 (HHV-8) in lymphocytes and macrophages

Activation of latent herpesvirus infections can cause symptomatic or asymptomatic recurrent infection. Physical trauma, stress, immunosuppression, immune dysfunction, and radiotherapy may trigger viral reactivation. Active herpesvirus infections may have particularly severe consequences in patients infected with human immuno-

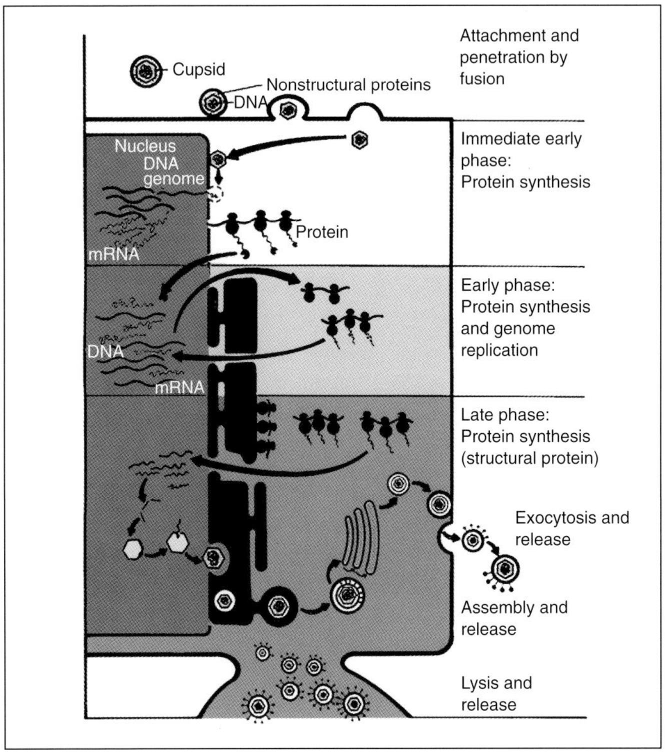

Fig 5-6 Schematic representation of the replication of herpesviruses. A virion initiates infection by fusion of the viral envelope with the plasma membrane after attachment to the cell surface. The capsid is transported to the nuclear pore, where viral DNA is released into the nucleus. Viral transcription and translation occur in three phases: immediate early, early, and late. Immediate early proteins shut off cell protein synthesis. Early proteins facilitate viral DNA replication. Late proteins are structural proteins of the virus that form empty capsids. Viral DNA is packaged into preformed capsids in the nucleus. Viral glycoproteins and tegument protein patches in cellular membranes and capsids are enveloped. Virions are transported via endoplasmic reticulum and released by exocytosis or cell lysis.

Table 5-2 The Human Herpesviruses

Human herpesvirus	Abbreviation	Herpes group	Most commonly associated illness
Herpes simplex virus type 1	HSV-1	α	Coldsores
Herpes simplex virus type 2	HSV-2	α	Genital lesions
Varicella-zoster virus	VZV	α	Chickenpox/shingles
Epstein-Barr virus	EBV	γ	Mononucleosis, Burkitt lymphoma, nasopharyngeal carcinoma
Human cytomegalovirus	HCMV	β	Congenital abnormalities
Human herpesvirus 6	HHV-6	β	Infant rash exanthem subitum
Human herpesvirus 7	HHV-7	β	Febrile illnesses
Kaposi sarcoma herpesvirus	KSHV, HHV-8	γ	Kaposi sarcoma

deficiency virus (HIV) and other immunocompromised individuals.

HSV-1, HSV-2, VZV, EBV, HCMV, and HHV-8 can cause oral disease.[115] Active herpesvirus infection in the oral cavity often involves ulceration of gingiva. Because Epstein-Barr virus type 1 (EBV-1) and HCMV have been implicated in the pathogenesis of human periodontal disease, these two herpesviruses are briefly described.

Epstein-Barr Virus[116]

At least two EBV types exist: type 1 and type 2. EBV-1 predominates in the Western hemisphere and EBV-2 in Africa. EBV infects and replicates in oral and oropharyngeal epithelia, as well as in B lymphocytes. Blood or saliva transmits EBV. In developing countries, EBV infects most children, usually asymptomatically, before the age of 2 years. In developed countries, primary EBV infection occurs mostly in adolescents, and sometimes in the form of infectious mononucleosis. Symptoms of infectious mononucleosis include fever, lymphadenopathy, malaise, and sore throat (pharyngitis). Oral ulcers and multiple palatal petechia have been reported and, infrequently, pericoronitis, acute ulcerative gingivitis, or gingival ulcerations as well. Individuals infected with HIV experience frequent EBV-2 infection or dual EBV-1 and EBV-2 infections.

Latent EBV infection can be reactivated, leading to viral shedding into oral mucosa. EBV-infected epithelial cells may cause oral hairy leukoplakia in HIV-positive patients, as evidenced by EBV replicating within epithelial cells of oral hairy leukoplakia lesions. The appearance of oral hairy leukoplakia in HIV-seropositive patients is often suggestive of the development of AIDS. However, oral hairy leukoplakia can appear in the absence of HIV infection and can be found in patients who are immunosuppressed for reasons other than HIV infection. Lesions similar to oral hairy leukoplakia can also occur in patients who show no evidence of EBV infection.

EBV can also cause malignancy, including nasopharyngeal carcinoma, Burkitt lymphoma, B-cell lymphoma, and oral carcinomas. Oral non-Hodgkin lymphoma may involve gingiva, causing tooth mobility and tooth exfoliation. Midline granuloma is an EBV-associated lymphoma that can cause severe gingival and periodontal destruction.

Human Cytomegalovirus[117]

HCMV is detected in blood and in many body secretions, including semen, maternal milk, and saliva. HCMV is a ubiquitous herpesvirus, usually acquired in early childhood. Most primary infections are asymptomatic. The site of HCMV latency is not known, although the virus is often recovered from salivary glands. HCMV may target endothelial and ductal epithelial cells and can also infect gingival macrophages and T lymphocytes. HCMV is emerging as an important opportunistic pathogen in immunocompromised individuals, especially in patients with AIDS and those who have had a transplant. People with AIDS may be infected with multiple HCMV strains and are at risk of disseminated HCMV infection.

HCMV infection produces three recognizable clinical syndromes: perinatal disease and HCMV inclusion disease, acute acquired HCMV infection, and disease in an immunocompromised host. Perinatal HCMV disease of infants whose mothers had a primary infection during pregnancy present microcephalia associated with mental retardation and hearing impairment. HCMV infection acquired neonatally resembles infectious mononucleosis or may progress asymptomatically. The second HCMV-related syndrome is similar to infectious mononucleosis except for the absence of pharyngitis and heterophilic antibodies. The third syndrome is observed in immunocompromised individuals, including HIV-infected individuals and patients who have had tissue and bone marrow transplants. HCMV infection can enhance the immunosuppressiveness of HIV and aggravate opportunistic infections.

Oral ulcerations in immunosuppressed patients are often related to HCMV. In HIV-positive patients, 53% of persistent ulcers showed HCMV, and another 28% showed HCMV and HSV co-infection. HCMV-related oral ulcers occasionally involve gingiva and periodontium with underlying bone destruction or osteomyelitis. HCMV infection may also give rise to gingival hyperplasia.

Association Between Herpesviruses and Periodontal Disease

Table 5-3 describes the distribution of herpesviruses in gingival biopsy specimens from 25 adult subjects.[118] Herpesviruses were rarely detected in specimens from healthy gingiva but were present in all gingival specimens from chronic periodontitis lesions. HSV, EBV-1, EBV-2, HCMV, and HHV-7 showed significant associations with periodontitis. HHV-8 was detected only in gingival specimens from HIV-infected patients.

Studies have revealed close relationships between EBV-1 and HCMV and chronic periodontitis, localized and generalized aggressive periodontitis, Papillon-Lefèvre syndrome periodontitis, Down syndrome periodontitis, HIV periodontitis, and acute necrotizing ulcerative gingivitis.[119] In periodontitis lesions, EBV infects B lymphocytes, and HCMV infects monocytes/macrophages and T lymphocytes.[120] Herpesvirus-infected inflammatory cells may have diminished ability to defend against bacterial challenge.

The study of localized aggressive periodontitis has demonstrated a relationship between active HCMV periodontal infection and initiation of the disease.[121] Also, localized aggressive periodontitis lesions showing HCMV activation had elevated levels of *A actinomycetemcomitans*, the major pathogenic bacterium of the disease. It appears that active HCMV periodontal infection initiates overgrowth of subgingival *A actinomycetemcomitans*, resulting in periodontal breakdown.

EBV-1 and HVMV occur more frequently in malnourished African children with acute necrotizing ulcerative gingivitis (ANUG) than in children without it.[122] Herpesviruses, together with malnutrition and pathogenic periodontal bacteria, may be important determinants in the development of some types of acute necrotizing ulcerative gingivitis.

As in medical infections in which herpesviruses reduce the host defense and give rise to overgrowth of pathogenic

Table 5-3 Herpesviruses in Gingival Biopsies from Periodontal Health and Periodontitis[118]

Herpesvirus	Periodontal health* (11 subjects)	Periodontitis* (14 subjects)	P values (chi-square test)
HSV	1 (9)	8 (57)	.04
EBV-1	3 (27)	11 (79)	.03
EBV-2	0 (0)	7 (50)	.02
HCMV	2 (18)	12 (86)	.003
HHV-6	0 (0)	3 (21)	.31
HHV-7	0 (0)	6 (43)	.04
HHV-8	0 (0)	4 (29)	.17

*Number (percentage) of virally positive samples.

microorganisms, herpesvirus-infected periodontal sites show elevated levels of periodontal pathogens. As described above, localized aggressive periodontitis lesions with active HCMV infection tend to yield high *A actinomycetemcomitans* counts. Many chronic periodontitis lesions showing EBV-1 and HCMV harbor high levels of the periodontal pathogens *P gingivalis, B forsythus, P intermedia, P nigrescens*, and *Treponema denticola*.[123]

Herpesviruses may also interfere with periodontal healing. A study of guided tissue regeneration showed that periodontal sites harboring either EBV-1 or HCMV had an average gain of clinical attachment of 2.3 mm compared with virally negative sites that showed a mean clinical attachment gain of 5.0 mm.[124] By infecting and altering functions of fibroblasts and other mammalian cells, herpesviruses may reduce the regenerating potential of the periodontal ligament.

Pathogenesis of Herpesvirus-Associated Periodontal Disease

Herpesviruses may cause periodontal pathology as a direct result of virus infection and replication, or as a result of virally induced damage to the host defense.[115] Herpesviruses may exert periodontopathic potential through at least five mechanisms, operating alone or in combination.

First, herpesviruses may have direct cytopathic effects on fibroblasts, keratinocytes, endothelial cells, inflammatory cells such as polymorphonuclear leukocytes, lymphocytes, macrophages, and possibly bone cells. Because these cells are key constituents of inflamed periodontal tissue, herpesvirus-induced cytopathic effects may hamper tissue turnover and repair.

Second, herpesvirus periodontal infections may impair cells involved in host defense, thereby predisposing the host to microbial superinfection. EBV-1 and HCMV can infect and/or alter functions of monocytes, macrophages, and lymphocytes in periodontitis lesions.

Third, gingival herpesvirus infection may promote subgingival attachment and colonization of periodontopathic bacteria, similar to the enhanced bacterial adherence to virus-infected cells observed in other infections. Viral proteins expressed on eukaryotic cell membranes can act as bacterial receptors and generate new bacterial binding sites. Also, loss of virus-damaged epithelial cells can expose the basement membrane and the surface of regenerating cells, providing new sites for bacterial binding.

Fourth, herpesvirus infections can give rise to altered inflammatory mediator and cytokine responses. In periodontitis, HCMV-induced expression of cytokines is particularly intriguing. HCMV infection can upregulate interleukin 1β and tumor necrosis factor (TNF)–α gene expression of monocytes and macrophages. In turn, IL-1β and TNF-α may upregulate matrix metalloproteinase, downregulate tissue inhibitors of metalloproteinase, and mediate periodontal bone destruction. Increased production of these proinflammatory cytokines by macrophages and monocytes has been associated with enhanced susceptibility to destructive periodontal disease.

Fifth, herpesviruses can produce tissue injury as a result of immunopathologic responses. EBV may trigger proliferation of cytotoxic T lymphocytes capable of recognizing and destroying virally infected cells. Moreover, acute EBV infection and infectious mononucleosis can induce polyclonal B-lymphocyte activation with generation of antineutrophil antibodies and neutropenia. EBV-infected B lymphocytes may shed viral structural antigens that result in production of blocking antibodies, immune complex formation, and T-suppressor cell activation. EBV can also suppress T-lymphocyte functions. Immunopathologic re-

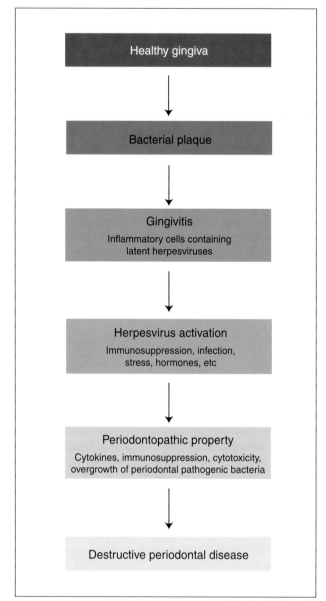

Fig 5-7 Model for herpesviruses-related periodontitis.

metabolic abnormalities in lymphocytes and monocytes. In addition, HCMV can suppress antigen-specific cytotoxic T-lymphocyte functions, resulting in decreases in circulating CD4+ cells and increases in CD8+ suppressor cells, which in turn may lead to global impairment of cell-mediated immunity.

Model for Herpesvirus-Mediated Periodontal Disease

Available data implicate certain herpesviruses in the etiology and/or pathogenesis of human periodontal disease based on the following:

1. Presence of nucleic acid sequences of EBV-1, HCMV, and other herpesviruses in aggressive and chronic periodontitis lesions
2. Association between herpesviruses and acute necrotizing gingivitis in malnourished African children
3. Detection of nucleic acid sequences of herpesviruses in inflammatory periodontal cells
4. Probable profound effect of herpesvirus infection on periodontal defense cells
5. Ability of herpesviruses to augment the expression of tissue-damaging cytokines in periodontal inflammatory cells
6. Increased frequency of periodontopathic bacteria in periodontitis lesions that test positive for herpesvirus
7. The apparent association between active HCMV infection and chronic and localized aggressive periodontitis

Figure 5-7 describes a model for herpesvirus-mediated periodontal disease. Initially, gingival inflammation permits herpesvirus-infected inflammatory cells to enter the periodontium. Herpesvirus reactivation in the periodontium may then occur spontaneously or as a result of concurrent infection, fever, drug use, tissue trauma, emotional stress, exposure to ultraviolet light, and other factors impairing the host immune defense. Active herpesvirus infection decreases the resistance of the periodontal tissues, thereby permitting subgingival overgrowth of periodontal pathogenic bacteria. Several recognized risk indicators for periodontal disease, including HIV infection, psychosocial and physical stress, pregnancy, and hormonal changes, have the potential to reactivate herpesviruses, which may be one important reason for their relationship to periodontal disease.

Herpesvirus reactivation in periodontal tissues resulting in transient immunosuppression may help explain the episodic, progressive nature of human periodontitis. Tissue tropism of herpesvirus infection may contribute to the localized pattern of tissue destruction in periodontitis. Absence of herpesvirus infection or reactivation in the peri-

actions similar to those associated with EBV infection have been implicated in the pathogenesis of human periodontal disease.

HCMV can induce cell-mediated immunosuppression by reducing the cell surface expression of major histocompatibility complex class I molecules, thereby interfering with T-lymphocyte recognition. HCMV can cause odontium may explain why some individuals carry peri-odontopathic bacteria in their subgingival microbiota while maintaining periodontal health.

If some types of periodontitis are indeed the result of herpesvirus-induced tissue destruction, a new direction in the prevention and treatment of periodontitis may focus on controlling the causative viruses. Vaccination against herpesviruses would then be an attractive approach to periodontal prophylaxis and treatment.

References

1. Moore WEC, Moore LVH. The bacteria of periodontal diseases. Periodontol 2000 1994;5:66–77.
2. Armstrong WG. Origin and nature of the acquired pellicle. Proc R Soc Med 1968;61:923–930.
3. Listgarten MA. Structure of surface coatings of teeth: A review. J Clin Periodontol 1976;47:139–147.
4. Newman HN. The organic films on enamel surfaces: The dental plaque. Br Dent J 1973;135:106–111.
5. Moore WE, Holdeman LV, Smibert RM, et al. Bacteriology of experimental gingivitis in young adult humans. Infect Immun 1982;38:651–667.
6. Syed SA, Loesche WJ. Bacteriology of human experimental gingivitis: Effect of plaque age. Infect Immun 1978;21:821–829.
7. Brecx M, Theilade J, Attstrom R. An ultrastructural quantitative study of the significance of microbial multiplication during early dental plaque growth. J Periodontal Res 1983;18:177–186.
8. Theilade E, Theilade J, Mikkelsen L. Microbiological studies on early dento-gingival plaque on teeth and Mylar strips in humans. J Periodontal Res 1982;17:12–25.
9. Listgarten MA. The structure of dental plaque. Periodontol 2000 1994;5:52–65.
10. Lang NP, Cumming BR, Löe H. Toothbrushing frequency as it relates to plaque development and gingival health. J Periodontol 1973;44:396–405.
11. Bostrom L, Bergstrom J, Dahlen G, Linder LE. Smoking and subgingival microflora in periodontal disease. J Clin Periodontol 2001;28:212–219.
12. Shiloah J, Patters MR, Waring MB. The prevalence of pathogenic periodontal microflora in healthy young adult smokers. J Periodontol 2000;71:562–567.
13. Zambon JJ, Grossi SG, Machtei EE, et al. Cigarette smoking increases the risk for subgingival infection with periodontal pathogens. J Periodontol 1996;67(suppl 10):1050–1054.
14. Socransky SS, Haffajee AD. Relationship of cigarette smoking to the subgingival microbiota. J Clin Periodontol 2001;28:377–382.
15. Costerton JW, Lewandowski Z, DeBeer D, et al. Biofilms, the customized microniche. J Bacteriol 1994;176:2137–2142.
16. Bryers JD. Bacterial biofilms. Curr Opin Biotechnol 1993;4:197–204.
17. Costerton JW, Lewandowski Z, Caldwell DE, et al. Microbial biofilms. Annu Rev Microbiol 1995;49:711–745.
18. Marsh PD, Bradshaw DJ. Dental plaque as a biofilm. J Ind Microbiol 1995;15:169–175.
19. Sissons CH, Wong L, Cutress TW. Patterns and rates of growth of microcosm dental plaque biofilms. Oral Microbiol Immunol 1995;10:160–167.
20. Bradshaw DJ, Marsh PD, Schilling KM, Cummins D. A modified chemostat system to study the ecology of oral biofilms. J Appl Bacteriol 1996;80:124–130.
21. Le Magrex E, Jacquelin LF, Carquin J, et al. Antiseptic activity of some antidental plaque chemicals on *Streptococcus mutans* biofilm. Pathol Biol 1993;41:364–368.
22. Wilson M. Susceptibility of oral bacterial biofilms to antimicrobial agents. J Med Microbiol 1996;44:79–87.
23. Socransky SS, Haffajee AD, Cugini MA, et al. Microbial complexes in subgingival plaque. J Clin Periodontol 1998;25:134–144.
24. Ximenez-Fyvie LA, Haffajee AD, Socransky SS. Microbial composition of supra- and subgingival plaque in subjects with adult periodontitis. J Clin Periodontol 2000;27:722–732.
25. Ximenez-Fyvie LA, Haffajee AD, Socransky SS. Composition of the microbiota of supra- and subgingival plaque in health and periodontitis. J Clin Periodontol 2000;27:648–657.
26. Patters MR, Landesberg RL, Johansson LA, et al. *Bacteroides gingivalis* antigens and bone resorbing activity in root surface fractions of periodontally involved teeth. J Periodontal Res 1982;17:122–130.
27. Slots J. Subgingival microflora in periodontal disease. J Clin Periodontol 1979;6:351–382.
28. Tanner ACR, Haffer C, Bratthall GT, et al. A study of the bacteria associated with advancing periodontitis in man. J Clin Periodontol 1979;6:278–307.
29. Loesche WJ, Syed SA. Bacteriology of human experimental gingivitis: Effect of plaque and gingivitis score. Infect Immun 1978; 21:830–839.
30. Listgarten M, Hellden L. Relative distribution of bacteria at clinically healthy and periodontally diseased sites in humans. J Clin Periodontol 1978;5:115–132.
31. Theilade E, Wright WH, Jensen SB, Löe H. Experimental gingivitis in man: A longitudinal clinical and bacteriological investigation. J Periodontal Res 1966:1–13.
32. White D, Mayrand D. Association of oral *Bacteroides* with gingivitis and adult periodontitis. J Periodontal Res 1981;16:259–265.
33. Kornman KS, Loesche WJ. The subgingival microbial flora during pregnancy. J Periodontal Res 1980;15:111.
34. Savitt E, Socransky S. Distribution of certain subgingival microbial species in selected periodontal conditions. J Periodontal Res 1984;19:111–123.
35. Haffajee AD, Socransky SS. Microbial etiological agents of destructive periodontal diseases. Periodontol 2000 1994;5:78–111.
36. Albandar JM, Olsen I, Gjermo P. Associations between six DNA probe-detected periodontal bacteria and alveolar bone loss and other clinical signs of periodontitis. Acta Odontol Scand 1990;48:415–423.
37. Choi JI, Nakagawa T, Yamada S, et al. Clinical, microbiological and immunological studies on recent periodontal disease. J Clin Periodontol 1990;17:426–434.
38. Dahlén G, Manji F, Baelum V, Fejerskov O. Putative periodontopathogens in diseased and non-diseased persons exhibiting poor oral hygiene. J Clin Periodontol 1992;19:35–42.
39. Dzink JL, Socransky SS, Haffajee AD. The predominant cultivable microbiota of active and inactive lesions of destructive periodontal diseases. J Clin Periodontol 1988;15:316–323.
40. Haffajee AD, Socransky SS, Ebersole JL, Smith DJ. Clinical, microbiological and immunological features of subjects with refractory periodontal diseases. J Clin Periodontol 1988;15:390.

41. Kornman KS, Newman MG, Moore DJ, Singer RE. The influence of supragingival plaque control on clinical and microbial outcomes following the use of antibiotics for the treatment of periodontitis. J Periodontol 1994;65:848–854.

42. Loesche WJ, Syed SA, Schmidt E, Morrison EC. Bacterial profiles of subgingival plaques in periodontitis. J Periodontol 1985;56:447–456.

43. Moore WEC, Moore LH, Ranney RR, et al. The microflora of periodontal sites showing active destructive progression. J Clin Periodontol 1991;18:729–739.

44. Slots J. The predominant cultivatable microflora of advanced periodontitis. Scand J Dent Res 1977;85:114.

45. Slots J. Bacterial specificity in adult periodontitis: A summary of recent work. J Clin Periodontol 1986;13:912–917.

46. Slots J, Bragd L, Wikström M, Dahlén G. The occurrence of Actinobacillus actinomycetemcomitans, Bacteroides gingivalis and Bacteroides intermedius in destructive periodontal disease in adults. J Clin Periodontol 1986;13:570–577.

47. Spiegel CA, Hayduk SE, Minah GE, Krywolap GN. Black-pigmented Bacteroides from clinically characterized periodontal sites. J Periodontol Res 1979;14:376–382.

48. Tanner ACR, Socransky SS, Goodson JM. Microbiota of periodontal pockets losing crestal alveolar bone. J Periodontal Res 1984;1:1.

49. Zambon JJ. Actinobacillus actinomycetemcomitans in human periodontal disease. J Clin Periodontol 1985;12:1–20.

50. Zambon JJ, Reynolds HS, Slots J. Black-pigmented Bacteroides spp in the human oral cavity. Infect Immun 1981;32:198–203.

51. Ali RW, Lie T, Skaug N. Early effects of periodontal therapy on the detection frequency of four putative periodontal pathogens in adults. J Periodontol 1992;63:540–547.

52. Gusberti FA, Syed SA, Lang NP. Combined antibiotic (metronidazole) and mechanical treatment effects on the subgingival bacterial flora of sites with recurrent periodontal disease. J Clin Periodontol 1988;15:353–359.

53. Kulkarni GV, Lee WK, Aitken S, et al. A randomized, placebo-controlled trial of doxycycline: Effect on the microflora of recurrent periodontitis lesions in high risk patients. J Periodontol 1991;62:197–202.

54. Nakagawa T, Yamada S, Tsunoda M, et al. Clinical, microbiological, and immunological studies following initial preparation in adult periodontitis. Bull Tokyo Dent Coll 1990;31:321–331.

55. Robertson PB, Buchanan SA, Armitage GC, et al. Evaluation of clinical and microbiological measures to predict treatment response in severe periodontitis. J Periodontal Res 1987;22:230–232.

56. Slots J, Emrich LJ, Genco RJ, Rosling BG. Relationship between some subgingival bacteria and periodontal pocket depth and gain or loss of periodontal attachment after treatment of adult periodontitis. J Clin Periodontol 1985;12:540–552.

57. Socransky SS, Haffajee AD. Effect of therapy on periodontal infections. J Periodontol 1993;64:754–759.

58. van Steenberghe D, Bercy P, Kohl J, et al. Subgingival minocycline hydrochloride ointment in moderate to severe chronic adult periodontitis: A randomized, double-blind, vehicle-controlled, multicenter study. J Periodontol 1993;64:637–644.

59. Topoll HH, Lange DE, Muller RE. Multiple periodontal abscesses after systemic antibiotic therapy. J Clin Periodontol 1990;17:268–272.

60. Papapanou PN, Sandros J, Lindberg K, et al. Porphyromonas gingivalis may multiply and advance within stratified human junctional epithelium in vitro. J Periodontal Res 1994;29:374–375.

61. Holt SC, Ebersole JL, Felton J, et al. Implantation of Bacteroides gingivalis in nonhuman primates initiates progression of periodontitis. Science 1988;239:55–57.

62. Kamma JJ, Nakou M, Manti FA. Predominant microflora of severe, moderate and minimal periodontal lesions in young adults with rapidly progressive periodontitis. J Periodontal Res 1995;30:66–72.

63. Gmür R, Strub JR, Guggenheim B. Prevalence of Bacteroides forsythus and Bacteroides gingivalis in subgingival plaque of prosthodontically treated patients on short recall. J Periodontal Res 1989;24:113–120.

64. Lai C-H, Listgarten MA, Shirakawa M, Slots J. Bacteroides forsythus in adult gingivitis and periodontitis. Oral Microbiol Immunol 1987;2:152–157.

65. Listgarten MA, Lai C-H, Young V. Microbial composition and pattern of antibiotic resistance in subgingival microbial samples from patients with refractory periodontitis. J Periodontol 1993;64:155–161.

66. Kornman KS, Robertson PB. Clinical and microbiological evaluation of therapy for juvenile periodontitis. J Periodontol 1985;56:443–446.

67. Moore WEC, Holdeman LV, Cato EP, et al. Comparative bacteriology of juvenile periodontitis. Infect Immun 1985;48:507–519.

68. Aass AM, Preus HR, Gjermo P. Association between detection of oral Actinobacillus actinomycetemcomitans and radiographic bone loss in teenagers. A 4-year longitudinal study. J Periodontol 1992;63:682–685.

69. Asikainen S, Alaluusua S, Kari K, Kleemola-Kujala E. Subgingival microflora and periodontal conditions in healthy teenagers. J Periodontol 1986;57:505–509.

70. Chung H-J, Chung C-P, Son S-H, Nisengard RJ. Actinobacillus actinomycetemcomitans serotypes and leukotoxicity in Korean localized juvenile periodontitis. J Periodontol 1989;60:506–511.

71. Delaney JE, Kornman KS. Microbiology of subgingival plaque from children with localized prepubertal periodontitis. Oral Microbiol Immunol 1987;2:71.

72. Ebersole JL, Sandoval MN, Steffen MJ, Cappelli D. Serum antibody in Actinobacillus actinomycetemcomitans infected patients with periodontal disease. Infect Immun 1991;59:1795–1802.

73. Kim KJ, Kim DK, Chung CP, Son S. Longitudinal monitoring for disease progression of localized juvenile periodontitis. J Periodontol 1992;63:806–811.

74. Mandell RL, Socransky SS. A selective medium for Actinobacillus actinomycetemcomitans and the incidence of the organism in juvenile periodontitis. J Periodontol 1981;52:593–598.

75. Newman M, Socransky S. Predominant cultivable microbiota in periodontosis. J Periodontal Res 1977;12:120–128.

76. Newman MG, Socransky SS, Savitt ED, et al. Studies of the microbiology of periodontosis. J Periodontol 1976;47:373–379.

77. Slots J. The predominant cultivable organisms in juvenile periodontitis. Scand J Dent Res 1976;84:1–10.

78. Slots J, Feik D, Rams T. Prevalence and antimicrobial susceptibility of Enterobacteriacease, Pseudomonadaceae and Acinetobacter in human periodontitis. Oral Microbiol Immunol 1990;5:149–154.

79. Slots J, Reynolds HS, Genco RJ. Actinobacillus actinomycetemcomitans in human periodontal disease: A cross-sectional microbiological investigation. Infect Immun 1980;29:1013–1020.

80. van der Velden U, Abbas F, van Steenbergen TJM, et al. Prevalence of periodontal breakdown in adolescents and presence of *Actinobacillus actinomycetemcomitans* in subjects with attachment loss. J Periodontol 1989;60:604–610.

81. van Steenbergen TJM, van der Velden U, Abbas F, de Graaff J. Microbiological and clinical monitoring of non-localized juvenile periodontitis in young adults: A report of 11 cases. J Periodontol 1993;64:40–47.

82. Zambon JJ, Christersson LA, Slots J. *Actinobacillus actinomycetemcomitans* in human periodontal disease: Prevalence in patient groups and distribution of biotypes and serotypes within families. J Periodontol 1983;54:707–711.

83. Bonta Y, Zambon JJ, Genco RJ, Neiders ME. Rapid identification of periodontal pathogens in subgingival plaque: Comparison of indirect immunofluorescence microscopy with bacterial culture for detection of *Actinobacillus actinomycetemcomitans*. J Dent Res 1985;64:793–798.

84. Papapanou PN, Sellen A, Wennstrom JL, Dahlen G. An analysis of the subgingival microflora in randomly selected subjects. Oral Microbiol Immunol 1993;8:24–29.

85. Wolff LF, Aeppli DM, Pihlstrom B, et al. Natural distribution of 5 bacteria associated with periodontal disease. J Clin Periodontol 1993;20:699–706.

86. Kornman KS, Newman MG, Alvarado R, et al. Clinical and microbiological patterns of patients with adult and refractory periodontitis, I. Clinical. J Periodontol 1991;62:634–642.

87. Mombelli A, Gmür R, Gobbi C, Lang NP. *Actinobacillus actinomycetemcomitans* in adult periodontitis, I. Topographic distribution before and after treatment. J Periodontol 1994;65:820–826.

88. Mombelli A, Gmür R, Gobbi C, Lang NP. *Actinobacillus actinomyceten*comitans in adult periodontitis, II. Characterization of isolated strains and effect of mechanical periodontal treatment. J Periodontol 1994;65:827–834.

89. Bragd L, Dahlén G, Wikström M, Slots J. The capability of *Actinobacillus actinomycetemcomitans*, *Bacteroides gingivalis* and *Bacteroides intermedius* to indicate progressive periodontitis: A retrospective study. J Clin Periodontol 1987;14:95–99.

90. Preus HR, Zambon JJ, Dunford RG, Genco RJ. The distribution and transmission of *Actinobacillus actinomycetemcomitans* in families with established adult periodontitis. J Periodontol 1994;65:2–7.

91. Moore WEC, Holdeman LV, Cato EP, et al. Comparative bacteriology of juvenile periodontitis. Infect Immun 1985;48:507–519.

92. Gharbia SE, Haapasalo M, Shah HN, et al. Characterization of *Prevotella intermedia* and *Prevotella nigrescens* isolates from periodontic and endodontic infections. J Periodontol 1994;65:56–61.

93. Asikainen S, Jousimies-Somer H, Kanervo A, Summanen P. Certain bacterial species and morphotypes in localized juvenile periodontitis and in matched controls. J Periodontol 1987;58:224–230.

94. Asikainen S, Lai CH, Alaluusua S, Slots J. Distribution of *Actinobacillus actinomycetemcomitans* serotypes in periodontal health and disease. Oral Microbiol Immunol 1991;6:115–118.

95. Kononen KS, Asikainen S, Alaluusua S, et al. Are certain oral pathogens part of normal oral flora in denture-wearing edentulous subjects? Oral Microbiol Immunol 1991;6:119–122.

96. Christersson LA, Slots J, Rosling BG, Genco R. Microbiological and clinical effects of surgical treatment of localized juvenile periodontitis. J Clin Periodontol 1985;12:465–476.

97. Christersson LA, Zambon JJ. Suppression of subgingival *Actinobacillus actinomycetemcomitans* in localized juvenile periodontitis by systemic tetracycline. J Clin Periodontol 1993;20:395–401.

98. Haffajee AD, Socransky SS, Ebersole JL, Smith DJ. Clinical, microbiological and immunological features associated with the treatment of active periodontosis lesions. J Clin Periodontol 1984;11:600–618.

99. Lindhe J, Liljenberg B. Treatment of localized juvenile periodontitis: Results after 5 years. J Clin Periodontol 1984;11:399–410.

100. Mandell RL, Socransky SS. Microbiological and clinical effects of surgery plus doxycycline on juvenile periodontitis. J Periodontol 1988;59:373–379.

101. Preus HR. Treatment of rapidly destructive periodontitis in Papillon-Lefevre syndrome. J Clin Periodontol 1988;15:639–643.

102. Saxen L, Asikainen S. Metronidazole in the treatment of localized juvenile periodontitis. J Clin Periodontol 1993;20:166–171.

103. Slots J, Rosling BG. Suppression of the periodontopathic microflora in localized juvenile periodontitis by systemic tetracycline. J Clin Periodontol 1983;10:465–486.

104. Christersson LA, Albini B, Zambon JJ, et al. Tissue localization of *Actinobacillus actinomycetemcomitans* in human periodontitis, I. Light, immunofluorescence and electron microscopic studies. J Periodontol 1987;58:529–539.

105. Saglie FR, Smith CT, Newman MG, et al. The presence of bacteria in the oral epithelium in periodontal disease, II. Immunohistochemical identification of bacteria. J Periodontol 1986;57:492–500.

106. Vandesteen GE, Williams BL, Ebersole JL, et al. Clinical, microbiological and immunological studies of a family with a high prevalence of early-onset periodontitis. J Periodontol 1984;55:159–169.

107. Walker C, Gordon J. The effect of clindamycin on the microbiota associated with refractory periodontitis. J Periodontol 1990;61:692–698.

108. Walker CB, Gordon JM, Magnusson I, Clark WB. A role for antibiotics in the treatment of refractory periodontitis. J Periodontol 1993;64:772–781.

109. Loesche WJ, Syed SA, Laughon BE, Stoll J. The bacteriology of acute necrotizing ulcerative gingivitis. J Periodontol 1982;53:223–230.

110. Haffajee AD, Socransky SS, Smith C, Dibart S. Relation of baseline microbial parameters to future periodontal attachment loss. J Clin Periodontol 1991;18:744.

111. Wennström JL, Heijl L, Dahlen G, Kerstin G. Periodic subgingival antimicrobial irrigation of periodontal pockets, I. Clinical observations. J Clin Periodontol 1987;14:541–550.

112. Listgarten MA, Slots J, Nowotny HH, et al. Incidence of periodontitis recurrence in treated patients with and without cultivable *Actinobacillus actinomycetemcomitans*, *Prevotella intermedia* and *Porphyromonas gingivalis*: A prospective study. J Periodontol 1991;62:377.

113. Feres M, Haffajee AD, Allard K, et al. Change in subgingival microbial profiles in adult periodontitis subjects receiving either systemically-administered amoxicillin or metronidazole. J Clin Periodontol 2001;28:597–609.

114. Roizman B. Herpesviridae. In: Fields BN, Knipe DM, Howley PM, et al (eds). Fields Virology, ed 3. Philadelphia: Lippincott-Raven, 1996:2221–2230.

115. Contreras A, Slots J. Herpesviruses in human periodontal disease. J Periodontal Res 2000;35:3–16.

116. Rickinson AB, Kieff E. Epstein-Barr virus. In: Fields BN, Knipe DM, Howley PM (eds). Fields Virology, ed 3. Philadelphia: Lippincott-Raven, 1996:2397–2446.

117. Britt WJ, Alford CA. Cytomegalovirus. In: Fields BN, Knipe DM, Howley PM (eds). Fields Virology, ed 3. Philadelphia: Lippincott-Raven, 1996:2493–2523.

118. Contreras A, Nowzari H, Slots J. Herpesviruses in periodontal pocket and gingival tissue specimens. Oral Microbiol Immunol 2000;15:15–18.

119. Slots J, Contreras A. Herpesviruses, a unifying etiological factor in periodontitis? Oral Microbiol Immunol 2000;15:277–280.

120. Contreras A, Zadeh HH, Nowzari H, Slots J. Herpesvirus infection of inflammatory cells in human periodontitis. Oral Microbiol Immunol 1999;14:206–212.

121. Ting M, Contreras A, Slots J. Herpesvirus in localized juvenile periodontitis. J Periodontal Res 2000;35:17–25.

122. Contreras A, Falkler WA Jr, Enwonwu CO, et al. Human *Herpesviridae* in acute necrotizing ulcerative gingivitis in children in Nigeria. Oral Microbiol Immunol 1997;12:259–265.

123. Contreras A, Umeda M, Chen C, et al. Relationship between herpesviruses and adult periodontitis and periodontopathic bacteria. J Periodontol 1999;70:478–484.

124. Smith MacDonald E, Nowzari H, Contreras A, et al. Clinical and microbiological evaluation of a bioabsorbable and a nonresorbable barrier membrane in the treatment of periodontal intraosseous lesions. J Periodontol 1998;69:445–453.

CHAPTER 6

The Biochemistry and Physiology of Periodontal Connective Tissues

P. Mark Bartold and A. Sampath Narayanan
- Biochemistry of Matrix Constituents
- Periodontal Connective Tissues
- Connective Tissue in Diseases of the Periodontium
- New Perspectives

Biochemistry of Matrix Constituents

The periodontium comprises the connective tissues around the teeth and consists of gingiva, periodontal ligament, cementum, and alveolar bone.[1] The epithelium (junctional, sulcular, and oral epithelia in normal periodontium and pocket epithelium in diseased tissue) is not strictly a connective tissue, but because of its unique relationship and functional demands, it must be considered a periodontal component. However, it will not be discussed in this section.

Several features distinguish the periodontium from other organs. For example, it is constantly subjected to mechanical and bacterial stress, yet it is remarkably efficient in maintaining its structural and functional integrity; this is due to the fast turnover and efficient remodeling of its component structures. The periodontium functions as a single unit, even though each of its components has a distinct composition and connective tissue architecture. Recent research has revealed that matrix constituents of one periodontal structure can influence the cellular activities of adjacent structures. Finally, its unique composition dic-

tates that maintenance, repair, and regeneration of periodontium require a variety of complex processes coordinating the synthesis and turnover of soft and hard tissues.[1]

The connective tissues of the periodontium consist of fibrous and nonfibrous molecular constituents. Fibrous components are collagens and elastin, and nonfibrous constituents are fibronectin, laminin, tenascin and other proteins, proteoglycans, tissue-bound growth factors, and lipid. In addition, calcified structures also contain osteopontin, bone sialoprotein (BSP), and minerals.

The objective of this chapter is to summarize currently available information on the periodontal connective tissue matrix in health and disease. To provide a perspective of matrix structure and function, first the biochemistry of matrix macromolecules is reviewed. Emphasis is on collagens, as these are the major constituents of all periodontal structures. This is followed by a description of connective tissue architecture in normal periodontium and how it is affected by inflammation and fibrotic diseases. Factors that cause pathological connective tissue alterations are outlined. Finally, emerging biologic principles of wound healing that are relevant to periodontal therapy are discussed. The chemistry and biology of periodontal connective tissues are discussed more extensively elsewhere.[2]

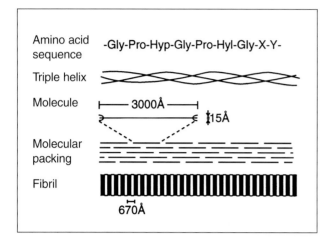

Fig 6-1 Structure of collagen fibrils formed from the basic gly-X-Y triple-helical unit. Three α chains with this amino acid sequence are assembled into the triple helix. Each triple-helical collagen molecule, represented as a line, is of size 3,000 × 15 Å. The molecules aggregate with a quarter stagger, which results in hole and overlap zones (alternating regions where there is a gap between ends of molecules and no gaps, respectively). These zones are responsible for the characteristic banding pattern in collagen fibers. The bands of a typical collagen fiber have a periodic spacing of 670 Å. (Modified from Byers,[5] with permission.)

Collagens

Collagens are the most abundant proteins in the animal kingdom. The word collagen is derived from the French word *collagene* (from the Greek *kolla* [glue] + *gen*) to designate connective tissue constituents that produce glue. The collagen molecule is rigid and resists stretching; therefore, it is utilized in tissues such as tendon, skin, and periodontal ligament, where mechanical force must be transmitted without loss. The organization of collagen depends upon the specific functional requirements in various tissues. For example, it forms branching and anastomosing fibers in skin, thick fibers oriented parallel to their long axes in tendons, and laminated sheets in the cornea.[3]

Structure and Types of Collagen

Several unique structural properties distinguish the collagen molecule from other proteins. First, three polypeptide chains, called α *chains*, form the collagen molecule. The α chains are left-handed helices that are assembled into a "triple helix" with a right-handed twist, and the molecule may be a homotrimer or a heterotrimer made up of similar or different α chains, respectively.[3,4] Second, a repeating gly-X-Y amino acid sequence forms the triple helix; the X and Y are usually amino acids other than glycine. In fibril-forming collagens, the helical domain is flanked at both ends by short nonhelical telopeptides. Short gly-X-Y repeats are also present in the complement component C1q, lung surfactant protein, and several other proteins; however, they are not considered collagens because they do not form part of the extracellular matrix. Third, collagen contains two unique amino acids, hydroxyproline (hyp) and hydroxylysine (hyl). In vertebrate collagens

these amino acids are present in the Y position. Fourth, collagen molecules are covalently linked through lysine-derived intrachain and interchain crosslinks. The hierarchical organization of collagen molecules into banded fibrils is schematically illustrated in Fig 6-1.

More than 19 different collagen types have been described.[5–7] These are divided into five groups. The first group includes those collagens that form banded fibrils in tissues; type I, II, III, V, and XI collagens belong to this group. In these collagens, called *fibril-forming collagens*, the triple-helical domain contains an uninterrupted stretch of 338 to 343 gly-X-Y triplets in each chain, and the molecule has the dimension 15 Å × 3,000 Å. The second group of collagens associates with the first group, forming connective tissue elements between banded fibrils and other components. This group is called *fibril-associated collagens with interrupted triple helices (FACITs)* and includes types IX, XII, XIV, XVI, and XIX. The third group, called *network-forming collagens*, includes type IV (basement membranes), type VIII (Descemet's membrane), and type X; these collagens form protein membranes. The fourth group forms beaded filaments and includes type VI (microfibrils) and type VII (anchoring fibrils). Type XIII and type XVII collagens are *transmembrane collagens*. Other collagens that do not fall into any of these groups include invertebrate collagens (which form cuticle).[7]

Tissues contain a mixture of collagen types. Type I collagen is the predominant kind in all connective tissues except cartilage, and it accounts for 65% to 95% of total collagens. Type III is the second major kind. The content of type III collagen in adult tissues ranges from 5% to 30%; however, it may be much higher in fetal and granulation tissues.[2] These two collagens are codistributed with types

Table 6-1 Vertebrate Collagen

Collagen type	Chain composition*	Gene†	Distribution
Fibrillar collagens			
Type I	$[(\alpha1)_2\alpha2]$	COL1A1, COL1A2	Soft tissues, bone
Type II	$[(\alpha1)_3]$	COL2A1	Cartilage, vitreous humor
Type III	$[(\alpha1)_3]$	COL3A1	All soft tissues
Type V	$[(\alpha1)_2\alpha2]$ $[\alpha1, \alpha2, \alpha3]$ $[(\alpha1)_3]$	COL5A1, COL5A2, COL5A3	Most soft tissues
Type XI	$[(\alpha1)_2\alpha2]$	COL11A1, COL11A2	Cartilage
FACIT collagens			
Type IX	$[\alpha1, \alpha2, \alpha3]$	COL9A1, COL9A2, COL9A3	Cartilage
Type XII	$[(\alpha1)_3]$	COL12A1	Soft tissues
Type XIV	$[(\alpha1)_3]$	COL14A1	All tissues
Network-forming collagens			
Type IV	$[(\alpha1)_2\alpha2]$	COL4A1, COL4A2	Basement membranes
Type VIII	$[(\alpha1)_3]$	COL8A1	Descemet's membrane
Type X	$[(\alpha1)_3]$	COL10A1	Cartilage
Beaded filament-forming collagens			
Type VI	$[\alpha1, \alpha2, \alpha3]$	COL6A1, COL6A2, COL6A3	Soft tissues
Type VII	$[(\alpha1)_3]$	COL7A1	Anchoring fibrils
Transmembrane collagens			
Type XIII	$[1(XIII)_3]$	COL1A13	Plasma membrane
Type XVII	$[\alpha1(XVII)_3]$	COL1A17	Hemidesmosomes

* The collagen molecule consists of three polypeptides called α chains. Each chain is identified by the arabic number that follows. The collagen molecule may be composed of same (homotrimers) or different (heterotrimers) α chains. Roman numerals indicate the collagen type. Thus, [α1(II)3] represents type II collagen composed of three α1(II) chains.

† COL represents collagen, and the arabic number that follows indicates its type. *A* and the number after it designates the α chain and its type. For example, COL5A2 is the gene for the α2(V) chain.

V, VI, and XII. In cartilage, type II is the major fibril-forming collagen, and it is present with FACIT types IX, XI, and XII. Type X is a short collagen with a 1,380-Å helix, and its distribution is limited to growing bones in the zone of hypertrophic chondrocytes.[6]

In type IV collagen, which is found only in basement membranes, triple-helical domains are interrupted by short nonhelical sequences. This collagen forms a fine, spiderlike network of cords, which is created by the assembly of N-terminal ends of four type IV molecules and dimerization of two nonhelical C-terminal ends. The type IV collagen binds to anchoring fibrils, which are structures attached by their extremities to epithelial basement membranes on one end and to anchoring plaques on the other end. The anchoring fibril consists of type VII collagen that contains a large 4,240-Å-long triple-helical region. In the

basement membrane zone, hemidesmosome contains type XVII collagen, also called *180-kd bullous pemphigoid antigen*, or BP 180. The features of various vertebrate collagen types and their tissue distribution are summarized in Table 6-1.

Biosynthesis of Collagens

The collagen molecule is insoluble under physiologic conditions. It contains several modified amino acids; the amino acid modifications can occur only on free α chains, because the enzymes responsible cannot act on the triple-helical molecule. For these and other reasons, collagen is first synthesized as a precursor in which the α chains have extra amino acid sequences at the N- and C-terminal ends. These "pro-α" chains undergo a series of well-coordinated biosynthetic reactions in the nucleus, cytoplasm, and ex-

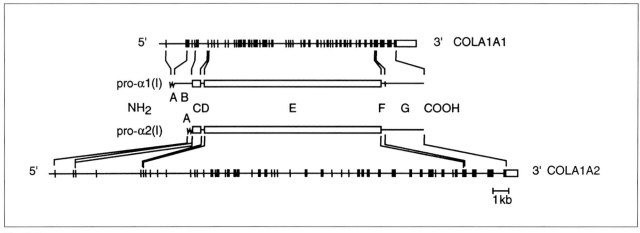

Fig 6-2 Structure of fibrillar collagen genes. The intron-exon organization of the prototype fibrillar collagen genes that encode for pro-α1(I) and pro-α2(I) are shown. The exons are designated by solid boxes or vertical lines. Exons 7 to 48 encode the triple-helical domain, and these start with a glycine codon and end with the codon for the Y amino acid. (A) to (G) designate various polypeptide domains in the molecule: (A) signal peptide, (B) N-terminal globular domain, (C) triple-helical domain of N-propeptide, (D) N-terminal telopeptide, (E) triple helix, (F) C-terminal telopeptide, and (G) C-terminal propeptide. (Modified from Byers,[5] with permission.)

tracellular space.[2,5] These reactions have been characterized for type I collagen, and most of them apply to other collagens as well. These events can be divided roughly into three groups associated with (1) gene expression, (2) translation and posttranslational cytoplasmic events, and (3) extracellular reactions.

Gene expression. The genes for collagens are large, ranging in size from 5 kilobases (kb) for COL10A1 to 100 kb for COL9A1 (see the footnote in Table 6-1 for terminology), and they are approximately 10 times the size of functional messenger ribonucleic acid (mRNA).[7,8] More than 27 genes have been described for collagen types I to XVII and their locations in human chromosomes identified. Although differences exist among various collagen genes, those for fibril-forming collagens have a similar arrangement of exons (coding sequences), and their exons for the triple-helical domain are of 54-bp size or its integral multiples. In contrast, exons for the type IV and VI collagen genes are in multiples of 9 bp. The type X collagen gene is unique because its triple-helical domain consists of a single exon.[8] The gene structure for type I collagen is shown schematically in Fig 6-2.

Translation and posttranslational events. Collagen mRNAs are transcribed in the nucleus, processed by splicing, capping, and polyadenylation, and then translocated to the cytoplasm. The translated α chains, called *pre-pro-α chains*, contain additional sequences at both N- and C-terminal ends and are approximately the length of 1,500 amino acids. After removal of signal sequences, the α chains, now called *pro-α chains*, reach the rough endoplasmic reticu-

lum (RER). As the pro-α chains are being translated, certain prolyl and lysyl residues at the "Y" position are oxidized to hyp and hyl, respectively, by the enzymes prolyl hydroxylase and lysyl hydroxylase. Prolyl hydroxylation occurs predominantly at the C-4 position of proline by prolyl-4-hydroxylase; however, it also occurs at C-3.

Hydroxylation of both prolyl and lysyl residues requires molecular O_2, Fe^{++}, α-ketoglutarate, and ascorbic acid as cofactors. Only nascent pro-α chains, not triple-helical molecules, are substrates for the hydroxylation reaction. Fully hydroxylated triple helix has a melting temperature (T_m, or the temperature at which the triple helix is denatured to individual α chains) of 39°C, while unhydroxylated molecules melt at 25°C[9]; therefore, prolyl hydroxylation is an essential step in collagen biosynthesis. The extent of hydroxylation varies with collagen types; for example, type IV collagen has a higher degree of 3-prolyl hydroxylation and up to 90% lysyl hydroxylation relative to types I and III. The pro-α chains are also glycosylated during translation at hyl and asparagine residues. Glycosylation occurs in the RER lumen and continues in the Golgi.

As soon as synthesis of pro-α chains is completed, globular domains at C-terminal ends fold, aided by intrachain disulfide bonds of cysteines. Triple helix formation is initiated and proceeds toward the N-terminal end. The triple helix is made up of three pro-α chains (two pro-α1 and one pro-α2 chains in type I collagen, along with three pro-α1 chains in homotrimers). The assembled "procollagen" molecule is then translocated to the Golgi (where additional glycosylation, sulfation, and phosphorylation occur), packaged into vesicles, and released into extracellular space.

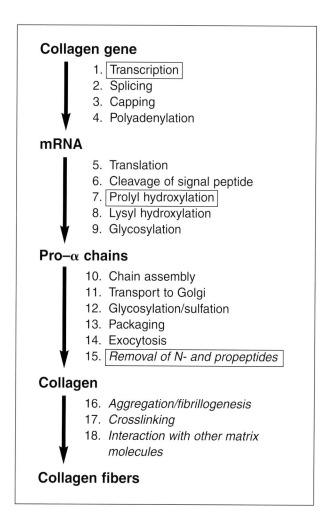

Fig 6-3 Collagen biosynthesis. Reactions occurring in the nucleus, cytoplasm, and extracellular space are shown in normal characters, bold, and italics, respectively, and boxed reactions are those associated with regulation of synthesis. The most significant point of regulation is the gene transcription stage. Prolyl hydroxylation determines the stability of the collagen molecule. N-propeptide can inhibit translation, causing a feedback inhibition of collagen biosynthesis. These reactions have been characterized for fibrillar collagens. Although this general scheme is common to all collagens, variations occur, especially in the removal of propeptide.

Extracellular events. The procollagen is then converted to collagen by removal of propeptide sequences at the N- and C-terminal ends. The enzymes responsible are N- and C-procollagen peptidases. Interestingly, bone morphogenetic protein-1 (BMP-1), a member of the bone-inducing factor family, is identical to the C-proteinase.[10] While removal of propeptides is necessary for type I, II, and III collagens, other collagens may not be processed similarly and some not at all. The "collagen" molecules formed then aggregate spontaneously into ordered fibrils, such that adjacent molecules are staggered by approximately one quarter of the length of the molecule (670 Å) (see Fig 6-1). Although the aggregation is nonenzymatic, the rate of fiber formation and diameter of the fibrils appear to be regulated by type V and III collagen and other macromolecules, notably decorin proteoglycan. Type IX and XI collagens appear to regulate the efficiency and lateral growth of type II collagen fibrils. Removal of propeptide extensions is necessary for ordered fibril organization in dermatosparaxis,[5] an inherited disease in cattle, sheep, and cats.

The collagen fibrillar array is then crosslinked by the enzyme lysyl oxidase. This enzyme oxidatively deaminates ε-amino groups of certain lysyl and hydroxylysyl residues. The products are allysyl and hydroxyallysyl residues, respectively. Aldehyde residues in allysines and hydroxyallysines condense spontaneously with each other or with unmodified lys or hyl residues in adjacent α chains, forming divalent crosslinks norleucine, hydroxynorleucine, and aldol condensation products. The crosslinks may join with additional residues, forming more complex crosslinks, merodesmosines and hydroxypyridiniums.[11] The reactions involved in collagen biosynthesis are summarized in Fig 6-3.

Regulation of Collagen Biosynthesis

Collagen biosynthesis is tightly regulated during normal development and homeostasis in a cell- and tissue-specific manner. Regulation of collagen synthesis can occur at the level of gene transcription or in posttranslational modification. The most significant point of regulation is at the gene transcription stage, and changes in its transcription

Table 6-2 Some Mediators Affecting Collagen Synthesis

Mediator*	Effect
TGF-β†	↑
PDGF	↑
IFN-γ	↓
IL-1α,β‡	↑
TNF-α	↓
PGE₂	↓
Glucocorticoids§	↓
Parathyroid hormone	↓
Vitamin D	↓

*PDGF = platelet-derived growth factor; IL = interleukin; PGE_2 = prostaglandin E_2.

†Also decreases synthesis of matrix metalloproteinases and increases production of proteoglycans and tissue inhibitors of metalloproteinases.

‡Enhances matrix degradation by stimulating MMP synthesis.

§Increases elastin and fibronectin synthesis.

rate are reflected in mRNA levels. The latter is also affected by the stability of mRNA. Posttranslationally, collagen production may be affected by the extent of prolyl hydroxylation, because underhydroxylation results in decreased stability of the collagen molecule, which is degraded. The prolyl hydroxylation is impaired in scurvy because of deficiency of vitamin C, which is a cofactor for prolyl hydroxylase. The biosynthetic steps at which regulation of collagen biosynthesis may occur are indicated in Fig 6-3.

The collagen genes, like other protein genes, contain cis-regulatory sequences, promoters, and enhancers.[12,13] Gene transcription is regulated through the binding of protein "transcription" factors to these sequences. For example, transforming growth factor β (TGF-β) activates collagen gene transcription through regulatory DNA sequence that binds to the nuclear factor NF-1.

The manner in which collagen genes are regulated differs for different collagen types. For example, in type IV collagen, genes for COL4A1 and COL4A2 are arranged head to head and separated by a short 130-bp segment. At the center of the intervening region is a regulatory sequence that participates in the regulation of both α1(IV) and α2(IV) genes.[12]

Developmental expression of collagens is regulated in a temporal, tissue-specific, and cell type–specific manner. For example, when the first intron of COL1A1 gene is interrupted in mouse germ line by integration of MoMLV viral gene, type I collagen is not made and the embryos die between 12 and 14 days. However, tooth rudiments synthesize normal amounts of type I collagen, indicating that in odontoblasts, unlike fibroblasts, this collagen is regulated by a site different from intron 1. In type IX col-

lagen, tissue-specific expression appears to be achieved by using different transcription initiation sites located 20 kb apart. Thus, in cartilage, its transcription starts in exon 1, whereas in cornea it starts downstream, at the the end of intron 6. Therefore, the corneal α1(IX) chain is shorter than cartilage α1(IX).[12]

A variety of growth factors and cytokines regulate collagen production during development, inflammation, and wound repair,[2] and in virtually all cases this is reflected in mRNA levels. Among the various molecules that affect collagen synthesis, TGF-β is an important mediator, as it enhances the synthesis of collagen and other matrix components. This polypeptide is believed to play a major role in wound repair and fibrosis. In contrast, tumor necrosis factor α (TNF-α) and interferon γ (IFN-γ) suppress collagen gene expression.[2] During inflammation and wound healing, these substances are secreted by platelets, macrophages, and other inflammatory cells. The action of some of these mediators on collagen synthesis is summarized in Table 6-2.

Inflammatory mediators may also regulate matrix composition through their effect on matrix-degrading enzymes. This is discussed in the following section.

Degradation and Remodeling of Collagens

Collagen undergoes degradation and remodeling during development, inflammation, and wound repair, and during resorption in bone. Collagen degradation requires special enzymes because the crosslinked molecules in fibers are resistant to most common proteinases. These enzymes, called collagenases, initiate collagen degradation by cleaving gly-ileu and gly-leu bonds in α1(I) and α2(I), respectively. These peptide bonds are located approximately one quarter of the length from the C-terminus, thus fragments of three-quarter and one-quarter size are released. The released fragments have a lower T_m than that of the native molecule, and thus they become denatured and are further degraded by other common tissue proteinases. Alternatively, collagens may be ingested via phagocytosis by macrophages and fibroblasts and hydrolyzed by lysosomal enzymes.

The enzymes responsible for degradation of collagen and other matrix molecules are a family of more than 20 metal-dependent enzymes called matrix metalloproteinases (MMPs) or matrixins. These are Zn^{++}-dependent endopeptidases that have related gene structures, and they share a basic structural organization consisting of propeptide, catalytic, hinge, and C-terminal hemopexin-like domains.[14,15] They play major roles in tissue remodeling during morphogenesis, inflammation, wound healing, angiogenesis, and apoptosis. Many of these enzymes have been implicated in diseases involving degradation, such as rheumatoid arthritis and tumor invasion and metastasis.

Table 6-3 Matrix Metalloproteinases

Enzyme	MMP*	Substrates
Interstitial collagenases		
Fibroblast type	MMP-1	Collagen types I to III, VII, VIII; aggrecan; serpin; α2m
PMN type	MMP-8	Same as MMP-1
Gelatinases/type IV collagenases		
72 kd	MMP-2	Gelatin; collagen types IV to VII, X, XI; elastin
92 kd	MMP-9	Same as MMP-2
Stromelysins		
Stromelysin 1	MMP-3	Aggrecan; fibronectin; nidogen; laminin; collagen types IV, V, IX, X
Stromelysin 2	MMP-10	Same as MMP-3
Stromelysin 3	MMP-11	α1-proteinase inhibitor
Other enzymes		
Putative metalloproteinase (PUMP-1)	MMP-7	Fibronectin, laminin, type IV collagen, gelatin
Telopeptidase	MMP-4	Collagen C-propeptide

* Classification based on Nagase et al.[16] Also see Birkedal-Hansen et al.[17]

These enzymes are divided into four groups (Table 6-3). The first group, interstitial collagenases, includes fibroblast-type (MMP-1) and polymorphonuclear-type (PMN-type) (MMP-8) collagenases. Collagen types I, II, III, VII, VIII, and X and gelatin are substrates for these enzymes. The fibroblast enzyme hydrolyzes type III fibers faster than type I, while the PMN enzyme hydrolyzes type I faster. The second group includes 72-kd (MMP-2) and 92-kd (MMP-9) gelatinases (also called *type IV collagenases*). These enzymes have a high affinity for gelatin and degrade gelatin; collagen types IV, V, VII, X, and XI; and elastin. They cleave gly-X-peptide bond where X = val, leu, glu, asn, or ser. Stromelysins 1, 2, and 3 (MMP-3, -10, and -11, respectively) form the third group, and these enzymes hydrolyze core proteins of proteoglycans; type IV, V, IX, and X collagens; and elastin. The fourth group is the membrane-type MMPs (MT-MMPs), and these enzymes are located on cell membranes. Apart from these MMPs, there are other enzymes that do not fall into these groups; these include the macrophage elastase (MMP-14), matrilysin (MMP-7), and enamelysin (MMP-20) (Table 6-3).

Fibroblasts, keratinocytes, monocytes/macrophages, and several other cells produce MMP, although MMP-2 has not been detected in PMN. The fibroblast and keratinocyte enzymes are regulated transcriptionally and synthesized in response to external stimuli; therefore, there is a time lag between exposure to an agent and release of active enzyme. Many inflammatory mediators and bacterial substances influence the MMP production by these cells.[17] In contrast, the PMN enzyme is released readily on demand, as it is stored in storage granules.

MMP activity is controlled in vivo in three ways.[14–18] First, the MMPs are synthesized and secreted as inactive precursors, and conversion to active form requires activation by plasmin, trypsin, or other proteinases. Second, production of MMP is regulated by several growth factors and cytokines and chemical agents (eg, phorbol esters). Proinflammatory cytokines interleukin 1 (IL-1) and TNF-α and phorbol esters stimulate MMP-1 gene expression, whereas TGF-β inhibits it. Regulation involves activator protein-1 (AP-1), AP-2, stimulating factor protein-1 (SP-1), and TPA responsive element (TRE) *cis*-regulatory elements. Certain signaling pathways lead to expression of a particular MMP gene; for example, activation of guanosine 5'-triphosphate (GTP)–binding protein Ras increases AP-1 levels and induces MMP-1 expression.[14] The IL-1 increases and TGF-β decreases MMP synthesis. Finally, the activity of MMPs is neutralized by serum and tissue inhibitors. A major serum inhibitor is α2-macroglobulin, which covalently crosslinks with susceptible proteolytic enzymes and inactivates them. The α2-macroglobulin is a potent inhibitor because it binds to MMP-1 with even greater avidity than its substrate, collagen. Tissues contain another group of protein inhibitors to MMP. Four such inhibitors—tissue inhibitor of metalloproteinases 1, 2, 3, and 4 (TIMP-1, TIMP-2, TIMP-3, and TIMP-4)—have been characterized. These inhibitors inactivate active MMPs and prevent their conversion to active forms from precursors. TIMP-1 and TIMP-2 are more effective toward interstitial collagenases and gelatinases, respectively.[18] The TIMPs are distributed widely in many tissues and fluids.

In contrast to the vertebrate enzymes, bacterial collagenases can degrade native collagen molecules to small peptides.

Diseases Associated with Collagen Alterations

Alterations either in the molecular structure or composition of collagens lead to functional abnormality of connective tissues. Collagen molecular structure is affected by mutations in both the collagen gene and genes of posttranslational processing enzymes. Such mutations could arise by nucleotide substitution, deletion, or insertion.

The severity of diseases caused by collagen molecular defects depends on several factors. Mutations that affect the structure of the pro-α1(I) gene are often lethal, whereas those affecting the pro-α2(I) chain are not; the reason is that when α2(I) cannot be produced because of a defect in its primary structure, homotrimers of α(I) can form, and these are stable. However, homotrimers of α2(I) chains are not stable, and they cannot assemble into functional trimers without α1(I). Therefore, large deletions, insertions, and mutations near the C-terminus of pro-α1(I) (which affect the assembly of pro-αI chains) are lethal. For example, in osteogenesis imperfecta II (OI-II), α1[I] glycine$_{988}$ is converted to cysteine; the mutated molecules cannot form trimers, so the condition is lethal.[5] OI-II is often associated with dentinogenesis imperfecta, as dentin contains type I collagen as a major component. In contrast to those on collagen genes, mutations of processing enzymes are usually not lethal, even though they could result in functional abnormalities of constituent tissues. Thus, defective lysyl oxidase and lysyl hydroxylation lead to loss of tensile strength of connective tissues and hypermobility of joints, respectively, in cutis laxa and Ehlers-Danlos syndrome.[6]

While diseases due to collagen molecular defects are inherited and rare, acquired diseases are much more common. The acquired diseases include chronic inflammatory diseases and fibroses. Many of these, especially systemic diseases affecting connective tissues, have manifestations in periodontium (eg, Crohn disease and progressive systemic sclerosis). Connective tissue alterations in acquired diseases differ from those in inherited diseases in several

respects. For instance, in acquired diseases gene expression is affected, but gene structure is not. The underlying causes of these diseases are often unknown, and they are multifactorial, with changes occurring in virtually all matrix components, including proteoglycans.[2] Proportions of collagen types may be affected in these diseases. In atherosclerosis, for example, type V collagen is enriched; in periodontal disease, type I and III collagens decrease, and type V increases (discussed later in the chapter).

Connective tissue alterations in acquired diseases are brought about by the interaction of connective tissue cells—chiefly fibroblasts—with numerous inflammatory mediators and cytokines present at the site of injury. These substances are released from damaged tissue and inflammatory cells.[2,19] Important among these substances are platelet-derived growth factor (PDGF) and TGF-β, which enhance cell growth and matrix synthesis, respectively, along with IFN-γ, TNF-α, and prostaglandin E$_2$ (PGE$_2$), which suppress collagen synthesis.[2] These substances may affect the synthesis activities of all resident cells. Alternatively, they may interact with a subpopulation of resident cells and selectively enrich it. The presence of such cells is believed to be one reason for the alterations of matrix constituents during wound repair in periodontal diseases and in scleroderma.[2] These mechanisms are discussed later in this chapter, in "Repair and Regeneration of Periodontal Connective Tissues."

Noncollagenous Proteins

Extracellular matrices of the periodontium and other connective tissues contain elastin, fibronectin, laminin, tenascin, thrombospondin, entactin, and other noncollagenous proteins. Quantitatively, the noncollagenous proteins are minor constituents relative to collagens, but they play a significant role in connective tissue integrity and function. Many of these proteins share several common features. For example, they are large molecules composed of multiple functional domains with distinct binding properties, they influence a variety of cellular activities, and they exist in multiple forms.

Elastin

Elastin is a unique rubberlike protein that is present in vertebrates in virtually every organ of the body. It is a major component of large arteries, vocal cords, elastic cartilage, and lungs, and it is important in nuchal ligaments in cows. Ultrastructurally, elastin fibers are composed of two morphologic components: an amorphous elastin component constituting 90% of the mature fiber and a 10- to 12-nm-diameter microfibrillar component. The latter is located around the periphery of the amorphous component.[20]

Elastin is the most insoluble protein known. Approximately 33% of the amino acids in elastin are glycine; however, unlike in collagen, glycine is not found regularly as every third amino acid. Elastin molecules are organized in such a manner that crosslink regions alternate with hydrophobic regions. The pentapeptide val-pro-gly-val-gly and hexapeptide pro-gly-val-gly-val-ala repeat several times in the hydrophobic regions. In the crosslink regions, lysine residues occur in sequences lys-ala-ala-ala-lys and lys-ala-ala-lys.[20]

Like collagen, elastin is first synthesized as an uncrosslinked precursor, tropoelastin. The elastin gene is approximately 40 kb long and contains 34 to 36 exons.[21] While organization of the exons may differ, there is considerable homology between human, porcine, bovine, and chicken genes. The tropoelastin mRNA is 3.5 kb long, and the overall size of tropoelastin is approximately 750 amino acids.

Elastin crosslinking is mediated by the enzyme lysyl oxidase, the same enzyme that acts on collagens.[11] The enzyme prefers the insoluble form of substrates, and it oxidatively deaminates lysines to allysines; the latter spontaneously condense to crosslinks. Elastin does not have hydroxylysine- and histidine-derived crosslinks, but it contains other crosslinks found in collagens. In addition, it has two unique crosslinks derived from four lysines each, desmosine and isodesmosine.[11] The desmosines connect two peptide chains each. The synthesis of elastin is regulated primarily at the transcriptional level.

Fibronectin

Fibronectin is a multifunctional adhesive glycoprotein that is codistributed with type I and III collagens in fibers. It is present in the extracellular matrix and various body fluids. It binds to fibroblasts and many other cell types and mediates their attachment, spreading, and migration. It also binds to collagens, heparin, fibrin, DNA, and bacteria. These properties allow fibronectin to participate in many biologic processes during growth, development, and repair. Fibronectin plays a prominent role in phagocytosis, hemostasis, thrombosis, and oncogenic transformation.[22]

Fibronectin is a large 540-kd dimer of two similar 230- to 270-kd polypeptide subunits, which are connected by disulfide bonds at the C-terminus. Two forms of fibronectins have been studied extensively, plasma fibronectin (pFN) and cellular fibronectin (cFN). Cellular fibronectin is a heterogeneous mixture of molecules assembled from eight different subunits, and pFN is from four. Plasma fibronectin is a major blood protein synthesized by hepatocytes, and cFN is produced by many cell types and incorporated into extracellular matrix.

Fibronectin gene and protein structures are highly conserved among species. The molecule is made up of three internally homologous repeats—types I, II, and III—which are assembled into globular domains with distinct biologic activities. The fibronectin gene ranges in size between 48 and 70 kb in different species and generates an 8-kb mRNA.[23] The gene contains 48 exons of similar size. The protein contains 12 type I repeats of approximately 45 amino acids coded by 12 exons. These repeats make up the fibrin-binding regions present at both N- and C-termini of the fibronectin molecule, and two repeats code for part of the gelatin-/collagen-binding domain. These repeats contain four cysteines each. However, no intrachain disulfide bonds are present in the type III repeats. There are 15 to 17 type III repeats, each with approximately 90 amino acids and coded by two exons. This domain contains binding sites for cells, heparin, and DNA and is highly conserved.

Fibronectin subunit variation is due to alternative mRNA splicing. Three variants in rats and five in humans arise because of a novel pattern of alternative splicing from a single exon in the V segment. This segment, which contains two splice sites, resides within the type III domain. This region is structurally different from other domains in amino acid distribution, and it contains glycosylation sites and the arg-gly-asp (RGD in the one-letter amino acid code) recognition sequence for cell attachment. Subunits also arise by alternative splicing at another type III repeat site designated as EIIIa and EIIIb; in this case an extra domain is either excluded or included in the fibronectin molecule. The inclusion occurs only in cFN.[23]

Thrombospondins

Thrombospondins are a family of large multidomain glycoproteins. They affect the migration, adhesion, and growth of many cells, especially the PMN and macrophages, and they participate in platelet aggregation, angiogenesis, and wound healing.[24]

Laminin

Laminin is a large 900-kd glycoprotein that is present only in basement membranes. It is composed of one heavy (400-kd) and two light (200-kd) chains assembled in a crosslike structure. It mediates many biologic functions associated with basement membranes, including cell attachment, migration, and differentiation, and it is expressed early in embryogenesis. Like fibronectin, laminin also interacts with other matrix components and cell surface molecules through specific sequence domains.[25] Several members of the laminin family have been identified.

Table 6-4 Integrin Receptors That Bind to Matrix Proteins and Serum Proteins

Class	Integrin	Binds to
β_1	$\beta_1\alpha_1$	Type I and IV collagens, laminin
	$\beta_1\alpha_2$	Same as above
	$\beta_1\alpha_3$	Types I to IV and VI collagens, laminin
	$\beta_1\alpha_4$	Fibronectin
	$\beta_1\alpha_5$	Fibronectin
	$\beta_1\alpha_6$	Laminin
	$\beta_1\alpha_v$	Vitronectin, fibronectin
β_2	$\beta_2\alpha_2$	ICAM-1, ICAM-2
	$\beta_2\alpha_M$	C3bi, factor X, fibrinogen
	$\beta_2\alpha_X$	P130/95 glycoprotein
β_3	$\beta_3\alpha_V$	Vitronectin, fibrinogen, von Willebrand factor, osteopontin, BSP-II
	$\beta_3\alpha_{IIb}$	Fibrinogen, vitronectin, fibronectin, von Willebrand factor
β_4	$\beta_4\alpha_6$	Basement membrane
β_5	$\beta_5\sigma_v$	Vitronectin

ICAM = intercellular adhesion molecule.

Tenascin

Tenascin (also called *cytotactin* and *hexabrachion*) is a star-shaped glycoprotein that consists of six disulfide subunits.[26,27] It is expressed selectively at mesenchyme condensations during development at sites of mesenchymal-epithelial interaction, and it is actively expressed during wound healing and tumorigenesis.

Entactin

Entactin (nidogen) is a 150-kd glycoprotein expressed in basement membranes, where it is present as a noncovalent complex with laminin. Entactin alone, and as a complex with laminin, binds to type IV collagen within basement membranes and contributes to the sievelike network in basement membranes.[28]

Cell-Surface/Matrix Interactions and Integrins

Within the primary structure of matrix proteins, the arg-gly-asp (RGD) amino acid sequence appears to be responible for many attachment interactions.[29] Attachment of the RGD recognition sequence is mediated by specific cell-surface receptors called *integrins*. The term *integrin* was first proposed in 1986 to describe those molecules on cell surfaces intimately involved in linking the extracellular matrix with the cytoskeleton. Integrins are heterodimers of α and β subunits and are classified on the basis of their β-subunit compostion (Table 6-4).[30] Each

chain is composed of three domains: a large extracellular domain, a membrane-spanning domain, and a short cytoplasmic domain. The amino acid sequence of the extracellular domain of α subunits contains Ca^{++} (or Mg^{++}) binding sites, which are homologous to similar sites in calmodulin. Seventeen α and eight β subunits have been described. Binding of integrins to matrix proteins is specific, is dictated by the α- and β-subunit composition (see Table 6-4), and depends on divalent cations. The binding induces signaling events such as activation of protein kinases, which are believed to mediate cell migration, attachment, growth, and other functions. The integrins provide a valuable link between extracellular matrix and cytoskeleton, and they are implicated in leukocyte migration, T cell–macrophage interactions, clot formation, epithelial cell migration, and fibroblast migration. They are expressed actively during wound healing, angiogenesis, and tumorigenesis.[19]

While the presence of the RGD sequence is necessary for many cell-matrix interactions, not all molecules that contain RGD sequences act as adhesion molecules. Sequence data banks indicate that hundreds of molecules contain such sequences, yet they do not play a significant role in cell adhesion. RGD-containing domains have also been identified in the bone matrix proteins osteopontin and BSP-II, which presumably function in regulating osteoblast adhesion. These proteins are discussed in chapter 8.

Table 6-5 Disaccharide Composition of Glycosaminoglycans

Glycosaminoglycan	Disaccharide subunit	Sulfate*
Hyaluronic acid	D-glucuronic acid, D-glucosamine	None
Chondroitin 4– and 6–sulfate	D-glucuronic acid, D-galactosamine	O-
Dermatan sulfate	D-glucuronic acid/L-iduronic acid, D-galactosamine	O-
Heparan sulfate	D-glucuronic acid/L-iduronic acid, D-glucosamine	N-, O-
Heparin	D-glucuronic acid/L-iduronic acid, D-glucosamine	N-, O-
Keratan sulfate	D-galactose, D-glucosamine	O-

* O- indicates O-sulfated through sugar; N- indicates N-sulfated through asparagine.

Proteoglycans

Proteoglycans are highly anionic molecules in which one or more hexosamine-containing polysaccharides called *glycosaminoglycans (GAGs)* are covalently attached to a protein core.[31] They are ubiquitous in all connective tissues and are located within the matrix as integral components, on cell surfaces, and within cell organelles.[32] By virtue of their high charge, they have been ascribed a variety of functions, including tissue hydration, retention and regulation of water flow, lubrication of synovial and mesothelial surfaces, regulation of collagen fiber formation, growth factor binding, cell adhesion, and growth.[33]

Glycosaminoglycans

The GAGs are composed of repeating, unbranched disaccharide units of uronic acid (either D-glucuronic acid or L-iduronic acid) and D-galactose or a hexosamine (either D-glucosamine or D-galactosamine) (Table 6-5). The GAG types include hyaluronan (hyaluronic acid, hyaluronate), chondroitin sulfates, dermatan sulfate, keratan sulfate, heparan sulfate, and heparin.[34] The specific composition of each of the GAGs is shown in Table 6-5.

Core Proteins

The exceptional diversity of proteoglycans is due to the number and posttranslational modifications of the core proteins, to which the GAGs are covalently bound. These polypeptides range in size from 10 to 300 kd and are rich in the amino acids serine, glycine, proline, and glutamic acid.[35] Various hydrophobic, hydrophilic, and globular domains are present within the molecules, and these correlate closely with the tissue location and function of pro-

teoglycans.[36] However, they do not appear to form a single supergene family.

Proteoglycan Synthesis

Like all proteins, the core proteins of proteoglycans are synthesized in the RER. All have a hydrophobic signal sequence at the N-terminal, which is removed as the protein is being translated. The addition of sulfated GAGs to the core protein occurs in the Golgi and is initiated by xylosyltransferase; this enzyme adds xylose to hydroxyl groups in acceptor serines. For GAG chain elongation to occur, up to six glucosyltransferases and two sulfotransferases are required.[35] First, xylose is added to the serine residue; this may occur either late in the RER or early in the Golgi. This is followed by sequential addition of galactose, glucuronic acid, and N-acetylglucosamine. Then the uronic acid and hexosamine are added sequentially to the nonreducing end of the growing chain. Sulfate esters are then added as the chain elongates. Additional modifications occur to dermatan sulfate, heparin, and heparan sulfate, either during or immediately after chain elongation. The modifications include epimerization of D-glucuronic acid to L-iduronic acid, 2-O-sulfation of L-iduronic acid, and N-deacetylation and N-sulfation of heparin and heparan sulfate.

Proteoglycan Types

Proteoglycans may be classified into three separate groups based on their location: *(1)* extracellular proteoglycans, which are matrix organizers and tissue space fillers; *(2)* cell-surface proteoglycans; and *(3)* intracellular proteoglycans of the hemopoietic cells (Table 6-6). A schematic representation of the structures of proteoglycans is provided in Fig 6-4.

Table 6-6 Composition and Distribution of Some Proteoglycans

Proteoglycan	GAG	Tissues	Interacts with
Extracellular proteoglycans			
Aggrecan	CS, KS	Cartilage	Hyaluronan
Versican	CS	Soft connective tissues, fibroblasts, gingiva, periodontal ligament, cementum	Hyaluronan
Perlecan	HS	Basement membranes	bFGF
Decorin	DS/CS	Soft connective tissues, bone, gingiva, periodontal ligament, cementum	Collagen types I and II, TGF-β, FN
Biglycan	DS/CS	Soft connective tissues, bone	Matrix components, not collagen, cell surface
Centoglycan	CS	Striated muscle, fibroblasts, bone	Collagen
Fibromodulin	KS	Skin, cementum, bone, cartilage, tendon	Collagen, TGF-β
Lumican	KS	Cornea, aorta, skin, cartilage	Collagen
Keratocan	KS	Cornea	Collagen
Cell surface proteoglycans			
Syndecan-1	CS/HS	Epithelium	Various growth factors (bFGF, EGF)
Syndecan-2	HS	Fibroblasts	Various growth factors (bFGF, EGF)
Syndecan-3	HS	Schwann cells, cartilage	Various growth factors (bFGF, EGF)
Syndecan-4	HS	Fibroblasts, endothelial and epithelial cells	Various growth factors (bFGF, EGF)
CD-44	CS/HS	Lymphocyte homing factor	Hyaluronan
Betaglycan	HS/CS	Cell surfaces	TGF-β receptor
Proteoglycans in hemopoietic cells			
Serglycine	CS	Secretory granules of mast cells, basophils, neutrophils, platelets, lymphocytes, NK cells	Intracellular enzymes

CS = chondroitin sulfate; KS = keratan sulfate; HA = hyaluronic acid; DS = dermatan sulfate; HS = heparan sulfate; FN = fibronectin; bFGF = basic fibroblast growth factor; EGF = epidermal growth factor; NK = natural killer.

Extracellular proteoglycans. Extracellular proteoglycans may be further subdivided into large and small species. Large extracellular proteoglycans include aggrecan, versican, and perlecan. Aggrecan is a large cartilage-specific proteoglycan bound to hyaluronan,[36] and it consists of approximately 100 chondroitin sulfate chains and approximately 100 keratan sulfate chains, together with numerous N- and O-linked oligosaccharides. Versican is the fibroblast equivalent of aggrecan, but it does not contain keratan sulfate. The protein core of this proteoglycan, like aggrecan, has a multidomain structure and can bind to hyaluronan to form large aggregates.[37] Perlecan, which is a basement membrane proteoglycan containing heparan sulfate, can aggregate with type IV collagen and laminin.[38]

Biglycan, decorin, fibromodulin, lumican, keratocan, epiphycan, osteoglycin, and centoglycan are all examples of leucine-rich repeat extracellular proteoglycans (LRRPs). The LRRPs include up to nine small proteoglycans forming three distinct subfamilies: class I contains decorin and biglycan; class II, lumican, fibromodulin, keratocan, and osteoadherin; and class III, epiphycan and osteoglycin.[31] Biglycan is a small dermatan sulfate–containing proteoglycan that has two sites for GAG attachment, and it is found in developing bone and cartilage.[39] It is localized in close association with keratinocytes and fibroblasts, and it binds to some matrix molecules, but not to collagens. Decorin is similar to biglycan in structure except that it has only one attachment site for the GAG chains and

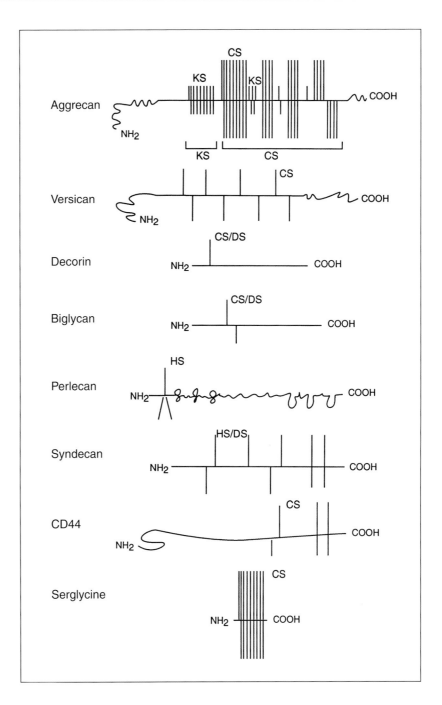

Fig 6-4 Composition of various proteoglycans. Each proteoglycan consists of a core protein (horizontal lines) covalently linked to glycosaminoglycan chains (vertical lines). (KS) keratan sulfate; (CS) chondroitin sulfates; (DS) dermatan sulfate; (HS) heparan sulfate.

shows a close association with collagen fibers localizing to the gap region of collagen fibrils.[39] Fibromodulin and lumican contain keratan sulfate chains and have been located in skin and cornea, as well as mineralized tissues such as cartilage and cementum.[31]

Cell-surface proteoglycans. Cell-surface proteoglycans are ubiquitous cell-surface components of all mammalian cells, and they are present on cell surfaces as integral components of membrane proteins spanning the lipid bilayer, by partial insertion into the lipid bilayer of a phosphatidyl inositol component of the proteoglycan, or by binding of a GAG side chain to specific plasma membrane receptors.[32,40]

Among the cell-surface proteoglycans, the syndecans are the best studied.[40] These molecules have a unique protein core composed of both hydrophobic and hydrophilic domains and substituted with heparan sulfate, chondroitin sulfate, or both. To date, four syndecans have been identified on the basis of their cDNA-derived amino acid sequence. Syndecan-1 is present in many cells, including epithelial cells, lymphocytes, and embryonic dental and lung mesenchyme. Syndecan-2 (fibroglycan) is like syndecan-1, and it can form large dimers or multimers. Syndecan-3 (N-syndecan) shares several structural features with syndecan-1 and fibroglycan, but it differs in extracellular domain in both amino acid sequence and location of the GAG attachment sites. It is expressed in high amounts during chondrogenesis and has numerous potential sites for mediating cell-matrix-cytoskeleton interactions. Syndecan-4 (ryudocan/amphiglycan) is an important component of most endothelial cells, epithelial cells, and fibroblasts. The syndecans have several functions. By virtue of their strategic location on the cell surface, they are believed to influence cell-cell, cell adhesion, and cell-matrix interactions.[40] The heparan sulfate chains of syndecan are believed to interact with growth factors, cytokines, extracellular matrix components, and protease inhibitors, and they even self-aggregate. The syndecans are differentially expressed during development and wound healing.

Other cell-surface proteoglycans include thrombomodulin; CD44, the lymphocyte homing factor; epican, a specialized form of CD44; glypican, which is intercalated to the cell membrane via a glycosylphosphatidylinositol membrane anchor; and betaglycan, which is a specific cell-surface proteoglycan.[40–44]

Proteoglycans of hemopoietic cells. Proteoglycans of hemopoietic cells are often found in secretory granules and are distinct from those residing in the matrix or cell surface.[45] Serglycine is the major proteoglycan of this type. It has a unique repeat sequence of serine and glycine residues in its protein core and is located in the secretory granules of mast cells, basophils, neutrophils, platelets, lymphocytes, and natural killer (NK) cells. The functions of proteoglycans belonging to this group remain largely unknown, although it has been speculated that they may be involved in enzyme packaging or as mediators of cellular activity.[45]

Hyaluronan

Hyaluronan (also called *hyaluaronic acid* or *hyaluronate*) has two distinguishing features: it is the only nonsulfated GAG, and it does not covalently associate with a protein to form a proteoglycan.[46] Nonetheless, it is considered part of the proteoglycan family by virtue of its ability to interact with the core proteins of several proteoglycans to form large aggregates. Hyaluronan also differs from proteoglycans in that it is synthesized in the plasma membrane by the addition of sugars to the reducing end of the molecule,

with the reducing end projecting into the pericellular environment. Hyaluronan is ubiquitous in all tissues and is synthesized by most cells. Its functions are many and varied, the most important being its association with tissue hydration; cell-surface matrix interactions; cell migration; tissue development; and aggregation with aggrecan, CD44, and other matrix components.[46,47]

Periodontal Connective Tissues

Normal Periodontium

Like all other connective tissues, the extracellular matrix of periodontal structures is made up of collagens, noncollagenous proteins, proteoglycans,[1,2] and several collagen types. The proportion of various matrix constituents, especially collagen types, and their organization differ in each periodontal component and are variably expressed during periodontal development.[48] These differences distinguish each component and determine its own characteristic structure and function, as well as the structure and function of the periodontium as a whole.

The integrity of the periodontium must be maintained to withstand tooth eruption and mesial drift, as well as to combat occlusal forces and microbial challenge; this challenge is met by the high turnover rate of connective tissue constituents. Experiments using marmoset and rat models have shown that the periodontal ligament and gingiva have high collagen turnover rates and that these are much higher than that of skin and other connective tissues. The primary cells responsible for synthesizing collagen and other matrix components are fibroblasts in soft tissues and osteoblasts in mineralized structures. Biosynthesis of collagens and proteoglycans by gingival and periodontal ligament fibroblasts has been studied extensively, and these cells have served as a model to examine mechanisms of connective tissue alterations in periodontal diseases and other acquired diseases.[2,49]

Recent ultrastructural studies by electron microscopy and immunocytochemistry have revealed that connective tissues are organized into distinct architectural patterns in gingiva, periodontal ligament, and cementum. The distribution of matrix proteins and proteoglycans in these structures and their organization are outlined in this section.

Gingiva

In the gingiva, collagen fibers form various groups that are classified based on location, origin, and insertion (see Fig 3-17b.[1] The *dentogingival* fibers arise from the cementum

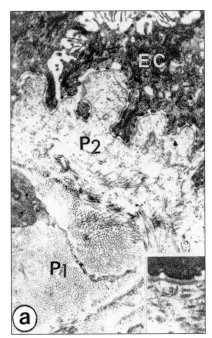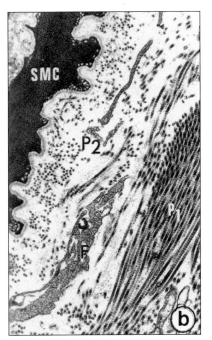

Fig 6-5 Distribution of dense (60- to 70-nm, P_1) and thinner (40- to 60-nm, P_2) collagen fibers at gingival lamina propria *(a)* and near a blood vessel *(b)*, respectively, viewed by electron microscopy ($\times$10,000). The P_2, which is a loose pattern of organization mixed with nonstriated fibrillar material, is found near basement membranes. (EC) epithelial cell; (SMC) smooth muscle cell; (F) fibroblast. The inset in *(a)* shows P_2 magnified $\times$20,000. (Reprinted from Chavrier et al,[50] with permission.)

immediately apical to the base of epithelial attachment and splay out into gingiva, while the *dentoperiosteal* fibers bend apically over the alveolar crest and insert into buccal and lingual periosteum. The *alveologingival* fibers originate from the crest of the alveolus, course coronally, and terminate in free and papillary gingiva, whereas the *circular* fiber group passes circumferentially around the cervical region of teeth in the free gingiva. The *semicircular* fibers traverse from cementum at the proximal root surface, extend into the free marginal gingiva, and insert into the corresponding position on the opposite side of the tooth. The *transgingival* fibers traverse between the cementoenamel junction to the free marginal gingiva of the adjacent tooth, and the *intergingival* fibers extend along the facial and lingual marginal gingiva from tooth to tooth. *Transseptal* fibers arise from the cementum surface just apical to the base of epithelial attachment, traverse the interdental bone, and insert into a comparable position on the opposite tooth. These various fiber groups are interdependent for function, and their anatomic relationship is believed to determine the pattern of spread of inflammatory periodontal diseases.[1]

Like other connective tissues, gingiva contains a heterotypic mixture of collagen types, with type I being the major one.[2,49] The ultrastructural distribution of collagen types has been studied using collagen-type–specific antibodies and electron microscopy. Type I collagen is the main collagen species in all layers of gingival corium. In the gingiva, collagen fibers are organized in two patterns; one consists of large, dense bundles of thick fibers, and the other is a loose pattern of short, thin fibers mixed with a fine reticular network (Fig 6-5). These fibers contain both type I and III collagens, of which type I is preferentially organized into denser fibrils in the lamina propria.[50–52] Although it is not restricted to any particular region, type III collagen appears to be localized mostly as thinner fibers in a reticular pattern near the basement membrane at the epithelial junction (Fig 6-6a). Type III collagen is a component of Sharpey's fibers (Fig 6-6b).

Immunostaining data have revealed that type V collagen has a parallel filamentous pattern, and it appears to coat dense fibers composed of type I and III collagens. The gingival connective tissue also contains type VI collagen, which is present as diffuse microfibrils in the lamina propria, around blood vessels, and near epithelial basement membrane and nerves.[53] It is intermingled with collagen fibrils and oxytalan and elastin fibers. In the gingiva, basement membrane is present at the epithelial junction, rete

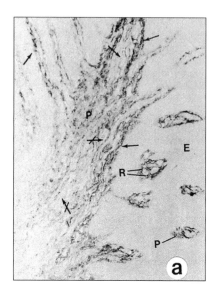 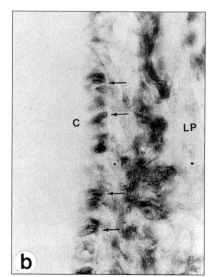

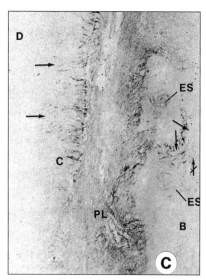 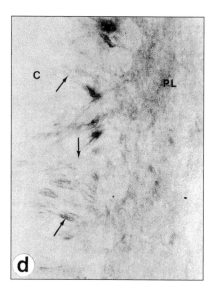

Fig 6-6 Distribution of type III collagen in the periodontium as revealed by an anti–type III collagen antibody. *(a)* Section of gingival papilla in which the antibody strongly stains areas adjacent to epithelium *(arrows)* and rete peg junctions, and blood vessel wall *(crossed arrows)*: (E) epithelium that is unstained, (P) papilla, and (R) reticular pattern of staining. *(b)* Junction between cementum (C) and lamina propria (LP) of gingiva; cementum is unstained, and strongly staining material *(arrows)* is Sharpey's fibers. *(c)* Alveolar bone and periodontal ligament: (B) alveolar bone, (PL) periodontal ligament, (C) cementum, (D) dentin, and (ES) endosteal spaces. Cementum and alveolar bone are largely unstained except at Sharpey's fibers *(arrows)*. *(d)* Higher magnification of Sharpey's fibers *(arrows)*. (Reprinted from Wang et al,[52] with permission.)

pegs, and nerves, as well as around blood vessels; like other basement membrane structures, it contains type IV collagen, laminin, and heparan sulfate proteoglycan.[2] The collagen-type composition of gingiva and other periodontal structures is summarized in Table 6-7.

The gingiva also contains fibronectin,[51] osteonectin,[55] tenascin,[56] and elastin.[57] Tenascin is present diffusely in the gingival connective tissue, and prominently near the subepithelial basement membrane in the upper connective tissue and capillary blood vessels. Although elastin is a minor constituent of gingival connective tissue, it is relatively more prominent in the submucosal tissues of the more movable and flexible alveolar mucosa (Fig 6-7).

The GAGs found in the gingival connective tissue include hyaluronan, heparan sulfate, dermatan sulfate, and chondroitin sulfate; dermatan sulfate and chondroitin sulfate are the predominant species.[58] Heparan sulfate is the predominant species in gingival epithelium. Gingival proteoglycans have been identified as decorin, biglycan, versican, and syndecan.[59] Immunohistochemical studies have shown that dermatan sulfate GAG and decorin proteoglycan are present within the gingival tissues closely associated with collagen fibers, especially in the subepithelial region (Fig 6-8). Biglycan is a relatively minor constituent of gingiva, but it appears to be localized in the matrix near the oral epithelium. Syndecan and CD44 have been localized mainly to epithelial cells. In the gingiva, the GAGs are largely made by fibroblasts, which may synthesize up to six different proteoglycans, including decorin, biglycan, versican, and syndecan.

Table 6-7 Distribution of Collagen Types in the Periodontium

Tissue	Collagen type*	Location
Healthy gingiva	I	Lamina propria
	III	Lamina propria
	IV	Basement membranes
	V	Collagen fibers, blood vessels
	VI	Microfibrils
Periodontal ligament	I	Principal, secondary fibers
	III	Same as type I
	V	Collagen fibers
Cementum	I	Sharpey's fibers, fibrillar cementum
	III	Sharpey's fibers
	V	Sharpey's fibers
Alveolar bone	I	Bone matrix, Sharpey's fibers
	III	Sharpey's fibers
Inflamed gingiva	I	Same as healthy gingiva
	III	Same as healthy gingiva
	V	Same as healthy gingiva
	IV, V, VI	Same as healthy gingiva
	$[\alpha 1(I)_3]$	Lamina propria
Edentulous ridge	I	Same as healthy gingiva
	III	Same as healthy gingiva
	V	Same as healthy gingiva

* In all structures, type I collagen is the major species, accounting for 80% to 85% in the gingiva to 99% in bone. Type III is the second most predominant collagen in gingiva and periodontal ligament, forming about 15% of the total. In alveolar bone and cementum, the type III is restricted to Sharpey's fibers. The content of all other collagens together in healthy tissues is less than 1%.

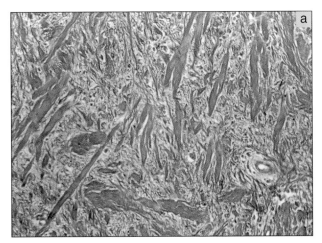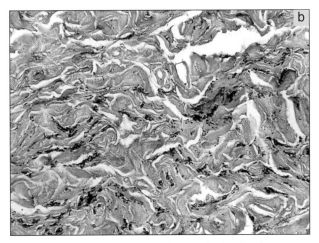

Fig 6-7 Elastin in human oral tissues: *(a)* attached gingiva and *(b)* alveolar mucosa. Note heavy deposits of elastin in the alveolar mucosa between collagen fibers and its virtual absence in attached gingival connective tissue. The tissue was treated with an antibody to tropoelastin and visualized by silver-intensified protein A-gold immunohistochemistry (×100). (Reprinted from Bartold,[54] with permission.)

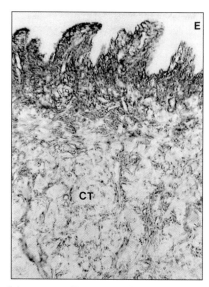

Fig 6-8 Distribution of dermatan sulfate proteoglycans in human gingival tissue. The tissue was reacted with a monoclonal antibody to dermatan sulfate and visualized by immunoperoxide procedure (×75). Note the intense staining in the immediate subepithelial connective tissue. (E) epithelium; (CT) connective tissue. (Reprinted from Bartold,[54] with permission.)

Periodontal Ligament

In mature periodontal ligament, collagen fibers are distinguished as *principal fibers* and *secondary fibers*. The principal fibers are dense bundles that traverse the periodontal space obliquely and insert into cementum and alveolar bone as Sharpey's fibers. In zones where extensive mesiodistal tooth movement has occurred, the Sharpey's fibers may continue from one tooth to another through interproximal bone. The secondary fibers are randomly oriented fibrils located between the principal fibers.

The principal collagen species in Sharpey's fibers and other collagen fibers of the periodontal ligament is type I, and this collagen also constitutes the fibrous component of endosteal spaces. Type III collagen appears to coat Sharpey's fibers (see Figs 6-6b to 6-6d). These two collagen types are codistributed with types V and XII[60] and fibronectin. During development, type XII collagen expression appears to be timed with the alignment and organization of ligament fibers to cells within the periodontal ligament,[61] and mutation affecting its function results in disorganization of fiber architecture in the periodontal ligament and skin.[62] Blood vessels contain type I, III, IV, and V collagens. The periodontal ligament also contains small amounts of elastin and tenascin, which are present in connective tissue and in zones along cementum and bone.

The types of proteoglycans present in periodontal ligament are similar to those in gingival tissue.[63] GAG components present are hyaluronate, heparan sulfate, dermatan sulfate, and chondroitin sulfate, of which dermatan sulfate is the principal species. The finding that dermatan sulfate is the principal GAG is consistent with the highly collagenous nature of the periodontal ligament. The two principal proteoglycans in the periodontal ligament are versican and decorin.

Cementum

Cementum is characterized by low metabolic turnover, lack of blood supply, lymph drainage, and innervation. It contains very few cells.[64] Collagen fibers are present as fine, randomly oriented fibrils embedded in granular matrix in primary cementum, which is devoid of cells. Secondary cementum contains cells, coarse collagen fibrils oriented parallel to the root surface, and Sharpey's fibers at right angles. The presence and organization of collagen fibers within cementum have formed the basis for a new classification of cementum.[65] Thus, the *acellular afibrillar cementum* located at the dentinoenamel junction does not contain collagen fibers or cells. *Acellular extrinsic fiber cementum* also does not have cells, but it contains large numbers of Sharpey's fibers. It is present in cervical to midroot areas, and it anchors teeth. Cellular cementum located at apical and interradicular root surfaces contains both extrinsic (Sharpey's) and intrinsic collagen fibers, while repair cementum has only the intrinsic fiber system. Intrinsic and extrinsic fibers differ in their orientation; the former occur randomly and parallel to the root surface, whereas extrinsic fibers are embedded at right angles. The Sharpey's fibers of cementum and alveolar bone are largely responsible for tooth anchorage.

Approximately 50% of the inorganic matrix in the cementum is hydroxyapatite, whereas the organic matrix is composed of predominantly type I and III collagens.[49] During tooth development in rats, two variant forms of α1(I) mRNA appear to be expressed in cementoblasts and osteoblasts.[66] The type III collagen is associated with Sharpey's fibers (see Fig 6-6b). A variety of nonfibrous proteins are also present in cementum; these include BSP, osteopontin, tenascin, fibronectin, osteonectin, and proteoglycans.[63,67] These proteins are expressed from early tooth development. Cementum also contains hyaluronate, dermatan sulfate, chondroitin sulfate, and keratan sulfate. These GAGs are closely associated with cementoblasts and lightly distributed throughout the matrix. A number of proteoglycans have been identified in cementum; they include fibromodulin, lumican, and syndecan.[68,69]

Two morphologically distinct cementoblasts appear to regulate the collagen fiber arrangement in the cementum.

Table 6-8 Glycosaminoglycans and Proteoglycans in the Periodontium

Tissue	GAGs[*]	Proteoglycans[†]
Gingiva	DS[‡], HA, CS, HS[§]	CS-PG, DS-PG, decorin, biglycan, versican, CD44
Periodontal ligament	DS[‡], CS, HA, HS	Decorin, biglycan, versican, syndecan-1
Alveolar bone	CS[‡], DS, HA, HS	Decorin, biglycan
Cementum	CS[‡], DS, HA	Lumican, fibromodulin, syndecan-2

[*]GAG = glycosaminoglycans; DS = dermatan sulfate; HA = hyaluronan; CS = chondroitin sulfate; HS = heparan sulfate; PG = proteoglycan.

[†]The localization of proteoglycans is as follows: CS = PG = general matrix in soft tissues and matrix and lacunae of bone and cementum; DS-PG and decorin = subepithelial matrix in the gingiva; decorin = predominantly at the subepithelial matrix; HA = mostly in the epithelium; CD44 = on epithelial cells. See text for references.

[‡]Major species. In the gingiva, DS is the major species in connective tissue.

[§]HS is the major GAG species in the gingival epithelium.

One type secretes intrinsic fibers to be incorporated into principal tooth support, and the other forms intrinsic fibers to adjust cementum thickness.[70]

Alveolar Bone

Collagens are major constituents of the alveolar bone matrix.[49,52,71] The bone is attached to principal fibers of periodontal ligament through Sharpey's fibers. As in the cementum, chondroitin sulfate is the major GAG species in the alveolar bone, and it is present along with heparan sulfate, dermatan sulfate, and hyaluronate.[72] Immunohistochemical localization studies have shown that these molecules are distributed on cells in their lacunae and in the mineralized matrix. Analysis of alveolar bone proteoglycans has identified a chondroitin sulfate–rich proteoglycan as the major species, which may be a mixture of decorin and biglycan.

The constituent collagen and proteoglycan types and their locations in various periodontal components are summarized in Tables 6-7 and 6-8.

Connective Tissue in Diseases of the Periodontium

The periodontium is the primary seat of several diseases, and many systemic and drug-induced diseases have manifestations in the periodontium, especially in the gingiva.[1] Gingivitis is one of the most common diseases of humans. In its lesions, gingival connective tissues are destroyed within 3 to 4 days after plaque accumulation, and this is associated with the migration of PMN into the junctional epithelium and gingival sulcus. The destruction begins at perivascular collagen bundles. Approximately 70% of collagen within the foci of inflammation is lost, mostly due to the activity of PMN. This lesion may remain established for years or decades and may be reversible. Gingivitis is common during pregnancy because sex hormones affect the inflammatory response and cellular metabolism during wound healing.

Chronic periodontitis leads to extensive destruction of gingival connective tissue, periodontal ligament, and alveolar bone, and it sometimes affects the root surfaces. Although plasma cells and lymphocytes are present in this lesion, macrophages and PMN are the major destructive cells. Large numbers of PMN may cause recurring destruction during times of cyclic disease. The amount of collagen is reduced, and fibrosis and scarring of the gingival tissue may occur at foci of inflammation. As the disease progresses, destruction may expand to alveolar bone housing and tooth roots; this causes the teeth to become loose and may lead to tooth loss. Gingival fibrosis, manifested by scarring of gingival tissues, is seen in chronic periodontitis and is common in baboons and chimpanzees; however, it is not seen in dogs, rodents, minks, or marmosets.[1] These changes are described in detail in chapter 4.

Quantitative and qualitative changes occur in the gingival collagen of patients with the above diseases.[2,49] In gingiva the collagen becomes more soluble, indicating active synthesis of new collagen and/or impaired crosslinking. The ratios of collagen types are altered; the amount of type V collagen increases and may exceed the amount of type III, and a new collagen—type I trimer—may appear (Fig 6-9).[51] Type I trimer is a homotrimer of $\alpha 1(I)$ chains that accumulates in certain hereditary collagen molecular diseases, embryonic tissues, and tumors. There is an in-

Fig 6-9 Distribution of type I and III collagens in normal and inflamed human gingiva. The collagens were visualized by indirect immunofluorescence using antibodies to these collagens. *(a)* Normal gingiva, anti–type I collagen antibody. *(b)* Inflamed gingiva, anti–type I collagen antibody. *(c)* Normal gingiva, anti–type III collagen antibody. *(d)* Inflamed gingiva, anti–type III antibody. (Ep) Epithelium. Note that the staining is considerably less in *(b)* and *(d)*, indicating loss of collagens. In *(a)* and *(c)*, arrows indicate bundles of collagen fibers. In *(b)* and *(d)*, small arrows indicate site of inflammation, and large arrows indicate remaining collagen fibers. (Reprinted from Narayanan et al,[51] with permission.)

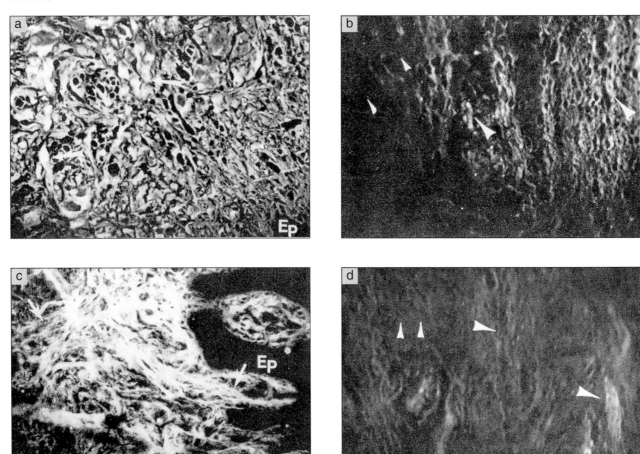

crease in the amount of type V collagen, which coats collagen fibrils composed of type I and III collagens, and this collagen may be present in greater proportion than type III. Type I and XII collagen mRNAs become undetectable.[73] Changes also occur in noncollagenous gingival constituents; in beagle dogs, noncollagenous proteins are lost from diseased gingiva.[59] Matrix proteoglycans are lost from the center of inflammatory foci but appear to be present in higher concentrations around the periphery. In inflamed gingival tissues, the amount of dermatan sulfate decreases while the content of chondroitin sulfate increases. Degradation of both proteoglycan core proteins and hyaluronan is characteristic of inflamed gingival connective tissues. The principal proteoglycan synthesized by inflammatory cells is chondroitin sulfate; therefore, in inflamed tissues, chondroitin sulfate levels increase at the expense of dermatan sulfate, which is lost along with collagenous components.

Excessive accumulation of connective tissue elements is a feature of drug-induced gingival hyperplasia and gingival fibromatosis.[74,75] Gingival hyperplasia is a common complication in patients who have been administered diphenylhydantoin (phenytoin), cyclosporin, nifedipine, and other drugs, affecting approximately 50%, 30%, and 20%, respectively, of patients. Ingestion of drugs alone is insufficient for the evolution of this lesion; genetics, age, and inflammation are other factors. In these lesions the gingival margin and interdental papillae overgrow; the overgrowth may become so extensive that teeth are displaced and their crowns covered with overgrown gingival tissues. Clinically these lesions have a cauliflower-like appearance with enlarged epithelium and foci of infiltrating leukocytes. Although during early stages these lesions are highly cellular, in mature lesions the matrix-to-cell ratio is close to normal. Excessive accumulation of gingival extracellular matrix and increased epithelial thickening are prominent features of these lesions.

The amount of noncollagenous proteins increases in phenytoin-induced gingival hyperplasia. The collagen content increases, and the ratio of type I to type III becomes different, with some loss of type I and elevated type III. It is interesting to note that the collagen composition of edentulous ridge resembles skin more than gingiva in both collagen-type ratios and hydroxy amino acid content.[2,49]

Gingival fibromatosis is an idiopathic progressive fibrous gingival enlargement that is inherited as an autosomal dominant disease. It may be focal or generalized and, unlike drug-induced gingival hyperplasia, does not have an inflammatory component.

Attempts have been made to utilize connective tissue alterations as indicators of periodontal disease. The gingival crevicular fluid (GCF) contains many breakdown products arising from inflammation; therefore, studies have focused on measuring the levels of plasma proteins, bacterial and host enzymes, and collagen degradation products such as hydroxyproline and $\alpha1(I)$-N-propeptide in the GCF.[2] However, differences between healthy and diseased tissues are subtle and do not appear to correlate well with the severity of disease.

Biochemistry of Periodontal Connective Tissue Alterations

The biochemical composition of diseased connective tissues is determined by various degradation and synthesis processes associated with inflammation and the healing response. The hallmark of inflammatory periodontal disease is connective tissue destruction. During inflammation, PMN and macrophages bring forth matrix degradation, and the degradation can occur either through phagocytosis or by MMP released by these cells. Enzymes involved in these processes have been discussed in an earlier section. Interstitial collagenases MMP-1 and MMP-8, as well as gelatinases MMP-2 and MMP-9, are important in this regard.[76,77] The PMN is capable of secreting large quantities of these enzymes from granules during acute inflammation, presumably causing extensive destruction in a short time. In addition, gingival sulcular epithelium also expresses a battery of MMPs, and MMP-13 and MMP-8 are expressed at greater levels in the gingiva of patients with chronic and localized aggressive periodontitis. The production of MMPs in the diseased tissue is affected by numerous cytokines present in the host tissue.[78] Differences in susceptibility of different collagen types may be one reason why differences occur in colla-

gen-type ratios in diseased gingiva. For example, greater susceptibility of type III and resistance of type V and type I trimer to proteinases may be one reason why the amounts of these collagens vary in inflamed tissues.[2,49]

Collagenase and gelatinase activities have been identified in GCF and saliva of patients with natural and experimental periodontitis. The major enzyme species present in the GCF are MMP-8 and MMP-9; however, neither 72-kd gelatinase (MMP-2) nor stromelysin-1 (MMP-3) has been identified. The activities of MMPs in GCF are inhibited by tetracycline, indicating that they are derived from PMN and leukocytes, not from fibroblasts. Fibroblast enzymes are not inhibited by this drug.[77] The collagenases of GCF from patients with chronic and diabetes-associated periodontitis are susceptible to tetracyclines, while those from patients with localized aggressive periodontitis are relatively more resistant. Attempts have been made to correlate GCF-collagenase activities to disease severity. However, although the overall activity is higher in periodontitis and decreases with treatment, there appears to be no good correlation with individual sites, disease severity, or bone loss.[2]

Collagenases in inflamed gingiva may also be derived from fibroblasts and epithelial cells.[76] Immunolocalization studies have shown that these cells express collagenases; however, they appear to be involved in remodeling rather than disease. Nevertheless, in the context of periodontal disease, enzyme production by these cells could be activated by inflammatory mediators and products of plaque bacteria. MMP expression is induced by IL-1, TNF-α, con A, cyclic adenosine monophosphate, and PGE$_2$, whereas it is repressed by TGF-β, steroids, and IFN-γ. These mediators can affect MMP activity through TIMPs as well; for example, TGF-β and IL-1 induce TIMP-1 expression, while TGF-β suppresses TIMP-2. Osteoclasts do not express MMP, and during bone resorption these cells appear to utilize acid hydrolases (cathepsins) for matrix degradation.

Many other hydrolytic enzymes have been identified in inflamed periodontal tissues. The most notable among these enzymes are β-glucuronidase, aryl sulfatase, and hyaluronidase.[79] The substrates for such enzymes would clearly be the carbohydrate components of the proteoglycans, as well as hyaluronan. However, in light of current biochemical analysis of inflamed tissues, there is little evidence to support a primary role for these enzymes in matrix degradation. More likely, these enzymes are involved in a secondary capacity in the breakdown of GAG chains after initial proteolytic cleavage of proteoglycans.

Another important source of matrix-degrading enzymes in inflamed gingiva is the microbial plaque.[79] In particular, the black-pigmented *Bacteroides* species synthesize numerous proteases capable of disrupting periodontal extracellular matrix. For example, *Porphyromonas gingi-*

valis, *Clostridium histolyticus*, and some facultative *Bacillus* species from dental plaque secrete collagen-degrading enzymes. Other enzymes with trypsinlike activities have been described in *P gingivalis*, *Treponema denticola*, and *Bacteroides forsythus*; although these enzymes degrade type I collagen and fibronectin, it is debatable whether they are involved in the initial phases of tissue destruction or later, once initial matrix destruction has been established.[79] Bacterial enzymes could also facilitate MMP activity by activating their inactive precursors and degrading MMP inhibitors. Alternatively, they can act as antigens, stimulating the cytokine production by host inflammatory cells. Although these mechanisms are a possibility, bacterial enzymes have not been detected in the GCF.[76]

Bacterial enzymes can also degrade proteoglycans. Oral bacteria synthesize hyaluronidase, neutral proteinases, heparinase, chondrosulfatase, and chondroitinase.[79] All these enzymes have the potential to degrade periodontal GAGs and to influence the matrix indirectly through activation of interleukins and by affecting fibroblast function. For instance, an enzyme released by *P gingivalis* has been found to have a significant effect on proteoglycan synthesis by periodontal ligament fibroblasts. A thiol proteinase from this bacterium induces the production of MMP-3 and MMP-13 by epithelial cells.

Changes in the production of MMPs have been implicated in the evolution of drug-induced gingival overgrowth and gingival fibromatosis. Evidence indicates that these changes are mediated through the levels of cytokines and growth factors such as IL-1, TGF-β, and basic fibroblast growth factor (bFGF).[74,75]

Although they have not been investigated actively, products of normal cell metabolism could also be agents of tissue destruction.[80] Oxygen-derived free radicals, such as hydroxyl and superoxide radicals, are integral reaction products of normal cellular metabolism, but these are active in cells undergoing respiratory bursts at inflammatory sites. These highly reactive molecules can damage bacteria; degrade macromolecules such as collagen, proteoglycans, and hyaluronan; promote degradation of polyunsaturated fatty acids; and lead to damage of structural membranes. In addition, free radicals can also inhibit the action of antiproteases and stimulate the production from the plasma of a factor chemotactic for neutrophils and prostaglandin synthesis. The role of these free radicals in periodontal tissue destruction has been largely overlooked in favor of the more commonly cited enzymatic degradation. However, given their highly reactive nature and abundance in inflamed periodontal tissues, their role in inflammation-mediated tissue destruction should not be discounted.[79] Studies on the effect of oxygen-derived free radicals on gingival proteoglycans and hyaluronan have

demonstrated a susceptibility of these molecules to depolymerization by such reactive molecular species in vitro.

Interaction Between Connective Tissue Cells and Mediators

Fibroblasts play a major role in normal connective tissue turnover, as well as in wound repair and regeneration. In inflamed gingival tissues, fibroblasts interact with numerous cytokines and growth factors derived from inflammatory cells, plasma serum, and the local environment.[49,78,79] These factors can affect the growth and synthesis activities of resident cells, thereby affecting the quantity and type of molecules produced in diseased gingiva. The effect may be on all cells or on only one or more subpopulations. In the latter case, the growth and products of a subpopulation of cells may be affected.[49] This appears to be one mechanism contributing to enhanced matrix accumulation in drug-induced gingival hyperplasia. These mechanisms are discussed in more detail in the next section.

Repair and Regeneration of Periodontal Connective Tissues

Repair of damaged tissues is a major biologic response of all animals. However, the nature of the repair process often leads to compromised function. In this respect the periodontium is no exception. Tissues affected by gingivitis usually regenerate to their complete form and function; however, this may not be the case with periodontitis. Once the destructive phase reaches the deeper periodontal structures, clinically predictable regeneration is less likely. A major goal of periodontal therapy is to reestablish soft tissue attachment and restore lost bone. Accomplishment of this goal requires matrix synthesis, regeneration of gingival connective tissues, formation of new cementum and bone, and restoration of the connective tissue attachment to the root surface.[65,81] Typically, a wound-healing response is initiated by inflammation when PMN migrates into the wound site that has been filled with fibrin clot. The PMN, and later monocyte-macrophages, removes damaged tissue and foreign matter, and this "demolition" phase is carried out through phagocytosis and by enzymes secreted by these cells. Organization of granulation tissue follows when endothelial cells actively divide, forming capillaries and myofibroblasts, and fibroblasts begin to synthesize matrix components. The granulation tissue is eventually remodeled and replaced by a permanent repair tissue.

These processes require the participation of a variety of cell types and molecules. During healing and repair, matrix synthesis begins when fibroblasts move into the wound site; the synthesis becomes significant at approximately 7 days, peaks at 3 weeks, and may continue for months until tensile strength of the tissue is restored. Healing takes place through a similar sequence of events in bone, although in this tissue, fibrous and bony calluses, instead of a granulation tissue, form the intermediate stage.

The course of wound-healing events is regulated by soluble mediators present at the site of injury.[19] These molecules include degradation products of fibrin clot and host tissue, along with growth factors, cytokines, and lymphokines secreted by platelets, macrophages, and other cells.[2] Prominent among these are PDGF, TGF-β, IL-1, IFN-γ, and TNF-α. A family of polypeptides collectively called *bone morphogenetic proteins (BMPs)* or *osteogenic proteins (OPs)* participate in the healing of bone; these molecules, along with several growth factors, are stored in the extracellular matrix of bone and are released when the matrix is degraded during inflammation.

Inflammatory mediators affect cells in a number of ways. These molecules influence cell migration, attachment, growth, and synthesis activities. PDGF is the major mitogen for mesenchymal cells. TGF-β activates the synthesis of collagen and other matrix components, while IFN-γ and TNF-α have the opposite effect. IL-1, as described previously, mediates matrix degradation through activation MMP synthesis (Fig 6-10; see also Table 6-2). In contrast to these molecules, the BMPs are unique in that they trigger inflammatory and wound-healing responses in injured bone and accomplish total healing of the injury.

The effect of these molecules may be broad and directed to all connective tissue cells, or it may be specific to certain cell types or subtypes. The latter type of interaction can result in selective proliferation and enrichment of certain cell populations (see Fig 6-10). By these activities, chemical mediators are believed to dictate the type and sequence of healing responses, and aberrations in any of these processes are likely to lead to pathological connective tissue alterations.[49]

Whether healing occurs by regeneration (new tissue is identical to old tissue) or repair (a wound is replaced by a scar) depends mostly on the participating cell type and the matrix scaffolding remaining after injury. Regeneration occurs when the "labile" cells carry out the healing. These are undifferentiated unipotent or pluripotent cells that have unlimited division potential. In contrast, repair occurs when fully differentiated "permanent" cells with no division capacity are to be replaced. Repair is carried out by "stable" cells. Mesenchymal cells such as fibroblasts, osteoblasts, and glial cells form the stable cell pool; these cells have a limited division potential, they normally remain quiescent, and they divide on demand in response to mediators such as PDGF.

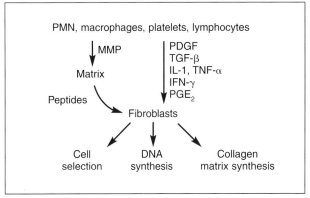

Fig 6-10 A scheme showing possible interactions between polypeptide mediators and resident cells during inflammation and wound repair. MMP and other hydrolytic enzymes released by inflammatory cells, and presumably by fibroblasts and epithelial cells through activation by bacterial substances, degrade the matrix. Cytokines, growth factors, and other molecules secreted by inflammatory cells and matrix degradation products affect the growth and synthesis activities of resident cells. These substances influence all the resident cells, or they may interact with and select one or more subpopulations and enrich these cells. Interference with any of these processes is likely to lead to aberrant healing or pathological alterations.

Presumably, several cell types are necessary for periodontal regeneration. These include fibroblasts for soft connective tissues, cementoblasts for cementogenesis, osteoblasts for bone, and endothelial cells for angiogenesis.[81] Where the regenerating cells are located or originate from is not yet clear, and this is especially true for the cementoblasts. Experiments in mice models indicate that these cells may be derived from precursor cells located paravascularly in periodontal ligament and in endosteal spaces of alveolar bone. Recent studies using cultured fibroblasts have indicated that in humans, such cells may be present as fibroblast subpopulations in the periodontal ligament and gingiva. Irrespective of their location, for regeneration to occur the cells responsible must participate at the right location and in the correct temporal sequence. More important for successful regeneration, certain cells—especially the epithelial cells—must be excluded from the healing site.

Attempts have been made to exploit some of the above principles in periodontal therapy. Early attempts used *root-surface conditioning* by demineralization, by coating with chemical agents such as fibronectin, or both. Demineralization was done to neutralize periodontitis-induced hypermineralization and to expose collagen fibers. Exposed collagen fibers were believed to discourage the attachment of unwanted epithelial cells but to favor fibroblasts to attach and help "splice" new with old collagen fibers. However, this procedure did not yield predictable regeneration, and it more likely caused ankylosis and root resorption.[81,82] The advantage of using fibronectin root-surface coating was also questionable because serum contains high fibronectin levels, and merely providing additional protein is unlikely to be beneficial.

A more recent procedure involves surgical placement of a physical barrier membrane between the connective tissue of a periodontal flap and the curetted root surface. The membrane was expected to prevent apical migration of gingival epithelial cells onto the root surface, exclude unwanted gingival connective tissues, and facilitate the repopulation of the wound site with periodontal ligament cells.[83] This *guided tissue regeneration procedure* demonstrated, for the first time, good potential for regeneration of root cementum, alveolar bone, and periodontal ligament, and it increased the incidence of new attachment formation. To date the clinical results of this method have been variable, and it may still not result in predictable periodontal regeneration. In another approach, growth factors or growth-promoting agents have been locally applied to the root surface to facilitate the cascade of wound-healing events that lead to new cementum and connective tissue formation.[84] Among the myriad factors currently characterized and available, epidermal growth factor (EGF), fibroblast growth factor, insulin-like growth factor (IGF), PDGF, TGFs, and an extract of enamel matrix protein have been proposed to be of potential use in relation to their regulatory effects of immune function, epithelium, bone, and soft connective tissues.

Role of Cementum in Periodontal Regeneration

An essential requirement for periodontal regeneration is the formation of new cementum into which new periodontal ligament fibers are to be inserted.[65] Although some information is available on the biology of cementogenesis in mice during development, how cementum formation is regulated in adult humans is not clear. The cementoblasts, cementum-forming cells, are unique, and only recently has it been possible to culture these cells and characterize their properties.[67,85] Recent studies indicate that the connective tissue matrix of cementum contains fibroblast growth factor, a battery of other growth factors, osteopontin, BSP, and an as-yet-unidentified polypeptide that mediates cell adhesion and spreading.[49,67] These molecules affect the migration, attachment, and proliferation of periodontal cells and their matrix synthesis; more important, they manifest cell specificity and tissue specificity among the same cell types. In addition to these soluble polypeptides, the extracellular matrix of cementum can also regulate the differentiation of precursor

cells into cementoblasts.[67] Thus, cementum appears capable of providing informational signals for the recruitment, proliferation, and differentiation of periodontal cells, and of regulating the regeneration of cementum as well as adjacent periodontal components.

New Perspectives

Significant information on the biochemistry of normal and diseased periodontal structures continues to be accrued. Studies are providing a more complete picture of the periodontium at the ultrastructural level. However, sufficient information on cementogenesis and the biochemical constituents of cementum is lacking. Efforts to characterize cementum components at the protein and gene levels are likely to open new avenues and make it possible to apply modern biotechnological approaches to future periodontal research. So far, satisfactory in vitro systems to study cementogenesis and to evaluate the function of cementum components have not been available; cultured cells from cementum will be useful in this regard.[85]

Although wound-healing models for other organs provide a wealth of information, the intricacies of periodontium may be unique in having to coordinate and integrate the processes involved in both soft and hard tissue healing. Specifically, the cell types and subtypes necessary for the regeneration of periodontal components need to be identified.[81]

In addition to inducing the tissues to regenerate, the control of tissue destruction is an important therapeutic goal in periodontitis. Whether degradation of periodontal tissues in advancing or aggressive periodontal diseases is due to accelerated breakdown or failure in normal regulation remains to be established. Advances have been made in the development of agents that block enzymatic activity, cytokine activity, and other inflammatory agents such as prostaglandins[77,78]; these advances have significant clinical ramifications.

Understanding the rational basis of therapeutic procedures requires knowledge about the variety of molecular and cellular processes associated with the formation of each periodontal component. Information is emerging on the availability of needed precursor cells, appropriate local environment, and biochemical signaling reactions that are conducive to regeneration processes. For example, cells with regeneration potential are available in all tissues, and their participation in healing and regeneration requires molecules that signal them to do their job.[86] Recruitment of these cells may require appropriate matrix components. It is becoming clear that matrix components are needed for cell division and differentiation, and integrins play a key role in this process.[49,81] Such processes and possible characteristic interactions between periodontal cells and matrix components are now being elucidated.[67,81] These processes and the molecules involved are yet to be identified, and it is necessary to determine how they interact with target cells and what signals are needed to trigger their biologic actions. This information will be useful in developing new techniques for periodontal regeneration, which is an integrated system of soft and hard tissue healing and restoration of bone loss. For example, approaches that could be useful to recruit cementoblasts for new attachment might use specific substances existing on healthy cementum surfaces and integrins or peptide sequences involved in binding cells to these substances.

Acknowledgments

This work was supported by United States NIH grants DE 08229, DE 10491, and DE13061, and by the National Health and Medical Research Council of Australia. We appreciate the help provided by Ms Theo Heinz and Mrs Glenda Maher in preparation of the manuscript.

References

1. Schluger S, Yuodelis RA, Page RC, Johnson R. Periodontal Disease, ed 2. Philadelphia: Lea & Febiger, 1990.
2. Bartold PM, Narayanan AS. Biology of Periodontal Connective Tissue. Chicago: Quintessence, 1998.
3. Piez KA. In: Ramachandran GN, Reddi AH (eds). Biochemistry of Collagen. New York: Plenum, 1976:1.
4. Ramachandran GN, Ramakrishnan C. In: Ramachandran GN, Reddi AH (eds). Biochemistry of Collagen. New York: Plenum, 1976:45.
5. Byers PH. Disorders of collagen biosynthesis and structure. In: Scriver C, Beudet AL, Sly WS, Valle D (ed). The Metabolic and Molecular Bases of Inherited Disease, ed 7. New York: McGraw-Hill, 1995:4029–4077.
6. Van Der Rest M, Garrone R. Collagen family of proteins. FASEB J 1991;5:2814.
7. Vuorio E, de Crombrugghe B. The family of collagen genes. Annu Rev Biochem 1990;59:837–872.
8. Sandell LJ, Boyd CD (eds). Extracellular Matrix Genes. San Diego: Academic Press, 1990:1.
9. Rosenbloom J, Harsch M, Jimenez S. Hydroxyproline content determines the denaturation temperature of chick tendon collagen. Arch Biochem Biophys 1973;158:478–484.
10. Li SW, Sieron AL, Fertala A, et al. The C-proteinase that processes procollagens to fibrillar collagens is identical to the protein previously identified as bone morphogenic protein-1. Proc Natl Acad Sci USA 1996;93:5127–5130.
11. Eyre DR, Paz MA, Gallop PM. Cross-linking in collagen and elastin. Annu Rev Biochem 1984;53:717–748.
12. Ramirez F, Di Liberto M. Complex and diversified regulatory programs control the expression of vertebrate collagen genes. FASEB J 1990;4:1616.
13. Karsenty G, Park RW. Regulation of type I collagen genes expression. Int Rev Immunol 1995;12:177–185.
14. Nagase H, Woessner JF Jr. Matrix metalloproteinases. J Biol Chem 1999;274:21491–21494.
15. Massova I, Kotra LP, Fridman R, Mobnashery S. Matrix metalloproteinases: Structures, evolution and diversification. FASEB J 1998;12:1075.
16. Nagase H, Barret AJ, Woessner JF Jr. Nomenclature and glossary of matrix metalloproteinases. Matrix Suppl 1992;1:421–424.
17. Birkedal-Hansen H, Moore WG, Bodden MK, et al. Matrix metalloproteinases: A review. Crit Rev Oral Biol Med 1993;4:197–250.
18. Gomez DE, Alonso DF, Yoshiji H, Thorgeirsson UP. Tissue inhibitors of metalloproteinases: Structure, regulation and biological functions. Eur J Cell Biol 1997;74:111–122.
19. Clark RAF, Henson PM (eds). The Molecular and Cellular Biology of Wound Repair. New York: Plenum, 1988.
20. Sandberg B, Soskel NT, Leslie JG. Elastin structure, biosynthesis, and relation to disease states. New Engl J Med 1981;304:566–579.
21. Indik Z, Yeh H, Ornstein-Goldstein N, Rosenbloom J. Structure of the elastin gene and alternative splicing of elastin mRNA. In: Sandell LJ, Boyd CD (eds). Extracellular Matrix Genes. San Diego: Academic Press, 1990:221–250.
22. Hynes RO, Yamada KM. Fibronectins: Multifunctional modular glycoproteins. J Cell Biol 1982;95:369–377.
23. Schwarzbauer J. The fibronectin gene. In: Sandell LJ, Boyd CD (eds). Extracellular Matrix Genes. San Diego: Academic Press, 1990:195–219.
24. Lawler J, Duquette M, Urry L, et al. The evolution of the thrombospondin family. J Mol Evol 1993;36:509–516.
25. Tryggvason K. The laminin family. Curr Opin Cell Biol 1993;5:877–882.
26. Chiquet-Ehrismann R. What distinguishes tenascin from fibronectin? FASEB J 1990;4:2598.
27. Erickson HP, Bourdon MA. Tenascin: An extracellular matrix protein prominent in specialized embryonic tissues and tumors. Annu Rev Cell Biol 1989;5:71–92.
28. Chung AE, Dong LJ, Wu C, Durkin ME. Biological functions of entactin. Kidney Int 1993;43:13–19.
29. Ruoslahti E, Pierschbacher MD. New perspectives in cell adhesion: RGD and integrins. Science 1987;238:491–497.
30. Albelda SM, Buck CA. Integrins and other cell adhesion molecules. FASEB J 1990;4:2868.
31. Hardingham TE, Fosang AJ. Proteoglycans: Many forms and many functions. FASEB J 1992;6:861.
32. Gallagher JT. The extended family of proteoglycans: Social residents of the pericellular zone. Curr Opin Cell Biol 1989;1:1201–1218.
33. Yanagishita M. Function of proteoglycans in the extracellular matrix. Acta Pathol Jpn 1993;43:283–293.
34. Roden L. Structure and metabolism of connective tissue proteoglycans. In: Lennarz W (ed). The Biochemistry of Glycoproteins and Proteoglycans. New York: Plenum, 1980:267–371.
35. Hassell JR, Kimura JH, Hascall VC. Proteoglycan protein families. Annu Rev Biochem 1986;55:539–567.
36. Margolis RU, Margolis RK. Aggrecan-versican-neurocan family proteoglycans. Methods Enzymol 1994;245:105–126.
37. Lebaron RG. Versican. Perspect Dev Neurobiol 1996;3:261–271.
38. Iozzo RV, Cohen IR, Grassel S, Murdock AD. The biology of perlecan: The multifaceted heparan sulfate proteoglycan of basement membranes and pericellular matrices. Biochem J 1994;302:625–639.

39. Fisher LW, Termine JD, Young MF. Deduced protein sequence of bone small proteoglycan I (biglycan) shows homology with proteoglycan II (decorin) and several nonconnective tissue proteins in a variety of species. J Biol Chem 1989;264:4571–4576.

40. Bernfield M, Götte M, Park PW, et al. Functions of cell surface heparan sulfate proteoglycans. Annu Rev Biochem 1999;68: 729–777.

41. Bourin M-C, Lundgren-Akerlund E, Lindahl U. Isolation and characterization of the glycosaminoglycan component of rabbit thrombomodulin proteoglycan. J Biol Chem 1990;265: 15424–15431.

42. Brown TA, Bouchard T, St John T, et al. Human keratinocytes express a new CD44 core protein (CD44E) as a heparan-sulfate intrinsic membrane proteoglycan with additional exons. J Cell Biol 1991;113:207–221.

43. David G, Lories V, Decock B, et al. Molecular cloning of a phosphatidylinositol-anchored membrane heparan sulfate proteoglycan from human lung fibroblasts. J Cell Biol 1990;111: 3165–3176.

44. Lopez-Casillas F, Wrana JC, Massague J. Betaglycan presents ligand to the TGF-beta signaling receptor. Cell 1993;73: 1435–1444.

45. Kolset SO, Gallagher JT. Proteoglycans in haemopoietic cells. Biochim Biophys Acta 1990;1032:191–211.

46. Laurent TC, Fraser JR. Hyaluronan. FASEB J 1992;6:2397.

47. Toole BP. Hyaluronan and its binding proteins, the hyaladherins. Curr Opin Cell Biol 1990;2:839–844.

48. Cho MI, Garant PR. Development and general structure of the periodontium. Periodontol 2000 2000;24:9–27.

49. Narayanan AS, Bartold PM. Biochemistry of periodontal connective tissues and their regeneration: A current perspective. Connect Tissue Res 1996;34:191–201.

50. Chavrier C, Couble ML, Magloire H, Grimaud JA. Connective tissue organization of healthy human gingiva: Ultrastructural localization of collagen types I-III-IV. J Periodontal Res 1984; 19:221–229.

51. Narayanan AS, Clagett JA, Page RC. Effect of inflammation on the distribution of collagen types I, III, IV, and V and type I trimer and fibronectin in human gingivae. J Dent Res 1985;64: 1111–1116.

52. Wang H-M, Nanda V, Rao LG, et al. Specific immunohistochemical localization of type III collagen in porcine periodontal tissues using the peroxidase-antiperoxidase method. J Histochem Cytochem 1980;28:1215–1223.

53. Everts V, Niehof A, Jansen D, Beertsen W. Type VI collagen is associated with microfibrils and oxytalan fibers in the extracellular matrix of periodontium, mesenterium and periosteum. J Periodontal Res 1998;33:118–125.

54. Bartold PM. Connective tissues of the periodontium. Research and clinical implications. Aust Dent J 1991;36:255–268.

55. Salonen J, Domenicucci C, Goldberg HA, Sodek J. Immunohistochemical localization of SPARC (osteonectin) and denatured collagen and their relationship to remodelling in rat dental tissues. Arch Oral Biol 1990;35:337–346.

56. Steffensen B, Duong AH, Milam SB, et al. Immunohistological localization of cell adhesion proteins and integrins in the periodontium. J Periodontol 1992;63:584–592.

57. Bourke KA, Haase H, Li H, et al. Distribution and synthesis of elastin in porcine gingiva and alveolar mucosa. J Periodontal Res 2000;35:361–368.

58. Bartold PM. Proteoglycans of the periodontium: Structure, role and function. J Periodontal Res 1987;22:431–444.

59. Bartold PM, Walsh LJ, Narayanan AS. Molecular and cell biology of the gingiva. Periodontol 2000 2000;24:28–55.

60. Karimbux NY, Rosenblum ND, Nishimura I. Site-specific expression of collagen I and XII mRNAs in the rat periodontal ligament at two developmental stages. J Dent Res 1992;71; 1355–1362.

61. MacNeil RL, Berry JE, Strayhorn CL, et al. Expression of type I and XII collagen during development of the periodontal ligament in the mouse. Arch Oral Biol 1998;43:779–787.

62. Reichenberger E, Baur S, Sukotjo C, et al. Collagen XII mutation disrupts matrix structure of periodontal ligament and skin. J Dent Res 2000;79:1962–1968.

63. Häkkinen L, Oksala O, Salo T, et al. Immunohistochemical localization of proteoglycans in human periodontium. J Histochem Cytochem 1993;41:1689–1699.

64. Bosshardt DD, Selvig KA. Dental cementum: The dynamic tissue covering of the root. Periodontol 2000 1997;13:41–75.

65. Schroeder HE. Biological problems of regenerative cementogenesis: Synthesis and attachment of collagenous matrices on growing and established root surfaces. Int Rev Cytol 1992; 142:1–59.

66. Brandsten C, Lundmark C, Christersson C, et al. Expression of collagen α1 (I) mRNA variants during tooth and bone formation in the rat. J Dent Res 1999;78:11–19.

67. Saygin NE, Giannobile WV, Somerman MJ. Molecular and cell biology of cementum. Periodontol 2000 2000;24:73–98.

68. Cheng H, Caterson B, Neame PJ, et al. Differential distribution of lumican and fibromodulin in tooth cementum. Connect Tissue Res 1996;34:87–96.

69. Worapamorn W, Li H, Pujic Z, et al. Expression and distribution of cell-surface proteoglycans in the normal Lewis rat molar periodontium. J Periodontal Res 2000;35:214–224.

70. Yamamoto T, Domon T, Takahashi S, et al. The regulation of fiber arrangement in advanced cellular cementogenesis of human teeth. J Periodontal Res 1998;33:83–90.

71. Sodek J, McKee MD. Molecular and cellular biology of alveolar bone. Periodontol 2000 2000;24:99–126.

72. Bartold PM. A biochemical and immunohistochemical study of the proteoglycans of alveolar bone. J Dent Res 1990;69:7–19.

73. Karimbux NY, Ramamurthy NS, Golub LM, Nishimura I. The expression of collagen I and XII mRNAs in *Porphyromonas gingivalis*–induced periodontitis in rats: The effect of doxycycline and chemically modified tetracycline. J Periodontol 1998;69: 34–40.

74. Seymour RA, Thomason JM, Ellis JS. The pathogenesis of drug-induced gingival overgrowth. J Clin Periodontol 1996;23: 165–175.

75. Marshall RI, Bartold PM. Medication induced gingival overgrowth. Oral Dis 1998;4:130–151.

76. Birkedal-Hansen H. Role of matrix metalloproteinases in human periodontal diseases. J Periodontol 1993;64:474–484.

77. Ryan ME, Golub LM. Modulation of matrix metalloproteinase activities in periodontitis as a treatment strategy. Periodontol 2000 2000;24:226–238.

78. Paquette DW, Williams RC. Modulation of host inflammatory mediators as a treatment strategy for periodontal diseases. Periodontol 2000 2000;24:239–252.

79. Bartold PM. Turnover in periodontal connective tissues: Dynamic homeostasis of cells, collagen and ground substances. Oral Dis 1995;1:238–253.

80. Henson PM, Johnston RB Jr. Tissue injury in inflammation: Oxidants, proteinases and cationic proteins. J Clin Invest 1987;79: 669–674.

81. Bartold PM, McCulloch CA, Narayanan AS, Pitaru S. Tissue engineering: A new paradigm for periodontal regeneration based on molecular and cell biology. Periodontol 2000 2000;24:253–269.

82. Marks SC Jr, Mehta NR. Lack of effect of citric acid treatment of root surfaces on the formation of new connective tissue attachment. J Clin Periodontol 1986;13:109–116.

83. Karring T, Nyman S, Gottlow J, Laurell L. Development of the biological concept of guided tissue regeneration—Animal and human studies. Periodontol 2000 1993;1:26–35.

84. Cochran DL, Wozney JM. Biological mediators for periodontal regeneration. Periodontol 2000 1999;19:40–58.

85. Grzesik WJ, Cheng H, Oh JS, et al. Cementum-forming cells are phenotypically distinct from bone-forming cells. J Bone Miner Res 2000;15:52–59.

86. McKay R. Stem cells in the central nervous system. Science 1997;276:66–71.

The Physiology of Bone

Zvi Schwartz, David D. Dean,
Christoph H. Lohmann, and Barbara D. Boyan

- Bone Structure and Remodeling
- The Osteoblast
- The Osteoclast
- Factors Regulating Bone Formation
- Factors Regulating Bone Resorption
- Regulation of Bone by Systemic Hormones

Bone Structure and Remodeling

Bone is a metabolically active organ, composed of both mineral and organic phases. It is exquisitely designed for its role as the load-bearing structure of the body. To accomplish its task, bone is formed from a combination of dense, compact bone and cancellous (trabecular) bone that is reinforced at points of stress. The mineral phase of the skeleton contributes about two thirds of its weight, while the remaining one third is organic matrix primarily consisting of collagen and small amounts of proteoglycan, lipid, and several noncollagenous proteins, such as osteopontin, osteonectin, osteocalcin (bone gla-protein), and matrix gla-protein.

Two major cell types are found in bone. The first is the osteoblast, whose function is to synthesize the organic matrix components and direct the events resulting in mineralization. The terminally differentiated osteoblast is the osteocyte, which is the major cell type in bone. The function of the osteocyte is to maintain bone homeostasis. It is believed that the osteocyte does this by sensing and responding to mechanical, electrical, and chemical stimuli. The second cell type is the osteoclast, whose function is to resorb both the mineral and organic phases of the bone. In a process known as *coupling*, cells in the osteoclast and osteoblast lineages remodel and maintain the skeleton throughout the life of the organism.

Bone consists of two macroscopically different envelopes: cortical bone, which is predominantly found in the long bones of the extremities, and cancellous bone, which is predominantly found in the vertebral column and the pelvis. Both types of bone are found in the maxilla and mandible, although cortical bone is more prominent in the mandible. Cortical bone makes up 80% of the bone in the body and cancellous bone, 20%. However, because cancellous bone is metabolically more active, skeletal metabolism is approximately equal between the two envelopes. The two envelopes are regulated by, and respond differently to, different hormones, factors, and treatment modalities.

When bone is studied under polarized light, a clear lamellar pattern is visible in both cortical and cancellous bone. However, if bone turnover is very high or disturbed—or during healing when primary bone is formed—the lamellar pattern disappears, and woven bone is formed.

Cortical bone is made up of the Haversian system (cortical osteon), which is found around central blood vessels and which may branch within the cortex of the bone. Spatially, the cells in the Haversian system cover a relatively small surface area, while cells in cancellous bone occupy a large portion of the surface. This observation may explain why cortical bone exhibits lower metabolic activity than cancellous bone.[1]

Cortical bone is delimited by the periosteum on the outside and the endosteum on the inside. The inner cortical

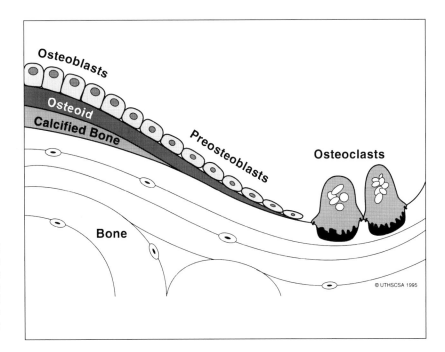

Fig 7-1 Modeling of bone by the concerted action of osteoclasts and osteoblasts. Bone is removed by osteoclasts and new bone synthesized by osteoblasts. The process is delicately balanced and regulated by local factors and hormones that act on the cells to ensure that bone resorption and formation are coupled with each other.

bone, the endosteal surface, exhibits pronounced osteoclastic and osteoblastic activity. The periosteum is important during growth, fracture repair, and healing around implants. During growth, the periosteum is important for bone modeling. Modeling is the process by which bone reshapes itself to create an organ with maximal compressive strength. Usually at the periosteal surface, bone formation exceeds bone resorption, creating a net increase in the outer diameter of bone with age. However, at the endosteum, modeling as well as remodeling occurs, and resorption generally exceeds bone formation, resulting in a net expansion of marrow capacity with age. It is important to note that this endocortical formation may become especially pronounced during states of high turnover, such as thyrotoxicosis and postmenopausal syndrome.

Cancellous bone consists of trabeculae with thicknesses ranging from 50 to 400 μm. The trabeculae are interconnected in a honeycomb pattern, maximizing the mechanical properties of the bone.

In bone, there is a constant process of modeling and remodeling. In this process, a constant resorption of the bone occurs on a particular bony surface, followed by a phase of bone formation (Fig 7-1). In normal adults, there is a balance between the amount of bone resorbed by osteoclasts and the amount of bone formed by osteoblasts.[2] Bone remodeling must be distinguished from bone modeling, which is the process associated with the formation and growth of bones in childhood and adolescence.[2] Bone modeling consists primarily of processes at the pe-

riosteum and endosteum, leading to changes in the shape of growing bone. During modeling, resorption and formation are spatially related and sometimes proceed in an uncoupled fashion. Moreover, modeling is continuous and covers a large surface, while remodeling is cyclical and usually covers only a small area.[1]

The current concept of bone remodeling is based on the hypothesis that osteoclastic precursors become activated and differentiate into osteoclasts, which begin the process of bone resorption. This phase is followed by a bone-formation phase. The number of sites entering the bone-formation phase, or activation frequency, together with the individual rates of the two processes, determines the rate of tissue turnover.[3,4] While resorption depth and mean wall thickness may vary by only 10% to 20% of normal in different diseases, activation frequency may vary by 50% to 100%. Thus, in most diseases, the activation frequency is the most important regulator of bone turnover and changes in bone mass.[3]

The termination of bone resorption and the initiation of bone formation in the resorption lacuna occur through a coupling mechanism.[5] The coupling process ensures that the amount of bone removed is similar to the amount of bone laid down during the subsequent bone-formation phase. The detailed nature of the activation and coupling mechanism is still unknown, although some growth factors, such as various lymphokines, fibroblast growth factor (FGF), transforming growth factor β (TGF-β), and prostaglandins, have been proposed.[6] Whether the activation of osteoblasts begins simultaneously with osteoclastic recruitment or at some later stage during lacunar development is still unsettled.

During aging, bone undergoes changes in its three-dimensional structure that have a profound impact on its physical characteristics. This process starts at approximately 25 to 30 years of age, when maximal bone formation is achieved. A steady decline in bone mass begins around 30 years of age for both men and women.[7,8] The decrease in bone mass leads to thinning of cortical bone due to tunneling, or trabeculation, of the endosteal cortical envelope, with expansion of the marrow cavity accompanied by some gain in bone diameter.[9]

Changes in cortical bone mass are sex dependent. Men exhibit an age-dependent increase in resorptive activity, leading to increased osteon diameter. Mean thickness of the bone formed in the osteon, however, remains constant with age. Thus, a trend toward a more negative balance between resorption and formation is reflected in increased Haversian canal diameter.[10] Women, in contrast, generally show reduced resorptive activity. This is reflected in decreases in osteon diameter with age, but unlike men, mean thickness of bone decreases with age, leading to a pronounced negative balance and increase in Haversian canal diameter.[10]

In cancellous bone of 20- to 80-year-old individuals, there is a decrease of about 45% in the fractional volume of trabecular bone; this is accompanied by a decrease in mean thickness of the horizontal trabeculae with no significant change in mean thickness of the vertically oriented trabeculae.[11] Furthermore, an increase in the distance between horizontal trabeculae during aging has been observed for both men and women, but the change is slightly greater for women. Histomorphometry of histologic sections of vertebra has shown an age-related decrease in mean trabecular bone thickness, with a decrease in trabecular volume. Moreover, a pronounced age-related increase in marrow space volume was also demonstrated, which was significantly greater for women than men.[12]

The Osteoblast

Cells of the osteoblast lineage occupy a central position in bone metabolism. Osteoblasts are cells with a number of functions. They are well known for synthesizing the organic matrix of bone and participating in its mineralization. In addition, they respond to circulating hormones, growth factors, and cytokines produced by themselves or other cells of the marrow, which play a major role in cell-to-cell communication and maintenance of bone. The formation of a structurally sound skeleton, with its strength and integrity conserved by constant remodeling, is the result of many direct and indirect influences on the osteoblast.

Types and Functions of Osteoblasts

The word *osteoblast* has traditionally been used to describe those cells in bone responsible for bone formation. Now, however, it is recognized that cells of the osteoblast lineage are also involved in a much larger number of functions. These include playing a role in the production of paracrine and autocrine factors (cytokines and growth factors), which profoundly influence bone resorption as well as bone formation. Osteoblasts also produce proteases, which are involved in matrix degradation and matrix maturation.

It is possible to separate mature osteoblasts into several main subpopulations: those that synthesize bone matrix; those that line trabeculae and endosteal surfaces; those that are called *osteocytes* and are buried in their lacunae, communicating with other osteocytes; and those on the surface of the bone.

Osteoblasts have been found to have gap junctions that connect them with neighboring osteoblasts and adjacent bone-lining cells,[13] providing an important mechanism for intercellular communication. Osteoblasts also communicate with osteocytes, below the bone surface, through a network of canalicular connections.

The osteoblast is an active cell, with a very prominent Golgi apparatus and extensive endoplasmic reticulum, reflecting its capacity for protein synthesis. It produces a bone-matrix–containing type I collagen as well as noncollagenous proteins, such as osteonectin, osteopontin, osteocalcin, and various proteoglycans. Osteoblasts control the process of bone mineralization at three levels: *(1)* in its initial phase, by production of an extracellular organelle called the *matrix vesicle*, which has a major role in primary calcification; *(2)* at a later stage, by controlling the ongoing process of mineralization by modifying the matrix through the release of different enzymes; and *(3)* by regulating the number of ions available for mineral deposition in the matrix.

Primary mineralization of bone occurs through a complex series of synthetic and regulatory events under the control of osteoblasts. This type of mineralized tissue is formed during embryonic and fetal bone development, postfetal bone growth, and bone repair and induction, either orthotopically or heterotopically. Matrix vesicles, organelles produced by osteoblasts and located in the extracellular matrix, are active in the initial phases of primary mineralization. This observation has been demonstrated repeatedly in developing tissue, in repair tissue, and in pathological processes. It is important to note, however,

Table 7-1 Some Noncollagenous Proteins in Bone Matrix

Protein	Known function	Regulation of production by osteoblasts
Osteocalcin	Inhibits mineralization, recruits bone-cell precursors	$1,25\text{-}(OH)_2D_3$, PTH, glucocorticoids
Osteonectin	Facilitates type I collagen mineralization, suppresses rate of hydroxyapatite crystal growth, modulates cell attachment and detachment	Glucocorticoids, TGF-β, IGF-1
Osteopontin	Cell-binding activity, osteoclast-anchoring activity, mineral-binding activity	$1,25\text{-}(OH)_2D_3$, TGF-β, retinoic acid, glucocorticoids, PTH
Bone sialoprotein	Cell-binding activity	Glucocorticoids, $1,25\text{-}(OH)_2D_3$
Bone proteoglycan (biglycan)	Function unclear	Not well characterized
Bone proteoglycan II (decorin)	Binds to collagen fibers, regulates fiber growth, binds/presents growth factors in matrix	Not well characterized
Thrombospondin	Binds and organizes matrix, cell attachment	TGF-β
Matrix gla-protein	Prevents growth plate mineralization	Retinoic acid, $1,25\text{-}(OH)_2D_3$
Latent TGF-β1 binding protein-1	Storage of latent TGF-β1	$1,25\text{-}(OH)_2D_3$

that calcification via matrix vesicles is not the only mechanism responsible for crystal formation in bone. The strategies used by cells to regulate events in the matrix are diverse and complex. However, careful regulation of the initial events helps to ensure that calcification is under cellular control. While it is accepted that mineral crystals are first seen in matrix vesicles, bulk-phase mineral deposition may not require matrix vesicles or their constituents.[14]

Because of their multiple functions, osteoblasts are under tight control by hormones such as parathyroid hormone (PTH), 1,25-dihydroxyvitamin D$_3$ [1,25-(OH)$_2$D$_3$] , 24,25-dihydroxyvitamin D$_3$ [24,25-(OH)$_2$D$_3$], estrogen, growth hormone, and thyroxin. They also respond to a number of growth factors and cytokines. In addition, some growth factors, such as TGF-β and insulin-like growth factor–1 (IGF-1), not only are produced by osteoblasts but also directly affect them, indicating both a paracrine and an autocrine role for these factors in bone.

Osteoblasts are thought to be derived from pluripotential stem cells present in the stromal fibroblastic system of bone marrow and other connective tissues, such as periosteum.[15] The stem cell from which osteoblasts arise is distinct from that giving rise to osteoclasts, which originate from the hematopoietic system.[16] Nevertheless, it is possible to draw analogies between the two pathways, since in both systems, stem cells are able to differentiate into cells of several lineages.[17] The osteoblast, at different stages of differentiation, will possess different properties,

depending on its location in bone and other local and humoral influences.

The entire developmental sequence of the osteoblast can be divided into three distinct phases.[18] Using a cell culture model, it has been shown that the initial, proliferative phase (days 0 to 15) is characterized by the synthesis of an organized, bone-specific extracellular matrix. After proliferation ceases, a second phase, characterized by matrix maturation (days 16 to 20), begins. This renders the matrix competent for the final phase of mineralization during days 20 to 25.

Osteoblasts synthesize a collagen-rich matrix, called *osteoid*, which mineralizes to form mature bone. Approximately 90% of the organic matrix of bone is collagen, and most of this is type I collagen. The correct transcription and translation of type I collagen by osteoblasts is necessary for normal bone formation; indeed, most of the genetic mutations identified in osteogenesis imperfecta are located on one of the two structural genes for type I collagen.[19] In bone matrix, there are also many noncollagenous proteins produced by osteoblasts. Several of these proteins have been characterized and cloned.[20] Table 7-1 summarizes our current knowledge of the major noncollagenous proteins in bone, their function, and what factors or hormones regulate their production.

The matrix produced by the osteoblast performs a number of functions, including structural support, orientation, and polarization of cells; binding of latent or active cytokines and growth factors; and regulation of adjacent cells. The matrix also participates in the mineralization process by providing the proper structure and regulatory signals.

The Osteocyte

Osteocytes are considered to be the "nerve cells" of the bone, maintaining the balance between resorption and remodeling.[21] The extracellular matrix of the osteocyte includes type I collagen, osteocalcin, osteopontin, and osteonectin. The cells are sensitive to mechanical strain and can transduce it into biochemical signals.[22] The osteocytes signal to neighboring cells through their extensive network of canaliculi via secretion of factors like prostaglandin E_2 (PGE_2) and nitric oxide.[23] Because they form gap junctions in response to mechanical stress, they are able to propagate signals over fairly large distances.

We are only beginning to understand the regulatory mechanisms that affect osteocyte behavior.[24] These cells appear to respond to systemic hormones like estrogen and $1,25\text{-}(OH)_2D_3$, but their responses differ from those of osteoblasts. Similarly, their production of autocrine and paracrine mediators differs from that of osteoblasts. Because osteocytes are the most abundant cell type in bone, increasing our knowledge of their role in bone homeostasis will help us build and maintain healthy tissue.

Hormones and Coupling

With the exception of calcitonin, all the hormones, cytokines, and growth factors that act on bone, as an organ, mediate their activity through osteoblasts.[25,26] Both PTH and PTH-related peptides have specific receptors on the osteoblast, and their effects are mediated by cyclic adenosine monophosphate (cAMP) at the postreceptor level. A similar effect has been observed with PGE_2. $1,25\text{-}(OH)_2D_3$ works through a specific nuclear receptor and affects osteoblast differentiation and matrix production. Studies also suggest that osteoblasts have membrane-associated receptors for $1,25\text{-}(OH)_2D_3$. Estrogen and growth hormone also work through a receptor in osteoblasts, although part of the effect observed with these hormones is mediated by the production of IGF-1, which by itself has a direct effect on osteoblasts. Several peptide growth factors, such as epidermal growth factor (EGF), TGF-α, TGF-β, and platelet-derived growth factor (PDGF), also evoke responses from osteoblasts through receptors. A family of cytokines that was initially thought to act on only the immune system has been found to contain several members that not only are produced by osteoblasts but also have substantial action on bone. This group includes interleukin 1 (IL-1), interleukin 6 (IL-6), and tumor necrosis factors α and β (TNF-α and TNF-β).

For many years, the activation of resorption was thought to be mediated by PTH, PGE_2, $1,25\text{-}(OH)_2D_3$, or IL-1 via direct action of these mediators on existing osteoclasts or on osteoclast precursors. Since the 1970s, however, a new concept has surfaced. According to this view, resorbing hormones act directly on osteoblasts, which then produce other factors that regulate osteoclast activity. This results in both bone formation and bone resorption being coupled. The coupling theory is based on the observation that once resorption occurs, osteoblasts respond by making more bone matrix. That is, any change in resorption or formation results in a change in the other. A hypothetical mechanism for explaining the coupling phenomenon is that resorbing bone produces a factor or factors that influence the rate and/or extent of osteoblastic activity.[27] It now seems likely that a discrete coupling factor does not exist but rather that the coupling process may be mediated by a number of factors.

TGF-β has been considered as one of the possible factors active in this process. Latent TGF-β is produced by osteoblasts and deposited in the extracellular matrix. As resorption takes place, latent TGF-β is released from the matrix. Concomitantly, PTH and other bone-resorbing hormones increase production and release of enzymes such as plasminogen activator by osteoblasts, which activate latent TGF-β. Alternatively, proteinases released by the osteoclast during resorption may also activate latent TGF-β. In either case, active TGF-β then enhances osteoblast differentiation and matrix formation and inhibits osteoclast activity. A scheme illustrating how TGF-β may regulate bone resorption and formation is shown in Fig 7-2.

Recent studies suggest that bone formation and bone resorption are coupled even more directly.[28,29] Osteoblasts and stromal cells express a member of the TNF-ligand family called *receptor activator of NFκB ligand (RANKL)* on their membranes. Osteoclast precursors that possess RANK, a TNF-receptor family member, recognize RANKL through cell-to-cell interaction with the osteoblasts. This causes them to differentiate into osteoclasts when macrophage colony-stimulating factor (CSF) is present. Mature osteoclasts also express RANK, and their bone-resorbing activity is stimulated by RANKL. In addition to RANKL, osteoblasts secrete a factor that inhibits osteoclastogenesis, called *osteoprotogerin (OPG)*. OPG is a "decoy" receptor for RANKL.[30] By binding RANKL, OPG prevents it from binding to RANK on the osteoclast or osteoclast precursor, and osteoclast formation and activity are prevented.

Proteolysis and increased cellular activity are found at sites of normal and pathological tissue remodeling. There is considerable evidence that osteoblasts are responsible for the production of proteinases, enzymes capable of mediating the localized turnover of both unmineralized and demineralized bone matrix. These enzymes are different

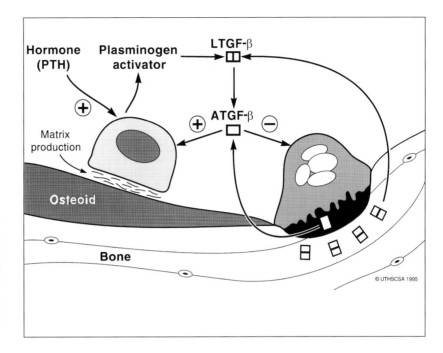

Fig 7-2 Osteoclasts secrete proteolytic enzymes, such as plasminogen activator, or acids that activate latent TGF-β (LTGF-β) in the extracellular matrix. Active TGF-β (ATGF-β) may then stimulate osteoblast differentiation and matrix formation and inhibit osteoclast activity. This model explains how TGF-β may act as a coupling factor to regulate osteoclast and osteoblast activities in bone modeling (see Fig 7-1).

from the enzymes produced by osteoclasts, which are responsible for direct action on bone matrix at acid pH. The proteinases that osteoblasts produce are active at neutral pH and include collagenase and plasminogen activator. Some of the proteinases produced by osteoblasts are present in extracellular matrix vesicles. Their release during maturation of osteoid may be important for mineralization of the matrix, as well as for latent growth factor activation.

The Osteoclast

The osteoclast is the cell responsible for resorption of the extracellular bone matrix. Under normal conditions, bone resorption plays a major role in the homeostasis of both the skeleton and serum calcium level. Further, bone resorption is also essential for the proper growth and remodeling of bone and is tightly coupled to the process of bone formation by osteoblasts. The correct functioning of this coupled process leads to the maintenance of the skeleton. When the balance between bone resorption and formation is disturbed during growth, repair after trauma, or regeneration during periodontal treatment, a change in size and shape of the individual bone will occur.

Changes in the coupling balance also result in various pathological conditions. For example, osteopetrosis and osteosclerosis are characterized by dense bone and osteoporosis, by porous bone. Faulty coupling can also result in high resorption, as seen in diseases of high bone turnover, such as hyperparathyroidism and Paget disease.

Characteristics of Osteoclasts

Osteoclasts have proven difficult to characterize. They are relatively rare in bone and cover only 1% of the bone surface; they are terminally differentiated and do not proliferate; they are attached to the mineralized matrix; and they are fragile due to their large size. Only recently have reliable methods been developed for the isolation and culture specimens of these cells from bone[31,32] or bone-marrow specimens.[33]

The osteoclast is a highly motile cell that attaches to, and migrates along, the interface between bone and the bone marrow (endosteum). It is generally a multinucleated cell (although mononuclear osteoclasts are also encountered), formed by the asynchronous fusion of mononuclear precursors derived from the bone marrow and differentiating within the granulocyte-macrophage lineage. Osteogenesis has become a topic of considerable interest in the study of prevention and treatment of metabolic bone disease. Osteoclasts can be derived from granulocyte-macrophage progenitor (colony-forming unit–granulocyte-macrophage) cells when cultured with RANKL, macrophage CSF, and dexamethasone.[34] Factors that increase the numbers of precursor cells, such as annexin II or IL-1, also result in a net increase in osteoclasts.[35] Many of these factors also activate committed osteoclasts. When activated, the osteoclast attaches to the mineralized bone matrix by forming a tight, ringlike zone of adhesion called the *sealing zone*, involving a specific interaction between the cell membrane and specific bone-matrix proteins (Fig 7-3).

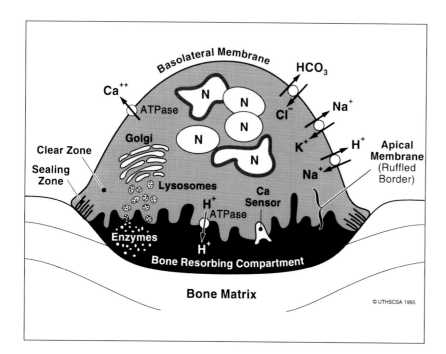

Fig 7-3 Longitudinal section through an activated osteoclast. Note the sealing zone, which delimits the bone-resorbing compartment along the apical membrane.

The space contained inside this ring of attachment and between the osteoclast and the bone matrix constitutes the bone-resorbing compartment. The osteoclast synthesizes several proteolytic enzymes, which are then vectorially transported and secreted into this extracellular bone-resorbing compartment. Simultaneously, the osteoclast lowers the pH of this compartment by extruding protons across its apical membrane (facing the bone matrix). The concerted action of the enzymes and the low pH in the bone-resorbing compartment lead to the dissolution of the mineral phase and digestion of the organic phase of the extracellular bone matrix. After resorbing to a certain depth, determined by mechanisms that remain to be elucidated, the osteoclast detaches and moves along the bone surface before reattaching and forming another resorption pit.

From this brief description, it is apparent that the activated osteoclast is a morphologically and functionally polarized cell, with one pole facing the bone matrix, toward which most of the secretion is targeted (the apical pole), and a pole facing the soft tissues in the local microenvironment (bone marrow or periosteum), which provides mostly regulatory functions (the basolateral pole).

The osteoclast is usually found singly or in low numbers at any one given time and site, characteristically at the interface between soft and calcified tissues, in an area where the bone matrix is fully mineralized. It is usually found on the periosteal surface, although most of the remodeling occurs along the endosteum. The osteoclast is easily characterized by its size, 50 to 100 μm, its multinucleation (usually 2 to 10 nuclei), and its presence within resorption lacuna at the calcified matrix–bone marrow in-

terface. The apical area of the cell, closest to the matrix, is characterized by a densely stained attachment apparatus and a lightly stained, highly vacuolated, and striated central area called the *ruffled border*. At the ultrastructural level, morphologic polarity of the cell is evident[36,37] (see Fig 7-3). The peripheral region of the apical membrane is tightly juxtaposed to the matrix (the sealing zone).[38] In the adjacent cytoplasm, an organelle-free area is found, called the *clear zone*, which is characteristically enriched in contractile protein. The osteoclast has an enlarged, well-developed Golgi apparatus that is actively engaged in biosynthesis and secretion of proteins.[37]

Activity of Osteoclasts

The structural features of the osteoclast that have been described above each reflect a specific function. The clear zone and the sealing zone are responsible for the attachment of the osteoclast to the bone matrix; the ruffled border corresponds to the area of ion transport and protein secretion; and the basolateral membrane is a major site for receipt and integration of regulatory signals.

Inside the osteoclast, an extensive cytoskeleton, composed of actin filaments and various actin-binding proteins, can be observed. This is involved in osteoclast migration and adhesion to bone and other surfaces. It has been reported that osteoclasts migrating across a surface (bone or glass) display a pattern characteristic of actin filaments.[39]

The cytoskeletal complex of the clear zone is necessary for anchoring and stabilizing the osteoclast on the bone surface. However, because the cytoskeletal complex is inside the cells, this complex is not directly responsible for that interaction. This role is filled by integral membrane proteins whose cytoplasmic domains interact with the cytoskeleton and whose extracellular domains interact with the appropriate bone-matrix proteins. These transmembrane proteins are members of the integrin family of adhesion molecules, which mediate cell-substratum and cell-cell interactions.[40] When osteoclasts are either activated or inhibited, rapid and dramatic changes occur in the cytoskeleton and attachment structures, further demonstrating the functional importance of these structures in bone resorption. Moreover, some of these changes might be associated with the regulation of the osteoclast's intracellular calcium level and/or pH.[41] Hence, the cytoskeleton and integral membrane receptors of the integrin family play essential roles in osteoclast motility, in specific attachment to the bone surface, in establishing the seal at the periphery of the extracellular bone-resorbing compartment, and in regulating the activity of the osteoclast.

The osteoclast is actively engaged in the synthesis of lysosomal enzymes that proceed through the Golgi and are transported from the trans-Golgi region to the ruffled-border apical membrane in coated transport vesicles. These transport vesicles then fuse exclusively with the ruffled border's plasma membrane and release their contents into the bone-resorbing compartment.[36,37] The enzymes secreted by the osteoclast into the bone-resorbing compartment participate in the degradation of the extracellular matrix and include acid phosphatase, aryl-sulfatase, β-glucuronidase, and several cysteine proteinases such as cathepsins B and L.[42] The major importance of these proteolytic enzymes is that they are capable of degrading helical collagen in an acidic environment.[43] Recently, it has also been found that tissue-plasminogen activator,[44] as well as collagenase (matrix metalloproteinase-1),[45] are produced by osteoclasts, suggesting a role for these two proteinases in bone resorption. In addition to the secretion of enzymes and protons, osteoclasts, like other cells in the monocyte-macrophage lineage, synthesize and secrete lysozyme.[46]

Acidification of the extracellular bone-resorbing compartment has emerged as one of the most important features of osteoclast biology.[47,48] The proton pumps in the osteoclast allow for acidification of extracellular fluids. During bone resorption, osteoclast-mediated acidification is required for the dissolution of the mineral phase and the enzymatic degradation of the organic phase of the extracellular matrix.[36,49] The acidification process directly involves two components: the apical electrogenic proton pump itself and carbonic anhydrase II. Briefly, the protons transported by the H^+ ATPase across the apical membrane are generated in the cytoplasm by the reversible hydration of carbon dioxide to produce carbonic acid, which ionizes to form protons and bicarbonate.[50] In conclusion, bone resorption includes an initial phase characterized by acidification, which is required for the dissolution of the mineral phase, followed by a degradation phase involving cysteine proteinases, which degrade the bulk of the collagen present in the acidified bone-resorbing compartment.

In contrast, collagenase and metalloproteinase action occurs at a more neutral pH. Consequently, if these enzymes are involved in bone resorption, it is likely that they are activated by enzymes released by the osteoclast or by the low pH in the resorption compartment. Alternatively, they may function after displacement of the cell from its previous resorbing site and subsequent neutralization of pH.

There are several obvious reasons why calcium is of major importance in the regulation of osteoclast function. First, the cell's activity is directly and indirectly regulated by several calciotropic hormones that function in calcium homeostasis. Second, the osteoclast is probably exposed to the highest local calcium concentrations of any cell in the body due to the dissolution of hydroxyapatite crystals in the acidic microenvironment of the bone-resorbing compartment. Third, bone resorption by the osteoclast is the major mechanism whereby calcium is mobilized from the skeleton, maintaining the correct calcium concentration in the extracellular fluids of the body.

In recent years, it has been suggested that hormones and/or local factors activate osteoclasts to start bone resorption. When the calcium concentration in the bone-resorbing compartment reaches a threshold level, calcium sensors open a novel type of calcium channel.[51,52] The increase in intracellular Ca^{+2} causes the osteoclasts to become inactivated, leading to osteoclast detachment. This allows the mobilized extracellular calcium to diffuse into the extracellular fluids. Later, the osteoclasts reattach and go through a second cycle of resorbing activity. This scenario provides a logical explanation for the cyclic activity of the osteoclast, as well as the multilacunar nature of resorption sites seen in vivo and in vitro.

Factors Regulating Bone Formation

The formation of new bone involves two major steps: *(1)* the production of a new organic matrix by the osteoblasts and *(2)* the mineralization of that matrix. Agents that regulate bone formation act on the osteoblast to either increase or decrease replication of cells in the osteoblastic lineage or to modify the differentiated function of the osteoblast. As outlined above, bone formation is controlled by systemic hormones and local factors. For the most part, the local regulators of bone formation are growth factors that act directly on cells of the osteoblastic lineage. These local factors may affect their cell of origin or different cells, and thus act as either autocrine or paracrine factors, respectively.[53]

While systemic hormones are likely to have direct effects on the bone-forming cells, they frequently act by stimulating the production of local growth factors. Systemic hormones can regulate growth-factor activity by one or more of four different mechanisms: (1) by regulating factor synthesis, as well as release from cells; (2) if the factor is released from the cell in a latent form, its physiologic effect can be regulated by controlling when the factor becomes activated; (3) by regulating receptor binding; and (4) by regulating the production of a binding protein that stabilizes the factor and promotes its binding to the receptor. Because the production of a particular growth factor is not unique to any specific tissue, it has been postulated that systemic hormones may provide target tissue specificity for a growth factor.

Growth factors that regulate bone formation have some common features: they are polypeptides; they exert their activity by binding to specific receptors on the cell surface; they primarily act locally; they are natural products of cells; and they are multifunctional in that they can stimulate a wide variety of cellular activities. In cases such as periodontal regeneration, the combined effect of many growth factors is involved.[54]

This section addresses the more "classic" growth factors synthesized by connective-tissue cells and includes PDGF, IGF-1 and IGF-2, TGF-β1 and TGF-β2, FGF, heparin-binding growth factors (HBGF) 1 and 2, and bone morphogenetic proteins (BMPs).

Platelet-Derived Growth Factor

PDGF is a cationic, heparin-binding polypeptide with a molecular weight of approximately 30,000 d. The active growth factor consists of a disulfide-linked dimer, which is the product of two distinct genes, PDGF-A and PDGF-B.[55] Three isoforms exist: PDGF-AA, PDGF-AB, and PDGF-BB. The most biologically active form in skeletal tissues is PDGF-BB. PDGF is produced by osteoblasts,[56,57] but much of the PDGF found in bone is probably derived from serum and platelets.

PDGF stimulates DNA synthesis and cell replication in osteoblasts,[53] as well as increases bone-collagen synthesis and the rate of bone-matrix apposition.[58] In addition to its effect on bone formation, PDGF has also been reported to increase bone resorption and collagen degradation,[53] although the mechanism for these effects is not clear.

A PDGF receptor containing two subunits has been found. PDGF binds to one or both subunits and forms a complex as part of the receptor-activation process. Only recently has it been found that a PDGF receptor is present in osteoblasts.[59] While little is known about the regulation of PDGF-AA synthesis, there is some evidence suggesting that PDGF-AA activity is regulated at the level of receptor binding. PDGF-BB might be critical in wound healing or fracture repair, since it is released after platelet aggregation. It may also play an entirely different role in bone-cell physiology than that of PDGF-AA.

Heparin-Binding Growth Factors

HBGFs are members of a family of seven related heparin-binding proteins.[60] Acidic fibroblast growth factor (aFGF) and basic fibroblast growth factor (bFGF) are the two better-known forms of the HBGFs and were the first to be purified, sequenced, and cloned.

Bone matrix is a rich source of FGFs, and bovine skeletal cells, expressing the osteoblastic phenotype, secrete basic, as well as acidic, FGF.[61] Both FGFs have been shown to be mitogenic for bone cells and to enhance collagen and noncollagen protein synthesis in bone culture. In bone cells, FGF interacts with heparin, which enhances the effect of FGF on bone-cell replication. Therefore, FGFs, and HBGFs generally, have significant effects on bone-cell replication, but their specific function in bone-cell biology and their role as therapeutic agents need further study.

Insulin-like Growth Factors

IGFs are nonglycosylated polypeptides with molecular weights of approximately 7,500 d. There are two forms of IGF: IGF-1, initially termed somatomedin C, and IGF-2, initially termed multiplication-stimulating activity. IGF-1 appears to be the principal growth regulator in bone and cartilage. The liver is the major source of circulating IGF-1 and is the target tissue for growth hormone that regulates IGF-1 production. The role of systemic IGF-1 is not entirely clear, since most tissues synthesize small amounts of this growth factor. In connective tissues, IGF-1 and IGF-2 are among the most abundant growth factors present[62] and are synthesized by most cell types present in skeletal tissue, including bone fibroblasts and osteoblasts.[63] Therefore, IGFs probably act as either paracrine or autocrine regulators of bone formation. Production of IGFs is increased by hormones such as growth hormone, estradiol, and local factors like PGE_2,[62] whereas production is inhibited by cortisol. Both forms of IGF increase preosteoblastic cell replication, have a stimulatory effect on osteoblastic collagen synthesis and bone-matrix apposition,[64] and decrease the degradation of collagen. IGFs play a major role in the maintenance of bone mass. Osteoblasts express both the IGF-β type 1 and IGF-β type 2 receptors,[65] and it has been suggested that the type 1 receptor mediates the effect of IGF on bone formation. IGF is probably one of the most important regulators of bone mass, because it is synthesized by bone cells and is present in substantial concentrations in the bone.

IGF-binding proteins modulate the effects of the IGFs on osteoblasts. Secreted IGF-binding proteins may be partitioned into separate compartments: proteins that are secreted into the interstitial fluid, proteins that remain cell associated, and proteins that are matrix bound.[66] These proteins act in multiple ways: by preventing binding of IGF to its receptors, by presenting the growth factor to its receptor, and by retaining IGF in the pericellular matrix. Thus, modulation of the IGF-binding proteins by growth factors, hormones, and cytokines fine-tunes the action of this important class of regulatory molecules in bone.[67]

Transforming Growth Factor β

TGFs are polypeptides that have been isolated from a variety of normal and malignant tissues. They were initially identified by their ability to stimulate in non-neoplastic cells what appears to be a growth habit characteristic of malignant cells. TGF-α is not synthesized by bone cells, but because it stimulates bone resorption, it may play a role in the development of hypercalcemia in some forms of malignancy. TGF-β is a polypeptide with an approximate molecular weight of 25,000 d that is synthesized by skeletal cells. It is one of the most abundant growth factors in bone matrix.[68] At present, several isoforms, as well as a number of polypeptides, have been identified that show significant homology with TGF-β and form the TGF-β superfamily of polypeptides. Among them are the bone morphogenetic proteins, the activins, and the inhibins. Activin and TGF-β have similar stimulatory effects on bone formation.[69]

This distribution of the TGF-β isoforms varies between tissues.[70] TGF-β1, TGF-β2, and TGF-β3 are detected at sites of endochondral and intramembranous ossification. At sites of endochondral bone formation, TGF-β1 is found in the proliferating cell zone and the prehypertrophic cell zone. TGF-β2 is distributed throughout the growth plate, but levels are highest in hypertrophic and calcifying cartilage. TGF-β3 is in the proliferating cell zone and hypertrophic cell zone. It is interesting to note that TGF-β3 is the most widely distributed form found in intramembranous bone; TGF-β1 and TGF-β2 are found primarily at sites where mineralization is occurring.

TGF-β is synthesized by osteoblasts in inactive (latent) form. A major step regulating TGF-β activity involves its conversion to a biologically active peptide; this can be accomplished in vivo and in vitro by brief acidification or proteolytic cleavage. TGF-β has been shown to stimulate preosteoblastic cell replication, osteoblastic collagen synthesis,[71] and bone-matrix apposition.

Bone cells have three discrete TGF-β receptors. The effects of TGF-β on bone-cell function can be regulated by altering the binding of the growth factor to its receptors.[69] Treatment with glucocorticoids decreases the effect of TGF-β on DNA and collagen synthesis in bone cells. The mechanism of this action seems to be related to shifting of TGF-β binding away from active receptors and toward the complex.[69]

In addition to its direct effect on bone-cell function, TGF-β has important interactions with other growth factors. TGF-β messenger RNA levels are increased by FGF, whereas TGF-β decreases PDGF-AA binding to its bone-cell receptor. TGF-β has been shown to initiate and regulate critical events during fracture repair.[72] Furthermore, cells within the fracture callus have been shown to express TGF-β messenger RNA, and this factor may be induced and act at the local level during fracture healing.

Bone Morphogenetic Proteins

During embryogenesis, new bone formation occurs through a complex series of cellular interactions. Most bones of the body initially go through a phase of cartilage formation and calcification, and then replacement by bone in a process known as *endochondral bone formation*. It is interesting to note that bone repair in adults is very similar to this process. During bone repair and bone-matrix destruction, many growth factors are released that affect the healing process. One of them, BMP, is a unique factor with osteoinductive activity. Since its original discovery, it has been found that what was originally believed to be one protein actually belongs to a family of proteins consisting of at least 15 different members (BMP-1 through BMP-15).

The implantation of BMP in ectopic sites, as well as in bone, induces the production of new bone through an endochondral pathway. BMP has a direct effect on osteoblasts by stimulating the differentiation of osteoblast precursor cells into more mature osteoblasts. BMP has also been shown to stimulate collagen production by mature osteoblasts. In the endochondral pathway, BMP induces chondrocyte differentiation and matrix mineralization.

Factors Regulating Bone Resorption

In recent years, it has become increasingly clear that many of the cellular events involved in bone resorption are modulated by a group of local factors (osteotropic cytokines), which have extremely potent effects on bone cells in both in vitro and in vivo systems. Many of the effects of local factors on bone resorption appear to overlap and are seemingly redundant; for example, IL-1, TNF-α, and lymphotoxin appear to affect bone resorption similarly. As more is learned about the mechanism of bone resorption, the role of each factor in the process will become clearer.

Cytokine regulation is likely to be more important for trabecular bone than for cortical bone, because trabecular bone is closer to the marrow, which is a rich source of cytokines. Many of the potent osteotropic cytokines, such as IL-1, IL-6, TNF-α, and TGF-β, mediate a multiplicity of effects in the body in addition to their effects on bone cells. However, there are other cytokines, such as BMP, that have relatively specific effects on bone cells. Most of the osteotropic cytokines, such as IL-1, TNF, lymphotoxin, and IL-6, are clearly products of immune cells that are present in regions where bone modeling is actively occurring. However, stromal cells, as well as bone cells, also produce these factors.[73] The production of cytokines by osteoblasts is regulated by bacteria, lipopolysaccharide, other cytokines, and different hormones (estrogen and steroids). It has also been observed that cytokines and hormones can have synergistic effects on bone resorption. For example, the effect of IL-1 together with PTH on bone resorption is greater than the additive effects of either IL-1 or PTH alone.[74]

The hypothesis that local factors play a major role in regulating bone remodeling has been strengthened by data that directly implicate at least one of these cytokines in normal osteoclastic bone resorption. In mice with the op/op variant of osteopetrosis, there is a defect in the region coding for CSF of the macrophage series (CSF-M), resulting in decreased CSF-M production. In this variant, the mice do not form functional osteoclasts. As a result, they do not form marrow cavities properly, and they develop osteopetrosis. If the mice are treated with CSF-M, the disease is reversed.[75]

Cytokines appear to play a major role in bone pathology. Solid tumors and carcinomas have been shown to produce IL-1.[76] Cytokines have also been associated with the bone destruction seen in chronic inflammatory conditions, such as rheumatoid arthritis and periodontal disease. The observed increase in cytokines during these diseases has been suggested as the cause of increased localized osteolytic bone destruction.

Interleukin 1

IL-1 is a powerful and potent bone-resorbing cytokine.[77] It has been found that IL-1α and IL-1β are equally potent in stimulating bone resorption and probably exert their effects on bone-resorbing cells in several ways. They stimu-late proliferation of precursor cells, but also probably act indirectly on mature cells to stimulate bone resorption.[78] The effects of IL-1 probably occur by two mechanisms. One mechanism is the stimulation of the production and release of PGE$_2$, which in turn stimulates bone resorption. The second mechanism involves the direct action of IL-1 on the osteoclast, which is independent of prostaglandin synthesis, through an 80,000-d receptor.

IL-1 has complex and apparently paradoxical effects on bone formation. The continued presence of IL-1 inhibits bone formation in vivo and in vitro.[79,80] IL-1 appears to stimulate proliferation of cells at early stages of differentiation in the osteoblast lineage, but it inhibits functions characteristic of the fully differentiated state. In contrast, transient exposure to IL-1 has been shown to stimulate bone formation by osteoblasts.

Interleukin 6

In some experimental models, IL-6 appears to have no effects on bone resorption. However, in others,[81] it stimulates bone resorption. IL-6 is also responsible for the formation of cells with an osteoclastic phenotype. Bone cells also have the ability to produce IL-6, which seems to be greater when the stimulus is by another cytokine.

Tumor Necrosis Factor and Lymphotoxin

Lymphotoxin and TNF are two closely related cytokines that have similar effects on bone cells. They are both multifunctional cytokines produced by activated lymphocytes, and they share the same receptor. Their major effect on bone is to stimulate osteoclastic bone resorption.[82] It has been suggested that part of the effect of TNF is mediated by PGE$_2$, as well as by IL-6. TNF also affects cells with osteoblast phenotypes, inhibiting differentiated function and stimulating cell proliferation. Production of TNF in some tumors, like squamous cell carcinomas, may be responsible for paraneoplastic syndromes.

Gamma Interferon

Gamma interferon (IFN-γ) is a multifunctional cytokine that in most biologic systems has effects similar to those of TNF or IL-1. However, it has an effect on bone resorption that is opposite that of IL-1 and TNF. IFN-γ is more effective in inhibiting IL-1β– or TNF-induced bone resorption than are systemic hormones like PTH or 1,25-(OH)$_2$D$_3$. Further, it has been found in long-term marrow cell cultures that IFN-γ inhibits the formation of cells with the osteoclast phenotype.

Colony-Stimulating Factors

CSFs have the ability to stimulate the differentiation of osteoclast precursors into mature osteoclasts. A number of human and animal tumors are associated with granulocytosis in which increased production of CSFs is involved. In many of these tumors, hypercalcemia is associated with increased bone resorption.

It is possible that CSFs mediate their effects on osteoclast formation indirectly. For example, early studies showed that CSF stimulates IL-1 production, which stimulates prostaglandin synthesis.

Prostaglandins and Other Arachidonic Acid Metabolites

A number of arachidonic acid metabolites act as modulators of bone-cell function. These factors are produced by immune, marrow, and bone cells. Prostaglandins of the E series were some of the first-described and best-tested stimulators of osteoclastic bone resorption. PGEs are slow-acting, but powerful, mediators of bone resorption, and they affect both active mature osteoclasts and differentiated osteoclast precursors. The effect of PGE is local and has been shown to mediate the effects of other factors, such as EGF and TGF-β. PGE is produced by osteoblasts and affects not just bone resorption but bone formation as well. In vitro and in vivo studies have found that high doses of PGE are inhibitory, while low doses stimulate bone formation. However, in vivo studies have shown that PGE increases periosteal bone formation.[83] There have also been reports that other arachidonic acid metabolites stimulate bone resorption as well. Arachidonic acid can be metabolized by an alternative enzyme system, 5-lipoxygenase, which also produces metabolites capable of stimulating bone resorption.

Regulation of Bone by Systemic Hormones

Parathyroid Hormone

It has been known for more than 70 years that PTH affects bone-cell function, may alter bone remodeling, and causes bone loss. It is now apparent that PTH acts on both bone-resorbing cells and bone-forming cells. The net effect of the hormone depends on whether it is administered continuously or intermittently. When administered continuously, it increases osteoclastic bone resorption and suppresses bone formation. However, when administered in low doses intermittently, its major effect is to stimulate bone formation, a response that has been called the *anabolic effect of PTH*.

PTH stimulates osteoclasts to resorb bone. In patients with primary hyperparathyroidism, there is a profound loss of bone associated with increased osteoclastic bone resorption (a disease referred to as *osteitis fibrosa cystica*). In organ cultures, PTH increases osteoclast activity, with resultant degradation of bone matrix and release of bone mineral.[84] In culture, parathyroid hormone produces a prolonged period of bone resorption after only 4 to 6 hours of treatment, while other agents, such as PGE_2 or $1,25\text{-}(OH)_2D_3$, require a longer period of incubation. These phenomena can be explained by the fact that PTH activates mature osteoclasts to resorb bone, whereas other agents exert their effects by increasing the formation of new osteoclasts.

In the in vivo situation, bone cells are never exposed to PTH alone, and other local factors and hormones are always present and interact with PTH. PTH probably acts at multiple points in the osteoclast lineage. It clearly stimulates mature, multinucleated osteoclasts to form ruffled borders and resorb bone. In addition, it has effects on cells earlier in the osteoclast lineage. However, the precise molecular mechanisms by which PTH exerts its effects on these cells are still not known. The effect of PTH on osteoclast precursors is combined with direct effects on the cell itself, with an indirect effect of regulating other cells to produce local factors that influence the osteoclast precursor cells, such as regulating cells of the granulocyte-macrophage type, to produce granulocyte-monocyte–colony-stimulating factor.

The effect of PTH on mature osteoclasts is also indirect because osteoclasts will not resorb bone unless osteoblasts are present, suggesting that PTH may stimulate osteoclastic bone resorption by interacting with cells in the osteoblast lineage.

PTH responsiveness is used as one of the criteria for characterizing cells of the osteoblast lineage. The response of osteoblasts to PTH includes an increase in adenylate cyclase activity, changes in proliferation, alkaline phosphatase activity, and production of type I collagen. The effect of PTH depends on its concentration. At low concentrations the effect is anabolic, and at high concentrations the effect is catabolic.[85] One way PTH enhances bone turnover or remodeling in vivo is by promoting the production of coupling factors.[27]

The mechanisms used by cells of the osteoblast phenotype to communicate with osteoclasts are still not known, but they may involve the production of soluble mediators. It has been suggested that osteoblasts may prepare the bone surface for osteoclastic bone resorption by producing proteolytic enzymes. However, this theory is questionable.

The effects of PTH on bone-forming and bone-resorbing cells are complex. Although much is known regarding the expression of PTH and regulation of PTH synthesis and secretion in the parathyroid cell, there is still much to be learned about the mechanisms by which PTH stimulates osteoclasts and osteoblasts and the relationship between these effects and maintenance of normal bone volume and control of calcium homeostasis.

1,25-Dihydroxyvitamin D₃

The active metabolites of vitamin D_3 have complex effects on calcium homeostasis and bone regulation. 1,25-$(OH)_2D_3$ and 24,25-$(OH)_2D_3$ are active metabolites of vitamin D that have been shown to directly affect bone-cell function. 1,25-$(OH)_2D_3$ has a catabolic effect on bone, while 24,25-$(OH)_2D_3$ has an anabolic effect. Both hormones promote the absorption of calcium and phosphate from the gut. 1,25-$(OH)_2D_3$ also stimulates osteoclastic bone resorption in vitro and in vivo. In the absence of 1,25-$(OH)_2D_3$ there is a failure of mineralization. This leads to rickets in children and osteomalacia in adults.

A nuclear receptor for 1,25-$(OH)_2D_3$ has been identified and characterized.[86] More recently, it has become clear that osteoblasts also possess membrane receptors for 1,25-$(OH)_2D_3$ that are distinct from the nuclear vitamin D receptor. The membrane receptor mediates rapid effects of the hormone on the cell, such as Ca^{++} ion flux and activation of the protein kinase C signal transduction pathway. The membrane receptor also mediates nuclear events resulting in gene transcription. There is now evidence from other systems that some of the effects of the membrane receptor–mediated pathway modulate the classic nuclear receptor–mediated regulation of gene transcription. The overall effect of 1,25-$(OH)_2D_3$ on osteoblasts is to decrease cell proliferation and stimulate osteoblast differentiation. However, excess 1,25-$(OH)_2D_3$ prevents terminal differentiation of the osteoblast, preventing mineralization.

The effect of 1,25-$(OH)_2D_3$ on osteoclastic bone resorption is different from that of other well-known bone-resorbing factors. 1,25-$(OH)_2D_3$ has a very slow onset of action, with a shallow dose-response curve. 1,25-$(OH)_2D_3$ increases both osteoclast number and activity, with an increase in ruffled-border size and clear-zone volume. Mature osteoclasts do not have nuclear receptors for 1,25-$(OH)_2D_3$; thus, the effects of this hormone on mature osteoclasts are most likely mediated indirectly through other cells.[87] The major effect of 1,25-$(OH)_2D_3$ on osteoclastic bone resorption may be to stimulate the fusion or differentiation of committed osteoclast progenitors to form mature cells. Use of 1,25-$(OH)_2D_3$ to treat infants with malignant osteopetrosis demonstrates that failure to form competent osteoclasts can be successfully treated. 1,25-$(OH)_2D_3$ also has other effects on bone cells that may be indirect.[88] For example, 1,25-$(OH)_2D_3$ influences and modulates cytokine production by immune cells. Given the potency of many cytokines as regulators of osteoclast function, the importance of 1,25-$(OH)_2D_3$ for osteoclastic bone resorption is probably great.

Calcitonin

Although calcitonin has been known for 30 years, there is little insight into its physiologic role in calcium homeostasis or its importance in bone remodeling. Friedman et al[89] demonstrated that calcitonin was able to inhibit osteoclastic bone resorption. The effect of calcitonin on osteoclasts is mediated through cAMP. Calcitonin decreases osteoclast activity, as can be seen within minutes after treatment by decreases in ruffled-border size and clear zone.[90] Other studies show that calcitonin inhibits the formation of new osteoclasts and may cause the separation of multinucleated osteoclasts into mononuclear cells.

The effects of calcitonin on bone resorption are short-lived, however. Osteoclasts eventually lose their responsiveness to calcitonin after continuous exposure, a phenomenon referred to as *escape*.[91] The molecular mechanism for escape has never been clearly demonstrated. One possible explanation for this phenomenon involves a decrease in receptor number after long periods of exposure. Another possible explanation is the emergence of a second population of osteoclasts that is not responsive to calcitonin.[92] Because calcitonin has only a transient effect on bone resorption, there has been considerable speculation as to whether it has an important role in calcium homeostasis. Today, it is believed that it inhibits bone resorption transiently when bone turnover is not needed for calcium homeostasis (as after a meal rich in calcium). A receptor for calcitonin has been identified in osteoclasts and has been shown to directly mediate the effect of calcitonin on these cells.[93]

Estrogens

Estrogen clearly inhibits the increase in bone resorption associated with menopause. Following estrogen withdrawal, an initial increase in bone turnover can be observed. Later, bone resorption occurs faster than bone formation, with a net effect of bone loss. Treatment with estrogen prevents these effects.[94,95]

The effects of estrogen in bone are mediated both directly by the action of the hormone on bone cells and indirectly by regulating nonbone cells to release factors that affect bone cells, such as growth hormone. The effects of estrogen on osteoclasts are in part direct and in part mediated through osteoblasts. The direct effect of estrogen is mediated by specific receptors found in cells of the osteoblast[96] and osteoclast[97] lineages. This results in increased expression of growth factors like IGF-1 and TGF-β and of cytokines. Estrogen inhibits prostaglandin production by bone cells, which can affect bone remodeling as well.

It is also possible that estrogen has a prolonged effect in stimulating bone formation. Low doses of estrogen increase skeletal growth in children, and it is clear that there is a marked increase in endosteal bone formation in rodents and birds treated with estrogens. Estrogen has been shown to enhance the expression of TGF-β and IGF-1 in cells with the osteoblast phenotype.[96,98] Studies have also shown that estrogen is produced by osteoblasts by the action of aromatase on androgen.[99] Moreover, production is regulated by glucocorticoid and 1,25-$(OH)_2D_3$.[100] This suggests that estrogen may also function as a local mediator of osteoblast function. Thus, the major effect of estrogen may be to inhibit osteoclastic bone resorption, but it may also have the additional effect of stimulating bone formation.

Androgen's effect on osteoclastic bone resorption is probably similar to estrogen's. Hypogonadal or castrated males have decreased bone mass associated with increased bone resorption.

Summary

Bone is a very active organ. In the adult, it is continuously renewed and capable of complete repair after injury. Both of these processes involve opposing events—the dissolution of existing mineral content with resorption of the extracellular matrix, and the formation of a new matrix. Distinct cell lineages are responsible for bone resorption and formation. The osteoclast lineage is of hematopoietic origin and includes the differentiated multinucleated osteoclast, which is the primary bone-resorbing cell. The osteoblast, which forms bone matrix, appears to originate from a stromal cell within the bone-marrow cavity. Mechanisms that couple osteoclastic and osteoblastic activities must exist within the bone. The process of bone resorption and bone formation are very carefully regulated by both systemic hormones and local factors. Changes in the normal balance of bone modeling and remodeling will cause diseases such as periodontal disease. In periodontal disease, the response of bone to local factors, produced by the inflammatory process, changes the bone-remodeling balance, with a net effect of bone resorption and loss of attachment.

Periodontal tissue can also repair and regenerate itself. Periodontal regeneration involves the reconstruction of lost supporting tissues, including alveolar bone, cementum, periodontal ligament, and gingival attachment. This process is regulated by the local production of growth factors. These factors stimulate the cellular events of regeneration, which potentially consist of cell chemotaxis, proliferation, differentiation, and formation of extracellular matrix, and will lead to new bone formation and new attachment.

Acknowledgments

This work was supported by United States NIH grants DE 05937 and DE 08603 and the Center for the Enhancement of the Biology/Biomaterials Interface at the University of Texas Health Science Center at San Antonio. The authors appreciate the assistance of Sandra Messier in the preparation of this manuscript.

References

1. Parfitt AM. The physiologic and clinical significance of bone histomorphometric data. In: Recker RR (ed). Bone Histomorphometry: Techniques and Interpretation. Boca Raton, FL: CRC Press, 1983:143–223.
2. Frost HM. Dynamics of bone remodeling. In: Frost HM (ed). Bone Biodynamics. Boston: Little, Brown, 1964:315–333.
3. Eriksen EF, Mosekilde L, Melsen F. Trabecular bone remodeling and balance in primary hyperparathyroidism. Bone 1986;7: 213–221.
4. Charles P, Eriksen EF, Mosekilde L, et al. Bone turnover and balance evaluated by a combined calcium balance and calcium-47 kinetic study and dynamic histomorphometry. Metabolism 1987;36:1118–1124.
5. Parfitt AM. The coupling of bone formation to bone resorption: A critical analysis of the concept and of its relevance to the pathogenesis of osteoporosis. Metab Bone Dis Relat Res 1982; 4:1–6.
6. Pilbeam CC, Klein-Nulend J, Raisz LG. Inhibition by 17β-estradiol of PTH-stimulated resorption and prostaglandin production in cultured neonatal mouse calvariae. Biochem Biophys Res Commun 1989;163:1319–1324.
7. Coupron P, Meunier PB, Bressot C, Giroux JM. Amount of bone iliac crest biopsy: Significance of the trabecular bone volume: Its value in normal and in pathological conditions. In: Meunier PJ (ed). Bone Histomorphometrie, Second International Workshop. Paris: Armour Montagu, 1977:39.
8. Melsen F, Mosekilde L. Tetracycline double-labeling of iliac trabecular bone in 41 normal adults. Calcif Tissue Res 1978;26: 99–102.
9. Sedlin ED. The ratio of cortical area to total cross section area in rib diaphysis. Clin Orthop 1964;36:161–168.
10. Broulik P, Kragstrup J, Mosekilde L, Melsen F. Osteon cross sectional size in the iliac crest: Variations in normals and patients with osteoporosis, hyperparathyroidism, acromegaly, hypothyroidism and treated epilepsia. Acta Pathol Microbiol Immunol Scand [A] 1982;90:339–344.
11. Mosekilde L. Iliac crest trabecular bone volume as predictor for vertebral compressive strength, ash density and trabecular bone volume in normal individuals. Bone 1988;9:195–199.

12. Vesterby A, Gundersen HJG, Melsen F, Mosekilde L. Marrow space star volume in iliac crest decreases in osteoporotic patients after continuous treatment with fluoride, calcium and vitamin D2 for five years. Bone 1991;12:33–37.

13. Doty SB. Morphological evidence of intercellular junctions between bone cells. Calcif Tissue Int 1981;33:509–512.

14. Sela J, Schwartz Z, Swain L, et al. Extracellular matrix vesicles in endochondral bone development and in healing after injury. Cells and Matrix 1992;2:153–161.

15. Friedenstein AJ. Precursor cells of mechanocytes. Int Rev Cytol 1976;47:327–359.

16. Ash P, Loutit JF, Townsend KMS. Osteoclasts derive from haematopoietic stem cells according to marker, giant lysosomes of beige mice. Clin Orthop 1981;155:249–258.

17. Caplan AI, Boyan BD. Endochondral bone formation: The lineage cascade. In: Hall B (ed). Bone. Boca Raton, FL: CRC Press, 1994:1–46.

18. Stein GS, Lian JB, Gerstenfeld LG, et al. The onset and progression of osteoblast differentiation is functionally related to cellular proliferation. Connect Tissue Res 1989;20:3–13.

19. Cole WG. Osteogenesis imperfecta. Baillieres Clin Endocrinol Metab 1988;2:243–265.

20. Gehron-Robey P. The biochemistry of the bone. Endocrinol Metab Clin North Am 1989;18:858–902.

21. Aarden EM, Burger EH, Nijweide PJ. Function of osteocytes in bone. J Cell Biochem 1994;55:287–299.

22. Klein-Nulend J, van der Plas A, Semeins CM, et al. Sensitivity of osteocytes to biomechanical stress in vitro. FASEB J 1995;9: 441–445.

23. Nijweide PJ, Burger EH, Klein-Nulend J, van der Plas A. The osteocyte. In: Bilezikian JP, Raisz LG, Rodan GA (eds). Principles of Bone Biology. San Diego, CA: Academic Press, 1996:115–126.

24. Bonewald LF. Establishment and characterization of an osteocyte-like cell line, MLO-Y4. J Bone Miner Metab 1999;17:61–65.

25. Partridge NC, Alcorn D, Michelangeli VP, et al. Functional properties of hormonally responsive cultured normal and malignant rat osteoblastic cells. Endocrinology 1981;108: 213–219.

26. Silve CM, Hradek GT, Jones AL, Arnaud CD. Parathyroid hormone receptor in intact embryonic chicken bone: Characterization and cellular location. J Cell Biol 1982;94:379–386.

27. Howard GA, Bottemiller BL, Turner RT, et al. Parathyroid hormone stimulates bone formation and resorption in organ culture: Evidence for a coupling mechanism. Proc Natl Acad Sci USA 1981;78:3204–3208.

28. Udagawa N, Takahashi N, Jimi E, et al. Osteoblasts/stromal cells stimulate osteoclast activation through expression of osteoclast differentiation factor/RANKL but not macrophage colony-stimulating factor: Receptor activator of NF-kappa B ligand. Bone 1999;25:517–523.

29. Hofbauer LC, Khosla S, Dunstan CR, et al. The roles of osteoprotegerin and osteoprotegerin ligand in the paracrine regulation of bone resorption. J Bone Miner Res 2000;15:2–12.

30. Yasuda H, Shima N, Nakagawa N, et al. Osteoclast differentiation factor is a ligand for osteoprotegerin/osteoclastogenesis-inhibitory factor and is identical to TRANCE/RANKL. Proc Natl Acad Sci USA 1998;95:3597–3602.

31. Zambonin-Zallone A, Teti A, Primavera MV. Isolated osteoclasts in primary culture: First observations on structure and survival in culture media. Anat Embryol (Berl) 1982;165:405–413.

32. Osdoby P, Martini MC, Caplan AI. Isolated osteoclasts and their presumed progenitor cells, monocytes, in culture. J Exp Zool 1982;224:331–344.

33. Udagawa N, Takahashi N, Akatsu T, et al. Origin of osteoclasts: Mature monocytes and macrophages are capable of differentiating into osteoclasts under a suitable microenvironment prepared by bone marrow-derived stromal cells. Proc Natl Acad Sci USA 1990;87:7260–7264.

34. Menaa C, Kurihara N, Roodman GD. CFU-GM–derived cells form osteoclasts at a very high efficiency. Biochem Biophys Res Commun 2000;267:943–946.

35. Uy HL, Dallas M, Calland JW, et al. Use of an in vivo model to determine the effects of interleukin-1 on cells at different stages in the osteoclast lineage. J Bone Miner Res 1995;10:295–301.

36. Baron R, Neff L, Louvard D, Courtov PJ. Cell-mediated extracellular acidification and bone resorption: Evidence for a low pH in resorbing lacunae and localization of a 100-kDa lysosomal membrane protein at the osteoclast ruffled border. J Cell Biol 1985;101:2210–2222.

37. Baron R, Neff L, Brown W, et al. Polarized secretion of lysosomal enzymes: Co-distribution of cation-independent mannose-6-phosphate receptors and lysosomal enzymes in the osteoclast exocytic pathway. J Cell Biol 1988;106:1863–1872.

38. Schenk R, Spiro D, Wiener J. Cartilage resorption in tibial epiphyseal plate of growing rats. J Cell Biol 1967;34:275–291.

39. Lakkakorpi P, Tuukkanen J, Hentunen T, et al. Organization of osteoclast microfilaments during the attachment to bone surface in vitro. J Bone Miner Res 1989;4:817–825.

40. Hynes RO. Integrins: A family of cell-surface receptors. Cell 1987;48:549–554.

41. Teti A, Marchisio PC, Zambonin-Zallone A. Clear zone in osteoclast function: Role of podosomes in regulation of bone-resorbing activity. Am J Physiol 1991;261:C1–C7.

42. Delaisse JM, Ledent P, Vaes G. Collagenolytic cysteine proteinases of bone tissue. Biochem J 1991;279:167–174.

43. Delaisse JM, Vaes G. Mechanism of mineral solubilization and matrix degradation in osteoblastic bone resorption. In: Rifkin BR, Gay CV (eds). The Biology and Physiology of the Osteoclast. Boca Raton, FL: CRC Press, 1992:328–337.

44. Grills BL, Gallagher JA, Allan EH, et al. Identification of plasminogen activator in osteoclasts. J Bone Miner Res 1990;5: 499–505.

45. Delaisse JM, Eeckhout Y, Neff L, et al. Procollagenase (matrix metalloproteinase 1) is present in rodent osteoclasts and in the underlying bone-resorbing compartment. J Cell Sci 1993;106: 1071–1082.

46. Hilliard TJ, Meadows G, Kahn AJ. Lysozyme synthesis in osteoclasts. J Bone Miner Res 1990;5:1217–1222.

47. Baron R. Molecular mechanisms of bone resorption by the osteoclast. Anat Rec 1989;224:317–324.

48. Arnett TR, Dempster DW. The effect of pH on bone resorption by rat osteoclasts in vitro. Endocrinology 1986;119:119–124.

49. Blair HC, Teitelbaum SL, Ghiselli R, Gluck S. Osteoclastic bone resorption by a polarized vacuolar proton pump. Science 1989; 245:855–857.

50. Gay CV, Mueller WJ. Carbonic anhydrase and osteoclasts: Localization by labelled inhibitor autoradiography. Science 1974; 183:432–434.

51. Zaidi M. "Calcium receptors" on eukaryotic cells with special reference to the osteoclast. Biosci Rep 1991;10:493–507.

52. Miyauchi A, Hruska KA, Greenfield EM, et al. Osteoclast cytosolic calcium, regulated by voltage-gated calcium channels and extracellular calcium, controls podosome assembly and bone resorption. J Cell Biol 1990;111:2543–2552.

53. Canalis E, McCarthy TL, Centrella M. Effects of platelet-derived growth factor on bone formation in vitro. J Cell Physiol 1989; 140:530–537.

54. Yu X, Antoniades HN, Graves DT. Expression of monocyte chemoattractant protein 1 in human inflamed gingival tissues. Infect Immunol 1993;61:4622–4628.

55. Heldin CH, Westermark B. PDGF-like growth factors in autocrine stimulation of growth. J Cell Physiol 1987;5(suppl):31–34.

56. Graves DT, Valentin-Opran A, Delgado R, et al. The potential role of platelet-derived growth factor as an autocrine or paracrine factor for human bone cells. Connect Tissue Res 1989;23:209–218.

57. Centrella M, McCarthy TL, Ladd C, Canalis E. Expression of platelet-derived growth factor (PDGF) and regulation of PDGF binding are both isoform specific in osteoblast-enriched cultures from fetal rat bone. J Bone Miner Res 1990;5(suppl 2):S86.

58. Pfeilschifter J, Oechsner M, Naumann A, et al. Stimulation of bone matrix apposition in vitro by local growth factors: A comparison between insulin-like growth factor I, platelet-derived growth factor, and transforming growth factor-beta. Endocrinology 1990;127:69–75.

59. Centrella M, Canalis E. Relative effects of hetero- and homodimeric isoforms of platelet-derived growth factors in fetal rat bone cells. In: Cohn DV, Glorieux FH, Martin TJ (eds). Calcium Regulation and Bone Metabolism, 10. Basic and Clinical Aspects. Amsterdam: Elsevier, 1990:324–329.

60. Burgess WH, Maciag TL. The heparin-binding (fibroblast) growth factor family of proteins. Annu Rev Biochem 1989;58:575–606.

61. Globus RK, Plouet J, Gospodarowicz D. Cultured bovine bone cells synthesize basic fibroblast growth factor and store it in their extracellular matrix. Endocrinology 1989;124:1539–1547.

62. Canalis E, McCarthy TL, Centrella M. Isolation and characterization of insulin-like growth factor I (somatomedin C) from cultures of fetal rat calvariae. Endocrinology 1988;122:22–27.

63. McCarthy TL, Centrella M, Canalis E. Cyclic AMP induces insulin-like growth factor I synthesis in osteoblast-enriched cultures. J Biol Chem 1990;265:15353–15356.

64. Hock JM, Centrella M, Canalis E. Insulin-like growth factor I (IGF-I) has independent effects on bone matrix formation and cell replication. Endocrinology 1988;122:254–260.

65. Centrella M, McCarthy TL, Canalis E. Receptors for insulin-like growth factors I and II in osteoblast-enriched cultures from fetal rat bone. Endocrinology 1990;126:39–44.

66. Chen Y, Shu H, Ji C, et al. Insulin-like growth factor binding proteins localize to discrete cell culture compartments in periosteal and osteoblast cultures from fetal rat bone. J Cell Biochem 1998;71:351–362.

67. Zhou Y, Mohan S, Linkhart TA, et al. Retinoic acid regulates insulin-like growth factor–binding protein expression in human osteoblast cells. Endocrinology 1996;137:975–983.

68. Seyedin SM, Thompson AY, Bentz H, et al. Cartilage-inducing factor-A: Apparent identity to transforming growth factor-beta. J Biol Chem 1986;261:5693–5695.

69. Centrella M, McCarthy TL, Canalis E. Glucocorticoid control of transforming growth factor β (TGFβ) binding and effects in osteoblast-enriched cultures from fetal rat bone. J Bone Miner Res 1990;5(suppl 2):S211.

70. Horner A, Kemp P, Summers C, et al. Expression and distribution of transforming growth factor beta isoforms and their signaling receptors in growing human bone. Bone 1998;23: 95–102.

71. Hock JM, Canalis E, Centrella M. Transforming growth factor-beta (TGF-beta 1) stimulates bone matrix apposition and bone cell replication in cultured fetal rat calvariae. Endocrinology 1990;126:421–426.

72. Joyce ME, Jingushi S, Bolander ME. Transforming growth factor-β in the regulation of fracture repair. Orthop Clin North Am 1990;21:199–209.

73. Gowen M, Chapman K, Littlewood A, et al. Production of tumor necrosis factor by human osteoblasts is modulated by other cytokines, but not by osteotropic hormones. Endocrinology 1990; 126:1250–1255.

74. Dewhirst FE, Ago JM, Peros WJ, Stashenko P. Synergism between parathyroid hormone and interleukin-1 in stimulating bone resorption in organ culture. J Bone Miner Res 1987;2: 127–134.

75. Felix R, Cecchini MG, Fleisch H. Macrophage colony stimulating factor restores in vivo bone resorption in the op/op osteopetrotic mouse. Endocrinology 1990;127:2592–2594.

76. Fried RM, Voelkel EF, Rice RH, et al. Two squamous cell carcinomas not associated with humoral hypercalcemia produce a potent bone resorption-stimulating factor which is interleukin-1 alpha. Endocrinology 1989;125:742–751.

77. Gowen M, Meikle MC, Reynolds JJ. Stimulation of bone resorption in vitro by a nonprostanoid factor released by human monocytes in culture. Biochim Biophys Acta 1983;762: 471–474.

78. Thomson BM, Saklatvala J, Chambers TJ. Osteoblasts mediate interleukin-1 stimulation of bone resorption by rat osteoclasts. J Exp Med 1986;164:104–112.

79. Canalis E. Interleukin-1 has independent effects on deoxyribonucleic acid and collagen synthesis in cultures of rat calvariae. Endocrinology 1986;118:74–81.

80. Smith D, Gowen M, Mundy GR. Effects of interferon gamma and other cytokines on collagen synthesis in fetal rat bone cultures. Endocrinology 1987;120:2494–2499.

81. Lowik CWGM, Van der Pluijm G, Bloys H, et al. Parathyroid hormone (PTH) and PTH-like protein (Plp) stimulate interleukin-6 production by osteogenic cells: A possible role of interleukin-6 in osteoclastogenesis. Biochem Biophys Res Commun 1989; 162:1546–1552.

82. Bertolini DR, Nedwin GE, Bringman TS, et al. Stimulation of bone resorption and inhibition of bone formation in vitro by human tumour necrosis factors. Nature 1986;319:516–518.

83. Jee WS, Ueno K, Kimmel DB, et al. The role of bone cells in increasing metaphyseal hard tissue in rapidly growing rats treated with prostaglandin E_2. Bone 1987;8:171–178.

84. Raisz LG. Bone resorption in organ culture: Factors influencing the response to parathyroid hormone. J Clin Invest 1965;44: 103–116.

85. Guinnes-Hey M, Hock JM. Increased trabecular bone mass in rats treated with human synthetic parathyroid hormone. Metab Bone Dis Relat Res 1984;5:177–181.

86. Haussler MR, Mangelsdorf DJ, Komm BS, et al. Molecular biology of the vitamin D hormone. Recent Prog Horm Res 1988;44: 263–305.

87. McSheehy PMJ, Chambers TJ. 1,25 dihydroxyvitamin D_3 stimulates rat osteoblastic cells to release a soluble factor that increases osteoclastic bone resorption. J Clin Invest 1987;80: 425–429.

88. Manolagas SC, Provvedini DM, Tsoukas C. Interactions of 1,25 dihydroxyvitamin D3 and the immune system. Mol Cell Endocrinol 1985;43:113–122.

89. Friedman JW, Au YW, Raisz LG. Responses of fetal rat bone to thyrocalcitonin in tissue culture. Endocrinology 1968;82: 149–156.

90. Holtrop ME, Raisz LG. Comparison of the effects of 1,25 dihydroxycholecalciferol, prostaglandin E_2, and osteoclast-activating factor with parathyroid hormone on the ultrastructure of osteoclasts in cultured long bones of fetal rats. Calcif Tissue Int 1979;29:201–206.

91. Binstock ML, Mundy GR. Effect of calcitonin and glucocorticoids in combination in malignant hypercalcemia. Ann Intern Med 1980;93:269–272.

92. Feldman R, Krieger N, Tashjian AJ. Effects of parathyroid hormone and calcitonin on osteoclast formation in vitro. Endocrinology 1980;107:1137–1143.

93. Forrest SM, Ng KW, Findlay DM, et al. Characterization of an osteoblast-like clonal cell line which responds to both parathyroid hormone and calcitonin. Calcif Tissue Int 1985;37:51–56.

94. Horsman A, Gallagher JC, Simpson M, Nordin BEC. Prospective trial of estrogen and calcium in postmenopausal women. Br Med J 1977;2:789–792.

95. Riis BJ, Thomsen K, Strom V, Christiansen C. The effect of percutaneous estradiol and natural progesterone on postmenopausal bone loss. Am J Obstet Gynecol 1987;156:61–65.

96. Eriksen EF, Colvard DS, Berg NJ, et al. Evidence of estrogen receptors in normal human osteoblast-like cells. Science 1988; 241:84–86.

97. Oursler MJ, Pyfferoen J, Osdoby P, et al. Osteoclasts express mRNA for estrogen receptor. J Bone Miner Res 1990;5:517.

98. Gray TK, Mohan S, Linkhart TA, Baylink DJ. Estradiol stimulates in vitro the secretion of insulin-like growth factors by the clonal osteoblastic cell line, UMR-106. Biochem Biophys Res Commun 1989;158:407–412.

99. Purohit A, Flanagan AM, Reed MJ. Estrogen synthesis by osteoblast cell lines. Endocrinology 1992;131:2027–2029.

100. Nawata H, Tanaka S, Tanaka S, et al. Aromatase in bone cell: Association with osteoporosis in postmenopausal women. J Steroid Biochem Mol Biol 1995;53:165–174.

CHAPTER 8

Immune Responses in Periodontal Diseases

Jeffrey L. Ebersole
- The Immune System
- Resistance to Infection
- Oral Immune Responses
- Periodontal Health
- Gingivitis
- Aggressive Periodontitis
- Chronic Periodontitis
- Severe Generalized Chronic Periodontitis
- Periodontitis Modified by Intrinsic or Extrinsic Factors

The Immune System

Organs and Tissues

The organs and tissues of the immune system are divided into two main categories: primary (central) and secondary (peripheral) lymphoid organs. The cells of the immune system are produced and mature in the primary lymphoid organs. Reticuloendothelial elements of bone marrow perform the function of hematopoiesis (the production of blood cells), as well as immune-related functions. Functional cells from these tissues are released into the circulation and populate the secondary lymphoid organs or tissues. The lymphatic vessels and the lymph nodes form a complete network that drains and filters the extravasated fluid (lymph) from the intercellular spaces of tissues. As lymphatic vessels leave lymph nodes, they coalesce to form a large lymphatic vessel, the thoracic duct. This duct receives lymph from the entire body and empties it into the bloodstream in one of the two veins that return blood to the heart for repeated circulation. The fluid and cells present in lymph mingle with the blood and re-enter the circulatory cycle.

Innate Resistance and Inflammation

The environment contains a large variety of infectious agents, including bacteria, viruses, fungi, and parasites. Most infections in normal individuals are of limited duration and leave little permanent damage due to the individual's immune system, which combats infectious agents. The immune system has two functional divisions: the innate immune system and the adaptive immune system. Innate immunity acts as a first line of defense against infections, and most potential pathogens are eliminated before they establish an overt infection. Ubiquitous nonspecific activities make up an innate physiologic process called *inflammation*. If these first defenses are unsuccessful, the adaptive immune system is activated and produces a specific reaction to each infectious agent, which normally annihilates that agent.

Inflammatory and Immune Mediators
Interleukin 1 (IL-1) has both local and systemic effects on cell metabolism and on immune and inflammatory reactions. IL-1 is considered an important mediator of inflammation, based on its presence at inflammatory sites and its ability to induce many of the hallmarks of the inflam-

Table 8-1 Identified Properties and Functions of Cytokines

Biologic property or function	IFN-α/-β	IFN-γ	TNF-α/-β	IL-1α/β	IL-2	IL-3	IL-4	IL-5	IL-6	IL-7	IL-8	IL-9	IL-10	IL-12	IL-13	IL-14	IL-15	CSF
Mitogenesis		+		+	+	+	+	+	+				+					+
Pyrogenicity	+	+	+	+	+													
Acute-phase reactant			+	+					+									
Macrophage functions	+	+			+			+					+					+
Antigen presentation/ MHC class II expression		+		+									+		+			
TNF receptor and TNF production		+			+													
Cytotoxicity			+											+				
PMN activation			+	+							+							+
NK activation	+	+			+									+				
B-cell activation		+		+			+	+										
B-cell proliferation	+	+		+	+	+	+	?							+	+		
B-cell differentiation	+	+		+	+	+	+	?	+	+			+					
Ig production & isotype switching	+	+					IgE; IgA IgG1					+	+		+	+		
T-cell activation				+	+		+										+	
T-cell proliferation	+			+	+		+			+			+	+			+	
T-cell differentiation				+	+		+		+			+					+	
PGE₂ production		+	+	+														
Metalloproteinase synthesis		+		+														
Bone resorption		+	+	+					+									

MHC = major histocompatibility complex; PGE$_2$ = prostaglandin E$_2$.

matory response. Microbial products such as endotoxins and exotoxins induce IL-1 production by monocytes. Finally, IL-1 has been shown to be a potent effector of bone resorption through stimulation of osteoblasts and the activity of osteoclasts.

Tumor necrosis factor α (TNF-α) is produced by activated macrophages and other cells and has a broad spectrum of biologic actions on many different immune and nonimmune target cells. TNF is an important inflammatory mediator and accounts for a cytokine-mediated wasting (cachexia), the induction of fever, and several of the acute-phase reactants. Tissue destruction induced by TNF-α resembles IL-1 activity, with bone resorption via the activation of osteoclasts and inhibition of bone synthesis.

IL-6 mediates communication between a large number of cell types by playing a role in the proliferation and differentiation of B lymphocytes, plasmacytomas and hybridomas, hematopoietic progenitors, hepatocytes, and T lymphocytes. Other activities overlap those of IL-1 and TNF-α, and thus IL-6 is considered a major immune and inflammatory mediator. Fibroblasts appear to produce IL-6 as an autocrine growth factor.

IL-8 is the best-characterized member of the chemokine family and is produced following activation of cells with lipopolysaccharide (LPS), TNF-α, and IL-1. This molecule activates and chemoattracts primarily neutrophils. Monocyte chemotactic peptide-1 (MCP-1) is also a member of this family and has activities similar to those of IL-8, except that the effects are limited to monocytes (Table 8-1).

Interferons (IFN-α and IFN-β) are peptides that promote antiviral activities in mammalian cells, which bind these peptides. They can regulate cytotoxic T-lymphocyte (CTL) activity and B-lymphocyte proliferation, promote antibody production and functions of macrophages, and enhance natural killer (NK)–cell activities.

Transforming growth factor β (TGF-β) has been most clearly demonstrated to affect cells involved in immunity and inflammation. TGF-β is a chemoattractant and promotes many functional activities of fibroblasts. TGF-β is a potential mediator of inflammation because it is a product of activated macrophages, and it is a potent chemoattractant for macrophages that can activate them to produce IL-1. Some of the other growth factors, such as platelet-derived growth factor (PDGF), epidermal growth factor (EGF), and fibroblast growth factor (FGF), also indirectly contribute to inflammation and immune responses by acting as chemotactic agents for monocytes and neutrophils, augmenting production of IFNs and antigen-presenting functions of macrophages.

Acute-Phase Response

The body responds to injury by increasing the hepatic synthesis of a number of plasma proteins, which increases their concentration in the plasma and at the site of injury. Fever is one of the first acute-phase responses that was described, and it may occur following many types of inflammatory stimuli. The cytokine IL-1 is now believed to be identical to the endogenous pyrogens that contribute to fever. Several components of the complement system are acute-phase reactants, as they increase during infection. C-reactive protein (CRP), when bound to bacteria, promotes the binding of complement, which facilitates the uptake of bacteria by phagocytes. Acute-phase reactants also include protease inhibitors in human plasma, which are involved in the inflammatory response by blocking proteases that degrade tissue surrounding an inflammatory process and cause damage leading to chronic inflammation. Various other acute-phase reactants bind iron and copper and contribute to wound healing.[1]

Cells of Innate Resistance

Inflammation provides an orderly sequence of coordinated events devised to protect the host from infections and minimize damage to host tissues. The vascular phase of inflammation primarily affects the microcirculation (ie, the capillaries, arterioles, and venules). A *transudate*, which is serum or other body fluids that have passed through basement membranes, is characterized by a low protein content and few cells; it contrasts with the polymorphonuclear leukocyte (PMN)–rich inflammatory exudate. PMNs (neutrophils) make up 60% to 70% of the total white blood cells in humans and are the hallmark of the acute inflammatory response in providing a primary, nonspecific, internal defense mechanism. They are the first cells to arrive at an inflammatory focus, appearing within a few hours.

In a healthy, nonallergic individual, *eosinophilic granulocytes* make up approximately 2% to 5% of circulating nucleated cells. Eosinophils appear to function by ingestion of immune complexes, limiting inflammatory reactions by antagonizing the effects of mediators. *Basophilic*

Table 8-2 Phenotypic Markers for Inflammatory/Immune Cells

Cell	Phenotypic marker
B cell	Ig, CD21 (C3d), CD23 (FcεR), HLA-DR (MHC II)
Plasma cell	Ig and isotypes
Pan T cells	CD3, HLA-DR (activated)
T helper cell	CD4⁺, CD8⁻, CD25 (IL-2R), CD45RO/RA, TCR-αβ or TCR-γδ
T cytotoxic/ suppressor cell	CD8⁺, CD4⁻, CD25 (IL-2R), CD45RO/RA, TCR-αβ or TCR-γδ
Natural killer cell	CD57, CD16 (FcγR), CD11b
Macrophage/ monocyte	CD64 (FcγR), CD14 (LPS receptor), CD89 (FcαR)
PMN	CD11/CD18, CD16 (FcγR), CD89 (FcαR)

granulocytes make up 0.5% to 2% of circulating leukocytes. Basophilic granules contain primarily histamine and leukotrienes LTC_4, LTD_4, and LTE_4 (ie, the slow-reacting substance of anaphylaxis), which are potent spasmogenic agents causing constriction of smooth muscle. Human skin and the gastrointestinal tract are particularly rich in *mast cells*; these contain granules with potent mediators, including histamine, heparin, serotonin, hyaluronic acid, and eosinophil chemotactic factor of anaphylaxis. *Platelets* contain heparin, serotonin, and lysosomal enzymes that are released from the granules during platelet aggregation and may contribute to the acute vascular phase of inflammation. However, the major role of platelets is to block damaged vessel walls and prevent hemorrhage.

In chronic inflammation, there is an emigration of mononuclear cells into the affected area. These monocytes represent approximately 4% to 10% of circulating nucleated cells. Differentiated cells of this series include macrophages (lymph nodes, peritoneal lining, pleural surfaces, joint linings, renal glomeruli, and inflammatory tissues), dendritic cells (lymph nodes), Kupffer cells (liver), Langerhans cells (skin), alveolar macrophages (lungs), osteoclasts (bone), microglia (central nervous system), and histiocytes (connective tissue). They play pivotal roles in both humoral and cell-mediated immune reactions to pathogens.

Approximately 5% of blood lymphocytes have neither the membrane immunoglobulin (Ig) characteristic of B cells nor phenotypes characteristic of T cells. These NK cells have on their membranes a high-affinity receptor for the Fc portion of the IgG, which enables them to play an important role in antibody-dependent cell-mediated cytolysis (Table 8-2).

Acquired Immune Responses

Acquired or adaptive immunity involves various molecules and cells that have the ability to recognize and discriminate foreignness (ie, "non-self"). Specific immune responses and specific immunity usually follow recovery from an infectious disease. The primary infection results in a state of decreased susceptibility to a subsequent attack by the microorganism that was responsible. This response encompasses a series of cellular interactions that involve and elaborate specific cell products.

It is common to divide immune reactions into two principal categories: *humoral* and *cell-mediated* responses. The hallmark of humoral immunity is production of antibodies, proteins uniquely constructed to interact with the stimulating material. Cell-mediated immunity includes a range of actions based upon the requirement that viable effector cells be present. The type of protective acquired immunity varies with different infectious agents. In general, protection mediated by humoral antibody (immunoglobulins) is effective against agents that exist extracellularly. In contrast, intracellular parasitic infections are principally resolved by cell-mediated immune reactions.

A material capable of eliciting immune response when introduced into an immunocompetent host is defined as an *immunogen* or *antigen*. There are unestimated numbers of non-self materials to which hosts potentially can be exposed. Some antigens are more effective than others in provoking an immune response; some individuals are more responsive than others to certain immunogens; and internal or external circumstances may influence the intensity of the immune response.

Cells of the immune system arise from pluripotent stem cells through the lymphoid lineage *(lymphocytes)* or myeloid lineage *(phagocytes)*. Descending from the lymphoid precursor are lymphocytes, which are further divided into T and B lymphocytes. Lymphocytes represent about 20% of the total white blood cell count.

Cellular Immune Responses

T cells and monocytes/macrophages. T cells make up 60% to 80% of the circulating lymphocytes. The T lymphocytes are associated with two types of immunologic functions, *effector* and *regulatory*. The effector functions include activities such as killing virally infected cells and tumors. The regulatory functions include the ability to amplify or suppress, through cytokines, other effector lymphocytes, including B and T cells. Subsets of helper T cells (T_H) and cytotoxic T cells (T_C) are involved in regulating immune responses, cooperating with B cells in the induction of antibody synthesis, releasing cytokines that can activate macrophages, and aiding in the elimination of many intracellular and viral pathogens.

Most circulating T cells express a combination of the cluster determinant (CD) markers CD2, CD3, CD4 (helper-inducer T cells), or CD8 (cytotoxic T cells), as well as a T-cell antigen receptor (TCR). As a population, T cells appear to be capable of synthesizing many cytokines, but individual T cells tend to produce a limited repertoire. In particular, CD4$^+$ T_H1 cells, which are largely involved in delayed-type hypersensitivity reaction, release IL-2, IFN-γ, and LT-α (TNF-β). In contrast, another subpopulation of CD4$^+$ T_H2 cells responsible for T-B cell cooperation secrete IL-4, IL-5, IL-6, and IL-10.

Monocytes/macrophages are responsible for antigen recognition, immune stimulation, and the tissue consequences that follow immune stimulation. Macrophages overlap as effectors of both natural and adaptive immunity. They can be involved in inflammatory responses and antigen presentation, and once activated by lymphokines, they demonstrate nonspecific cytotoxicity to altered cells by both direct contact and by cytolytic factors (ie, TNF-α) (see Table 8-2).

Cytokines that develop, regulate, and activate lymphocytes. Cytokines are nonantibody substances that influence activities of other cells. They are generated following the specific or nonspecific activation of lymphocytes or other cell types, which then can act as cellular mediators of the inflammatory and immune response.

Interleukins. The major function of IL-2 is to enhance proliferation of activated T lymphocytes, NK cells (enhancing NK activity of that portion of the large granular lymphocyte population that expresses the IL-2 receptor after contact with IL-1), and macrophages (stimulating already activated macrophages to increased tumor-killing capacity).

IL-3 is responsible for promoting proliferation of earlier-lineage pluripotent stem cells in the bone marrow, which can lead to a rise in peripheral leukocyte counts.

IL-4 is a CD4$^+$ T cell–derived cytokine that stimulates resting B cells. IL-4 has been found to induce expression of major histocompatibility complex (MHC) class II genes on the surface of resting B lymphocytes and to enhance the production of immunoglobulin (particularly IgG and IgE) from activated B cells.

IL-5 is a cytokine produced by activated CD4$^+$ T cells and activated mast cells that acts as a co-stimulator for the growth of antigen-activated B cells. IL-5 has also been shown to act on mature B cells to cause increased synthesis of IgA.

IL-7 is produced by bone marrow stroma. It not only promotes the growth of immature B cells but also appears to be a most potent stimulator of proliferation of the most immature T-cell population (CD4$^-$, CD8$^-$ thymocytes).

IL-9 is a multifunctional cytokine produced by naive CD4$^+$ T cells and T_H2 lymphocytes. IL-9 acts as a co-stimulator of fetal thymocytes, erythroid precursor cells, and mast cells.

IL-10 is considered a cross-regulatory cytokine of T cells. It is produced by T_H2 cells and inhibits cytokine synthesis by T_H1 cells upon antigen stimulation. The effect appears to be via inhibition of macrophage functions, including antigen presentation to the T cells, as well as cytokine production following stimulation with LPS.

IL-12 is a cytokine produced by monocytes/macrophages, B cells, and other accessory cells in response to bacteria or their products. This cytokine acts on NK cells and T cells by inducing transcription and secretion of cytokines, increasing cytotoxic activity, and inducing proliferation of these cell types following activation by other cytokines (eg, IL-2).

IL-13 is a cytokine secreted by activated T lymphocytes that increases MHC class II expression on B cells and monocytes/macrophages related to antigen presentation and responsiveness. This molecule decreases proinflammatory cytokine and chemokine production by monocytes/macrophages and increases the synthesis of IL-1 receptor antagonist, thus suggesting an anti-inflammatory function for this cytokine. Additionally, IL-13 increases proliferation and Ig switching of B cells.

IL-15 is a cytokine produced by activated monocytes/macrophages and some epithelial cell lines. This cytokine binds to various cell lines, human mononuclear cells (especially NK cells), and activated T cells. It induces proliferation, cytotoxic activity, and cytokine production by NK cells.[2]

IL-16 is a soluble ligand for CD4; it is derived from activated T cells and is a potent chemoattractant for CD4+ T cells, eosinophils, and monocytes. It also induces proinflammatory cytokines, inhibits human immunodeficiency virus 1 replication, and plays a key role in asthma.[3]

IL-17 is a CD4+ T cell–restricted proinflammatory cytokine secreted by activated memory T cells. It has effects like those of a T_H1 cytokine, and it stimulates hematopoiesis and causes neutrophilia.[4]

IL-18 plays a critical role in the development of T_H1 responses and immunity to intracellular pathogens. It is considered a proinflammatory cytokine that activates NK and T_H1 cells by inducing IFN-γ.[5]

Lymphotoxin, interferon, and colony-stimulating factor (CSF). Lymphotoxin is produced by activated T lymphocytes and is frequently coordinated with IFN-γ. The lymphotoxin complex is a heterotrimer that consists of LT-α (formerly TNF-β) and LT-β chains. LT-β is a membrane-bound protein that anchors the complex to the surface of activated lymphocytes and contributes to normal lymphoid tissue development. It is a potent activator of neutrophils, as well as activating endothelial cells for increased leukocyte adherence and initiating cellular changes that allow emigration from the vasculature. IFN-γ, which appears after activation of specific T cells, modulates the nature and intensity of both the inflammatory and immune

responses. Like IFN-γ, granulocyte-macrophage colony-stimulating factor (GM-CSF) has been shown to be a potent activator of macrophage function. Monocyte/macrophage colony-stimulating factor (M-CSF) is produced by macrophages, fibroblasts, and endothelial cells. This molecule acts primarily on a stem cell that is already committed to differentiate into monocytes. Granulocyte colony-stimulating factor (G-CSF) is produced by endothelial cells, fibroblasts, and macrophages. This factor acts on marrow stem cells already committed to development into granulocytes (see Table 8-1).

Humoral Immune Responses

B lymphocytes and plasma cells. B cells are derived from the bone marrow, which remains the major repository of stem cells for B lymphocytes throughout life. Mature B lymphocytes are the products of lymphoid stem cells that undergo a sequence of differentiation under the influence of a special microenvironment. In mammals, the differentiation occurs first in the fetal liver and subsequently in the bone marrow. The B-cell development can be divided into two stages, antigen dependent and antigen independent. B lymphocytes make up approximately 5% to 15% of circulating nucleated cells of normal human blood. They are classically identified by their cell surface immunoglobulin.

One of the most fascinating aspects of B lymphocytes is their heterogeneity; they differ in terms of the specificity of their antibody-combining sites. While there are hundreds of gene segments corresponding to the variable regions of antibodies, relatively few encode constant regions that result in heavy chains for the major classes or isotypes (IgM, IgD, IgG1, IgG2, IgA, IgE, etc) and light-chain types (κ or γ). Plasma cells can produce and release thousands of molecules per second, and the C-terminal portion of such secreted Ig is different from the membrane form of Ig made by B cells.

There are many molecules detectable on B cells. One, CD21, is the receptor for Epstein-Barr virus. Another, CD23, acts as a receptor for the Fc portion of IgE. There are receptors for a number of regulatory molecules (eg, IL-1, IL-2, IL-3, IL-4, IFN-γ, and TGF-β). Contact with antigen generates strong Fc-combining capacity. Finally, B cells have membrane receptors for several proteins of the complement system.

The fully differentiated plasma cell presents different membrane markers than B cells and is specialized to manufacture and secrete immunoglobulins with no further need for environmental stimulation or regulation. After several days of manufacturing and releasing immunoglobulin molecules, the individual plasma cell, which is a terminally differentiated B cell, dies without reproducing (see Table 8-2).

Immunoglobulins. Immunoglobulins (antibodies) are glycoproteins representative of the adaptive immune system that are present in the serum and fluids of all mammals. These molecules bind specifically to foreign antigens such as bacteria, viruses, parasites, and toxins. Five distinct classes of immunoglobulins are identified in most higher mammals: IgG, IgA, IgM, IgD, and IgE. These are identified by differences in size, charge, amino acid composition, and carbohydrate content, particularly on the heavy chains of the molecules. The constant regions of the human heavy chains also define four subclasses of IgG and two subclasses of IgA in humans. Additionally, a unique structural variant of IgA exists in exocrine secretions; this variant is a dimer of IgA with an attached J (joining) chain and secretory component (SC).

IgM is the first immunoglobulin class to appear in the immune response, the first antibody formed by the neonate, and the predominant antibody in a primary immune response. The IgM molecule exhibits potent fixation of complement, and the pentameric nature of IgM results in a high capacity for agglutination/aggregation of bacteria. IgM is also the antibody most frequently observed in autoimmune disorders (ie, rheumatoid factor).

IgG makes up 75% of serum immunoglobulin. IgG is the most important serum immunoglobulin, and after prolonged exposure to most antigens, antibody activity is mainly associated with this isotype. Thus, it is the predominant antibody in a secondary immune response and as such is the majority of the immune response. This immunoglobulin isotype exists in both intravascular and extravascular spaces. Due to differences in antigen epitopes on the heavy chains of the molecules, there are four subclasses of IgG: IgG1, IgG2, IgG3, and IgG4.

IgA is primarily a monomeric immunoglobulin in serum, and it is the predominant Ig in secretions existing as a dimeric molecule with a J chain and SC. Serum IgA responses to both protein and carbohydrate antigens have been identified, but the function of these antibodies is not clear. They may help limit inflammation by blocking IgG/IgM binding to antigens and thus interfering with fixation of complement and amplification of the inflammatory response. A major protective role in external secretions is played by secretory IgA (SIgA). The structure of the molecule makes it especially resistant to proteolytic degradation. IgA is the most abundant antibody in secretions (tears, saliva, gut secretions, milk, and nasal mucus), although it also makes up 10% to 15% of the circulating immunoglobulins. It has been shown to be composed of two subclasses, IgA1 and IgA2.

IgD, in association with IgM, is found on the surface of B lymphocytes. It is suggested that IgD is important in B-cell differentiation.

The serum concentration of *IgE* is very low, about 0.004% of the total immunoglobulin. This immunoglobulin isotype increases dramatically in atopic (allergic) individuals. The antibody functions by arming mast cells and basophils for a role in allergic reactions. As a protective antibody, IgE appears to be important in response to certain parasitic diseases, resulting in an allergic type of parasite expulsion.

Hypersensitivity reactions. Under certain circumstances, exposure to antigen can result in complex immunologic events that are deleterious to the host. These reactions, which take place in an exaggerated or inappropriate manner and may involve both lymphocytes and antibodies, are termed *hypersensitivity reactions.* The tissue damage from hypersensitivity reactions is primarily due to inflammation, which, if not exaggerated, would be beneficial. Hypersensitivity reactions can be separated into two types: immediate hypersensitivities mediated by antibodies and delayed hypersensitivities mediated by T lymphocytes. There is little difference between immunity and hypersensitivity other than a qualitative one. Three types of immediate hypersensitivity have been described: type I (anaphylactic), type II (cytotoxic), and type III (immune complex). Type IV is a delayed-type hypersensitivity.

Anaphylactic (type I) hypersensitivity. Type I hypersensitivity, or allergy, occurs when an IgE antibody response is formed against frequently innocuous antigens (eg, pollen). IgE hypersensitivity in humans can be either localized or systemic. Local allergic reactions include hay fever (allergic rhinitis) in response to plant pollens, industrial chemicals, microbial spores, and insects contained in household dust. Asthma, a complex condition that sometimes has an immunologic basis, is generally directed toward similar allergens as hay fever. Systemic allergic reactions (anaphylaxis) result from the allergen reaching the blood or lymph circulation. The ensuing reaction involves several organs and may be triggered by insect venoms, drugs, or even certain foods. Each of these allergic reactions can have severe consequences.

Cytotoxic (type II) hypersensitivity. Type II hypersensitivity is characterized by antibody binding to cell-surface or tissue antigens. Binding of IgM or IgG antibody to the antigens on the cell surface activates the classic complement pathway leading to cytolysis. The release of complement components can trigger the influx of phagocytic cells. The mechanism of phagocytic damage to cells is similar to the manner by which phagocytes deal with infectious pathogens.

Several human syndromes have been associated with cytotoxic hypersensitivity. Transfusion reactions to various blood-group antigens on erythrocytes arise from antibody directed to surface antigens on the red blood cells. Hemolytic disease of the newborn is a cytotoxic hypersensitivity whereby antibody from the maternal circulation is directed to incompatible Rh antigens on the fetal erythrocytes. Autoimmune hemolytic anemias occur when patients produce antibodies to their own erythrocytes. Drugs eliciting an allergic reaction against erythrocytes or platelets provoke drug-induced reactions. Hyperacute graft rejection results when the recipient has preformed antibodies to antigens on the graft. Patients with myasthenia gravis demonstrate antibodies to the acetylcholine receptor on the surface of muscle membranes. Thyroiditis and diabetes involve antibodies directed to thyroid cells and pancreatic islet cells.

Immune-complex–mediated (type III) hypersensitivity. Immune-complex disorders are a type of hypersensitivity initiated by antigen-antibody complexes that form in solution rather than on a cell surface. Immune complexes are produced each time antibody reacts with antigen, but because the concentration of antigen in the circulation is usually low, they are usually effectively removed by the reticuloendothelial system. However, under certain circumstances, the antigen-antibody complexes persist in high concentrations and cause tissue damage by sticking to the walls of capillary vessels, depositing on basement membranes, or both. The complexes bind complement and release both C3a and C5a, which are chemotactic for polymorphonuclear leukocytes. The attracted cells phagocytize the complexes and release hydrolytic enzymes into the intercellular spaces, resulting in tissue destruction, inflammation, and sometimes local hemorrhage and organ dysfunction. Disease resulting from immune-complex hypersensitivity can be separated into three major categories: *(1)* persistent infection with microbial antigens; *(2)* autoimmune reactions to self antigens; and, *(3)* responses to extrinsic environmental antigens.

Delayed-type (type IV) hypersensitivity. Type IV hypersensitivity is a cell-mediated hypersensitivity initiated by lymphocytes rather than antibody. As such, it cannot be transferred by serum but only by T lymphocytes. The T cells involved have been sensitized by previous contact with the antigen. Although these sensitized T cells are critical in producing delayed-type reactions, a major portion of the reaction involves nonsensitized cells that are recruited by the antigen-specific T lymphocytes. The prototypical reaction is the detection of challenge with *Mycobacterium tuberculosis*, which is elicited by intradermal injection of the microorganism or, more commonly, antigens from the mycobacteria (purified protein derivative).

Numerous chronic diseases elicit delayed hypersensitivity. Among them are diseases caused by mycobacteria (tuberculosis and leprosy), bacteria (listeriosis), fungi (blastomycosis), and parasites (leishmaniasis and schistosomiasis). In all of these infections, the agent provides a persistent, chronic antigenic stimulation to the host.

Resistance to Infection

Immune responses of mammals and the pathogenic/virulence capabilities of microorganisms have evolved together, each producing selective pressures on the other. For a pathogen to produce disease, it must have two attributes: *(1)* it must be able to metabolize and multiply in or upon host tissues, and *(2)* it must be able to resist host defense mechanisms for sufficient time to reach the numbers required to produce overt disease.

Many bacteria produce infection by multiplying primarily outside phagocytic cells. Generally, when these types of bacteria are ingested, they are readily killed by the phagocytes. These microorganisms produce infection and disease under only two general circumstances: *(1)* when the bacteria possess a structure or a mechanism that prevents their being readily phagocytized and *(2)* when any impairment of host mechanisms for intracellular killing promotes disease by these bacteria. These types of bacteria may cause mucosal surface infections, systemic infections, or local infections. Colonization and infection of a mucous membrane depends on the adhesive properties of the bacteria. Systemic infections are characterized by bacteremia. Local infections are generally acute infections with an extensive amount of inflammation (Table 8-3).

Cellular Resistance

Intracellular Bacterial Pathogens

Both facultative and obligate intracellular bacterial pathogens have been identified. *Facultative* pathogens are usually readily phagocytized by neutrophils and other phagocytic cells but are resistant to intracellular killing. *Obligate* pathogens cannot multiply unless they are within cells. They generally utilize part of the metabolic apparatus of the host cell, either for nutritional purposes or to supply energy.

Mycotic Infections

There is an increased incidence of fungal infections in immunocompromised hosts, and these infections are frequently identified as opportunistic. All mycotic infections that limit their disease potential to the cornified layers of the epidermis and the superfollicular portion of the hair have been termed *superficial mycoses.* Recovery is generally associated with some resistance to reinfection and appears to correlate with the development of a positive delayed-type hypersensitivity reaction to the microorganism. Cutaneous mycoses are infections of the epidermal

Table 8-3 Immunity to Bacterial, Viral, and Mycotic Infections

Pathogen	Nonspecific	Specific	
		Humoral	Cellular
Bacterial			
Extracellular			
Gram positive	+++ (PMNs)	++ (opsonins, antitoxins, anticapsule, SIgA)	... + (mø in *Salmonella typhi*)
Gram negative	+ (PMNs + C')	+++ (opsonins, antitoxins, anticapsule, anti-LPS, SIgA)	
Spirochetes	...	+++ (agglutinins, opsonins, immobilization, lysins)	+ (latency in 2° syphilis)
Mycoplasma species	...	++ (opsonins, SIgA)	
Intracellular			
Facultative	...	++ (opsonins)	+++
Obligate	...	++ (opsonins)	++
Viral			
Cytolytic	++ (IFN)	+++ (opsonins, ADCC, C', SIgA)	...
Persistent			
Latent	+ (NK)	++ (opsonins)	++
Chronic	...	++ (opsonins, SIgA)	+++
Slow	...	?	?
Integrated	+ (NK)	+ (ADCC)	+++
Fungal			
Superficial and cutaneous	... (antifungals)	...	+
Subcutaneous	+++	...	++
Systemic	... (amphotericin)	...	+++
Opportunistic	+ (mucormycosis)	+ (allergy)	+++

+ to +++ denote increasing contribution of host response components to resistance to infection by the pathogen.

Ellipses denote that this form of host response does not contribute to immunity.

tissues by fungi classified as dermatophytes. Recovery is usually not immunologically mediated but occurs by active treatment with topical antifungal agents. However, chronic infections despite treatment by these agents have been associated with absent or abnormal cell-mediated immune responsiveness.

The agents that cause subcutaneous mycoses, including chromomycosis and phycomycosis, are saprophytic fungi that cause chronic nodules or ulcers if they gain access to the subcutaneous tissues following trauma. Natural resistance to this infection is high, particularly after full maturation of the immune system during the teenage years. The primary immune mechanism for interfering with these pathogens appears to be delayed-type hypersensitivity cellular immune reactions that involve both eosinophils and macrophages that are activated so as to kill the fungi.

Viral Infections

Viruses have been classified into two general categories based on the nucleic acid composition of their genome,

DNA or RNA, which controls their method of multiplication. Numerous members of both types cause a variety of human diseases resulting from cytolytic, persistent, or integrated viral infections. Immune responses and effective immunity to these infections are determined by the ability of the host to interact with the extracellular virus particles or the host cells infected by the virions. Immune responses to viruses can be directed to antigens on the viral particle or to host cells infected with the virus. Immunity to viruses is highly dependent on T lymphocytes, both as direct effector cells expressing cell-mediated immune functions and as a requirement for B-cell responses and antibody formation to the viral antigens. Thus, individuals with immunodeficiencies characterized by T-cell dysfunctions are exceptionally predisposed to severe viral pathogenesis.

Cell-mediated responses that provide immunity against viral infections are characterized by T lymphocytes, NK cells, macrophages, and killer (K) cells. Generally, cellular immunity is considered to be a principal component in recovery from viral infections, as well as subsequent resistance of the host. These cell-mediated responses are particularly critical in elimination of infected cells, while the antiviral antibodies are of primary importance in neutralizing extracellular viruses. T cells are essential for eliminating primary infection with many viruses. The cells are able to lyse virus-infected cells; secrete lymphokines that activate macrophages; and secrete immune IFN-γ, which protects adjacent cells and activates NK cells. T lymphocytes have been detected in various viral infections, and their pivotal role in immunity is demonstrated by the frequency and severity of viral diseases in T cell–immunodeficient individuals. NK cells are involved in natural cell-mediated cytotoxicity. These cells are capable of lysing a wide variety of host cells, including virus-transformed cells, cells (particularly fibroblasts) that are acutely infected with certain viruses, and persistently infected cells. The contribution of NK cells to viral immunity is increased following activation by IFN released by T lymphocytes.

Humoral Resistance

Gram-Positive Bacterial Infections

Various gram-positive cocci cause disease in humans as extracellular pathogens. Principal immunity to these bacteria appears to derive from PMN phagocytosis. Systemic opsonic antibody, including anticapsular, anti–type specific (M protein), and anticellular antibody, contributes to immune protection. Immunity to *Streptococcus mutans* appears to be primarily via secretory antibodies of the IgA isotype, which act to decrease the ability of the microorganism to colonize the teeth. Gram-positive rod-shaped bacteria are also etiologic for various human diseases. Systemic antibodies are produced that can agglutinate these bacteria and activate complement. There is some evidence that antibody levels decrease after recovery from disease; however, no immunity to reinfection has been identified. Immunity to toxigenic infections by these bacteria is strictly related to the production of antitoxin antibodies, which generally results from active immunization with a toxoid or an avirulent strain of the microorganisms.

Gram-Negative Bacterial Infections

Antibody to either the *Escherichia coli* enterotoxin or colonization factors such as pili appears to provide protection against this gram-negative bacterial infection. Enteric fever provides some protection against the infecting serotype of *Salmonella typhosa*, presumably from antibody production in response to the microorganism. People in areas where *Shigella dysenteriae* infection is endemic acquire some immunity to the disease through both anticell antibody (as opsonin for phagocytosis) and antitoxin anti-

body. Immunity to *Klebsiella pneumoniae* is afforded by the production of anticapsule antibody, which enhances phagocytosis and killing. The host produces circulating vibriocidal *(Vibrio cholerae)* antibody and local secretory IgA to the bacteria and antibodies to the enterotoxin. The IgA antibody prevents attachment of the vibrio to the gut; however, this response is generally short-lived. The systemic antibacterial responses may enhance local phagocytosis and killing of the bacteria in the gut.

Generally, immunity to *Pseudomonas aeruginosa* appears to be via antibody production to both the extracellular slime and LPS, which both enhance phagocytosis and killing under normal circumstances. Successful protection from the *Bordetella pertussis* infection has been accomplished by parenteral immunization with whole-cell vaccines. Immunity results from the formation of IgG opsonic antibody, which enhances phagocytosis and killing. Anticapsular antibody that opsonizes *Haemophilus influenzae* and promotes phagocytosis appears to be the active agent in vivo. Antibodies against the capsule of *Neisseria* organisms are bactericidal (with complement) and enhance phagocytosis and intracellular killing by PMNs. Most frequently, the polymicrobic diseases are treated with antibiotics; however, opsonic antibody responses to the microorganisms can provide some protection. Systemic antibodies are formed to *Actinobacillus actinomycetemcomitans*, but their protective capacity is unknown.

Finally, bacterial sepsis and endotoxic shock are associated with numerous gram-negative bacterial infections. Generally, these are manifested in individuals with defective functions of PMNs. The toxic activity is caused by the lipopolysaccharide (endotoxin) that is an integral component of all gram-negative bacterial cell walls. Protection from this substance is via the production of antibodies to the core glycolipid of the LPS and has been exemplified in human studies by the administration of monoclonal anti-LPS antibodies during sepsis.

Spirochetal Infections

Syphilis is an infectious disease of humans caused by the spirochete *Treponema pallidum*. Following primary syphilis, most patients have antibodies to *T pallidum* that will fix complement, inhibit the motility, and eliminate the infectious nature of the spirochete. Delayed-type hypersensitivity to treponemal antigens occurs late in secondary syphilis and may cause the onset of latency of the disease. Immunity to extracellular spirochetes has been correlated with agglutinating antibodies. These antibodies provide both agglutinating and opsonizing properties and promote destruction by phagocytes. Humoral immunity appears to protect against the *Borrelia* spirochetes (eg, those that cause Lyme disease, or borreliosis) by agglutinating, immobilizing, and/or lysing the borreliae.

Table 8-4 Oral Cavity Immune Components

Immune system	Inflammatory/Innate	Cellular	Humoral
Saliva	Amylase, lysozyme lactoferrin	Epithelial cells	SIgA/IgG, mucins, PRP, histatins
Serum	Acute-phase proteins, IL-1β, IL-6, TNF-α, transferrin	PMN, monocytes, T cells, B cells, NK cells	IgG/IgA/IgM, C'
GCF	Prostaglandins, leukotrienes, IL-1α/β, IL-2, IL-6, IL-8, IFN-γ CSF, TNF-α, acute-phase proteins, transferrin	PMN, monocytes, T cells, B cells	IgG/IgA/IgM, C'

Mycoplasma Infections

Mycoplasmas lack a cell wall and can cause pneumonia and urogenital infections. Serum antibodies of both the IgM and IgG isotypes are produced to the infection; however, these do not provide full protection. Additionally, cell-mediated immunity does not appear to provide adequate protection. It does appear that secretory IgA antibody in the lung secretions may provide protection by minimizing attachment and colonization by the pathogen.

Viral Infections

Mammalian antiviral immunity is demonstrated in both the humoral and cellular aspects of the immune response. Antibody can function alone in antiviral immunity, with activation of the complement system, or in concert with K cells in antibody-dependent cellular cytotoxicity. Viral antibody is often composed of IgG, IgA, and IgM isotypes. IgG antibody can neutralize viruses by blocking the interactions of the viral adsorption to host cells, by blocking the penetration of the cells, and by blocking uncoating of the virion. Antibody attached to the virus enhances the ingestion of the complex by PMNs and macrophages via their Fc receptor. Additionally, the antibody can agglutinate the virus so that clumping reduces the density of infectious particles and enhances phagocytosis. Complement-fixing antibody (IgG and IgM) can affect viral pathogenesis by binding to the antigen and increasing the size of the complex to trigger phagocytosis. Antibody and complement can result in lysis of viruses with envelopes by damaging the lipid membrane of the pathogen. Antibody and complement may also function by lysing virus-infected host cells manifesting viral or altered host antigens. Complement alone has been demonstrated to kill certain viruses and cells infected with certain viruses by activation of the alternative pathway, which can lead to direct lysis or increased phagocytosis of the coated material. IgA, particularly SIgA found in external secretions, has been shown to be very effective in blocking the initial colonization potential of many viruses and thus preventing disease. Finally, under certain conditions, IgG anti-body bound to virus-infected cells has been shown to interact with certain Fc receptor–bearing lymphocytes (K cells) and lead to host cell lysis and inhibition of virus multiplication.

Oral Immune Responses

The oral cavity represents the entry portal for a wide array of antigenic challenges, both transient and more permanent. The more permanent challenges are represented by the substantial bacterial colonization in the oral cavity. This environment presents a variety of niches for the establishment of unique microbial ecologies, including the oral mucosa, tongue, tooth surface, and gingival sulcus. Many members of the complex oral microbiota maintain a symbiotic relationship with the host; however, select individual species (eg, *S mutans* and *A actinomycetemcomitans*) clearly represent pathogens within this environment. For the host to maintain homeostasis within the oral cavity, three distinct but interrelated immune response systems contribute to controlling the microbial colonization. They are the salivary, systemic (serum), and gingival tissue (gingival crevicular fluid, or GCF) immune systems (Table 8-4).

Local Contribution

Salivary Glands

The salivary domain of the oral cavity represents those structures bathed by products of the salivary glands. Whole saliva in the oral cavity is composed of secretions of both major and minor salivary glands, components derived from the oral mucosa, and fluid derived from the gingival sulcus.

In addition to the epithelial barrier of the mucosa, from which cells are sloughed (which removes adhered bacteria), various innate immune molecules contribute to these secretions. Mucins are high-molecular-weight glycoproteins that lubricate the oral surfaces and exhibit some specificity for complexing oral bacteria, enhancing elimination. Lactoferrin can be derived from both the serous cells of the glands and the gingival fluid, which mediates its antibacterial effects through binding iron necessary for bacterial metabolism. Salivary peroxidase acts on substrates in the saliva to form hypothiocyanate ions, which are toxic to certain bacteria. Lysozyme derives from the ductal epithelium of the salivary glands and enzymatically attacks the peptidoglycans of bacterial cell walls. Histidine-rich proteins (histatins) from the salivary glands are antifungal, particularly against *Candida albicans*. The proline-rich proteins exhibit selective binding of certain oral species, which may be beneficial to blocking more pathogenic species.

The primary acquired immune component in saliva is SIgA antibody. This molecule is formed by a cooperative cellular interaction of IgA plasma cells in the salivary gland tissues and the epithelial cells producing the SC necessary for transporting the immune molecule to the external lumen. SIgA antibodies are found at all mucosal surfaces of the body and have been identified to have specificity for various bacterial, fungal, and viral pathogens. Studies have also indicated that active immunization enhances the levels and protective capacity of this immune component. In addition to SIgA, whole and glandular saliva has been shown to contain both IgG and IgM antibodies. IgG is a minor constituent of whole saliva and appears to be primarily derived from gingival fluid. IgM is present in low concentrations in saliva from normal subjects and has been shown to have the SC associated with the pentameric structure. However, approximately 1 in 500 to 700 individuals are selectively IgA deficient, and nearly one third of this deficient group exhibits increased SIgM in saliva as a compensatory mechanism of immunity.

The salivary glands are a component of the common mucosal immune system and thus demonstrate homing of IgA cells from other mucosal sites. Therefore, research in humans and animal models has shown that salivary antibody can be elicited by local challenge of the glands, as well as by oral stimulation of the gut-associated lymphoid tissue (GALT). This knowledge is currently being used to explore the development of oral vaccines for dental caries and other mucosal infections.

Gingival Tissue

Gingival crevicular fluid exhibits an exceedingly more complex array of immune components than does glandular saliva, and the fluid flow contributes many antibacterial mechanisms to the oral cavity.[6] GCF is derived from gingival capillary beds (serum components) and resident and emigrating inflammatory cells. Both IgG and IgA are present in the GCF and are derived from serum and plasma cells in the gingival tissues. This immunoglobulin has been shown to have antigenic specificity for local bacterial antigens, as well as a substantial portion that appears to be derived from polyclonal B-cell activation. Additionally, numerous studies have confirmed that significant local elevations in Ig occur in periodontitis resulting from extensive local production. Numerous complement components are detected in GCF, which can be derived from serum, as well as local synthesis. Both C3 and C4 are present in GCF from healthy subjects; however, with gingivitis and periodontitis, activation products that include C4a, C3b, and C5a are found consistent with activation of both the classic and alternative complement pathways. In addition to these components of the acquired immune response, an extensive profile of inflammatory/immune mediators and cytokines, including prostaglandins, leukotrienes, IL-1, IL-6, TNF-α, and IL-8, have also been identified in GCF and the adjacent gingival tissues. Thus, these components would be expected to contribute to local immune regulations in this local environment.

The GCF also contains a variety of inflammatory and immune cells associated with increasing inflammation. Neutrophils make up the majority of sulcal leukocytes irrespective of the stage of periodontal destruction. However, mononuclear white blood cells, including T cells, B cells, and monocyte/macrophages, are also detected and appear to increase with greater emigration of these cells into the inflamed tissues. In general, GCF contains approximately 95% PMNs, 2% to 3% monocytes, and 1% to 2% lymphocytes. Finally, both bacterial products that can modify host responses and host regulatory molecules that can alter the cellular distribution in the GCF and contiguous tissues can be detected.

Systemic Contribution

The oral epithelium is the only site in the body in which the epithelial barrier is deliberately breached by hard tissues (cementum and enamel). This breach must be sealed from the external milieu. Even in gingival health, a fluid transudate flows from the site of this seal, presumably as a mechanical factor in minimizing bacterial accumulation. This fluid also contains a variety of macromolecular components that are derived from serum and the interstitia of the gingiva. The concentration of these components appears to be related to the size of the molecules, suggesting a passive filtering system of the intact gingival tissues. The levels of these molecules, including protease inhibitors, β_2-microglobulin, fibrinogen, albumin, and lipoproteins, appear proportional to serum levels. Similarly, IgG and IgA are contained in this transudate in a ratio comparable to serum. Thus, in addition to the mechanical cleansing action of the fluid flow, these innate and acquired immune molecules may contribute to healthy homeostasis.

As inflammation of the gingiva increases, the transudate changes to an inflammatory exudate composed of higher levels of serum-derived molecules, vascular-derived cellular components of inflammation, and locally derived molecules from the gingival tissues. Because the macromolecules from serum and gingival tissues are identical species, it has been difficult to accurately determine the contribution of each to the exudate. However, there clearly are unique molecules produced in the local tissues.

Periodontal Health

Local Responses

Gingival health can be characterized by an absence of an inflammatory infiltrate; however, this usually represents subjects who have continual and extensive mechanical prophylaxis and may be considered "supernormal." Histologically, gingival health usually represents a balance between the existing subgingival microbiota and host resistance factors. Thus, there is some minimal inflammation with an associated flow of fluid into the healthy sulcus, as well as some inflammatory cells in the tissues. In this state, the gingival tissues contain low numbers of leukocytes that are primarily classified as lymphocytes. These lymphocytes appear to be primarily T cells, and findings indicate that T-cell clonotypes, as determined by TCR characteristics, are different in healthy gingiva compared with skin and peripheral blood from the same individuals.[7] Further studies have provided the concept that these types of local T cells may be critical to maintaining a homeostasis between the host periodontal tissues and the bacterial plaque. Data have indicated that more than 30% of leukocytes in normal gingival tissue are TCR-$\alpha\beta$, as well as being mostly CD4$^-$, CD8$^-$, and CD45RA$^+$. This phenotype indicates naive/unprimed cells and may be the first line of immune regulatory defense in the local tissues.[8]

Consistent with the low level of inflammation in the healthy gingiva, most studies of inflammatory mediators have shown low levels of these factors, and many healthy sites are devoid of prostaglandin E$_2$ (PGE$_2$) as a marker of inflammation.[9] Furthermore, low or no IL-1β is detected in tissue extracts from healthy sites,[10] and low numbers of cells containing TGF-β1 are found in healthy gingiva.[11] Mediator profiles have been examined in clinically healthy sites from normal subjects, as well as from patients with periodontitis or following treatment (adult maintenance). These results showed higher PGE$_2$ and lower IgA levels in adult maintenance patients and higher PGE$_2$, LTC$_4$, and IL-1β levels in adult refractory patients when compared with healthy sites from normal subjects. Thus, even in clinically healthy sites, it appears that the host controls the local response capabilities, which may indicate some intrinsic control of the inflammatory response.[12] One report has found that IL-8 message is increased in healthy tissues compared with periodontitis tissues.[13] This characteristic might be expected to influence a more robust emigration of neutrophils into the local tissue. Resident gingival fibroblasts have been identified to produce IL-8 when stimulated with bacterial products,[14] and this finding may indicate a local activation of these structural cells in normal tissue remodeling.

In addition to inflammatory cells and mediators, products of the humoral immune response have also been identified locally. Although complement activation is generally considered a protective mechanism in antibacterial immunity, products of this pathway clearly have proinflammatory activities that can lead to tissue destruction. While even in health the gingival sulcus contains bacteria, data have indicated that conversion of C3 is minimal in GCF during health. These findings suggest that the intact epithelium provides an effective barrier or that the bacteria associated with healthy plaque are not particularly active in stimulating alternative complement fixation.[15] Finally, immunoglobulins and antibodies of all isotypes are generally low in GCF from healthy sites, minimizing the potential for various hypersensitivity reactions that could contribute to local tissue destruction.

Systemic Responses

Systemic immune responses in periodontal health would be expected to reflect the lack of local inflammation and immune stimulation, and T-cell sensitization to plaque antigens, in fact, is low in healthy subjects.[16] Serum antibodies to most oral bacteria are detected in healthy subjects. Responses of the IgG, IgM, and IgA isotypes are quite variable with respect to the microorganisms that colonize the supragingival and subgingival plaque in health (eg, oral *Streptococcus* and *Actinomyces* organisms). Additionally, serum antibodies to these bacteria have been found to be significantly lower in periodontally normal adolescents when compared with healthy adults,[17] suggesting a continuum of stimulation by the plaque, even in health. Finally, antibody levels to putative periodontopathogens are usually quite low in health when compared with all other groups (10% to 20% of levels in gingivitis or periodontitis). An interesting report by Schenkein et al[18] indicated that black subjects with a healthy gingiva have a decreased neutrophil chemotaxis when compared with a similar group of white subjects. Therefore, there may exist certain markers, either genetically or environmentally determined, that could indicate increased risk in even healthy individuals.

Gingivitis

Local Responses

Gingivitis is primarily a response to the bacteria in plaque. It includes a vascular response with increased fluid accumulation and inflammatory-cell infiltration. The early response is mostly lymphocytic, represented by T cells; however, advanced and more chronic gingivitis can contain plasma cells. The predominant cell type in inflamed gingiva from adolescents has been identified as the T cell.[19] These local tissue responses are not associated with bacteria in tissues, but are in response to products that appear to traverse the gingival epithelium that has lost some of its innate protective barrier functions. Epithelial cells of the gingival tissues were determined to produce thromboxane B_2 (TXB_2). Histologically, the TXB_2 was significantly increased (10 times) in gingivitis over health, but it remained intracellular.[20] In experimental gingivitis, the inflammatory lesion remains dominated by lymphocytes.[19] Moreover, total T-cell and PMN levels peak early in experimental gingivitis and then decrease, which would be consistent with the B-cell infiltrate noted in more advanced periodontitis tissues.[21]

Acute-phase proteins, including α_2-macroglobulin, α_1-antitrypsin, and transferrin, are increased with gingival inflammation, reflecting the locally stressed environment.[21] Additionally, cleaved C3—indicating conversion of this molecule, presumably through the alternative pathway—is increased in the GCF of gingivitis patients.[22] Cytokines play crucial roles in the maintenance of tissue homeostasis, a process that requires a delicate balance between anabolic and catabolic activities. However, there is little doubt that excessive and/or continuous production of cytokines in inflamed periodontal tissues is responsible for the progression of periodontitis.[23]

Investigations continue to characterize the profile of host responses in gingivitis. The goal of these studies is the ability to identify individuals or sites at risk for transition from gingivitis to destructive disease. Increased levels of IL-1 activity are found in inflamed sites of chronic gingivitis[24] and in experimental gingivitis accompanying increased expression of human leukocyte antigen-DR (HLA-DR).[21] Results by Kinane et al[21] indicate that IL-1 levels in GCF increase with plaque, and peak levels of this mediator precede clinical signs of inflammation in experimental gingivitis. Additionally, both IL-8 protein and message are higher in GCF from inflamed sites.[25]

While it has been suggested that PGE_2 is related to periodontitis and exhibits bone-resorptive capabilities in vitro,[26] numerous reports indicate an initial increase in this mediator in the transition from health to gingivitis. It was recently reported that in experimental gingivitis, PGE_2

levels decreased in GCF through day 21, and TCR-Vβ genes were expressed in both healthy tissues and peripheral blood. However, a restricted expression of the Vβ repertoire was suggested during gingivitis similar to that described in chronic periodontitis.[27] GCF contains increased levels of tissue plasminogen activator in sites with gingivitis. The role of this biomarker as a clinical marker of inflammation was proposed.[28] Cathepsin G in GCF, derived from neutrophils, was also evaluated in experimental gingivitis. The results suggested a rapid increase during experimental gingivitis and an additional increase during the 2- to 3-week interval of study.[29]

Examination of local inflammatory responses in experimental gingivitis has demonstrated some differences between young and old subjects. Variations in acute-phase reactants and some immunoglobulins were noted, as well as an increase in B cells and a decrease in PMNs in old subjects. The results imply some changes in the characteristics of the host response to plaque associated with aging.[30] The level of inflammatory/immune mediators in gingivitis sites from healthy and periodontally diseased patients was also examined. The results showed higher PGE_2, LTC_4, and IL-1β levels in gingivitis sites compared with healthy sites of normal subjects. Additionally, similar levels of IL-2 and IgG, along with lower IgA levels, were noted in the gingivitis sites.[12] In GCF from gingivitis sites of chronic periodontitis patients, PGE_2, LTC_4, IL-1β, IL-2, and IgG levels were increased, while lower IgA levels were noted.

Finally, a report by Grbic et al[31] demonstrated that IgA levels were significantly increased in GCF from gingivitis sites when compared with periodontitis sites, suggesting the potential for IgA to function as a protective factor in this local environment. These findings suggested that inflammation of the periodontium, clinically identified as gingivitis, may express an inflammatory profile that depends on the clinical characteristics of the patient.

Systemic Responses

In general, levels of systemic T-cell responses in gingivitis patients are slightly higher than those in healthy subjects. Increases have been noted in the T-cell response to some of the members of the microbiota that appear to increase in supragingival and subgingival plaque associated with gingivitis (ie, *Streptococcus*, *Actinomyces*, and *Fusobacterium* organisms). The results suggest that antigens from this bacterial accumulation have greater access to the systemic circulation, presumably through a break in the integrity of the epithelial barrier of innate defense.

Similarly, serum antibodies to these types of bacteria are also noted in gingivitis patients. Levels of SIgG antibody to *Actinomyces* species were found to be higher in gingivitis, and antibodies to at least three bacteria (*Actino-*

myces species, *Bacterionema matruchotii*, and *Leptotrichia buccalis*) were detected in gingivitis patients, with a wide variation in levels.[17] Okuda and colleagues[32] examined gingivitis patients and showed a positive correlation between age and increased IgG antibody to *Porphyromonas gingivalis* until puberty. Furthermore, they reported a positive correlation between increased IgG antibody and infection with gingivitis, including increased IgG antibody to *A actinomycetemcomitans* and infection with serotype c in gingivitis. Similar results reported by Danielsen[33] showed that patients with high levels of gingival inflammation had higher levels of serum antibody to *P gingivalis* and *Prevotella intermedia*. In the same study, levels of SIgG antibody to *P intermedia*, *Fusobacterium nucleatum*, and *Streptococcus sanguis* did not change during experimental gingivitis, although levels of IgG to *P gingivalis* decreased with improved oral hygiene and during the development of gingivitis.

Bimstein and Ebersole[34] have examined the serum antibody response patterns in children and young adults to a group of oral microorganisms and related those levels to the severity of gingival disease. Serum IgG and IgM antibody to 14 gram-positive and gram-negative bacteria were examined in children (younger than 12 years) and young adults (older than 20 years). Additionally, the subjects were stratified into those with minimal or no gingival inflammation and those with severe gingivitis. The antibody levels exhibited an age-related increase to most microorganisms. Significant differences in IgM antibody levels to many bacteria were observed between the child and adult groups with gingivitis. The IgM antibody levels also could be used to discriminate between adults with and without gingivitis. In contrast, the IgG levels were unrelated to disease in the adult groups, but they did help to distinguish between the children with and without gingivitis. In both children and adults, the levels of antibody to many of the proposed periodontopathogens were dramatically different than the levels detected in periodontitis patients. Since the bacterial composition of dental plaque has been suggested to be related to the serum antibody levels, these findings may be related to changes in the dental plaque composition associated with gingivitis, as well as the host-bacterial interactions that arise from this inflammatory response.

Many studies have examined serum antibodies to a wide variety of oral bacteria as a control for changes in response in periodontitis. Generally, the gingivitis patients exhibit antibody to an array of these bacteria; however, the levels of antibody to suspected periodontopathogens are uniformly and significantly lower than those seen in periodontitis patients.[35,36] Recently, subjects with gingival recession were noted to have increased levels of SIgG2 antibody to phosphorylcholine (a common bacterial antigen) in comparison with individuals with no attachment loss, supporting a systemic challenge even in the absence of destructive disease.[37] Because T-cell function has been suggested to make an important contribution to immunoregulation in gingivitis and periodontitis, the capacity of T cells derived from patients with gingivitis or periodontitis to proliferate following triggering of the CD3 receptor and interaction with extracellular matrix was evaluated. The results indicated that experimental gingivitis patients showed the highest response to this type of stimulus. Thus, this type of host response activity may help maintain periodontal homeostasis.[38]

Genetic Concepts in Gingivitis

It has long been recognized that, within populations, there appear to be measurable differences in individual responses to plaque accumulation, a noxious challenge to the periodontal tissues. Thus, certain individuals appear to produce a rapid and robust inflammatory response to plaque, while others generate an observably slower clinical inflammatory response. Lang and colleagues (personal communication, 1999) have conducted well-controlled experimental gingivitis studies over many years. Some of these studies have been performed on multiple occasions in the same healthy subjects. These evaluations suggest a rapid development of clinical inflammation during experimental gingivitis.

Ebersole et al[39] have analyzed local host responses during experimental gingivitis in subjects grouped according to high or low response to plaque accumulation. The results suggested differences in levels of local inflammatory mediators and immunoglobulins between the groups. Moreover, the high-responder group demonstrated numerous positive correlations among the host response parameters compared with the low-responder group. One interpretation is that the differences reflect a genetic contribution to the responses and a greater level of immunoregulation in the high responders, potentially related to resistance to destructive disease.[39]

Aggressive Periodontitis

Local Responses

The term *early-onset periodontitis* was used in the periodontal literature for many years to identify a group of diseases in which the periodontal destruction was evident in childhood or the disease appeared to be occurring more rapidly than one would expect from the clinical levels of bacterial plaque. Early-onset periodontitis (EOP) included localized and generalized prepubertal periodontitis (PPP), localized juvenile periodontitis (LJP), generalized juvenile periodontitis (GJP), and rapidly progressive periodontitis (RPP). Nomenclature has recently changed for this group of diseases, since evidence of the time of disease initiation was often not available when the patient was seen clinically for therapy. These diseases are currently included under the term *aggressive periodontitis*. Many of the research studies on aggressive cases, however, used very specific criteria for selecting patients and noted distinct differences in the biology of the different patterns of disease. For example, GJP cases tend to have different antibody responses than LJP cases. This chapter uses the specific disease terms from the original research publications to allow the reader to appreciate some of the biologic distinctions that have been described.

These diseases appear to occur in a high-risk group,[40] and their hallmark is a periodontal destruction that is initiated at an early age; the rapidity of progression is often not commensurate with the level of local inciting factors. The immune-response characteristics of this group are relatively heterogeneous, but a few typical characteristics can be discerned from the literature. The inflammatory cellular infiltrate in the gingival tissues and GCF is predominately PMNs. B cells and plasma cells make up a substantial proportion of the mononuclear-cell infiltrate in lesions of EOP. The plasma cells are predominantly IgG, with lower numbers of IgA cells. Mackler et al[41] also described the subclass distribution of the IgG plasmacytes and suggested an enrichment for IgG4 cells in the diseased tissues. The T cells identified in EOP lesions have been shown to have a decreased T_H/T_C ratio when compared with normal gingival tissues or peripheral blood from the same patients, suggesting an altered immunoregulation that may contribute to periodontal pathology.[42]

Much of the research on inflammatory mediators in periodontitis has been directed toward studies of adult periodontitis.[43] However, some reports have specifically addressed these factors in patients with early-onset disease. Although PGE_2 levels have been noted to increase with gingival inflammation, higher levels are noted in GCF from diseased sites of EOP, particularly at sites exhibiting active attachment loss.[9] IL-1α and IL-1β are detected in 90% of GCF samples from EOP, and the levels of these proinflammatory mediators decreased after treatment,[44] which may contribute to the bone loss in this disease.[45] Manhart et al[46] demonstrated increases in IL-4–producing cells in EOP gingival tissues compared with tissues from gingivitis sites with and without stimulation by *P gingivalis*. Additionally, they noted higher IL-2 levels in EOP than in gingivitis cultures after *P gingivalis* stimulation. Thus, they suggested that altered IL-2/IL-4 levels and associated activities may relate to periodontitis. However, as IL-2 and IL-4 have not been strongly associated with other

forms of periodontitis, this finding will require further investigation. Recently, IL-8 levels in GCF showed a negative correlation with the gingival index in LJP patients. In addition, no significant differences were noted in local IL-8 levels between subjects with LJP and healthy subjects, suggesting an altered ability to produce this neutrophil chemokine in spite of substantial local challenge.[47] Finally, there is evidence that both C3 and C4 components of the complement system are cleaved in GCF from EOP,[22,48] indicating the potential of antigen-antibody complexes to contribute to local immune modulation.

A wealth of evidence supports the existence of local specific antibody production by plasma cells present in inflamed tissues of the periodontal pocket.[49,50] Likewise, a proportion of GCF samples within a given subject have local antibody levels significantly greater than can be accounted for by a serum contribution.[49,50] Similar findings were reported by Johnson et al[51]; GCF antibody levels to *P gingivalis* were often increased in EOP patients, although the site levels varied substantially within the same patient.

Recent findings have used gingival explant cultures to examine local humoral responses. In these studies, nearly 50% of gingival explant cultures from subjects with juvenile periodontitis and RPP, 40% of cultures from subjects with chronic periodontitis, and only 17% of cultures from subjects with healthy tissue made antibody to *A actinomycetemcomitans*.[52] Additionally, gingival explant cultures from subjects with juvenile periodontitis produced IgG antibody most frequently to *E notatum* and *A actinomycetemcomitans*, although more cultures were positive for anti–*P intermedia*, *Capnocytophaga ochracea*, and *Peptostreptococcus micros* than were healthy tissues. These data suggest that this local host response may reflect the potential for multiple bacterial etiologies in juvenile periodontitis.[53]

Cross-sectional studies have suggested that GCF samples with increased antibody levels frequently harbor the homologous bacteria, and that a combination of the antigen and the host response is frequently associated with progressing disease.[50] Studies of GCF from RPP patients showed that sites infected with *P gingivalis* had high levels of specific GCF antibody to this microorganism, which was related to clinical status. After treatment, these local antibody levels decreased with pocket depth, attachment level stabilized, and inflammation resolved.[51]

Extensive studies on EOP patients infected with *A actinomycetemcomitans* demonstrated increased levels of GCF antibodies to *A actinomycetemcomitans* in 90% of the patients, although only 16% of samples had increased IgG antibody to this bacterium. Moreover, approximately 15% of the patients had more than 20% of samples showing increased levels of IgG antibody to *A actinomycetemcomi-*

tans. This prevalence data is substantially greater than previous frequencies reported on general periodontitis populations. The presence of increased levels of IgA antibody to *A actinomycetemcomitans* was also noted in approximately 3% of the sites, which is consistent with previous data reported by Smith et al.[54] However, in this population, no instance of increased IgM antibody to *A actinomycetemcomitans* was demonstrated in any of the 547 sites. This agrees with previous studies that demonstrated a general lack of local production of IgM, as well as IgM plasmacytes in the gingival tissues.[55] The presence of all subclasses of IgG have been identified in GCF, with IgG1 and/or IgG4 levels in GCF increased relative to serum concentrations.[56,57]

These findings also indicated some selectivity in the local IgG antibody response to *A actinomycetemcomitans* in these patients. Examination of absolute levels of antibody in the GCF demonstrated all subclasses; however, IgG3 and IgG4 subclasses were particularly increased relative to comparable serum levels. While nearly 30% of the samples showed antibody levels that were below the level in serum, the antibody pattern was unique and suggested a major contribution of IgG2 in sites with this profile. Approximately 57% of GCF samples exhibited antibody that was within the range of the homologous serum sample and demonstrated a striking increase in IgG1 relative to the other subclasses. Finally, in GCF samples that showed increased antibody relative to serum, the most dramatic changes were in the levels of IgG3 and IgG4. The majority of sites with increased IgG3 and IgG4 antibody were also colonized by the microorganism. The results support the existence of a unique local response in individual sites within certain patients and are consistent with a progression of subclass responses at sites of infection and disease.

An intriguing facet of host responses in periodontitis has been the relationship between local and systemic antibodies. The general paradigm exists that GCF is composed primarily of a serum transudate at the site of inflammation.[58,59] The results showed excellent positive correlations between IgG3, IgG4, and IgG2 levels in serum and GCF when comparing samples demonstrating increased antibody in each of these subclasses.[17] These findings are consistent with the idea of systemic antibody being a manifestation of the local antibody responses in the gingival tissues, and the idea that a portion of serum antibody may be derived from local gingival responses to this infection. In contrast, IgG1 showed a very low correlation and may indicate a different mechanism of antigen processing and presentation for the synthesis of this subclass in local versus systemic tissues.

The studies described above document some characteristics of the local immune response and their relationship

to infection and clinical presentation in EOP patients, particularly periodontitis patients infected with *A actinomycetemcomitans*. The findings are consistent with the potential to utilize antibodies or local mediators in GCF as adjuncts in the diagnosis of periodontitis and in defining the mechanisms of disease.

Systemic Responses

One of the primary features of EOP patients, particularly the LJP subset, is alterations in neutrophil functions, including chemotaxis, phagocytosis, superoxide production, and bactericidal mechanisms.[60,61] Moreover, some patients with RPP[62] and generalized PPP[63] demonstrate these neutrophil dysfunctions. Initially, these dysfunctions emphasized an intrinsic or genetic defect that appeared to be associated with alterations in membrane receptors involved in signaling the neutrophil.[64] However, recently it has been suggested that both local[65] and systemic neutrophils from these diseased patients may exhibit a state of "hyperactivation" resulting in increased adherence and changes in functional capacity.[15]

Furthermore, serum from LJP patients appeared to decrease chemotaxis and formylmethionyl-leucylphenylalanine (FMLP) responses of PMNs.[66] Specifically, neutrophils from LJP patients with decreased chemotaxis and increased adherence showed increased expression of the CD11/CD18 family of adherence molecules. Treatment of normal neutrophils with sera from the LJP patients increased the expression of these molecules, and pretreatment of the LJP sera with anti–TNF-α or anti–IL-1β partially inhibited this activity. Thus, the upregulation of adherence molecules on neutrophils by LJP sera suggested the importance of circulating cytokines in modulating neutrophil functions in these patients.[67] Variable and sometimes abnormal circulating T_H/T_C ratios have been noted in EOP or RPP.[19] Nagai et al[68] have reported abnormal proportions of γ∂ T cells in EOP and chronic periodontitis patients when compared with healthy subjects. These alterations in T-cell phenotypes may relate to the decreased autologous mixed leukocyte reaction (AMLR) activity in GJP or RPP patients.[19]

In addition to the T-cell alteration, there has been reported a hyperresponsiveness of peripheral blood mononuclear cells to B-cell mitogens in GJP.[19] Recently, T-cell responses to peptides from a 53-kd antigen of *P gingivalis* were evaluated in EOP and healthy subjects. The findings indicated that a peptide fragment with amino acids from positions 141 to 161 contained a major T-cell epitope recognized by EOP patients but not by healthy subjects.[69] A single report examined acute-phase proteins or cytokines in serum from EOP patients and showed that their TNF-α levels were similar to those of normal subjects.[70]

Accompanying the documentation of specific infections in periodontitis patients has been the definition of active host systemic immune responses to these bacteria.[17] Previous studies have suggested that serum antibody specificities may reflect a local gingival response to plaque bacteria, including *A actinomycetemcomitans*, and the presence of increased serum IgG antibody to *A actinomycetemcomitans* in periodontitis patients.[17] In particular, it appears clear that in most populations, patients with LJP exhibit increased serum IgG antibody to *A actinomycetemcomitans*.[71] These results have been derived from cross-sectional studies and have demonstrated some correlation with the ability to identify the homologous microorganism in the subgingival plaque.[72,73]

In longitudinal studies, serum antibody reactivity to individual antigens suggested a variation in response over time in individual patients, consistent with antigenic diversity.[74] Findings of one study suggested that human serum antibody reactivities to *A actinomycetemcomitans* are observed to a wide variety of antigens derived from the outer membrane of this pathogen. The results indicated a response to certain antigens that were distinctive in active disease patients. They may do the following: *(1)* indicate changes in antigen expression by *A actinomycetemcomitans*,[75] *(2)* reflect the overall increase in serum antibody levels noted in active disease patients, or *(3)* relate to the increase in the *A actinomycetemcomitans* burden resulting in greater antigenic load. Similarly, a relationship was reported between individual antibody reactivities to outer membrane antigens of *A actinomycetemcomitans* and the extent of existing disease.[76]

Questions have arisen as to why periodontal disease can have periods of exacerbation in patients with a substantial host local[77-79] and systemic[80-84] antibody response. Although serum IgG antibodies to *A actinomycetemcomitans* have been shown to have a protective function, as evidenced by a negative correlation with disease severity, a more complicated relationship between the antibody and infection with *A actinomycetemcomitans* has been indicated.[85-88] Current data[77] are consistent with the idea that serum antibody produced during infection successfully lowers the infection to a threshold that is at or below the level necessary for destructive processes.

Studies on SIgG antibody to *A actinomycetemcomitans* or antigens isolated from the bacteria have found a diversity of responses, as indicated by different IgG subclass patterns. The significance of these differences is not yet understood.

Longitudinal investigations of host immune responses in periodontal disease have generally been directed toward use of these response characteristics to acquire a clearer understanding of the mechanisms resulting in tissue destruction, or as a method for correlation with disease activity and assessment of treatment outcomes.[89,90] Previous studies using heterogeneous populations of patients with periodontal diseases have suggested some relationship between antibody levels and disease activity; however, consistent findings have not been provided.[17] In one early study of 22 patients monitored for up to 5 years, 14 of the patients showed episodes of active disease.[91] Two thirds of the patients demonstrated increased serum antibody to the same bacteria during multiple phases of disease. Additionally, it appeared that multiple treatment procedures were required to affect the level of antibody in the serum.

A separate study noted that patients with increased SIgG antibody showed the homologous microorganism in 80% of active sites, suggesting that the increased antibody is a response to an active infection and accompanying disease.[92] A complex association has recently been shown between the distribution of *A actinomycetemcomitans* infection (ie, the number of teeth infected and the proportion of *A actinomycetemcomitans* per tooth) and the antibody levels to the intact bacteria in both serum[92] and GCF.[77] In other studies, approximately 70% of the patients with active disease showed an increase in IgG antibody level by 2 to 4 months prior to clinical evidence of disease activity. Patients with the greatest frequency of active disease appeared to show a general decrease in the recognition of the *A actinomycetemcomitans* outer membrane antigens. Thus, it appeared that *A actinomycetemcomitans* infection relates to a particular type of disease with accompanying antibody responses that reflect periods of active disease. The dynamics of this infection and the systemic antibody responses to this pathogen indicate that the immune response is critical to managing this infection.

It appears clear that *P gingivalis* is highly correlated with a subset of patients diagnosed as having RPP, and it may be an important etiologic agent in disease progression. The level of antibodies to this microorganism is generally low in younger individuals and increases dramatically in some cases of generalized EOP.[93,94] Geographic differences in antibody responses have also been reported. For example, a higher number of Turkish LJP and RPP patients exhibited increased antibody to *P gingivalis* compared with US patients. The findings suggested potential differences in subgingival colonization by suspected periodontal pathogens and/or antigenic composition of the strains from varying geographic regions.[95]

In conclusion, while *A actinomycetemcomitans* and *P gingivalis* appear to be predominant pathogens in EOP, other bacteria, including *P intermedia*, *Eubacterium corrodens*, and *Campylobacter rectus*, have been implicated based on both microbiologic and immunologic studies.[17,96,97] A detailed study of serum antibody responses to various spirochetes showed a higher frequency of seropositive juvenile periodontitis patients, while patients with severe EOP had a uniformly low level or absence of antibody to the treponemes, although they were cultivated from these patients.[98] Similarly, serum antibody to *Bacteroides forsythus*, a major pathogen in chronic periodontitis, is found at low levels and low frequency in EOP patients.

Genetic Concepts in Aggressive Periodontitis

Numerous studies have shown that EOP clearly aggregates within families.[99] This finding has spurred research to explore the potential genetic control of this disease.[100,101] HLA A9, B15, A28, and DR4 positively associated with EOP (both RPP and LJP), and HLA A2 and A10 negatively associated.[99,102,103] Furthermore, various reports have described an HLA linkage to generalized periodontitis (ie, RPP), but not as strong a linkage to LJP.[99,100,102–104] HLA A9 and B15 associated with generalized, but not localized, EOP.[102] Early studies identified a female preponderance of EOP; however, recent information has suggested this to be an ascertainment bias. Furthermore, Marazita et al[104] defined an autosomal major locus with dominant transmission in both blacks and nonblacks, with penetrance of approximately 70% in EOP.

How this genetic predisposition may contribute to susceptibility to EOP remains ill defined. As described previously, there is some indication that neutrophils from these patients may show an intrinsic functional defect or may respond abnormally to challenge with certain pathogens.[60,61,67,105] Various studies have identified transmission of *A actinomycetemcomitans* within families with EOP, suggesting increased susceptibility to infection as a predisposing factor.[106,107] Moreover, evidence has shown an increased incidence of LJP and GJP in black individuals who exhibit increased SIgG2 levels, increased IgG2 antibody to *A actinomycetemcomitans*, and neutrophil alterations.[99,108]

A recent investigation has identified an increased frequency of the HLA *DRB1*1501-DQB1*0602* genotype in EOP patients.[103] This HLA genotype has an altered amino acid, which may enhance its ability to bind certain bacterial antigens. Additionally, a strong T-cell response to a *P gingivalis* antigen was noted with this genotype, suggesting that an altered T-cell response could increase susceptibility to periodontitis.[109] Finally, significant evidence of a linkage disequilibrium in the IL-1 genetic polymorphism was found in EOP patients, irrespective of smoking. The IL-1 alleles associated with high risk in EOP were those identified with low risk in adult periodontitis patients. The overall findings suggested that EOP is a complex, oligogenic disorder and that IL-1 genetic variation may contribute to this.[110] Summarizing

these findings would support some likelihood of a genetic control of host immune responses to infection, with this microorganism contributing to decreased resistance and disease susceptibility.

Chronic Periodontitis

Local Responses

Extensive studies have been performed examining the characteristics of the inflammatory infiltrate in chronic periodontitis (CP). The distribution of gingival mononuclear cells includes plasma cells (5% to 15%), lymphocytes (30% to 35%), and macrophages (40% to 55%) in CP.[111] The T_H/T_C ratios are reduced in adult periodontal lesions when compared with homologous peripheral blood and normal/chronic gingivitis tissues.[46,63,112] The proportions of infiltrating mononuclear inflammatory cells in granulation from chronic periodontitis and EOP patients were evaluated. B cells predominated in chronic periodontitis lesions but not in EOP lesions, while T cell levels were lower. No differences in macrophages were noted. The ratio of macrophages to T cells was also increased in CP lesions. No differences were noted in proportions of memory T cells, nor in the CD4/CD8 in the disease categories.[113]

The plasma cells are predominately IgG, followed by IgA; no IgM cells are found in tissues from CP.[114] Moreover, IgG cells in the gingival tissues were identified as IgG1 > IgG2 > IgG3 ≅ IgG4 and IgA1, with high levels of IgA2 cells in advanced lesions.[114] Kinane and coworkers[115] demonstrated histologically that IgG, IgA, and J chains can be locally produced in periodontitis tissues. They noted that IgG1 was the predominant IgG-expressing plasma cell in gingiva and granulation tissues. In contrast, IgA was primarily expressed in the gingiva, with IgA1 predominating, although IgA2 and J chain–positive cells were enriched in the gingiva. It is interesting to note that deeper tissues contain IgM plasma cells, with lower levels of other isotypes.

Extensive studies have examined the presence of levels of inflammatory/immune mediators in GCF and gingival tissues of chronic periodontitis.[116] Clearly, PGE_2 levels are increased in periodontitis when compared with healthy sites, and evidence has been provided that sites with active attachment loss exhibit even higher levels.[9] With respect to IL-1, investigations have shown the following: *(1)* IL-1α and IL-1β activity were found in more than 70% of GCF[44,117–119]; *(2)* IL-1β levels appear higher in GCF from CP when compared with healthy sites and in active sites versus inactive sites,[12,118,120,121] which decrease after treatment[44]; *(3)* IL-1β and cells producing this cytokine are increased in tissues of CP and are detected in the lamina propria of these tissues[121–123]; and (4) most studies were unable to document a relationship between IL-1β and the clinical parameters (ie, pocket depth, gingival index, and bone resorption) of the site.[10,119,122] Although a recent study suggested that GCF collected from periodontitis patients exhibited an increased activity for stimulating osteoclastic bone resorption, biologic evaluation of the samples demonstrated this activity as IL-1α.[124]

Low and inconsistent levels of IL-2 have been detected in GCF, with levels lower in CP than in normal sites.[2,15] Additionally, lymphocytes from periodontitis patients with slight inflammation appear to produce detectable IL-2.[123] Consistent with these findings in the fluid are few or no IL-2–producing cells within the gingival mononuclear cell population.[114,125,126]

Similarly, the literature consistently supports a lack of IL-4 product in GCF or cells in gingival tissues of CP patients.[63,114,126] However, a report by Seymour et al[126] suggested that subjects susceptible to breakdown have an increase in IL-4 (type 2)–producing T cells, and nonsusceptible subjects exhibit an enrichment of 1 IL-2 (type 1)/IFN-γ–producing T cells in gingiva. In contrast, high levels of IL-5–producing cells have been detected in CP gingival tissues.[63,114]

Because B lymphocytes and plasma cells have been identified as significant components of the cellular infiltrate in progressing periodontitis, numerous studies have examined IL-6 production in these tissues as a regulator of B-cell expansion.[127] These studies have shown the following: (1) IL-6–producing mononuclear cells are increased in inflamed gingival tissue of CP when compared with healthy tissue,[63,114,123,128] and gingival mononuclear cells from CP tissues produce IL-6 at higher levels than do peripheral mononuclear cells from the same patients[123]; (2) IL-6 levels in GCF are correlated with bleeding and pocket depth, and these IL-6 levels were higher in active disease active sites[129]; (3) IL-6 message in the inflamed gingival tissues is detected in lymphoid cells (macrophages) and nonlymphoid cells (endothelial cells and fibroblasts) but is absent in healthy tissues[128]; (4) local B-cell increases in differentiation into plasma cells would correlate with high local IL-6 levels[130]; and (5) IL-6R (receptor) is increased in gingival mononuclear cells of CP patients.[111]

A recent study demonstrated that both IL-6 and IL-10 were also locally increased in inflamed tissues compared with peripheral blood. TNF-α has been detected in GCF and tissues from patients with CP[123,124]; however, this cytokine has not been found to be related to Gingival or Plaque Index or pocket depth.[123]

Calprotectin, a zinc-binding protein, is a major cytosol protein of leukocytes that increases at sites of inflammation and has antimicrobial activities. Calprotectin levels in GCF were significantly correlated with GCF volume, the degree of gingival inflammation, collagenase levels, and aspartate aminotransferase levels.[131] GCF cathepsin G was also positively correlated with periodontitis and was decreased by initial treatment.[29]

Exudates from periapical periodontitis patients were evaluated for the production of nitric oxide (NO) by PMNs. The findings indicated that inflammatory cytokines produced by stimulated mononuclear cells can trigger PMNs to produce NO at the site of chronic periodontal infections. The NO levels would alter vascular function and could be involved in regulating chronic inflammation.[132]

The increased levels of tissue plasminogen activator (TPA) in GCF from periodontitis sites were significantly decreased after periodontal therapy. The role of TPA in periodontal tissue destruction and tissue remodeling, as well as a clinical marker of inflammation and treatment, was proposed.[28] The neuropeptide substance P was detected in GCF and related to various host-response biomarkers and clinical presentations. Substance P was correlated with probing depth, but it appeared unrelated to gingival inflammation. This molecule was also correlated with PGE_2, aspartate aminotransferase, alkaline phosphatase, myeloperoxidase, IL-1β, TNF-α, IL-8, and MCP-1 levels, suggesting a coupling of this molecule with the general local host inflammatory response.[133] Therefore, it appears that developing profiles of the proinflammatory and anti-inflammatory cytokines/mediators and other biomarkers in the local environment, as well as gaining insight into the dynamics of their formation and regulation, should lead to a better understanding of mechanisms contributing to tissue destruction or maintenance of gingival health.

Numerous studies have identified the presence of Ig in GCF and the cells within inflamed gingival tissues producing immunoglobulins.[45,78,134] Recently, studies of the regulatory aspects of the cells in the gingival tissues have shown that Ig production by GMC is suppressed after in vitro stimulation,[125] but can be increased after removal of $CD8^+$ cells.[42] These results suggested that B cells in the gingival tissues are already stimulated, which is consistent with increased IgG levels in GCF from CP patients with active disease.[135] Furthermore, IgG1 and IgG4[56,136,137] appear to be specifically increased in GCF in active sites of CP patients. Soluble Fcγ-binding components (eg, Fcγ receptor III) have been detected in GCF from periodontal lesions.[138] Additionally, GCF and serum from periodontitis patients were analyzed for soluble Fcγ receptor III. The results showed increased local levels of this molecule when compared with matched sera, suggesting a potential contribution to disruption of local homeostasis.[139] IgA levels have been routinely negatively correlated with attachment level, pocket depth, and bleeding before and after treatment.[31] Because IgA synthesis is highly dependent on T_H

cells, the lower number of these regulatory cells in destructive disease would provide a link in the T-cell–B-cell progression in disease.

In addition to Ig levels in GCF of CP patients, various studies have examined specific antibody responses in these fluids. As such, sites with greater pocket depth and higher levels of inflammation showed lower GCF antibody to *P gingivalis*.[140] A significant frequency of GCF samples with increased antibody to *P gingivalis* in periodontitis sites of CP patients compared with normal sites has been found.[141]

Systemic Responses

Early studies indicated that T cells in the periphery are sensitized to antigens from oral bacteria in adult periodontitis patients.[16] However, the data concerning whether these responses are antigen specific or mitogenic have been ambiguous. More recent data examining cytokine production as a marker of T-cell activation have also provided varied results. Levels of IL-2, IL-2R, and IL-4 have been reported to be higher in sera of subjects with CP compared with healthy subjects.[123] The allogeneic mixed leukocyte reaction (MLR), an indicator of T-cell function, was found to be altered—both high and low—in individual CP patients, with circulating CD4+/CD45R+ T cells significantly reduced in those patients with depressed allogenic MLR and IL-2 generation. It is interesting that both the allogenic MLR and T-cell phenotypes were restored to normal following successful clinical treatment.[16] CTLA-4+ cells (expressed at the late phase of T-cell activation) within the CD4+ T-cell population were increased in periodontitis patients following stimulation with outer membranes of *P gingivalis*. Additionally, IL-10 messenger RNA was increased in the diseased patients following the outer membrane stimulation. These findings lend additional support to the importance of local immune regulation in health and disease. Moreover, CD5 and HLA-DR cells appear to be increased in peripheral blood of periodontitis patients compared with healthy patients.[142] Both TNF-α and IL-6 levels were similar in serum from patients with CP and normal subjects,[70,128] while IL-6 and antigen-specific–antibody plasma cells were detected in the periphery of CP patients only with stimulation. Sensitization of patients with periapical periodontitis was examined by stimulation of blood cultures to produce proinflammatory cytokines. *Prevotella melaninogenica* elicited increased levels of IL-6 from patients with multilesional disease in comparison with other groups. Therefore, it appears that characterization of these cytokines/mediators supports the local nature of host-parasite interactions in periodontitis, without strong evidence for generalized stimulation of inflammatory responses like those noted in diseases such as rheumatoid arthritis.

In contrast to results noted with cytokines/mediators, increased systemic antibody levels have routinely been noted in CP patients.[17,96] Although polyclonal B-cell activation has been found to be increased in some periodontitis patients,[143] the majority of reports in CP have substantiated a specific immune response. Black-pigmented bacteria are frequently members of the microbial ecology in subgingival plaque at sites of periodontitis lesions in adults.

It now appears clear that *P gingivalis* is highly correlated with adult periodontitis and probably other clinical types of periodontitis, and it may be an important etiologic agent in disease progression.[144,145] As in most bacterial infections, various investigations have identified increased systemic antibody responses to *P gingivalis* in periodontal disease.[17] Levels of antibodies to this microorganism are generally low in younger individuals and increase dramatically in many cases of adult periodontitis.[93]

A report by DeNardin et al[146] compared serum IgG antibody levels to various *P gingivalis* isolates between younger and older adult periodontitis patients. The findings indicated that both older and younger patients with periodontitis exhibited increased serum IgG antibody to *P gingivalis*. While IgG is a distinctive immune response to *P gingivalis*, increased levels of both IgM and IgA isotypes have been shown in CP patients.[147] Additionally, IgG and IgM antibody avidity to *P gingivalis* was higher in subjects with CP compared with RPP controls.[148] This finding was generally supported by Lopatin and Blackburn,[149] who found a low avidity in CP patients and suggested a potential low function for these antibodies. Furthermore, serum anti–*P gingivalis* antibody level and avidity were noted to change following therapy.[150] Kinane et al[140] identified serum IgG and serum IgA antibody levels to *P gingivalis*, which correlated with GCF antibody levels in CP patients.

Examination of *P gingivalis* has shown that the microorganism contains a variety of potential virulence factors and structures that may be crucial to its pathogenicity.[151] In many bacterial infections, the host response to antigens from pathogens may provide some measure of protection from disease progression induced by the microorganisms. Thus, knowledge of the specificity of the host antibody responses could be important as a diagnostic tool and/or in understanding the protective nature of the response.

Various studies have identified human antibody responses in periodontitis to some of these factors,[32,152–154] although recent investigations have demonstrated the complexity of human antibody responses to surface antigens of *P gingivalis*.[155,156] Adult patients seropositive for P gingivalis were used to examine the characteristics of serum antibody to *P gingivalis* serotypes K1 to K6, representing the capsular antigens. There were correlations of antibody levels to the various K antigens within the population. The primary antibody was IgG2, and a relationship was noted between smoking and decreased antibody to the K2 serotype. The results suggested that having antibodies to multiple serotypes is common in adult periodontitis patients.[157] The avidity of the IgG antibody to whole-cell antigens, LPS, and fimbriae of P gingivalis was determined in periodontitis and healthy subjects. The patient sera with high antibody levels had low-avidity antibody compared with the sera of healthy subjects, suggesting that a lack of function of the humoral immune response in periodontitis may contribute to susceptibility to this pathogen.[158] Evaluation of patients with periapical periodontitis lesions demonstrated that LPS from suspected periodontal pathogens elicited higher IL-8 levels, and the diseased patients exhibited increased antibody to P gingivalis LPS.[159] Finally, a novel approach to identifying immunodominant antigens from P gingivalis used a panel of murine monoclonal antibodies and delineated the ability of sera from patients to block binding to specific antigens. The results identified an antigen defined as PF18, which was identified by antibody in sera of patients but was absent from sera of all healthy subjects. The antibody in the patients' sera was predominantly the IgG2 subclass.[160]

Additional studies[161,162] have shown IgG2 as the principal subclass response to LPS from P gingivalis (IgG2 > IgG4 > IgG3 > IgG1 and IgA2 > IgA1), and IgG3 was the predominant response to fimbriae from the microorganism (IgG3 > IgG1 > IgG2 > IgG4 and IgA1 > IgA2). Recent data indicated that particular antigen bands were indicative of early responses to the P gingivalis serotypes; however, as higher levels of antibody were produced, reactions to additional antigens appeared and may be indicative of a more advanced infectious process.[155]

Longitudinal studies have suggested that individuals have unique P gingivalis responses and that the levels are modulated by episodes of disease activity and treatment. Various other investigations have also shown that treatment of periodontitis often results in decreases of systemic antibody to P gingivalis after an interval of time.[163-165] It also has been noted in both AP and EOP subjects that treatment can decrease SIgG antibody levels to certain microorganisms, but these changes were noted to take as long as 8 to 10 months after treatment and were specific for selected bacteria in individual patients.[35]

Thus, the current knowledge about antibody levels in periodontitis and changes associated with treatment appears to be dependent on patient selection, antibody specificity examined, and study design. It is clear that a subpopulation of periodontitis patients develop an extensive serum antibody response, which can recognize multiple serotypes of P gingivalis and may define a patient population with a P gingivalis disease.[155] It has been reported that human immune responses to outer-envelope antigens from A actinomycetemcomitans exhibit substantial heterogeneity in quality and quantity,[76] suggesting the potential for antigenic diversity among A actinomycetemcomitans infections. In contrast, other results indicate a more consistent antigenic composition for P gingivalis as recognized by humans, which may enhance the potential for strategies to immunologically interfere with disease caused by this microorganism.[155] Serum antibody levels and avidity to A actinomycetemcomitans and P gingivalis were related to clinical parameters of periodontitis. A negative correlation between probing depth and antibody level and avidity was observed using A actinomycetemcomitans and the antigen. A positive correlation was noted with the level and avidity of antibody to P gingivalis and probing depth. Additionally, the antibody characteristics were negatively correlated with A actinomycetemcomitans infection and positively correlated with P gingivalis infection. These results suggested that the relationship of periodontitis severity, antibody responses, and infection varied with these two pathogens and may relate to the effectiveness of the humoral immune response in controlling the infections.

While P gingivalis appears to play a prominent role in periodontitis in adults, it is clear that other putative periodontopathogens make up a distinct proportion of the population that in most cases is not colonized by P gingivalis. In one study in which adult periodontitis patients were stratified according to the frequency of active disease episodes, the results indicated that increased antibody to P intermedia, E corrodens, and C rectus was correlated with more severe disease.[83] Consequently, this type of study supports the potential for serum antibody to be used as an indicator of disease in selected patients, in addition to identifying potential etiologic agents.

Okuda et al[32] have shown a positive correlation between increased IgG to A actinomycetemcomitans and infection in adult periodontitis. Studies of SIgG antibody in AP to LPS and fimbriae of A actinomycetemcomitans showed that increased antibody levels and avidity to fimbriae were related to lack of cultivable A actinomycetemcomitans.[166,167] No difference in antibody avidity to A actinomycetemcomitans was noted in CP patients compared with other groups.[168] Serum antibody responses to A actinomycetemcomitans outer-membrane antigens were studied in infected adult patients. The results demonstrated antibody to approximately 40% of the antigens, which was significantly greater than that noted in healthy subjects. Moreover, selected antigens were dominant, as well as being distributed differently in adult versus EOP patients.

Serum antibody reactivity to individual antigens suggested a variation in response over time in individual patients, consistent with antigenic diversity.[74] Chronic periodontitis patients exhibit significantly increased serum IgG and serum IgA antibody to most *Eubacterium* species compared with healthy subjects. This is consistent with the available evidence linking *Eubacterium* species with the biofilm of periodontitis patients. A cell-surface protein of *B forsythus* was identified as a 98-kd protein (BspA) and the gene (bspa) sequenced. Adult periodontitis patients exhibit antibody to this protein, which may contribute to the ability of the pathogen to interact with extracellular matrix and clotting factors.[169]

The characteristics of *P micros* in chronic periodontitis patients showed a higher proportion of smooth strains in periodontitis, although the levels of serum antibody were not different in periodontitis versus gingivitis, nor in smokers versus nonsmokers.[170] In contrast, Mangan et al[171] reported that serum antibody to treponemes was lower in patients with AP than in controls, with little relationship to the spirochete proportions in plaque. Similar results were noted with antibody to *B forsythus*, which was at low levels and low frequency in chronic periodontitis patients, suggesting that this microorganism may be poorly immunogenic or less capable of interacting with the systemic immune response apparatus.[172] These findings support the concept that the quality of humoral immune response to suspected periodontopathogens should have an effect on the etiology of periodontitis. They also support the need to further study this host-parasite interaction.

Genetic Concepts in Chronic Periodontis

Numerous recent studies have begun to define and evaluate potential genetic contributions to the risk of developing adult periodontitis. A study by Kornman and di Giovine[173] examined IL-1 polymorphisms in chronic periodontitis. The results indicated that, excluding smokers, a particular IL-1 allele genotype was significantly correlated with severe adult periodontitis. A further investigation observed that the composite IL-1 genotype was significantly associated with the severity of adult periodontitis in a study of a clinical practice population. Additionally, smoking was a significant response modifier in this population. The results suggest that IL-1 genotyping and smoking history can be objective risk factors for periodontal disease.[174] Similarly, the distribution of bi-allelic IL-1β and TNF-α genotypes was determined in adult periodontitis and healthy subjects. One allele for each of these cytokines was significantly increased in advanced periodontitis patients when compared with either healthy or gingivitis subjects. However, there appeared to be no correlation of the genotypes with cytokine production in the patients.[174]

Severe Generalized Chronic Periodontitis

Local Responses

Immunologic data describing host responses in refractory periodontitis patients are sparse. One reason for this lack of information is the difficulty in documenting this disease, as well as in attempting to generate a homogenous group in which to assess the characteristics of the host local and systemic responses. Additionally, because the pathogens associated with disease in this patient group appear similar to those in other forms of periodontitis, the suggestion has been made that this patient group may represent a host defect in response to these bacteria. Sites in refractory periodontitis patients with the highest total cytokine level demonstrated that refractory patients had higher IL-6 levels than stable patients.[175] Moreover, the presence of *P gingivalis*, *E corrodens*, or *A actinomycetemcomitans* correlated with only increased GCF IL-1 levels. Thus, local IL-1 and IL-6 production may be in response to different factors, and IL-6 may play a role in refractory periodontitis.[175]

Systemic Responses

As has been mentioned, there is a paucity of data describing systemic immune responses in patients with refractory periodontitis. Recent findings indicate that CD4-to-CD8 ratios are decreased in refractory periodontitis.[176] Additionally, *P gingivalis* LPS stimulation of monocytes from refractory patients caused a change in monocyte phenotype and increased IL-1β and PGE$_2$ secretion compared with subjects with gingivitis or normal subjects.[176] There is preliminary evidence that serum from refractory periodontitis patients demonstrates elevations in IgG antibody to multiple periodontopathogens. However, the variability in the population was extensive and diminished statistical significance.

Refractory periodontitis patients were denoted as a heterogeneous group using serum antibody levels to a large battery of subgingival bacterial species. In general, the refractory patients exhibited higher numbers and levels of serum antibody reactions than those noted in successfully treated or healthy subjects. The results demonstrated that high levels of serum antibody to a select group of bacteria identified patients with an increased likelihood of being refractory to conventional periodontal therapy.[177] A discriminant analysis used by Colombo and colleagues[178] included plaque composition, serum antibody levels, genetic haplotypes, and clinical measures to characterize refractory periodontitis patients. The results indicated that a combination of 17 predictor variables, including serum antibody levels, could be used to discriminate refractory periodontitis patients with robust sensitivity and specificity. Refractory adult patients infected with *A actinomycetemcomitans* were evaluated for the genotype of the microorganism and antigenic specificity of serum antibody prior to and following therapy. The results indicated that each patient was infected with a single genotype, which persisted throughout the study. No differences in antibody activity were noted to outer-membrane antigens from baseline or 24-month isolates. Finally, it appeared that only certain genotypes were associated with refractory disease.[179]

Studies examining the development of treatment modalities for these patients suggested altered host defenses, particularly cell-mediated defenses in patients with severe forms of periodontitis that do not respond to treatment.[180] Thus, the lack of response to treatment may result from impaired host defense or exaggerated inflammatory responses.[180] Clearly, additional studies are required to identify unique or common components of local and systemic inflammatory/immune responses in these patients.

Periodontitis Modified by Intrinsic or Extrinsic Factors

Individuals with congenital and acquired alterations in immune functions should provide models to aid in delineating the cellular mechanisms contributing to periodontitis. Frequently these individuals suffer from severe systemic medical complications, and thus the maintenance of general health supersedes oral concerns and often complicates interpretation of host-parasite interactions at local sites of disease activity. However, there do exist some data that describe the frequency and severity of periodontitis in subjects who are compromised by these immune alterations.

Patients with Immunodeficiencies

Substantial literature exists concerning increased periodontitis in patients with neutrophil dysfunction. Disease in these patients may present as unusually severe periodontitis ranging from marginal gingivitis to rapidly progressive periodontal disease with advancing bone loss affecting both deciduous and permanent teeth.[181] This relationship has been described in detail previously,[61] so the following sections will concentrate on deficiencies that affect the acquired immune system functions.

Congenital Deficiencies

A variety of genetically determined syndromes or diseases alter the normal functions of the host immune system. The congenital changes are brought about by numerous alterations in the host genome and are manifest at various stages in the ontogenic development of the immune apparatus. The genetic lesions that affect the earliest stages of stem cell differentiation are often fatal in infancy due to broad-based systemic viral, bacterial, or fungal infections. However, as medical care capabilities increase, individuals with congenital immune abnormalities are surviving and may be subject to severe oral complications that could pose a threat to compromised systemic management. Various investigations have been performed to document the prevalence and severity of periodontal disease in these affected individuals and to use the information to explain the cellular mechanisms controlling susceptibility or resistance to this oral disease.

There is a range of immune dysfunctions that alter B-cell, T-cell, complement, and phagocytic cell functions. In general, studies that have included patients with decreased B- or T-cell numbers and/or functions have suggested that the severity of periodontal disease is similar to that in normal individuals.[182–185] These observations have been interpreted to mean that the acquired immune system has minimal involvement in the development of, or protection from, periodontal disease. However, these studies are not straightforward in design and usually include populations that are under extensive medical care. This care often includes the chronic administration of prophylactic antibiotics or routine injection of gamma globulin to prevent life-threatening complications of the immune deficiencies.

Furthermore, a number of these investigations have included both gingival inflammation associated with gingivitis and the destructive forms of periodontal disease in assessing clinical parameters of these individuals. These "experiments of nature" have not been exceptionally useful in clarifying the mechanisms of disease and presumably reinforce the complexity of host-parasite interactions that occur in the disease. They are also consistent with the view that maintaining periodontal health is the ultimate requirement for maintenance of immune regulation and disease prevention at the local site.

Acquired Deficiencies

A variety of extrinsic factors can also result in transient or chronic immunosuppression. These include various malignant changes; anticancer chemotherapy; immunosuppressive agents used in tissue transplantation; radiation therapy; bone-marrow transplantation; autoimmune diseases;

and bacterial, viral, and fungal diseases. Studies of patients receiving immunosuppressive drugs have generally noted no more disease than normal.[186,187] However, as with congenitally immunocompromised patients, these individuals are often under varied and extensive medical coverage, which makes interpretation of direct host-parasite relationships difficult.

Kristoffersen[188] reviewed the possible relationship of serum antibody responses and immunosuppression by periodontopathic bacteria in the initiation and progression of periodontitis. Additionally, it has been reported that several plaque components can suppress immune responses.[189–192] Some of the reports of lower antibody levels in periodontitis (compared with healthy controls) are consistent with this in vivo functional activity. It has also been suggested that increased antibody levels after treatment could be due to removal of immunosuppressive factors. There have likewise been reports of decreased lymphoproliferative responses, particularly in severe periodontitis.[193]

These suppressive factors in periodontitis could have the following: (1) a normal regulatory role in modulating immune response to indigenous flora, (2) a pathogenic role for evasion of host responses, (3) a role in protection by limiting inflammatory response, or (4) a diagnostic/prognostic value, where depressed antibody and/or lymphoproliferation could identify subjects at risk. Extension of results derived from human studies and animal models should allow a more decisive approach to the immunologic interference with bacterial infections.

Patients with Diabetes Mellitus

Type I Diabetes Mellitus

Type 1 diabetes mellitus (T1DM, or insulin-dependent diabetes mellitus) and type 2 diabetes mellitus (T2DM, or non–insulin-dependent diabetes mellitus) have both been shown to be major risk factors for the development of periodontal disease.[194–196] Earlier studies of the influence of diabetes on periodontal disease progression make it difficult to discriminate between patients with T2DM and T1DM, except on the basis of age of onset, since few clinical data were provided other than for hyperglycemia. Hyperglycemia progressively glycates proteins in T1DM patients. These altered proteins can stimulate phagocytes to release greater levels of proinflammatory mediators when challenged, thus exacerbating inflammatory tissue destruction.[197]

Studies from Finland have indicated that patients with poorly controlled T1DM and T2DM, demonstrated more gingival bleeding,[198] more periodontal pockets,[199] and an increased prevalence and severity of periodontitis and calculus formation.[200] The investigators concluded that duration and quality of diabetic control, combined with the presence of calculus at periodontal sites, were important risk factors for periodontal disease in diabetics. Furthermore, more severe periodontitis was noted when the amount of plaque was the same as that present in nondiabetic controls.

Studies of oral biomarkers to discriminant susceptible patients have shown salivary peroxidase activity in subjects with T1DM and healthy subjects. Clinical measures of plaque and inflammation were increased in the T1DM patients, which appeared to be related to significantly increased levels of this biomarker.[201] T1DM patients with periodontitis also appear to have increased levels of fragmented serum α1-proteinase inhibitor compared with orally healthy patients, although levels of functional α1-proteinase inhibitor were similar among the patients.[202]

Preliminary evidence has suggested that the HLA-DR4 genotype is associated with diabetes and periodontitis.[203] Recently, selected HLA-DR alleles were associated with impaired neutrophil chemotaxis in T1DM patients with increased risk for EOP.[204] An interesting study explored the relationship among T1DM, periodontitis, and HLA haplotype of antibody response characteristics to *Capnocytophaga* species antigens. The results identified antibody response profiles related to T1DM, periodontitis, or both. Furthermore, specific HLA-DR,DQ haplotypes were related to T1DM and/or periodontitis, as well as correlating with the IgG reactivity patterns. Generally, the responses to this bacterial genus were depressed in T1DM and periodontitis. The conclusions also suggested that periodontitis in T1DM may be related more to the HLA-D haplotype and altered immune responses than to the diabetes itself.[205]

Periodontal therapy had a negligible effect on medical parameters of T1DM or T2DM patients. Moreover, the oxidative burst of PMNs following stimulation with either TNF-α or FMLP was similar in patients with diabetes or normal patients, suggesting that well-controlled diabetics should respond well to nonsurgical periodontal therapy.[206] Substantial evidence indicates that patients with diabetes have recurrent bacterial and mycotic infections and immune alterations.[207–211] These include decreased T-cell proliferation and IL-2 production,[203] as well as defects in chemotaxis, phagocytosis, and bacterial killing by PMNs.[212] Various reports have described the predominant microorganisms in periodontitis sites from T1DM subjects.[213–215] However, evidence for alterations in serum antibody levels to periodontopathogens in diabetes is sparse. Morinushi et al[216] showed that antibody to *Actinomyces naeslundii* and *F nucleatum* increased with age in T1DM subjects and related these findings to oral microbial changes with puberty. A further study in T1DM patients with periodontitis demonstrated few antibody responses to *P gingivalis*; however, five of nine patients had increased antibody to *A actinomycetemcomitans* that correlated with *A actinomycetemcomitans* infection.[217]

A variety of studies have evaluated potential alterations in host-based responses as contributing to the increased risk of periodontal destruction in T1DM. T1DM patients exhibit significantly elevated GCF levels of PGE_2 and IL-1β compared with healthy subjects with a similar level of periodontitis. T1DM patients also exhibit an upregulated monocyte response to LPS, resulting in increased levels of PGE_2, IL-1β, and TNF-α compared with nondiabetic controls. Moreover, within the T1DM population, those patients with the greatest periodontitis demonstrated an enhanced monocyte responsiveness.[218] High GCF and monocytic secretion of PGE_2 and IL-1β in T1DM patients may be a consequence of a systemic response trait. The presence of chronic gram-negative bacterial infections that accompany periodontitis may elicit high levels of local mediators and increase the severity of disease.[219] Similarly, T1DM patients exhibit significantly higher TNF-α responses of monocytes to P gingivalis LPS. Moreover, T1DM patients with periodontitis were more responsive to the LPS, suggesting an upregulation of the host response compared with both adult periodontitis and T1DM patients with gingivitis or periodontal health.[220] A subset of T1DM patients have the following: (1) an extremely robust IL-10 response to P gingivalis LPS; (2) higher levels of CD5 B cells, which are related to autoantibody production; and (3) a higher frequency of anti–collagen-secreting cells in peripheral blood. This hyperresponsive phenotype could predispose the individual to periodontitis through autoimmune mechanisms.[221]

Type 2 Diabetes Mellitus

T2DM is a heterogeneous disorder characterized by diminished tissue sensitivity to insulin and impaired β-cell function. It accounts for about 90% of the diabetic patients in the United States. The prevalence of T2DM is markedly increased among Native Americans, African Americans, and Hispanics. Patients with T2DM may demonstrate normal or increased basal insulin concentrations combined with insulin resistance and diminished tissue sensitivity to insulin that progressively leads to impaired β-cell function. T2DM is usually diagnosed after the age of 30 years and is frequently observed as part of a multifaceted syndrome that includes obesity, hypertension, dyslipidemia, and atherosclerotic cardiovascular disease. Insulin deficiency, combined with insulin resistance, leads to the hyperglycemia associated with advanced T2DM. Substantial evidence indicates a genetic predisposition to T2DM, as well as environmental familial influences, such as diet and obesity.

Rosette-forming T cells appear similar in T2DM and normals subjects, while IgG, IgA, IgM, and IgE were increased in serum of periodontitis patients with and without T2DM.[209] Analysis of clinical periodontal data from the Pima Indian study[144,222] demonstrated that there was an increased prevalence of periodontal destruction in the diabetic group and that this had led to a greater degree of tooth loss in this population. Further analysis of the relationships between T2DM and oral health status in this population[223] revealed that only diabetic status, age, and the presence of subgingival calculus were significantly associated with increased severity and prevalence of periodontal destruction. Diabetes increased the risk of developing destructive periodontal disease about threefold.

Data have suggested a model whereby severe periodontitis increases the severity of diabetes by complicating metabolic control. The infection associated with periodontitis upregulates cytokine synthesis by chronic stimulation. These factors can modify the effects of the advanced-glycation end product on cytokine responses and synergize in disease expression.[224] Circulating immune complexes have been reported to be increased in the serum of T2DM patients with periodontitis compared with nondiabetics.[208]

Data are available concerning the bacterial specificity of T2DM-associated periodontal disease. Studies of T2DM in the Pima Indians suggested that P gingivalis from disease sites of this high-risk group was a different serotype than that found in periodontitis patients who did not have T2DM.[144,215] The higher prevalence of periodontal destruction in diabetics has also been confirmed by Grossi et al,[196] who showed that age, diabetes, smoking, and the presence of the periodontal pathogens P gingivalis and B forsythus were the major clinical determinants for periodontal destruction. The extent of control of the diabetic condition appeared to have minimal impact on the characteristics of the pathogens present at disease sites. P gingivalis, P intermedia, C rectus, F nucleatum, and E corrodens could be identified at disease sites in T2DM subjects, and diabetes control had no effect on the distribution of these bacteria.[215] Thus, it would appear that periodontitis in diabetics is characterized by a similar set of putative pathogens as those noted in adult periodontitis. A single study showed increased serum IgG antibody to P intermedia and P gingivalis in T2DM periodontitis and suggested a role for these pathogens in disease in this type of high-risk patient.[215] Another study has been initiated to investigate serum antibody responses to oral bacteria in Hispanic subjects with T2DM and periodontitis. The results indicated that serum IgG antibody to both P gingivalis and C rectus is significantly increased in periodontitis T2DM patients. Additional information is required to delineate the host responses in T2DM periodontitis, as well as the relationship of these responses to subgingival microbial colonization.

IL-6 levels were significantly increased in GCF from T2DM subjects when compared with adult periodontitis and healthy subjects. No correlation was noted between IL-6 levels and clinical parameters. The elevation of IL-6 in T2DM could indicate a different microbial challenge or altered host responses in the local environment.[225] Clinical indices of periodontitis are significantly increased in patients with poorly controlled and well-controlled T2DM versus systemically healthy patients. There were significant positive correlations between GCF IL-1β, gingival tissue IL-1β, and IL-6 with periodontal inflammation. Additional variations were noted in the oral and systemic environments related to diabetic control.[226]

Environmental Factors

Smoking

Numerous reports have documented a relationship between smoking and periodontal disease. Tobacco smoking is probably the most important, controllable environmental risk factor in periodontitis.[227] The effect of smoking on gingivitis appears to be a function of smoking exposure and the amount of local plaque challenge. In virtually all populations studied, there was a significantly increased frequency of periodontitis in patients who smoked.[144] Young adults with EOP had advanced periodontal destruction prior to referral for specialist care. Smoking was strongly correlated with severe bone destruction in these EOP patients, particularly in patients with generalized disease.[228]

Bergström and Preber[229] provided data indicating that smokers and nonsmokers exhibit similar periodontopathogens, thus supporting a role for altered host responses in susceptibility to increased disease. With gingival health, GCF volume is decreased with smoking, although no differences are noted in a variety of inflammatory mediators in the GCF.[230] Cigarette smoking resulted in lowered elastase and neutrophil levels in the oral cavity, suggesting a lack of correlation of these measures with the severity of periodontitis in smokers.[231] In contrast, PGE_2 and matrix metalloproteinase-8 levels were increased with probing depth in periodontitis, and elastase levels were increased in diseased sites of smokers.[232]

It is interesting to note that nicotine and smokeless tobacco increased the inflammatory response of peripheral blood mononuclear cells to stimulation with oral bacterial products. However, these materials did not alter the response of gingival mononuclear cells, suggesting that the local cells were already maximally stimulated.[233] Peripheral neutrophil responsiveness to opsonized bacteria was increased in periodontitis patients but was unaffected by smoking. CRP levels were also increased in periodontitis. The neutrophil count, haptoglobin levels, and α1-antitrypsin levels were altered by smoking.[234] In measurements of various acute-phase proteins in the serum of

these patients, there was extensive variation in both the diseased and healthy subjects, although C-reactive protein appeared to be increased in smokers with EOP.[235]

There appears to be some relationship between serum cotinine levels (as a measure of smoking) and soluble intercellular adhesion molecule 1, which has been linked to cardiovascular disease and could affect periodontal health.[227] A study examining smokers with EOP compared with healthy nonsmokers and healthy smokers with only gingivitis demonstrated that total IgG and IgA were significantly increased compared with both healthy nonsmokers and healthy smokers, while IgA was significantly decreased in the healthy smoker group. These findings suggest that smoking may negatively affect the systemic immune system.[235] IgG antibody to only P gingivalis was increased in the EOP group versus the other groups. Moreover, IgG2 levels were lower in periodontitis patients, and this effect was compounded by smoking.[234] Smoking was correlated with a decrease in SIgG2 levels and increased periodontal destruction in white subjects. This relationship was not observed in black adult periodontitis. patients.[236] Additionally, smoking was associated with a reduction in SIgG2 antibody to A actinomycetemcomitans in generalized EOP patients, although IgG2 antibody to other antigens appeared unaffected.[237] These results suggest that smoking may contribute to host immune alteration and susceptibility to colonization by, and infection with, certain pathogens. When the capacity of oral bacteria to exhibit toxicity in the presence of cotinine was evaluated, cotinine appeared to synergize toxic activities exhibited by the periodontal pathogens.[238]

The genetic relationship of this environmental risk was noted in studies examining IL-1 polymorphism in adult periodontitis. The results indicated that, excluding smokers, a particular IL-1 allele genotype was significantly correlated with severe adult periodontitis. It was suggested that smoking and the IL-1 genotype are independent risk factors in severe periodontitis.[173] The composite IL-1 genotype was significantly associated with the severity of adult periodontitis in a study of a clinical practice population. Additionally, smoking was a significant response modifier in this population. The results suggested that IL-1 genotyping and smoking history can be objective risk factors for periodontal disease.[174]

Conclusions

This chapter has attempted to describe the broad armamentarium that the host can mount both to maintain homeostasis in the face of pathogenic agents from the environment and to exist as part of the commensal ecology of humans. There do appear to be strategies used by the host to protect itself specifically against extracellular (humoral immune strategies), intracellular (cell-mediated immune strategies), and toxin-producing (humoral immune strategies) pathogens. These defense strategies have generally been delineated for acute or chronic medical infections. For more than two decades, studies of periodontal disease have been oriented toward an infectious process with some apparent specific pathogens. This concept has resulted in investigations to develop immunologic strategies for interfering with tissue destruction in the periodontium. Because the majority of proposed periodontopathogens appear to be extracellular pathogens that in some cases produce toxins, the humoral immune response has been emphasized in these studies.

The recognition of both local and systemic immune responses in periodontal disease also prompted comparisons in attempting to elucidate mechanisms for protection or destruction of host tissues. Investigations of both humans and animal models have also demonstrated a sequence of cellular infiltrates into the inflamed tissues that appears to reflect the critical nature of PMNs in providing primary protection, and of T lymphocytes as the local immunoregulators in maintaining a healthy periodontium. It is clear that specific pathogens or consortia of microorganisms initiate an immunoinflammatory process, which is the major contributor to tissue destruction in periodontitis. Kornman[239] recently suggested that specific targeting of tissue-destructive enzymes, inflammatory mediators, and/or selected cytokines may be an important future strategy for reducing periodontitis.

The increasing significance of oral disease as a manifestation of systemic compromise in patients, as well as the potential for oral disease to adversely affect the medical condition, must also be recognized. These concepts could thus be formulated into a characterization of "high-risk" patients for periodontitis within the population. The contribution of innate and acquired immune responses in each of these populations will vary, and the complex of host resistance/susceptibility and microbial virulence will be a challenge for general practitioners and periodontists in the future.

References

1. Ebersole JL, Cappelli D. Acute phase reactants in infections and inflammatory diseases. Periodontol 2000 2000;23:19–49.
2. Yoshikai Y, Nishimura H. The role of interleukin-15 in mounting an immune response against microbial infections. Microbes Infect 2000;2:381–389.
3. Mathy NL, Scheuer W, Lanzendorfer M, et al. Interleukin-16 stimulates the expression and production of pro-inflammatory cytokines by human monocytes. Immunology 2000;100:63–69.
4. Schwarzenberger P, Huang W, Ye P, et al. Requirement of endogenous stem cell factor and granulocyte-colony-stimulating factor for IL-17-mediated granulopoiesis. J Immunol 2000;164:4783–4789.
5. Okamura H, Tsutsui H, Kashiwamura S-I, et al. Interleukin-18: A novel cytokine that augments both innate and acquired immunity. Adv Immunol 1998;70:281–312.
6. Cimasoni G. Crevicular Fluid Updated. Basel, Switzerland: Karger, 1983.
7. Kinane DF, Karin SN, Garioch JJ, et al. Heterogeneity and selective localization of T cell clones in human skin and gingival mucosa. J Periodontal Res 1993;28:497–499.
8. Lundqvist C, Hammarström M-L. T-cell receptor-expressing intraepithelial lymphocytes are present in normal and chronically inflamed human gingiva. Immunology 1993;19:38–45.
9. Offenbacher S, Heasman PA, Collins JG. Modulation of host PGE₂ secretion as a determinant of periodontal disease. J Periodontol 1993;64:432–444.
10. Honig J, Rordorf AC, Siegmund C, et al. Increased IL-1 beta concentration in gingival tissues of periodontitis patients. J Periodontal Res 1989;24:362–367.
11. Steinsvoll S, Halstensen TS, Schenck K. Extensive expression of TGF-beta1 in chronically-inflamed periodontal tissue. J Clin Periodontol 1999;26:366–373.
12. Ebersole JL, Singer RE, Steffensen B, et al. Inflammatory mediators and immunoglobulins in GCF from healthy, gingivitis, and periodontitis sites. J Periodontal Res 1993;28:543–546.
13. Tonetti MS, Freiburghaus K, Lang NP, Bickel M. Detection of interleukin-8 and matrix metalloproteinases transcripts in healthy and diseased gingival biopsies by RNA/PCR. J Periodontal Res 1993;28:511–513.
14. Dongari-Bagtzoglou AI, Ebersole JL. Production of inflammatory mediators and cytokines by human gingival fibroblasts following bacterial challenge. J Periodontal Res 1996;31:90–98.
15. Lamster IB, Novak MJ. Host mediators in gingival crevicular fluid: Implications for the pathogenesis of periodontal disease. Crit Rev Oral Biol Med 1992;3:31–60.
16. Okada H. T cell functions in periodontal diseases. In: Hamada S, Holt S, McGhee J (eds). Periodontal Disease: Pathogens and Host Immune Responses. Chicago: Quintessence, 1991:223–236.
17. Ebersole JL. Systemic humoral immune responses in periodontal disease. Crit Rev Oral Biol Med 1990;1:283–331.
18. Schenkein HA, Best AM, Gunsolley JC. Influence of race and periodontal clinical status on neutrophil chemotactic responses. J Periodontal Res 1991;26:272–275.
19. Ranney RR. Immunologic mechanisms of pathogenesis in periodontal diseases: An assessment. J Periodontal Res 1991;26:243–254.
20. Bons-Sicard C, Choquet A, Escola R. Localization and quantification of TXB2 in human healthy and inflammatory gingival mucosa. J Periodontal Res 1998;33:27–32.
21. Kinane DF, Adonogianaki E, Moughal N, et al. Immunocytochemical characterization of cellular infiltrate, related endothelial changes and determination of GCF acute-phase proteins during human experimental gingivitis. J Periodontal Res 1991;26:286–288.
22. Patters MR, Neikrash CE, Lang NP. Assessment of complement cleavage in gingival fluid during experimental gingivitis in man. J Clin Periodontol 1989;16:33–37.
23. Okada H, Murakami S. Cytokine expression in periodontal health and disease. Crit Rev Oral Biol Med 1998;9:248–266.

24. Charon JA, Luger TA, Mergenhagen SE, Oppenheim JJ. Increased thymocyte-activating factor in human gingival fluid during gingival inflammation. Infect Immun 1982;38:1190–1195.

25. Bickel M. The role of interleukin-8 in inflammation and mechanisms of regulation. J Periodontol 1993;64:456–460.

26. Offenbacher S, Collins JG, Yalda B, Haradon G. Role of prostaglandins in high-risk periodontitis patients. In: Genco R (ed). Molecular Pathogenesis of Periodontal Disease. Washington, DC: American Society of Microbiology, 1994:203–213.

27. Preshaw PM, Geatch DR, Lauffart B, et al. Longitudinal changes in TCRβ variable gene expression and markers of gingival inflammation in experimental gingivitis. J Clin Periodontol 1998; 25:774–780.

28. Yin X, Bunn CL, Bartold PM. Detection of tissue plasminogen activator (t-PA) and plasminogen activator inhibitor 2(PAI-2) in gingival crevicular fluid from healthy, gingivitis and periodontitis patients. J Clin Periodontol 2000;27:149–156.

29. Kunimatsu K, Mine N, Muraoka Y, et al. Identification and possible function of cathepsin G in gingival crevicular fluid from chronic adult periodontitis patients and from experimental gingivitis subjects. J Periodontal Res 1995;30:51–57.

30. Fransson C, Mooney J, Kinane DF, Berglundh T. Differences in the inflammatory response in young and old human subjects during the course of experimental gingivitis. J Clin Periodontol 1999;26:453–460.

31. Grbic JT, Singer RE, Jan HH, et al. Immunoglobulin isotypes in gingival crevicular fluid: Possible protective role of IgA. J Periodontol 1995;66:55–61.

32. Okuda K, Saito A, Hirai K, et al. Role of antibodies in periodontopathic bacterial infections. In: Genco R (ed). Molecular Pathogenesis of Periodontal Disease. Washington, DC: American Society for Microbiology, 1994:257–265.

33. Danielsen B, Wilton JMA, Baelum V, et al. Serum immunoglobulin G antibodies to Porphyromonas gingivalis, Prevotella intermedia, F nucleatum and Streptococcus sanguis during experimental gingivitis in young adults. Oral Microbiol Immunol 1993;8:154–160.

34. Bimstein E, Ebersole JL. Serum antibody levels to oral microorganisms in children and young adults with relation to the severity of gingival disease. Pediatr Dent 1991;13:267–272.

35. Ebersole JL, Holt SC. Immunological procedures for diagnosis and risk assessment in periodontal diseases. In: Johnson N (ed). Periodontal Diseases: Markers of Disease Susceptibility and Activity. Cambridge, England: Cambridge University Press, 1991:203–227.

36. Ebersole JL, Holt SC, Cappelli D, Kesavalu L. Significance of systemic antibody responses in the diagnostic and mechanistic aspects of progressing periodontitis. In: Hamada S, Holt S, McGhee J (eds). Periodontal Disease: Pathogens and Host Immune Responses. Chicago: Quintessence, 1991:343–357.

37. Schenkein HA, Gunsolley JC, Best AM, et al. Antiphosphorylcholine antibody levels are elevated in humans with periodontal diseases. Infect Immun 1999;67:4814–4818.

38. Slotwinska SM, Gorski A, Wierzbicka M, et al. T-cell interactions with extracellular matrix proteins in periodontal disease. Immunol Lett 1998;63:131–134.

39. Ebersole JL, Lang NP, Singer RE. Inflammatory profile of gingival crevicular fluid in experimental gingivitis [abstract 514]. J Dent Res 2001;80:100.

40. Johnson NW, Griffiths GS, Wilton JM, et al. Detection of high-risk groups and individuals for periodontal diseases: Evidence for the existence of high-risk groups and individuals and approaches to their detection. J Clin Periodontol 1988;15:276–282.

41. Mackler BE, Waldrop TC, Schur P, et al. IgG subclass bearing lymphocytes and plasma cells. J Periodontal Res 1978;13: 109–119.

42. Taubman MA, Wang HY, Lundquist CA, et al. The cellular basis of host responses in periodontal diseases. In: Hamada S, Holt S, McGhee J (eds). Periodontal Disease: Pathogens and Host Responses. Chicago: Quintessence, 1991:199–208.

43. Page RC. The role of inflammatory mediators in the pathogenesis of periodontal disease. J Periodontal Res 1991;26:230–242.

44. Masada MP, Persson R, Kenney JS, et al. Measurement of interleukin-1alpha and -1beta in gingival crevicular fluid: Implications for the pathogenesis of periodontal disease. J Periodontal Res 1990;25:156–163.

45. Mundy GR. Inflammatory mediators and the destruction of bone. J Periodontal Res 1991;26:213–217.

46. Manhart SS, Reinhardt RA, Payne JB, et al. Gingival cell IL-2 and IL-4 in early-onset periodontitis. J Periodontol 1994;65: 807–813.

47. Ozmeric N, Bal B, Balos K, et al. The correlation of gingival crevicular fluid interleukin-8 levels and periodontal status in localized juvenile periodontitis. J Periodontol 1998;69: 1299–1304.

48. Schenkein HA, Genco RJ. Gingival fluid and serum in periodontal diseases, II. Evidence for activation of complement components C3, C3 proactivator and C4 in gingival fluid. J Periodontol 1977;48:778–784.

49. Ebersole JL, Taubman MA, Smith DJ, Goodson JM. Gingival crevicular fluid antibody to oral microorganisms, I. Method of collection and analysis of antibody. J Periodontal Res 1984;19: 124–130.

50. Ebersole JL, Taubman MA, Smith DJ. Local antibody responses in periodontal diseases. J Periodontol 1985;56:51–55.

51. Johnson V, Johnson BD, Sims TJ, et al. Effects of treatment of antibody titer to Porphyromonas gingivalis in gingival crevicular fluid of patients with rapidly progressive periodontitis. J Periodontol 1993;64:559–565.

52. Hall ER, Falkler WA, Martin SA, Suzuki JB. The gingival immune response to Actinobacillus actinomycetemcomitans in juvenile periodontitis. J Periodontol 1991;62:792–798.

53. Hall ER, Martin SA, Suzuki JB, Falkler WA Jr. The gingival immune response to periodontal pathogens in juvenile periodontitis. Oral Microbiol Immunol 1994;9:327–334.

54. Smith D, Gadalla L, Ebersole J, Taubman M. Gingival crevicular antibody to oral microorganisms. III. Association of gingival homogenate and gingival crevicular fluid antibody levels. J Periodontal Res 1985;20:357–367.

55. Sandholm L, Saxen L. Local immunoglobulin synthesis in juvenile and adult periodontitis. J Clin Periodontol 1984;11:459–466.

56. Reinhardt RA, McDonald TL, Bolton RW, et al. IgG subclasses in gingival crevicular fluid from active versus stable periodontal sites. J Periodontol 1989;60:44–50.

57. Powell JR. Mediators of inflammation and tissue destructive metabolism in gingival crevicular fluid (GCF). J Dent Res 1992;72: 1848.

58. Cimasoni G. Crevicular fluid updated. In: Myers H (ed). Monographs in Oral Science. Basel, Switzerland: Karger, 1983:45–102.

59. Challacombe SJ, Russell MW, Hawkes J. Passage of intact IgG from plasma to the oral cavity via crevicular fluid. Clin Exp Immunol 1978;34:417–422.

60. Kalmar JR. Antimicrobial dysfunction in localized juvenile periodontitis neutrophils. In: Genco R (ed). Molecular Pathogenesis of Periodontal Disease. Washington, DC: American Society for Microbiology, 1994:337–349.

61. Van Dyke TE. Role of neutrophils in host defense to periodontal infections. In: Hamada S, Holt S, McGhee J (eds). Periodontal Disease: Pathogens and Host Immune Responses. Chicago: Quintessence, 1991:251–261.

62. Page RC, Altman LC, Ebersole JL, et al. Rapidly progressive periodontitis: A distinct clinical condition. J Periodontol 1983; 54:197–209.

63. Van Dyke TE, Lester MA, Shapira L. The role of the host response in periodontal disease progression: Implications for future treatment strategies. J Periodontol 1993;64:792–806.

64. DeNardin E. Neutrophil receptors: N-formyl-l-methionyl-l-leucyl-l-phenylalanine and interleukin-8. In: Genco R (ed). Molecular Pathogenesis of Periodontal Disease. Washington, DC: American Society for Microbiology, 1994:351–361.

65. Wilton JMA. Crevicular neutrophils: Protective or damaging? In: Lehner T, Cimasoni G (eds). The Borderland Between Caries and Periodontal Disease. Geneva: Editions Medecine et Hygiene, 1986:71–85.

66. Agarwal S, Suzuki JB, Piesco NP, Aichelmann-Reidy MB. Neutrophil function in juvenile periodontitis: Induction of adherence. Oral Microbiol Immunol 1994;9:262–271.

67. Agarwal S, Suzuki JB. Altered neutrophil function in localized juvenile periodontitis: Intrinsic cellular defect or effect of immune mediators. J Periodontal Res 1991;26:276–278.

68. Nagai A, Takahashi K, Sato N, et al. Abnormal proportion of ys T cells in peripheral blood is frequently detected in patients with periodontal disease. J Periodontol 1993;64:963–967.

69. Ohyama H, Matsushita S, Kato N, et al. T cell responses to 53-kDa outer membrane protein of Porphyromonas gingivalis in humans with early-onset periodontitis. Hum Immunol 1998;59: 635–643.

70. Meyle J. Neutrophil chemotaxis and serum concentration of tumor-necrosis-factor-α (TNFα). J Periodontal Res 1993;28: 491–493.

71. Cappelli D, Ebersole JL, Kornman KS. Early-onset periodontitis in Hispanic adolescents associated with A actinomycetemcomitans. Community Dent Oral Epidemiol 1994;22:116–121.

72. Ebersole JL, Taubman MA, Smith DJ, et al. Human serum antibody responses to oral microorganisms, IV. Correlation with homologous infection. Oral Microbiol Immunol 1987;2:53–59.

73. Tew JG, Marshall DR, Moore WEC, et al. Serum antibody reactive with predominant organisms in the subgingival flora of young adults with generalized severe periodontitis. Infect Immun 1985;48:303–311.

74. Ebersole JL, Steffen MJ, Cappelli D. Longitudinal human serum antibody responses to outer membrane antigens of Actinobacillus actinomycetemcomitans. J Clin Periodontol 1999;26:732–741.

75. Hall E, Ebersole JL, Prihoda TJ, Steffen MJ. Antigenic diversity in Actinobacillus actinomycetemcomitans: Presumptive identification. J Dent Res 1993;72:244.

76. Ebersole JL, Cappelli D, Sandoval M-N, Steffen MJ. Antigen specificity of serum antibody in Actinobacillus actinomycetemcomitans–infected periodontitis patients. J Dent Res 1995;74: 658–666.

77. Ebersole JL, Cappelli D. Gingival crevicular fluid antibody to Actinobacillus actinomycetemcomitans in periodontal disease. Oral Microbiol Immunol 1994;9:335–344.

78. Genco RJ, Zambon JJ, Murray PA. Serum and gingival fluid antibodies as adjuncts in the diagnosis of A. actinomycetemcomitans-associated periodontal disease. J Periodontol 1985;56: 41–50.

79. Tew JG, Marshall DR, Burmeister JA, Ranney RR. Relationship between gingival crevicular fluid and serum antibody titers in young adults with generalized and localized periodontitis. Infect Immun 1985;49:487–493.

80. Ebersole JL, Taubman MA, Smith DJ, et al. Human immune responses to oral micro-organisms, I. Association of localized juvenile periodontitis (LJP) with serum antibody responses to Actinobacillus actinomycetemcomitans. Clin Exp Immunol 1982; 47:43–52.

81. Ebersole JL, Sandoval M-N, Steffen MJ, Cappelli D. Serum antibody in A. actinomycetemcomitans-infected patients with periodontal disease. Infect Immun 1991;59:1795–1802.

82. Wilton JMA, Johnson NW, Curtis MA, et al. Specific antibody responses to subgingival plaque bacteria as aids to the diagnosis and prognosis of destructive periodontitis. J Clin Periodontol 1991;18:1–15.

83. Ebersole JL, Cappelli D, Steffen MJ. Characteristics and utilization of antibody measurements in clinical studies of periodontal disease. J Periodontol 1992;63:1110–1116.

84. Genco RJ. Host responses in periodontal diseases: Current concepts. J Periodontol 1992;63:338–355.

85. Califano JV, Schenkein HA, Tew JG. Immunodominant antigens of Actinobacillus actinomycetemcomitans serotype b in early-onset periodontitis patients. Oral Microbiol Immunol 1992;7: 65–70.

86. Page RC, Sims TJ, Engel LD, et al. The immunodominant outer membrane antigen of A. actinomycetemcomitans is located in the serotype-specific high-molecular-mass carbohydrate moiety of lipopolysaccharide. Infect Immun 1991;59:3451–3462.

87. Tsai C-C, McArthur WP, Baehni PC, et al. Serum neutralizing activity against Actinobacillus actinomycetemcomitans leukotoxin in juvenile periodontitis. J Clin Periodontol 1981;8:338–348.

88. Underwood K, Sjöström K, Darveau R, et al. Serum antibody opsonic activity against Actinobacillus actinomycetemcomitans in human periodontal diseases. J Infect Dis 1993;168: 1436–1443.

89. Taubman MA, Haffajee AD, Socransky SS, et al. Longitudinal monitoring of humoral antibody in subjects with destructive periodontal diseases. J Periodontal Res 1992;27:511–521.

90. Ebersole JL, Cappelli D, Steffen MJ, et al. Host response assessment in recurring periodontitis. J Clin Periodontol 1996;23: 258–262.

91. Ebersole JL, Holt SC. Serum antibodies to periodontopathic microorganism: Specific induction. In: Guggenheim B (ed). Periodontology Today. Basel, Switzerland: Karger, 1988:169.

92. Ebersole JL, Cappelli D, Sandoval M-N. Subgingival distribution of A. actinomycetemcomitans in periodontitis. J Clin Periodontol 1994;21:65–75.

93. Mouton C, Hammond PG, Slots J, Genco RJ. Serum antibodies to oral Bacteroides asaccharolyticus (Bacteroides gingivalis): Relationship to age and periodontal disease. Infect Immun 1981;31:182.

94. Ebersole JL, Taubman MA, Smith DJ, Frey DE. Human immune responses to oral microorganisms: Patterns of systemic antibody levels to Bacteroides species. Infect Immunol 1986;51:507.

95. Celenligil H, Ebersole JL. Analysis of serum antibody responses to periodontopathogens in early-onset periodontitis patients from different geographical locations. J Clin Periodontol 1998; 25:994–1002.

96. McArthur WP, Clark WB. Specific antibodies and their potential role in periodontal diseases. J Periodontol 1993;64:807–818.

97. Ebersole JL, Taubman MA. The protective nature of host responses in periodontal diseases. Periodontol 2000 1994;5:112–141.

98. Tew JG, Smibert RM, Scott EA, et al. Serum antibodies in young adult humans reactive with periodontitis associated treponemes. J Periodontal Res 1985;20:580–590.

99. Schenkein HA. Genetics of early-onset periodontal diseases. In: Genco R (ed). Molecular Pathogenesis of Periodontal Disease. Washington, DC: American Society for Microbiology, 1994:373–386.

100. Wilton JMA. Unchanging, subject-based risk factors for destructive periodontitis: Race, sex, genetic, congenital and childhood systemic diseases. In: Johnson N (ed). Periodontal Diseases: Markers for Disease Susceptibility and Activity. Cambridge, England: Cambridge University Press, 1991:109–138.

101. Hart TC. Genetic considerations of risk in human periodontal disease. Curr Opin Periodontol 1994;3–11.

102. Shapira L, Eizenberg S, Sela MN, et al. A9 and B15 are associated with the generalized form, but not the localized form, of early-onset periodontal diseases. J Periodontol 1994;65:219–223.

103. Takashiba S, Noji S, Nishimura F, et al. Unique intronic variations of HLA-DQB gene in early-onset periodontitis. J Periodontol 1994;65:379–386.

104. Marazita ML, Burmeister JA, Gunsolley JC, et al. Evidence for autosomal dominant inheritance and race-specific heterogeneity in early-onset periodontitis. J Periodontol 1994;65:623–630.

105. Van Dyke TE, Duncan RL, Cutler CW, et al. Mechanisms and consequences of neutrophil interaction with subgingival microbiota. Periodontol Today 1988:209–217.

106. Alaluusua SS, Asikainen SM, Lai C-H. Intrafamilial transmission of Actinobacillus actinomycetemcomitans. J Periodontol 1991;62:207–210.

107. Zambon JJ, Christersson LA, Slots J. Actinobacillus actinomycetemcomitans in human periodontal disease: Prevalence in patient groups and distribution of biotypes and serotypes within families. J Periodontol 1983;54:707–712.

108. Gunsolley JC, Tew JG, Gooss CM, et al. Effects of race and periodontal status on antibody reactive with Actinobacillus actinomycetemcomitans strain Y4. J Periodontal Res 1988;54:303–307.

109. Karimzadeh K, Morrison J, Zadeh HH. Comparison of gingival and peripheral blood T cells among patients with periodontitis suggests skewing of the gingival T cell antigen receptor V beta repertoire. J Periodontal Res 1999;34:445–456.

110. Diehl SR, Wang Y, Brooks CN, et al. Linkage disequilibrium of interleukin-1 genetic polymorphisms with early-onset periodontitis. J Periodontol 1999;70:418–430.

111. Fujihashi K, McGhee JR, Yamamoto M, et al. Cytokine networks and immunoglobulin synthesis in inflamed gingival tissues. In: Genco R (ed). Molecular Pathogenesis of Periodontal Disease. Washington, DC: American Society for Microbiology, 1994:135–145.

112. Okada H. Phenotypic and functional characterization of peripheral blood T cells in adult periodontitis. J Periodontal Res 1991;26:289–292.

113. Lappin DF, Koulouri O, Radvar M, et al. Relative proportions of mononuclear cell types in periodontal lesions analyzed by immunohistochemistry. J Clin Periodontol 1999;26:183–189.

114. Fujihashi K, Kono Y, Beagley KW, et al. Cytokines and periodontal disease: Immunopathological role of interleukins for B cell responses in chronic inflamed gingival tissues. J Periodontol 1993;64:400–406.

115. Kinane DF, Lappin DF, Koulouri O, Buckley A. Humoral immune responses in periodontal disease may have mucosal and systemic immune features. Clin Exp Immunol 1999;115:534–541.

116. Lamster IB, Smith QT, Celenti RS, et al. Development of a risk profile for periodontal disease: Microbial and host response factors. J Periodontol 1994;65:511–520.

117. Tatakis DN. Interleukin-1 and bone metabolism: A review. J Periodontol 1993;64:416–431.

118. Priess DS, Meyle J. Interleukin-1B concentration of gingival crevicular fluid. J Periodontol 1994;65:423–428.

119. Wilton JMA, Bampton JLM, Hurst TJ, et al. Interleukin-1B and IgG subclass concentrations in gingival crevicular fluid from patients with adult periodontitis. Arch Oral Biol 1993;38:55–60.

120. Stashenko P, Nguyen L, Li Y-P. Mechanisms of regulation of bone formation by proinflammatory cytokines. In: Genco R (ed). Molecular Pathogenesis of Periodontal Disease. Washington, DC: American Society for Microbiology, 1994:171–181.

121. Jandinski JJ, Stashenko P, Feder LS, et al. Localization of interleukin-1B in human periodontal disease. J Periodontol 1991;62:36–43.

122. Kabashima J, Maeda K, Iwamoto Y, et al. Partial characterization of an interleukin-1-like factor in human gingival crevicular fluid from patients with chronic inflammatory periodontal disease. Infect Immun 1990;58:2621–2627.

123. Kjeldsen M, Holmstrup P, Bendtzen K. Marginal periodontitis and cytokines: A review of the literature. J Periodontol 1993;64:1013–1022.

124. Rasmussen L, Hanstrom L, Lerner UH. Characterization of bone resorbing activity in gingival crevicular fluid from patients with periodontitis. J Clin Periodontol 2000;27:41–52.

125. Taubman MA, Eastcott JW, Shimauchi H, et al. Modulatory role of T lymphocytes in periodontal inflammation. In: Genco R (ed). Molecular Pathogenesis of Periodontal Disease. Washington, DC: American Society for Microbiology, 1994:147–157.

126. Seymour GJ, Gemmell E, Reinhardt RA, et al. Immunopathogenesis of chronic inflammatory periodontal disease: Cellular and molecular mechanisms. J Periodontal Res 1993;28:478–486.

127. Le J, Vilcek J. Interleukin 6: A multifunctional cytokine regulating immune reactions and the acute phase protein response. Lab Invest 1989;6:588–602.

128. Takahashi K, Takashiba S, Nagai A, et al. Assessment of interleukin-6 in the pathogenesis of periodontal disease. J Periodontol 1994;65:147–153.

129. Geivelis M, Turner DW, Pederson ED, Lamberts BL. Measurements of interleukin-6 in gingival crevicular fluid from adults with destructive periodontal disease. J Periodontol 1993;64:980–983.

130. Kono Y, Ogawa T, Beagley KW, et al. Immunopathology of periodontal disease: Studies with interleukins which mediate both immunoglobulin synthesis and inflammation in disease gingiva. In: Hamada S, Holt S, McGhee J (eds). Periodontal Disease Pathogens and Host Immune Response. Chicago: Quintessence, 1991:209–221.

131. Nakamura T, Kido J, Kido R, et al. The association of calprotectin level in gingival crevicular fluid with gingival index and the activities of collagenase and aspartate aminotransferase in adult periodontitis patients. J Periodontol 2000;71:361–367.

132. Takeichi O, Saito I, Okamoto Y, et al. Cytokine regulation on the synthesis of nitric oxide in vivo by chronically infected human polymorphonuclear leucocytes. Immunology 1998; 93:275–280.

133. Hanioka T, Takaya K, Matsumori Y, et al. Relationship of the substance P to indicators of host response in human gingival crevicular fluid. J Clin Periodontol 2000;27:262–266.

134. Holmberg K, Killander J. Quantitative determination of immunoglobulins (IgG, IgA and IgM) and identification of IgA-type in the gingival fluid. J Periodontal Res 1971;6:1–8.

135. Lamster IB, Oshrain RL, Celenti RS, et al. Indicators of the acute inflammatory and humoral immune responses in gingival crevicular fluid: Relationship to active periodontal disease. J Periodontal Res 1991;26:261–263.

136. Page RC. Host response tests for diagnosing periodontal diseases. J Periodontol 1992;63:356–366.

137. Powell JR, Caves J, Austin A, Wilton JMA. Interrelationships of crevicular fluid inflammatory markers in adult periodontitis. J Dent Res 1994;73:2332.

138. Yuan ZN, Tolo K, Helgeland K. Soluble Fc gamma receptors in periodontal lesions. Oral Microbiol Immunol 1998;13: 310–314.

139. Yuan ZN, Tolo K, Schenck K, Helgeland K. Increased levels of soluble Fc gamma receptor III in gingival fluid from periodontal lesions. Oral Microbiol Immunol 1999;14:172–175.

140. Kinane DF, Mooney J, MacFarlane TW, McDonald M. Local and systemic antibody response to putative periodontopathogens in patients with chronic periodontitis: Correlation with clinical indices. Oral Microbiol Immunol 1993;8:65–68.

141. Suzuki JB, Martin SA, Vincent JW, Falkler WA. Local and systemic production of immunoglobulins to periodontopathogens in periodontal disease. J Periodontal Res 1984;19:599–603.

142. Berglundh T, Liljenberg B, Tarkowski A, Lindhe J. Local and systemic TCR V gene expression in advanced periodontal disease. J Clin Periodontol 1998;25:125–133.

143. Donaldson SL, Ranney RR, Tew JG. B-lymphocyte blastogenesis in response to periodontitis-associated bacteria: Kinetics and proportion of total response. J Periodontol 1984;55:359–363.

144. Genco RJ. Assessment of risk of periodontal disease. Compen Contin Educ Dent 1994;18:S678–S683.

145. Van Winkelhoff AJ, Van Steenbergen TJM, De Graaff J. The role of black-pigmented Bacteroides in human oral infections. J Clin Periodontol 1988;15:145.

146. DeNardin AM, Sojar HT, Grossi SG, et al. Humoral immunity of older adults with periodontal disease to Porphyromonas gingivalis. Infect Immun 1991;59:4363–4370.

147. Taubman MA, Ebersole JL, Smith DJ. Association between systemic and local antibody and periodontal disease. In: Genco R, Mergenhagen S (eds). Host-Bacterial Interactions in Periodontal Diseases. Washington, DC: American Society for Microbiology, 1982:283–298.

148. Mooney J, Adonogianaki E, Kinane DF. Relative avidity of serum antibodies to putative periodontopathogens in periodontal disease. J Periodontal Res 1993;28:444–450.

149. Lopatin DE, Blackburn E. Avidity and titer of immunoglobulin G subclasses to Porphyromonas gingivalis in adult periodontitis patients. Oral Microbiol Immunol 1992;7:332–337.

150. Chen HA, Johnson BD, Sims TJ, et al. Humoral immune responses to Porphyromonas gingivalis before and following therapy in rapidly progressive periodontitis patients. J Periodontol 1991;62:781–791.

151. Holt SC, Bramanti TE. Factors in virulence expression and their role in periodontal disease pathogenesis. Crit Rev Oral Biol Med 1991;2:177–281.

152. Schenck K, Helgeland K, Tollefsen T. Antibodies against lipopolysaccharide from Bacteroides gingivalis before and after periodontal treatment. Scand J Dent Res 1987;95:112–119.

153. Ogawa T, Kiyono H, Kusumoto Y, et al. Immune responses to Porphyromonas (Bacteroides) gingivalis in various human periodontal diseases. In: Hamada S, Holt S, McGhee J (eds). Periodontal Disease: Pathogens and Host Immune Responses. Chicago: Quintessence, 1991:187–198.

154. Yoshimura F, Toshikazu S, Kawanami M, et al. Detection of specific antibodies against fimbriae and membrane proteins from the oral anaerobe Bacteroides gingivalis in patients with periodontal disease. Microbiol Immunol 1987;31:935–941.

155. Ebersole JL, Steffen MJ. Human antibody responses to outer envelope antigens of Porphyromonas gingivalis serotypes. J Periodontal Res 1995;30:1–14.

156. Naito Y, Okuda K, Takazoe I. Detection of specific antibody in adult human periodontitis sera to surface antigens of Bacteroides gingivalis. Infect Immun 1987;55:832–834.

157. Califano JV, Schifferle RE, Gunsolley JC, et al. Antibody reactive with Porphyromonas gingivalis serotypes K1-6 in adult and generalized early-onset periodontitis. J Periodontol 1999; 70:730–735.

158. Takahashi J, Saito A, Nakagawa T, et al. Dynamics of serum immunoglobulin G avidity for Porphyromonas gingivalis in adult periodontitis. J Periodontol 1998;69:367–373.

159. Matsushita K, Tajima T, Tomita K, et al. Inflammatory cytokine production and specific antibody responses to lipopolysaccharide from endodontopathic black-pigmented bacteria in patients with multilesional periapical periodontitis. J Endod 1999;25:795–799.

160. Kawai T, Ito HO, Sakato N, Okada H. A novel approach for detecting an immunodominant antigen of Porphyromonas gingivalis in diagnosis of adult periodontitis. Clin Diagn Lab Immunol 1998;5:11–17.

161. Schenck K, Michaelsen TE. IgG subclass distribution of serum antibodies against lipopolysaccharide from Bacteroides gingivalis in periodontal health and disease. Acta Pathol Microbiol Immunol Scand 1987;95:41–46.

162. Ogawa T, Kusumoto Y, Hamada S, et al. Bacteroides gingivalis-specific serum IgG and IgA subclass antibodies in periodontal diseases. Clin Exp Immunol 1990;82:318–325.

163. Mouton C, Deslauriers M, Allard H, Bouchard M. Serum antibodies to Bacteroides gingivalis in periodontitis: A longitudinal study. J Periodontal Res 1987;22:426–430.

164. Aukhil I, Lopatin DE, Syed SA, et al. The effects of periodontal therapy on serum antibody (IgG) levels to plaque microorganisms. J Clin Periodontol 1988;15:544–550.

165. Ebersole JL, Taubman MA, Smith DJ, Haffajee AD. Effect of subgingival scaling on systemic antibody responses to oral microorganisms. Infect Immun 1985;48:534–539.

166. Saito A, Hosaka Y, Nakagawa T, et al. Significance of serum antibody against surface antigens of Actinobacillus actinomycetemcomitans in patients with adult periodontitis. Oral Microbiol Immunol 1993;8:146–153.

167. Saito A, Hosaka Y, Nakagawa T, et al. Relative avidity of immunoglobulin G antibody for the fimbria antigen of *Actinobacillus actinomycetemcomitans* in patients with adult periodontitis. Infect Immun 1993;61:332–334.

168. Mooney J, Kinane DF. Humoral immune responses to *Porphyromonas gingivalis* and *Actinobacillus actinomycetemcomitans* in adult periodontitis and rapidly progressive periodontitis. Oral Microbiol Immunol 1994;9:321–326.

169. Sharma A, Sojar HT, Glurich I, et al. Cloning, expression, and sequencing of a cell surface antigen containing a leucine-rich repeat motif from *Bacteroides forsythus* ATCC 43037. Infect Immun 1998;66:5703–5710.

170. Kremer BH, Loos BG, van der Velden U, et al. *Peptostreptococcus micros* smooth and rough genotypes in periodontitis and gingivitis. J Periodontol 2000;71:209–218.

171. Mangan DF, Laughon BE, Bower B, Lopatin DE. In vitro lymphocyte blastogenic responses and titers of humoral antibodies from periodontitis patients to oral spirochete isolates. Infect Immun 1982;37:445–451.

172. Califano JV, Gunsolley JC, Schenkein HA, Tew JG. A comparison of IgG antibody reactive with *Bacteroides forsythus* and *Porphyromonas gingivalis* in adult and early-onset periodontitis. J Periodontol 1997;68:734–738.

173. Kornman KS, di Giovine FS. Genetic variations in cytokine expression: A risk factor for severity of adult periodontitis. Ann Periodontol 1998;3:327–338.

174. McDevitt MJ, Wang HY, Knobelman C, et al. Interleukin-1 genetic association with periodontitis in clinical practice. J Periodontol 2000;71:156–163.

175. Reinhardt RA, Masada MP, Daldahl WB, et al. Gingival fluid IL-1 and IL-6 levels in refractory periodontitis. J Clin Periodontol 1993;20:225–231.

176. Hernichel-Gorbach E, Kornman KS, Holt SC, et al. Host responses in patients with generalized refractory periodontitis. J Periodontol 1994;65:8–16.

177. Colombo AP, Sakellari D, Haffajee AD, et al. Serum antibodies reacting with subgingival species in refractory periodontitis subjects. J Clin Periodontol 1998;25:596–607.

178. Colombo AP, Haffajee AD, Smith CM, et al. Discrimination of refractory periodontitis subjects using clinical and laboratory parameters alone and in combination. J Clin Periodontol 1999;26:569–576.

179. Ehmke B, Schmidt H, Beikler T, et al. Clonal infection with *Actinobacillus actinomycetemcomitans* following periodontal therapy. J Dent Res 1999;78:1518–1524.

180. Collins JG, Offenbacher S, Arnold RR. Effects of combination therapy to eliminate *Porphyromonas gingivalis* in refractory periodontitis. J Periodontol 1993;64:998–1007.

181. Kirstilä V, Sewon L, Laine J. Periodontal disease in three siblings with familial neutropenia. J Periodontol 1993;64:566–570.

182. Dahlen G, Bjorklander J, Gahnberg L, et al. Periodontal disease and dental caries in relation to primary IgG subclass and other humoral immunodeficiencies. J Clin Periodontol 1993;20:7–13.

183. Leggot PJ, Robertson RB, Greenspan D, et al. Oral manifestations of primary and acquired immunodeficiency diseases in children. Pediatr Dent 1987;2:98–104.

184. Robertson PB, Wright TEI, Mackler BF, et al. Periodontal status of patients with abnormalities of the immune system. J Periodontol Res 1978;13:37–45.

185. Robertson PB, Mackler BR, Wright TE, Levy BM. Periodontal status of patients with abnormalities of the immune system, II. Observations over a 2-year period. J Periodontol 1980;51:70–73.

186. Tollefsen T, Saltvedt E, Koppang HS. The effect of immunosuppressive agents on periodontal disease in man. J Periodontal Res 1978;13:240–250.

187. Tollefsen T, Schenck K, Tolo K. Cross-sectional study of the effects of immunosuppressive agents on humoral immune responses to 6 oral microorganisms in humans. J Periodontal Res 1986;21:553–562.

188. Kristoffersen T. Host responses to bacteria and bacterial products in periodontal disease: Immunosuppressive effects of periodontitis-related microorganisms? Scand J Dent Res 1985;93:112–118.

189. Boehringer H, Taichman NS, Shenker BJ. Suppression of fibroblast proliferation by oral spirochetes. Infect Immun 1984;45:155–159.

190. Kurita-Ochiai T, Ochiai K, Ikeda T. Immunosuppressive effect inducted by *Actinobacillus actinomycetemcomitans*: Effect on immunoglobulin production and lymphokine synthesis. Oral Microbiol Immunol 1992;7:338–343.

191. Shenker BJ, Slots J. Immunomodulatory effects of *Bacteroides* products on in vitro human lymphocyte functions. Oral Microbiol Immunol 1989;4:24–29.

192. Shenker BJ, DiRienzo JM. Suppression of human peripheral blood lymphocytes by *Fusobacterium nucleatum*. J Immunol 1984;132:2357–2362.

193. Ivanyi L. Immunosuppression in severe periodontitis. In: Lehner T, Cimasoni G (eds). The Borderland Between Caries and Periodontal Disease. Geneva: Editions Medecine et Hygiene, 1986:223–232.

194. Oliver RC, Tervonen T. Periodontitis and tooth loss: Comparing diabetics with the general population. J Am Dent Assoc 1993;124:71–76.

195. Oliver RC, Tervonen T. Diabetes: A risk factor for periodontitis in adults? J Periodontol 1994;65:530–538.

196. Grossi SG, Zambon JJ, Ho AW, et al. Assessment of risk for periodontal disease, I. Risk indicators for attachment loss. J Periodontol 1994;65:260–267.

197. Nishimura F, Takahashi K, Kurihara M, et al. Periodontal disease as a complication of diabetes mellitus. Ann Periodontol 1998;3:20–29.

198. Ervasti T, Knuuttila M, Pohjamo L, et al. Relation between control of diabetes and gingival bleeding. J Periodontol 1985;56:154–157.

199. Tervonen T, Knuuttila M. Relation of diabetes control to periodontal pocketing and alveolar bone level. Oral Surg Oral Med Oral Pathol 1986;61:346–349.

200. Tervonen T, Oliver RC. Long-term control of diabetes and periodontitis. J Clin Periodontol 1993;20:431–435.

201. Guven Y, Satman I, Dinccag N, Alptekin S. Salivary peroxidase activity in whole saliva of patients with insulin-dependent (type-1) diabetes mellitus. J Clin Periodontol 1996;23:879–881.

202. Bristow CL, Di Meo F, Arnold RR. Specific activity of alpha1proteinase inhibitor and alpha2macroglobulin in human serum: Application to insulin-dependent diabetes mellitus. Clin Immunol Immunopathol 1998;89:247–259.

203. Alley CS, Reinhardt RA, Maze CA, et al. HLA-D and T lymphocyte reactivity to specific periodontal pathogens in type 1 diabetic periodontitis. J Periodontol 1993;64:974–979.

204. Gustke CJ, Stein SH, Hart TC, et al. HLA-DR alleles are associated with IDDM, but not with impaired neutrophil chemotaxis in IDDM. J Dent Res 1998;77:1497–1503.

205. Grossi SG, Genco RJ. Periodontal disease and diabetes mellitus: A two-way relationship. Ann Periodontol 1998;3:51–61.

206. Christgau M, Palitzsch KD, Schmalz G, et al. Healing response to non-surgical periodontal therapy in patients with diabetes mellitus: Clinical, microbiological, and immunological results. J Clin Periodontol 1998;25:112–124.

207. Anil S, Beena VT, Remani P, et al. Total hemolytic complement (CH50) and its fractions C3 and C4 in the sera of patients with localized juvenile periodontitis. Ann Dent 1993;52:18–20.

208. Anil S, Remani P, Ankathil R, Vijayakumar T. Circulating immune complexes in diabetic patients with periodontitis. Ann Dent 1990;49:3–5.

209. Anil S, Remani P, Vijayakumar T, Hari S. Cell-mediated and humoral immune responses in diabetic patients with periodontitis. Oral Surg Oral Med Oral Pathol 1990;70:44–48.

210. Delesphesse G, Duchateau J, Bastenie PA, et al. Cell mediated immunity in diabetes mellitus. Clin Exp Immunol 1974;18:461–465.

211. Rossini AA, Mordes JP, Like AA. Immunology of insulin-dependent diabetes mellitus. Annu Rev Immunol 1985;3:289–320.

212. Cutler CW, Eke P, Arnold RR, Van Dyke TE. Defective neutrophil function in an insulin-dependent diabetes mellitus patient. J Periodontol 1991;62:394–401.

213. Feitosa AC, de Uzeda M, Novaes AP Jr. *Actinobacillus actinomycetemcomitans* in Brazilian insulin-dependent individuals with diabetes mellitus. Braz Dent J 1992;3:25–31.

214. Mashimo PA, Yamamota Y, Slots J, et al. The periodontal microflora of juvenile diabetics: Culture, immunofluorescence and serum antibody studies. J Periodontol 1983;54:420–430.

215. Zambon JJ, Reynolds H, Fisher JG, et al. Microbiological and immunological studies of adult periodontitis in patients with noninsulin-dependent diabetes mellitus. J Periodontol 1988;59:23–31.

216. Morinushi T, Lopatin DE, Syed SA, et al. Humoral immune response to selected subgingival plaque microorganisms in insulin-dependent diabetic children. J Periodontol 1989;60:199–204.

217. Mandell RL, Dirienzo J, Kent R. Microbiology of healthy and diseased periodontal sites in poorly controlled insulin dependent diabetics. J Periodontol 1992;63:274–279.

218. Salvi GE, Beck JD, Offenbacher S. PGE2, IL-1 beta, and TNF-alpha responses in diabetics as modifiers of periodontal disease expression. Ann Periodontol 1998;3:40–50.

219. Salvi GE, Yalda B, Collins JG, et al. Inflammatory mediator response as a potential risk marker for periodontal diseases in insulin-dependent diabetes mellitus patients. J Periodontol 1997;68:127–135.

220. Salvi GE, Collins JG, Yalda B, et al. Monocytic TNF alpha secretion patterns in IDDM patients with periodontal diseases. J Clin Periodontol 1997;24:8–16.

221. Stein SH, Hart TE, Hoffman WH, et al. Interleukin-10 promotes anti-collagen antibody production in type I diabetic peripheral B lymphocytes. J Periodontal Res 1997;32:189–195.

222. Schlossman M, Knowler WC, Pettitt DJ, Genco RJ. Type 2 diabetes mellitus and periodontal disease. J Am Dent Assoc 1990;121:532–536.

223. Emrich LJ, Schlossman M, Genco RJ. Periodontal disease in non-insulin dependent diabetes mellitus. J Periodontol 1991;62:123–130.

224. Dyer JK, Peck MA, Reinhardt RA, et al. HLA-D types and serum IgG responses to *Capnocytophaga* in diabetes and periodontitis. J Dent Res 1997;76:1825–1832.

225. Kurtis B, Develioglu H, Taner IL, et al. IL-6 levels in gingival crevicular fluid (GCF) from patients with non-insulin dependent diabetes mellitus (NIDDM), adult periodontitis and healthy subjects. J Oral Sci 1999;41:163–167.

226. Cutler CW, Machen RL, Jotwani R, Iacopino AM. Heightened gingival inflammation and attachment loss in type 2 diabetics with hyperlipidemia. J Periodontol 1999;70:1313–1321.

227. Palmer RM, Scott DA, Meekin TN, et al. Potential mechanisms of susceptibility to periodontitis in tobacco smokers. J Periodontal Res 1999;34:363–369.

228. Mullally BH, Breen B, Linden GJ. Smoking and patterns of bone loss in early-onset periodontitis. J Periodontol 1999;70:394–401.

229. Bergström J, Preber H. Tobacco use as a risk factor. J Periodontol 1994;65:545–550.

230. Persson L, Bergström J, Gustafsson A, Asman B. Tobacco smoking and gingival neutrophil activity in young adults. J Clin Periodontol 1999;26:9–13.

231. Pauletto NC, Liede K, Nieminen A, et al. Effect of cigarette smoking on oral elastase activity in adult periodontitis patients. J Periodontol 2000;71:58–62.

232. Soder B. Neutrophil elastase activity, levels of prostaglandin E2, and matrix metalloproteinase-8 in refractory periodontitis sites in smokers and non-smokers. Acta Odontol Scand 1999;57:77–82.

233. Bernzweig E, Payne JB, Reinhardt RA, et al. Nicotine and smokeless tobacco effects on gingival and peripheral blood mononuclear cells. J Clin Periodontol 1998;25:246–252.

234. Fredriksson MI, Figueredo CM, Gustafsson A, et al. Effect of periodontitis and smoking on blood leukocytes and acute-phase proteins. J Periodontol 1999;70:1355–1360.

235. Mathys EC. Host Factors and Generalized Early Onset Periodontitis. San Antonio, TX: University of Texas Health Science Center at San Antonio, 1993.

236. Quinn SM, Zhang JB, Gunsolley JC, et al. The influence of smoking and race on adult periodontitis and serum IgG2 levels. J Periodontol 1998;69:171–177.

237. Tangada SD, Califano JV, Nakashima K, et al. The effect of smoking on serum IgG2 reactive with *Actinobacillus actinomycetemcomitans* in early-onset periodontitis patients. J Periodontol 1997;68:842–850.

238. Sayers NM, James JA, Drucker DB, Blinkhorn AS. Possible potentiation of toxins from *Prevotella intermedia, Prevotella nigrescens,* and *Porphyromonas gingivalis* by cotinine. J Periodontol 1999;70:1269–1275.

239. Kornman KS. Host modulation as a therapeutic strategy in the treatment of periodontal disease. Clin Infect Dis 1999;28:520–526.

CHAPTER

9

Inflammatory Response in Periodontal Diseases

Steven P. Engebretson, Gülnur Emingil, and Ira B. Lamster
- Vascular Events in Acute Inflammation
- Cellular Events in Acute Inflammation
- The Macrophage and Chronic Inflammation
- Indicators in Gingival Crevicular Fluid
- Influence of Periodontal Infection and Inflammation on Systemic Diseases

The inflammatory response is a series of vascular and cellular events that characterize the initial reaction of an organism to a biologic, physical, or chemical insult. Inflammation is associated with wound healing and repair of damaged and altered tissue, as well as elimination of foreign microorganisms that infect the host.

There are five cardinal signs of the inflammatory response. The first four, originally defined by Celsius in the first century, include *rubor* (redness), *calor* (heat), *tumor* (swelling), and *dolor* (pain). Later, Galen added the fifth sign, *functio laesa* (loss of function). These signs are associated with specific changes that accompany acute inflammation. Rubor indicates increased blood flow into an area. Calor is due to an increase in local temperature that occurs with increased blood flow. Tumor is the swelling that results when vascular fluid (serum) moves from capillaries and postcapillary venules into the extravascular tissues. Dolor results from the release of neurogenic mediators in the inflamed area. Functio laesa is the result of the first four signs. While all five signs may be present together in a single lesion, all five are not necessarily observed in every inflammatory response.

Acute inflammatory gingivitis illustrates the signs of acute inflammation. The patients in Figs 9-1a and 9-1b have erythematous (red) and edematous (swollen) interdental papillae. The use of an intracrevicular temperature probe would indicate that the temperature in the inflamed area is increased, and periodontal probing of the sulcus would elicit pain. As a result of these changes, the tissue does not function properly; the papillae does not deflect food debris, and the patient may not be able to perform routine oral hygiene. The inflammatory response can be observed clinically and histologically through all phases of periodontal disease.[1]

Vascular Events in Acute Inflammation

The acute inflammatory response begins with alteration of vascular permeability. Serum moves from the capillaries and postcapillary venules of the gingival plexus into the surrounding connective tissue, and then into the gingival

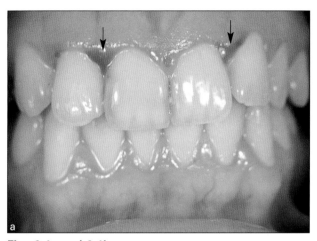 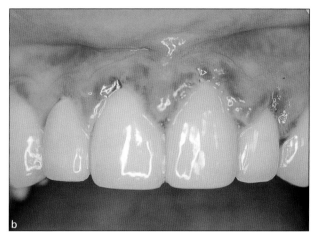

Figs 9-1a and 9-1b Patients with gingivitis demonstrating aspects of acute inflammation, including tissue swelling (edema) and color changes (erythma). *(a)* The interdental papillae are inflamed *(arrows)*. *(b)* A patient with pregnancy gingivitis. The marginal and papillary tissues display pronounced inflammation.

crevice[2,3] This phenomenon is closely associated with the accumulation of plaque bacteria at the interface of the tooth and gingiva and with the development of gingival inflammation.[4,5]

The facultative aerobic and anaerobic bacteria present at the gingival margin and in the gingival crevice release a variety of substances that can initiate the vascular events of acute inflammation (Fig 9-2). These substances include metabolic acids, extracellular enzymes, volatile sulfur compounds, lipoteichoic acid, and lipopolysaccharides. These factors can directly or indirectly damage the sulcular epithelium and underlying connective tissue and disrupt the microvasculature. The initial host response to the insult is characterized by the release of a number of vasoactive mediators.

Histamine is released from mast cells, possibly as a direct result of bacterial mediators such as lipopolysaccharide, or via complement activation. This mediator causes increased vascular permeability and is important early in the acute inflammatory response. The complement cleavage products C3a and C5a can be generated in response to the formation of an antigen/antibody complex (the classic pathway) or lipopolysaccharide and trypsinlike enzymes released from bacteria (the alternate pathway). These mediators can cause release of mast-cell granules that contain histamine and other vasoactive mediators.

Bradykinin is another potent mediator of vascular permeability. It is released as a result of the activation of a cascade of enzymes present in serum. The production of bradykinin begins when Hageman factor (factor XII in the coagulation pathway) is cleaved to its active form. This happens in response to tissue and vascular injury. The action of bradykinin is believed to be important following the action of histamine.

Plasmin is part of the fibrinolytic system. Activation of the Hageman factor begins this cascade. The generation of this mediator results in fibrin degradation and the production of fibrin-split products. These split products promote vascular permeability. Plasmin is also involved in a positive feedback loop by promoting cleavage of both Hageman factor and kininogen. This activity is believed to occur later in the acute inflammatory response.

Other mediators can contribute to the development of the vascular component of acute inflammation in the periodontal tissues. Cell membranes of human cells contain phospholipids. When sensing a cellular perturbation, enzymes known as *phospholipases* generate arachidonic acid from the membrane phospholipids. Steroids block the conversion of phospholipids to arachidonic acid. In turn, the enzymes cyclooxygenase and lipoxygenase act on arachidonic acid to produce a wide variety of mediators that can affect many aspects of the inflammatory response. The cyclooxygenase pathway leads to formation of the prostaglandins (ie, PGE_2) and prostacyclin (PGI_2).

These mediators produce vasodilation, as well as other proinflammatory effects on many cell types. The cyclooxygenase pathway is blocked by aspirin and other nonsteroidal anti-inflammatory drugs, such as ibuprofen. The lipoxygenase pathway leads to the formation of other biologically important mediators known as *leukotrienes (LTs)*. LTB_4 can induce neutrophil chemotaxis. The combination of LTC_4, LTD_4, and LTE_4 is released from mast cells; this combination was formerly known as *slow-reacting substance of anaphylaxis (SRS-A)*. Among other effects, SRS-A was shown to induce vascular permeability.[6]

Platelet aggregation and granule release play an important role in the early development of the vascular and cellular aspects of the inflammatory response. Release of

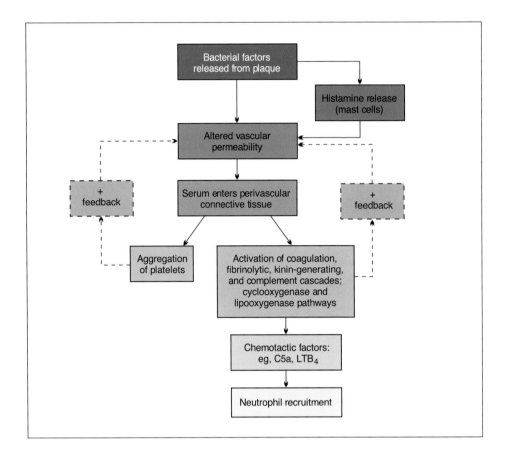

Fig 9-2 Vascular events in acute inflammation.

granules from platelets can help initiate vascular permeability. Mediators released from platelets include serotonin, several factors in the coagulation cascade, platelet-derived growth factor, and thromboxane A_2.

Ultimately, a change occurs in the gingival vascular plexus. The vessels proliferate, and a distinct loop formation develops in the small vessels directly below the basement membrane of the sulcular epithelium.[7] The vasodilation of the gingival vasculature, the presence of specific mediators released from bacteria, and the activation of enzyme cascades present in serum all promote the recruitment and activation of neutrophils and macrophages.

Cellular Events in Acute Inflammation

The cellular hallmark of the acute inflammatory response is the polymorphonuclear leukocyte, or neutrophil. Neutrophils account for 50% to 60% of the circulating leukocyte pool in humans. They are characterized by a multilobed nucleus, lysosomal granules (which do not stain

with hematoxylin and eosin), and glycogen granules in the cytoplasm. The purpose of the multilobed nucleus has not been defined, but this nuclear morphology may assist the cell in its passage between endothelial cells into the inflammatory focus. The lysosomal granules contain a large variety of enzymes that can degrade host tissue as part of normal tissue turnover and wound healing, as well as a variety of antimicrobial mechanisms that can kill ingested (phagocytosed) microorganisms. The presence of glycogen in the cytoplasm of these cells allows them to be independent of external sources of energy during phagocytosis.

Neutrophil emigration follows a defined series of events.[8] These cells respond to a chemotactic gradient by lining the surface of the endothelial cells. Adhesion molecules become more abundant on the surface of the endothelial lumen as a result of increased levels of these vasoactive substances and inflammatory cytokines.[9] These molecules promote adherence of neutrophils to the endothelial surface. The neutrophils move along the endothelial cells until they encounter an interendothelial cell junction, and then move from the vessel into the surrounding connective tissue. This movement of neutrophils to the extravascular milieu is called *diapedesis*. The movement through the endothelial basement membrane is accom-

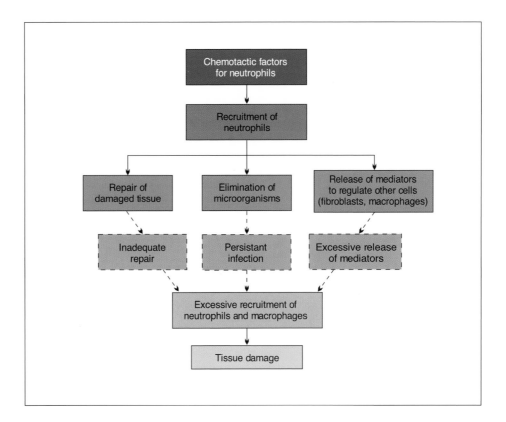

Fig 9-3 Cellular events in acute inflammation.

plished by the release of lysosomal granules and the action of degradative enzymes such as collagenase and elastase. Chemoattractants for neutrophils include the complement component C5a, small peptides released from bacteria (eg, N-formyl-methionyl-leucyl-phenylalanine), the arachidonic acid metabolite LTB$_4$,[10] and the chemokine interleukin 8 (IL-8) (Fig 9-3). Movement of neutrophils in the direction of a chemotactic gradient is independent of, but enhanced by, the action of vasodilating agents such as histamine and bradykinin. The accumulation of neutrophils in the gingival crevice is one important way to define inflammation of the periodontal tissues.[11,12]

There are specific receptors on the surface of neutrophils that mediate the chemotactic response. These include receptors for the small peptides derived from bacteria[13,14] and for C5a. Other receptors on the neutrophil surface allow binding to the constant region or stem portion of the immunoglobulin G (IgG) molecule (known as *CR1 receptors*), as well as the C3b component of complement (known as *CR3 receptors*). These receptors are important in phagocytosis, the process of ingesting foreign microorganisms.[15]

Phagocytosis provides a mechanism for these cells to eliminate organisms that invade the host. In an inflammatory response, the major phagocytes are the neutrophil (during acute inflammation) and the macrophage (during chronic inflammation). Phagocytosis is enhanced when the target cell, usually a bacterium, is opsonized. *Opsonization* is a word derived from the Greek and means "preparation to dine." Opsonins of primary importance in the elimination of bacteria include IgG antibody and the complement component C3b. In the case of an IgG molecule, the immunoglobulin binds to the microorganism via the antigen-specific or Fab portion of the molecule. The other part of the molecule (referred to as the *Fc portion*) is available for binding, and the CR1 surface receptors bind this part of the IgG molecule.

Ingestion of bacteria by neutrophils is an energy-dependent process.[6] The energy for phagocytosis is supplied by metabolism of glycogen. Both oxygen-independent and oxygen-dependent metabolism by neutrophils can occur.

After phagocytosis a foreign microorganism is contained in a phagosome. The killing of the engulfed microorganism is accomplished after the fusion of the phagosome with one or more lysosomal granules. These granules contain a variety of antimicrobial compounds for elimination of harmful microorganisms, as well as enzymes that can degrade host tissue. Four types of lysosomal granules have been identified in the cytoplasm of neutrophils. The two major types are referred to as the *primary* and *secondary granules*. The primary granules contain antimicro-

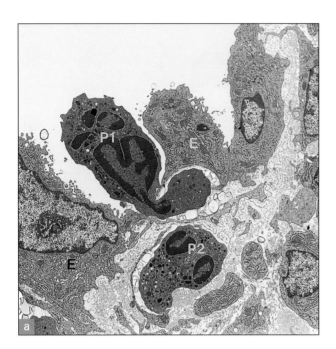

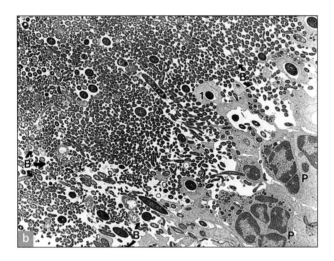

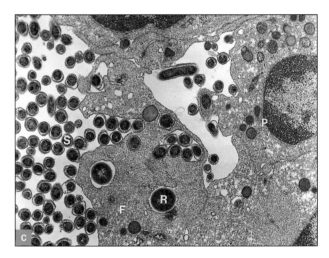

Figs 9-4a to 9-4c Electron micrographs illustrating polymorphonuclear leukocyte activity in the crevicular environment of squirrel monkeys. *(a)* Polymorphonuclear leukocytes (P) in the gingival lamina propria. P1 is in the process of emigrating from the lumen of a venule. P2, located in the connective tissue, contains a full complement of lysosomal granules. (E), Endothelial cells (5,000×). *(b)* The interface between bacterial plaque (B) and polymorphonuclear leukocyte (P). Note the reduction in lysosomal granules in the polymorphonuclear leukocytes and the phagocytosis (1) of bacteria only at the leading edge of the accumulated leukocytes. *(c)* Higher magnification of bacterial phagocytosis by polymorphonuclear leukocytes. Note the dense filamentous nature of the cytoplasm in the zone of phagocytosis (F). Spirochetes (S) and rod-shaped bacteria (R) can be seen in cross section (15,000×). (All electron micrographs courtesy of Dr Philias Garant, School of Dental Medicine, SUNY at Stony Brook.)

bial substances such as myeloperoxidase and lysozyme, along with tissue-degrading enzymes such as elastase, cathepsin, and β-glucuronidase.[16] Similarly, the secondary granules contain antimicrobial factors such as lysozyme and lactoferrin, as well as matrix metalloproteinases (MMPs) such as MMP-8 (collagenase) and MMP-9 (gelatinase).[17,18]

With the fusion of a phagosome and lysosomal granules, the antimicrobial factors in the granules come in contact with the organism, and microbial killing will normally result. The killing is the consequence of a number of systems, but perhaps the most potent is generation of reactive oxygen metabolites as end products of aerobic glycolysis or as a result of activation of the hydrogen peroxide/halide/myeloperoxidase system.

Phagocytosis by neutrophils occurs in the gingival crevice, but it is not an important mechanism in controlling the accumulation of subgingival plaque microorganisms.[19] Neutrophils, however, do provide a barrier between the plaque mass and the crevicular epithelium (Figs 9-4a to 9-4c).

If the neutrophil influx in the crevice is overwhelmed by the bacterial challenge, an abscess can develop (Figs 9-5a and 9-5b). An abscess is the result of degranulation of large numbers of neutrophils in a confined area. With the extracellular release of the lysosomal granules present in neutrophils, enzymes such as MMP-8, MMP-9, elastase, β-glucuronidase, and arylsulfatase (which participate in degradation of the ground substance) can attack host tissue and cause pronounced localized tissue damage. Re-

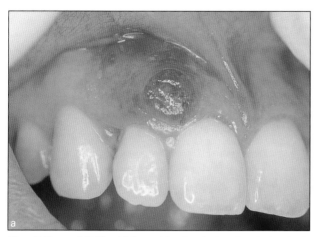
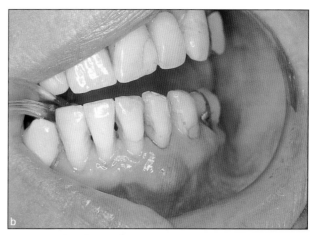

Figs 9-5a and 9-5b *(a)* A combined periodontal-endodontic abscess on the buccal surface between the maxillary central and lateral incisors. *(b)* A periodontal abscess on the buccal surface of the mandibular lateral incisor.

active oxygen metabolites are also believed to have an important detrimental effect.

Blockage of the orifice of the gingival crevice can lead to the formation of an abscess by preventing the flow of gingival fluid from the apex of the crevice into the oral cavity proper. Normally this flow prevents the accumulation of bacteria and host cells in the crevice. A blockage may result if a deep crevice lacks tissue turgor at the orifice, or when mechanical closure of the orifice occurs as a result of the accumulation of food or other debris.

The Macrophage and Chronic Inflammation

The macrophage (or tissue monocyte) is the cell that characterizes classic chronic inflammation. Lymphocytes and plasma cells are also part of the infiltrate in chronic inflammation. The distinction between chronic inflammation and immunity, however, is often blurred. While it is recognized that macrophages have an important role in antigen processing as part of the development of an immune response, a subset of these cells have impressive phagocytic capability. Furthermore, these cells are capable of synthesizing a large array of molecules that contribute to repair, but they can also have proinflammatory effects. In long-standing inflammatory lesions the number of macrophages is increased, and this is seen in periodontal disease.[20,21]

Monocytes respond to the same chemotactic factors as neutrophils (ie, C5a and IL-8). In addition, the cytokine transforming growth factor β (TGF-β) is recognized as a very important chemoattractant for monocytes. This mediator is released from a variety of cells, including platelets, neutrophils, and monocytes. Macrophages have very specific receptors for TGF-β, and very low concentrations of this cytokine will induce a chemotactic gradient. Higher concentrations of TGF-β will lead to metabolic activation of the cells, with production of a number of other mediators that can participate in both tissue repair and propagation of the inflammatory response.[22] Macrophages are believed to be an important source of reactive oxygen metabolites, including superoxide anion (O_2^-), hydrogen peroxide (H_2O_2), the hydroxyl radical (–OH), and hypochlorous acid (HOCl).[6] All these metabolites are potentially microbicidal, but they can also be toxic to host cells. Macrophages can also be an important source of arachidonic acid metabolites such as PGE_2 and LTB_4.[23] PGE_2 has many regulatory effects. This product of the cyclooxygenase pathway can decrease adherence and migration of macrophages while also stimulating both production and release of collagenase, phagocytosis, and bone resorption. PGE_2 can suppress lymphocyte function. Macrophages also can modify neutrophil function. LTB_4 can attract neutrophils into the area, as well as cause metabolic activation of these cells as measured by increased microbicidal activity. LTB_4 also has an inhibitory effect on lymphocyte activity. PGE_2 is regulated by PGE synthase; it also influences the production of both the constitutively expressed type of cyclooxygenase (COX-1) and the induced type (COX-2).[24] These enzymes are also elevated in inflamed gingival tissues.

Macrophages have an impressive capacity to produce inflammatory mediators that can influence the development of an inflammatory lesion. While all of the mediators described in the following discussion are considered proinflammatory and their roles in the development of the periodontal lesion have begun to be examined, low concentrations of these mediators also play a role in tissue repair. It is important to remember that while macrophages are an important source of the cytokines described below, many other cell types have also been shown to produce these mediators.

Interleukin 1 (IL-1) is perhaps the most studied monokine. IL-1 occurs in two forms: IL-1α and IL-1β. These proteins are synthesized with a molecular weight of 31,000 d, but the active form has a molecular weight of 17,000 d. IL-1α and IL-1β share only about one third of their amino acid sequence, but their biologic activities are very similar, since they bind to the same receptor. IL-1 is recognized to have biologic activities associated with tissue repair, including enhancement of fibroblast function. It is likely, however, that overstimulation of macrophages will lead to production of excessive amounts of IL-1. Proinflammatory effects associated with IL-1 include induction of fever, stimulation of collagenase production, and the sharing of an amino acid sequence with osteoclast-activating factor. The last characteristic is potentially very important for the bone loss seen in periodontitis. Elevated levels of IL-1β have been demonstrated in tissue collected from patients with chronic periodontitis,[25] and both IL-1α and IL-1β have been identified in gingival crevicular fluid (GCF).[26,27] IL-1 also influences the expression of COX-2 messenger RNA.[28]

Tumor necrosis factor (TNF) is a 17,000-d monokine that was originally described as causing necrosis of tumor cells in culture. The biologic activities of TNF are similar to those of IL-1. This monokine can both act with IL-1 in a synergistic fashion and cause production of IL-1 by different cell types. TNF has been studied in GCF.[29–31]

Interleukin 6 (IL-6) is another proinflammatory cytokine with activities similar to those of IL-1. This inflammatory mediator can act in synergy with IL-1, particularly in relation to production of acute-phase proteins (serum components that are important in inflammatory response). Several reports describing IL-6 in GCF have been published.[31,32]

Interleukin-8 (IL-8) is a chemoattractant called a *chemokine* because of its potent ability to attract neutrophils. Elevated levels of IL-8 in GCF have been described in patients with periodontitis.[33]

Indicators in Gingival Crevicular Fluid

More than 60 years ago, it was demonstrated that fluid could be collected from the orifice of the gingival crevice. Subsequently, GCF was recognized as an inflammatory exudate derived from the periodontal tissues. The fluid component is derived primarily from serum. Fluid constituents originate from serum; structural cells of the periodontium; inflammatory and immune cells in the connective tissue, epithelium, and gingival crevice; and subgingival bacteria.[34] GCF can be collected by several techniques. The most common procedure employs small, precut strips of methylcellulose filter paper placed at the orifice or in the gingival crevice (Fig 9-6). The generation of GCF is associated with microleakage from the gingival vascular plexus. As noted earlier, vascular permeability is a characteristic of the inflammatory response.

Many inflammatory mediators have been identified in GCF, including products of the four interrelated serum enzyme cascades (coagulation,[35] fibrinolytic,[36] kinin-generating,[37] and complement systems[38–40]). Of these, the complement cascade has been the most intensely studied. The conversion of C3 (the point at which the classic and alternate pathways converge) to its cleavage product C3c was observed in GCF from 13% of healthy subjects, 40% of gingivitis patients, 69% of chronic adult periodontitis patients, and 90% of patients with juvenile periodontitis (now called aggressive periodontitis).[40] Longitudinally, C3 cleavage in GCF was observed to increase with the development of gingivitis,[38] and therapy reduced C3 conversion in patients with periodontitis.[39] Furthermore, the data suggest that in gingivitis and chronic adult periodontitis, activation of the complement cascade is via the alternate pathway. In juvenile periodontitis, the classic pathway is activated.[40] As noted earlier, activation has an important role in the development of the inflammatory response by, for example, causing the release of vasoactive amines from mast cells, as well as recruitment of neutrophils and macrophages into the inflammatory focus.

Studies examining the relationship of markers of inflammatory-cell activity in GCF to the progression of periodontal disease have provided an improved understanding of the pathogenesis of periodontitis. Following the progression of periodontal disease over defined intervals of time, specific mediators in GCF have been examined to determine their relationship to the progression of disease. This progression can be measured in humans by an increase in the probing attachment level or an increase in the amount of bone loss seen radiographically. Longitudinal studies have suggested that elevated levels of the inflammatory mediators PGE$_2$,[41] neutrophil elastase,[42] and β-glucuronidase (a lysosomal enzyme considered a marker of neutrophil activity in the crevicular environment[43]) all can identify an increased risk for active periodontal disease. PGE$_2$ is a more general inflammatory marker, with macrophages, fibroblasts, and neutrophils contributing to its presence in GCF. The lysosomal enzymes are indicative of neutrophil activity. Recently, certain gene polymorphisms for IL-1 have been shown to be associated with increased risk for severe periodontitis.[44] Elevated IL-1β in GCF was also shown in these patients.[45] Cumulatively, these data strongly suggest that an exuberant inflammatory response is associated with progression of disease in patients with chronic adult periodontitis.

MMPs are also critical to the development of the periodontal lesion.[46] The expression of proinflammatory cytokines induces connective tissue and bone resorption primarily through the MMP family of host-derived collagenases. The cellular source of gingival crevicular fluid MMP is thought to be the polymorphonuclear leukocyte, but many cell types increase MMP expression in response to the inflammatory cytokines.

In certain aggressive forms of periodontitis, such as localized juvenile periodontitis, there is a documented reduction in peripheral blood neutrophil function (chemotaxis).[15] This may seem to conflict with the concept that elevated levels of inflammatory mediators derived from neutrophils and macrophages are involved in the progression of chronic adult periodontitis. However, aggressive periodontitis is clinically different from chronic periodontitis. The GCF studies reflect local inflammatory-cell activity. Nevertheless, it now appears that an inappropriate inflammatory response, be it inadequate or exuberant, can be associated with disease progression.[16]

The function of both neutrophils and macrophages in the periodontal environment is directed toward containment of the microbial challenge. The involvement of these cells in the progression of periodontal disease may appear to be a contradiction. In many of the studies cited above, GCF samples from patients who did not have disease progression contained detectable levels of the mediators. Under these conditions, the neutrophils and macrophages are functioning normally to contain the microbial challenge. By contrast, a periodontal abscess involves a large influx of neutrophils and is associated with localized tissue destruction. Excessive neutrophil influx and metabolic activation have also been associated with certain systemic disorders (eg, emphysema).[47] Hence, it appears that neutrophils and macrophages, when activated by bacterial products and cytokines, may play an unwitting role in the nonmineralized and mineralized tissue destruction observed in periodontitis.

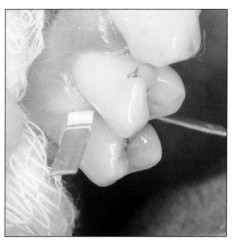

Fig 9-6 Collection of gingival crevicular fluid using precut strips of methylcellulose filter paper. Sample collected from the mesial surface of the maxillary second premolar using strips placed from the buccal and palatal directions.

The complexity of the inflammatory response in periodontal disease continues to unravel. A more complete picture is emerging of how an appropriate inflammatory response associated with containment of a microbial challenge can become an excessive response associated with tissue destruction. This appears to be a multifactorial process involving, for example, the nature of the subgingival microflora and the intensity of the individual's inflammatory response to a challenge. Ultimately, these studies will offer new strategies for evaluating patients with periodontal disease.[48–50]

Influence of Periodontal Infection and Inflammation on Systemic Diseases

Until recently, the inflammatory response in the context of periodontal disease was considered to have only local consequences. That is, inflammation in the periodontal tissues has been studied in relation to the loss of supporting tissues of the teeth. However, there is now considerable interest in the association between periodontal disease, periodontal infection, inflammatory sequelae, and systemic illness.

This concept is not new. In the late 1800s a number of prominent clinicians wrote that periodontal disease had a negative influence on systemic health.[51] Scientific evidence for this purported association was lacking at the time. Since the late 1980s, however, a number of properly performed studies have confirmed this relationship. The study of the association between periodontitis and systemic disease is called *periodontal medicine*.[52] As this association continues to be defined, it will become increasingly important for practitioners to be aware of the mechanisms involved in the host inflammatory response to periodontal pathogens in the context of an anatomically localized infectious disease with potentially significant systemic sequelae.

What, then, are the systemic effects of periodontitis? Periodontitis is a low-grade chronic polymicrobial infection of the supporting hard and soft tissues of the teeth. An increasing number of studies are investigating the periodontal disease–systemic health association as related to ischemic cerebrovascular/cardiovascular disease, diabetes mellitus, and preterm/low-birth-weight infants. This field is evolving, and new developments will likely occur over the next several years.

Periodontitis and Ischemic Cerebrovascular/Cardiovascular Disease

A growing body of evidence suggests a role for infection and inflammation in the pathophysiology of ischemic vascular disease, including stroke and myocardial infarction (MI).[53] It has long been observed that stroke and MI rates increase in a population following influenza epidemics.[54] Indeed, it has been noted that the beginning of the decline in atherosclerosis-related deaths corresponds with the start of the common use of antibiotics. Other evidence suggests increased risk of stroke in conjunction with infectious and inflammatory processes.[55] Several types of infectious agents have been proposed to be causally related to atherosclerosis on the basis of epidemiologic and pathologic studies; they include *Helicobacter pylori*,[56] cytomegalovirus,[57] and *Chlamydia pneumonia*.[58]

Mattila et al[59] and Syrjanen et al[60] published cross-sectional studies in 1989 that indicated that dental disease was an important risk indicator for both cerebrovascular accidents (CVAs) and acute MI. In a case-control study, Syrjanen et al[60] compared the level of dental disease in 40 patients with CVAs with 40 randomly selected community controls matched for gender and age. In that study, severe chronic dental infection was shown to be an important type of infection associated with cerebral infarction in males younger than 50 years. In two separate case-control studies, Mattila[61] examined 100 patients with acute MI and 102 controls for the association between poor dental health and acute MI. Dental health was graded by using two indices, one of which was assessed blindly. Based on

these indices, dental health was significantly worse in patients with acute MI than in controls. The association remained valid after adjustment for age, social class, smoking, serum lipid concentrations, and the presence of diabetes mellitus. DeStefano et al[62] analyzed the National Health and Nutrition Examination Survey (NHANES) database and used a prospective cohort study design involving data from 9,760 subjects examined from 1971 to 1987. They found that individuals with periodontal disease, as measured by the Periodontal Index (an epidemiological instrument that does not include probing or attachment measurements[63]), had a nearly twofold higher risk of coronary heart disease than did individuals with no periodontal disease.

Beck et al[64] conducted a cohort study using data combined from the Normative Aging Study and the Dental Longitudinal Study sponsored by the Department of Veterans Affairs. This data set consisted of 1,147 subjects who were medically healthy at baseline. Of these subjects, 207 developed coronary heart disease over an average follow-up time of 18 years. Radiographic evidence of bone loss around teeth (an indicator of chronic periodontal disease) was used to stratify the subjects according to severity of bone loss. The results, presented as incidence odds ratios adjusted for age and race, showed a significant association between advanced bone loss and total coronary heart disease, fatal coronary heart disease, and stroke. Additional support for this association is provided in a recent study examining the association of periodontal disease and the risk for cerebrovascular disease/cerebrovascular accidents using the data from the first NHANES. Wu and colleagues[65] determined that periodontitis was a significant risk factor for a first nonfatal or fatal CVA. This was particularly true for nonhemorrhagic stroke. As compared with a healthy periodontium, the relative risk for nonhemorrhagic stroke associated with periodontitis was 2.11; for all CVAs, the relative risk was 1.66.

Taken together, these studies strongly suggest that periodontal disease may be a significant independent risk factor for cardiovascular/cerebrovascular disease. Nevertheless, caution is urged; a recent study by Hujoel and colleagues[66] failed to identify periodontal disease as a significant risk factor for coronary heart disease (defined as hospitalization or death from coronary heart disease, or the need for a revascularization procedure). Any discrepancies will be resolved only by development of appropriate animal models and prospective studies relating the development of cardiovascular/cerebrovascular disease to periodontal disease and the presence of periodontal infections.

Transient Bacteremia

The proposed basis for the association of periodontal disease and cardiovascular disease is either the direct contribution of the subgingival bacteria or the inflammatory response to the persistent infection. Periodontal bacteria and bacterial products may gain access to the peripheral circulation following its contact with inflamed tissue. Many dental procedures cause a transient bacteremia. Transient bacteremia can also occur as a result of toothbrushing, flossing, and even chewing.[67,68] The severity of dental plaque, probing depth, and gingival inflammation appear to correlate positively with incidence and magnitude of bacteremia.[69] In patients with periodontitis, gingival bleeding is common in association with toothbrushing and flossing. While a single tooth may accumulate bacterial levels as high as 10^9,[70] the oral bacterial load is influenced by salivary flow, mastication, nutrient availability, and oral hygiene. Poor oral hygiene can account for a 10-fold increase in oral bacterial load.

The predominant subgingival microorganisms in both health and gingivitis are gram-positive aerobes, while those in the subgingival environment of periodontitis patients are gram-negative anaerobes.[71] Species that have been isolated from the blood during transient bacteremia of oral origin include gram-positive and gram-negative aerobes and anaerobes.[72] Frequent transient gram-negative bacteremias occur in individuals with periodontitis.[69] Some of the subgingival gram-negative anaerobes also display tissue-invasion properties,[73,74] which could contribute to inflammation at distal sites. As an example, *Porphyromonas gingivalis* was recently shown to invade bovine and human endothelial cells, as assessed by an antibiotic protection assay and transmission and scanning electron microscopy.[75]

It appears that the acute and chronic effects of transient bacteremia as a result of dental manipulations are benign for most individuals, because within 30 minutes of such manipulations the blood is again found to be sterile.[76] However, patients with untreated existing periodontal disease have a larger intraoral bacterial load and hence larger and more frequent transient bacteremias. These transient bacteremias occur many times a day for many years. The frequency of these events suggests a chronic challenge to the vascular endothelium, which may alter rheologic and hemostatic parameters.

C-reactive Protein and Fibrinogen

From the preceding discussion it seems clear that individuals with periodontitis have frequent transient systemic exposure to gram-negative microbes. The chronic effects of these repeated bacteremia have not been studied. What is known, however, is that patients with periodontal disease appear to have higher levels of serum C-reactive protein (CRP) and fibrinogen, the so-called acute-phase proteins, as well as higher white blood cell counts.[77] These proteins are elevated in patients with in-

flammation or infection, and each has been associated in epidemiologic studies with increased risk for cardiovascular disease. A high white blood cell count likewise has long been considered a risk factor for cardiovascular disease. The rise of acute-phase proteins and other blood markers of infection is collectively referred to as the *acute-phase response*.

CRP was discovered 50 years ago as a serum protein that reacts with C-polysaccharide derived from the cell wall of pneumococcus.[78] CRP is synthesized only by hepatocytes, and production is regulated by IL-6. IL-6 is a cytokine with procoagulant and proinflammatory activity often isolated from bacteremic patients.[79] CRP may rise in the sera of normal patients within 6 to 12 hours after injury or infection. CRP serum levels (the half-life of CRP is 19 hours) may increase 100-fold, and fibrinogen levels may increase 10-fold in response to a microbial challenge.[80] Elevated CRP levels are considered a marker for systemic inflammation and as such have been evaluated by Ridker et al[81] using the Physician's Health Study database. CRP was found to be independently associated with risk for MI in apparently healthy men. Increased levels of CRP and fibrinogen may be predictors of future MI and stroke, even in individuals who do not have elevated cholesterol or total serum lipid levels.[82]

Fibrinogen, a pivotal component of the coagulation cascade, participates in platelet function and is the substrate for fibrin formation. Fibrinogen is a plasma protein that is converted from a soluble protein to an insoluble polymer by the action of thrombin, resulting in the formation of a fibrin clot. Fibrinogen is also an acute-phase protein, which may become elevated as a consequence of systemic infection.[83–85] An elevated fibrinogen level may predispose an individual to thrombosis and is an indicator of risk for coronary heart disease.[86]

The absence of an identifiable source of infection in cases of elevated CRP and fibrinogen levels has led some investigators to speculate that the elevated serum levels of inflammatory mediators are due to infection of "unknown origin," or subclinical infection.[81] Chronic periodontal disease is common in the population and often overlooked by medical examiners. Consequently, this undiagnosed and untreated infection could contribute to the increased CRP and fibrinogen levels and white blood cell counts that have been found to be predictors of MI and stroke. Ebersole et al[87] have shown CRP to be present and elevated in the serum of patients with periodontal disease. In addition, Kweider et al[77] have demonstrated an increase in the number of white blood cells and level of fibrinogen in periodontitis patients, further indicating periodontal disease as a systemic modifier.

This indirect evidence does not define causality; it may be, in fact, a casual relationship. While bacteremia of

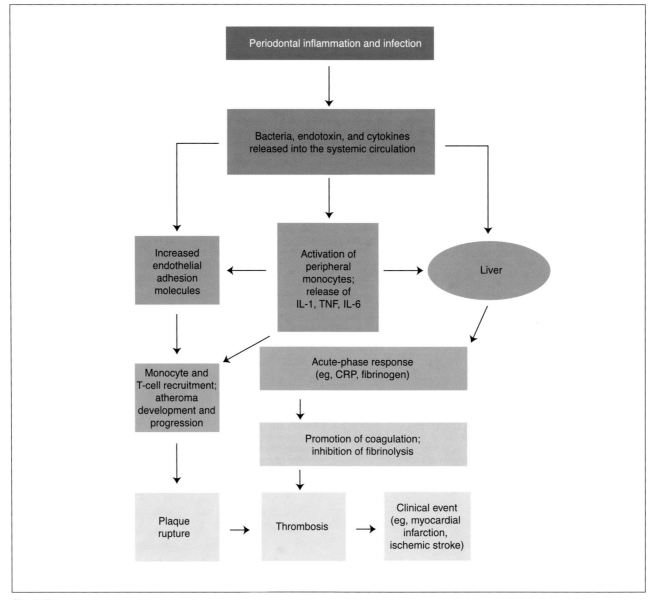

Fig 9-7 Proposed mechanisms to explain the association between periodontal disease and cardiovascular disease.

oral origin may provide the impetus for systemic inflammation, the chronically inflamed peripheral vasculature is also a potent source of proinflammatory cytokines and prostaglandins.[88] Because these mediators are found at high levels within the inflamed periodontium, they may enter the circulation and further contribute to endothelial dysfunction.

Hence, evidence from experimental and epidemiologic studies, taken together, indicates that chronic periodontal disease may play a role in the etiology of cardiovascular disease. These findings support a biologically plausible model for the pathogenesis of atherosclerosis in which periodontal infection may be a source of endotoxin and inflammatory mediators, which may have adverse effects on the vascular endothelium and the liver (Fig 9-7).

Periodontitis and Pregnancy

The preceding discussion sets the stage for understanding how the effects of periodontitis may influence different organ systems and systemic diseases. If bacteria and endotoxin can gain access to the peripheral blood, what are the potential ramifications for the maternal-fetal circulation during pregnancy? This section will discuss the potential influence of periodontitis on pregnancy.

Preterm birth/low birth weight secondary to the onset of preterm labor remains the leading cause of morbidity and mortality among neonates,[89] especially those of young minority mothers of low socioeconomic status.[90] Approximately 1 in 10 births in the United States results in preterm birth/low birth weight.[91] Preterm birth/low birth weight accounts for 62% to 75% of all prenatal deaths and 85% of nonanomalous prenatal deaths.[92] Preterm/low-birth-weight infants face life-long morbidity and have high mortality rates. Specific treatments to prevent preterm birth/low birth weight have met with limited success,[93] and many mothers of these infants have no known risk factor. However, a substantial body of evidence links maternal infection with the pathophysiology of preterm birth/low birth weight.[94]

How might infectious microorganisms influence the developing fetus? In bacterial vaginosis, microorganisms from the cervix or the vagina are believed to colonize the lower poles of the fetal membranes, resulting in inflammation (chorioamnionitis) with premature rupture of the membranes and release of the arachidonic acid metabolite PGE_2.[95] Uterine contractions and premature labor ensue. Infection of the chorion and amnion (chorioamnionitis) is diagnosed clinically by gravida pyrexia, uterine tenderness, maternal tachycardia, and fetal tachycardia.[96] The diagnosis of chorioamnionitis can also be made histologically by examining the postpartum placenta.[97] Histologic observation of these placental tissues reveals a chronic inflammatory cell infiltrate. Bacteria, however, are not always found in the tissues of the chorion and amnion.[98] The diagnosis of histologic chorioamnionitis is frequently made in the absence of clinical chorioamnionitis, suggesting that this infection is often "silent." The chronically inflamed chorion is a potent source of proinflammatory cytokines and prostaglandins.[99,100] Elevated levels of cytokines and prostaglandins have been found in the amniotic fluid of patients with both clinical and histologic chorioamnionitis.[101,102] These increased levels have frequently been associated with preterm labor.[103]

Endotoxin and lipopolysaccharide (LPS), products of cell walls of gram-negative bacteria, elicit an inflammatory response involving the cytokines IL-1β and TNF.[104] IL-1β and TNF act synergistically to induce PGE_2 in many tissue types, including the placenta.[99,105] There are data to suggest that IL-1β and PGE_2 levels are increased in, and predictive of, preterm delivery.[106] Additionally, increased amniotic levels of TNF and PGE_2 are associated with physiologic labor.[99] It is believed that increased levels of IL-1β and TNF, along with PGE_2, act on the surrounding maternal tissues to induce cervical ripening, uterine contractility, and premature rupture of membranes.[107] IL-6 has also been isolated routinely from the amniotic fluid of women in preterm labor.[108] It has been linked repeatedly with infection and appears to follow IL-1β and TNF in the sequence of events that begin with LPS-induced inflammation.[104] However, despite evidence of an association between chorioamnionitis and preterm birth/low birth weight, 18% to 49% of placentas showing signs of inflammation are culture negative.[109] The absence of an identifiable source of infection of the fetal-placental unit in many cases of chorioamnionitis has led some investigators to speculate that the elevated amniotic levels of inflammatory mediators are due to infection of "unknown origin."[100]

Subclinical infection has been speculated to be an adverse influence on birth outcome.[110] In 1988, McGregor et al[111] proposed that chronic maternal infections such as periodontal disease should be considered as a possible influence. The first direct evidence for this theory was provided in 1998 by Hill,[112] who determined that the subspecies of *Fusobacterium nucleatum* most commonly isolated from the amniotic fluid were not commonly found in the vaginal flora but were common in the oral flora. Hill concluded that some amniotic bacterial isolates may be hematogenous and of oral origin. *F nucleatum* is a ubiquitous periodontal pathogen.[71]

In 1996, Offenbacher and colleagues[113] observed a significantly greater extent and severity of periodontal disease in women with preterm birth/low-birth-weight infants than in controls. The multivariate logistic regression model used in this study controlled for other risk factors for preterm birth/low birth weight and demonstrated that periodontal disease is a statistically significant independent risk factor with an adjusted odds ratio of 7.9. This high odds ratio exceeds by several fold that of other known risk factors for preterm birth/low birth weight, including smoking, bacterial vaginosis, and history of urinary tract infection.

Taken together, the findings of Hill[112] and Offenbacher et al[113] support a model for the pathogenesis of preterm birth/low birth weight in which periodontal infection may be considered the source of bacteria, LPS, and inflammatory mediators that may have adverse effects on pregnancy outcome via a hematogenous route (Fig 9-8). Furthermore, studies have shown that during pregnancy there can be an increase in the number of some black-pigmented anaerobes in the gingival crevice. The increase in these organisms has been attributed to changing estrogen levels. Specifically, certain black-pigmented subgingival bacteria utilize estrogen as a growth factor.[114] This overgrowth may further contribute to the intraoral bacterial load during pregnancy.

Periodontitis and Diabetes Mellitus

Individuals with diabetes mellitus have an increased incidence of atherosclerotic cardiovascular, peripheral vascular, and cerebrovascular disease. Neuropathy, retinopathy, and nephropathy are also common in individuals with diabetes mellitus. Furthermore, people with diabetes mellitus have an increased incidence and severity of periodontal disease.[115] The prevalence of diabetes mellitus is 10% in the population, while the prevalence of severe peri-

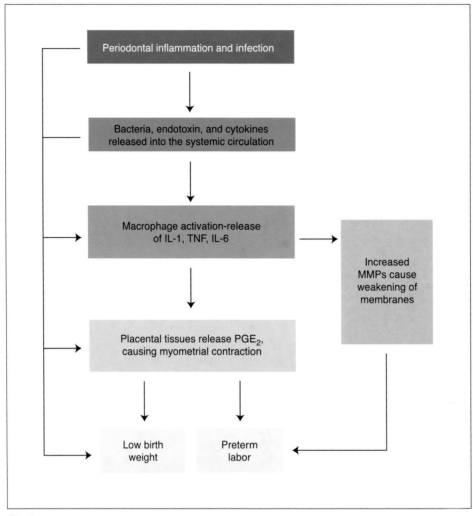

Fig 9-8 Proposed mechanisms to explain the association between periodontal disease and preterm birth/low-birth-weight infants.

odontal disease is 15%.[116] The prevalence of severe periodontal disease among people with diabetes mellitus, however, has been reported to be as high as 40%.[115] Thus, periodontal disease is a major complication of diabetes mellitus.[117] Indeed, periodontal disease has been recognized as the sixth complication of the disease.[117]

The molecular mechanisms of diabetic periodontitis remain unclear, but researchers have developed an animal model that has provided new insights into this problem.[118] Studies have demonstrated that the hyperglycemia that characterizes diabetes mellitus results in the nonenzymatic glycation of proteins, an example of which is glycosylated hemoglobin, used as a clinical marker of long-term glucose control in patients with diabetes mellitus. Further molecular rearrangements of these glycosylated proteins result in the formation of advanced glycation end products (AGEs). AGEs can interact with distinct

cellular receptors, the best characterized of which is the receptor for AGEs, or RAGE. The AGE-RAGE interaction on target cells in the periodontium of diabetics can lead to sustained inflammation and an exaggerated response to periodontal pathogens (Fig 9-9). This model suggests that a persistent inflammatory response will result in the increased gingival inflammation and alveolar bone loss observed in diabetic patients.

An exaggerated inflammatory response may contribute to local periodontal tissue destruction, but inflammation in the patient with diabetes mellitus may have other consequences as well. Chronic infection may alter blood glucose levels. Infection deteriorates the metabolic status in patients with diabetes mellitus, resulting in the need for higher insulin doses or insulin injections in patients normally receiving medication orally. Uncontrolled periodontal disease may interfere with glycemic control.[119] As

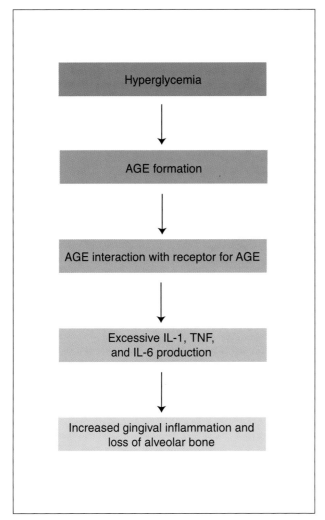

Fig 9-9 A possible mechanism to explain periodontitis associated with diabetes mellitus. AGE indicates advanced glycation end product.

noted, bacteremia is common in patients with periodontal disease. Transient bacteremias result when the highly vascular, chronically inflamed gingiva is irritated by daily mechanical perturbations of the bacterial plaque (eg, chewing and toothbrushing). The resulting release of bacteria and LPS into the circulation may play a role in the insulin resistance seen in diabetes mellitus patients with infection.[120]

A recent clinical report suggested that the treatment of existing periodontal disease in the diabetic patient can lead to a statistically significant reduction in the level of serum glycosylated hemoglobin (HbA1C).[121] Serum HbA1C, a laboratory measure of relatively short-term glucose control, has become the measurement of choice in monitoring the treatment of diabetes mellitus and making decisions on when and how to implement therapy. Hence, HbA1C is a valuable tool for monitoring glycemia.

In a case-control study, Grossi et al[121] used HbA1C as the outcome variable of interest in reporting on the treatment of 113 periodontitis patients with diabetes mellitus. Patients were divided into one of five treatment groups. Each group received scaling and root planing, as well as irrigation with either water, chlorhexidine, or providone-iodine. In addition, three of the five groups received systemically administered doxycycline (100 mg/day for 2 weeks), and the other two groups received a placebo. The results showed that patients in the doxycycline groups achieved a 10% reduction in HbA1C at 3 months following therapy, while patients in the scaling and root planing plus placebo groups experienced no reduction. A reduction of 10% in HbA1C is meaningful. For example, in the UK Prospective Diabetes Study,[122] an 11% reduction in HbA1C resulted in 25% fewer diabetes mellitus–related complications and 10% fewer diabetes mellitus–related deaths over a 10-year period.[123]

Conclusions

Inflammatory mechanisms associated with human periodontal disease have been defined. Periodontal infections and the resulting inflammatory response appear to have both local and distant sequelae.

The widespread and growing interest in the relationship between periodontal disease and systemic illness has important implications for the dental profession. Long-term longitudinal studies that examine the development of cardiovascular/cerebrovascular disease and the metabolic control of diabetes mellitus in the presence of periodontal disease are required to critically assess the impact of oral infections on systemic disease. Appropriate animal models are also needed to clarify the specific cellular events that account for these conditions. Nevertheless, the association data appear quite strong, and this information emphasizes the importance of regular oral examinations and appropriate dental and periodontal treatment. As these associations are defined, dental health care will increasingly be considered in the context of general health care.

References

1. Page RC, Schroeder HE. Pathogenesis of inflammatory periodontal disease: A summary of current work. Lab Invest 1976; 34:235–249.
2. Brill N. Influence of capillary permeability on flow of tissue fluid into gingival pockets. Acta Odontol Scand 1959;17:277–284.
3. Cimasoni G. Crevicular Fluid Updated, ed 2, monograph 12, Monographs in Oral Science. New York: Karger, 1983.
4. Poulsen S, Holm-Pedersen P, Kelstrup J. Comparison of different measurements of development of plaque and gingivitis in man. Scand J Dent Res 1979;87:178–183.

5. Lamster IB, Hartley LJ, Vogel RI. Development of a biochemical profile for gingival crevicular fluid: Methodological considerations and evaluation of collagen-degrading and ground substance-degrading enzyme activity during experimental gingivitis. J Periodontol 1985;56:13–21.

6. Gallin JI, Goldstein IM, Snyderman R. Inflammation: Basic Principles and Clinical Correlates. New York: Raven, 1988.

7. Hock J, Niki K. A vital microscopy study of the morphology of normal and inflamed gingiva. J Periodontal Res 1971;6:81–88.

8. Murphy P. The neutrophil. New York: Plenum Medical Book, 1976.

9. Bevilacqua MP, Pober JS, Wheeler ME, et al. Interleukin 1 acts on cultured human vascular endothelium to increase the adhesion of polymorphonuclear leukocytes, monocytes, and related leukocyte cell lines. J Clin Invest 1985;76:2003–2011.

10. Gimbrone MA Jr, Brock AF, Schafer AI. Leukotriene B4 stimulates polymorphonuclear leukocyte adhesion to cultured vascular endothelial cells. J Clin Invest 1984;74:1552–1555.

11. Kowashi Y, Jaccard F, Cimasoni G. Sulcular polymorphonuclear leucocytes and gingival exudate during experimental gingivitis in man. J Periodontal Res 1980;15:151–158.

12. Klinkhamer JM, Zimmerman S. The function and reliability of the orogranulocytic migratory rate as a measure of oral health. J Dent Res 1969;48:709–715.

13. Schiffmann E, Corcoran BA, Wahl SM. N-formylmethionyl peptides as chemoattractants for leucocytes. Proc Natl Acad Sci USA 1975;72:1059–1062.

14. Sklar LA, Jesaitis AJ, Painter RG. The neutrophil N-formyl peptide receptor: Dynamics of ligand-receptor interactions and their relationship to cellular responses. Contemp Top Immunobiol 1984;14:29–82.

15. Van Dyke TE, Hoop GA. Neutrophil function and oral disease. Crit Rev Oral Biol Med 1990;1:117–133.

16. Lamster IB, Novak MJ. Host mediators in gingival crevicular fluid: Implications for the pathogenesis of periodontal disease. Crit Rev Oral Biol Med 1992;3:31–60.

17. Ding Y, Uitto VJ, Haapasalo M, et al. Membrane components of *Treponema denticola* trigger proteinase release from human polymorphonuclear leukocytes. J Dent Res 1996;75:1986–1993.

18. Ding Y, Haapasalo M, Kerosuo E, et al. Release and activation of human neutrophil matrix metallo- and serine proteinases during phagocytosis of *Fusobacterium nucleatum, Porphyromonas gingivalis* and *Treponema denticola.* J Clin Periodontol 1997; 24:237–248.

19. Garant PR. Plaque-neutrophil interaction in monoinfected rats as visualized by transmission electron microscopy. J Periodontol 1976;47:132–138.

20. Topoll HH, Zwadlo G, Lange DE, Sorg C. Phenotypic dynamics of macrophage subpopulations during human experimental gingivitis. J Periodontal Res 1989;24:106–112.

21. Zappa U, Reinking-Zappa M, Graf H, Espeland M. Cell populations and episodic periodontal attachment loss in humans. J Clin Periodontol 1991;18:508–515.

22. Wahl SM, Hunt DA, Wakefield LM, et al. Transforming growth factor type beta induces monocyte chemotaxis and growth factor production. J Immunol 1987;139:1342–1347.

23. Wahl L, Wahl S. Inflammation. In: Cohen IK, Diegelmann RF, Lindblad WJ (eds). Wound Healing: Biochemical and Clinical Aspects. Philadelphia: Saunders, 1992:40–62.

24. Newton R, Kuitert LM, Slater DM, et al. Cytokine induction of cytosolic phospholipase A2 and cyclooxygenase-2 mRNA is suppressed by glucocorticoids in human epithelial cells. Life Sci 1997;60:67–78.

25. Stashenko P, Jandinski JJ, Fujiyoshi P, et al. Tissue levels of bone resorptive cytokines in periodontal disease. J Periodontol 1991; 62:504–509.

26. Masada MP, Persson R, Kenney JS, et al. Measurement of interleukin-1 alpha and -1 beta in gingival crevicular fluid: Implications for the pathogenesis of periodontal disease. J Periodontal Res 1990;25:156–163.

27. Matsuki Y, Yamamoto T, Hara K. Localization of interleukin-1 (IL-1) mRNA-expressing macrophages in human inflamed gingiva and IL-1 activity in gingival crevicular fluid. J Periodontal Res 1993;28:35–42.

28. Ristimaki A, Garfinkel S, Wessendorf J, et al. Induction of cyclooxygenase-2 by interleukin-1 alpha: Evidence for post-transcriptional regulation. J Biol Chem 1994;269:11769–11775.

29. Rossomando EF, Kennedy JE, Hadjimichael J. Tumour necrosis factor alpha in gingival crevicular fluid as a possible indicator of periodontal disease in humans. Arch Oral Biol 1990;35: 431–434.

30. Rossomando EF, White LB, Hadjimichael J. Immunomagnetic separation of tumor necrosis factor alpha. II: In situ procedure for the human gingival space. J Chromatogr 1992;583:19–26.

31. Salvi GE, Brown CE, Fujihashi K, et al. Inflammatory mediators of the terminal dentition in adult and early onset periodontitis. J Periodontal Res 1998;33:212–225.

32. Reinhardt RA, Masada MP, Kaldahl WB, et al. Gingival fluid IL-1 and IL-6 levels in refractory periodontitis. J Clin Periodontol 1993;20:225–231.

33. Tsai CC, Ho YP, Chen CC. Levels of interleukin-1 beta and interleukin-8 in gingival crevicular fluids in adult periodontitis. J Periodontol 1995;66:852–859.

34. Lamster IB, Grbic JT. Diagnosis of periodontal disease based on analysis of the host response. Periodontol 2000;7:83–99.

35. Gustafsson G, Nilsson L. Fibrinolytic activity in fluid from gingival crevice. Proc Soc Exp Biol Med 1961;106:277–280.

36. Hidaka N, Maeda K, Kawakami C, et al. Fibrinolytic activity in periodontal disease: The relationship between fibrinolytic activity and severity of periodontal disease. J Periodontol 1981;52: 181–186.

37. Montgomery EH, White RR. Kinin generation in the gingival inflammatory response to topically applied bacterial lipopolysaccharides. J Dent Res 1986;65:113–117.

38. Niekrash CE, Patters MR, Lang NP. The relationship of complement cleavage in gingival fluid to periodontal diseases. J Periodontal Res 1984;19:622–627.

39. Niekrash CE, Patters MR. Simultaneous assessment of complement components C3, C4, and B and their cleavage products in human gingival fluid, II. Longitudinal changes during periodontal therapy. J Periodontal Res 1985;20:268–275.

40. Niekrash CE, Patters MR. Assessment of complement cleavage in gingival fluid in humans with and without periodontal disease. J Periodontal Res 1986;21:233–242.

41. Offenbacher S, Odle BM, Van Dyke TE. The use of crevicular fluid prostaglandin E2 levels as a predictor of periodontal attachment loss. J Periodontal Res 1986;21:101–112.

42. Palcanis KG, Larjava IK, Wells BR, et al. Elastase as an indicator of periodontal disease progression. J Periodontol 1992;63: 237–242.

43. Lamster IB, Holmes LG, Gross KB, et al. The relationship of beta-glucuronidase activity in crevicular fluid to probing attachment loss in patients with adult periodontitis: Findings from a multicenter study. J Clin Periodontol 1995;22:36–44.

44. Kornman KS, Crane A, Wang HY, et al. The interleukin-1 genotype as a severity factor in adult periodontal disease. J Clin Periodontol 1997;24:72–77.

45. Engebretson SP, Lamster IB, Herrera-Abreu M, et al. The influence of interleukin gene polymorphism on expression of interleukin-1beta and tumor necrosis factor-alpha in periodontal tissue and gingival crevicular fluid. J Periodontol 1999;70:567–573.

46. Birkedal-Hansen H. Role of matrix metalloproteinases in human periodontal diseases. J Periodontol 1993;64:819–827.

47. Weiss SJ. Tissue destruction by neutrophils. N Engl J Med 1989; 320:365–376.

48. Ebersole JL, Singer RE, Steffensen B, et al. Inflammatory mediators and immunoglobulins in GCF from healthy, gingivitis and periodontitis sites. J Periodontal Res 1993;28:543–546.

49. Heasman PA, Collins JG, Offenbacher S. Changes in crevicular fluid levels of interleukin-1 beta, leukotriene B4, prostaglandin E2, thromboxane B2 and tumour necrosis factor alpha in experimental gingivitis in humans. J Periodontal Res 1993;28: 241–247.

50. Lamster IB, Smith QT, Celenti RS, et al. Development of a risk profile for periodontal disease: Microbial and host response factors. J Periodontol 1994;65:511–520.

51. Nash HS. Loosening Teeth, or, Chronic Alveolitis: Its Causes, Clinical History and Treatment. New York: Horton F Welles, 1897.

52. Offenbacher S. Periodontal diseases: Pathogenesis. Ann Periodontol 1996;1:821–878.

53. Loesche WJ, Lopatin DE. Interactions between periodontal disease, medical diseases and immunity in the older individual. Periodontol 2000 1998;16:80–105.

54. Tillett HE, Smith JW, Gooch CD. Excess deaths attributable to influenza in England and Wales: Age at death and certified cause. Int J Epidemiol 1983;12:344–352.

55. Grau AJ, Buggle F, Becher H, et al. Recent bacterial and viral infection is a risk factor for cerebrovascular ischemia: Clinical and biochemical studies. Neurology 1998;50:196–203.

56. Whincup PH, Mendall MA, Perry IJ, et al. Prospective relations between Helicobacter pylori infection, coronary heart disease, and stroke in middle aged men. Heart 1996;75:568–572.

57. Nieto FJ, Adam E, Sorlie P, et al. Cohort study of cytomegalovirus infection as a risk factor for carotid intimal-medial thickening, a measure of subclinical atherosclerosis. Circulation 1996;94:922–927.

58. Saikku P, Leinonen M, Tenkanen L, et al. Chronic Chlamydia pneumoniae infection as a risk factor for coronary heart disease in the Helsinki Heart Study. Ann Intern Med 1992;116:273–278.

59. Mattila KJ, Nieminen MS, Valtonen VV, et al. Association between dental health and acute myocardial infarction. Br Med J 1989;298:779–781.

60. Syrjanen J, Peltola J, Valtonen V, et al. Dental infections in association with cerebral infarction in young and middle-aged men. J Intern Med 1989;225:179–184.

61. Mattila KJ. Dental infections as a risk factor for acute myocardial infarction. Eur Heart J 1993;14(suppl K):51–53.

62. DeStefano F, Anda RF, Kahn HS, et al. Dental disease and risk of coronary heart disease and mortality. Br Med J 1993;306: 688–691.

63. Burt BA. The distribution of periodontal destruction in the populations of industrialized countries. In: Johnson NW (ed). Risk Markers for Oral Diseases, vol 3. Cambridge, England: Cambridge University Press, 1991:9–26.

64. Beck J, Garcia R, Heiss G, et al. Periodontal disease and cardiovascular disease. J Periodontol 1996;67:1123–1137.

65. Wu T, Trevisan M, Genco RJ, et al. Periodontal disease and risk of cerebrovascular disease: The first national health and nutrition examination survey and its follow-up study. Arch Intern Med 2000;160:2749–2755.

66. Hujoel PP, Drangsholt M, Spiekerman C, DeRouen TA. Periodontal disease and coronary heart disease risk. JAMA 2000; 284:1406–1410.

67. Hockett RN, Loesche WJ, Sodeman TM. Bacteraemia in asymptomatic human subjects. Arch Oral Biol 1977;22:91–98.

68. Roberts GJ, Holzel HS, Sury MR, et al. Dental bacteremia in children. Pediatr Cardiol 1997;18:24–27.

69. Silver JG, Martin AW, McBride BC. Experimental transient bacteraemias in human subjects with varying degrees of plaque accumulation and gingival inflammation. J Clin Periodontol 1977; 4:92–99.

70. Loesche WJ, Syed SA, Schmidt E, Morrison EC. Bacterial profiles of subgingival plaques in periodontitis. J Periodontol 1985; 56:447–456.

71. Haffajee AD, Socransky SS. Microbial etiological agents of destructive periodontal diseases. Periodontol 2000 1994;5:78–111.

72. Pallasch TJ, Slots J. Antibiotic prophylaxis and the medically compromised patient. Periodontol 2000 1996;10:107–138.

73. Christersson LA, Wikesjo UM, Albini B, et al. Tissue localization of Actinobacillus actinomycetemcomitans in human periodontitis, II. Correlation between immunofluorescence and culture techniques. J Periodontol 1987;58:540–545.

74. Madianos PN, Papapanou PN, Nannmark U, et al. Porphyromonas gingivalis FDC381 multiplies and persists within human oral epithelial cells in vitro. Infect Immunol 1996;64:660–664.

75. Deshpande RG, Khan MB, Genco CA. Invasion of aortic and heart endothelial cells by Porphyromonas gingivalis. Infect Immunol 1998;66:5337–5343.

76. Durack DT. Prevention of infective endocarditis. N Engl J Med 1995;332:38–44.

77. Kweider M, Lowe GD, Murray GD, et al. Dental disease, fibrinogen and white cell count: Links with myocardial infarction? Scott Med J 1993;38:73–74.

78. Tillet WS, Francis T. Serological reactions in pneumonia with a non-protein somatic fraction of pneumococcus. J Exp Med 1930;52:561–571.

79. Blackwell TS, Christman JW. Sepsis and cytokines: Current status. Br J Anaesth 1996;77:110–117.

80. Vigushin DM, Pepys MB, Hawkins PN. Metabolic and scintigraphic studies of radioiodinated human C-reactive protein in health and disease. J Clin Invest 1993;91:1351–1357.

81. Ridker PM, Cushman M, Stampfer MJ, et al. Inflammation, aspirin, and the risk of cardiovascular disease in apparently healthy men. N Engl J Med 1997;336:973–979.

82. Berk BC, Weintraub WS, Alexander RW. Elevation of C-reactive protein in "active" coronary artery disease. Am J Cardiol 1990; 65:168–172.

83. Vasse M, Paysant J, Soria J, et al. Regulation of fibrinogen biosynthesis by cytokines, consequences on the vascular risk. Haemostasis 1996;26(suppl 4):331–339.

84. Szirmai IG, Kamondi A, Magyar H, Juhasz C. Relation of laboratory and clinical variables to the grade of carotid atherosclerosis. Stroke 1993;24:1811–1816.

85. Ernst E, Resch KL. Fibrinogen as a cardiovascular risk factor: A meta-analysis and review of the literature. Ann Intern Med 1993; 118:956–963.

86. Grau AJ, Buggle F, Becher H, et al. The association of leukocyte count, fibrinogen and C-reactive protein with vascular risk factors and ischemic vascular diseases. Thromb Res 1996; 82:245–255.

87. Ebersole JL, Machen RL, Steffen MJ, Willmann DE. Systemic acute-phase reactants, C-reactive protein and haptoglobin, in adult periodontitis. Clin Exp Immunol 1997;107:347–352.

88. Kinlay S, Selwyn AP, Libby P, Ganz P. Inflammation, the endothelium, and the acute coronary syndromes. J Cardiovasc Pharmacol 1998;32:S62–S66.

89. Goldenberg RL, Rouse DJ. Prevention of premature birth. N Engl J Med 1998;339:313–320.

90. Hogue CJ, Hargraves MA. Class, race, and infant mortality in the United States. Am J Public Health 1993;83:9–12.

91. Copper RL, Goldenberg RL, Das A, et al. The preterm prediction study: Maternal stress is associated with spontaneous preterm birth at less than thirty-five weeks' gestation: National Institute of Child Health and Human Development Maternal-Fetal Medicine Units Network. Am J Obstet Gynecol 1996;175: 1286–1292.

92. McCormick MC. The contribution of low birth weight to infant mortality and childhood morbidity. N Engl J Med 1985;312: 82–90.

93. Rust OA, Bofill JA, Arriola RM, et al. The clinical efficacy of oral tocolytic therapy. Am J Obstet Gynecol 1996;175:838–842.

94. Gomez R, Romero R, Edwin SS, David C. Pathogenesis of preterm labor and preterm premature rupture of membranes associated with intraamniotic infection. Infect Dis Clin North Am 1997;11:135–176.

95. Gravett MG, Witkin SS, Haluska GJ, et al. An experimental model for intraamniotic infection and preterm labor in rhesus monkeys. Am J Obstet Gynecol 1994;171:1660–1667.

96. Tan BP, Hannah ME. Prostaglandins for prelabour rupture of membranes at or near term [review]. Cochrane Database Syst Rev 2000;2:CD000178.

97. Beebe LA, Cowan LD, Hyde SR, Altshuler G. Methods to improve the reliability of histopathological diagnoses in the placenta. Paediatr Perinat Epidemiol 2000;14:172–178.

98. Hillier SL, Krohn MA, Kiviat NB, et al. Microbiologic causes and neonatal outcomes associated with chorioamnion infection. Am J Obstet Gynecol 1991;165:955–961.

99. Mitchell MD, Romero RJ, Edwin SS, Trautman MS. Prostaglandins and parturition. Reprod Fertil Dev 1995;7:623–632.

100. Romero R, Mazor M, Wu YK, et al. Bacterial endotoxin and tumor necrosis factor stimulate prostaglandin production by human decidua Prostaglandins Leukot Essent Fatty Acids 1989;37:183–186.

101. Hirst JJ, Teixeira FJ, Zakar T, Olson DM. Prostaglandin H synthase-2 expression increases in human gestational tissues with spontaneous labour onset. Reprod Fertil Dev 1995;7:633–637.

102. Keelan JA, Coleman M, Mitchell MD. The molecular mechanisms of term and preterm labor: Recent progress and clinical implications. Clin Obstet Gynecol 1997;40:460–478.

103. Calder A, Embrey MP. Prostaglandins and the unfavourable cervix [letter]. Lancet 1973;2:1322–1323.

104. Dinarello CA. Interleukin-1 and interleukin-1 antagonism. Blood 1991;77:1627–1652.

105. Kelly RW, Carr GG, Elliott CL, et al. Prostaglandin and cytokine release by trophoblastic villi. Hum Reprod 1995;10:3289–3292.

106. Halgunset J, Johnsen H, Kjollesdal AM, et al. Cytokine levels in amniotic fluid and inflammatory changes in the placenta from normal deliveries at term. Eur J Obstet Gynecol Reprod Biol 1994;56:153–160.

107. Mercer BM, Lewis R. Preterm labor and preterm premature rupture of the membranes: Diagnosis and management. Infect Dis Clin North Am 1997;11:177–201.

108. Weimann E, Reisbach G, Reinsberg J, Lentze MJ. IL-6 and G-CSF levels in amniotic fluid during the second trimester in normal and abnormal pregnancies. Arch Gynecol Obstet 1995; 256:125–130.

109. Hillier SL, Martius J, Krohn M, et al. A case-control study of chorioamnionic infection and histologic chorioamnionitis in prematurity. N Engl J Med 1988;319:972–978.

110. Gibbs RS, Romero R, Hillier SL, et al. A review of premature birth and subclinical infection. Am J Obstet Gynecol 1992; 166:1515–1528.

111. McGregor JA, French JI, Lawellin D, Todd JK. Preterm birth and infection: Pathogenic possibilities. Am J Reprod Immunol Microbiol 1988;16:123–132.

112. Hill GB. Preterm birth: Associations with genital and possibly oral microflora. Ann Periodontol 1998;3:222–232.

113. Offenbacher S, Katz V, Fertik G, et al. Periodontal infection as a possible risk factor for preterm low birth weight. J Periodontol 1996;67:1103–1113.

114. Kornman KS, Loesche WJ. The subgingival microbial flora during pregnancy. J Periodontal Res 1980;15:111–122.

115. Glavind L, Lund B, Loe H. The relationship between periodontal state and diabetes duration, insulin dosage and retinal changes. J Periodontal Res 1969;4:164–165.

116. Oliver RC, Brown LJ, Loe H. Periodontal diseases in the United States population. J Periodontol 1998;69:269–278.

117. Loe H. Periodontal disease: The sixth complication of diabetes mellitus. Diabetes Care 1993;16:329–334.

118. Lalla E, Lamster IB, Feit M, et al. A murine model of accelerated periodontal disease in diabetes. J Periodontal Res 1998; 33:387–399.

119. Taylor GW, Burt BA, Becker MP, et al. Severe periodontitis and risk for poor glycemic control in patients with non-insulin-dependent diabetes mellitus. J Periodontol 1996;67:1085–1093.

120. Blackard WG, Anderson JH Jr, Spitzer JJ. Hyperinsulinism in endotoxin shock dogs. Metabolism 1976;25:675–684.

121. Grossi SG, Skrepcinski FB, DeCaro T, et al. Treatment of periodontal disease in diabetics reduces glycated hemoglobin. J Periodontol 1997;68:713–719.

122. Intensive blood-glucose control with sulphonylureas or insulin compared with conventional treatment and risk of complications in patients with type 2 diabetes (UKPDS 33). UK Prospective Diabetes Study (UKPDS) Group. Lancet 1998;352:837–853.

123. Stratton IM, Adler AI, Neil HA, et al. Association of glycaemia with macrovascular and microvascular complications of type 2 diabetes (UKPDS 35): Prospective observational study. Br Med J 2000;321:405–412.

Aging of the Periodontium

Olav F. Alvares and Bradley D. Johnson

- Types of Aging
- Age Changes in the Oral Mucosa
- Age Changes in the Periodontium
- Predisposing Factors for Periodontitis
- Management of Periodontitis in the Elderly

The average age of the US population has increased in recent years and will continue to do so. By the year 2020, about one in five Americans will be over 65 years of age.[1] Meeting the oral health needs of the elderly requires understanding the biology of aging in the oral cavity. Demographic change makes this requirement increasingly urgent.

Types of Aging

The aging of an organ may be defined as the postmaturational deteriorative changes that, with time, lead to an increased vulnerability to challenges, thereby decreasing the functional ability of the organ. It is imperative to distinguish between changes brought about by cumulative environmental insults and those associated with intrinsic or chronologic aging. This concept is certainly applicable to an organ such as the skin and, in all probability, to the oral mucosa as well. In skin, the clinical and cellular features associated with intrinsic aging (ie, those in sun-protected areas) are different from those seen in photoaging (ie, those in sun-exposed areas).[2] For example, intrinsic aging in the skin is clinically characterized by fine wrinkling, atrophy of the dermis, reduction of the subcutaneous tissue, and

fragility of blood vessels. Sun-damaged skin appears thickened and leathery and is characterized by coarse wrinkling and furrowing.[3] The fact that some older individuals resemble younger ones in biologic processes such as wound healing[4] brings into focus another distinction—that between biologic and chronologic aging. Rates of biologic aging differ among individuals at any given age, and this could partly account for the variability (which can be considerable) observed within and between different age groups. Finally, regional (eg, palate versus floor of mouth) differences in histologic and biochemical traits are known to exist in the oral mucosa. These regional differences should be borne in mind in any consideration of age-related changes in the oral mucosa.

Age Changes in the Oral Mucosa

A 1992 symposium titled "The Effects of Aging in Skin and Oral Mucosa" provided a forum for experts to critically assess the current state of knowledge on the effects of aging on both skin and oral mucosa. It led to the following main conclusions with respect to oral mucosa.[5]

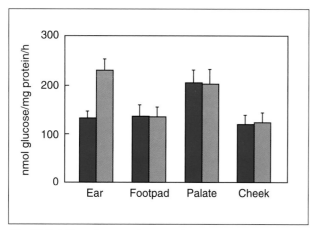

Fig 10-1 Effect of age on the rate of anaerobic glycolysis in epithelia from different regions. Dark bars represent results from young animals (mean ± standard deviation); light bars show results from old animals. (Reprinted from Wertz et al,[7] with permission.)

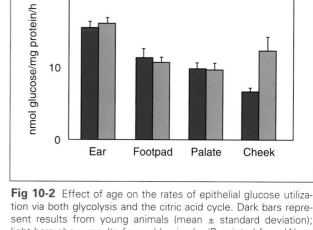

Fig 10-2 Effect of age on the rates of epithelial glucose utilization via both glycolysis and the citric acid cycle. Dark bars represent results from young animals (mean ± standard deviation); light bars show results from old animals. (Reprinted from Wertz et al,[7] with permission.)

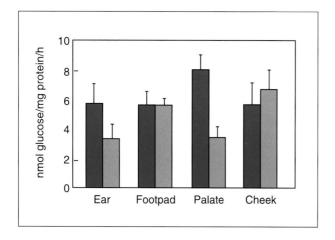

Fig 10-3 Effect of age on the rates of epithelial glucose utilization via the hexose monophosphate shunt. Dark bars represent results from young animals (mean ± standard deviation); light bars show results from old animals. (Reprinted from Wertz et al,[7] with permission.)

Histologic Changes

A hallmark of epithelial differentiation is the synthesis of a family of proteins referred to as *cytokeratins*. It is not known if the pattern of cytokeratin expression in oral mucosa—or for that matter, other markers of epithelial differentiation, such as filaggrin or involucrin—is altered with age. In the skin and oral mucosa of experimental animals, the activities of the major biochemical pathways (protein synthesis, anaerobic glycolysis, and hexose monophosphate shunt) that drive the process of epithelial differentiation remain intact with increasing age.[6] Wertz and coworkers[7] have suggested that the regional differences in carbohydrate and lipid metabolism (Figs 10-1 to 10-3) in oral mucosal epithelia of older animals may be secondary to changes in the underlying mesenchymal connective tissue. Epithelial-mesenchymal interactions initiated during embryogenesis continue to prevail in the maintenance of adult tissues. There are some clues in the literature that these interactions may be altered with increasing age.

The studies of Gilchrest[8] and Yaar and Gilchrest[9] have shown that there is a significant decrease in the mitogenic response of adult keratinocytes in culture to epidermal growth factor and a 29-kd fibroblast growth factor—like protein as compared with cells obtained from newborns and young adults. Conversely, keratinocytes elaborate an array of cytokines, including interleukin 1 (IL-1). In addition to modulating the inflammatory-immune response, IL-1 influences fibroblast and endothelial cell behavior.[10]

When compared with newborn donors, the production of IL-1 by adult human keratinocytes is markedly reduced.[9] Is the production of other cytokines and growth factors (eg, transforming growth factor β, platelet-derived growth factor, and tumor necrosis factor α) altered with increasing age? Insufficient or excessive production of these factors may contribute to the pathogenesis of autoimmune and infectious disorders of the oral mucosa in the elderly.

Studies of autopsy material reveal some structural changes (in epithelial thickness, as well as in size and number of fibroblasts) in the oral mucosa of the elderly, but in this tissue it has proven difficult to distinguish the effects of environmental insults from those associated with intrinsic aging.[11] Regional differences in age-associated changes in the oral mucosa further complicate this distinction. The barrier function of the oral mucosa, and its vascular supply, might be expected to have important clinical implications. Unfortunately, the available data for human oral mucosa for both of these cellular traits are inconclusive, although in experimental animals, some oral sites (palate, dorsal surface of tongue) do exhibit a decrease in blood flow.[12]

Whether or not delayed wound healing as related to epithelial involvement is an intrinsic impairment associated with the aging process is still debatable. In experimental animal models, where the environmental effects can be controlled, Hill[13] found that there was an initial delay in epithelial proliferation and migration in older animals, but that the skin and oral mucosa of young and old animals ultimately exhibit a similar response to tissue injury. The molecular basis for the early epithelial alteration is not known.

Maintenance of epithelial cell proliferation is vital for epithelial homeostasis and optimal wound healing. After a critical evaluation of published studies and the researcher's own animal data, Hill[13] concluded that aging has a minor influence on the rate of epithelial cell proliferation in skin and oral mucosa, regardless of the species investigated. Thus, it is conceivable that the delayed wound healing in the skin of the elderly is the result of environmental influences, such as loss of hydration and ultraviolet damage, rather than the effect of an intrinsic aging process.

Clinical Changes

The impact of intrinsic aging on the clinical status of the oral mucosa is of particular interest. While the prevalence of oral mucosal lesions in individuals in nursing homes is higher than in noninstitutionalized individuals,[14] additional epidemiologic data are needed to establish the true prevalence of oral pathosis and its relationship to intrinsic aging in the elderly.

To reiterate, it is important to distinguish between changes accompanying intrinsic aging, if any, and those brought about by chronic exposure to risk factors. If one excludes risk factors such as denture wear, alcohol abuse, smoking, and prolonged medication, the oral mucosa in the elderly has a clinical appearance similar to that in younger individuals.[15] Beliefs that the oral mucosa in the elderly, in general, is "thinned, red, dry, and easily friable" or exhibits "delayed wound healing" are no longer tenable. The findings reported at the 1992 Iowa Conference suggest that aging per se produces very little change in human oral mucosa. A recent cross-sectional clinical study supports this viewpoint.[15] Increasing age does not necessarily produce global alteration in human cell systems and processes. For example, well-designed studies reveal a lack of age-related changes in amino acid metabolism in healthy, nonobese, and nondiabetic men,[16] and salivary flow rates in nonmedicated aging individuals also remain unaltered with increasing age.[17] The oral mucosa may be one of those organs that are little affected by age.

The oral cavity, with its mucosal lining and attendant organs (salivary glands, taste buds), is the portal of entry to the gastrointestinal tract. This confers on it a significant role in the preliminary processing of nutrients necessary for the survival of the organism. The minor changes that do occur in the oral mucosa of the elderly might represent an important adaptation phenomenon contributing to survival. The notion that the oral mucosa is immune to age-related changes as such still deserves close scrutiny. Past studies on age-related changes in oral mucosa have not employed the sensitive techniques of molecular biology that are available today. Modern technological tools, combined with in vivo, in vitro, accelerated, and decelerated models,[18,19] are in place for the study of age-related changes in oral mucosa. What remains is to identify the important questions.

Age Changes in the Periodontium

A plethora of studies dating back to the 1960s (reviewed by Johnson et al[20]) have yielded a detailed account of age-related changes in the periodontium. With increasing age, there is an increase in the width of the gingiva,[21] a change that can be attributed to the eruptive movement of teeth rather than to an intrinsic aging phenomenon. Aging also brings an increased prevalence of gingival recession. This finding appears to be largely due to the cumulative environmental effects of vigorous toothbrushing rather than to inflammatory periodontal disease or aging. Tissue culture studies on gingival fibroblasts obtained from donors 12 to 68 years old have revealed a reduction in the rate of cell proliferation, a reduction in the quantity and quality of

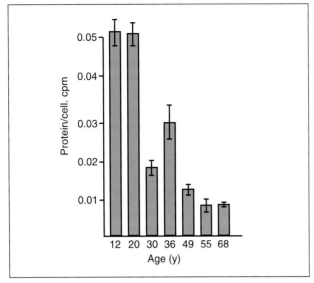

Fig 10-4 Protein production by cultures of fibroblasts from donors of various ages, as assessed by measuring uptake and incorporation of [³H]proline into precipitable material. Cultures were labeled for 24 hours, and the results are expressed as the mean counts from triplicate cultures with the scanning electron microscope. (Reprinted from Johnson et al,[23] with permission from Williams & Wilkins.)

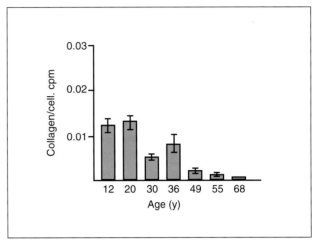

Fig 10-5 Collagen production by cultures of fibroblasts from donors of various ages, as assessed by measuring the incorporation of [³H]proline into precipitable material digested by highly purified collagenase. Cultures were labeled for 24 hours, and the results are expressed as the mean counts from triplicate cultures with the scanning electron microscope. (Reprinted from Johnson et al,[23] with permission from Williams & Wilkins.)

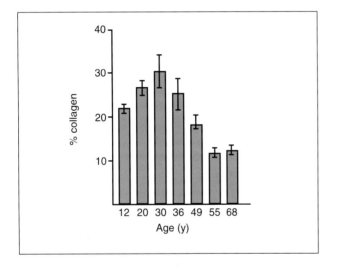

Fig 10-6 The percentage of total protein production committed to collagen production by cultures of fibroblasts from donors of various ages, measured as the percentage of total incorporated counts digested by highly purified collagenase and reported as the mean counts from triplicated cultures with the scanning electron microscope. (Reprinted from Johnson et al,[23] with permission from Williams & Wilkins.)

proteoglycans,[22] and diminished protein and collagen production[23] (Figs 10-4 to 10-6) with increasing donor age. The fibroblasts that make up the gingival connective tissue are heterogeneous with respect to their biochemical traits. It may be that with increasing age, selective pressures favor the predominance of fibroblast subpopulations with the aforementioned phenotypic expression.

Other tissues of the periodontium also exhibit changes with aging. Both in laboratory animals and humans, the thickness of the cementum along the entire root surface increases with age, and this thickening is more pronounced at the apical third of the root.[24] This change may be attributable to occlusal wear and eruption of teeth, though it has also been noted in impacted teeth. Along with an increase in the thickness of cementum in aging, there is increased fibrosis and decreased cellularity of the periodontal ligament.[24,25] There is, however, no consistent agreement with respect to a change in the width of the periodontal ligament with increasing age.[26]

Dental plaque is the major causal factor for inflammatory periodontal disease. The sparse data that exist suggest that there may be some age-associated changes in the bacterial composition of dental plaque.[27,28] In addition, in laboratory animals, the inflammatory response to plaque accumulation tends to be more "acute" (greater number of polymorphonuclear neutrophils [PMNs]) in the younger than in the older animal.[28] While individuals 65 years and older, as a group, exhibit more bone and attachment loss than younger individuals, this clinical finding probably reflects the cumulative effects of plaque-induced insults spanning several decades rather than an increased propensity for disease. In fact, clinical studies have led investigators to conclude that chronologic aging per se does not inevitably lead to attachment loss or decrease in alveolar bone support.[29–31]

Predisposing Factors for Periodontitis

Studies have found that 75% of people over 65 years old suffer from a chronic disease[32] and so may be taking a number of medications that in turn adversely modify host response or resistance to disease. The question arises whether there are factors that place the older person at greater risk for a chronic infection like periodontitis.

Inflammatory-Immune Response

Abundant data underscore the important host defense function of the PMN. It is noteworthy that in circumstances where PMNs exhibit impaired chemotaxis (such as agranulocytosis, cyclic neutropenia, and Chediak-Higashi syndrome), individuals are prone to more severe periodontal disease.[33,34] There are data showing that a general decrease in function occurs in neutrophils taken from healthy older individuals, including decreased superoxide production, chemotaxis, phagocytic activity, cytotoxicity, and lysosomal enzyme activity.[35] It may be that this compromise in PMN function with increasing age, in apparently healthy individuals, is associated with a predisposition to a chronic infection such as periodontitis. This would be difficult to prove, however, because severity of periodontitis in an older individual could simply be explained as the cumulative effect of years of disease activity rather than as a result of a relatively short period of

PMN dysfunction. In addition, other components of the inflammatory-immune system may offset, to some extent, this age-associated compromise in PMN function.

The elderly show an increased incidence of infections, which are often treated with antibiotics. Mandell's[36] data show that erythromycin, chloramphenicol, penicillin G, cephalothin, vancomycin, tetracycline, and rifampin all inhibit PMN chemotaxis. The myeloperoxidase–halide–hydrogen peroxide complex is an important bactericidal system in PMNs. Ampicillin has been shown to depress myeloperoxidase activity. The possible clinical significance of these effects of antibiotics on PMN function vis-à-vis periodontal disease remains to be determined.

The Langerhans cell is regarded as the outermost sentry of the immunosurveillance system. Although there is a decrease in the number of Langerhans cells in the oral mucosa of aged experimental animals,[37] no significant changes in their number have been reported in human oral mucosa with increasing age.[38] There does appear to be a general agreement that a decrease in cell-mediated, as opposed to humoral, immunity is a primary manifestation of aging. This is manifested by a decreased response to foreign antigens and an increased response to self antigens.[39]

While the total number of T cells is not altered with age,[40,41] only one half of these cells respond to mitogens in older individuals.[39] Further, the reduced proliferative capacity in T cells is exhibited principally by the cytotoxic/suppressor (CD8 + ve) subset rather than the helper/inducer subset (CD4 + ve).[42] IL-2 is a crucial factor for T-cell proliferation. The decrease in T-cell proliferative capacity may be the result of decreased secretion of IL-2 by T cells,[43] a reduction in the number of T cells expressing the IL-2 receptor, and/or a reduction in IL-2 receptor density.

A compromise in cell-mediated immunity could have an impact on oral health, since this aspect of the immune system plays an important role in the prevention of viral and fungal infections. It may partly account for the increased prevalence of oral mucosal infections, such as herpes zoster and candidosis, in the elderly. However, an impairment in T-cell function does not appear to be accompanied by an increased prevalence and severity of periodontal disease, either in man or in experimental animals.[44,45] Nevertheless, immune changes among older patients[46] may help explain the clinically significant difference in their periodontal tissue response to plaque accumulation and therapy.[47,48]

Nutrition

A steady and adequate supply of a number of nutrients is required for the important physiologic processes in the periodontal tissues. Cell division requires proteins, folic acid, and zinc; epithelial differentiation requires proteins, iron, ascorbic acid, and zinc; clot formation requires vitamin K; phagocytic activity requires protein, ascorbic acid, and zinc; collagen synthesis requires acsorbic acid, iron, and vitamins A and B complex; and synthesis of interstitial material requires manganese and vitamin A.

Clinically overt nutrition deficiency is very rarely encountered in industrialized societies. However, marginal, subclinical, or secondarily induced nutrition deficiency states may be seen in the United States. One measure of an individual's nutrition status is how best he or she meets the recommended dietary allowances developed by the National Academy of Sciences. Concerted efforts are in progress to more clearly define the recommended dietary allowances (at least of vitamins) for the elderly.[49] One study showed that 5% to 9% of noninstitutionalized elderly people (aged 65 to 85 years) exhibited low serum concentrations of vitamin B_6, vitamin B_{12}, and folate.[50] Still others have reported that noninstitutionalized elderly people are at risk for a deficiency of, or exhibit a compromised nutrition status with respect to, vitamin D, vitamin E (less than 2.5% of the elderly exhibit a deficiency), thiamin (15%), riboflavin (10%), and iron (1% to 6%).[49,51] An age-related decline in calcium absorption has also been reported to occur in the normal nonosteoporotic elderly.[52] The elderly, then, are at risk for a deficiency of a number of nutrients that are essential for the homeostasis of the periodontal tissues.

Low socioeconomic status, chronic alcohol abuse (5% to 10% of the elderly), and gastrointestinal disorders are factors that can affect the nutrition status of the elderly.[32] Another factor, for the polymedicated elderly, is drug-nutrient interactions. A 1980 report[53] indicated that while, at that time, the elderly accounted for 11% of the population, they consumed 22% of all prescription drugs. A significant number of the elderly take more than one drug—in some cases, from four to nine prescribed medications.[54] The antirheumatoid drug, colchicine, may damage intestinal mucosa and thereby impair the absorption of vitamin B_{12}, carotene, and magnesium.[55] By a similar mechanism, corticosteriods may impair zinc, calcium, and potassium metabolism; long-term use of cholestyramine can lead to a subclinical deficiency of vitamins A, D, E, and K. Phenytoin is reported to interfere with the metabolism of vitamin D and folic acid.[55]

Inadequate nutrition is accompanied by an increased susceptibility to infections. Further, there is a synergistic interaction between inadequate nutrition and infections.[56] Invariably, this increased susceptibility to infections has been due to a compromise in host defense mechanisms. In this way, the elderly may be put at risk for infections such as plaque-induced periodontitis.

Management of Periodontitis in the Elderly

Effective and judicious management of periodontal disease in the older patient requires a clear understanding of the many facets of overall health care provision for the elderly. The older periodontal patient comes with a lifetime of physiologic, psychologic, and social "baggage" that must be taken into consideration when planning dental and periodontal treatment that is effective and appropriate for the individual.

Physiologic changes can also affect the manner in which the elderly patient copes with stress or adapts to changes; these changes can influence attitude, endurance, motivation, and expectation of results.[57–60] Age-related sensory changes and loss of mobility or dexterity can hamper adaptation and aggravate stress. As many older individuals have fixed incomes but greater-than-ever out-of-pocket expense for dental care,[61] financial stress may have to be considered along with the patient's medical and psychosocial situation in the formulation of a rational dental treatment plan.[62] Treatment that meets the patient's functional and esthetic demands, even though it is less than the "ideal" therapy, should not be classed as substandard. It may be appropriate given the circumstances, and it may permit the patient to function comfortably for an extended time.

In contrast, some elderly people have significant disposable income for the first time in their lives, and they may desire extensive therapy. It has been suggested that there is an increased demand for cosmetic care among older patients,[63] and studies on the elderly have indicated a significant correlation between self-esteem and perception of oral health.[64,65] Each of these factors is an important consideration in the management of the elderly periodontal patient.

Medication

Older patients have more chronic diseases for which numerous medications may be prescribed[66,67] than do their younger counterparts.[68] Many of these medications may have a potential impact on dental and periodontal conditions, which must be taken into account in managing the problems of these patients. Side effects such as xerostomia may have a devastating effect on the dentition and can occur secondarily to anticholinergic, antihypertensive, antidepressant, or anxiolytic medications. The reduction in salivary buffering and flushing action leads to greater plaque accumulation and an attendant increase in caries incidence, in addition to exacerbation of plaque-induced gingival inflammation and mucosal disturbances. The side effect of prolonged bleeding should be noted in those taking aspirin for cardiac/stroke prophylaxis and those taking nonsteroidal anti-inflammatory preparations, frequently in large doses, for degenerative osteoarthritis or other inflammatory or painful changes associated with aging. These medications should be discontinued, after consultation with the patient's physician, for 7 to 10 days prior to planned dental surgery to ensure adequate hemostasis.

Some medications used in dentistry may be directly contraindicated for elderly patients with certain medical conditions or may conflict with pre-existing drug regimens. For example, the use of vasoconstrictors in patients with cardiovascular disease should be minimized. Also, renal and hepatic degeneration with aging may influence the metabolism (serum levels or duration of action) of drugs used in dental care.[68] In this event, dosages should be adjusted to prevent oversedation or toxic drug levels. The effects of drug interactions, such as the increased theophylline levels seen in patients with concomitant erythromycin administration, should always be considered, especially with the polymedicated older patient.

Gingival Recession

Gingival recession, possibly secondary to periodontal therapy, may have additional significance in the older patient—namely, increased risk for cervical abrasion; dentinal sensitivity; and most important, predisposition to root caries. Although details of root-caries management are not within the scope of this discussion, development of an effective management plan for the older patient who is prone to root caries is an integral component of periodontal care. Owing to increased secondary dentin formation, dentinal sensitivity in the older periodontal patient is much less a problem than gingival recession. It can frequently be treated by conservative methods such as the use of desensitizing toothpastes or fluoride gels, or by office applications of potassium oxylate solutions or fluoride varnish.

Intractable situations may require root-coverage procedures such as gingival grafting or use of unfilled-dentin–bonding resins. Significant unresponsive dentinal sensitivity, as well as a high root-caries rate, may influence the use of periodontal surgical techniques aimed at pocket reduction, since such therapeutic procedures may promote gingival recession. Effective instruction in nonabusive oral hygiene techniques incorporating soft brushes, nonabrasive dentifrices, and gentle yet thorough techniques should be the mainstay in dealing with the older patient with significant recession or cervical abrasion. These concepts may be in conflict with the patient's habitual practices and may require significant instruction

and reinforcement. Unless restoration would contribute to the patient's sense of oral health or facilitate plaque control, a healthy, clean area of dentinal abrasion may not need to be restored in the older patient.

In the treatment of gingival recession in the older patient, control of causal factors such as inflammation and abusive oral hygiene should be addressed first. While areas of recession with minimal gingiva may remain stable for some time, gingival augmentation of teeth that have no keratinized gingiva may stabilize recession or promote more comfortable oral hygiene practices. Absence of gingiva in an area planned for subgingival restoration would also suggest the need for gingival augmentation prior to restoration. Careful documentation of recession can assist in identifying areas of progressive recession, where gentle oral hygiene practices should be reinforced or gingival augmentation performed (see chapter 32).

Individualized Treatment

It is of paramount importance to tailor periodontal treatment to the individual needs of the older patient. The older patient with sensory limitations and diminished dexterity may require additional support, additional aids, or modifications of conventional aids to assist in oral hygiene performance. With respect to oral hygiene aids, it is important to note that many powered toothbrushes may be too heavy and large to be held by some people with arthritis. Individual assessment and the provision of a number of available options will help the patient achieve and maintain an acceptable level of oral hygiene. In elderly people who are physically unable to achieve acceptable levels of oral hygiene, the use of chlorhexidine rinses once or twice daily may improve oral health.

Rates of edentulism are decreasing, and many elderly people are retaining more teeth for longer periods. The more teeth that are retained, the greater the number of teeth that are at risk for periodontal disease. The lack of effective preventive measures has been suggested as the single greatest weakness in programs dealing with periodontal disease in the elderly.[69] Although opinions vary on the therapy level required to control periodontal destruction, it is generally accepted that the plaque-induced chronic periodontitis typically seen in the older patient is less destructive than aggressive forms of periodontitis.

The available data suggest that therapy directed toward improving oral hygiene, along with quality periodontal debridement, may be of significant benefit in periodontal disease control in the older patient. The quality of the debridement, rather than the particular mode of therapy, is of greatest importance. However, in the absence of medical contraindications, open debridement should be employed where closed debridement has yielded an inadequate result or where regenerative techniques are deemed necessary. Resective techniques (pocket elimination) may be employed in the event of a prosthetic need. Site-specific antimicrobial therapy may be used to advantage in controlling inflammation and disease progression in those for whom surgical therapy is medically or otherwise contraindicated, or in localized postsurgical disease progression.

Finally, several studies of osseointegrated implant use showed that implant survival rates were as high in older patients as in younger ones followed for an equal time.[70,71] Another investigation revealed problems with adaptation and muscle control in older implant patients.[71]

Many factors complicate the management of periodontal disease in the older patient. Thus, it is important to bear in mind that the prognosis for tooth retention in the older patient is in general—and especially with therapy—better than that for a younger person with the same degree of disease severity. This is not to say that dramatic episodes of disease progression may not occur in the older periodontal patient. Vigilant periodontal monitoring is as necessary for the elderly as for any other patients. So is aggressive management, consistent with the patient's general physiologic status, when disease activity is observed. The fundamental aspects of all periodontal therapy—those of consistent personal and professional debridement—are the essentials in management of periodontal disease in the elderly. When conscientiously applied, they have been shown to significantly promote increased long-term tooth retention.

Conclusions

Epidemiologists, clinicians, and researchers continue to seek insights into the nature of periodontal diseases in older adults,[72] but substantive progress in our understanding of key issues in this area has been slow. For example, Moxham et al,[73] employing a panel of monoclonal antibodies, showed age-related alterations in the cytoskeletal components of rat periodontal ligament fibroblasts. However, the clinical significance of this finding is not clear. Some interesting data have recently emerged on the potential role of inflammatory mediators in the pathogenesis of experimental gingivitis in the elderly. In their experimental gingivitis study, Fransson et al[74] have reported that the elderly are at risk for more severe gingivitis. The gingival crevicular fluid in these older individuals had higher levels of alpha$_2$-macroglobulin, a molecule that can contribute to gingival redness via an increase in the vascular permeability. In addition, this reported increased risk for gingivitis in the elderly may have a basis in animal and in vitro studies that have shown that compared with young cells, aged gingival and periodontal ligament fibroblasts

produce higher levels of prostaglandin E$_2$ and IL-1β.[75,76] These two inflammatory mediators can potentially influence the severity of inflammation and bone resorption in the elderly. Finally, we are currently witnessing an exponential growth in interest in the association, and possible causal relationships, between periodontal diseases and age-related systemic diseases such as coronary heart disease or aspiration pneumonia; determination of cause-effect relationships, however, will require additional investigations.[77,78]

References

1. US Bureau of the Census. Projections of the population of the US by age, sex, and race: 1988–2000. Washington, DC: US Department of Commerce, 1989.
2. Kligman AM, Lavker RM. Cutaneous aging: The differences between intrinsic aging and photoaging. J Cutan Aging Cosmet Dermatol 1988;1:5–11.
3. Webster GF, Uitto J. Pharmacology of the aging skin. In: Mukhtar H (ed). Pharmacology of the Skin. Boca Raton, FL: CRC Press, 1992:203–212.
4. Grove GL. Age related differences in healing of superficial skin wounds in humans. In: Squier CA, Hill MW (eds). The Effect of Aging in Oral Mucosa and Skin. Boca Raton, FL: CRC Press, 1994:121–127.
5. Alvares O. Effects of aging on oral mucosa and skin—Perspectives and future studies. In: Squier CA, Hill MW (eds). The Effect of Aging in Oral Mucosa and Skin. Boca Raton, FL: CRC Press, 1994:151–155.
6. Hill MW, Karthigasan J. Glucose metabolism and protein synthesis in stratified epithelia of young and old mice. Exp Gerontol 1989;24:331–340.
7. Wertz PW, Karthigasan J, Hill MW. Effects of aging on epithelial metabolism. In: Squier CA, Hill MW (eds). The Effect of Aging in Oral Mucosa and Skin. Boca Raton, FL: CRC Press, 1994: 107–112.
8. Gilchrest B. In vitro studies of aging human epidermis 1975–1900. Rev Biol Res Aging 1990;4:281–289.
9. Yaar M, Gilchrest BA. Cellular and molecular mechanisms of cutaneous aging. J Dermatol Surg Oncol 1990;16:915–922.
10. Lugar TZ, Schwarz T. Evidence for an epidermal cytokine network. J Invest Dermatol 1990;95:1005–1045.
11. Williams DM, Cruchley AT. Structural aspects of aging in oral mucosa. In: Squier CA, Hill MW (eds). The Effect of Aging in Oral Mucosa and Skin. Boca Raton, FL: CRC Press, 1994: 65–74.
12. Hill MW, Squier CA, Preston P. Blood flow in skin and oral mucosa of young and old rats. J Dent Res 1987;66(special issue): 1053.
13. Hill MW. Epithelial proliferation and turnover in oral epithelium and epidermis with age. In: Squier CA, Hill MW (eds). The Effect of Aging in Oral Mucosa and Skin. Boca Raton, FL: CRC Press, 1994:75–83.
14. McIntyre RJ, Jackson M, Shosenburg JW. Dental health status and treatment needs of institutionalized seniors. Ont Dent 1986;63:12–17.
15. Ship JA, Baum BJ. Old age in health and disease: Lesions from the oral cavity. Oral Surg Oral Med Oral Pathol 1993;76:40–44.

16. Finch CE. Gene expression and macromolecular biosynthesis. In: Finch CE (ed). Longevity, Senescence and the Genome. Chicago: University of Chicago Press, 1990.

17. Ship JA, Baum BJ. Is reduced salivary flow rate normal in old people? Lancet 1990;336:1507.

18. Masoro EJ. Use of rodents as models for the study of "normal aging": Conceptual and practical issues. Neurobiol Aging 1991; 12:639–643.

19. Philips PD, Cristfalo VJ. A review of recent research on cellular aging in culture. Rev Biol Res Aging 1987;3:385–415.

20. Johnson BD, Mulligan K, Kiyak AH, Marder M. Aging or disease? Periodontal changes and treatment considerations in the older dental patient. Gerodontology 1989;8:109–118.

21. Ainamo A, Ainamo J, Poikkens R. Continuous widening at the band of attached gingiva from 23 to 65 years of age. J Periodontal Res 1981;16:595–599.

22. Bartold PM, Boyd RR, Page RC. Proteoglycans synthesized by gingiva fibroblasts derived from donors of different ages. J Cell Physiol 1986;126:37–46.

23. Johnson BD, Page RC, Narayanan AS, Pieters HP. Effect of donor's age on protein and collagen synthesis in vitro by human diploid fibroblasts. Lab Invest 1986;55:490–496.

24. Berglundh T, Lindhe J, Sterett JD. Clinical and structural characteristics of periodontal tissues in young and old dogs. J Clin Periodontol 1991;18:616–623.

25. Grant D, Bernick S. The periodontium of aging humans. J Periodontol 1972;43:600–667.

26. Van der Velden U. Effect of age on the periodontium. J Clin Periodontol 1994;11:281–294.

27. Savitt ED, Kent RL. Distribution of *Actinobacillus actinomycetemcomitans* and *Porphyromonas gingivalis* by subject age. J Periodontol 1991;62:490–494.

28. Berglundh T, Lindhe J. Gingivitis in young and old dogs. J Clin Periodontol 1993;20:179–185.

29. Burt B. Periodontitis and aging: Reviewing recent evidence. J Am Dent Assoc 1994;125:273–279.

30. Papapanou PN, Lindhe J, Sterrett JD, Eneroth L. Considerations on the contribution of aging to loss of periodontal tissue support. J Clin Periodontol 1991;18:611–615.

31. Papapanou PN, Lindhe J. Preservation of probing attachment and alveolar bone levels in two random population samples. J Clin Periodontol 1992;19:583–588.

32. Lamy PP. Drug nutrient interactions in the aged. In: Watson RR (ed). Handbook of Nutrition in the Aged. Boca Raton, FL: CRC Press, 1985:249–278.

33. Van Dyke TE, Levine M, Genco RJ. Neutrophil function and oral disease. J Oral Pathol 1985;14:95–120.

34. Page RC, Beatty P, Waldrop TC. Molecular basis for the functional abnormality in neutrophils from patients with generalized prepubertal periodontitis. J Periodontal Res 1987;22:182–183.

35. Lipschitz DA, Udupa KB, Ingelicato SR, Das M. Effect of age on second messenger generation in neutrophils. Blood 1991;78: 1347–1354.

36. Mandell LA. The effects of antibacterial, antiviral and antifungal drugs on the phagocytic, microbicidal and chemotactic functions on human polymorphonuclear leukocyte. In: Eikenberg HV, Hahn H, Opferkuch W (eds). The Influence of Antibiotics on the Host-Parasite Relationship. Berlin: Springer-Verlag, 1982:40–54.

37. Rittman BR, Hill MW, Rittman GA, Mackenzie IC. Age associated changes in Langerhans cell of murine oral epithelium and epidermis. Arch Oral Biol 1987;32:885–889.

38. Crutchley AT, Williams DM, Farthing P, et al. Langerhans cell density in normal human oral mucosa and skin: Relationship to age, smoking and alcohol consumption. J Oral Pathol Med 1994;23:55–59.

39. Weksler ML. Immune senescence in man. In: Febris N (ed). Immunology and Aging. Boston: Martinus Nijhoff, 1982: 165–186.

40. Beregi E, Regius O, Rajczy K. Comparative study of the morphological changes in lymphocytes of elderly individuals and centenarians. Age Ageing 1991;20:55–59.

41. Brill S, Kukulansky T, Tal E, et al. Individual changes in T lymphocyte parameters of old human subjects. Mech Aging Dev 1987;40:71–79.

42. Grossman A, Ledbetter JA, Rabinovitch PS. Reduced proliferation in T lymphocytes in aged humans is predominantly in the CD8+ subset and is unrelated to defects in transmembrane signaling which are predominantly in the CD4+ subset. Exp Cell Res 1989;180:367–382.

43. Barcellini W, Borghi MO, Sguotti C, et al. Heterogeneity of immune responsiveness in healthy, elderly individuals. Clin Immunol Immunopathol 1988;47:142–151.

44. Robertson PB, Mackler BR, Wright TE, Levy BM. Periodontal status of patients with abnormalities of the immune system, II. Observations over a 2-year period. J Periodontol 1980;51: 70–73.

45. Page RC, Schroeder HE. Periodontitis in Man and Other Animals: A Comparative Review. New York: Karger, 1982.

46. Kay MMB, Baker LS. Cell changes associated with declining immune function. In: Cherkin A, Finch CE, Kharasch N, et al (eds). Physiology and Cell Biology of Aging. New York: Raven Press, 1979:27–49.

47. Holm-Pederson P, Agerbaek N, Theilade E. Experimental gingivitis in young and elderly individuals. J Clin Periodontol 1975;2:14–24.

48. Lindhe J, Socransky S, Nyman S, et al. Effect of age on healing following periodontal therapy. J Clin Periodontol 1985;12: 774–787.

49. Russell RM, Suter PM. Vitamin requirements of elderly people: An update. Am J Clin Nutr 1993;58:4–14.

50. Joosten E, Van den Berg A, Riezler R, et al. Metabolic evidence that deficiencies of vitamin B-12 (cobalamin), folate and vitamin B-6 occur commonly in the elderly. Am J Clin Nutr 1993; 58:468–476.

51. Johnson MA, Fischer JG, Bowman BA, Gunter EW. Iron nutriture in elderly individuals. FASEB J 1994;8:609–621.

52. Gallagher JC, Riggs BL, Eisman J, et al. Intestinal calcium absorption and serum vitamin D metabolites in normal subjects and osteoporotic patients: Effect of age and dietary calcium. J Clin Invest 1979;64:729–736.

53. Drug Utilization in Office Practice by Age and Sex of the Patient: National Ambulatory Medical Care Survey. US Dept Health and Human Services, publication 82-1250. Government Printing Office, 1980.

54. Schwartz D. Medication errors made by elderly, chronically ill patients. Am J Public Health 1962;52:2018–2029.

55. Chernoff R. Aging and nutrition. Nutr Today 1987;22:4–10.

56. Gontzea I. Nutrition and Anti-Infectious Defense. New York: Karger, 1974:49–53.

57. Laskin DM. Age: A barrier to oral surgery? Int Dent J 1983;33: 313–316.

58. Davidoff A, Sinkler S, Lee MHM. Dentistry for the Special Patient: The Aged, Chronically Ill and Handicapped. Philadelphia: Saunders, 1972:1–12.

59. Franks AST, Hedegard B. Geriatric Dentistry. Oxford, England: Blackwell Scientific, 1973.

60. Jette AM, Feldman HA, Douglass C. Oral disease and physical disability in community dwelling older persons. J Am Geriatr Soc 1993;41:1102–1108.

61. Dolan TA, Atchison KA. Implications of access, utilization and need for health care by the non-institutionalized and institutionalized elderly on the dental delivery system. J Dent Educ 1993;57:876–887.

62. Ettinger RL. Clinical decision making in the dental treatment of the elderly. Gerodontology 1984;3:157–165.

63. Carlson DS. Orthodontics in an Aging Society, monograph 22, Craniofacial Growth Monograph Series. Ann Arbor, MI: Center for Human Growth, 1989.

64. Kiyak HA. Clinical test: Preventive dentistry for the elderly. Final report submitted to NIDR (Grant No. R23-DE05235), 1980.

65. Kiyak HA, Mulligan K. Studies of the relationship between oral health and physical well being. Gerodontics 1987;3:109–112.

66. Baker KA, Levy SM, Chrischille EA, Kohout FJ. Medications with dental significance: Use in nursing home population. Spec Care Dentist 1991;11:19–25.

67. Picozzi A, Neidle EA. Geriatric pharmacology for the dentist: An overview. Dent Clin North Am 1984;28:581–593.

68. National Center for Health Statistics. Current Estimates from the National Health Interview Survey: US 1981. National Health Survey Series 10 #141. US Dept Health and Human Services, publication 82-1569. Government Printing Office, 1982.

69. Robinson PJ. Periodontal therapy for the aging mouth. Int Dent J 1979;29:220–225.

70. Knodell PA, Nordenran A, Landt H. Titanium implants in the treatment of edentulousness: Influence of patient's age on prognosis. Gerodontics 1988;4:280–284.

71. Jemt T. Implant treatment in the elderly. Int J Prosthodont 1993; 6:456–461.

72. Ellen RP. Periodontal diseases among older adults: What is the issue? Periodontol 2000 1998;16:7–8.

73. Moxham BJ, Webb PP, Benjamin M, Ralph JR. Changes in the cytoskeleton of the cells within the periodontal ligament and dental pulp of the rat first molar tooth during aging. Eur J Oral Sci 1998;106:376–383.

74. Fransson C, Mooney J, Kinane DF, Berglundh T. Differences in the inflammatory response in young and old human subjects during the course of experimental gingivitis. J Clin Periodontol 1999;26:453–460.

75. Okamura H, Yamaguchi M, Abiko Y. Enhancement of lipopolysaccharide-stimulated PGE 2 and IL-1 beta production in gingival fibroblast cells from old rats. Exp Gerontol 1999; 34:379–392.

76. Abiko Y, Shimizu N, Yamaguchi M, et al. Effect of aging on functional changes of periodontal tissue cells. Ann Periodontol 1998;3:350–369.

77. Loesche WJ, Lopatin DE. Interactions between periodontal disease, medical diseases and immunity in the older individual. Periodontol 2000 1998;16:80–105.

78. Slots J. Casual or causal relationship between periodontal infection and non-oral disease? J Dent Res 1998;77:1764–1765.

Genetics and Periodontal Diseases

Kenneth S. Kornman
- Some Patients Are at Greater Risk for Severe Destruction
- Leading Periodontal Disease Concepts
- Modifying Factors
- Genetics Primer
- Determining Genetic Variations Involved in Periodontal Diseases
- Aggressive Periodontitis
- Chronic Periodontitis

Why does a book about periodontics have a chapter on genetics? Although it has been known for many years that bacterial plaque accumulating on the teeth leads to periodontal disease, our understanding of that process has changed dramatically in the past few years. Bacteria cause periodontal disease, but other factors determine how severe that disease will become and how a specific patient responds to therapy. It is still true, however, that periodontal disease will not develop in a perfectly clean mouth.

Approximately 70% of the population has some periodontal disease, most of which is gingivitis. The most common form of periodontitis, chronic periodontitis, is usually not detectable until after age 35, and it affects approximately 30% of adults in the United States and Europe. Most individuals with chronic periodontitis have only one to two affected teeth, with minimal periodontal destruction. Multiple studies, however, have shown that 8% to 13% of adults in the United States, Europe, and much of the world have severe generalized periodontitis. In contrast, a substantial number of adults—approximately 10% of the population—with the same oral hygiene will develop severe generalized destruction of bone and connective tissue attachment. Of perhaps greater concern is that these same individuals appear to respond less predictably to periodontal therapy.

Recently, the clinical severity of periodontal disease was evaluated for 117 sets of adult identical (monozygous) and fraternal (dizygous) twins. It was determined that between 48% and 59% of the clinical severity of disease was explainable by genetic factors.[1] The similarity in disease between monozygous twins could not be explained by smoking or other behavioral factors.

Some Patients Are at Greater Risk for Severe Destruction

As was seen in Fig 1-4, bacteria are still required to initiate the patient's inflammatory response, but other factors modulate or amplify that inflammatory response to change the clinical presentation of disease. Some data suggest that smoking, diabetes, and genetic influences put certain individuals at a high risk for severe periodontitis. The bacterial challenge initiates inflammation in the tissues, and then genetic risk factors and acquired risk factors, such as smoking, amplify the inflammatory response in the tissues and determine the resulting disease progression and severity that is seen clinically. The effective management of periodontal disease therefore requires the control of bacterial plaque and the identification and management of the modifying factors that affect disease severity and response to therapy.

Everyone who does not maintain proper oral hygiene gets periodontal disease, but not everyone gets the same severity of disease. However, because the evidence is very clear that bacteria accumulating on the teeth as dental plaque are essential for the initiation of adult periodontal disease, it was quite reasonable to extend this fact to several concepts that guided prevention and therapy in the past.

Leading Periodontal Disease Concepts

1965 to 1995

Between 1965 and 1995, three popular assumptions guided periodontal treatment:

1. Populations with poor plaque control and limited professional dental care have widespread severe periodontitis.
2. Individuals with poor plaque control for many years have severe generalized periodontitis.
3. The severity of disease depends on the combination of the bacterial challenge (ie, plaque control) and the length of time of exposure to the bacterial challenge.

Given these assumptions, individual patient differences in disease susceptibility were of limited concern; clinicians believed that the clinical variability in disease expression was almost entirely explainable by oral hygiene and time. However, with the improvement of oral hygiene habits in the population and the evolution of the ability to monitor clinical signs of periodontitis, including better ways to measure tissue destruction, clinicians and researchers began to notice that not everyone appeared to be equally susceptible to periodontitis.

A few classic observations demonstrated the apparent variability in host susceptibility to the bacterial challenge. Lindhe and coworkers,[2] in an experimental periodontitis study in dogs, noted that with long-term plaque accumulation and gingivitis development, some of the dogs developed only minimal loss of attachment or none at all. Similarly, in tea plantation workers in Sri Lanka,[3] with no oral hygiene or professional dental care, three distinct patterns of periodontitis were evident, including some individuals who developed only minimal disease (11% of the population) and some who developed severe generalized periodontitis (8% of the population).

For several years, researchers attempted to determine whether the different susceptibilities to destructive periodontitis were the result of specific bacteria or unique host responses to the bacterial challenge. It is now evident that both specific bacteria and unique host responses contribute in the periodontal cases that present real clinical problems.

Today

The following insights have contributed to the concepts of periodontal disease today:

1. Periodontitis requires specific bacteria for the initiation and progression of attachment loss and bone loss.
2. There is a "normal" host response to this bacterial challenge.
3. Although the normal host response is primarily protective, it also causes tissue destruction.
4. Healing and repair are constantly going on in the periodontal tissues.
5. In the majority of individuals with a moderate bacterial challenge, protection and repair dominate destruction, and very little disease is clinically evident prior to age 60.
6. Some patients have "altered" host responses and develop more severe destruction.
7. Altered host responses may result from (a) heavy bacterial challenges overwhelming the protective and repair mechanisms or (b) the presence of disease modifiers that reduce the protective component of the host response or amplify the destructive component. Examples of disease modifiers include smoking, diabetes, and the interleukin 1 (IL-1) genetic variations (see Fig 1-4).

Modifying Factors

The factors that determine severity and response to treatment are often called *disease modifiers*. Disease modifiers, when present in a patient, change the trajectory of the clinical disease expression over time (Fig 11-1), so an individual with a disease modifier is at increased risk for more severe signs and symptoms at any given time in the disease, as compared with an individual without that modifier. Most disease modifiers in a multifactorial chronic disease exhibit an interaction with the major causative factors. This is very different from the way clinicians have been trained to think about risk factors.

The effects of risk factor interaction may be explained by considering the effect of smoking on periodontitis. If the effect of smoking on periodontal disease is independent of the effect of bacterial plaque, the risk for periodontitis due to smoking will be additive to the risk due to

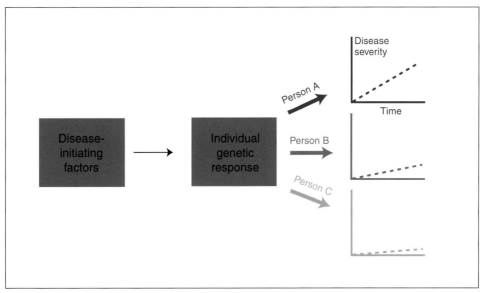

Fig 11-1 Disease trajectories for patients with different disease-modifying factors. The severity of clinical disease over time varies substantially because of the different ways people respond to challenges.

plaque levels. In that situation, the curve for risk of disease due to plaque plus smoking will be parallel to the curve for risk of disease due to plaque alone. This means that even with excellent plaque control, there would be a measurable effect of smoking on periodontitis. It also implies that smoking may be a "cause" of periodontal destruction even when there is no bacterial challenge. Clinical data over many years indicate that smoking is not a direct cause of periodontitis—ie, smoking will not produce periodontitis in a perfectly clean mouth—but it is an amplifier of disease.

Most data indicate that smoking, as well as other risk factors that are nonbacterial, is a disease modifier, not the cause of disease. Disease modifiers in periodontal disease usually interact in some way with the bacterial challenge to produce a risk curve that is not parallel to the curve showing risk without the modifying factor; thus, at higher bacterial levels, the effects of smoking on disease are actually multiplicative, not just additive. Because very few patients maintain perfect bacterial control over long periods of time, the prevention and therapeutic strategies described in this book focus on controlling the bacterial cause of disease and determining and reducing the disease modifiers.

With this new understanding of how disease-modifying factors are involved in the prevention and management of periodontal disease, it is essential to consider the role of inherited risk.

Genetics Primer

Although the Human Genome Project has introduced some genetics terminology to the common language, the current science of genetics was not part of the training of dental practitioners and physicians prior to the mid-1990s. This section is provided as a brief introduction to some of the new information that is important in understanding the genetics of periodontal diseases.

What Is DNA?

To a great extent, the structure and function of the body and all its systems are directed by *proteins*. Proteins are the building blocks of the structure of the body itself. For example, collagen is one of the major structural proteins of gingival connective tissue and bone. Enzymes are proteins that direct all the metabolic activities of the body, such as energy metabolism, replication of cells, protective mechanisms, synthesis of tissues, or breakdown of tissues. For example, cyclooxygenase 2 is an enzyme that makes prostaglandin E_2 (PGE_2), which is prominently involved in inflammation.

Each protein is a series of chemical units, called *amino acids*, and the specific order of amino acids in the protein chain defines the protein's structure and function. The instructions for making a specific protein in the body are

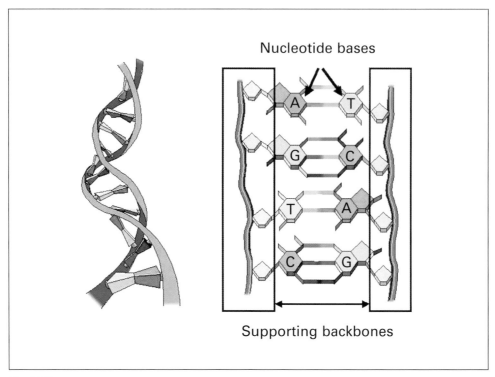

Fig 11-2 Schematic illustrations of DNA structure. (A) Adenine, (T) thymine, (C) cytosine, and (G) guanine.

written on a specific segment of the human genome, and the segment of the genome that carries the instructions for a specific protein is the *gene* for that protein.

All the genes necessary to define the structure and function of the entire body—ie, the *human genome*—are contained in each cell of the body. The genome is made up of *deoxyribonucleic acid (DNA)*. Just before each cell undergoes division, the DNA condenses to form distinct units called *chromosomes*.

Humans have 23 pairs of chromosomes. One chromosome in each cell comes from an individual's mother and one from the father. Twenty-two of these chromosomes are *autosomes* (not linked to transmission of the sex of the individual) and are labeled from 1 to 22. The 23rd chromosome determines the sex of the individual.

The DNA is a twisted ladder, a double helix in which the rungs of the ladder are pairs of compounds, called *nucleotide bases*, attached to two supporting backbones (Fig 11-2). There are four nucleotide bases, and each nucleotide base can physically pair up with only one other specific nucleotide; ie, thymine (T) pairs up only with adenine (A), and cytosine (C) pairs up only with guanine (G). If the ladder were split longitudinally so that each rung was split between the *base pairs*, there would be a specific sequence of nucleotides on each of the two backbones,

eg, A-G-C-T-T- and so on. It is this sequence of nucleotides that provides the instructions to produce a protein. Thus, the nucleotide sequence of a gene defines the sequence of amino acids that will be put together to make a specific protein. Most of the nucleotide sequences in the genome do not produce proteins. Only the sequences that do produce a protein are called genes.

A specific nucleotide base location within a specific gene is called a *genetic locus*, and it may be identified physically by an address that represents the number of nucleotide bases from the point on the gene where the cell starts reading the protein instructions (ie, the *transcription start site*). A locus of +3954 for the IL-1β gene that makes IL-1β refers to the 3,954th base pair of nucleotides past the transcription start site of gene IL-1β. A locus of –511 refers to the 511th base pair *preceding* the transcription start site on gene IL-1β.

Does Everyone Have the Same Genes?

All humans have essentially the same set of genes. Everyone has a gene for IL-1β and a gene for cyclooxygenase 2. However, individuals obviously differ in both physical characteristics and in susceptibility to diseases.

Differences among individuals are both genetically and environmentally determined, of course. Differences due to genetics arise primarily because the same gene may differ in DNA sequence (ie, nucleotide sequence) between two individuals. The different sequences are termed *alleles*. Because there are two copies of each chromosome, there are two copies of each gene. Therefore, at a specific genetic locus, an individual may have one nucleotide sequence (eg, "allele 1") on one chromosome and another sequence (eg, "allele 2") on the other chromosome. The alleles present at a specific locus are called the individual's *genotype*. In the example above, the individual has an allele 1 and an allele 2 at the specific locus in question, so the genotype would be 1.2 (the individual is said to be *heterozygous*). If the genotype is 1.1, the individual is *homozygous* for allele 1 at that locus. In its simplest form, eye color is the result of different alleles in the genes responsible for eye color.

All variations in the DNA sequence are the result of *mutations*. Some mutations occur in cells of the body that do not produce eggs or sperm, so those mutations are not passed on to the children of that individual. Other mutations that do alter sperm and eggs may produce some biologic advantage or disadvantage to the children. If a mutation produces some survival advantage, the number of individuals with that mutation will tend to selectively increase over many years. When a mutation increases to a level involving more than 1% of the population, it is referred to as a *polymorphism*, which merely means that there are multiple forms *(poly + morphic)* of the specific nucleotide sequence that may be found at that genetic locus. Humans have many polymorphisms in their genome that are passed on to their children. Some of the polymorphisms produce no changes at all; some produce differences that are evident, such as eye color; and some produce differences in a biochemical path that is important to protection against a specific microbial pathogen. Some polymorphisms, however, produce biochemical changes that contribute to susceptibility to certain diseases, and that represents the "family history" of disease that is of increasing interest.

Gene Polymorphisms and Differences Among Ethnic Groups

Most population groups were physically isolated and separated for many thousands of years, so local environmental influences could selectively increase polymorphisms in one population and not in others. For example, there is a genetic polymorphism that appears to protect some individuals from becoming infected with the human immunodeficiency virus in spite of repeated exposure. Current data suggest that polymorphism also pro-

tected some individuals against the plague (black death) in the 13th and 14th centuries. In places where the plague was especially bad, people without the protective polymorphism were more likely to die, and the surviving population became enriched for the protective polymorphism. In populations with minimal exposure to the plague, such enrichment for this polymorphism did not occur. Therefore, there is a different distribution of this polymorphism throughout the world.

Most ethnic differences evolved in response to local environmental pressures, such as the black death. Thus, ethnic differences are, to a great extent, a collection of genetic polymorphisms that provided some selective advantage to the individuals in that specific geographic location.

How Are Genotypes Identified?

At a specific locus in a gene, the nucleotide variations that are commonly found in the population may be described by the actual nucleotide sequence or by a number that refers to how commonly that sequence is found in the population; allele 1 is, by standard convention, always listed as the most common variation. However, there are two copies of each chromosome, and therefore two copies of each gene, so the alleles found on each chromosome at a specific locus are listed. For example, say the genotype at locus IL-1α (+4845) = 1.2. That means that at the +4845 position in the IL-1α gene, one chromosome has an allele 1, and the other chromosome has an allele 2.

Single-Gene Disorders versus Multifactorial Diseases

The genetic mechanisms under discussion do not explain the rare severe genetic disorders commonly studied in school, such as Down syndrome. Instead, they relate to common multifactorial diseases that have a genetic or "family history" component, such as coronary artery disease. These common multifactorial genetic conditions involve interactions between the genes and the environment and, often, multiple genes. The clinical effects are usually seen in adulthood with a midlife onset, and an initiating factor must exist. These genetic disorders are not the cause of disease; rather, they are amplifiers of the disease process.

Much of the literature about genetic diseases involves major genetic disorders in which the genetic factor is sufficient by itself to cause the disease. These conditions are usually *single-gene diseases*, such as Tay-Sachs disease and familial hypercholesterolemia, or *chromosome abnormalities* involving an altered number or an altered structure of chromosomes, such as Down syndrome (trisomy 21). In both single-gene diseases and chromosomal abnormalities, the disease is usually clinically evident in childhood or produces some pathology in childhood.

When physicians ask about a family history of coronary artery disease, they are not concerned about unusual single-gene disorders. They are trying to determine if a patient has inherited a genetic variation that subtly modifies how the body develops heart disease.

Most common diseases, such as heart disease and periodontitis, have substantial genetic components, but they behave differently from single-gene or chromosomal disorders. These diseases are called *multifactorial diseases*, because they involve complex interactions among multiple genes and environmental factors. In multifactorial diseases the genetics by themselves are not sufficient to cause the disease; the clinical signs and symptoms are not usually evident until adulthood; and there must be some other disease-initiating factor. The genetic disorders are not the cause of the disease; they are an amplifier of the disease process.

Disease traits that may be measured on a continuous scale, such as hypertension or low bone density, are often multifactorial, because they depend on the cumulative function of multiple genetic and environmental influences. It is likely that periodontal disease in adults is a multifactorial disease. Early-onset forms of periodontitis, such as localized aggressive periodontitis and generalized aggressive periodontitis, may be more consistent with single-gene disorders.

Thus, multifactorial diseases have one or more genetic polymorphisms that interact with other factors to make subtle changes in the disease process. In most cases these differences may not be evident for several years, but in certain situations the differences appear rapidly.

What is Genetic Testing?

Because almost all cells (except platelets) have a copy of the individual's DNA, any cellular material, including a blood sample or a scraping of cells from the inside of the cheek, may be examined for specific genetic factors. There are three main types of genetic testing:

1. *Testing for chromosomal abnormalities, such as trisomy 21.* Chromosomal abnormalities are often evaluated by examining DNA under a microscope for abnormalities in number of chromosomes.
2. *Testing for unusual mutations, such as BRCA1 as a risk for breast cancer.* Because different mutations in the same gene may produce similar problems, the genetic testing requires an analysis of the actual gene sequence of a certain segment of the genome.
3. *Testing for common polymorphisms, such as those being studied for risk of severe periodontal disease.* These single-nucleotide polymorphisms (SNPs) are usually assayed in the laboratory by very simple techniques that analyze the presence of specific nucleotides at one location in the genome. There are several techniques for this type of analysis.

Determining Genetic Variations Involved in Periodontal Diseases

There are undoubtedly thousands of genes involved in the development of the periodontium, in the normal remodeling of bone and connective tissues, and in the inflammatory and immune mechanisms that protect the tissues from external challenges. While these genes are most certainly involved in periodontal disease, they also determine the "normal" biochemical processes involved in the development of the periodontium and the tissue responses that essentially all individuals express. The primary question appears to be which genes have specific variations that determine how rapidly individuals develop signs of disease and how they respond to therapy.

Three major approaches are available to identify the genetic variations of importance to periodontal patients. The first approach involves the use of candidate genes; the second is a genomic scan; and the third involves proteomics.

The first approach to finding which genetic factors are associated with periodontal disease is to use *candidate genes*, which are genes known to influence some key aspect of the biology involved in the disease. Because everyone has the same genes, there are two basic questions relative to the role of genetics in periodontal disease: First, is gene x critical to the development of disease? If so, it may lead to approaches to alter the action of that gene, or the gene itself, to prevent disease. The second, and more likely, question for common diseases is, What genetic variations produce differences in disease among different individuals? This question is studied by looking for variations in the candidate genes. There may be many variations in a specific gene, most of which are of no consequence. Some of these variations are SNPs, which are simply a change in one nucleotide. Some SNPs alter the amount of protein produced by the gene; others alter when the protein is produced (ie, the conditions under which the gene is activated). SNPs in candidate genes are studied for association with disease.

The second approach to studying the genetics of periodontal disease involves *genomic scans*. A genomic scan starts with specific variations in the nucleotide sequence (genetic markers) that are located at intervals along the entire genome. The association of each genetic marker with measures of a disease is determined for groups of families. Using complicated statistical approaches, it is possible to determine whether some of the markers are significantly associated with disease. The markers that are found to be associated with disease define the physical locations in the genome that are more likely than others to influence that disease. Each physical location that is identified on the genomic scan must then be explored for potential genes of importance. In some cases, that location will contain candidate genes that have already been identified. In other cases, the physical location must be extensively analyzed to find new candidate genes that may be involved in the disease. Once candidate genes have been identified, additional association studies must be performed to confirm and better understand the relationship of those candidate genes and disease susceptibility. The role of candidate genes in disease is studied as discussed above.

A third approach to studying the genetics of periodontal disease is *proteomics*, which involves the analysis of those genes that are more activated during disease. By comparing which proteins are expressed in diseased tissue as compared with healthy tissue, one can develop a list of the proteins that are critical to disease, as well as many others that are not. The specific proteins that are thought to be critical to disease development or progression can then be used to find their genes. Most genes that are activated during disease represent normal biologic processes that are switched on by the bacterial challenge. To find genes that lead to more rapid disease destruction or a poor response to therapy, researchers must compare protein levels in tissues from sites with moderate disease and sites with generalized severe disease.

Which Genes Are Important to Periodontal Diseases?

Of course, many different genes are involved in the development of the periodontium and periodontal disease. If one were to study the genes involved in the structure of connective tissue and bone, one would find a specific set of genes. If one were to study the immune response in periodontitis, one would find another set of genes. If one is interested in just the genetic factors that contribute to the rate of disease progression, one should be able to use the extensive research from the past 20 years to focus on genes that are more likely to be involved in regulating disease progression. These are the candidate genes that may be involved in the variations in disease progression seen within the population in the Western world.

Many studies throughout the world have shown that three chemicals in the tissues are consistently associated with more severe disease or actively progressing disease. Those chemicals are IL-1, PGE_2, and the enzymes that de-stroy collagen and bone (matrix metalloproteinases).[4,5] These chemicals are important mediators of the inflammatory response and appear to play a central role in bone loss. IL-1 is a primary regulator of both PGE_2 and matrix metalloproteinases. There are excellent reviews dealing with the roles of PGE_2 and matrix metalloproteinases in periodontitis. This discussion will focus on IL-1, the genetic factors that regulate IL-1 levels, and what that information means to the management of individual patients in clinical practice.

There are many reports associating IL-1 levels in tissue and gingival crevicular fluid with bone loss and more advanced or severe periodontitis.[6–10] For example, recent studies[11] looking at the severity of bone loss compared with gingival crevicular fluid levels of IL-1 show essentially a straight-line relationship—ie, the higher the levels of IL-1 in the crevicular fluid, the more severe the bone loss. Other studies[12] showed that specific blocking of IL-1 and tumor necrosis factor α (TNF-α) in the gingival tissues, without any plaque-control measures, blocked a substantial part of the bone loss in a monkey model of periodontal disease.

The extensive research of the past 20 years may be applied to the identification of candidates for genetic studies. It seems reasonable to consider the following as candidates for genetic influences on periodontal disease differences among individuals: *(1)* IL-1; *(2)* TNF-α; *(3)* PGE_2; *(4)* other cytokines that regulate immunoinflammatory processes—eg, IL-10, IL-4, IL-13, and IL-12; and *(5)* growth factors involved in wound healing and connective tissue and bone metabolism.

In summary, most severe periodontal disease is concentrated in a limited segment of the population. A small set of identifiable risk factors, of which genetics is one, appear to define which patients are most likely to develop severe generalized periodontitis and to have a less predictable response to therapy. Current knowledge of the biology of periodontal diseases suggests a few specific genes that are appropriate starting points—ie, candidates—for a genetic influence in periodontitis.

Evidence for a Genetic Influence on Periodontal Diseases

Evidence for a genetic influence on periodontitis comes from multiple sources, including familial aggregation and formal genetic studies of aggressive forms of periodontitis, the association of periodontitis with certain Mendelian inherited diseases, and twin studies of chronic periodontitis. Several reviews have discussed the specific data supporting a genetic role in periodontal disease.[13–16]

Aggressive Periodontitis

Genetic disorders in which a single gene has a major effect on the clinical expression of the condition are usually evident in childhood or early adulthood. For this reason, it was reasonable to investigate a potential role for genetics in periodontal disease by first focusing on the childhood periodontal diseases, such as localized and generalized aggressive periodontitis (formerly referred to as localized juvenile periodontitis and prepubertal periodontitis). Much of the support for a genetic role in periodontitis has come from studies of aggressive forms of the disease, which have been studied by classic genetic techniques. Considerable evidence suggests some genetic basis for aggressive periodontal disease,[17–18] and the data are consistent with what one would expect if a major part of the genetic effects were due to variations in a single gene.

Commonly occurring chronic diseases tend to aggregate in families. This familial aggregation is often due to many factors that are not inherited, such as common local customs and socioeconomic influences and transmission of bacteria within the family, but familial aggregation of disease is one reflection of a strong genetic influence. Numerous studies have reported familial aggregation for aggressive periodontitis.[17,19–27] This aggregation is certainly consistent with a heritable component of the disease; however, other factors may also affect such a disease pattern.[28,29]

Other studies, using a technique called *segregation analysis*, attempt to determine if the family patterns of disease are consistent with known patterns of how genes are transmitted through families. Although all segregation analyses for aggressive periodontitis have supported the finding that this clinical condition is genetically transmitted, their conclusions differed in terms of the pattern of inheritance. Interpretation of family studies is complicated by difficulties in determining whether an older family member actually had an aggressive form of periodontitis and by the selection of specific genetic patterns for analysis. When these issues were carefully considered, the earlier data appear to support an autosomal dominant inheritance for aggressive periodontitis.[30]

Marazita and coworkers[24] have evaluated more than 100 US families with aggressive periodontitis and found the data to be most consistent with an autosomal dominant transmission for this type of disease. However, autosomal recessive inheritance patterns have been reported for aggressive periodontitis in certain northern European and South American populations. It is likely that the clin-ical cases that are now categorized as aggressive periodontitis (or localized or generalized aggressive periodontitis) may represent multiple biologic patterns influenced by different genes.

Another approach to studying the genetics of disease is *genetic linkage analysis*. This method attempts to determine the chromosomal location of a gene that affects specific observable traits in the disease that is being studied. For a gene that influences the disease to be identified by this technique, it must have a substantial effect on the disease (ie, be a gene of major effect), and its effects must be independent of other genetic and environmental factors.

The use of this technique in cases of aggressive periodontitis has been reviewed.[14,31] Boughman and coworkers[17] reported genetic linkage for a localized type of juvenile periodontitis (LJP, now called localized aggressive periodontitis) in an extended family from the Brandywine population in eastern Maryland. They localized a major gene for LJP to the vicinity of the vitamin D–binding protein on chromosome 4q. Subsequent linkage studies performed for 19 African-American and Caucasian families did not confirm the initial linkage localization reported on chromosome 4.[31] Candidate genes in the chromosome 9q32–33 region include one of the genes for prostaglandin synthesis (cyclooxygenase 1). In addition, certain genetic variations that affect the immune response (eg, human leukocyte antigen genes on chromosome 6) have been associated with aggressive periodontitis.

More recently, a powerful linkage analysis technique called *transmission disequilibrium testing* was used with aggressive periodontitis cases and found a significant role for polymorphisms in the IL-1 genes on chromosome 2q. Diehl and coworkers[32] evaluated 28 African-American and 7 Caucasian families in which at least two family members had aggressive periodontitis. Very careful diagnostic criteria were used to define the cases. Polymorphisms in the genes for IL-1α (IL-1α[–889]) and IL-1β (IL-1β[+3954]) were significantly associated with aggressive periodontitis, with the strongest effect for IL-1β. Of interest was the finding that the genetic variation most commonly found in the population (allele 1) was the variation associated with risk for aggressive periodontitis. This finding is in contrast to the association of the IL-1 gene polymorphisms with severity of chronic periodontitis, in which the less common variation (allele 2) is associated with the greatest risk for disease in adults. Diehl and coworkers concluded that the data are consistent with aggressive periodontitis being a multifactorial disorder in which IL-1 gene polymorphisms are one of the significant influences on disease expression.

Antibody Genetics (Immunoglobulin G2 and Fcγ Receptors)

Other candidate genes have been evaluated primarily in aggressive periodontitis. The serum immunoglobulin response to specific microbes is an important determinant in limiting and controlling microbial infection, and the immunoglobulin (Ig) subclasses (eg, IgG1, IgG2, and IgG3) are known to have somewhat different functional roles in the host defense system. Selective immunoglobulin subclass deficiencies are frequently found in association with recurrent infections in childhood, and IgG2 deficiency in particular has been associated with recurrent infections with encapsulated bacteria such as *Haemophilus influenzae* and *Streptococcus pneumoniae*.[33]

Serum IgG2 levels in localized aggressive periodontitis cases are higher than in generalized aggressive periodontitis cases and age-matched controls with no disease,[34] a finding that supports the concept that a robust serum antibody response is associated with protection in aggressive periodontitis cases.[35]

Most of the bacterial removal in the gingival area that is not the result of mechanical removal is by means of polymorphonuclear neutrophil leukocytes (PMNs), which constantly flood the gingival crevice. Antibody is critical to the efficiency of removing bacteria by specific binding to the bacterial cell and binding to the surface receptors on PMNs. The antibody, therefore, amplifies the effectiveness of PMNs by targeting specific bacteria.

The effectiveness of antibody is primarily a function of how much high-quality antibody is present and how well it binds to the receptors on the PMN. A number of different biologic mechanisms may be involved in variations in antibody levels, including genetics and smoking. One known genetic variation appears to influence the amount of IgG2 antibody[36]: G2m(23), also referred to as G2m(n). Young Caucasians of the low-responder variation (G2m[null]), which is synonymous with G2m("), G2m(–n), and G2m(–23), are predisposed to specific bacterial infections.[37]

Segregation analysis studies[38] of IgG2 levels for members of 123 families with aggressive periodontitis support the association between antibody levels and disease and strongly support a role for both genetic control of IgG2 and antibody genetics in aggressive periodontitis.

The surface receptor that allows the PMN to bind the IgG antibody and then phagocytose the bacterial cell is called the *Fcγ receptor*. Polymorphisms in Fc receptors[39,40] expressed on the surface of phagocytic cells recently have been shown to be important determinants of susceptibility to infection.[41] The FcγRIIa (CD32) receptor recognizes the IgG2 antibody, and therefore neutrophils expressing this receptor are capable of recognizing bacteria that have been bound by IgG2.

The immunoglobulin FcγRII genes are found on chromosome 1, and the FcγRIIa polymorphism has two variations, R131 and H131. The R131 variation binds significantly less antibody than the H131 variation.[42]

Wilson and coworkers[43] have shown that in patients with localized aggressive periodontitis, serum containing IgG2 antibodies is effective in phagocytosing *Actinobacillus actinomycetemcomitans* when employed in conjunction with neutrophils that express Fcγ receptors capable of recognizing this antibody. IgG2 was significantly more effective in mediating phagocytosis of *A actinomycetemcomitans* when used with human neutrophils that were homozygous for the H131 receptor, as compared with neutrophils from individuals homozygous for the R131 receptor. The genetic polymorphism that defines FcγRII, therefore, appears to be a promising marker for susceptibility to localized aggressive periodontitis.

The candidate genes that have been evaluated for influences on aggressive periodontitis are summarized in Table 11-1.

Chronic Periodontitis

Genetics has only recently emerged as a major consideration in chronic periodontitis. One reason is advances in the techniques available to study the disease. Another reason is the improved conceptual understanding of periodontal disease, which has come about primarily through two kinds of observations. First, although bacterial plaque is essential for the initiation and progression of periodontitis, the amount of plaque is not a good predictor of the severity of destruction. Second, studies of identical twins who were separated at birth and raised in different families show that they develop similar levels of periodontitis as adults.

The prevalence of severe generalized periodontitis in a specific country is very consistent throughout the world and is not explainable by oral hygiene levels and access to dental care. In the past, the prevailing view was that periodontitis was ubiquitous in human populations, so there was not much value in looking for factors that determined why individual patients were more or less susceptible to the disease. This is true in some regards; if individuals do not brush their teeth, they will develop gingivitis and some signs of periodontitis. However, researchers now know that in many populations in the world, the prevalence of severe generalized periodontitis actually involves a rather small percentage of the population, so the prevalence of periodontal disease can be described by the following statements: *(1)* Approximately 70% of the population will have some form of periodontal disease, mostly gingivitis; *(2)* approximately 30% of the population will have at least

Table 11-1 Candidate Genes Evaluated for Influence on Aggressive Periodontitis

Candidate gene evaluated	General findings	References
IL-1α and IL-1β	Significant association	Diehl et al[32]
N-formyl peptide receptor*	Significant association	Gwinn et al[44]
Diacylglycerol kinase[†]	Significant association	Hurttia et al[45,46]
Cytokeratin genes	No association with Papillon-Lefèvre syndrome[‡]	Hart et al[47]
Cathepsin C	Significant association with Papillon-Lefèvre syndrome and aggressive periodontitis	Fischer et al[48] Laass et al[49] Hart et al[50–52]
Vitamin D receptor[§]	Significant association	Hennig et al[53]
FcγRIIIb[‖]	Significant association	Kobayashi et al[54]
IL-10[¶]	No association	Kinane[55]
TNF-α[¶]	No association	Kinane[55]

* N-formyl-1-methionyl-1-leucyl-1-phenylalanine (FMLP) is a special peptide produced by microorganisms. The PMN receptors for FMLP are involved in the activation and response to chemotactic stimuli. Gwinn and colleagues[44] sequenced the FMLP genes and found that two single-nucleotide polymorphisms (+329 T→C and +378 C→G) were common in subjects with localized aggressive periodontitis but not in controls or subjects with chronic periodontitis.

† Diacylglycerol kinase[45,46] activity appears to be reduced within the PMN, and this decreased activity seems to contribute to adhesion of the cells. The gene for diacylglycerol kinase has been localized to chromosome 17q22.

‡ Papillon-Lefèvre syndrome involves palmoplantar hyperkeratosis and early loss of teeth. Recent studies show no association with cytokeratin genes.[47] The syndrome has been mapped to chromosome 11q14–21 and appears to involve mutations that result in loss of cathepsin C activity.[48–51,56] Aggressive periodontitis in young children has recently been associated with the same gene.[52]

§ Vitamin D receptor gene polymorphism is associated with localized aggressive periodontitis but not aggressive periodontitis in general.[53]

‖ Antibody genes, such as those that influence IgG levels, and genes for Fcγ receptors influence the quality of binding between IgG and PMNs. FcγRIIIb is one of the genetic variations in receptors for IgG that is found on PMNs.

¶ This study used microsatellite markers in genes for TNF-α and IL-10 and found no association with aggressive periodontitis.[55]

one detectable site of periodontitis; and (3) somewhere between 8% and 15% will have what would be classified as severe periodontitis in multiple areas of the mouth.

Many practitioners noticed that although most of their patients maintained fair to good plaque control, the amount of periodontal destruction varied greatly among patients. One of the most impressive demonstrations of this phenomenon occurred with Löe's studies in Sri Lanka.[3] One population group included workers in tea plantations. They had no routine dental cleaning devices and no professional dental care, so they generally had heavy accumulations of plaque and calculus. Researchers first reported that the tea workers developed severe periodontitis at an early age, but further analysis, surprisingly, identified three distinct groups. One group had severe tooth loss and severe attachment loss at a very early age, with loss of all teeth by age 40 to 45. A second group, despite not brushing their teeth and never seeing a practitioner, had essentially no periodontitis and no tooth loss. The third group had mild to moderate periodontitis, a level of disease much like most populations in the United States today who brush

their teeth regularly and see a practitioner once or twice a year. Of great interest is the number of tea workers in each of the three groups. About 8% to 10% had severe generalized periodontitis, and a comparable number had minimal to no periodontitis. Eighty-one percent of the Sri Lankan individuals had mild to moderate disease, even with minimal oral hygiene.[3] Studies of twins raised together and twins separated at birth found that 30% to 60% of the variability in their periodontal condition as adults, as measured by routine clinical parameters such as gingival bleeding and probing depths, could be explained entirely by genetic factors.[57,58] It is therefore now clear that bacteria cause chronic periodontitis, but other factors, including genetics, are likely to determine the severity of disease. Periodontal disease, therefore, appears to be affected by a range of different host responses to pathogenic bacteria. Certain individuals are at relatively high risk for a more destructive response and, therefore, more severe clinical disease. A few specific risk factors appear to play an important role in determining the severity of chronic periodontitis, and at least part of that risk is controlled by genetics.

Candidate Genes in Chronic Periodontitis

The earlier concepts related to major-gene defects have guided most of the genetic studies on the aggressive forms of periodontitis. Because chronic periodontitis did not seem to fit that concept and was very difficult to study using that concept, little work has been done in this area. One set of genetic factors that regulate IL-1, however, appears to have a significant influence on the severity of chronic periodontitis and the response to treatment.

IL-1 Genotype

Patients who are IL-1 genotype positive have an increased inflammatory response in the presence of bacteria. Some individuals produce higher levels of IL-1 than others. The high producers on one day will also be high producers if examined again at a later date, and high production of IL-1 tends to run in families. It is now known that specific IL-1 gene variations cause high production of IL-1 when that individual is exposed to a bacterial challenge. Approximately 30% of Caucasians have these genetic factors.

In some, but not all, studies, peripheral white blood cells[59–62] incubated in the laboratory with bacterial products from gram-negative bacteria produced significantly more IL-1β if the white blood cells came from a person with a specific variation in the IL-1 genes (genotype positives). Perhaps most important, however, the levels of IL-1 are higher in the periodontal tissues of genotype positives. In a recent study, the IL-1β level was significantly higher in the gingival crevicular fluid of genotype-positive patients than genotype-negative patients.[63] In fact, the greatest difference between genotype-positive and genotype-negative patients was found in sites with minimal pocket depth (less than 4 mm). Sites of mild and moderate disease are the major concern in disease progression, and in patients with these types of sites, those who were genotype positive showed 2.5 to 3 times more IL-1β than did those who were genotype negative. Another study has shown that crevicular fluid levels of IL-1α are higher in patients carrying one of the IL-1 gene variations.[64]

In addition, bleeding on probing is a good clinical indicator of the inflammatory response. In a longitudinal study on the association of bleeding on probing and genotype, Lang and coworkers[65] evaluated more than 320 randomly selected patients in a clinical recall program. Out of 139 nonsmokers, genotype-positive patients were significantly more likely than genotype-negative patients to have an increase in bleeding sites during four maintenance visits. In summary, IL-1 genotype–positive patients have increased IL-1 from the white blood cells, increased IL-1 in the gingival crevicular fluid, and increased bleeding on probing.

Patients who are IL-1 genotype positive have increased bacterial counts and more pathogens associated with active periodontal disease. At the Forsyth Institute in Boston, Socransky and colleagues[66] have studied the role of specific bacteria in periodontal disease for many years. They have identified groups of specific bacteria that are found together in progressive periodontal disease. The bacterial species most commonly associated with progressing periodontal disease have been called the *red* and *orange complexes* (see Fig 5-4).

In recent studies by these researchers, IL-1 genotype–positive patients were found to have higher total numbers of the red and orange complex bacteria than genotype-negative patients.[66] The bacteria in the red and orange complexes depend on tissue products to grow and multiply. One possible explanation for these findings is that the bacteria in the red and orange complexes activate inflammation in the tissues, and then in IL-1 genotype–positive individuals, the exaggerated inflammation and bleeding may provide extra nutrients for growth of the pathogens. This explanation suggests that in IL-1 genotype–positive patients the pieces will be in place for a more chronic persistent infection and resultant inflammation.

Patients who are IL-1 genotype positive are at increased risk for severe periodontal disease. Individuals who are positive for the IL-1 genotype are more likely to have generalized severe periodontitis.[67,68] In a recent study, McDevitt·and collaborators[69] examined 90 subjects with no or minimal smoking history. Multivariate logistic regression models demonstrated that a patient's age, former smoking history, and IL-1 genotype were significantly associated with the severity of periodontal bone loss in adults. For nonsmokers or former light smokers (less than 5 pack-years), IL-1 genotype–positive patients had increased odds of developing moderate to severe periodontal disease of 3.75 (P = .043) to 5.27 (P = .026), depending on ethnicity, compared with IL-1 genotype–negative patients.

Patients who are IL-1 genotype positive are less likely to respond favorably to periodontal therapy. In a study on a periodontal maintenance patient population, McGuire and Nunn[70] examined patients who had been followed for 5 to 14 years after periodontal therapy. The occurrence of tooth loss was evaluated after completion of active periodontal treatment and during the periodontal maintenance phase. The investigators found that only two predictors, IL-1 genotype and heavy smoking (more than 40 pack-years), were significantly related to tooth loss. The IL-1 genotype increased the risk of tooth loss by 2.7, and heavy smoking increased the risk of tooth loss by 2.9. Patients who were genotype positive and also were heavy smokers had an increased risk of tooth loss of 7.7. The clinical parameters traditionally used to assign prognosis were found to be valuable only in IL-1 genotype–negative patients who were nonsmokers.

In another study, predictors of treatment outcomes were evaluated after guided tissue regeneration surgery to regenerate the destroyed periodontal attachment.[71] In 40 patients treated with this surgery, there was no difference in the clinical outcomes after 1 year. Four years after the surgery, although the treated sites remained stable (lost less than 1 mm of clinical attachment) in 73% (19 of 26) of the IL-1 genotype–negative patients, sites were stable in only 21.4% (3 of 14) of the genotype-positive patients.

It is important to emphasize that chronic diseases such as periodontitis involve complex biologic interactions over time. The relationship between IL-1 gene expression and a few single-nucleotide polymorphisms describes only one dimension of the biology. On a clinical level, the actual expression of IL-1 at a specific site in a specific patient undoubtedly involves complex interactions among many local and systemic factors.

Fcγ Receptors on PMNs

The serum Ig response to specific microbes is an important determinant in limiting and controlling microbial infection. Most of the bacterial removal in the gingival area that is not the result of mechanical removal is by means of PMNs, which constantly flood the gingival crevice. Antibody is critical to the efficiency of removing bacteria through specific binding to the bacterial cell and binding to the surface receptors on PMNs. Polymorphisms have been associated with an increased risk for recurrent and more severe disease in Japanese adults[72,73] but not in US Caucasians.[74]

Antibody and PMNs play a critical role in protecting periodontal tissues from bacteria. It is reasonable to assume that subtle variations in antibody binding to PMNs and antibody levels may alter bacterial control.

1. In a Japanese population, the polymorphisms for FcγRIIa and FcγRIIIb receptors showed no difference between controls and individuals with chronic periodontitis, but the FcγRIIIb (NA2) was associated with increased rate of disease recurrence.[72]
2. In FcγRIIIa, one polymorphism, 158V, has greater affinity for antibody than 158F; 158F was significantly overrepresented in adult Japanese individuals with disease recurrences.[74]

HLA-DR Antigens

Genetic differences in major histocompatibility antigens (the HLA system) have long been known to influence response to various immunoinflammatory diseases, including graft rejection and arthritis. This system has been studied relative to risk for aggressive periodontitis and severe chronic periodontitis. Some studies have shown an association between one HLA locus (DR4) and severe chronic periodontitis.[75] This finding is interesting because the same locus is associated with more severe arthritis and is also strongly linked to TNF-α genetic variations.

Summary

Recent studies from multiple groups have clearly shown that genetics are a major determinant of the severity of chronic periodontitis in adults. All of the current information indicates that the role of genetics in complex diseases, such as chronic periodontitis, is as a disease "modifier." In periodontitis, this means that the bacteria must be present for disease initiation and progression, but that modifiers, including smoking, diabetes, and certain genetic variations, alter the body's response to the bacterial challenge. The severity, rate of disease progression, and response to therapy are therefore influenced by the modifiers. It must be emphasized that this type of genetic influence is different from the "single-gene" defects (Tay-Sachs) or chromosome abnormalities (Down syndrome) in which a genetic factor causes the disease.

Extensive work is in progress to define which genetic variations are important in chronic forms of periodontitis. It is likely that a few genetic variations with a high prevalence in the population will be found to influence chronic periodontitis. Currently, the presence of interleukin 1 genetic variations appears to identify individuals who are at increased risk for more severe disease and for a less predictable response to therapy.

References

1. Michalowicz BS, Diehl SR, Gunsolley JC, et al. Evidence of a substantial genetic basis for risk of adult periodontitis. J Periodontol 2000;71:1699–1707.
2. Lindhe J, Hamp SE, Löe H. Plaque induced periodontal disease in beagle dogs: A 4-year clinical, roentgenographical and histometrical study. J Periodontal Res 1975;10:243–255.
3. Löe H, Ånerud A, Boysen H, Morrison E. Natural history of periodontal disease in man: Rapid, moderate and no loss of attachment of Sri Lankan laborers 14–46 years of age. J Clin Periodontol 1986;13:431–440.
4. Page RC, Kornman KS. The pathogenesis of periodontitis. Periodontol 2000 1997;14:112–157.
5. Offenbacher S. Periodontal diseases: Pathogenesis. Ann Periodontol 1996;1:821–878.
6. Liu C-M, Hou L-T, Wong M-Y, Rossomando EF. Relationships between clinical parameters, interleukin-1B and histopathologic findings of gingival tissue in periodontitis patients. Cytokine 1996;8:161–167.

7. Preiss DS, Meyle J. Interleukin-1 beta concentration of gingival crevicular fluid. J Periodontol 1994;65:423–428.

8. Yavuzyilmaz E, Yamalik N, Bulut S, et al. The gingival crevicular fluid interleukin-1 beta and tumour necrosis factor-alpha levels in patients with rapidly progressive periodontitis. Aust Dent J 1995;40:46–49.

9. Salvi GE, Brown CE, Fujihashi K, et al. Inflammatory mediators of the terminal dentition in adult and early onset periodontitis. J Periodontal Res 1998;33:212–225.

10. Stashenko P, Fujiyoshi P, Obernesser MS, et al. Levels of interleukin-1β in tissue from sites of active periodontal disease. J Clin Periodontol 1991;18:548–554.

11. Cavanaugh PF Jr, Meredith MP, Buchanan W, et al. Coordinate production of PGE2 and IL-1β in the gingival crevicular fluid of adults with periodontitis: Its relationship to alveolar bone loss and disruption by twice daily treatment with ketorolac tromethamine oral rinse. J Periodontal Res 1998;33:75–82.

12. Assuma R, Oates T, Cochran D, et al. IL-1 and TNF antagonists inhibit the inflammatory response and bone loss in experimental periodontitis. J Immunol 1998;160:403–409.

13. Hart TC, Kornman KS. Genetic factors in the pathogenesis of periodontitis. Periodontol 2000 1997;14:202–215.

14. Hart TC. Genetic considerations of risk in human periodontal disease. Curr Opin Periodontol 1994:3–11.

15. Hassell TM, Harris EL. Genetic influences in caries and periodontal diseases. Crit Rev Oral Biol Med 1995;6:319–342.

16. Michalowicz BS. Genetic and heritable risk factors in periodontal disease. J Periodontol 1994;65:479–488.

17. Boughman JA, Halloran SL, Roulston D, et al. An autosomal-dominant form of juvenile periodontitis: Its localization to chromosome 4 and linkage to dentinogenesis imperfecta and Gc. J Craniofac Genet Dev Biol 1986;6:341–350.

18. Hart TC. Genetic risk factors for early-onset periodontitis. J Periodontol 1996;67:355–366.

19. Beaty TH, Boughman JA, Yang P, et al. Genetic analysis of juvenile periodontitis in families ascertained through an affected proband. Am J Hum Genet 1987;40:443–452.

20. Benjamin SD, Baer PN. Familial patterns of advanced alveolar bone loss in adolescence (periodontosis). Periodontics 1967;5:82.

21. Boughman JA, Astemborski JA, Suzuki JB. Phenotypic assessment of early onset periodontitis in sibships. J Clin Periodontol 1992;19:233–239.

22. Jorgenson RJ, Levin LS, Hutcherson ST, Salinas CE. Periodontitis in sibs. Oral Surg Oral Med Oral Pathol 1975;39:396–402.

23. Long JC, Nance WE, Waring P, et al. Early onset periodontitis: A comparison and evaluation of two proposed modes of inheritance. Genet Epidemiol 1987;4:13–24.

24. Marazita ML, Burmeister JA, Gunsolley JC, et al. Evidence for autosomal dominant inheritance and race-specific heterogeneity in early-onset periodontitis. J Periodontol 1994;65:623–630.

25. Ohtonen S, Kontturri-Narki L, Markkanen H, Synjanen S. Juvenile periodontitis—a clinical and radiological familial study. J Pedod 1983;8:28–33.

26. Saxen I, Nevalinna HR. Autosomal recessive inheritance of juvenile periodontitis: Test of a hypothesis. Clin Genet 1984;25:332–335.

27. Van Dyke T, Finlay C, Levine AJ. A comparison of several lines of transgenic mice containing the SV40 early genes. Cold Spring Harbor Symposia on Quantitative Biology 1985;50:671–678.

28. Alaluusua S, Asikainen S, Lai C. Intrafamilial transmission of Actinobacillus actinomycetemcomitans. J Periodontol 1991;62:207–210.

29. Petit MDA, van Steenbergen TJM, de Graff J, van der Velden U. Epidemiology and transmission of Porphyromonas gingivalis and Actinobacillus actinomycetemcomitans among children and their family members. J Clin Periodontol 1993;20:641–650.

30. Hart TC, Marazita ML, Schenkein HA, Diehl Sr. Reinterpretation of the evidence of X-linked dominant inheritance of juvenile periodontitis. J Periodontol 1992;63:169–173.

31. Hart TC, Marazita ML, McCanna KM, et al. Re-evaluation of the chromosome 4q candidate region for early onset periodontitis. Hum Genet 1993;91:416–422.

32. Diehl SR, Wang Y, Brooks CN, et al. Linkage disequilibrium of interleukin-1 genetic polymorphisms with early-onset periodontitis. J Periodontol 1999;70:418–430.

33. Bradwell AR. IgG subclasses in childhood infections. Acta Paediatr Sin 1995;36:164–169.

34. Lu H, Wang M, Gunsolley JC, et al. Serum immunoglobulin G subclass concentrations in periodontally healthy and diseased individuals. Infect Immun 1994;62:1677–1682.

35. Gunsolley JC, Burmeister JA, Tew JG, et al. Relationship of serum antibody to attachment level patterns in young adults with juvenile periodontitis or generalized severe periodontitis. J Periodontal Res 1987;58:314–320.

36. Oxelius VA. Serum IgG and IgG subclass contents in different Gm phenotypes. Scand J Immunol 1993;37:149–153.

37. Ambrosino DM, Schiffman G, Gotschlich EC, et al. Correlation between G2m(n) immunoglobulin allotype and human response and susceptibility to polysaccharide encapsulated bacteria. J Clin Invest 1985;75:1935–1942.

38. Marazita ML, Lu H, Cooper ME, et al. Genetic segregation analyses of serum IgG2 levels. Am J Hum Genet 1996;58:1042–1049.

39. Bredius RGM, de Vries CEE, Troelstra A, et al. Phagocytosis of Staphylococcus aureus and Haemophilus influenzae type Bna opsonized with polyclonal human IgG1 and IgG2 antibodies: Functional hFc-gamma-RIIa polymorphism to IgG2. J Immunol 1993;151S:1463–1472.

40. Sanders LA, van de Winkel JG, Rijkers GT, et al. Fcγ receptor IIa (CD32) heterogeneity in patients with recurrent bacterial respiratory tract infections. J Infect Dis 1994;170:854–861.

41. Sanders LA, Feldman RG, Voorhorst-Ogink MM, et al. Human immunoglobulin G (IgG) Fc receptor IIA (CD32) polymorphism and IgG2-mediated bacterial phagocytosis by neutrophils. Infect Immun 1995;63:73–81.

42. Salmon JE, Millard S, Schachter LA, et al. Fc-gamma-RIIA alleles are heritable risk factors for lupus nephritis in African Americans. J Clin Invest 1996;97:1348–1354.

43. Wilson ME, Bronson PM, Hamilton RG. Immunoglobulin G2 antibodies promote neutrophil killing of Actinobacillus actinomycetemcomitans. Infect Immun 1995;63:1070–1075.

44. Gwinn MR, Sharma A, De Nardin E. Single nucleotide polymorphisms of the N-formyl peptide receptor in localized juvenile periodontitis. J Periodontol 1999;70:1194–1201.

45. Hurttia HM, Pelto LM, Leino L. Evidence of an association between functional abnormalities and defective diacylglycerol kinase activity in peripheral blood neutrophils from patients with localized juvenile periodontitis. J Periodontal Res 1997;32:401–407.

46. Hurttia H, Saarinen K, Leino L. Increased adhesion of peripheral blood neutrophils from patients with localized juvenile periodontitis. J Periodontal Res 1998;33:292–297.

47. Hart TC, Stabholz A, Meyle J, et al. Genetic studies of syndromes with severe periodontitis and palmoplantar hyperkeratosis. J Periodontal Res 1997;32:81–89.

48. Fischer J, Blanchet-Bardon C, Prud'homme JF, et al. Mapping of Papillon-Lefevre syndrome to the chromosome 11q14 region. Eur J Hum Genet 1997;5:156–160.

49. Laass MW, Hennies HC, Preis S, et al. Localisation of a gene for Papillon-Lefevre syndrome to chromosome 11q14-q21 by homozygosity mapping. Hum Genet 1997;101:376–382.

50. Hart TC, Pallos D, Bowden DW, et al. Genetic linkage of hereditary gingival fibromatosis to chromosome 2p21. Am J Hum Genet 1998;62:876–883.

51. Hart TC, Hart PS, Bowden DW, et al. Mutations of the cathepsin C gene are responsible for Papillon-Lefevre syndrome. J Med Genet 1999;36:881–887.

52. Hart PS, Zhang Y, Firatli E, et al. Identification of cathepsin C mutations in ethnically diverse Papillon-Lefevre syndrome patients. J Med Genet 2000;37:927–932.

53. Hennig BJ, Parkhill JM, Chapple IL, et al. Association of a vitamin D receptor gene polymorphism with localized early-onset periodontal diseases. J Periodontol 1999;70:1032–1038.

54. Kobayashi T, Sugita N, van der Pol WL. The Fcgamma receptor genotype as a risk factor for generalized early-onset periodontitis in Japanese patients. J Periodontol 2000;71:1425–1432.

55. Kinane D. Blood and lymphoreticular disorders. Periodontol 2000 1999;21:84–93.

56. Toomes C, James J, Wood AJ, et al. Loss-of-function mutations in the cathepsin C gene result in periodontal disease and palmoplantar keratosis. Nat Genet 1999;23:421–424.

57. Michalowicz BS, Aeppli D, Kuba RK, et al. A twin study of genetic variation in proportional radiographic alveolar bone height. J Dent Res 1991;70:1431–1435.

58. Michalowicz BS, Aeppi D, Virag JG, et al. Periodontal findings in adult twins. J Periodontol 1991;62:293–299.

59. Mark LL, Haffajee AD, Socransky SS, et al. Effect of the interleukin-1 genotype on monocyte IL-1beta expression in subjects with adult periodontitis. J Periodontal Res 2000;35:172–177.

60. di Giovine FS, Cork MJ, Crane A, et al. Novel genetic association of an IL-1β gene variation a +3953 with IL-1β protein production and psoriasis. Cytokine 1995;7:606.

61. Pociot F, Molvig J, Wogensen L, et al. A TaqI polymorphism in the human interleukin-1 beta (IL-1 beta) gene correlates with IL-1 beta secretion in vitro. Eur J Clin Invest 1992;22:396–402.

62. Galbraith GM, Hagan C, Steed RB, et al. Cytokine production by oral and peripheral blood neutrophils in adult periodontitis. J Periodontol 1997;68:832–838.

63. Engebretson SP, Lamster IB, Herrera-Abreu M, et al. The influence of interleukin gene polymorphism on expression of interleukin-1beta and tumor necrosis factor-alpha in periodontal tissue and gingival crevicular fluid. J Periodontol 1999;70:567–573.

64. Shirodaria S, Smith J, McKay IJ, et al. Polymorphisms in the IL-1A gene are correlated with levels of interleukin-1alpha protein in gingival crevicular fluid of teeth with severe periodontal disease. J Dent Res 2000;79:1864–1869.

65. Lang NP, Tonetti MS, Suter J, et al. Effect of interleukin-1 gene polymorphisms on gingival inflammation assessed by bleeding on probing in a periodontal maintenance population. J Periodontal Res 2000;35:1027.

66. Socransky SS, Haffajee AD, Smith C, Duff GW. Microbiological parameters associated with IL-1 gene polymorphisms in periodontitis patients. J Clin Periodontol 2000;27:810–818.

67. Kornman KS, Crane A, Wang HY, et al. The interleukin 1 genotype as a severity factor in adult periodontal disease. J Clin Periodontol 1997;24:72–77.

68. Gore EA, Sanders JJ, Pandey JP, et al. Interleukin-1β +3953 allele 2: Association with disease status in adult periodontitis. J Clin Periodontol 1998;25:781–785.

69. McDevitt MJ, Wang HY, Knobelman C, et al. Interleukin-1 genetic association with periodontitis in clinical practice. J Periodontol 2000;71:156–163.

70. McGuire MK, Nunn ME. Prognosis versus actual outcome, IV. The effectiveness of clinical parameters and IL-1 genotype in accurately predicting prognoses and tooth survival. J Periodontol 1999;70:49–56.

71. DeSanctis M, Zuchelli G. Interleukin-1 gene polymorphisms and long-term stability following guided tissue regeneration. J Periodontol 2000;71:606–613.

72. Kobayashi T, Westerdaal NA, Miyazaki A, et al. Relevance of immunoglobulin G Fc receptor polymorphism to recurrence of adult periodontitis in Japanese patients. Infect Immun 1997;65:3556–3560.

73. Sugita N, Kobayashi T, Ando Y, et al. Increased frequency of FcgammaRIIIb-NA1 allele in periodontitis-resistant subjects in an elderly Japanese population. J Dent Res 2001;80:914–918.

74. Colombo AP, Eftimiadi C, Haffajee AD, et al. Serum IgG2 level, Gm(23) allotype and FcgammaRIIa and FcgammaRIIIb receptors in refractory periodontal disease. J Clin Periodontol 1998;25:465–474.

75. Bonfil JJ, Dillier FL, Mercier P, et al. A "case control" study on the role of HLA DR4 in severe periodontitis and rapidly progressive periodontitis: Identification of types and subtypes using molecular biology. J Clin Periodontol 1999;26:77–84.

Tobacco Use and Its Relation to Periodontal Diseases

Mark I. Ryder
- Effect of Tobacco Smoking on the Prevalence and Severity of Periodontal Diseases
- Alterations to Periodontal Treatment Response in Smokers
- Underlying Mechanisms of Tobacco Smoking in Periodontal Diseases
- Cigar Smoking, Pipe Smoking, and Smokeless Tobacco Products
- Applications to Clinical Practice

There is an increasing awareness of the role of tobacco use in the prevalence and severity of periodontal diseases and subsequent tooth loss.[1,2] Cigarette smoking is one of the most important risk factors in the development of a variety of periodontal diseases, including various forms of chronic periodontitis, aggressive periodontitis, and necrotizing periodontal disease.[3–5] More important is the fact that among the major risk factors, cigarette smoking and the use of other tobacco products is perhaps the only *preventable* risk factor for periodontal diseases. In the United States, where in 1997 approximately 25% of the adult population smoked cigarettes,[6] and in other countries where the percentage of smokers may be higher,[7,8] this link between cigarette smoking and periodontal diseases presents a serious public health problem. Although the rates of smoking among adults appear to be gradually declining in the United States and some other countries,[6,7] these rates are rising among young people, women, and certain minorities. In addition, the use of other smoking products, such as cigars and pipes, has increased in recent years. Finally, the use of smokeless tobacco products, particularly among young people, appears to be on the rise.[9] The use of all these types of tobacco products may affect periodontal health.

This chapter focuses on five central questions: *(1)* What evidence supports the role of tobacco smoking in periodontal diseases? *(2)* Can smoking alter the response to periodontal treatment? *(3)* What underlying factors alter the progression of periodontal diseases in smokers? *(4)* What are the effects of other tobacco products such as pipes, cigars, and smokeless tobacco products on periodontal tissues? and *(5)* How can we apply current knowledge of the relationship of tobacco use and periodontal disease to clinical practice and prevention?

Effect of Tobacco Smoking on the Prevalence and Severity of Periodontal Diseases

As early as 1946, a direct relationship was demonstrated between the amount of smoking and the prevalence of necrotizing ulcerative gingivitis (NUG).[10,11] More recently, a similar relationship has been shown between tobacco smoking and the "NUG-like" lesions in individuals infected with human immunodeficiency virus.[12] However, prior to the 1980s, epidemiological studies on the relationship of smoking to other periodontal diseases did not

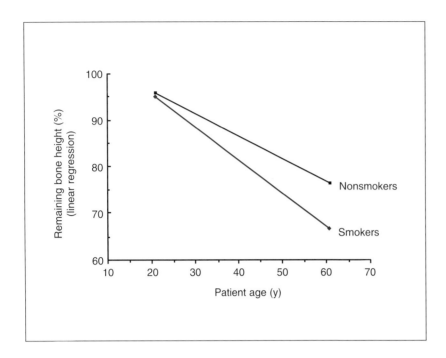

Fig 12-1 In this cross-sectional study of 72 smokers and 163 nonsmokers, both groups had a high standard of oral hygiene (average plaque index, 0.9). However, when bone height was examined for subjects at different ages and a linear regression analysis was performed, older smokers had more bone loss. (Modified from Bergström and Eliasson[29] with permission.)

demonstrate any clear trend. With a few exceptions,[13] these studies were cross-sectional rather than longitudinal. Some of these earlier studies reported either less gingival inflammation or no difference in smokers when compared with nonsmokers.[14,15] However, other studies demonstrated greater gingival inflammation in smokers.[16-18] Some studies demonstrated either an increase[14,17-20] or no difference[21,22] in the amounts of plaque in smokers versus nonsmokers. While some studies reported a direct relationship between smoking and an increase in average pocket depth and bone loss,[14,23-25] other studies reported no clear relationship.[17,18] Some investigators suggested that the difference in attachment loss between smokers and nonsmokers was probably due to poorer home care in smokers, which would result in greater accumulations of plaque.[13,18,20] Thus, the effect of smoking on periodontal diseases would be a secondary effect that could be corrected with plaque-control measures.

However, in the past 15 years, several large cross-sectional and longitudinal studies of chronic periodontitis have been conducted in which plaque accumulation levels were either adjusted between smokers and nonsmokers, or plaque accumulation was kept to a minimum in both smokers and nonsmokers.[13,26-29] In these "plaque-adjusted" studies, smokers demonstrated a greater general periodontal disease severity and had more sites with deeper pockets.[26-28] In addition, alveolar bone loss was greater in smokers than in nonsmokers, especially in older

subjects (Fig 12-1).[29,30] Similar findings have been reported from other large cross-sectional population studies.[31] Furthermore, other studies have investigated the influence of the quantity of tobacco smoke consumed as measured in pack-years[32,33] (packs per day times years smoked) or serum cotinine levels[34] (the serum level of cotinine, a breakdown product of nicotine in tobacco, is related to long-term tobacco consumption). These studies have demonstrated a direct relationship between levels of tobacco consumption and the severity of periodontal disease. From these studies, a general pattern has emerged: smokers have more bone loss, increased numbers of deep pockets, and increased calculus formation, but they have the same or less gingival inflammation and the same levels of plaque accumulation.

In addition to the risk of smoking in chronic periodontitis, smoking is a major risk factor in the development of forms of aggressive periodontitis[35,36] that are characterized by generalized or localized rapid loss of periodontal support in comparatively younger populations. A relatively high proportion of smokers with both chronic and aggressive forms of periodontitis show no discernible improvement when treated by conventional periodontal therapies, and their condition may continue to rapidly deteriorate. Several studies have shown that an unusually high percentage of patients resistant to therapy are smokers (85% to 90%) when compared with the percentage of smokers in the general population.[37,38]

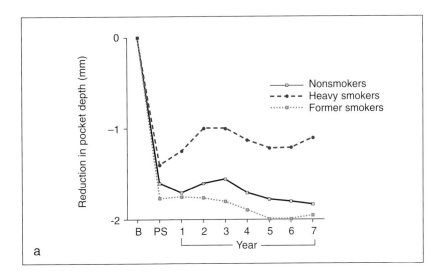

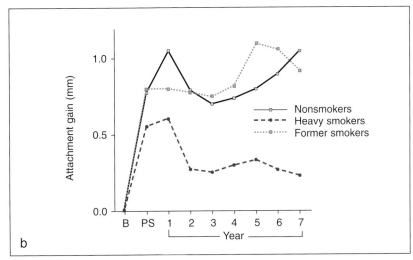

Figs 12-2a and 12-2b A longitudinal study comparing clinical attachment gain in heavy smokers, light smokers (not shown), former smokers, and nonsmokers after initial debridement, flap surgery, and 3- to 6-month maintenance therapy. From the period 10 weeks to 7 years after surgery, there was a significantly greater reduction in pocket depth *(a)* and a significantly greater gain in attachment level *(b)* in nonsmokers compared with smokers. Moreover, when comparing the group of former smokers with the nonsmokers, the reductions in pocket depth and gains in clinical attachment were similar. The results of this study point to the benefits of smoking cessation prior to periodontal therapy. (B) baseline; (PS) postsurgical. (Modified from Kaldahl et al[43] with permission.)

Alterations to Periodontal Treatment Response in Smokers

There seems to be a strong relationship between smoking and periodontal diseases, so one would expect that smokers would require more periodontal treatment. It has been shown that the percentage of patients seen in periodontal practices in the United States and other countries who are smokers is significantly higher than the percentage of smokers in the general population.[22,27] In addition, smokers appear to require more extensive periodontal treatment when a standard treatment needs index is used.[39] Current smokers are far more likely to present with moderate to advanced periodontal disease in US periodontal

practices when compared with former smokers or nonsmokers.[40]

When providing care for the smoking patient, the practitioner should bear in mind that smoking may alter the response to various forms of periodontal therapy. For example, reduction of probing depths following flap surgery procedures has been reported to be significantly less in smokers (Fig 12-2a).[41–43] In addition, gains in clinical attachment (a critical criterion in evaluating the success of periodontal procedures) following flap surgery are significantly less in smokers when compared with nonsmokers (Fig 12-2b).[42–44]

Smoking may also affect other forms of periodontal therapy. For example, in scaling and root planing, the subsequent reductions in bleeding on probing, pocket depths, and periodontal flora are poorer in smokers,[45–47] particularly in anterior areas, where there is more direct contact of the tissues with smoke.[48] In periodontal maintenance patients treated with systemic antibiotics and scaling and root planing, smokers had significantly less reduction in probing depth than did nonsmokers, even when the smokers exhibited good plaque control.[49] Poorer results in smokers have also been observed in both soft tissue and bone graft procedures,[50–53] as well as in guided tissue regeneration procedures in the treatment of bony defects and furcations.[53,54] In addition, smoking may be the most significant risk factor in bone loss around dental implants and in implant failure.[55–57]

However, poorer results of these therapeutic approaches in current smokers can be almost completely avoided with some form of smoking cessation. In both long- and short-term studies involving a variety of surgical and nonsurgical therapies, when smokers quit just prior to therapy, the results were comparable to those seen in nonsmokers (see Figs 12-2a and 12-2b).[43,58]

The use of systemic and local controlled delivery of antimicrobials has become more common in treatment of periodontal diseases. In several studies, smoking has been shown to adversely affect the treatment outcomes of scaling and root planing coupled with systemic metronidazole.[59,60] Smokers also had less pocket reduction when treated with locally delivered tetracycline fibers, minocycline gel, or metronidazole gel.[61] In contrast, no differences in treatment outcomes were observed between smokers and nonsmokers when a controlled delivery system with doxycycline was used.[62]

Underlying Mechanisms of Tobacco Smoking in Periodontal Diseases

Microbiology

One hypothesis regarding the role of tobacco smoking in periodontal disease is that smokers have either greater amounts of plaque accumulation or differences in the types of plaque microbiota compared with nonsmokers. However, most recent studies have shown that there is generally very little difference in the level of plaque accumulation in smokers versus nonsmokers.[27,29,31] Furthermore, as discussed in the first section, in studies where plaque levels were kept at a minimum in both smokers and nonsmokers, alveolar bone loss was greater in smokers.[29] Several studies have shown that smokers seem to have greater accumulations of calculus.[10,11,28,31,63] Calculus may act as a local tissue irritant and/or create a local environment conducive to certain kinds of bacterial colonization and growth. In addition, the periodontal pockets

of smokers are more anaerobic.[64,65] This anaerobic environment may promote the growth of periodontopathic anaerobic gram-negative species in subgingival plaque.

Thus, smoking may create an environment that is more conducive to the colonization and growth of periodontopathic bacteria. However, the relationship between smoking and the prevalence of specific periodontal pathogens remains unclear. While several studies have found no significant differences in the recovery of selected periodontal organisms,[66–68] others have found increased recovery and detection rates of these harmful organisms.[69–72] Some of these differences may be due to the deeper pocket probing depths found in smokers, which could lead to a local anaerobic environment conducive to the growth of these organisms. However, in some studies where the levels of pocket depth and attachment loss have been taken into account,[71] as well as in studies of the microbial flora in periodontal health,[73] significant differences between smokers and nonsmokers were still noted.

Host Response

The effects of smoking on the periodontal bacterial flora remain unresolved, but other investigations have focused on the role of smoking in altering the periodontal host response. Tobacco products could exert effects on the host response both locally at higher concentrations due to direct exposure to cigarette smoke and systematically at lower concentrations due to circulation of tobacco products in the bloodstream, saliva, and so on. In general, two types of changes in the host response due to smoking could lead to increased periodontal destruction: (1) tobacco smoking could impair the normal function of the host response in neutralizing infection and (2) tobacco smoking could overstimulate the host to destroy the surrounding healthy tissue. Cigarette smoking may exert both of these types of effects on the host response.

Several lines of evidence demonstrate the effects of smoking on impairing the normal function of the host response. For example, smokers have decreased amounts of salivary antibodies (immunoglobulin A, or IgA, which is necessary to neutralize bacteria in the mouth)[74] and a decreased serum IgG antibody response to *Prevotella intermedia* and *Fusobacterium nucleatum*.[75] In addition to this general decrease in antibodies, smokers also have decreases in specific subtypes of antibodies that may be of particular importance in dealing with the most potentially harmful periodontal bacteria. These depressed antibodies include IgG2[76–78] and antibodies to more harmful strains of *Porphyromonas gingivalis*.[79] In addition, smokers appear to have fewer helper T lymphocytes, which are necessary in combating a variety of infections.[80,81] One of the most extensively studied cells in the host response is the neutrophil. Whole tobacco smoke has been shown to impair both oral and peripheral (blood) neutrophil chemotaxis and phagocytosis.[82–86] Similar effects have been observed with higher concentrations of individual tobacco components such as nicotine, acrolein, and cyanide.[87,88]

Evidence also supports the role of smoking in overstimulating the host response, resulting in destruction of the surrounding periodontal tissues. For example, while smoke exposure may impair the neutrophils' ability to combat periodontal microorganisms, it also may stimulate the release of oxidative burst products and enzymes that could break down periodontal tissue.[89,90] Smoke may also promote an accumulation of neutrophils in periodontal tissues by stimulating a change in the level of adhesion molecules that control the migration and accumulation of neutrophils and other inflammatory cells in tissue.[91,92] These other inflammatory cells include monocytes and lymphocytes, which secrete potentially destructive inflammatory cytokines such as interleukin 1β (IL-1β) and tumor necrosis factor α (TNF-α). Recent studies have shown that the high concentrations of nicotine in smokeless tobacco product exposure can stimulate IL-β secretion,[93,94] and TNF-α levels are significantly elevated in the gingival crevicular fluid in smokers.[95,96] Furthermore, smokers who carry the genetic marker for elevated IL-1β production have an increased probability of 7.7 of losing teeth and alveolar bone support when compared with nonsmokers without this genetic marker.[97] Finally smoke exposure may lead to the local release of collagenase, elastase, and other enzymes from inflammatory cells, which may break down periodontal tissue. The effect of smoke on various enzymes remains inconclusive, with some studies showing an elevation of elastase levels in crevicular fluid[98] and other studies showing no significant differences in crevicular fluid elastase or collagenase levels.[99,100] Local controlled delivery of doxycycline may protect against some of the damaging effects of tobacco smoke on periodontal tissues by inhibiting some of these enzymes and other products of inflammation.[62]

Direct Effects on Periodontal Tissues

Tobacco products such as nicotine may also affect the progression of periodontal diseases by directly damaging the normal cells of the periodontal tissues. For example, nicotine can be stored in, and released from, periodontal fibroblasts.[101] These nicotine-exposed fibroblasts have an altered morphology[102] and an impaired ability to attach to root surfaces, to proliferate, and to synthesize collagen.[103–106] In addition, nicotine can impregnate the root surface itself.[107] These nicotine effects on both fibroblasts and root surfaces may in turn impair normal wound healing and regeneration.

Another area of investigation into the underlying causes of periodontal diseases in smokers is the possible alteration of gingival blood flow from tobacco smoke. As early as 1946, several investigators proposed that the increased incidence of NUG in smokers may be due to reduced blood flow that could lend to cytotoxic effects and necrosis.[10,11] However, gingival blood flow studies have been inconclusive. An earlier study using a heat diffusion technique to measure blood flow demonstrated a decrease in gingival blood flow in smokers.[108] However, more recent studies using laser Doppler probes to measure blood flow have not found decreased blood flow in smokers.[109,110] Other investigators have hypothesized that cigarette smoke may cause heat damage to periodontal tissues. However, studies have not found a significant difference in the heat delivered to periodontal tissues[111] or an elevation in periodontal pocket temperature[112] in smokers versus nonsmokers.

Cigar Smoking, Pipe Smoking, and Smokeless Tobacco Products

From the preceding discussion of the possible mechanisms of tobacco smoking on periodontal destruction, it is evident that tobacco products can have both local and systemic harmful effects on normal tissues and the host response. This concept is important to keep in mind when discussing the effects of cigar smoking, pipe smoking, and smokeless tobacco use on periodontal diseases. Whereas cigarette smoke is taken into the mouth, airways, and lungs and there is considerable absorption of tobacco products into the bloodstream, these other products are primarily taken into the mouth, with much less uptake into the bloodstream. Therefore, the effects of cigar smoking, pipe smoking, and smokeless tobacco products are primarily due to the acute local exposure of these products in the mouth during use. Nevertheless, cigar and pipe smoking can significantly increase the risk for alveolar bone loss and tooth loss[31,113] (Fig 12-3) and should *not* be considered a safer alternative method of tobacco consumption to prevent periodontal diseases.

Smokeless tobacco products, such as snuff and chewing tobacco, are popular among young adults, participants in certain sports on both the academic and professional levels, and older women in the rural southeastern United States.[114–117] The relationship of smokeless tobacco and oral carcinoma has been well documented.[115] However, the relationship of smokeless tobacco and various forms of periodontal disease is less clear. Recent large-scale studies of athletes who use smokeless tobacco demonstrated a

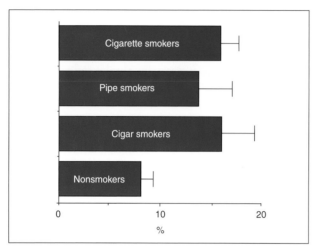

Fig 12-3 A longitudinal study conducted on 690 dentate males over a 23-year period that compared alveolar bone loss among cigarette smokers, cigar smokers, pipe smokers, and nonsmokers. The percentage of sites with bone loss of 40% or more during the 23-year period is greater in cigar smokers (P < .05), cigarette smokers (P < .001), and pipe smokers (P = .17) when compared with nonsmokers. (Modified from Krall et al[113] with permission.)

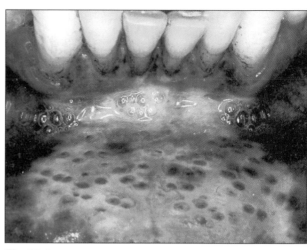

Fig 12-4 Buccal vestibule area from a long-term smokeless tobacco user. Note the marked leukoplakia and gingival recession in the area where the smokeless tobacco product was placed. (Courtesy of Dr John Greenspan.)

significantly higher prevalence of oral leukoplakia.[114,116] These leukoplakia lesions are commonly found in areas of the mouth where smokeless tobacco products are placed (Fig 12-4). Although individual cases of aggressive NUG, gingivitis, gingival recession, and periodontitis have been reported in smokeless tobacco users,[117–121] a relationship between smokeless tobacco use and generalized periodontal conditions has not been clearly demonstrated. In recent studies of smokeless tobacco users, a significant increase in the incidence of localized oral lesions accompanied by localized periodontal attachment loss and gingival recession was reported.[117] These localized areas of attachment loss were especially noted in the mandibular buccal areas. This local attachment loss and recession corresponded to the site of placement of the smokeless tobacco in the adjacent buccal vestibule (see Fig 12-4). As discussed in the previous section, local exposure to high concentrations of tobacco products may play a role in this localized attachment loss.[114,117]

Applications to Clinical Practice

As previously discussed, the severity of periodontal disease appears to be related to the quantity and duration of smoking. It also appears to be greater in current smokers when compared with patients who have quit smoking or never smoked (Fig 12-5).[1,40,122,123] These studies imply that

current smokers may reduce the severity of their periodontitis (but not eliminate their disease) by stopping smoking. To date there have been no published studies on the effectiveness of smoking cessation programs and resolution of periodontal diseases. However, as previously mentioned, several studies have shown that smokers who quit prior to therapy have treatment results as favorable as nonsmokers (see Fig 12-2). From this recent evidence, the American Academy of Periodontology recommends smoking cessation programs as an integral part of periodontal therapy.[124]

Evidence from a large body of epidemiological research has shown that tobacco use is directly related to a variety of medical problems, including pulmonary, cardiovascular, and gastrointestinal diseases.[125] In addition, there is evidence of possible harmful effects of secondhand smoke (tobacco smoke inhaled by nonsmokers in the vicinity of smokers). For example, in the United States it is estimated that 53,000 nonsmokers died from diseases related to inhalation of secondhand smoke in 1991.[126] While these smoking effects may be more life-threatening than periodontal conditions, smokers who are medically healthy may be more likely to visit their dentists than their physicians. Smoking advice—whether it is from a dentist regarding periodontal disease or from a physician regarding pulmonary diseases, cardiovascular diseases, gastrointestinal diseases, or other medical conditions related to smoking—may benefit both the smoking patient and the general population.

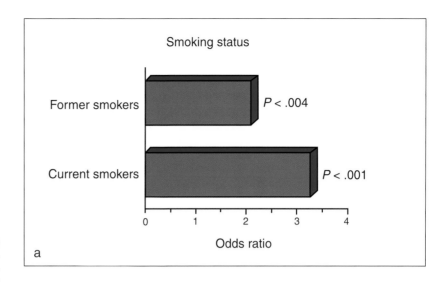

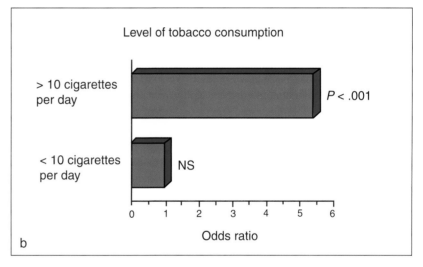

Figs 12-5a and 12-5b A study of 196 smokers and 209 nonsmokers from five general practices (patients with no prior treatment for periodontal disease) and from one periodontal practice (patients with moderate to advanced periodontal disease). These data compare the prevalence of moderate to advanced periodontal disease in the periodontal practice with the relatively periodontally healthy patients in the five general dental practices (as expressed by an age and sex adjusted summary odds ratio). It can be seen that current smokers have a higher prevalence of moderate to severe periodontal disease when compared with former smokers (Fig 12-5a). In addition, heavy smokers (> 10 cigarettes per day) have a higher prevalence of moderate to severe periodontal disease when compared with lighter smokers (< 10 cigarettes per day) (Fig 12-5b). Results of studies like these point to the long-term benefits of smoking cessation and the reduction of the severity of periodontal diseases. (Data from Haber and Kent.[40])

Summary

A large body of evidence testifies to the role of tobacco use in periodontal diseases. At comparable plaque levels, cigarette smokers have greater pocket depths, attachment loss, and bone loss than do nonsmokers or former smokers. In addition, smokers do not respond as well to conventional periodontal therapy. Smoking has been implicated as a major risk factor in the development of a variety of periodontal diseases, including forms of slowly progressing chronic periodontitis and more rapidly progressing aggressive periodontitis. Furthermore, cigarette smoking may play a harmful role in almost all forms of periodontal disease and adversely affect the outcomes of almost all forms of periodontal treatment. Both cigar and pipe smoking also have similar harmful effects on periodontal tissues. Smokeless tobacco products damage periodontal tissues locally at the site at which they are placed in the mouth. Tobacco products may induce or exacerbate various forms of periodontal disease by direct local damage to periodontal tissues and/or by altering the host response. The changes in the host response may impair neutralization of infection and/or give rise to enhanced destruction of healthy periodontal tissues. The severity of periodontal disease appears to be related to the smoking status of the patient. Therefore, in a patient who smokes, cessation of smoking may improve the periodontal status and the outcome of periodontal treatment.

References

1. Haber J, Wattles J, Crowley M, et al. Evidence for cigarette smoking as a major risk factor for periodontitis. J Periodontol 1993;64:16–23.

2. Research, Science and Therapy Committee of the AAP. Position paper: Tobacco use and the periodontal patient. J Periodontol 1999;70:1419–1427.

3. Locker D, Leake JL. Risk indicators and risk markers for periodontal disease experience in older adults living independently in Ontario, Canada. J Dent Res 1992;72:9–17.

4. Grossi SG, Zambon JJ, Ho AW, et al. Assessment of risk for periodontal disease, I. Risk indicators for attachment loss. J Periodontol 1994;65:260–267.

5. Bergström J, Preber H. Tobacco use as a risk factor. J Periodontol 1994;65:545–550.

6. Garfinkel L. Trends in cigarette smoking in the United States. Prev Med 1997;26:447–450.

7. Jha P, Ranson MK, Nguyen SN, Yach D. Estimates of global and regional smoking prevalence in 1995, by age and sex. Am J Public Health 2002;92:1002–1006.

8. Council on Scientific Affairs. The worldwide smoking epidemic: Tobacco trade, use, and control. JAMA 1990;263:3312–3318.

9. Centers for Disease Control and Prevention. Tobacco use among high school students—United States. MMWR Morb Mortal Wkly Rep 1989;40:617–619.

10. Pindborg JJ. Tobacco and gingivitis, I. Statistical examination of the significance of tobacco in the development of ulceromembranous gingivitis and in the formation of calculus. J Dent Res 1947;26:261–264.

11. Pindborg JJ. Tobacco and gingivitis, II. Correlation between consumption of tobacco, ulcero-membranous gingivitis and calculus. J Dent Res 1949;28:460–463.

12. Swango PA, Kleinman DV, Konzelman JL. HIV and periodontal health: A study of military personnel with HIV. J Am Dent Assoc 1991;122:49–54.

13. Ismail II, Burt BA, Eklund SA. Epidemiologic patterns of smoking and periodontal disease in the United States. J Am Dent Assoc 1983;106:617–623.

14. Bergström J, Floderus-Myrhed B. Co-twin control study of the relationship between smoking and some periodontal disease factors. Community Dent Oral Epidemiol 1983;11:113–116.

15. Ludwick W, Massler M. Relation of dental caries experience and gingivitis to cigarette smoking in males 17 to 21 years old. J Dent Res 1952;31:319.

16. Arno A, Waehaug J, Lovda A, Schei O. Incidence of gingivitis as related to sex, occupation, tobacco consumption, toothbrushing and age. Oral Surg 1958;11:587–595.

17. Preber H, Kant T. Effects of tobacco smoking on periodontal tissue of 15-year-old school children. J Periodontal Res 1973;8:278.

18. Preber H, Kant T, Bergstrom J. Cigarette smoking, oral hygiene and periodontal health in Swedish army conscripts. J Clin Periodontol 1980;7:106.

19. Bergström J. Short term investigation on the influence of cigarette smoking upon plaque accumulation. Scand J Dent Res 1981;89:235–238.

20. Sheiham A. Periodontal diseases and oral cleanliness in tobacco smokers. J Periodontol 1971;42:259–263.

21. Macgregor IDM, Edgar WM, Greenwood AR. Effects of cigarette smoking on the rate of plaque formation. J Clin Periodontol 1985;12:35.

22. Preber H, Bergström J. Cigarette smoking in patients referred for periodontal treatment. Scand J Dent Res 1986;94:102–108.

23. Arno A, Schei O, Lovdal A, Waerhaug J. Alveolar bone loss as a function of tobacco consumption. Acta Odontol Scand 1959;17:3–10.

24. Herulf G. On the marginal alveolar ridge in adults. Sven Tandlak Tidskr 1968;3:675–703.

25. Solomon HA, Prior RL, Bross IDJ. Cigarette smoking and periodontal disease. J Am Dent Assoc 1968;77:108.

26. Bergström J, Eliasson S. Noxious effect of cigarette smoking on periodontal health. J Periodontal Res 1987;22:513–517.

27. Bergström J. Cigarette smoking as risk factor in chronic periodontal disease. Community Dent Oral Epidemiol 1989;17:245–247.

28. Linden GJ, Mullally BH. Cigarette smoking and periodontal destruction in young adults. J Periodontol 1994;65:718–728.

29. Bergström J, Eliasson S. Cigarette smoking and alveolar bone height in subjects with high standard of oral hygiene. J Clin Periodontol 1987;14:466–469.

30. Axelsson P, Paulander J, Lindhe J. Relationship between smoking and dental status in 35-, 50-, 65-, and 75-year-old individuals. J Clin Periodontol 1998;25:297–305.

31. Feldman RS, Bravacos JS, Rose CL. Associations between smoking, different tobacco products and periodontal disease indexes. J Periodontol 1983;54:481–488.

32. Grossi SG, Genco RJ, Machtei EE, et al. Assessment of risk for periodontal disease, II. Risk indicators for attachment loss. J Periodontol 1994;65:260–267.

33. Martinez-Canut P, Lorca A, Magan R. Smoking and periodontal disease severity. J Clin Periodontol 1995;22:743–749.

34. Gonzalez YM, DeNardin A, Grossi SG, et al. Serum cotinine levels, smoking and periodontal attachment loss. J Dent Res 1996;75:796–802.

35. Mullally BH, Breen B, Linden GJ. Smoking and patterns of bone loss in early-onset periodontitis. J Periodontol 1999;70:394–401.

36. Schenkein HA, Gunsolley JC, Koertge TE, et al. Smoking and its effects on early-onset periodontitis. J Am Dent Assoc 1992;126:1107–1113.

37. MacFarlane GD, Herzberg MC, Wolff LF, Hardie NA. Refractory periodontitis associated with abnormal polymorphonuclear leukocyte phagocytosis and cigarette smoking. J Periodontol 1992;63:908–913.

38. Bergström J, Blomhof L. Tobacco smoking is a major risk factor associated with refractory periodontal disease [abstract 1530]. J Dent Res 1992;71(special issue):297.

39. Goultschin J, Sgan Cohen HD, Donchin M, et al. Association of smoking with periodontal treatment needs. J Periodontol 1990;61:364–367.

40. Haber J, Kent RL. Cigarette smoking in periodontal practice. J Periodontol 1992;63:100–106.

41. Preber H, Bergström J. Effect of cigarette smoking on periodontal healing following surgical therapy. J Clin Periodontol 1990;17:324–328.

42. Ah MKB, Johnson GK, Kaldahl WB, et al. The effect of smoking on the response to periodontal therapy. J Clin Periodontol 1994;21:91–97.

43. Kaldahl WB, Johnson GK, Patil KD, Kalkwarf KL. Levels of cigarette consumption and response to periodontal therapy. J Periodontol 1996;67:675–681.

44. Boström L, Linder LE, Bergström J. Influence of smoking on the outcome of periodontal surgery: A 5-year follow-up. J Clin Periodontol 1998;25:194–201.

45. Preber H, Bergstrom J. Effect of non-surgical treatment on gingival bleeding in smokers and non-smokers. Acta Odontol Scand 1986;44(2):85–89.

46. Haffajee AD, Cugini MA, Divart S, et al. The effect of SRP on the clinical and microbiological parameters of periodontal diseases. J Clin Periodontol 1997;24:324–334.

47. Renvert S, Dahlen G, Wikström M. The clinical and microbiological effects of non-surgical periodontal therapy in smokers and non-smokers. J Clin Periodontol 1998;25:153–157.

48. Preber H, Bergström J. The effect of nonsurgical treatment on periodontal pockets in smokers and non-smokers. J Clin Periodontol 1986;13:319–323.

49. Kornman K, Newman M, Choi J-I. Smoking effects on clinical and microbial outcomes of periodontal therapy [abstract 641]. J Dent Res 1993;72(special issue):184.

50. Miller PD. Root coverage with the free gingival graft: Factors associated with incomplete coverage. J Periodontol 1987;58:674–681.

51. Harris RJ. The connective tissue with partial thickness double pedicle graft: The results of 100 consecutively-treated defects. J Periodontol 1994;65:448–461.

52. Rosen PS, Marks MH, Reynolds MA. Influence of smoking on long-term clinical results of intrabony defects treated with regenerative therapy. J Periodontol 1996;67:1159–1163.

53. Tonetti MS, Pini-Prato G, Cortellini P. Effect of cigarette smoking on periodontal healing following GTR infrabony defects: A preliminary retrospective study. J Clin Periodontol 1995;22:229–234.

54. Cortellini P, Pini Prato GP, Tonetti MS. Long-term stability of clinical attachment following guided tissue regeneration and conventional therapy. J Clin Peridontol 1996;23:106–111.

55. De Bruyn H, Collaert B. The effect of smoking on early implant failure. Clin Oral Implants Res 1994;5:260–264.

56. Lindquist LW, Carlsson GE, Jemt T. Association between marginal bone loss around osseointegrated mandibular implants and smoking habits: A 10-year follow-up study. J Dent Res 1997;76:1667–1674.

57. Sbordone L, Barone A, Ciaglia RN, et al. Longitudinal study of dental implants in a periodontally compromised population. J Periodontol 1999;70:1322–1329.

58. Grossi SG, Zambon J, Machtei EE, et al. Effects of smoking and smoking cessation on healing after mechanical therapy. J Am Dent Assoc 1997;128:599–607.

59. Palmer RM, Matthews JP, Wilson RF. Non-surgical periodontal treatment with and without adjunctive metronidazole in smokers and non-smokers. J Clin Periodontol 1999;26:158–163.

60. Söder B, Nedlich U, Jin LJ. Longitudinal effect of non-surgical treatment and systemic metronidazole for 1 week in smokers and non-smokers with refractory periodontitis: A 5-year study. J Periodontol 1999;70:761–771.

61. Kinane DF, Radvar M. The effect of smoking on mechanical and antimicrobial periodontal therapy. J Periodontol 1997;68:467–472.

62. Ryder MI, Pons B, Adams D, et al. Effects of smoking on local delivery of controlled-release doxycycline as compared to scaling and root planing. J Clin Periodontol 1999;26:683–691.

63. Bergström J. Tobacco smoking and supragingival dental calculus. J Clin Periodontol 1999;26:541–547.

64. Kenney EB, Saxe SR, Bowles RD. The effect of cigarette smoking on anaerobiosis in the oral cavity. J Periodontol 1975;46:82.

65. Hanioka T, Tanaka M, Takaya K, et al. Pocket oxygen tension in smokers and non-smokers with periodontal disease. J Periodontol 2000;71:550–554.

66. Preber H, Bergström J, Linder LE. Occurrence of periopathogens in smoker and non-smoker patients. J Clin Periodontol 1992;19:667–671.

67. Stoltenberg JL, Osborn JB, Pihlstrom BL, et al. Association between cigarette smoking, bacterial pathogens, and periodontal status. J Periodontol 1993;64:1225–1230.

68. Darby IB, Hodge P, Riggio MP, Kinane DF. Microbial comparison of smoker and non-smoker adult and early-onset periodontitis patients by polymerase chain reaction. J Clin Periodontol 2000;27:417–424.

69. Edwardsson S, Bing M, Axtelius B, et al. The microbiota of periodontal pockets with different depths in therapy-resistant periodontitis. J Clin Periodontol 1999;26:143–152.

70. Kazor C, Taylor WG, Loesche WJ. The prevalence of BANA-hydrolyzing periodontopathic bacteria in smokers. J Clin Periodontol 1999;26:814–821.

71. Zambon JJ, Grossi SG, Machtei AW, et al. Cigarette smoking increases the risk for subgingival infection with periodontal pathogens. J Periodontol 1996;67:1050–1054.

72. Kamma JJ, Nokou M, Baehni PC. Clinical and microbiological characteristics of smokers with early onset periodontitis. J Periodontal Res 1999;34:25–33.

73. Shiloah J, Patters MR, Waring MB. The prevalence of pathogenic periodontal microflora in healthy young adult smokers. J Periodontol 2000;71:562–567.

74. Bennet KR, Read PC. Salivary immunoglobulin A levels in normal subjects, tobacco smokers, and patients with minor aphthous ulceration. Oral Surg Oral Med Oral Pathol 1982;53:461–465.

75. Haber J, Grinnel C, Crowley M, et al. Antibodies to periodontal pathogens in cigarette smokers [abstract 1126]. J Dent Res 1993;71(special issue):244.

76. Quinn SM, Zhang JB, Gunsolley JC, et al. The influence of smoking and race on adult periodontitis and serum IgG2 levels. J Periodontol 1998;69:171–177.

77. Tangada SD, Califano JV, Nakashima K, et al. The effect of smoking on serum IgG2 reactive with *Actinobacillus actinomycetemcomitans* in early-onset periodontitis patients. J Periodontol 1997;68:842–850.

78. Fredriksson MI, Figueredo CMS, Gustafsson A, et al. Effect of periodontitis and smoking on blood leukocytes and acute-phase proteins. J Periodontol 1999;70:1355–1360.

79. Califano JV, Schifferle RE, Gunsolley JC, et al. Antibody reactive with *Porphyromonas gingivalis* serotypes K1-6 in adult and generalized early-onset periodontitis. J Periodontol 1999;70:730–735.

80. Costabel U, Bross KJ, Reuter C, et al. Alterations in immunoregulatory T-cell subsets in cigarette smokers: A phenotypic analysis of bronchoalveolar and blood lymphocytes. Chest 1986;90:39–44.

81. Ginns LC, Goldenheim PD, Miller LG, et al. T-lymphocyte subsets in smoking and lung cancer. Am Rev Respir Dis 1982;126:265–269.

82. Kenney EG, Kraal JH, Saxe SR, Jones J. The effect of cigarette smoke on human oral polymorphonuclear leukocytes. J Periodontal Res 1977;12:227–234.

83. Kraal JH, Chancellor MB, Bridges RB, et al. Variations in the gingival polymorphonuclear leukocyte migration rate in dogs induced chemotactic autologous serum and migration inhibition from tobacco smoke. J Periodontal Res 1977;12:242–249.

84. Lannan S, McLean A, Drost E, et al. Changes in neutrophil morphology and morphometry following exposure to cigarette smoke. Int J Exp Pathol 1992;73:183–191.

85. Ludwig PW, Hoidal JR. Alterations in leukocyte oxidative metabolism in cigarette smokers. Am Rev Respir Dis 1982;126:977–980.

86. Selby C, Drost E, Brown D, et al. Inhibition of neutrophil adherence and movement by acute cigarette smoke exposure. Exp Lung Res 1992;18:813–827.

87. Eichel B, Shahrik HA. Tobacco smoke toxicity: Loss of human oral leukocyte function and fluid cell metabolism. Science 1969;166:1424.

88. Ryder MI. Nicotine effects on neutrophil F-actin formation and calcium release: Implications for tobacco use and pulmonary diseases. Exp Lung Res 1994;20:283–296.

89. Kalra J, Chandhary AK, Prasad K. Increased production of oxygen free radicals in cigarette smokers. Int J Exp Pathol 1991;72:1–7.

90. Ryder MI, Fujitaki R, Johnson G, Huynh W. Alterations of neutrophil oxidative burst by in vitro smoke exposure: Implications for oral and systemic diseases. Ann Periodontol 1998;3:76–87.

91. Ryder MI, Fujitaki R, Lebus S, et al. Alterations of neutrophil L-selectin and CD18 expression by tobacco smoke: Implications for periodontal diseases. J Periodontal Res 1998;33:359–368.

92. Palmer RM, Scott DA, Meekin TN, et al. Potential mechanisms of susceptibility to periodontitis in tobacco studies. J Periodontal Res 1999;34:363–369.

93. Bernzweig E, Payne JB, Reinhardt RA, et al. Nicotine and smokeless tobacco effects on gingival and periodontal blood mononuclear cells. J Clin Periodontol 1998;25:246–252.

94. Johnson GK, Poore TK, Payne JB, Organ CC. Effect of smokeless tobacco extract on human gingival keratinocyte levels of prostaglandin E2 and interleukin-1. J Periodontol 1996;67:116–124.

95. Boström L, Linder LE, Bergström J. Smoking and crevicular fluid levels of IL-6 and TNF-α in periodontal disease. J Clin Periodontol 1999;26;352–357.

96. Boström L, Linder LE, Bergstrom J. Smoking and GCF levels of IL-1β and IL-1ra in periodontal disease. J Clin Periodontol 2000;27:250–255.

97. McGuire MK, Nunn ME. Prognosis versus actual outcome, III. The effectiveness of clinical parameters and IL-1 genotype in accurately predicting prognosis and tooth survival. J Periodontol 1999;79:49–56.

98. Söder B. Neutrophil elastase activity, levels of prostaglandin E2, and matrix metallo-proteinase-8 in refractory periodontitis sites in smokers and non-smokers. Acta Odontol Scand 1999;57:77–82.

99. Persson L, Bergström J, Gustafsson A, Åsman B. Tobacco smoking and gingival neutrophil activity in young adults. J Clin Periodontol 1999;26:9–13.

100. Pauletto NC, Liede K, Nieminen A, et al. Effect of cigarette smoking on oral elastase activity in adult periodontitis patients. J Periodontol 2000;71:58–62.

101. Hanes PJ, Schuster GS, Lubas S. Binding, uptake, and release of nicotine by human gingival fibroblasts. J Periodontol 1991;62:147–152.

102. Raulin L, McPherson J, McQuade M, Hanson B. The effect of nicotine on the attachment of human fibroblasts to glass and human root surfaces in vitro. J Periodontol 1989;59:318–325.

103. Cattaneo V, Cetta G, Rota C, et al. Volatile components of cigarette smoke: Effect of acrolein and acetaldehyde on human gingival fibroblasts in vitro. J Periodontol 2000;71:425–432.

104. Checchi L, Ciapetti G, Monaco G, Ori G. The effects of nicotine and age on replication and viability of human gingival fibroblasts in vitro. J Clin Periodontol 1999;26:636–642.

105. Giannopoulou C, Geinoz A, Cimasoni G. Effects of nicotine on periodontal ligament fibroblasts in vitro. J Clin Periodontol 1999;26:49–55.

106. James JJ, Sayers NM, Drucker DB, Hull PS. Effects of tobacco products on the attachment and growth of periodontal ligament fibroblasts. J Periodontol 1999;70:518–525.

107. Cuff MJ, McQuade MJ, Scheidt MJ, et al. The presence of nicotine on root surfaces of periodontally diseased teeth in smokers. J Periodontol 1989;60:564–569.

108. Clarke NG, Shephard BC, Hirsch RS. The effects of intraarterial epinephrine and nicotine on gingival circulation. Oral Surg Oral Med Oral Pathol 1981;52:577–582.

109. Baab DA, Oberg PA. The effect of cigarette smoking on gingival flow in humans. J Clin Periodontol 1987;14:418–424.

110. Meekin TN, Wilson RF, Scott DA, et al. Laser Doppler flowmeter measurement of relative gingival and forehead skin blood flow in light and heavy smokers during and after smoking. J Clin Periodontol 2000;27:236–242.

111. Bastian RJ. The effects of tobacco smoking on periodontal tissues. Periodontol Abstr 1979;27:120–125.

112. Trikilis N, Rawlinson A, Walsh TF. Periodontal probing depth and subgingival temperature in smokers and non-smokers. J Clin Periodontol 1999;26:38–43.

113. Krall EA, Garvey AJ, Garcia RI. Alveolar bone loss and tooth loss in male cigar and pipe smokers. J Am Dent Assoc 1999;130:57–64.

114. Ernster V, Grady DG, Greene JC, et al. Smokeless tobacco use and health effects among baseball players. JAMA 1990;264:218–224.

115. Wray A, McGuirt F. Smokeless tobacco usage associated with oral carcinoma. Arch Otolaryngol Head Neck Surg 1993;119:929–933.

116. Creath CJ, Cutter G, Bradley DH, Wright, JT. Oral leukoplakia and adolescent smokeless tobacco use. Oral Surg Oral Med Oral Pathol 1991;72:35–41.

117. Robertson PB, Walsh M, Greene J, et al. Periodontal effects associated with the use of smokeless tobacco. J Periodontol 1990;61:438–443.

118. Hoge HW, Kirkham DB. Clinical management and soft tissue reconstruction of periodontal damage resulting from habitual use of snuff. J Am Dent Assoc 1983;107:744–745.

119. Offenbacher S, Weathers DR. Effects of smokeless tobacco on the periodontal, mucosal and caries status of adolescent males. J Oral Pathol 1985;14:169.

120. Christen AG, Armstrong WR, McDaniel RK. Intraoral leukoplakia, abrasion, periodontal breakdown and tooth loss in a snuff dipper. J Am Dent Assoc 1979;98:584.

121. Cullen JW, Blot JS, Henninfield J, et al. Health consequences of using smokeless tobacco: Summary of the Advisory Committee's Report to the Surgeon General. Public Health Rep 1986;101:355.

122. Krall EA, Dawson-Hughes B, Garvey AJ, Garcia RI. Smoking, smoking cessation and tooth loss. J Dent Res 1997;76:1653–1659.

123. Bergström J, Eliasson S, Dock J. Exposure to tobacco smoking and periodontal health. J Clin Periodontol 2000;27:61–68.

124. American Academy of Periodontology. Parameters of care. J Periodontol 2000;71(5 suppl):i–ii, 847–883.

125. Smoking and Health Report of the Surgeon General. Washington, DC: US Dept Health, Education and Welfare, 1979:5–7.

126. Glantz SA, Parmley WW. Passive smoking and heart disease: Epidemiology, physiology and biochemistry. Circulation 1991;83:1–12.

CHAPTER 13

Endocrine Disorders

Terry D. Rees
- Hyperparathyroidism
- Alterations in Sex Hormones

William W. Hallmon
- Diabetes Mellitus

Endocrine glands secrete hormones that are integrally involved in the regulation of cell metabolism and the maintenance of physiologic homeostasis. The pituitary gland is a three-lobed structure resting in the sella turcica at the base of the brain. Hormonal secretions from the anterior lobe of the pituitary gland exert profound effects on several other hormone-producing organs, such as the adrenal cortex, thyroid gland, and sex hormone organs. In addition, the pituitary gland secretes somatotropins, which markedly affect all animal growth and development. The pituitary is controlled by the hypothalamus, and its function is mediated by a complex feedback mechanism via the hypothalamus–pituitary–adrenal cortex axis. Thyroid hormones help to control the basic metabolic rate of the body and influence bone metabolism, while the adrenal cortex produces gonadotrophic hormones, mineralocorticoids, and glucocorticoids. In a broad sense, endocrine abnormalities of any kind may adversely affect periodontal tissues either directly or secondarily by contributing to neutrophil dysfunction or by altering wound healing.[1]

Endocrine dysfunctions, such as hyperparathyroidism and diabetes mellitus, are associated with an increased susceptibility to periodontitis or to accelerated destruction in coexistent periodontal diseases. Additionally, physiologic fluctuations of sex hormones during various life stages may exert direct effects on the tissues of the periodontium, perhaps altering patient response to plaque-induced periodontal inflammation.[1,2]

Hyperparathyroidism

The role of parathyroid hormone in helping control calcium metabolism is also discussed in chapter 14. Calcium metabolism involves a complex interaction among vitamin D; calcitonin; parathormone; and calcium intake, absorption, and excretion.[1]

Primary hyperparathyroidism most often occurs as the result of a benign adenoma or a malignancy of the parathyroid gland leading to excessive secretion of parathormone. This hormonal excess mobilizes calcium in bone and releases it into serum, leading to osteoporosis. The affected bone is often replaced by fibrous tissue (osteitis fibrosa cystica). Jaw radiographs may reveal multilocular, radiolucent lesions (the brown tumor of hyperparathyroidism); loss of the lamina dura; and a ground-glass appearance of the alveolar bone, suggesting demineralization. Demineralized alveolar bone may be destroyed more rapidly in the presence of periodontitis.[3,4]

Secondary hyperparathyroidism occurs when renal disease results in excessive excretion of calcium in urine and retention of serum phosphorus. This initiates a reactive parathyroid hyperactivity in an effort to sustain adequate serum calcium levels. Any oral manifestations are indistinguishable from those of primary hyperparathyroidism. Treatment is directed toward elimination of the underlying factors with a resultant return of normal radiographic appearance of the jaws.[1,2]

Alterations in Sex Hormones

An enhanced response to bacterial plaque and increased susceptibility to gingivitis in relation to pregnancy was recognized more than 100 years ago, long before gonadotrophic sex steroid hormones were identified.[5,6] Today it is generally recognized that the body content of sex hormones fluctuates markedly during various periods of life, especially in women, and there is some evidence that these variations, although physiologic, may have an adverse effect on the gingival response to bacterial plaque. The possible relationships between periodontal diseases and puberty, menstruation, pregnancy, oral contraceptives, and menopause are discussed in this section.

Puberty

Peripubertal children have been reported to have a relatively high incidence of gingivitis, although the condition is usually not associated with loss of attachment or bone.[7–11] The severity of gingival inflammation is believed to coincide with increases in circulating sex hormones associated with puberty and its immediate aftermath.[9–12] These changes do not cause gingivitis, but they may lead to altered capillary permeability and increased fluid accumulation in the gingival tissues,[13–17] resulting in an edematous, hemorrhagic, hyperplastic gingivitis in the presence of dental plaque. This inflammatory gingivitis is believed to be transient as the body accommodates to the ongoing presence of the sex hormones. Pubertal gingivitis occurs equally often in girls and boys.[11,12] An increase in circulating androgens (male sex hormones) has been demonstrated during puberty in boys, and gingival hyperplastic enlargement has been reported in patients treated with androgenic sex hormones.[18] There is also some evidence that androgens may affect gingival tissue by suppressing cellular immunity.[19]

Some investigators dispute the occurrence of a hormonally mediated gingival response in puberty. Instead, they conclude that inadequate oral hygiene is a greater contributor to gingivitis among young teenagers than is the stage of sexual maturation.[20,21] A marked increase in periodontopathogenic microorganisms occurs in the dental plaque of children and adolescents after puberty.[22–24] This finding and other evidence suggest that sex hormones may alter the microbial environment of dental plaque and offer a nutrient source for anaerobic microorganisms such as *Prevotella intermedia* and *Bacteroides, Eikenella,* and *Capnocytophaga* species, all of which are potential periodontopathogens.[25–28]

Menstruation

The normal menstrual cycle is associated with fluctuations in the female sex hormones estrogen, progesterone, and chorionic gonadotropins. During ovulation, estrogen and progesterone levels are high, and there is an increase in gingival crevicular fluid exudate in humans and other animals, especially if gingivitis is already present.[29–32] Changes during the menstrual cycle, however, did not alter tooth mobility among 31 females studied.[33] Fluctuations in gingival crevicular fluid flow at various stages of the menstrual cycle have been reported in women who had poor oral hygiene, but no fluctuations were found among women with good oral hygiene and good gingival health.[30] To summarize, available evidence suggests that the normal menstrual cycle has little effect on gingival health, although gingival crevicular exudation may peak during ovulation and may increase slightly at various points in the cycle among women with preexistent gingivitis.[29–33]

Pregnancy

Gingival changes associated with pregnancy have been observed for many years, usually manifesting as an increased incidence or severity of gingivitis. Gingival enlargement and formation of pyogenic granulomas may occur in association with the presence of local irritants.[1,34] Clinical changes include a fiery red, edematous, easily bleeding, hyperplastic gingivitis that is often most pronounced in the anterior gingiva.[2] Severity of the gingival inflammation is exacerbated by inadequate oral hygiene. There is some evidence that gingival changes occur in all pregnant women.[6,17,35] Gingival inflammation increases in pregnant women in the presence of small amounts of plaque,[36–40] but in most instances the clinical changes occur only in tissues with preexistent gingivitis, while healthy gingiva remains free of clinical inflammation as long as effective plaque control is maintained.[17,30,41,42] Increased probing depth and tooth mobility—perhaps due to the protective decrease in immune responsiveness associated with the fetus in the womb—have also been described.[43,44]

Increased signs of gingival inflammation appear after the second month of gestation or later and peak during the eighth month. Following this, the inflammatory response stabilizes and subsequently gradually diminishes following parturition.[45] These changes most closely correlate with progesterone levels during these time periods.[17,46,47]

Gingival tissue contains both estrogen and progesterone receptors.[48] Progesterone, however, appears to exert the most marked effect on the gingival microvasculature, altering capillary permeability and inducing increased crevicular fluid flow.[6,49] Tissue metabolism also may be altered, and some evidence suggests that the cellular immune response is diminished during pregnancy.[14,50,51] This may partially explain the increase in gingival inflammation sometimes reported despite low levels of plaque formation.[52]

Severity of gingival inflammation in pregnancy may also be influenced by the development of an anaerobic crevicular microbial flora. This microbial shift appears to occur because estrogen and progesterone provide essential growth factors for periodontopathogens such as *P intermedia*, although not all studies confirm this association.[27,53]

Oral Contraceptives

Oral contraceptives contain synthetic progesterone and estrogen and create a physiologic state in women that has been described as mimicking pregnancy.[54] Although the commercially available contraceptive preparations vary significantly in content of the two hormonal groups, a possible relationship between oral contraceptives and hyperemic gingivitis was suspected soon after the drugs became available. Several early studies found gingivitis and gingival enlargement to be more common in women taking oral contraceptives,[55–62] and animal studies supported these findings.[63] Some studies indicated that gingival inflammation increased in direct relationship to the duration of oral contraceptive use.[55,64,65] Others, however, suggested that oral contraceptive use was associated with an initial surge of gingival inflammation and exudation but that later the tendency for gingival changes subsided to a level approximating that in early pregnancy.[54,56] Kalkwarf found higher levels of gingival inflammation among women using various oral contraceptives, but he was unable to correlate the degree of inflammation with oral debris levels or with the duration of use of the drug.[62] The incidence of alveolar osteitis following tooth extraction has also been reported to be higher in women using oral contraceptives.[66]

The quantity of synthetic hormones contained in most oral contraceptives has decreased in recent years. Thus, current oral contraceptive agents may no longer affect the gingiva to the same degree as previously reported, and basic studies should probably be repeated.

Reduced effectiveness of oral contraceptives potentially leading to breakthrough pregnancy has been reported when certain drugs are taken simultaneously with oral contraceptives. These drugs include antibiotics such as rifampin, ampicillin and other penicillins, and tetracyclines; antihistamines; anticonvulsants; and some analgesics.[65,67,68] Although this adverse effect is probably highly unlikely, the prudent practitioner should advise patients to use additional means of birth control when such drugs are being prescribed.

Menopause

Menopause is associated with the loss of ovarian function and the ability of women to reproduce. It usually occurs between the ages of 45 and 55, but a surgically complete hysterectomy can induce artificial menopause at any age. Some women undergoing the climacteric may experience transient or prolonged somatic disorders such as flushing, sweating, headaches, burning sensations in the oral cavity, and altered taste sensations.[1] For many years a menopausal or desquamative gingivitis has occasionally been described among postmenopausal women.[69] The condition is similar histologically to the atrophic vaginitis that is sometimes experienced by the same group. Available evidence, however, suggests that atrophic gingivitis found in this age group is more likely to be a feature of a mucocutaneous disorder, such as erosive lichen planus or mucous membrane pemphigoid. The concept of a hormonally induced desquamative gingivitis cannot be totally ruled out, however. This topic has been reviewed in detail by Mariotti.[64]

Diabetes Mellitus

Diabetes mellitus is a diverse, genetically associated endocrine disorder characterized by glucose intolerance.[70] A cardinal sign of this disease is an increased blood glucose level, which may be the result of decreased production of insulin, insulin dysfunction, or lack of insulin-receptor responsiveness at the cell surface.[71] Diabetes mellitus is generally regarded as a debilitating disease that profoundly affects a variety of host systems. Its effects include vascular disease (microangiopathy and atherosclerosis), retinopathy, nephropathy, neuropathy, and reduced host resistance.[71–74] Effects on the oral tissues, including dry mouth, infection, and an increased incidence of periodontal disease, have also been observed. Diabetes mellitus is considered a strong predictor for the development of periodontal disease.[75,76] It is important for the practitioner to have a basic understanding of diabetes mellitus and its systemic and oral impacts to provide more effective preventive and therapeutic dental care.

Classification and Epidemiology

Two major types of diabetes mellitus have been described. Type 1 diabetes mellitus (formerly insulin-dependent diabetes mellitus) commonly develops in individuals younger than 30 years but may occur at any age.[72] Insulin therapy is required for all patients with type 1 diabetes mellitus, and failure to receive insulin will result in systemic ketosis or acidosis.[72–75] This form of diabetes mellitus accompanies the destruction of the beta cells of the pancreatic islets of Langerhans. This event appears to be related to a genetic predisposition and may be mediated by a host autoimmune response associated with viral infection. Effective control and stabilization may be difficult in these patients. It is estimated that type 1 diabetes accounts for 5% to 15% of all cases of diabetes mellitus.[70,75,77,78]

Type 2 diabetes mellitus (formerly non–insulin-dependent diabetes mellitus) is the most common form of the disease. It usually begins in middle age (40 years) but may occur earlier or later. Individuals with type 2 diabetes mellitus are often obese and require dietary control and oral hypoglycemic agents (eg, sulfonylureas) to regulate blood glucose levels. Patients with this type of diabetes mellitus are usually resistant to the development of ketoacidosis.[70,72,79] Type 2 diabetes mellitus results from insulin dysfunction or insulin resistance associated with a lack of insulin-receptor responsiveness at the cell surface.[79–81] It is estimated that this form of the disease accounts for 85% to 90% of all cases of diabetes mellitus.[75]

The American Diabetes Association has developed a classification scheme for diabetes mellitus based on its etiology and/or pathogenesis. In addition to type 1 and type 2 diabetes mellitus, this scheme includes conditions of impaired glucose tolerance and impaired fasting glucose; gestational diabetes mellitus; and other types of diabetes mellitus resulting from exocrine pancreatic diseases, endochrinopathics, drugs and chemicals, infections, and genetic disorders.[82] There are an estimated 12 million to 14 million people with diabetes mellitus in the United States. Approximately 2% to 4% of people in the United States have been diagnosed with diabetes mellitus, and it is suggested that an equal number of people remain undiagnosed.[83,84]

Clinical Features

The classic signs and symptoms of diabetes mellitus include polydipsia (increased thirst), polyuria (increased urination), and polyphagia (increased hunger). These are more commonly observed in type 1 diabetes mellitus. Weight loss, restlessness, increased irritability, and ketoacidosis accompanied by vomiting and nausea may also be observed.[79,83] While these signs and symptoms may also be manifested with type 2 diabetes mellitus, occurrence is more variable and slower in onset. However, obesity is more common in type 2 diabetes mellitus. Other indications of diabetes mellitus may include peripheral numbness, blurred vision, delayed healing, infection, and oral manifestations.[77,79] Regardless of type, diabetes mellitus is generally regarded as a debilitating disease with far-reaching effects on a variety of host systems as a result of unrelenting hyperglycemia and lack of metabolic control. As previously noted, complications of diabetes mellitus may include vascular disease, retinopathy, nephropathy, neuropathy, and reduced host resistance. The end result is an increased incidence of cardiovascular disease, increased susceptibility to infection, necrosis of digits, renal failure, sensory deficits, and blindness.[71,72,74,85]

Oral Manifestations

Oral manifestations that have been reported in association with diabetes mellitus include xerostomia,[75] burning mouth, altered taste (neuropathy),[86] candidiasis,[75] increased caries rate,[87,88] and progressive periodontitis.[76,89–91] The level of metabolic control, duration of the disease, and age of the individual appear to influence these manifestations to a greater extent than does the type of diabetes mellitus.[92–94]

Periodontal disease has been said to be the sixth complication of diabetes mellitus.[90] While some studies have clearly validated an increased incidence of gingivitis and periodontitis among people with diabetes mellitus, others fail to do so.[95,96] Studies prior to 1980 often failed to clearly define and classify the diabetic status of study populations. More recently, studies have sought to delineate the type of diabetes mellitus (ie, type 1 or type 2) and the degree of metabolic control, affording more accurate insight into the interrelationship and impact of this systemic disease on the host periodontium.[97,98] Although variable results persist, there is a preponderance of evidence supporting a direct relationship between diabetes mellitus and periodontal disease. Increased incidence and severity of gingivitis[99–107] and periodontitis[89–91,93,100,103–105,107–114] have been observed in people with diabetes compared with people who do not have the disease. There is some indication that the severity of periodontal destruction may be related to the type of diabetes mellitus (type 1 versus type 2), the degree of metabolic control, the duration of the disease, and the presence of other complications.[91,94,107,115–117]

Specific details concerning the association between periodontal disease and diabetes mellitus remain to be elucidated, but proposed mechanisms of diabetic influence include microangiopathy of the periodontal tissues,[118–120] altered collagen metabolism,[121] microbial alterations,[122–124] and defective polymorphonuclear leukocyte chemotaxis.[76,125–128] Based on these observations, it may be speculated that the diabetic host periodontium may be at risk for disease as a result of vascular compromise. As glucose levels in the gingival crevicular fluid increase,[129] selective overgrowth of putative periodontal pathogens may be favored and facilitated by decreased tissue oxygen diffusion. As a result of polymorphonuclear leukocyte compromise, the individual with diabetes mellitus may be unable to provide an effective host response against the destructive microflora and its associated toxic products. The periodontium, adversely affected by impaired collagen metabolism, may sustain the cumulative effects of the destructive disease process.[75,97,130]

A key development related to complications associated with diabetes mellitus is the role of advanced glycation end products (AGEs). AGEs result from glycation of proteins in the presence of elevated blood glucose levels (hyperglycemia). In chronic hyperglycemia, AGEs increase and appear capable of adversely altering extracellular matrix–cell function and interaction. They may also bind with receptors on macrophages and monocytes and initiate a cascade of cytokine-mediated events that play a principal role in pathogenesis of diabetic complications. AGEs are also believed to affect the periodontal tissues, increasing susceptibility for periodontal destruction in the individual with diabetes mellitus.[131,132]

Clinical periodontal changes often associated with uncontrolled diabetes mellitus include proliferative tissue at the gingival margin; enlarged red velvety gingival tissues that bleed easily; periodontal abscesses (often multiple); and loose teeth, which often reflect a rapid and disproportionate loss of the supporting tissues.[75,97,102] Marked improvement of oral health may accompany effective metabolic regulation of the patient, and there are reports of reduction of insulin requirements following periodontal therapy.[75,133–135]

Patient Treatment

Diabetes mellitus has a significant effect on the diagnosis, treatment planning, and treatment of the patient with extensive dental needs. Conversely, a thorough oral examination may lead the practitioner to suspect undiagnosed or uncontrolled diabetes mellitus.

Patients with rapid or disproportionate loss of periodontal support in the absence of significant local factors (eg, bacterial plaque or calculus) should alert the clinician to possible underlying systemic disorders.[102] A comprehensive medical history may facilitate a tentative diagnosis of diabetes mellitus and may be effectively complemented

by appropriate laboratory tests. Reliable patient screening tests for diabetes mellitus include tests of sequential fasting blood glucose (FBG) levels, FBG levels plus a 2-hour postprandial test, and the glycosylated hemoglobin test. As opposed to the point-in-time values of the first two tests, the glycosylated hemoglobin test affords a global view of diabetic status and control for the previous 8 weeks. Self-monitoring devices may also be used for rapid disclosure of blood glucose values and serve as a valuable adjunct for patient diabetic control and for a quick check in the office.[77,83,136]

It is extremely important that the undiagnosed diabetic or inadequately controlled diabetic be referred to a physician for care before dental treatment begins. All routine dental care should be deferred until the diabetic status is determined and effectively controlled. Addressing diabetic control up front often results in improved oral health and affords a more accurate assessment of actual treatment needs. The dentist is in a perfect position to encourage patient compliance and control.[97]

A patient with diabetes mellitus who has acceptable control and no underlying systemic complications (eg, renal disease) has no greater predisposition for untoward dental treatment sequelae than do patients who do not have the disease. Key considerations relative to the dental treatment of the patient with diabetes mellitus include stress reduction, appointment times, inpatient versus outpatient care, and antibiotic use.[137–139]

A stress-reduction protocol may help stabilize the patient's insulin requirements and assist in maintenance of metabolic homeostasis. Efforts directed at allaying patient apprehension and minimizing discomfort may include pretreatment sedation and analgesia. Local anesthetics may contain varying concentrations of epinephrine, but this has not proven to have a significant diabetogenic effect. Practically speaking, stress-induced endogenous epinephrine is probably more significant, but it can be minimized by stress-reduction pain control measures.[97]

Dental appointments scheduled early in the day usually result in well-rested diabetes mellitus patients with maximum tolerance for potentially stressful dental procedures. These patients should be encouraged to take their usual medications and to schedule their dental appointments approximately 1½ hours after medications and breakfast. While patients receiving intermediate or long-acting insulin may be treated in the afternoon, extensive dental procedures (eg, surgery) are best completed in the early morning, providing an opportunity to monitor food intake and posttreatment status in the afternoon.[97]

Periodontal treatment often includes surgical procedures that are accompanied by mild to moderate posttreatment discomfort. As a result of compromised chewing and swallowing that often accompany such procedures, modification of the patient's diet may be required. It may be necessary to consult the patient's physician before the appointment to determine diet modifications (eg, liquid/semisolid dietary alternatives).[97]

Most diabetic patients can be effectively treated in the dental office on a routine outpatient basis. However, inpatient management may be considered for the poorly controlled patient or one whose treatment will unduly alter insulin and dietary schedules for extended periods. Diabetic patients with severe infections or significant medical complications should be hospitalized to avoid potentially life-threatening sequelae.[75,97] The incidence of postoperative infection following periodontal surgical procedures in a healthy population is less than 1%.[140] As in this group, prophylactic antibiotics are generally not necessary for well-controlled diabetics, but may be considered on the basis of the extent of the anticipated surgical procedure or the potential for infection related to elevated blood glucose levels.[79,97]

Diabetic Emergencies

Insulin shock (hypoglycemia) is the most likely diabetic emergency that the practitioner will encounter. It occurs when blood glucose levels are 40 mg/dL or less and may result from failure to adequately balance medication and diet, excessive insulin intake, exercise, or stress. Insulin shock is characterized by confusion, sweating, nausea, tachycardia, cold and clammy skin, belligerent behavior, and loss of consciousness if untreated. Treatment should be rendered immediately and should consist of orally administered carbohydrates (eg, orange juice, candy, or soft drink with sucrose) where possible. Dextrose may also be administered intravenously or glucagon (1 mg) given intramuscularly. The patient should be observed closely until stabilized, and his or her physician should be notified. Patients with diabetes mellitus should bring their glucometers to their appointments so that blood glucose values can be determined at that time. It is very important to be alert to the possibility of hypoglycemia and to avoid it. A review of the patient's dietary intake, medication (type and timing), and blood glucose levels will be most helpful in preventing hypoglycemia.[75,77,79]

Diabetic hyperglycemia generally develops more slowly, usually being manifested in the person with uncontrolled diabetes mellitus. As this condition proceeds, the individual becomes disoriented and takes rapid, deep breaths (Kussmaul-Kien respiration), which may have an acetone odor. Hypotension and loss of consciousness (blood glucose levels, 300 to 600 mg/dL) may ensue. Treatment consists of emergency medical services activation for hospital transport, basic life support, maintenance of an airway, provision of 100% oxygen, and intravenous

fluids. If there is any question whether the emergent condition is hypoglycemia or hyperglycemia, it should be managed as hypoglycemia initially, since this management is less invasive to the patient and will not significantly worsen an existing hyperglycemia.[77,79]

References

1. Ferguson MM, Silverman S Jr. Endocrine disorders. In: Jones JH, Mason DK (eds). Oral Manifestations of Systemic Disease, ed 2. London: Bailliere Tindall, 1990:593–615.

2. Rees TD. Systemic factors in periodontal disease. In: Newman HN, Rees TD, Kinane DF (eds). Diseases of the Periodontium. Northwood: Science Reviews Limited, 1993:67–72.

3. Eversole LR. Clinical Outline of Oral Pathology, ed 3. Philadelphia: Lee and Febiger, 1992:266–267.

4. Knezevic G, Uglesic V, Kobler P, et al. Primary hyperparathyroidism: Evaluation of different treatments of jaw lesions based on case reports. Br J Oral Maxillofac Surg 1991;29:185–187.

5. Pinard A. Gingivitis in pregnancy. Dent Register 1877;31: 258–259.

6. Löe H. Periodontal changes in pregnancy. J Periodontol 1965; 36:37–44.

7. Russell AL. The prevalence of periodontal disease in different populations during the circumpubertal period. J Periodontol 1971;42:508–512.

8. Blankenstein R, Murray JJ, Lind OP. Prevalence of chronic periodontitis in 13 to 15 year-old children. A radiographic study. J Clin Periodontol 1978;5:285–292.

9. Parfitt GJ. A five year longitudinal study of the gingival condition of a group of children in England. J Periodontol 1957;42: 26–32.

10. Massler M, Schour I, Chopra B. Occurrence of gingivitis in suburban Chicago school children. J Periodontol 1950;21: 146–164.

11. Sutcliffe PJ. A longitudinal study of gingivitis and puberty. J Periodontal Res 1972;7:52–58.

12. Stamm JW. Epidemiology of gingivitis. J Clin Periodontol 1986; 13:360–366.

13. Mohamed AH, Waterhouse JP, Friederici HHR. The microvasculature of the rabbit gingiva as affected by progesterone: An ultrastructural study. J Periodontol 1974;45:50–60.

14. Nyman S. Studies on the influence of estradiol and progesterone on granulation tissue. J Periodontal Res 1971;7(suppl): 1–24.

15. Lindhe J, Brånemark PI. The effects of sex hormones on vascularization of granulation tissue. J Periodontal Res 1968;3:6–11.

16. Lindhe J, Sonesson B. The effect of sex hormones on inflammation, II. Progestogen, oestrogen and chronic gonadotropin. J Periodontal Res 1967;2:7–12.

17. Lindhe J, Birch J, Brånemark P-I. Vascular proliferation in pseudo-pregnant rabbits. J Periodontal Res 1968;3:12–20.

18. Hugoson A. Gingival inflammation and female sex hormones. J Periodontal Res 1970;5(suppl):1–18.

19. Michaelides PL. Treatment of periodontal disease in a patient with Turner's syndrome. J Periodontol 1981;2:386–389.

20. Vittek J, Rappaport SC, Gordon GG, et al. Concentration of circulating hormones and metabolism of androgens by human gingiva. J Periodontol 1979;50:254–264.

21. Tianinen L, Asikainen S, Saxen L. Puberty-associated gingivitis. Community Dent Oral Epidemiol 1992;20:87–89.

22. Yanover L, Ellen RP. A clinical and microbiologic examination of gingival disease in parapubescent females. J Periodontol 1986;57:562–567.

23. Mombelli A, Lang NP, Burgin WB, Gusberti FA. Microbial changes associated with the development of puberty gingivitis. J Periodontal Res 1990;25:331–338.

24. Gusberti FA, Mombelli A, Lang NP, Minder CE. Changes in subgingival microbiota during puberty: A four year longitudinal study. J Clin Periodontol 1990;17:685–692.

25. Moore WEC, Burmeister JA, Brook CN, et al. Investigation of the influences of puberty, genetics and environment on the composition of subgingival periodontal floras. Infect Immun 1993; 61:2891–2898.

26. Wojcicki CJ, Harper DS, Robinson PJ. Differences in periodontal disease–associated microorganisms of subgingival plaque in prepubertal, pubertal and postpubertal children. J Periodontol 1987;58:219–223.

27. Kornman K, Loesche WJ. Effects of estradiol and progesterone on *Bacteroides melaninogenicus* and *Bacteroides gingivalis*. Infect Immun 1982;35:256–263.

28. Kornman K, Loesche WJ. The subgingival microflora during pregnancy. J Periodontal Res 1980;5:111–122.

29. Holderman LV, Moore WEC, Cato EP, et al. Distribution of *Capnocytophaga* in periodontal microfloras. J Periodontal Res 1985; 20:475–483.

30. Lindhe J, Attstrom R, Bjorn AL. Influence of sex hormones on gingival exudation in dogs with chronic gingivitis. J Periodontal Res 1968;3:279–283.

31. Holm-Pedersen P, Löe H. Flow of gingival exudate as related to menstruation and pregnancy. J Periodontal Res 1967;2:13–20.

32. Lindhe J, Attstrom R. Gingival exudation during the menstrual cycle. J Periodontal Res 1967;2:194–198.

33. Larato DC. Oral tissue changes during menstruation. J Oral Med 1971;26:27–29.

34. Friedman LA. Horizontal tooth mobility and the menstrual cycle. J Periodontal Res 1972;7:125–130.

35. Rothwell BR, Gregory CEB, Sheller B. The pregnant patient: Considerations in dental care. Spec Care Dent 1987;7: 124–129.

36. Löe H, Silness J. Periodontal disease in pregnancy, I. Prevalence and severity. Acta Odontol Scand 1963;21:533–551.

37. Löe H. Periodontal changes in pregnancy. J Periodontol 1965; 36:209–217.

38. Silness J, Löe H. Periodontal disease in pregnancy, II. Correlation between oral hygiene and periodontal condition. Acta Odontol Scand 1964;22:120–135.

39. Arafat AH. Periodontal status during pregnancy. J Periodontol 1974;45:641–643.

40. Adams D, Carney JS, Dicks DA. Pregnancy gingivitis: A survey of 100 antenatal patients. J Dent 1974;2:106–110.

41. Samant A, Malik CP, Chabra SK, Devi PK. Gingivitis and periodontal disease in pregnancy. J Periodontol 1976;47:415–418.

42. O'Neil TCA. Plasma female sex hormone levels and gingivitis in pregnancy. J Periodontol 1979;50:279–282.

43. Silness J, Löe H. Periodontal disease in pregnancy, III. Response to local treatment. Acta Odontol Scand 1966;24:747–759.

44. Rateitschak KH. Tooth mobility changes in pregnancy. J Periodontal Res 1967;2:199–206.

45. Lopatin DE, Kornman KS, Loesche WJ. Modulation of immunoreactivity to periodontal disease–associated microorganisms during pregnancy. Infect Immunol 1980;28:713–718.

46. Hugoson A, Lindhe J. Gingival tissue regeneration in female dogs treated with sex hormones: Histologic observations. Odontol Rev 1971;22:425–439.

47. Cohen W, Shapiro J, Friedman L, et al. Longitudinal investigation of the periodontal changes during pregnancy and fifteen months post–partum, II. J Periodontol 1971;42:653–657.

48. Shklar G, Glickman I. The effect of estrogenic hormone on the periodontium of white mice. J Periodontol 1965;27:16–23.

49. Ojanotko A, Harri MP. Progesterone metabolism by rat oral mucosa, II. The effect of pregnancy. J Periodontal Res 1982;17: 196–201.

50. Vittek J, Hernandez MR, Wenk EJ, et al. Specific estrogen receptors in human gingiva. J Clin Endocrinol Metab 1982;54: 608–612.

51. Hugoson A. Gingivitis in pregnant women. Odontol Rev 1970; 21:1–20.

52. Lindhe J, Sonesson B. The effect of sex hormones on inflammation, I. The effect of progestogen. J Periodontal Res 1966;1:212–217.

53. O'Neil TCA. Maternal T-lymphocyte response and gingivitis in pregnancy. J Periodontol 1979;50:178–184.

54. Kornman KS, Loesche WJ. The subgingival microflora during pregnancy. J Periodontal Res 1980;5:111–122.

55. Jonsson R, Howland BE, Bowden GHW. Relationship between periodontal health, salivary steroids and *Bacteroides intermedius* in males, pregnant and non-pregnant women. J Dent Res 1988;67:1062–1069.

56. El-Ashiry GM, El-Kafrawy AH, Naser MG, Younis N. Oral symptomatology during pregnancy and oral contraceptive therapy. Egypt Dent J 1969;110:116–119.

57. Knight GM, Wade AB. The effects of hormonal contraceptives on the human periodontium. J Periodontal Res 1974;9:18–22.

58. Lindhe J, Bjorn AL. Influence of hormonal contraceptives on the gingiva of women. J Periodontal Res 1967;2:1–6.

59. Lynn BD. "The pill" as an etiologic agent in hypertrophic gingivitis. Oral Surg Oral Med Oral Pathol 1967;24:333–334.

60. Sperber GH. Oral contraceptive hypertrophic gingivitis. J Dent Assoc S Africa 1969;24:37–40.

61. Pearlman BA. An oral contraceptive drug and gingival enlargement; the relationship between local and systemic factors. J Clin Periodontol 1974;1:47–51.

62. Kalkwarf KL. Effect of oral contraceptive therapy on gingival inflammation in humans. J Periodontol 1978;49:560–563.

63. Roth GD, Lin HS, Liu FTY. Effect of contraceptives on the periodontal tissue of rats. J Periodontal Res 1972;7:315–322.

64. Mariotti A. Sex steroid hormones and cell dynamics in the periodontium. Crit Rev Oral Biol Med 1994;5:27–53.

65. Pankhurst CL, Waite IM, Hicks KA, et al. The influence of oral contraceptive therapy on the periodontium—Duration of drug therapy. J Periodontol 181;52:617–620.

66. Sweet JB, Butler DP. Increased incidence of postoperative localized osteitis in mandibular third molar surgery associated with patients using oral contraceptives. Am J Obstet Gynecol 1977;127:518–519.

67. Barnett ML. Inhibition of oral contraceptive effectiveness by concurrent antibiotic administration—A review. J Periodontol 1984;56:18–20;

68. van Minden F. Use of female sex hormones in the treatment of chronic desquamative gingivitis. J Am Dent Assoc 1946;33: 1294–1297.

69. Kennon S, Tasch EG, Arm RN. Considerations in the management of patients taking oral contraceptives. J Am Dent Assoc 1978;97:641–643.

70. Rose LF, Kaye D. Internal Medicine for Dentistry. St Louis: Mosby, 1983:1259.

71. Schwartz S, Schwartz J. Management of Diabetes Mellitus. Durant, OK: Essential Medical Information Systems, 1993:10–47.

72. American Academy of Periodontology. Position paper: Diabetes and periodontal diseases. J Periodontol 1999;70:935–949.

73. Merimee TJ. Diabetic retinopathy: A synthesis of perspectives. N Engl J Med 1990;322:978–983.

74. Selby JV, Fitzsimmons SC, Newman JM, et al. The natural history and epidemiology of diabetic nephropathy: Implications for prevention and control. JAMA 1990;263:1954–1960.

75. Rees TD. The diabetic dental patient. Dent Clin North Am 1994;38:447–463.

76. Genco RJ, Löe H. The role of systemic conditions and disorders in periodontal disease. Periodontol 2000 1993;2:98–116.

77. Rees TD, Otomo-Corgel J. The diabetic patient. In: Wilson TG, Kornman KS, Newman MG (eds). Advances in Periodontics. Chicago: Quintessence, 1992:278–295.

78. Krolewski AS, Warram JH, Rand LI, Kahn CR. Epidemiologic approach to the etiology of type I diabetes mellitus and its complications. N Engl J Med 1987;317:1390–1398.

79. Montgomery MT, Rees TD, Moncrief JW. The diagnosis and management of the diabetic patient: Implications for dentistry. Austin, TX: Department of Health, 1992.

80. Smith U. Insulin action—Chemical and clinical aspects. Acta Med Scand 1987;222:7–13.

81. Lillioja S, Mott DM, Howard BV, et al. Impaired glucose tolerance as a disorder of insulin action. N Engl J Med 1988;318:1217–1224.

82. American Diabetes Association. Report of the Expert Committee on the Diagnosis and Classification of Diabetes Mellitus. Diabetes Care 1997;20:1183–1197.

83. Nathan DM. Diabetes mellitus. In: Rubenstein E, Federman DD (eds). Scientific American Medicine. New York: Scientific American, 1993:1–27.

84. Diabetes in America: Diabetes data compiled 1984. NIH publication 85-1268. Washington, DC: National Diabetes Data Group, 1985.

85. Defronzo RA, Farrannini E. Insulin resistance: A multifaceted syndrome responsible for NIDDM, hypertension, dyslepidemia and atherosclerotic cardiovascular disease. Diabetes Care 1991;14:173–195.

86. Hardy SL, Brennand CP, Wyse BW. Taste thresholds of individuals with diabetes mellitus and on control subjects. J Am Diabetic Assoc 1981;79:286–289.

87. Falk H, Hugoson A, Thorstensson H. Number of teeth, prevalence of caries and periapical lesions in insulin-dependent diabetes. Scand J Dent Res 1989;97:198–206.

88. Goteiner D, Vogel R, Deasy M, Goteiner C. Periodontal and caries experience in children with insulin-dependent diabetes mellitus. J Am Dent Assoc 1986;113:277–279.

89. Schlossman M. Diabetes mellitus and periodontal disease—A current perspective. Compend Contin Educ Dent 1994;15:1018–1032.

90. Löe H. Periodontal disease: The sixth complication of diabetes mellitus. Diabetes Care 1993;16:329–334.

91. Oliver RC, Tervonen T. Diabetes—A risk factor for periodontitis in adults? J Periodontol 1994;65:530–538.

92. Bacic M, Plancak D, Granic M. CIPTN assessment of periodontal status in diabetics. J Periodontol 1988;59:816–822.

93. Hugoson, A, Thorstensson H, Falk H, Kuylensturma J. Periodontal conditions in insulin-dependent diabetics. J Clin Periodontol 1989;16:215–223.

94. Glavind L, Lund B, Löe H. The relationship between periodontal state and diabetes duration, insulin dosage and retinal changes. J Periodontol 1968;39:341–347.

95. Hove KA, Stallard RE. Diabetes and the periodontal patient. J Periodontol 1970;41:713–718.

96. Barnett ML, Baker RL, Yancey JM, et al. Absence of periodontitis in a population of insulin-dependent diabetes mellitus (IDDM) patients. J Periodontol 1984;55:402–405.

97. Hallmon WW, Mealey BL. Implications of diabetes mellitus and periodontal disease. Diabetes Educator 1992;18:310–315.

98. Soskolne WA. Epidemiological and clinical aspects of periodontal diseases in diabetics. Ann Periodontol 1998;3:3–12.

99. Sandholm L, Swanljung O, Rytomaa I, et al. Periodontal status of Finnish adolescents with insulin-dependent diabetes mellitus. J Clin Periodontol 1989;16:617–620.

100. Rylander H, Ramburg P, Blotime G, Lindhe J. Prevalence of periodontal disease in young diabetics. J Clin Periodontol 1987;17:38–43.

101. Bernick S, Cohen DW, Bakers L, Laster L. Dental disease in children with diabetes mellitus. J Periodontol 1975;46:241–245.

102. Cianciola LJ, Park BH, Bruck E, et al. Prevalence of periodontal disease in insulin-dependent diabetes mellitus (juvenile diabetes). J Am Dent Assoc 1982;104:653–660.

103. De Pommereau V, Dargent-Paré C, Robert JJ, Brion M. Periodontal status in insulin-dependent adolescents. J Clin Periodontol 1992;19:628–632.

104. Ervash T, Knuuttila M, Pohjamo L, Haukiparo K. Relation between control of diabetes and gingival bleeding. J Periodontol 1985;56:154–157.

105. Gusberti FA, Syed SA, Bacon G, et al. Puberty gingivitis in insulin-dependent diabetic children, I. Cross sectional observations. J Periodontol 1983;54:714–720.

106. Cohen DW, Friedman L, Shapiro J, et al. Diabetes mellitus and periodontal disease: Two-year longitudinal observations. J Periodontol 1970;41:709–712.

107. Belting CM, Hiniker JJ, Dumme HCO. Influence of diabetes mellitus on the severity of periodontal disease. J Periodontol 1964;35:476–480.

108. Bartolucci E, Parkes RB. Accelerated periodontal breakdown in uncontrolled diabetes. Oral Surg Oral Med Oral Pathol 1981;52:387–389.

109. Seppala B, Seppala M, Ainamo J. A longitudinal study on insulin-dependent diabetes mellitus and periodontal disease. J Clin Periodontol 1993;20:161–165.

110. Schlossman M, Knowler WC, Pettitt D, Genco RJ. Type 2 diabetes mellitus and periodontal disease. J Am Dent Assoc 1990;121:532–536.

111. Emrich LJ, Schlossman M, Genco RJ. Periodontal disease in non–insulin-dependent diabetes mellitus. J Periodontol 1991;62:123–130.

112. Mandell RL, DiRienzo J, Kent R, et al. Microbiology of healthy and diseased periodontal sites in poorly-controlled insulin-dependent diabetes. J Periodontol 1992;63:274–279.

113. Novaes AB Jr, Pariera A, deMoraes N, Novaes AB. Manifestations of insulin–dependent diabetes mellitus in the periodontium of young Brazilian patients. J Periodontol 1991;62:116–122.

114. Firatli E. The relationship between clinical periodontal status and insulin-dependent diabetes mellitus. J Periodontol 1997;68:136–140.

115. Safkan-Seppala B, Ainamo J. Periodontal conditions in insulin-dependent diabetes mellitus. J Clin Periodontol 1992;63:843–848.

116. Tervonen T, Oliver GC. Long-term control of diabetes mellitus and periodontitis. J Clin Periodontol 1993;20:431–435.

117. Karjalainen KM, Knuuttila MLE, von Dickhoff KJ. Association of the severity of periodontal disease with organ complications in type 1 diabetic patients. J Periodontol 1994;65:1067–1072.

118. Frantzis TG, Reeve GM, Brown AL. The ultra-structure of capillary basement membranes in the attached gingiva of diabetic and non-diabetic patients with periodontal disease. J Periodontol 1971;42:406–411.

119. Listgarten MA, Ricker FH, Laster L, et al. Vascular basement lamina thickness in the normal and inflamed gingiva of diabetics and non-diabetics. J Periodontol 1974;45:676–684.

120. Ketcham BS, Cobb CM, Denys FR. Comparison of the capillary basal lamina width in marginal gingiva of diabetic and non-diabetic patients. Ala J Med Sci 1975;12:295–301.

121. Rumamurthy NS, Golub LM. Diabetes increases collagenase activity in extracts of rat gingiva and skin. J Periodontal Res 1983;18:23–30.

122. Sandholm L, Swanljung O, Rytomaa I, et al. Morphotypes of the subgingival microflora in diabetic adolescents in Finland. J Periodontol 1989;60:526–528.

123. Mashimo PA, Yumamoto Y, Slots J, et al. The periodontal microflora of juvenile diabetes: Culture, immunofluorescence and serum antibody studies. J Periodontol 1983;54:420–430.

124. Zambon JJ, Reynolds H, Risher JG, et al. Microbiological and immunological studies of adult periodontitis in patients with non–insulin-dependent diabetes mellitus. J Periodontol 1988;59:23–31.

125. Genco RJ, Slots J. Host responses in periodontal diseases. J Dent Res 1984;63:441–451.

126. Cutler C, Eke P, Arnold RR, Van Dyke TE. Defective neutrophil function in an insulin-dependent diabetes mellitus patient: A case report. J Periodontol 1991;62:394–401.

127. Ueta E, Osaki T, Yoneda K, Yamamoto T. The prevalence of diabetes mellitus in odontogenic infections and oral candidiasis: An analysis of neutrophil suppression. J Oral Pathol Med 1993;22:168–175.

128. Manouchehr-Pour M, Spagnuolo PJ, Rodman HM, Bissada NF. Comparison of neutrophil chemotactic response in diabetic patients with mild and severe periodontal disease. J Periodontol 1981;52:167–173.

129. Ficara, AJ, Levin MP, Grower MF, Kramer GD. A comparison of the glucose and protein content of gingival fluid from diabetics and non-diabetics. J Periodontal Res 1973;10:171–175.

130. Manouchehr-Pour M, Bissada NF. Periodontal disease in juvenile and adult diabetic patients: A review of the literature. J Am Dent Assoc 1983;107:766–770.

131. Lalla E, Lamster IB, Schmidt AM. Enhanced interaction of advanced glycation end products with their cellular receptor RAGE: Implications for the pathogenesis of accelerated periodontal disease in diabetes. Ann Periodontol 1998;3:13–19.

132. Grossi S, Genco R. Periodontal disease and diabetes mellitus: A two-way relationship. Ann Periodontol 1998;3:51–61.

133. Williams RC, Mahan CJ. Periodontal disease and diabetics in young adults. JAMA 1960;172:776–778.

134. Miller LS, Manwell MA, Newbold D, et al. The relationship between reduction in gingival inflammation and diabetes control: A report of 9 cases. J Periodontol 1992;63:843–848.

135. Grossi S, Skrepcinski F, Decaro T, et al. Treatment of periodontal disease in diabetics reduces glycated hemoglobin. J Periodontol 1997;68:713–719.

136. Kesson CM, Young RE, Talwar D, et al. Glycosylated hemoglobin in the diagnosis of non–insulin-dependent diabetes mellitus. Diabetes Care 1982;5:395–398.

137. Malamed JS. Handbook of Medical Emergencies in the Dental Office, ed 3. St Louis: Mosby, 1987:198–214.

138. Ryan DE. Dentistry and the diabetic patient. Dent Clin North Am 1982;26:105–112.

139. Rhodus NL. Detection and management of the diabetic patient. Compend Contin Educ Dent 1987;8:73–79.

140. Pack PD, Haber J. The incidence of clinical infection after periodontal surgery: A retrospective study. J Periodontol 1983;54:441–443.

Other Systemic Modifiers

Terry D. Rees
- Psychosomatic Factors and Stress
- Nutrition Deficiencies and Metabolic Disorders

Michael Glick
- Human Immunodeficiency Virus Disease

Mark R. Patters
- Neutrophil Abnormalities

Thomas J. Pallasch and Tommy W. Gage
- Adverse Drug Reactions

Tremendous progress has been made in understanding the causative factors in the development of periodontal diseases. It has been clearly established that these conditions are infectious and predicated on the presence of bacterial plaque accretions in the supragingival or subgingival areas of the teeth. Consequently, bacterial plaque is the primary causative factor in periodontal disease.

Not all plaque accumulations lead to the development of periodontal disease, however, even when large numbers of periodontopathogens are present. Additionally, the presence of untreated gingivitis does not always lead to periodontal destruction, and the degree of destruction that does occur varies markedly from one individual to another.[1] These findings have led to the recognition that factors other than plaque play a significant role in determining why some individuals are more susceptible than others to periodontal destruction. The search for periodontitis susceptibility (risk) factors is complex, because multiple factors may need to be present to significantly alter host resistance, and these factor combinations may vary at different times in the life cycle of an individual.[2]

Strong evidence suggests that genetically derived immunologic deficiencies are risk factors for periodontal disease.[3–9] However, externally created risk factors may also be important, especially in chronic periodontitis. Host response to periodontal infections may be affected by an in-

tricate combination of external factors such as use of tobacco; the use of certain medications; or the presence of debilitating systemic diseases, stress, or malnutrition—any or all of which may modify the systemic neuroendocrine-immunologic mechanisms that make up host defenses.[9] Other systemic factors such as age, race, or sex may have an effect on the progression of periodontal disease in an individual or in specific groups of individuals.[10,11] Some evidence suggests that, in turn, an increased incidence of periodontal disease may be a risk factor for cardiovascular disease and cerebral infarction.[12] This chapter will review some of the putative and established host resistance factors that may be involved in the progression of periodontal diseases.

Psychosomatic Factors and Stress

The relationship of a sound mind to the maintenance of a healthy body has been recognized throughout most of recorded history. The ancient Romans and Greeks discussed the importance of the patient's mental attitude and temperament in the treatment of physical disease.[13] In 1936, Selye developed the concept that physical or mental stress can have a profound detrimental effect on the human body.[14] This concept later evolved into Selye's general adaptation syndrome (GAS),[15] which was based on the observation that stress significantly influences endocrine function through the hypothalamus and anterior pituitary gland, leading to enlargement and increased function of the adrenal cortex. The first phase of the GAS (alarm reaction) activates the adrenal cortex to release corticosteroids to better prepare the body to adapt to and resist the stressful incident (resistance stage). If the causative stressful event is not suppressed, the third stage of GAS occurs (exhaustion stage). At this point, the body's ability to resist is overwhelmed, and damage occurs to target tissues. Thus, the GAS initially exerts a beneficial effect but becomes harmful if the stress continues unabated. This response is further modified by extraneous factors such as the patient's immunologic and nutrition status, medications, age, and the presence or absence of coexistent systemic diseases.[16–18]

The possible interrelationship between stress and periodontal disease was identified more than 50 years ago.[19] Subsequently, several human and animal studies have supported the relationship, although the mechanism of action has not been fully determined.[20–23] Increased susceptibility to and severity of periodontal disease have been reported in the presence of unwelcome life events, including financial and occupational stress and noise.[24–27]

Several animal and human studies suggest that the ability to cope with stress may be more important than the nature of the stressful situation experienced. Poor coping skills are often manifested as depression.[27] Depression may affect host resistance factors, but depression may also induce negligence in oral hygiene procedures, increased smoking and alcohol use, decreased salivary flow, and bruxism.[28] Certain personality traits and psychiatric disturbances have also been implicated.[29–34] In 1976, De Marco[35] presented a series of case reports describing severe alveolar bone loss in 11 soldiers who had experienced severe wartime emotional stress. He proposed that in the absence of other obvious causative factors, these cases represented a disease entity that he called *periodontal emotional stress syndrome*.

The effects of stress have also been studied in animals. In a sophisticated series of evaluations, Riley[36] demonstrated that stress can be induced in animals by factors such as noise, increased population density, male-female proximity, handling by animal keepers, and deliberate trauma. These effects may stimulate a variety of neuroimmunologic phenomena in multiple organs and tissues, and they confirm that the study of stress is very complex. In a low-stress environment, however, Riley was able to demonstrate that plasma corticosteroid levels were significantly increased by single, slightly stressful stimuli, and

that these increased levels adversely affected the immune response of the animals.

Other animal studies have assessed the effects of stress on the periodontium.[37–41] These studies suggest that the exhaustion stage of the GAS is associated with osteoporosis of alveolar bone, degeneration of the periodontal ligament, delayed wound healing, and apical migration of the epithelial attachment with pocket formation. Animal studies, however, do not confirm that a similar response occurs in humans. For example, the administration of corticosteroids or other immunosuppressive agents in humans has not been found to be associated with an increased incidence of periodontal disease. However, this may relate to the fact that agents such as corticosteroids and azathioprine have anti-inflammatory, as well as immunosuppressive, effects in humans.

The strongest correlation between stress and periodontal disease is found in acute necrotizing ulcerative gingivitis (ANUG).[34,42,43] This condition occurs more commonly in young adults under stress, such as college students at examination time,[44] individuals entering military service, or soldiers experiencing stress in relation to military life.[45–47] Davis and Baer[48] reported about two drug addicts who experienced ANUG, possibly due to the stress of withdrawal from their addictive habit. Presumably, the neuroendocrine mechanism is activated under stressful conditions, but stress-induced vasoconstriction may also induce local tissue ischemia and predispose the periodontal tissues to microbial invasion. Both of these effects could be enhanced by tobacco smoking, which is a nearly universal habit among individuals with ANUG.[12]

Measurement of serum and urinary cortisol levels has been used in the assessment of stress in relation to periodontal disease or its treatment.[34,49–51] These studies affirm an increase in corticosteroid levels in patients with ANUG, and these findings are supported by animal studies. They offer a partial explanation for the possible role of stress in periodontal disease.[34,36,39,52] Corticosteroids and other drugs, including drugs of abuse, have been demonstrated to adversely affect the neuroendocrine system, as well as the function of immunocompetent cells, leading to lymphocytopenia, alterations in chemotaxis, phagocytosis and killing of polymorphonuclear leukocytes, and macrophage dysfunction.[32,52,53] Other conditions, such as blood dyscrasias, malnutrition, malignancies, and other severe debilitating diseases, may also have a similar effect on the immunologic system. These conditions have all been associated with an increased incidence of ANUG.[52,54–56] Successful treatment of ANUG, however, is predicated on control of bacterial plaque, even in circumstances in which stressful or debilitating conditions and smoking persist,[34] suggesting that stress and related conditions have a limited role as etiologic factors in periodontal disease.

Nutrition Deficiencies and Metabolic Disorders

The importance of adequate nutrition in overall health is well recognized. It is logical to anticipate that tissues of the oral cavity are also affected by nutrition deficiencies; this can be demonstrated by the development of cancrum oris in association with severe protein deficiency (kwashiorkor) or of scurvy in long-standing vitamin C deficiency.[57–59] The importance of sound nutrition in prevention of disease is currently a topic of great discussion in medicine, and the prophylactic use of nutrition supplements to prevent cancer, cardiovascular disease, or other systemic disorders has been the target of considerable interest in recent years in the professional and lay literature.[60–62]

In the United States, nutrition deficiencies are found most commonly in the elderly, those of low socioeconomic status, and individuals addicted to drugs or alcohol.[63,64] The conditions may also occur, however, in edentulous patients or those with severe painful dental disease, food faddists, or strict vegetarians.[65] In theory, poor nutrition lowers resistance to periodontal disease, making an individual more susceptible to infection and the damage from periodontitis more severe. In fact, though, very few patients experience a demonstrable negative periodontal effect due to deficiency of a specific nutrient.[66,67] In general, efforts to associate periodontal disease with nutrition deficiencies have yielded conflicting results, with deficiency studies occasionally demonstrating profound effects in animals but not humans.[68,69]

The consistency of food would logically be assumed to have an effect on plaque accumulation and, subsequently, periodontal disease. A soft, sticky diet promotes plaque accumulation in animals, while firm, resistant foods that require vigorous chewing would be expected to be self-cleansing and to better stimulate salivary flow. These results have not been confirmed in humans, however, although a diet higher in fiber is probably desirable in maintaining periodontal health.[70]

Nutrition requirements change during various stages of life, such as the growth years; old age; puberty; pregnancy and lactation; and times of injury, infection, or surgery.[65] The effects of sex hormones on the periodontium, as discussed in chapter 13, may in fact relate to nutrition abnormalities occurring during life periods in which nutrition requirements are altered. Elderly individuals may be especially prone to nutrition deficiency because of partial or complete edentulism, difficulty in wearing dental appliances, altered susceptibility to soft tissue injury, altered muscle function, reduced salivary flow, altered taste sen-

sation, decreased appetite, and diseases that are more common in the elderly (eg, Alzheimer disease and Parkinson disease).[71] Despite these factors, a National Oral Health Survey failed to identify an increased tendency for tooth loss among the elderly when compared with younger individuals over a 10-year period.[69]

Wound healing initiates an increased nutrition requirement, and failure to supply dietary needs may slow the healing process. The stress of an injury or surgical procedure may further compromise the patient's nutrition status. The dental patient may have difficulty meeting increased nutrition needs following oral trauma or surgery because of discomfort associated with eating, and as a consequence, nutrition supplementation with multivitamins and proteins may be indicated during prolonged healing of an oral wound.[65,72]

Infections, including those of the oral cavity, tend to increase nutrition needs but are often associated with reduced dietary intake following oral injury due to mouth discomfort. Conversely, infections superimposed on malnutrition tend to be more severe because of the profound effect of the nutrition deficiency on the immunologic system.

Effects of Specific Nutrition Deficiencies

Vitamin Deficiency

Vitamins are coenzymes that are essential for health. They are classified as water soluble (vitamins B and C) and fat soluble (vitamins A, D, E, and K). In general, fat-soluble vitamins are stored in the body, while water-soluble agents are not. Vitamin A is involved in the synthesis of epithelial cells and proteoglycans, as well as in the expression of fibronectin and type 1 procollagen.[65] Vitamin A deficiency in animals alters epithelial integrity, induces keratinization of normally nonkeratinized mucosa, and stimulates cemental resorption and osseous changes.[73,74] There is no current evidence of an association between vitamin A deficiency and periodontal disease in humans, but vitamin A (retinol) is under intense study today as an antioxidant agent, which may have beneficial effects in prevention of malignancy, cardiovascular disease, and perhaps even periodontitis. This will be discussed in more detail in following sections.

The B-complex vitamins are water-soluble agents involved as a group in enzymatic activities necessary for energy production and cell division and growth. Thiamin (vitamin B_1) deficiency may lead to degeneration of the myelin sheath of peripheral nerve fibers and to beriberi. Riboflavin (vitamin B_2) deficiency may induce a seborrheic dermatitis, and it causes angular cheilitis, glossitis, and ulcerations in the oral cavity. Pyridoxine (vitamin B_6) is involved in carbohydrate metabolism. Deficiency may occur because of alcoholism or severe nutrition deprivation and may induce a generalized stomatitis, glossitis, or gingivitis, among other oral symptoms. Anemia, peripheral neuropathy, and dermatitis may result from prolonged deficiency. There is little evidence to suggest that administration of dosages greater than the minimal daily requirements of B vitamins is of benefit.[65,75]

Cobalamin (vitamin B[12]) deficiency may occur as the result of reduced dietary intake or secondary to altered gastrointestinal absorption, such as that which occurs in pernicious anemia. Vitamin B[12] deficiency is associated with epithelial cell abnormalities of oral mucous membranes, including epithelial thinning and increased mitotic activity. In such circumstances, affected gingival epithelia may be more susceptible to epithelial dysplasia or malignant transformation.[76,77]

Folic acid, or folate, is a component of amino acid that is attached to a B vitamin residue. In concert with vitamin B[12] deficiency, a folate deficiency may lead to megaloblastic anemia, and both deficiencies may result from pernicious anemia. Supplementation of folic acid without concomitant vitamin B[12] supplementation will reduce symptoms but will not prevent the onset of subacute combined degeneration of the spinal cord sometimes associated with pernicious anemia.[64,65,75] Folic acid is of interest to periodontists because some evidence suggests that folate supplementation or topical application may be of benefit in reducing gingivitis or phenytoin-induced gingival enlargement.[78] These findings, however, have not been duplicated in all studies.[79,80]

Vitamin C (ascorbic acid) is essential to collagen biosynthesis, and deficiency may adversely affect periodontal connective tissues, capillary integrity, and wound healing. Scurvy, or prolonged deprivation of ascorbic acid, will induce severe periodontal changes in humans, probably as a result of altered immune function, increased permeability of gingival sulcus epithelium, increased levels of glycosaminoglycans, and retention of extracellular fluid related to the altered capillary permeability.[65] Mild to moderate gingivitis may occur as an early feature of scurvy, suggesting a slight alteration in host resistance to plaque-induced disease possibly due to diminished chemotactic and phagocytic activities of polymorphonuclear leukocytes.[65,81,82] Later, generalized gingival changes occur, including acutely inflamed, edematous, hemorrhagic, gingival enlargement. After prolonged vitamin C deprivation, oral symptoms are accompanied by systemic features of frank scurvy, including lassitude, weakness, malaise, sore joints, ecchymosis, and weight loss. As the condition worsens, severe periodontal pathoses develop, including increased tooth mobility, increased destruction of the periodontal ligament, osseous abnormalities, and ultimately exfoliation of the teeth.[59,82,83] Frank scurvy is preceded by many months of severe ascorbic acid deficiency, and there is no evidence to indicate that mild vitamin C deficiency initiates periodontitis.[84] However, Nishida et al identified a weak but statistically significant increase in periodontitis among current and former smokers with low levels of daily dietary intake of vitamin C.[85] Vitamin C is yet another antioxidant agent believed by some to have preventive powers if taken in doses that exceed established minimum daily requirements.

Vitamin D is a fat-soluble vitamin that is composed of at least 16 steroid hormones involved in maintenance of bone quality throughout the body. The primary compound, cholecalciferol (vitamin D[3]), forms in the skin in response to the ultraviolet rays of the sun. It is concentrated in the liver and undergoes metabolic conversion in the kidneys to form the active hormone, 1,25-dihydroxycholecalciferol. The substance acts to regulate plasma calcium levels by promoting calcium absorption from the intestine, by helping to regulate kidney reabsorption of calcium, and by controlling alkaline phosphatase activity within bone. This vitamin works in concert with parathyroid hormone to mobilize calcium release from bone to maintain plasma levels.

Vitamin D deficiency or other factors that disrupt plasma calcium or phosphorus levels interfere with normal mineralization of organic bone matrix and lead to replacement of normal bone with osteoid. This condition is termed *rickets* in children and *osteomalacia* in adults.[65,75] Vitamin D–resistant rickets occurs as a result of defective receptors for vitamin D metabolites. In the elderly, osteomalacia is most commonly caused by defective liver or kidney function. The same effect can be initiated by primary hyperparathyroidism or by hyperparathyroidism induced secondary to renal failure. Rickets features retarded skeletal development and malformation of long bones. In the oral cavity, rickets is associated with radiographic changes in the alveolus, including loss of the lamina dura, thinning of the cortical plates of the jaws, and indistinct trabeculae. Dental anomalies are common, including delayed development of the permanent dentition, enamel hypoplasia, cemental resorption, open apical foramina, enlarged pulp chambers, and frequent pulp stones. In adults, osteomalacia may result in destruction of the periodontal ligament, resorption of alveolar bone, and replacement fibrous dysplasia.[86–88] Recent evidence suggests that low daily calcium intake, without regard to vitamin D deficiency, may be a minor risk factor for increased severity of periodontitis, especially in younger females (aged 20 to 39).[89] Osteoporosis is the loss of bone mass due to an imbalance of the plasma calcium-phosphorus levels with resultant release of calcium from bone. It may occur in a primary form (postmenopausal or senile osteoporosis) or secondarily as a result of calcium deficiency, hyperparathyroidism, or osteomalacia.[90] Fractures of vertebrae or long bones are common, but any bone may be involved. Several animal and human studies indicate that the severity of alveolar bone loss increases if periodontitis is present in individuals or animals suffering from estrogen deficiency–induced osteopenia or osteoporosis.[91–95] The severity of loss of alveolar bone density and clinical attachment levels may be greater among estrogen-deficient women who smoke.[96,97] These findings support other studies that associate increased tooth loss and more rapid resorption of edentulous alveolar ridges in osteoporotic individuals or in postmenopausal patients without estrogen supplementation.[93,98–103] The incidence of osteoporosis increases with age, and the condition is more common in women than men. Treatment in women includes estrogen replacement therapy; supplementation of vitamin D and calcium; exercise; and the administration of fluorides, calcitonin, and diphosphonates.[98] Results of therapy may be equivocal, and prevention of osteoporosis continues to be an important goal in medicine.

Trace metals such as zinc, copper, iron, and selenium are involved in several intracellular enzymatic functions and protein synthesis. Trace metal deficiencies have been reported to impair immunologic and inflammatory reactions, contribute to tissue destruction, and delay wound healing.[104,105] Studies of the effects of zinc deficiency on the periodontium suggest that a deficiency may increase susceptibility to plaque-induced disease and delay wound healing, but there is no evidence that zinc deficiency directly induces periodontal destruction.[106,107]

Protein Deficiency

Most of the 20 amino acids in protein can be synthesized by the body, yet severe protein deficiency will retard growth, alter physiologic functions, and significantly reduce host defenses and wound healing. Protein deprivation adversely affects immunoglobulin A in saliva, polymorphonuclear leukocyte phagocytosis and complement activation, and cell-mediated and humoral immune responses.[65] Severe protein deficiency (kwashiorkor) or general starvation (marasmus) has long been associated with oral changes, including glossitis, angular cheilitis, xerostomia, increased gingival inflammation, and periodontal bone loss.[57,58] As previously described, kwashiorkor is associated with an increased incidence and severity of necrotizing gingivitis, periodontitis, and cancrum oris. These effects may occur because of altered cell-mediated and humoral immune and inflammatory responses in the presence of plaque-associated disease. In animals, protein deprivation will lead to alveolar osteoporosis, reduced deposition of cementum, degeneration of the periodontal ligament, and delayed wound healing, but periodontal pocketing does not occur in the absence of plaque.[108,109]

Some authors have attributed altered resistance to periodontal disease to subtle protein deficiency, but there is little evidence to support this conclusion on a clinical basis.[98,110,111]

Antioxidants

Over the past 25 years or so, research regarding the relationship between diet and health has increased. Considerable attention has been directed toward free oxygen radicals, which are toxic molecular fragments capable of causing DNA mutation, changes in enzymatic activities, peroxidation of lipid membranes, and cell death. Free radicals appear to be involved in cancer, heart disease, and some forms of lung congestion.[60,61,112,113] Many studies have been directed toward the use of antioxidant agents such as betacarotene, retinol (vitamin A), ascorbic acid (vitamin C), alpha-tocopherol (vitamin E), and selenium in the prevention of these diseases. The use of antioxidants in the treatment of human oral leukoplakia and perhaps oral cancer shows promise, but to date, results are inconclusive.[60,61,112,113] There is evidence that free oxygen radicals are involved in the tissue destruction associated with chronic inflammatory osteoarthritis and periodontitis.[114,115] In periodontal diseases, proteases released from inflammatory cells, especially polymorphonuclear leukocytes, contain free oxygen radicals, which may damage adjacent periodontal tissues. Ongoing research is under way to determine whether or not antioxidant nutrition supplements are of benefit in reducing the tissue destruction occurring in plaque-induced periodontal diseases.[115]

Nutrient Excesses

Excessive intake of vitamins and minerals, including the antioxidants, may have toxic effects in humans. Excess water-soluble vitamins are excreted, whereas fat-soluble vitamins may be retained and stored in the body. There is evidence, however, that water-soluble vitamins may be toxic if ingested in large quantities for prolonged periods.[57] Toxic overdoses have been described in response to prolonged excessive daily ingestion of vitamin A. Symptoms include dry, coarse, scaly skin; hair loss; fissuring of the lips; and pruritus. Oral changes may include gingival inflammation and ulceration, loss of keratinization in tissues that are normally keratinized, and desquamation of lips and other tissues.[116–118]

Iron overload may increase susceptibility to infectious diseases, perhaps including periodontal infections, and bacterial sepsis has been reported following toxic overdose of iron. This may be due to the use of iron as an essential growth factor for enterobacteria.[119–122]

Several studies have noted a possible relationship between hyperlipidemia and periodontitis, especially among individuals with diabetes mellitus. On rare occasions gingival xanthomas may be present in individuals with elevated serum lipid levels.[123] It is not clear if hyperlipidemia contributes to susceptibility to periodontitis or if periodontitis contributes to hyperlipidemia. Hyperlipidemia is also considered a risk factor for vascular atheroma formation, and its presence may in part explain the possible association of periodontitis with poor diabetes mellitus control and increased risk of cardiovascular disease.[124–128]

Human Immunodeficiency Virus Disease

Human immunodeficiency virus (HIV) disease is characterized by progressive immune deterioration resulting in the development of opportunistic infections, including pathologic conditions in the oral cavity. The epidemiology of oral lesions is closely related to the overall health of patients and is consequently strongly associated with the efficacy of anti-HIV drug therapy. Since the introduction of new and more powerful antiretroviral medications in the mid-1990s a significant change in the prevalence of oral lesions has been noted. A retrospective study of lesions diagnosed between 1990 and 1999 revealed a significant decrease in the occurrence of oral candidiasis, oral hairy leukoplakia, and Kaposi sarcoma.[129] However, there was a significant increase in salivary gland disease and oral warts. Interestingly, even though there has been dramatic change in the prevalence and incidence of oral lesions since the introduction of medications such as protease inhibitors, the significance of oral changes as they relate to the level of immune suppression remains the same.[130]

Oral lesions found in individuals infected with HIV have been classified according to whether they have a pathogenic origin or lack a pathogenic origin (eg, fungal, viral, bacterial, or nonspecific ulcers) or according to how suggestive a lesion is for HIV disease (eg, a lesion such as oral hairy leukoplakia is a stronger indicator for HIV infection than is an aphthous ulcer).[131–134] It is interesting to note that many oral lesions found in HIV-infected individuals have been documented in periodontal tissues[135] (Tables 14-1 and 14-2). Some of these lesions can mimic periodontal conditions and must be excluded from a diagnosis of periodontal disease.

Periodontal disease among HIV-infected individuals can be manifested differently than in immunocompetent individuals. Furthermore, during progression of HIV disease, periodontal disease may become more rapidly progressive and more aggressive, or be manifested as a characteristic HIV-associated periodontal entity.

This section summarizes periodontal disease conditions that have been described as being associated with HIV in-

Table 14-1 HIV-Associated Oral Manifestations Observed in Periodontal Tissue

Fungal
   Candidiasis
   Geotrichosis
   Histoplasmosis
   Cryptococcosis

Viral
   Herpes simplex virus
   Cytomegalovirus
   Human papillomavirus

Bacterial
   Bacillary epithelioid angiomatosis
   Periodontal disease
      Linear gingival erythema
      Necrotizing ulcerative gingivitis
      Necrotizing ulcerative periodontitis

Neoplastic
   Kaposi sarcoma
   Non-Hodgkin lymphoma
   Squamous cell carcinoma

Without pathogenic origin
   Necrotizing stomatitis

fection, periodontal microbial flora in HIV-infected individuals, treatment of HIV-associated periodontal disease, and the association between periodontal disease and progressive immune deterioration seen during the course of HIV disease.

In 1987 Winkler and Murray described a periodontal condition they named *AIDS virus–associated periodontitis*, or *AVAP*.[136] This lesion was clinically similar to ANUG lesions superimposed on generalized aggressive periodontitis. The characteristic features of the lesion included generalized aggressive periodontitis; interproximal necrosis and ulcerations; marked edema and intense erythema of marginal and attached gingiva; deep-seated, bony pain; and spontaneous, often nocturnal, gingival bleeding. Some patients experienced an attachment loss of 90% in as short a time as 3 to 4 months. The cause of this clinical condition, initially described in homosexual men with HIV disease, was not clear and was not associated with unique periodontal pathogens. However, immunologic changes in the periodontium, such as an enhanced polymorphonuclear leukocyte response, and a shift in the periodontal flora were put forth as likely causes for this condition.

Another periodontal condition associated with HIV disease, but limited to soft tissues, was later identified. This entity was described as distinctive erythema of the free and attached gingiva and alveolar mucosa, and it was manifested as an intensely red linear band (2 to 3 mm) ex-

Table 14-2 HIV-Associated Periodontal Lesions

Classification	Clinical findings	Radiographic findings	Treatment
Linear gingival erythema (LGE, formerly known as HIV-associated gingivitis [HIV-G])	Distinct, 2- to 3-mm, intensely red band along the margin of the gingiva; petechia-like patches or punctuated lesion on the attached gingiva that blanches upon pressure; spontaneous or easily induced gingival bleeding; poor response to conventional periodontal therapy.	No evidence of alveolar bone loss	Systemic antibiotics and antibacterial mouthrinses in conjunction with scaling and curettage
Necrotizing ulcerative gingivitis	Ulcerative and necrotic destruction of one or more dental papillae; easily induced gingival bleeding; fetid breath.	No evidence of alveolar bone loss	Systemic antibiotics and antibacterial mouthrinses in conjunction with scaling and curettage
Necrotizing ulcerative periodontitis (NUP, formerly known as HIV-associated periodontitis [HIV-P] or AIDS virus–associated periodontitis [AVAP])	General or localized rapid soft and hard tissue destruction; possible bone sequestration; possible tooth mobility; spontaneous, usually nocturnal, gingival bleeding; fetid breath; intense deep-seated pain.	Rapid alveolar bone loss in affected areas	Systemic antibiotics and antibacterial mouthrinses in conjunction with scaling and curettage
Necrotizing stomatitis	Localized, acute necrotic area of the oral mucosa, usually overlying bone; exposure and sequestration of bone.	Rapid alveolar bone destruction	Systemic antibiotics, antibacterial mouthrinses, and systemic or local glucocorticosteroids, in conjunction with an occlusal dressing

tending apically from the marginal gingiva into the alveolar mucosa. It appeared as petechia-like patches on the attached gingiva that blanched upon pressure, exhibited spontaneous gingival bleeding, and typically did not respond to conventional periodontal therapy. This condition was called *HIV-associated gingivitis (HIV-G)*. Accordingly, the periodontitis first described as AVAP was renamed *HIV-associated periodontitis (HIV-P)*.[137]

A more severe form of HIV-P, extending beyond periodontal tissues into the oral mucosa, has also been described and was named *necrotizing stomatitis* or *necrotizing ulcerative stomatitis (NUS)*.[138,139] NUS is defined as a localized, acute, painful ulceronecrotic lesion that exposes underlying bone or penetrates or extends into contiguous tissues without the presence of an identifiable etiologic agent. A recent study demonstrated that NUS is an inflammatory disease and is not always associated with progression of necrotizing ulcerative periodontitis (NUP).[140]

Attempts have been made to characterize and describe periodontal conditions found in individuals with HIV disease, but there is still confusion concerning appropriate terminology and diagnostic criteria.[141,142] This confusion is mainly due to the lack of understanding of the cause of these lesions, which forces clinicians to make a diagnosis based purely on clinical impressions. Because many of the periodontal conditions found in HIV-infected individuals are also found in other immune-suppressed individuals,[143,144] recent reclassifications of these lesions have excluded references to HIV.[134] This has resulted in the classification of lesions based on clinical descriptions, such as linear gingival erythema (LGE) instead of HIV-G, and NUP instead of HIV-P. Presently four basic periodontal conditions are described as associated with HIV disease: LGE, necrotizing ulcerative gingivitis (NUG), NUP, and necrotizing stomatitis. It is thought that NUG may be an earlier stage of NUP, so these two conditions are often not differentiated in epidemiological and bacteriologic studies. The most recent classification of periodontal diseases and conditions groups NUG and NUP under the heading of "Necrotizing Periodontal Diseases" as two separate entities.[145] This classification will probably remain until the relationship between these two entities and their association with systemic conditions have been further elucidated.

In an attempt to validate diagnostic criteria for HIV-associated periodontal disease, Robinson studied periodontal conditions in both HIV-positive and HIV-negative men in the United Kingdom.[146] He found that erythema of the attached gingiva, necrotizing periodontal disease, and interdental craters were highly predictive of HIV disease.

Epidemiology of Periodontal Conditions

Few studies have evaluated the prevalence of conventional gingivitis in the HIV-infected population. However, the few studies that have been performed could not detect any difference in incidence between HIV-infected individuals and the general population.[147–150]

A study of a large cohort of HIV-positive adults in North Carolina looked at the severity and extent of periodontitis and the prevalence of HIV-associated periodontal disease.[151] Sixty-two percent of the subjects had probing depths greater than 5 mm, while 66% exhibited attachment levels greater than or equal to 5 mm. Only 15 of 316 dentate subjects were classified as having HIV-associated periodontal disease. This low prevalence was further attenuated by antiretroviral medications.

Controversy still surrounds the prevalence of LGE. Studies have suggested rates ranging from 4% to 50%.[152,153] Two of only a few studies performed on HIV-infected children found an LGE prevalence rate of 30% to 37%.[154,155] Others have concluded that LGE is very rare and might not be more prevalent among HIV-infected individuals than among the general population.[147,148] It is not possible to determine the true prevalence of this lesion, but the prevalence rate may differ greatly between different geographic areas using different medical treatment standards, as well as between different patient populations.

The prevalence rate of NUP is also hard to determine, mainly because of a lack of consensus among examiners,[142] as well as not taking into account patient medications that can influence the development of this lesion. Swango et al reported a prevalence rate of 6% among 189 HIV-infected military recruits,[156] which is similar to a rate of 4% to 10% among a cohort of 136 individuals (134 males) reported by Masouredis et al from an AIDS clinic in San Francisco.[153] These rates are higher than those reported by Riley et al, whose cohort of 200 individuals revealed a prevalence of NUP of only 1%.[157] The reason for this low prevalence rate is not clear. One of the largest studies on NUP, including 700 HIV-infected patients, found a prevalence rate of 6.3%.[158] The same study indicated that NUP was more common among homosexual/bisexual men than among other individuals with HIV infection. Furthermore, patients taking trimethoprim-sulfamethoxazole (Bactrim) had a much lower prevalence of this lesion compared with a control group.

Too few cases of necrotizing stomatitis have been documented to determine the prevalence of this lesion.

Periodontal Microflora in HIV-Infected Individuals

On the basis of a study of 39 HIV-positive patients with gingivitis or periodontitis, Moore et al concluded that there was no major difference in the microbial composition of periodontal lesions in HIV-positive and HIV-negative patients.[159] Only *Mycoplasma salivarium* was found in significantly increased numbers in HIV-infected individuals. The conclusion of these researchers was based in part on previously published data for HIV-negative patients, as their study population lacked HIV-negative controls. Other reports propose that although the periodontal flora do not differ significantly from that of non-HIV individuals, progression of periodontal disease in HIV-infected patients is associated with immune competence, or the lack thereof, as well as the local inflammatory response.[160] Specifically, it has been proposed that a reduced Th 1 lymphocyte response results in inadequate priming of polymorphonuclear cells. This may allow for subgingival colonization of pathogens such as *Candida* species; when in concert with subgingival bacterial pathogens, it may also increase the occurrence of periodontal attachment loss.[161]

The pathogens for HIV-associated periodontal disease have not yet been defined. However, the fact that antimicrobial agents and mechanical debridement are usually successful in treating these conditions is highly suggestive of a bacterial origin. In addition to bacteria, a dysfunctional immune response is probably necessary to achieve the extensive tissue destruction.

Several investigators have described the prevalent flora in both LGE and NUP to be *Actinobacillus actinomycetemcomitans*, *Bacteroides* (now *Porphyromonas*) *gingivalis*, *Bacteroides intermedius* (now *Prevotella intermedia*), and *Fusobacterium nucleatum*.[162–165] These suspected pathogens were not found in statistically significantly greater numbers in LGE and NUP than in control gingivitis and periodontitis sites or healthy sites, regardless of HIV status. While the periodontal microbiota of LGE and NUP sites resembled that of conventional periodontitis, the LGE microbiota differed significantly from that in conventional gingivitis. Similar studies, in which the bacterial monitoring was conducted with DNA probes, yielded essentially identical results.[166] These findings suggested that LGE is more aggressive than conventional gingivitis and that LGE lesions may be precursors of NUP. Furthermore, Grbic and coworkers have reported a statistically significant association between LGE and the presence of oral candidiasis among homosexual men.[149] The presence of oral candidiasis in association with a local immunosuppressive effect on CD4 T-lymphocytes has also been suggested to predispose HIV-infected individuals to gingival ulcerations.[167]

However, some studies have demonstrated a few differences in bacterial flora between LGE and NUP. *Wolinella recta* was four times more prevalent in NUP than in LGE; subgingival *Candida albicans* was recovered in 62% of AIDS patients[164] compared with less than 17% in non–HIV-infected patients with severe chronic periodontitis.[168] Some enterics, including *Enterococcus*, *Clostridium*, and *Klebsiella* species, were also recovered in these patients.

The previously described studies provide important information about the undisturbed microbiota of patients with HIV-associated periodontal disease and suggest that periodontitis lesions in HIV-positive and HIV-negative individuals differ little in their associated microbiota. It is not clear from existing studies whether periodontal treatments affect the composition of the microbiota in these patients, or to what extent changes in the microbial composition are accompanied by changes in the clinical status of the periodontal lesions.

Microbial studies of necrotizing stomatitis have found no unique pathogens that can explain the morbidity of this lesion.

The association between periodontal disease and herpes viruses has also been investigated. In a study of 21 HIV-positive and 14 HIV-negative adults, Mardirossian and colleagues found human herpes virus type 6 (HHV-6), human herpes virus type 7 (HHV-7), or human herpes virus type 8 (HHV-8) in 90% of gingival biopsies in HIV-positive subjects but in only 43% of biopsies from HIV-negative subjects.[169] The significance of this finding is not clear.

Treatment of HIV-Associated Periodontal Conditions

One characteristic feature of LGE is its poor response to conventional therapy. Normal scaling and curettage will not resolve the lesion. Instead, systemic antibiotics and antibacterial mouthrinses must be instituted, as for treatment of NUP.

Treatment for both NUG and NUP consists of mechanical debridement, antibiotic therapy, and antibacterial mouthrinse.[170] It is interesting to note that the pain associated with NUP usually disappears within 24 to 36 hours after the institution of antibiotic therapy.[135]

Initial debridement of the lesion can be accomplished with povidone-iodine irrigation and light mechanical debridement. The most commonly used antibiotic is metronidazole, but tetracycline is also being used. The routine metronidazole dosage is 250 mg given three to four times per day. Tetracycline hydrochloride may be used in a dosage of 250 mg four times per day or doxycycline in a dosage of 100 mg twice a day. The antibiotics should be used for 5 to 7 days. The emergence of *Candida* infection is much more likely with the tetracy-

clines than with metronidazole. When clinical candidiasis develops, an antifungal medication can be prescribed concurrently. An antimicrobial mouthrinse such as 0.12% chlorhexidine gluconate is administered twice daily, and the patient is rescheduled for a follow-up appointment within 3 days. Although resolution of the lesion is rapid, recurrence is not uncommon.

Treatment for necrotizing stomatitis is similar to that for NUP. However, sometimes resolution can be achieved only after the use of a protective mouthguard covering the lesion, with topical antibiotics and glucocorticosteroid preparations placed inside the mouthguard.[171]

Periodontal Health and the Course of HIV Disease

The relationship between periodontal health and the prevalence and severity of conventional gingivitis and conventional periodontal disease among immunosuppressed HIV-infected individuals is still not known. Some reports have indicated an increased prevalence of periodontitis among HIV-seropositive individuals compared with comparable HIV-seronegative cohorts.[172] A more progressive periodontal disease has also been described in an 18-month longitudinal study of 30 HIV-seropositive individuals.[173] This study noted a strong correlation between progression of HIV disease and increased attachment loss in patients with preexisting periodontitis, despite a lack of plaque buildup.

An increased incidence of attachment loss was also noted by Barr et al[174] in homosexual and bisexual HIV-infected men with more depressed immune status. Individuals with $CD4^+$ cell counts below 200 cells/mm^3 had more than six times more frequent relative attachment loss of at least 3 mm compared with individuals with $CD4^+$ cell counts above 200 cells/mm^3 (normal $CD4^+$ cell count is 600 to 1,000 cells/mm^3). Similarly, a rapid attachment loss has been documented with defects in neutrophil functions.[175] Another study of 30 HIV-infected individuals correlated a more progressive periodontal disease with decreasing numbers of $CD4^+$ cells and more advanced stages of HIV infection.[176] These and other cross-sectional studies suggest that severity of periodontal conditions in HIV-infected individuals is manifested with increased attachment loss but seldom with increased gingival or plaque indices. As previously mentioned, other studies have not reported any differences between periodontal health in HIV-infected individuals, usually in the early stages of HIV disease, compared with that in the general population.[147,148] However, generalized aggressive periodontitis may still be an early marker for HIV disease.[177]

The presence of LGE and necrotizing stomatitis has been associated with severely depressed immune status, but cohort studies have not been large enough to determine if these findings are statistically significant.[171,178]

A strong correlation between severe immune suppression and the presence of NUP has been documented.[129,137,158] A study from the mid-1990s documented the presence of NUP as a significant marker for both AIDS and an extremely low CD4+ cell count (below 100 CD4+ cells/mm³).[158] The same study indicated that patients presenting with NUP had a cumulative probability of death of 60% within 18 months of a diagnosis of NUP.

In summary, HIV-infected patients may have more progressive periodontal disease compared with non–HIV-infected individuals. The periodontal flora is similar in both kinds of patients, but may be present in higher numbers in HIV patients. When the patient's immune status deteriorates, more severe periodontal manifestations may occur. These lesions are associated with a high incidence of morbidity and are often early signs of immune deterioration and HIV disease progression.

Neutrophil Abnormalities

An overwhelming abundance of evidence has confirmed that the cause of inflammatory gingivitis and periodontitis is bacteria. However, many factors can modify the response of the host to microbial infection and influence the conversion of gingivitis to periodontitis, and thus the progression of periodontal disease. Clearly, the defense systems of the host have a major effect on the oral microflora and establish a balance between the pathogenic bacteria of dental plaque and the host during disease quiescence. This equilibrium can be altered by several factors, including changes in the flora and/or alterations in the host's defenses, such that periods of disease progression result until the balance can be restored.

Chief among defense mechanisms available to the host is the polymorphonuclear neutrophil (PMN), which has been shown to be the first line of host defense to combat acute bacterial infection. A characteristic morphologic feature of all stages of gingivitis and periodontitis is the accumulation of PMNs in the gingival connective tissue, junctional epithelium, and gingival crevice or periodontal pocket.[179] Given the intimate relationship between PMNs and the periodontal microflora, it would not be surprising that a decrease in neutrophil function might result in increased severity of periodontal destruction. This section will explore the relationship between neutrophil abnormalities and periodontal diseases.

Neutropenias

Effects of neutropenia, a decrease in systemic neutrophils, on the oral cavity were noted in the early 20th century. Early literature described numerous manifestations of diminished circulating PMNs that included skin infections, upper respiratory infections, otitis media, stomatitis, early exfoliation of teeth, and severe gingivitis with ulceration. Most cases were manifested in infancy, and severe PMN disorders often had a fatal outcome. The cause of neutropenias, when known, can vary widely and include drug-induced (associated with antithyroid drugs, phenothiazines, quinidine, penicillin, sulfonamides, and other antibiotics), radiation-induced, disease-induced (diabetes mellitus; Down syndrome; Felty syndrome; tuberculosis; leukemia; aplastic anemia; and other viral, bacterial, rickettsial, and protozoan infections), and autoimmune conditions. Most systemic neutropenias appear to be idiopathic, but a genetic factor may be important.

Chronic idiopathic neutropenia ranges in severity from mild (1,000 to 2,000 PMN/mm³) to severe (< 500 PMN/mm³), with the degree of neutrophil suppression correlating with the extent and severity of systemic symptoms. Oral manifestations of chronic neutropenia include gingivitis, aggressive periodontitis, and oral ulcerations.[180]

Cyclic neutropenia, first recognized by Leale in 1910, is a rare condition that exhibits neutropenic episodes of 1 week's duration every 3 weeks. Although the cause is unknown, a regulatory defect in hematopoietic stem cells has been postulated. Dental symptoms include sore gingivae, aphthous ulcers, and early-onset periodontal destruction.[181]

Neutrophil Dysfunctions

The normal response of the neutrophil to microbial invasion is migration to the site of infection, followed by phagocytosis and killing of the invading microorganism. For this to occur, the following events must transpire:

1. Stem cells of the bone marrow differentiate into PMNs.
2. Mature neutrophils are released from the bone marrow to the bloodstream.
3. PMNs marginate and adhere to the endothelium of blood vessels.
4. Neutrophils migrate from the blood vessel into the connective tissue.
5. Neutrophils migrate through the connective tissue to the site of infection.
6. PMNs identify, attach, and engulf foreign material (bacteria).
7. The bacteria are killed and digested by the neutrophil.

An appropriate response of the PMN to microbial invasion requires that several biologic processes of neutrophils operate unimpaired. These processes include (1) adherence, the binding of PMNs to endothelial cells via specific adherence molecules on the PMN surface; (2) chemotaxis, the directed migration of cells toward a gradient of chemotactic molecules, such as complement cleavage products (C5a) or bacterial peptides (formylmethionyl peptides); (3) phagocytosis, the engulfment of foreign material into a phagolysosome by invagination of the cell membrane following recognition of specific host-derived molecules bound to the bacterial surface (opsonins, eg, immunoglobulin G and C3b); and (4) bacterial killing, the destruction of the microorganism by release of lysosomal constituents into the phagolysosome.

Techniques have been developed that allow in vitro measurement of these biologic processes of PMNs. Using these assays, defects in human PMN function have been identified and characterized.

Adherence Defects

Glycoprotein molecules have been identified on the PMN surface that are critical for the adhesion of PMNs to endothelial cells. These glycoproteins, termed LFA-I, Mac-1, and p150,95, are members of the integrin family of adhesion proteins and are composed of distinct α and common β subunits. A deficiency of these molecules, termed leukocyte adherence defect (LAD), has been identified in patients whose clinical condition is characterized by recurrent bacterial infections, diminished pus formation, prolonged wound healing, and leukocytosis.[182] Dentally, the disease is characterized by generalized periodontitis, progressive alveolar bone loss, premature exfoliation of deciduous and permanent teeth, and severe gingival inflammation.[183,184] Genetic study of affected patients has identified a heritable autosomal recessive defect of a gene on chromosome 21 that codes for the common β subunit of the adhesion molecules.[185]

The severity of the clinical manifestations of LAD is directly related to the degree of glycoprotein deficiency. Patients with severe LAD (> 0.3% of normal glycoprotein adherence molecules) have life-threatening systemic infections and often die in infancy. The moderate phenotype (2.5% to 30% of normal) has an increased survival rate. The dental conditions observed include rapid horizontal and vertical bone loss following the eruption of the primary teeth, fiery red gingiva, marginal gingival proliferation, recession, clefting, and bleeding.[183] Gingival biopsy specimens reveal a marked peripheral blood leukocytosis, but minimal infiltration of PMNs into the connective tissue.[183]

Thus, LAD represents a clinical disease entity for which the underlying biochemical, molecular, and genetic basis is known. As previously described, defective adhesion molecules prevent successful margination of PMNs, thus trapping them in the peripheral circulation and preventing their emigration to the site of infection.

Chemotaxis Defects

Chemotaxis, the directional migration of cells toward higher concentrations of attracting molecules, is a critical biologic function of host defense cells. Attracting molecules, either bacterial or host derived, are detected by specific receptors on the PMN surface.[186] The binding of a chemotactic molecule to the specific receptor results in internalization of the receptor-substrate complex. This initiates a complex series of reactions known collectively as signal transduction, involving Ca^{2+}, phosphoinosotides, and phospholipids, and it results in a respiratory burst and cell locomotion. Cell movement involves the polarization of the cell with the development of a receptor-rich lamellipodium and a thin uropod that attaches to the substrate, reorganization of the cytoskeletal structure of microtubules and microfilaments, and replacement of chemotactic receptors by fusion of receptor-bearing specific granules with the cell membrane.

Several rare diseases and syndromes that involve defects in neutrophil locomotion and chemotaxis have been documented in the literature. Many of these entities have severe periodontal consequences (Table 14-3).

The best-characterized periodontal disease associated with a neutrophil chemotactic defect is localized aggressive periodontitis, which is distinguished by vertical bony lesions affecting the first molars and incisors and is seen in adolescents and young adults. The disease is believed to have an onset around the time of puberty. The majority of cases have a characteristic saccharolytic microflora in which A actinomycetemcomitans is predominant. The PMN chemotactic defect occurs in approximately 75% of cases[188] and is intrinsic to the PMN.[189] The defect is not reversible with treatment and occurs within families.[190] The cause of the defect has been identified as a reduced number of chemotactic receptor molecules on the PMN surface[191] and an associated reduction in a surface glycoprotein known as GP110, thought to be involved in signal transduction.[192]

The interrelationship between the PMN chemotaxis defect in localized aggressive periodontitis and the predominance of A actinomycetemcomitans in the subgingival flora remains to be explained. Several strains of A actinomycetemcomitans are known to produce a leukotoxin or leucocidin, a protein that has direct lytic effects on human neutrophils.[193] Observation of the leukotoxic strains present in the flora of subjects with localized aggressive periodontitis and healthy subjects has revealed a significantly higher proportion of leukotoxin-producing isolates in the former group,[194] suggesting that the leukotoxin is an important virulence factor in periodontitis.

Defects in Phagocytosis and Killing

As discussed previously, the relationship between the neutrophil defect and *A actinomycetemcomitans* requires further study. However, recent experiments have examined the ability of neutrophils to phagocytose and kill *A actinomycetemcomitans* in vitro. Results of this work show that localized aggressive periodontitis neutrophils can internalize *A actinomycetemcomitans* but fail to kill the internalized organism.[195] In contrast, *A actinomycetemcomitans* is easily killed by normal neutrophils, and localized aggressive periodontitis neutrophils kill other species readily. If confirmed, this finding has widespread implications regarding a quantitative defect in the ability to kill a specific pathogen and may explain the lack of systemic disease in patients with localized aggressive periodontitis.

Interaction of the neutrophil chemotactic receptors with chemotactic molecules stimulates a strong respiratory burst in the cell. This respiratory burst yields superoxide ions (O_2^-), hydroxyl radicals (OH^-), and hydrogen peroxide (H_2O_2), all of which are toxic to bacteria. Superoxide is generated by the interaction of molecular oxygen with the plasma membrane enzyme nicotinamide adenine dinucleotide phosphate (NADPH) as follows:

$$NADPH + 2O_2 \rightarrow NAPD + 2O_2^- + H^+$$

In the presence of the enzyme superoxide dismutase, superoxide ions are converted to hydrogen peroxide, which is degraded by catalase. Although O_2^- and H_2O_2 are toxic at high concentrations, myeloperoxidase present in neutrophil azurophilic granules can react with H_2O_2 and halide to form hypochlorite (OCl^-), which is highly toxic to bacteria, fungi, viruses, and mycoplasma.

Polymorphonuclear neutrophils can also kill bacteria in an anaerobic environment, where oxygen is unavailable. Several substances contained in the lysosomal granules, including lysozyme, proteases, and lactoferrin, have direct toxic effects on bacteria.

Chronic granulomatous disease is an inherited disorder of dysfunctional PMN killing due to lack of production of bactericidal oxygen reagents.[196] Most cases have been shown to be X-chromosome linked and characterized by the absence of cytochrome c, which prevents NADPH synthesis. The disease is characterized by recurrent bacterial infections, including periodontitis and formations of neutrophil-containing granulomatous lesions.

The observation that neutrophil disorders reduce the protective response of the host has increased our understanding of the pathology of infectious disease. It has

Table 14-3 Neutrophil Locomotion Abnormalities with Oral Manifestations*

Condition	Random locomotion	Chemotaxis
Chediak-Higashi syndrome	Unknown	Depressed
Diabetes mellitus	Normal	Depressed
Prediabetes	Normal	Depressed
Down syndrome	Normal	Depressed
Ulcerative colitis	Increased	Depressed
Job syndrome	Normal	Depressed
Lazy leukocyte syndrome	Depressed	Depressed
Papillon-Lefèvre syndrome	Unknown	Depressed
Malnutrition	Depressed	Depressed

*Adapted from Van Dyke.[187]

been clearly demonstrated that PMN disorders increase susceptibility to infection and that the periodontium, given the large number of microorganisms present, is extremely sensitive to such pathological alterations. Severe periodontal destruction is seen in cases of severe neutrophil dysfunction, such as LAD, and in cases of subtle disturbance, such as localized aggressive periodontitis. With an increased appreciation of the molecular and genetic bases of these diseases, a greater understanding of the infectious disease process is at hand.

Adverse Drug Reactions

The oral cavity can be the site of a wide spectrum of reactions evoked by a variety of drugs. It appears that systemic medications usually have little direct effect on periodontal health,[197] but if locally irritating, they may significantly affect plaque control. The local or systemic adverse effects of medications on the oral cavity may generally be placed into seven categories: gingival enlargement, abnormal pigmentation, oral mucosal lesions, allergic reactions, cancer chemotherapy toxicity, salivary gland disorders, and oral manifestations of substance abuse. Because it is common for patients to take a wide variety and large number of prescribed drugs, an appreciation of the adverse effects of oral drugs is important. A review of the adverse effects of medication in the oral cavity is available.[198]

Gingival Enlargement

Gingival enlargement or overgrowth may be the result of a variety of causes, including inflammatory gingival disease and systemic modifiers. The inflammatory and systemic components usually occur together, exaggerating the overall gingival response. Systemic conditions that may be associated with gingival enlargement include, but are not limited to, selected drugs, leukemia, and multisystem syndromes.

Many medications are associated with the induction of gingival enlargement. The mechanism by which this adverse effect occurs is not well understood; therefore, approaches to treatment and subsequent results have been somewhat variable. Among the drugs and substances associated with gingival enlargement are anticonvulsants, cyclosporine, calcium channel antagonists, cannabis, and erythromycin (a single but documented report).[199–201] Regardless of causes or mechanisms, the resultant gingival enlargement has progressive and dynamic adverse effects on function, esthetics, and phonetics.

Anticonvulsants

Phenytoin is one of the most common drugs used to treat major seizure disorders in both adults and children. Its proposed anticonvulsant action is believed to consist of stabilizing damaged neuronal discharge and limiting progression of neuronal excitation by blocking calcium ion influx across cell membranes.[202] Phenytoin-associated gingival overgrowth was reported within a year of its introduction.[203] Reports of overgrowth range from 0% to 84%, with an average incidence of approximately 50%.[204,205] The mechanism by which associated gingival enlargement occurs is unknown, but it may involve stimulation of selected subpopulations of fibroblasts and may be genetically influenced.[206] The study of connective tissue from phenytoin-associated gingival tissues indicates that there may be a significant increase in the noncollagenous matrix and a corresponding decrease in the collagenous matrix.[207] A decrease in collagenase activity has also been suggested.[208,209] Conflicting results of the effects of phenytoin and its metabolites on fibroblasts in tissue cell cultures have been reported.[210]

Clinical gingival manifestations range from a granular, pebbly surface to extensive outgrowths affecting the interdental and marginal tissues. The anterior facial gingiva is affected most often. The gingival enlargement may interfere with normal tooth eruption and oral hygiene efforts, and it may cause tooth migration.[211] The magnitude of overgrowth may be related to serum drug levels.[209]

Histologically, gingival overgrowth specimens are typically characterized by epithelial hyperplasia with deeply penetrating, tubular rete ridges. The underlying connective tissue is usually inflamed and quite fibrotic.[205]

Treatment and prevention of the phenytoin-induced overgrowth is based on effective plaque control. Chlorhexidine mouthrinses may be valuable adjuncts to mechanical oral hygiene methods.[212–214] Alternative medications less likely to be associated with gingival enlargement may be prescribed by the patient's physician if seizure control can be maintained. While these approaches may decrease or eliminate the overgrowth, surgical correction is often required to restore acceptable tissue contour.[215,216] Other anticonvulsant agents that have been associated with gingival overgrowth include ethosuximide, mephenytoin, ethotoin, phenobarbital, and valproic acid.[217,218]

Cyclosporine

Cyclosporine is an immunosuppressant drug used extensively by organ and bone marrow transplant recipients and for a variety of other systemic diseases. It has selective inhibitory effects on T lymphocytes. It also suppresses interleukin 2 and calcineurin activity and has been shown to increase expression of transforming growth factor β. Adverse effects include nephrotoxicity, neurotoxicity, hepatotoxicity, hypertrichosis, and gingival overgrowth.[219] Associated gingival enlargement was first reported in 1983 and occurs in approximately 8% to 70% of patients taking the medication, with an overall incidence of approximately 25%.[202,220–223] Cyclosporine is often used in combination with calcium channel antagonists, such as nifedipine. The combined use of cyclosporine with nifedipine has been suggested to produce greater gingival overgrowth than the use of each drug alone.[224]

Clinically and histologically, cyclosporine-induced gingival enlargement resembles that associated with phenytoin. It affects the interproximal papillae initially, resulting in lobulations that disfigure the marginal gingiva and interfere with normal function.[225–227] The altered tissues are influenced by plaque-associated inflammation and can make oral hygiene maintenance difficult, if not impossible. Gingival enlargement is more common anteriorly than posteriorly and usually affects labial surfaces.[225] Although a threshold dose of cyclosporine necessary to trigger gingival enlargement no doubt exists, efforts to relate dosage and blood levels of the drug in patients with and without gingival enlargement have failed to establish a predictable relationship.[228] Cyclosporine-induced gingival enlargement does not seem to affect tissues in edentulous areas.[221] Patients receiving cyclosporine therapy may be at increased risk of developing Kaposi sarcoma and squamous cell carcinoma.[229,230]

Histologically, affected tissues reveal an abundance of amorphous connective tissue substance without a significant increase in the numerical density of fibroblasts.[231] The connective tissue is often highly vascularized, exhibits inflammatory cell infiltration, and manifests deeply penetrating epithelial ridges.[232]

Treatment of cyclosporine-induced gingival enlargement is extremely challenging. Patients receiving the medication are often medically compromised, and consultation with the patient's physician is required to ensure safe and effective management. Treatment consists of a multiphasic approach combining mechanical and chemical plaque control, scaling and root planing, and surgical reduction of residual tissue enlargement.[216] The patient must be advised of the likelihood of recurrence of the gingival overgrowth following treatment. Periodontal maintenance and recall on a regular basis (eg, every 3 months) are extremely important in these patients. If possible, the physician should consider selection of an alternative immunosuppressant drug.[233] Withdrawal of the drug may not be possible, however, because it is usually essential to patient survival.

Calcium Channel Antagonists

Calcium channel antagonists have gained widespread use in the treatment of cardiovascular diseases. This drug class consists of the dihydropyridines (eg, felodipine, nitrendipine, isradipine, nifedipine, nicardipine, and amlodipine), benzothiazine derivatives (eg, diltiazem), and phenylalkylamine derivatives (eg, verapamil). These agents have proven extremely effective in the management of hypertension, angina pectoris, and cardiac arrhythmias by antagonism of the slow calcium channels in the cell membrane.[201,234]

A principal concern to the practitioner is the gingival overgrowth that may accompany the use of most of these agents. Nifedipine is most often implicated in gingival overgrowth, with initial associations being reported in 1984.[235] Although the overgrowth may be generalized, the most dramatic changes affect the anterior gingiva.[236–239] Incidence data suggest that some degree of associated gingival overgrowth will develop in 10% to 20% of patients taking nifedipine.[221,234,236,240,241] While the occurrence does not appear to be dose related, discontinuation of the medication has been associated with improvement of the gingival overgrowth[242]; however, the patient must be advised that this response is not always predictable.[238]

Gingival Enlargement Unrelated to Drugs or Medications

Leukemia. Practitioners should be aware that the gingival tissues may be affected in patients with leukemia. Leukemia is a generalized neoplastic disorder of the blood-forming tissues, primarily those of the leukocyte series.[257] Leukemias may be categorized based on cell type (granulocytes, monocytes, and lymphocytes) and course of the disease (acute or chronic). The most common leukemia is the chronic lymphocytic form. Regardless of type, impaired marrow function is often accompanied by anemia, thrombocytopenia, and increased susceptibility to infection.[258]

Gingival enlargement has been reported in 10% of patients with chronic forms and 36% of patients with acute forms of leukemia.[259] Of patients with leukemia examined during the course of their disease, 65% had some oral signs or symptoms.[260] Clinically, the enlargement is usually generalized[259]; histologically, it is a combination of inflammation and infiltration by the leukemic cells.[261] Leukemic infiltration is more often associated with the acute monocytic form, but infiltration may accompany other forms of the disease.[262,263] Gingival bleeding is common in patients with leukemia.[260]

Compromised host defense may lead to infection, a problem often associated with the patient's resident flora. Dental treatment should be carefully coordinated with the patient's physician. Courses of chemotherapy must be considered, and oral care must emphasize prevention, which may incorporate mechanical plaque control and adjunctive antimicrobial rinses (eg, chlorhexidine).[264] Where possible, oral sources of infection should be eliminated prior to chemotherapy in acute leukemia.[265] Incipient periodontal disease should be treated and any surgical treatment planned during remission of the disease, using antibiotic coverage. Oral infection should be actively and aggressively treated in these patients.[264] Once again, staged periodontal maintenance and recall are extremely important.

Multisystem syndromes. Gingival fibromatosis has been observed in association with a variety of conditions, including mental retardation, epilepsy, deafness, stunted growth, and hypertrichosis.[266–270] This condition may be generalized or localized. Gingival fibromatosis has also been reported with soft tissue and skeletal anomalies, as well as splenomegaly, described as Laband syndrome.[267,268] This gingival enlargement has also been associated with other conditions, including Cowden syndrome, Rutherfurd syndrome, and Murray-Puretic-Descher syndrome (juvenile hyaline fibromatosis).[270] Histologically, hyperplasia of mature collagenous connective tissue predominates. Treatment consists of surgical correction that is complemented by an effective program of oral hygiene. Despite treatment, there is no assurance that the gingival enlargement will not recur.

The practitioner may encounter gingival fibromatosis as part of a multisystem syndrome, but these disorders are rare. The cause of this gingival enlargement is unknown.

Histologic observations of nifedipine-associated gingival overgrowth tissues are consistent with those reported with phenytoin.[202,243,244] Ultrastructural studies indicate that these drug-associated gingival enlargements may be the result of increased ground substance production by activated fibroblasts.[202,218,239]

Treatment is initially directed toward effective plaque control (mechanical and chemical), since plaque-associated inflammation characteristically accompanies the nifedipine-induced gingival enlargement. These efforts may be combined with scaling and root planing to help reduce the severity of the gingival response.[245–247] Surgical reduction is usually required to correct the gingival deformity, and the patient should be advised of the tendency for recurrence. Supportive periodontal treatment and monitoring of the gingival tissues are essential for these patients.

As previously noted, other calcium channel antagonists have been associated with gingival enlargement. These include verapamil,[234,248] nitrendipine,[249] diltiazem,[241,242,250,251] felodipine,[252] isradipine,[253] nimodipine,[206] nisoldipine,[206] and oxodipine.[252] At least one report has suggested that the extent of the gingival overgrowth may be reduced in patients switching to isradipine.[254]

Cannabis

Excessive use of marijuana has been associated with gingival enlargement. This may resemble other forms of drug-induced overgrowth and may be accompanied by gingivitis and alveolar bone loss. As with other drug-associated gingival enlargement, the causative mechanism is unknown.[255]

Erythromycin

A single report in the literature has identified a patient with gingival enlargement while using the macrolide antibiotic erythromycin. The case involved a 6-year-old boy who presented with gingival overgrowth and itching of the oral tissues. The enlargement began within a week after he began taking erythromycin for treatment of tonsillitis. The enlargement involved the anterior gingiva, as well as palatal and lingual gingiva. After he stopped taking the erythromycin, the condition cleared in few weeks. The patient was rechallenged with erythromycin, and the gingival overgrowth recurred.[256]

Abnormal Pigmentation

A number of chemicals and diseases may induce unusual pigmentation in the oral cavity. Implicated drugs include minocycline (Minocin), bismuth, conjugated estrogens (Premarin), antimalarials (hydroxychloroquine), zidovudine (azidothymidine, or AZT), phenothiazines, gold salts,

and anticancer drugs (doxorubicin, busulfan, and cisplatin).[271] More recently, clofazimine and ketoconazole have been associated with pigmentation.[272] Drug-induced pigmentation must be distinguished from various syndromes accompanied by oral pigmentation, including Addison disease, Peutz-Jeghers syndrome, melanoma, neurofibromatosis, hemochromatosis, metallic pigmentation (amalgam tattoo), pituitary adenoma, and gingival melanosis.[271]

Minocycline may induce a gray-blue-black pigmentation of alveolar mucosa and attached gingiva, a dark gray-green discoloration of bone, and a blue-gray discoloration of the skin, particularly in areas of scarring and inflammation.[273] Bismuth produces a gray discoloration at the mucogingival line and a gray skin color.[274] Conjugated estrogens may induce dark brown melanin macules in the mucosal surfaces of the lips, cheeks, and floor of the mouth[271]; antimalarials cause a blue-gray pigmentation of the gingiva[275]; and zidovudine induces hyperpigmented macules in the soft palate, gingiva, lips, tongue, and torso.[276]

Oral Mucosal Lesions

Stevens-Johnson syndrome (SJS), erythema multiforme (EM), and toxic epidermal necrolysis (TEN) are related mucocutaneous disorders characterized by purulent conjunctivitis, bullae and vesicles of the skin and mucous membranes with the presence of Nikolsky sign (separation of the epidermis from the dermis), and a sheetlike loss of the epidermis in severe cases of SJS and TEN.[277,278] Fortunately, all three diseases are rare, with an incidence of 1.2 cases per million persons per year for TEN and 2.6 to 7.1 cases per million persons per year for SJS.[277] Only 10% of EM cases are associated with drug use (it is more common with herpes or mycoplasma infections), in contrast to 50% of SJS cases and 95% of TEN cases.[277,278] More than 100 different drugs have been potentially implicated in the causation of these three disorders, the most common drugs being the sulfonamides, antiepileptics (phenytoin, carbamazepine), barbiturates, nonsteroidal anti-inflammatory drugs (NSAIDs), and aminopenicillins; cephalexin, quinolones, and vancomycin are less often involved.[278]

Oral drug-induced lichenoid lesions have been associated with mercury in dental amalgam and methylmethacrylate denture materials.[279] Many drugs, including methyldopa (Aldomet), gold salts, diuretics, nystatin, ketoconazole, penicillamine, angiotensin-converting enzyme (ACE) inhibitors, sulfonylurea antidiabetic agents, cefaclor, and the NSAIDs may induce nonspecific oral ulcerations.[280–282] The ACE inhibitors (captopril, enalapril, and lisinopril) may cause painful, burning tongue (glossodynia or glossopyrosis) and facial angioedema.[283,284] Corticosteroid inhalers may induce oral vesicles and ulcers, as well as angina bullosa hemorrhagica (benign subepithelial blood-filled vesicles).[285,286] Nicorandil (currently not available in the United States) has been reported to cause severe oral ulcerations. It belongs to a new class of drugs, identified as potassium channel activators, for use in the treatment of angina pectoris.[287] Drugs are apparently not a common cause of burning mouth syndrome except as a sign of contact allergy to dental materials or when xerostomia exacerbates the condition.[288]

Dental Materials Allergy

Contact lesions of the oral mucosa (analogous to contact dermatitis of the skin) caused by allergy to dental amalgam—principally its mercury component—are very rare, with an estimated incidence in a general population of 0.04% to 0.00001%, with 27 case reports in the literature as of 1984.[289,290] The rate of allergy to mercury in the general population is estimated to be 3.2% to 4.9%. Most amalgam reactions are Gell-Coombs type IV delayed contact dermatitis allergic reactions; type I (immunoglobulin E–mediated) acute allergic reactions are very rare.[289]

Allergic reactions to amalgam are manifested as erythematous, eczema-like lesions resembling lichen planus (12% to 62% of persons with lichen planus are allergic to mercury).[289,291] Lesions are located near freshly placed or corroded amalgam restorations.[292] These allergic symptoms may extend also to the face, neck, and trunk.[290] Skin patch tests are useful in determining the particular metal allergy, because the tin, copper, zinc, and silver in dental amalgam may also be allergenic.[289] These amalgam reactions are self-limiting and resolve within 2 to 3 weeks after removal of the restoration.[293]

Mucosal contact lesions to the polymethyl methacrylate of denture materials are also rare, with 150 to 200 case reports in the literature from 1940 to 1980.[289] The symptoms are similar to those seen with dental amalgam: erythema, edema, and eczema-like lesions in prosthesis contact areas.[294–296]

Allergic Reactions to Dental Hygiene Products

There are increasing reports in the literature of oral mucosal reactions to new products for home care dental hygiene. These products include the newer formulations of toothpaste that claim to reduce tartar and gingivitis, with or without whitening agents. However, mouthrinses with sanguinarine, chlorhexidine, and essential oils have also been implicated. This reaction is usually manifested in the anterior oral mucosa but can include other tissues, such as the tongue and lip mucosa. Tissue response includes intraoral burning, erythematous tissues, cracked and pealing

lips, and angular cheilitis. Sloughing of the oral mucosa without pain, perhaps the most common reaction, may be the only sign.[198,296,297]

Specific chemical agents identified or suspected as being the potential allergen in these reactions include peppermint, spearmint,[298] and cinnamon flavors[198]; sodium lauryl sulfate[299]; anethole[300]; L-carvone[301]; hexylresorcinol; menthol; thymol; propolis; and azulene.[302] Reactions have been suggested to be the result of allergies or direct irritation and could be confused with desquamative gingival diseases. Histologic examination of tissues reveals a characteristic allergic reaction.[303]

Treatment includes carefully gathering a history of product use in relation to the onset of symptoms. When assessing the history, keep in mind that patients may be allergic to other products, such as cosmetics and foods. Patient discomfort can be managed with systemic antihistamines for the immediate period. The offending agent should be withdrawn immediately, and tissues will return to normal within a few days.[297]

Cancer Chemotherapy

Acute or chronic oral adverse reactions develop in approximately 40% of all cancer patients receiving chemotherapy; rates range from 12% of patients with carcinoma/sarcoma to 80% of those with leukemia.[304,305] The most common complaints following cancer chemotherapy are altered taste sensations and mucositis (a mucosal burning sensation accompanied by erythema, erosions, and ulcerations followed by xerostomia, bleeding, and infection).[304,306] Dental preoperative and postoperative care of such patients has recently been reviewed.[304]

Salivary Gland Disorders

Medications may affect the salivary glands in three ways: enlargement (usually inflammatory) of the gland (sialadenitis), increased salivary secretions (hypersalivation), and reduced salivary secretions (hyposalivation, xerostomia).

Enlargement of the salivary glands, particularly the parotid gland (parotitis), may be induced by various drugs, including nifedipine (Procardia), methyldopa (Aldomet), L-asparaginase, doxycycline, iodine (radiocontrast material), antipsychotic agents, H_2-receptor antagonists, nitrofurantoin (Furadantin), and propranolol (Inderal).[307–310] The mechanisms involved may include allergic reactions and inflammation leading to reduced salivary flow and xerostomia.[310] Parotid gland enlargement has also been reported in alcoholics and in cocaine/alcohol users who also have extensive masseter muscle enlargement from bruxism.[311,312]

Hypersalivation is seen with the use of clozapine (Clozaril), an atypical antipsychotic agent with anticholinergic actions,[313,314] which should induce hyposalivation. As many as 31% of patients receiving clozapine exhibit hypersalivation, which may be mediated through adrenergic mechanisms.[315]

More than 400 drugs have been implicated as causing hyposalivation or xerostomia,[316] with the majority possessing some anticholinergic activity. These anticholinergic drugs include, among others, atropine, diphenoxylate, antihypertensive agents, antipsychotic neuroleptics, antidepressants, antiparkinsonians, benzodiazepines, antihistamines, and diuretics.[316-318] As many as 74% of the drugs used in the elderly may induce xerostomia,[319] and the incidence of dry mouth in the elderly population is 16% to 28%, and 44% to 71% in those who are institutionalized.[317,320] This reduction in salivary flow has been associated with increased cervical and root caries, gingivitis, oral infections, decreased taste acuity and denture retention, mucosal erythema, soreness and burning, angular cheilosis, parotitis, candidiasis, and difficulties in speech and mastication.[317,321] Several excellent reviews are available on the treatment of patients with reduced salivation.[320,322]

Substance (Chemical) Abuse

The recognition and management of the chemically dependent patient[255,323] may be easy, difficult, or essentially impossible, depending on the state of deterioration of the individual and the magnitude of the denial associated with the chemical dependency. The patient with chronic alcoholic deterioration is easy to identify, but the early cocaine abuser may readily escape detection.

Some general characteristics of substance abuse are general health neglect, poor oral hygiene, advanced caries and periodontal disease, xerostomia, bruxism, reduced tolerance to pain, an inordinate fear of needles, a history of hepatitis and/or AIDS, and a low-grade septicemia (from intravenous injections).[323] The dental caries pattern in opioid-dependent individuals tends to be localized on the labial or buccal aspects of the teeth rather than interproximally.[324] Diffuse gingival hyperplasia, extensive caries and periodontal disease, and increased carriage of *Candida albicans* have been ascribed to marijuana (cannabis) use.[255,324-326]

The oral manifestations of cocaine abuse include xerostomia, bruxism, temporomandibular joint/myofascial pain disorders, cervical tooth abrasion from pathological brushing, angular cheilosis, glossodynia (painful tongue), and gingival lacerations.[255,324,327,328] An unusual case of generalized dental erosion on the facial/buccal aspects of the teeth both coronally and cervically has been described in cocaine abuse.[329] In the mistaken belief that the practice is harmless, people have rubbed cocaine into the gingival tissues, resulting in vasculitis, ulceration, and necrosis resembling necrotizing ulcerative gingivitis or herpetic gingivostomatitis.[328,330-332]

Detection of the chemically dependent patient is important, as many of these individuals have significant health problems that can affect dental treatment. In the cocaine-dependent patient, coronary artery spasm, myocardial infarction, and stroke may occur without warning, even in young and apparently otherwise healthy individuals.[323,327,333]

References

1. Löe H. Periodontal disease as we approach the year 2000. J Periodontol 1994;65(suppl):464–467.
2. Beck J. Methods of assessing risk for periodontitis and developing multifactorial models. J Periodontol 1994;65(suppl):468–478.
3. Michalowicz B. Genetic and heritable risk factors in periodontal disease. J Periodontol 1994;65(suppl):479–488.
4. Cutler C, Wasfy M, Ghaffar K, et al. Impaired bactericidal activity of PMN from two brothers with necrotizing ulcerative gingivo-periodontitis. J Periodontol 1994;65:357–363.
5. Ishikawa I, Umeda M, Laosrisin N. Clinical, bacteriological, and immunological examinations and the treatment process of two Papillon-Lefevre syndrome patients. J Periodontol 1994;65: 364–371.
6. Katsuragi K, Takashiba S, Kurihara H, Murayama Y. Molecular basis of leukocyte adhesion molecules in early-onset periodontitis patients with decreased CD11/CD18 expression on leukocytes. J Periodontol 1994;65:949–957.
7. Lehner T. Immunoglobulin abnormalities in ulcerative gingivitis. Br Dent J 1969;127:165–169.
8. Hernichel-Gorbach E, Kornman K, Holt S, et al. Host responses in patients with generalized refractory periodontitis. J Periodontol 1994;65:8–16.
9. Seymour G. Importance of the host response in the periodontium. J Clin Periodontol 1991;18:421–426.
10. Hart T, Shapira L, Van Dyke T. Neutrophil defects as risk factors for periodontal diseases. J Periodontol 1994;65:521–529.
11. Wheeler T, McArthur W, Magnusson I, et al. Modeling the relationship between clinical, microbiologic and immunologic parameters and alveolar bone levels in an elderly population. J Periodontol 1994;65:68–78.
12. Loesche W. Periodontal disease as a risk factor for heart disease. Compend Contin Educ Dent 1994;15:976–991.
13. Landa J. Psychosomatics in relation to periodontics. J Periodontol 1954;25:209–215.
14. Selye H. A syndrome produced by diverse noctious agents. Nature 1936;138:32.
15. Selye H. What is stress? Metabolism 1956;5:525–530.
16. Gupta O. Psychosomatic factors in periodontal disease. Dent Clin North Am 1966;Mar:11–19.
17. Pennell BM, Keagle JG. Predisposing factors in the etiology of chronic inflammatory periodontal disease. J Periodontol 1977; 48:517–532.
18. Gupta O. Psychosomatic factors in periodontal disease. J Indian Dent Assoc 1968;40:101–107.
19. Dean MT, Dean RD. Gingival symptom complexes. Am J Orthodontol Oral Surg 1945;31:473–486.

20. Ballieux R. Impact of mental stress on the immune response. J Clin Periodontol 1991;18:427–430.
21. Breivik T, Sluyter R, Hof M, Cools A. Differential susceptibility to periodontitis in genetically selected Wistar rat lines that differ in their behavioral and endocrinological response to stressors. Behav Genet 2000;30:123–130.
22. Shapira L, Frolov I, Halabi A, Ben-Nathan D. Experimental stress suppresses recruitment of macrophages but enhanced their *P. gingivalis* LPS-stimulated secretion of nitric oxide. J Periodontol 2000;71:476–481.
23. Deinzer R, Kottmann W, Forster P, et al. After-effects of stress on crevicular interleukin-1beta. J Clin Periodontol 2000;27:74–77.
24. Freeman R, Goss S. Stress measures as predictors of periodontal disease—A preliminary communication. Community Dent Oral Epidemiol 1993;21:176–177.
25. Green L, Tryon WB, Huryn J. Periodontal disease as a function of life events stress. J Human Stress 1986;12:32–36.
26. Haskell B. Association of aircraft noise stress to periodontal disease in aircrew members. Aviat Space Environ Med 1975;46:1041–1043.
27. Genco RJ, Ho AW, Grossi SG, et al. Relationship of stress, distress and inadequate coping behaviors to periodontal disease. J Periodontol 1999;70:711–723.
28. Lamey PJ, Linden GJ, Freeman R. Mental disorders and periodontics. Periodontol 2000 1998;18:71–80.
29. Manhold J. Report of a study on the relationship of personality variables to periodontal conditions. J Periodontol 1953;24:248–251.
30. Miller S, Thaller J, Soberman A. The use of the Minnesota multiphasic personality inventory as a diagnostic aid in periodontal disease—Preliminary report. J Periodontol 1956;27:44–46.
31. Formicola A, Witte E, Curran P. A study of personality traits and acute necrotizing ulcerative gingivitis. J Periodontol 1970;41:36–38.
32. Baker E, Crook G, Schwabacher E. Personality correlates of periodontal disease. J Dent Res 1961;40:396–403.
33. Friedlander A, West L. Dental management of the patient with major depression. Oral Surg Oral Med Oral Pathol 1991;71:573–578.
34. Cohen-Cole S, Cogen R, Stevens J, et al. Psychiatric, psychosocial, and endocrine correlates of acute necrotizing ulcerative gingivitis (trench mouth): A preliminary report. Psychiatr Med 1983;1:215–220.
35. De Marco T. Periodontal emotional stress syndrome. J Periodontol 1976;47:67–68.
36. Riley V. Psychoneuroendocrine influences on immunocompetence and neoplasia. Science 1981;212:1100–1109.
37. Gupta O, Blechman H, Stahl S. Effects of stress on the periodontal tissues of young adult male rats and hamsters. J Periodontol 1960;31:413–417.
38. Shklar G. Periodontal disease in experimental animals subjected to chronic cold stress. J Periodontol 1966;37:377–383.
39. Cohen M, Shusterman S, Shklar G. The effect of stressor agents on the gray lethal mouse strain periodontium. J Periodontol 1969;40:462–466.
40. Ratcliff P. The relationship of the general adaptation syndrome to the periodontal tissues in the rat. J Periodontol 1956;27:40–43.
41. Stahl S. Healing gingival injury in normal systemically stressed young adult male rats. J Periodontol 1961;32:63–73.
42. Rowland RW. Necrotizing ulcerative gingivitis. Ann Periodontol 1999;4:65–73.
43. Murayama Y, Kurihara H, Nagai A, et al. Acute necrotizing ulcerative gingivitis: Risk factors involving host defense mechanisms. Periodontol 2000 1994;6:116–124.
44. Giddon D, Goldhaber P, Dunning J. Prevalence of reported cases of acute necrotizing ulcerative gingivitis in a university population. J Periodontol 1963;34:366–371.
45. Schluger S. Osseous resection—A basic principle in periodontal surgery. Oral Surg Oral Med Oral Pathol 1949;2:316–325.
46. Pindborg J. Influence of service in the armed forces on incidence of gingivitis. J Am Dent Assoc 1951;42:517–522.
47. Grupe H, Wilder L. Observations of necrotizing gingivitis in 870 military trainees. J Periodontol 1956;45:255–266.
48. Davis R, Baer P. Necrotizing ulcerative gingivitis in drug addict patients being withdrawn from drugs. Oral Surg Oral Med Oral Pathol 1971;31:200–204.
49. Shannon I, Kilgoe W, O'Leary T. Stress as a predisposing factor in necrotizing ulcerative gingivitis. J Periodontol 1969;40:240–242.
50. Maupin C, Bell B. Relationship of 17-hydroxycorticosteroid to acute necrotizing ulcerative gingivitis. J Periodontol 1975;46:721–722.
51. Shepherd S, Sims T, Johnson B, Hershman J. Assessment of stress during periodontal surgery with intravenous sedation and with local anesthesia only. J Periodontol 1988;59:147–154.
52. Cogen R, Stevens AW Jr, Cohen-Cole S, et al. Leukocyte function in the etiology of acute necrotizing ulcerative gingivitis. J Periodontol 1983;54:402–407.
53. Rees T. Oral effects of drug abuse. Crit Rev Oral Biol Med 1992;3:163–184.
54. Wilton J, Griffiths G, Curtis M, et al. Detection of high-risk groups and individuals for periodontal diseases. J Clin Periodontol 1988;15:339–346.
55. Johnson B, Engel D. Acute necrotizing ulcerative gingivitis: A review of diagnosis, etiology and treatment. J Periodontol 1986;57:141–149.
56. Sabiston CB Jr. A review and proposal for the etiology of acute necrotizing gingivitis. J Clin Periodontol 1986;13:727–734.
57. Enwonwu C. Epidemiological and biochemical studies of necrotizing ulcerative gingivitis and noma (cancrum oris) in Nigerian children. Arch Oral Biol 1972;17:1357–1371.
58. Pindborg J, Bhat M, Roed-Petersen B. Oral changes in south Indian children with severe protein deficiency. J Periodontol 1967;38:218–221.
59. Charbeneau T, Hurt W. Gingival findings in spontaneous scurvy: A case report. J Periodontol 1983;53:694–697.
60. The Alpha-Tocopherol BCCPSG. The effect of vitamin E and beta carotene on the incidence of lung cancer and other cancers in male smokers. New Engl J Med 1994;330:1029–1035.
61. Hennekens C, Buring J. Antioxidant vitamins—Benefits not yet proved. New Engl J Med 1994;330:1080–1081.
62. Toufexis A. New scoop on vitamins. Time 1992 Apr 6:36.
63. Rees T. Systemic factors in periodontal disease. In: Newman H, Rees T, Kinane D (eds). Diseases of the Periodontium. Northwood, England: Science Reviews, 1993.
64. Rees T. Oral effects of drug abuse. Crit Rev Oral Biol Med 1992;3:163–184.
65. Speirs R, Beeley J. Food and oral health, II. Periodontium and oral mucosa. Dent Update 1992;19:161–167.
66. Touyz LZ. Oral scurvy and periodontal disease. J Can Dent Assoc 1997;63:837–845.
67. Abrams RG, Romberg E. Gingivitis in children with malnutrition. J Clin Periodontol 1999;23:189–194.

68. O'Leary T, Rudd K, Crump P, Krause R. The effect of ascorbic acid supplementation on tooth mobility. J Periodontol 1969;40:284–286.

69. Eklund S, Burt B. Risk factors for total tooth loss in the United States: Longitudinal analysis of national data. J Public Health Dent 1994;54:5–14.

70. Alfano M. Controversies, perspectives, and clinical implications of nutrition in periodontal disease. Dent Clin North Am 1976;20:519–548.

71. Nizel A. Role of nutrition in the oral health of the aging patient. Dent Clin North Am 1976;20:569–584.

72. Navia J, Menaker L. Nutritional implications in wound healing. Dent Clin North Am 1976;20:549–567.

73. Miglani D. The effect of vitamin A deficiency on the periodontal structures of rat molars, with emphasis on cementum resorption. Oral Surg Oral Med Oral Pathol 1954;12:1372–1376.

74. Dreizen S, Levy B, Bernick S. Studies on the biology of the periodontium of marmosets, XI. Histopathologic manifestations of spontaneous and induced vitamin A deficiency in the oral structures of adult marmosets. J Dent Res 1973;52:803–809.

75. Ferguson M. Nutritional disorders. In: Jones J, Mason D (eds). Oral Manifestations of Systemic Disease. London: Brailliere Tindall, 1990:300–310.

76. Mitchell K, Ferguson M, Lucie N, MacDonald D. Epithelial dysplasia in the oral mucosa associated with pernicious anemia. Br Dent J 1986;161:259–260.

77. Theaker J, Porter S, Fleming K. Oral epithelial dysplasia in vitamin B12 deficiency. Oral Surg Oral Med Oral Pathol 1989;67:81–83.

78. Vogel R, Fink R, Schneider L, et al. The effect of folic acid in gingival health. J Periodontol 1976;47:667–668.

79. Brown R, DiaStanislau P, Beaver W, Bottomley W. The administration of folic acid to institutionalized epileptic adults with phenytoin-induced gingival hyperplasia. Oral Surg Oral Med Oral Pathol 1991;71:565–568.

80. Poppell T, Keeling S, Collins J, Hassell T. Effect of folic acid on recurrence of phenytoin-induced gingival overgrowth following gingivectomy. J Clin Periodontol 1991;18:134–139.

81. Vogel R, Lamster I, Wechsler S, et al. The effects of megadoses of ascorbic acid on PMN chemotaxis and experimental gingivitis. J Periodontol 1986;57:472–479.

82. Leggott P, Robertson P, Rothman D, et al. The effect of controlled ascorbic acid depletion and supplementation on periodontal health. J Periodontol 1986;57:480–485.

83. Dreizen S, Levy B, Bernick S. Studies on the biology of the periodontium of marmosets. J Periodontal Res 1969;4:274–280.

84. Ismail A, Burt A, Eklund S. Relation between ascorbic acid intake and periodontal disease in the United States. J Am Dent Assoc 1983;107:927–931.

85. Nishida M, Grossi SG, Dunford RG, et al. Dietary vitamin C and the risk for periodontal disease. J Periodontol 2000;71:1215–1223.

86. Laufer D, Benderly A, Hochberg Z. Dental pathology in calcitriol resistant rickets. J Oral Med 1987;42:272–275.

87. Weinmann J, Schour I. Experimental studies in calcification: Effect of rachitogenic diet on dental tissues of white rats. Am J Pathol 1945;21:821–831.

88. Bissada N, Demarco J. The effect of a hypocalcemic diet on the periodontal structure of the adult rat. J Periodontol 1974;45:739–745.

89. Nishida M, Grossi SG, Dunford RG, et al. Calcium and the risk for periodontal disease. J Periodontol 2000;71:1057–1066.

90. Kanis J. Calcium nutrition and its implications for osteoporosis, I. Children and healthy adults. Eur J Clin Nutr 1994;48:757–767.

91. Payne JB, Reinhardt RA, Nummikoski PV, Patil KD. Longitudinal alveolar bone loss in postmenopausal osteoporotic/osteopenic women. Osteoporos Int 1999;10:34–40.

92. Payne JB, Zachs NR, Reinhardt RA, et al. The association between estrogen status and alveolar bone density changes in postmenopausal women with a history of periodontitis. J Periodontol 1997;68:24–31.

93. Birkenfeld L, Yemini M, Dase NG, Birkenfeld A. Menopause-related oral alveolar bone resorption: A review of relatively unexplored consequences of estrogen deficiency. Menopause 1999;6;129–133.

94. Johnson RB, Gilbert JA, Cooper RC, et al. Alveolar bone loss one year following ovariectomy in sheep. J Periodontol 1997;68:846–871.

95. Tezal M, Wactawski-Wende J, Grossi SG, et al. The relationship between bone mineral density and periodontitis in postmenopausal women. J Periodontol 2000;71:1492–1498.

96. Reinhardt RA, Payne JB, Maze CA, et al. Influence of estrogen and osteopenia/osteoporosis on clinical periodontitis in postmenopausal women. J Periodontol 1999;70:823–828.

97. Hildebolt CF, Pilgram TK, Yokoyama-Crothers N, et al. Alveolar bone height and postcranial bone mineral density: Negative effects of cigarette smoking and parity. J Periodontol 2000;71:683–689.

98. Zachariasen R. Oral manifestations of metabolic bone disease: Vitamin D and osteoporosis. Compend Contin Educ Dent 1990;11:612–618.

99. Taguchi A, Suei Y, Ohtsuka M, et al. Relationship between bone mineral density and tooth loss in elderly Japanese women. Dentomaxillofac Radiol 1999;28:219–223.

100. Bando K, Nitta H, Matsubara M, Kshikawa I. Bone mineral density in periodontally healthy and edentulous postmenopausal women. Ann Periodontol 1998;3:322–326.

101. Streckfus CF, Johnson RB, Nick T, et al. Comparison of alveolar bone loss, alveolar bone density and second metacarpal bone density, salivary and gingival crevicular fluid interleukin-6 concentrations in healthy premenopausal and postmenopausal women on estrogen therapy. J Gerontol A Biol Sci Med Sci 1997;52:M343–M351.

102. Krall EA, Garcia RI, Bawson-Hughes B. Increased risk of tooth loss is related to bone loss at the whole body, hip, and spine. Calcif Tissue Int 1996;59:433–437.

103. Grodstein F, Colditz GA, Stampfer MJ. Post-menopausal hormone use and tooth loss: A prospective study. J Am Dent Assoc 1996;127:370–377.

104. Agren M, Stromberg H, Rindby A, Hallmans G. Selenium, zinc, iron and copper levels in serum of patients with arterial and venous leg ulcers. Acta Derm Venereol 1986;66:237–240.

105. Hansen M, Fernandes G, Good R. Nutrition and immunity: The influence of diet on autoimmunity and the role of zinc in the immune response. Annu Rev Nutr 1982;2:151–177.

106. Joseph C, Ashrafi S, Steinberg A, Waterhouse J. Zinc deficiency changes in the permeability of rabbit periodontium to c-phenytoin and c-albumin. J Periodontol 1981;53:251–256.

107. Williamson C, Yukna R, Gandor D. Zinc concentration in normal and healing gingival tissues in beagle dogs. J Periodontol 1984;55:170–174.

108. Frandsen A, Becks H, Nelson M, Evans H. The effects of various levels of dietary protein on the periodontal tissues of young rats. J Periodontol 1953;24:135–142.

109. Stahl S. The healing of experimentally induced gingival wounds in rats on prolonged nutritional deprivation. J Periodontol 1965;36:283–287.

110. Cheraskin E, Ringsdorf WM Jr, Setyaadmadija A, Ray D. An ecologic analysis of tooth mobility: Effect of prophylaxis and protein supplementation. J Periodontol 1967;38:227–236.

111. Cheraskin E, Ringsdorf WM Jr, Setyaadmadija A, Barrett R. An ecologic analysis of gingival state: Effect of prophylaxis and protein supplementation. J Periodontol 1968;39:316–321.

112. Garewal H, Meyskens JF, Friedman S, et al. Oral cancer prevention: The case for carotenoids and anti-oxidant nutrients. Prev Med 1993;22:701–711.

113. Kaugers G, Silverman S Jr, Lovas J, et al. A review of the use of antioxidant supplements in the treatment of human oral leukoplakia. J Cell Biochem 1993;suppl 17F:292–298.

114. Jacoby B, Davis W. The electron microscopic immunolocalization of a copper-zinc superoxide dismutase in association with collagen fibers of periodontal soft tissues. J Periodontol 1991;62:413–430.

115. Asman B, Wijkander P, Hjerpe A. Reduction of collagen degradation in experimental granulation tissue by vitamin E and selenium. J Clin Periodontol 1994;21:45–47.

116. de Menezes A, Costa I, El-Guindy M. Clinical manifestations of hypervitaminosis A in human gingiva: A case report. J Periodontol 1984;55:474–476.

117. Toxic effects of vitamin overdosage. Med Letter 1984;26:73–74.

118. Rhodus N. Zinc, impaired immunity and oral disease in the geriatric patient. Gerodontology 1987;3:141–145.

119. Ackerman Z, Seidenbaum M, Loewenthal E, Rubinow A. Overload of iron in the skin of patients with varicose ulcers. Arch Dermatol 1988;124:1376–1378.

120. Burnett J. Cutaneous abnormalities induced by aluminum, iron and silica. Cutis 1991;47:391–392.

121. Mofenson H, Caraccio T, Sharieff N. Iron sepsis: *Yersinia enterocolitica* septicemia possibly caused by an overdose of iron. New Engl J Med 1987;316:1092–1093.

122. Brock J. Iron and the outcome of infection. Br Med J 1986;293:518–520.

123. Warnock GR, Correll RW, Schorn V. Multiple asymptomatic yellowish-white nodules on the free ginviva. J Am Dent Assoc 1987;114:367–368.

124. Loesche W, Karapetow F, Pohl A, Kocher T. Plasma lipid and blood glucose levels in patients with destructive periodontal disease. J Clin Periodontol 2000;27:537–541.

125. Noack B, Jachmann I, Roscher S, et al. Metabolic diseases and their possible link to risk indicators of periodontitis. J Periodontol 2000;71:898–903.

126. Cutler CW, Shinedling EA, Nunn M, et al. Association between periodontitis and hyperlipidemia: Cause or effect? J Periodontol 1999;70:1429–1434.

127. Cutler CW, Machen RL, Jotwani R, Iacopino AM. Heightened gingival inflammation and attachment loss in type 2 diabetics with hyperlipidemia. J Periodontol 1999;70:1313–1321.

128. Iacopino AM. Diabetic periodontitis: Possible lipid-induced defect in tissue repair through alternation of macrophage phenotype and function. Oral Dis 1995;1:214–229.

129. Greenspan D, Canchola AJ, MacPhail LA, et al. Effect of highly active antiretroviral therapy on frequency of oral warts. Lancet 2001;357:1411–1412.

130. Patton LL. Sensitivity, specificity, and positive predictive value of oral opportunistic infections in adults with HIV/AIDS as markers of immune suppression and viral burden. Oral Surg Oral Med Oral Pathol Oral Radiol Endod 2000;90:182–188.

131. Scully C, Laskaris G, Pindborg J, et al. Oral manifestations of HIV infection and their management, I. More common lesions. Oral Surg Oral Med Oral Pathol 1991;71:158–166.

132. Scully C, Laskaris G, Pindborg J, et al. Oral manifestations of HIV infection and their management, II. Less common lesions. Oral Surg Oral Med Oral Pathol 1991;71:167–171.

133. Greenspan JS, Barr CE, Sciubba JJ, et al. Oral manifestations of HIV infection: Definitions, diagnostic criteria and principles of therapy. Oral Surg Oral Med Oral Pathol 1992;73:142–144.

134. EEC Clearinghouse on Oral Problems Related to HIV Infection and WHO Collaborating Centre on Oral Manifestations of the Human Immunodeficiency Virus: Classification and diagnostic criteria for oral lesions in HIV infection. J Oral Pathol Med 1993;22:289–291.

135. Glick M. Dental Management of Patients with HIV. Chicago: Quintessence, 1994.

136. Winkler JR, Murray PA. Periodontal disease: A potential intra-oral expression of AIDS may be rapidly progressive periodontitis. J Calif Dent Assoc 1987;15:20–24.

137. Winkler JR, Grassi M, Murray PA. Clinical description and etiology of HIV-associated periodontal disease. In: Robertson PB, Greenspan JS (eds). Perspectives on Oral Manifestations of AIDS. Littleton, MA: PSG, 1988:119–130.

138. Winkler JR, Murray PA, Hammerle C. Gangrenous stomatitis in AIDS. Lancet 1989;2:108.

139. Williams CA, Winkler JR, Grassi M, Murray PA. HIV-associated periodontitis complicated with necrotizing stomatitis. Oral Surg Oral Med Oral Pathol 1990;69:351–355.

140. Jones AC, Gulley ML, Freedman PD. Necrotizing ulcerative stomatitis in human immunodeficiency virus-seropositive individuals: A review of the histopathologic, immunohistochemical, and virologic characteristics of 18 cases. Oral Surg Oral Med Oral Pathol Oral Radiol Endod 2000;89:323–332.

141. Robinson PG. Periodontal diseases and HIV infection: A review of the literature. J Clin Periodontol 1992;119:609–614.

142. Robinson PG, Winkler JR, Palmer G, et al. The diagnosis of periodontal conditions associated with HIV infection. J Periodontol 1994;65:236–243.

143. Glick M, Garfunkel AA. Common oral findings in two different diseases—Leukemia and AIDS, I. Compend Contin Educ Dent 1992;13:432–450.

144. Garfunkel AA, Glick M. Common oral findings in two different diseases—Leukemia and AIDS, II. Compend Contin Educ Dent 1992;13:550–562.

145. Armitage GC. Development of a classification system for periodontal diseases and conditions. Ann Periodontol 1999;4:1–6.

146. Robinson PG. Which periodontal changes are associated with HIV infection? J Clin Periodontol 1998;25:278–285.

147. Drinkard CR, Decker L, Little JW, et al. Periodontal status of individuals in early stages of human immunodeficiency virus infection. Community Dent Oral Epidemiol 1991;19:97–100.

148. Friedman RB, Gunsolley J, Gentry A, et al. Periodontal status of HIV-seropositive and AIDS patients. J Periodontol 1991;62:623–627.

149. Grbic JT, Mitchell-Lewis DA, Fine JB, et al. The relationship of candidiasis to linear gingival erythema in HIV-infected homosexual men and parenteral drug users. J Periodontol 1995;66:30–37.

150. Robinson PG, Boulter A, Birnbaum W, Johnson NW. A controlled study of relative periodontal attachment loss in people with HIV infection. J Clin Periodontol 2000;27:273–276.

151. McKaig RG, Thomas JC, Patton LL, et al. Prevalence of HIV-associated periodontitis and chronic periodontitis in a southeastern US study group. J Public Health Dent 1998;58:294–300.

152. Laskaris G, Hadjivassiliou M, Stratigos J. Oral signs and symptoms in 160 Greek HIV-infected patients. J Oral Pathol Med 1992;21:120–123.

153. Masouredis CM, Katz MH, Greenspan D, et al. Prevalence of HIV-associated periodontitis and gingivitis in HIV-infected patients attending an AIDS clinic. J Acquir Immune Defic Syndr 1992;5:479–483.

154. Schoen D, Murray P, Jandinski J, et al. Periodontal status of HIV-positive children. J Dent Res 1994;73:2003A.

155. San Martin T, Jandinski JJ, Palumbo P, et al. Periodontal disease in children infected with HIV. J Dent Res 1992;71:366A.

156. Swango PA, Kleinman DV, Konzelman JL. HIV and periodontal health: A study of military personnel with HIV. J Am Dent Assoc 1991;122:49–54.

157. Riley C, London JP, Burmeister JA. Periodontal health in 200 HIV-positive patients. J Oral Pathol Med 1992;21:124–127.

158. Glick M, Muzyka BC, Salkin LM, Lurie D. Necrotizing ulcerative periodontitis: A marker for immune deterioration and a predictor for the diagnosis of AIDS. J Periodontol 1994;65:393–397.

159. Moore LVH, Moore WEC, Riley C, et al. Periodontal microflora of HIV positive subjects with gingivitis or adult periodontitis. J Periodontol 1993;64:48–56.

160. Lamster IB, Grbic JT, Bucklan RS, et al. Epidemiology and diagnosis of HIV-associated periodontal disease. Oral Dis 1997;3(Suppl 1):S141–S148.

161. Lamster IB, Grbic JT, Mitchell-Lewis DA, et al. New concepts regarding the pathogenesis of periodontal disease in HIV infection. Ann Periodontol 1998;3:62–75.

162. Murray PA, Winkler JR, Sadowski L, et al. Microbiology of HIV-associated gingivitis and periodontitis. In: Robertson PG, Greenspan JS (eds). Perspectives on Oral Manifestations of AIDS. Littleton, MA: PSG, 1988:105–118.

163. Murray PA, Grassi M, Winkler JR. The microbiology of HIV-associated periodontal lesions. J Clin Periodontol 1989;16:636–642.

164. Zambon JJ, Reynolds HS, Genco RJ: Studies of the subgingival microflora in patients with acquired immunodeficiency syndrome. J Periodontol 1990;61:699–704.

165. Rams TE, Andriolo MJ, Feik D, et al. Microbiological study of HIV-related periodontitis. J Periodontol 1991;62:74–81.

166. Murray PA, Winkler JR, Peros WJ, et al. DNA probe detection of periodontal pathogens in HIV-associated periodontal lesions. Oral Microbiol Immunol 1991;6:34–40.

167. Robinson PG, Sheiham A, Challacombe SJ, et al. Gingival ulceration in HIV infection. A case series and a case control study. J Clin Periodontol 1998;25:260–267.

168. Slots J, Rams TE, Listgarten MA. Yeasts, enteric rods and pseudomonads in the subgingival flora of severe adult periodontitis. Oral Microbiol Immunol 1988;3:47–52.

169. Mardirossian A, Contreras A, Navazesh M, et al. Herpesvirus 6, 7, and 8 in HIV- and non–HIV-associated periodontitis. J Periodontal Res 2000;35:278–284.

170. Murray PA. HIV disease as a risk factor for periodontal disease. Compend Contin Educ Dent 1994;15:1052–1064.

171. Muzyka BC, Glick M. Necrotizing stomatitis and AIDS. Gen Dent 1994;42:66–68.

172. Melnick SL, Engel D, Truelove E, et al. Associations with the presence of antibodies to the human immunodeficiency virus. Oral Surg Oral Med Oral Pathol 1989;68:37–43.

173. Yeung SCH, Stewart GJ, Cooper DA, Sindhusake D. Progression of periodontal disease in HIV seropositive patients. J Periodontol 1993;64:651–657.

174. Barr C, Lopez MR, Rua-Dobles A. Periodontal changes by HIV serostatus in a cohort of homosexual and bisexual men. J Clin Periodontol 1992;19:794–801.

175. Ryder M, Winkler JR, Weinreb RN. Elevated phagocytosis, oxidative burst, and F-actin formation in PMNs from individuals with intraoral manifestations of HIV infection. J Acquir Immune Defic Syndr 1988;1:346–353.

176. Lucht E, Heimdahl A, Nord CE. Periodontal disease in HIV-infected patients in relation to lymphocyte subsets and specific micro-organisms. J Clin Periodontol 1991;18:252–256.

177. Levine RA, Glick M. Rapidly progressive periodontitis as an important clinical marker for HIV disease. Compend Contin Educ Dent 1991;12:478–488.

178. Glick M, Pliskin ME, Weiss RC. The clinical and histologic appearance of HIV-associated gingivitis. Oral Surg Oral Med Oral Pathol 1990;69:395–398.

179. Page RC, Schroeder HE. Pathogenesis of inflammatory periodontal disease: A summary of current work. Lab Invest 1976;34:235–249.

180. Kalkwarf KL, Gutz DP. Periodontal changes associated with chronic idiopathic neutropenia. Pediatr Dent 1981;3:189–195.

181. Gorlin RJ, Chandhry AP. The oral manifestations of cyclic (periodic) neutropenia. Arch Dermatol 1960;82:344–348.

182. Anderson DC, Schmalstieg FC, Feingold MJ, et al. The severe and moderate phenotypes of heritable Mac-1 LFA-I p150,95 deficiency: Their quantitative definition and relation to leukocyte dysfunction and clinical features. J Infect Dis 1985;152:668–689.

183. Waldrop TC, Anderson DC, Hallmon WW. Periodontal manifestations of the heritable Mac-1 LFA-I deficiency syndrome: Clinical histopathologic and molecular characteristics. J Periodontol 1987;58:400.

184. Page RC, Beatty P, Waldrop TC. Molecular basis for the functional abnormality in neutrophils from patients with generalized prepubertal periodontitis. J Periodontal Res 1987;22:182.

185. Springer TA, Thompson WS, Miller LJ, et al. Inherited deficiency of the -1 Mac-1 p150,95 glycoprotein family and its molecular basis. J Exp Med 1984;160:1901–1908.

186. Williams LT, Snyderman R, Pike MC, Lefkowitz RJ. Specific receptor sites for chemotactic peptides on human polymorphonuclear leukocyte. Proc Natl Acad Sci USA 1977;74:1204–1208.

187. Van Dyke TE. Receptor deficiency in leukocytes from patients with juvenile periodontitis. Rev Infect Dis 1985;7:419–423.

188. Van Dyke TE, Levine M, Genco RJ. Neutrophil function and oral disease. J Oral Pathol 1985;14:95–120.

189. Van Dyke TE, Horoszewicz HU, Cianciola LJ, Genco RJ. Neutrophil chemotaxis dysfunction in human periodontitis. Infect Immun 1980;27:124–132.

190. Suzuki JB, Risom M, Falker WA, et al. Effect of periodontal therapy on lymphocyte response and neutrophil chemotaxis in localized and generalized juvenile periodontitis patients. J Clin Periodontol 1985;12:124–134.

191. Van Dyke TE, Horoszewicz HU, Cianciola LJ, Genco RJ. Reduced chemotactic peptide binding in juvenile periodontitis: A model for neutrophil function. Biochem Biophys Res Commun 1981;10:1278–1284.

192. Genco RJ, Van Dyke TE, Levine MJ, et al. Molecular factors influencing neutrophil defects in periodontal disease. J Dent Res 1986;65:1379–1391.

193. Tsai C-C, MacArthur WP, Baehni PC, et al. Extraction and partial characterization of a leukotoxin from a plaque-derived gram-negative microorganism. Infect Immun 1979;25:427–439.

194. Zambon JJ, Deluca C, Slots J, Genco RJ. Studies of leukotoxin from *Actinobacillus actinomycetemcomitans* using the promyclocytic HL-60 cell line. Infect Immun 1983;40:205–212.

195. Kalmar JR, Arnold RR, Van Dyke TE. Direct interaction of *Actinobacillus actinomycetemcomitans* with normal and defective (LJP) neutrophils. J Periodontal Res 1987;22:179–181.

196. Boxer LA, Morganroth ML. Neutrophil function disorders. Dis Mon 1987;33:681–780.

197. McClain DL, Bader JD, Daniel SJ, Sams DH. Gingival effects of prescription medications among adult dental patients. Spec Care Dentist 1991;11:15–18.

198. Rees TD. Drugs and oral disorders. Periodontol 2000 1998:18: 21–36.

199. Hallmon WW, Rossman JA. The role of drugs in the pathogenesis of gingival overgrowth: A collective review of current concepts. Periodontol 2000 1999;21:176–196.

200. Mathews TG. Medication side effects of dental interest. J Prosthet Dent 1990;64:219–226.

201. Hassell T, Hefti A. Drug-induced overgrowth: Old problem, new problem. Crit Rev Oral Biol Med 1991;2:103–137.

202. Seymour R, Heasman P. Drugs and the periodontium. J Clin Periodontol 1988;15:1–16.

203. Kimball O. The treatment of epilepsy with sodium diphenyl hydantoinate. JAMA 1939;112:1244–1245.

204. Angelopoulos A, Goaz P. Incidence of diphenylhydantoin gingival hyperplasia. Oral Surg Oral Med Oral Pathol 1972;34: 898–906.

205. Peñarrocha-Diago M, Bagan-Sebastian J, Vera-Sempere F. Diphenylhydantoin-induced gingival overgrowth in man: A clinico-pathological study. J Periodontol 1990;61:571–574.

206. Hassell T, Harris E, Broughman J, Cockey G. Gingival overgrowth: Hereditary considerations. Compend Contin Educ Dent Suppl 1990;14:S511–S514.

207. Dahlof G, Reinholt R, Hjerpe A, Modeer T. A quantitative analysis of connective tissue components in phenytoin-induced gingival overgrowth in children. J Periodontal Res 1984;19:401.

208. Vernillo A, Schwartz N. The effects of phenytoin (5,5-diphenylhydantoin) on human gingival fibroblasts in culture. J Periodontal Res 1987;22:307–312.

209. Stinnett E, Rodu B, Grizzle W. New developments in understanding phenytoin-induced gingival hyperplasia. J Am Dent Assoc 1987;114:814–816.

210. Vijayasingham S, Dykes P, Marks R. Phenytoin has little effect on in vitro models of wound healing. Br J Dermatol 1991;125: 136–139.

211. Jones J, Weddell J, McKown C. Incidence and indications for surgical management of phenytoin-induced gingival overgrowth in a cerebral palsy population. J Oral Maxillofac Surg 1988;46:385–390.

212. O'Neal T, Figures K. The effects of chlorhexidine and mechanical methods of plaque control on recurrence of gingival hyperplasia in young patients taking phenytoin. Br Dent J 1982;152:130–133.

213. Pihlström B, Carlson J, Smith Q, et al. Prevention of phenytoin-associated gingival enlargement: A 15-month longitudinal study. J Periodontol 1980;51:311–317.

214. Tal H, Littner S, Gordon M. Effect of oral hygiene on phenytoin-induced gingival hyperplasia. Dent Med 1988;6:10–13.

215. Swenson H. Case report: A nineteen year study of dilantin hyperplasia. Periodontal Case Rep 1984;6:31–33.

216. Rossman J, Ingles E, Brown R. Multimodal treatment of drug-induced gingival hyperplasia in a kidney transplant patient. Compend Contin Educ Dent 1994;15:1266–1274.

217. Leppik I. Antiepileptic medications. Compend Contin Educ Dent 1990;14(suppl):S490–S496.

218. Syrjanen S, Syrjanen K. Hyperplastic gingivitis in a child receiving sodium valproate treatment. Proc Finn Dent Soc 1979;75:95–98.

219. Boltchi FE, Rees TD, Iacopino AM. Cyclosporine A-induced gingival overgrowth: A comprehensive review. Quintessence Int 1999;30:775–783.

220. Williamson M, Miller E, Plemons J, et al. Cyclosporin-A upregulates interleukin-6 gene expression in human gingiva: Possible mechanism of gingival overgrowth. J Periodontol 1994; 65:895–903.

221. Lundergan W. Drug-induced gingival enlargements: Dilantin hyperplasia and beyond. J Calif Dent Assoc 1989;17:48–52.

222. Stone C, Eshenour A, Hassell T. Gingival enlargement in cyclosporine-treated multiple sclerosis patients. J Dent Res 1989;68:285–289.

223. Palestine A, Nussenblatt R, Chan C. Side effects of systemic cyclosporine in patients not undergoing transplantation. Am J Med 1984;7:652–656.

224. Jackson C, Babich S. Gingival hyperplasia: Interaction between cyclosporine A and nifedipine? A case report. NY State Dent J 1997;63:46–48.

225. Dary T, Wysocki G. Cyclosporin therapy: Its significance to the periodontium. J Periodontol 1984;55:708–712.

226. Butler RT, Kalkwarf KL, Kaldahl WB. Drug-induced gingival hyperplasia: Phenytoin, cyclosporine, and nifedipine. J Am Dent Assoc 1987;114:56–60.

227. Wysocki G, Gretzinger H, Laupacis A, et al. Fibrotic enlargement of the gingiva: A side effect of cyclosporin. Oral Surg Oral Med Oral Pathol 1983;55:274–278.

228. Seymour R, Smith D, Rogers S. The comparative effects of azathioprine and cyclosporin on some gingival health parameters of renal transplant patients: A longitudinal study. J Clin Periodontol 1987;14:610–613.

229. Varga E, Tyldesley W. Carcinoma arising in cyclosporin-induced gingival hyperplasia. Br Dent J 1991;171:26–27.

230. Qunibi W, Aktitar M, Ginn E, Smith P. Kaposi's sarcoma in cyclosporin-induced gingival hyperplasia. Am J Kidney Dis 1988;11:349–352.

231. McGaw T, Porter H. Cyclosporin-induced gingival overgrowth: An ultrastructural streologic study. Oral Surg Oral Med Oral Pathol 1988;65:186–190.

232. Rateitschak-Pluss E, Jefti A, Lortschar R, Thiel G. Initial observation that cyclosporin-A induces gingival enlargement in man. J Clin Periodontol 1983;10:237–246.

233. Dodd DA. Rapid resolution of gingival hyperplasia after switching from cyclosporine A to tacrolimus. J Heart Lung Transplant 1997;16:579.

234. Seymour R. Calcium channel blockers and gingival overgrowth. Br Dent J 1991;170:376–379.

235. Lederman D, Lumerman H, Reuben S, Fredman P. Gingival hyperplasia associated with nifedipine therapy: Report of a case. Oral Surg Oral Med Oral Pathol 1984;57:620–622.

236. Tagawa T, Nakamura H, Murata M. Marked gingival hyperplasia induced by nifedipine. Int J Oral Maxillofac Surg 1989;19:72–73.

237. Van der Wall E, Tuinzing D, Hes J. Gingival hyperplasia induced by nifedipine, an arterial vasodilating drug. Oral Surg Oral Med Oral Pathol 1985;60:38–40.

238. Lainson P. Gingival overgrowth in a patient treated with nifedipine (Procardia). Periodontal Case Rep 1986;8:64–66.

239. Lucas R, Howell L, Wall B. Nifedipine-induced gingival hyperplasia: A histochemical and ultrastructure study. J Periodontol 1985;56:211–215.

240. Slavin J, Taylor J. Cyclosporin, nifedipine and gingival hyperplasia. Lancet 1987;320:739.

241. Fattore L, Stablein M, Bredfeldt G, et al. Gingival hyperplasia: A side effect of nifedipine and diltiazem. Spec Care Dent 1991;11:107–109.

242. Colvard M, Bishop J, Weissman D, Garguilo A. Cardizem-induced gingival hyperplasia: A report of two cases. Periodontal Case Rep 1986;8:67–68.

243. Nishikawa S, Tada H, Hamasaki A, Ishida H. Nifedipine-induced gingival hyperplasia: A clinical and in vitro study. J Periodontol 1991;62:30–35.

244. Barak S, Engelberg I, Hiss J. Gingival hyperplasia caused by nifedipine: Histopathologic findings. J Periodontol 1987;58:639–642.

245. Yusof W. Nifedipine-induced gingival hyperplasia. J Can Dent Assoc 1989;55:389–391.

246. Puolijoki H, Siitonen L, Saha H, Suojanen I. Gingival hyperplasia caused by nifedipine. Proc Finn Dent Soc 1988;84:311–314.

247. Hancock R, Swan R. Nifedipine-induced gingival overgrowth: Report of a case treated by controlling plaque. J Clin Periodontol 1992;19:12–14.

248. Cucchi G, Guistaniani S, Robustelli F. Hypertrophic gingivitis caused by verapamil. G Ital Cardiol 1985;15:556–557.

249. Heijl L, Sundin Y. Nitrendipine-induced gingival overgrowth in dogs. J Periodontol 1988;60:104–112.

250. Giusstiniani S, della Cuna F, Marieni M. Hyperplastic gingivitis during diltiazem therapy. Int J Cardiol 1987;15:247–249.

251. Bowman J, Levy B, Grubb R. Gingival overgrowth induced by diltiazem. Oral Surg Oral Med Oral Pathol 1988;65:183–185.

252. Lombardi T, Fiore-Donno G, Belser U, Dia' FR. Felodipine-induced gingival hyperplasia: A clinical and histologic study. J Oral Pathol Med 1991;20:89–92.

253. Medical Letter T: Isradipine for hypertension. Med Lett Drugs Ther 1991;33:51–54.

254. Westbrook P, Bednarczyk EM, Carlson M, et al. Regression of nifedipine-induced gingival hyperplasia following switch to a same class calcium channel blocker, isradipine. J Periodontol 1997;68:645–650.

255. Rees TD. Oral effects of drug abuse. Crit Rev Oral Biol Med 1992;3:163–184.

256. Valsecchi R, Cainelli T. Gingival hyperplasia induced by erythromycin. Acta Derm Venereol (Stockh) 1992;72:157.

257. American Academy of Periodontology. Glossary of Periodontal Terms. Chicago: American Academy of Periodontology, 1992.

258. Newman H, Rees T, Kinane D. Diseases of the Periodontium. Northwood, England: Science Reviews, 1993.

259. Lynch M, Ship I. Initial oral manifestations of leukemia. J Am Dent Assoc 1967;75:932–940.

260. Stafford A, Sonis S, Lockart P, Sonis A. Oral pathoses as diagnostic indicators in leukemia. Oral Surg Oral Med Oral Pathol 1980;50:134–139.

261. Burket L. A histopathologic explanation of the oral lesions in the acute leukemias. Am J Orthod 1944;30:516.

262. Sydney S, Serio F. Acute monocytic leukemia diagnosed in a patient referred because of gingival pain. J Am Dent Assoc 1981;103:886–887.

263. Presant C, Safdar S, Cherrick H. Gingival leukaemic infiltration in chronic lymphocytic leukaemia. Oral Surg Oral Med Oral Pathol 1973;36:672–674.

264. Fischman S. The patient with cancer. Dent Clin North Am 1983;27:235–246.

265. Greenberg M, Cohen S, McKitrick J, Cassileth P. The oral flora as a source of septicemia in patients with acute leukemia. Oral Surg Oral Med Oral Pathol 1982;53:32–36.

266. James P, Prasad S. Gingival fibromatosis: Report of a case. J Oral Surg 1971;29:55.

267. Laband P, Habib G, Humphreys G. Hereditary gingival fibromatosis: Report of an affected family with associated splenomegaly and skeletal and soft-tissue abnormalities. Oral Surg Oral Med Oral Pathol 1964;17:339.

268. Oikawa K. Laband syndrome: Report of a case. Oral Surg Oral Med Oral Pathol 1979;37:120–122.

269. Horning G, Fisher J, Barker B, et al. Gingival fibromatosis with hypertrichosis. J Periodontol 1985;56:344–347.

270. Sciubba J, Niebloom T. Juvenile hyaline fibromatosis (Murray-Puretic-Descher syndrome): Oral and systemic findings in siblings. Oral Surg Oral Med Oral Pathol 1986;62:397–409.

271. Perusse R, Morency R. Oral pigmentation induced by Premarin. Cutis 1991;48:61–64.

272. Porter SR, Scully C. Adverse drug reactions in the mouth. Clin Dermatol 2000;18:525–532.

273. Siller GM, Tod MA, Savage NW. Minocycline-induced oral pigmentation. J Am Acad Dermatol 1994;30:350–354.

274. Zala L, Hunziker T, Braathen LR. Pigmentation following long-term bismuth therapy for pneumatosis cystoides intestinalis. Dermatology 1993;187:288–289.

275. Veraldi S, Schianchi-Veraldi R, Scarabelli C. Pigmentation of the gum following hydroxychloroquine therapy. Cutis 1992;49:261–262.

276. Merenich JA, Hannon RN, Gentry RH, Harrison SM. Azidothymidine-induced hyperpigmentation mimicking primary adrenal insufficiency. Am J Med 1989;86:469–470.

277. Breathnach SM, Phillips WG. Epidemiology of bullous drug eruptions. Clin Dermatol 1993;11:441–447.

278. Roujean JC, Stern RS. Severe adverse cutaneous reactions to drugs. N Engl J Med 1994;331:1272–1285.

279. Bircher AJ, von Schulthess A, Henning G. Oral lichenoid lesions and mercury sensitivity. Contact Dermatitis 1993;29:275–276.

280. Halevy S, Shai A. Lichenoid drug eruptions. J Am Acad Dermatol 1993;29:249–255.

281. Blignaut E. Cefaclor associated with intraoral ulceration. S Afr Med J 1990;77:426–427.

282. Siegel MA, Balciunas BA. Medication can cause severe ulcerations. J Am Dent Assoc 1991;122:75–77.

283. Drucker CR, Johnson TM. Captopril glossopyrosis. Arch Dermatol 1989;125:1437.

284. Candelaria LM, Huttula CS. Angioedema associated with angiotensin-converting enzyme inhibitors. J Oral Maxillofac Surg 1991;49:1237–1239.

285. Pillans P. Mouth blistering and ulceration associated with inhaled steroids [letter]. Respir Med 1994;88:159–160.

286. Higgins EM, Du Vivier AWP. Angina bullosa haemorrhagica—A possible relation to steroid inhalers. Clin Exp Dermatol 1991;16:244–246.

287. Scully S, Azul AM, Crighton A, et al. Nicorandil can induce severe oral ulceration. Oral Surg Oral Med Oral Pathol Oral Radiol Endod 2001;91:189–193.

288. Tourne LPM, Fricton JR. Burning mouth syndrome: Critical review and proposed clinical management. Oral Surg Oral Med Oral Pathol 1992;74:158–167.

289. Kaaber S. Allergy to dental materials with special reference to the use of amalgam and polymethylmethacrylate. Int Dent J 1990;40:359–365.

290. White IR, Smith BGN. Dental amalgam dermatitis. Br Dent J 1984;156:259–260.

291. Bolewska J, Holmstrup P, Moller-Madsen B, et al. Amalgam associated mercury accumulation in normal oral mucosa, oral mucosal lesions of lichen planus and contact lesions associated with amalgam. J Oral Pathol Med 1990;19:39–42.

292. Veien NK. Stomatitis and systemic dermatitis from mercury in amalgam dental restorations. Dermatol Clin 1990;8:157–160.

293. Holmstrup P. Reactions of the oral mucosa related to silver amalgam: A review. J Oral Pathol Med 1991;20:1–7.

294. Agner T, Menne T. Sensitization to acrylates in a dental patient. Contact Dermatitis 1994;30:249–250.

295. Olveti E. Contact dermatitis from an acrylic metal dental prosthesis. Contact Dermatitis 1991;24:57.

296. Torres V, Mano-Azul AC, Correia T, Soares AP. Allergic contact cheilitis and stomatitis from hydroquinone in an acrylic dental prosthesis. Contact Dermatitis 1993;29:102–103.

297. Holmes G, Freeman S. Chelitis caused by contact urticaria to mint flavoured toothpaste. Australas J Dermatol 2001;42:43–45.

298. Skrebova N, Brocks K, Karlsmark T. Allergic contact cheilitis from spearmint oil. Contact Dermatitis 1998;39:35.

299. Lee AY, Yoo SH, Oh JG, Kim YG. Two cases of allergic contact cheilitis from sodium lauryl sulfate in toothpaste. Contact Dermatitis 2000;42:111.

300. Franks A. Contact allergy to anethole in toothpaste associated with loss of taste. Contact Dermatitis 1988;38:354.

301. Worm M, Jeep S, Sterry W, Zuberbier T. Perioral contact dermatitis caused by L-carvone in toothpaste. Contact Dermatitis 1998;38:338.

302. Francalanci S, Sertoli A, Giorgini S, et al. Multicenter study of allergic contact cheilitis from toothpastes. Contact Dermatitis 2000;43:216–222.

303. Rees TD. Drugs and the periodontium. In: Newman HN, Rees TD, Kinane DF (eds). Diseases of the Periodontium. Northwood, England: Science Reviews, 1993:109–134.

304. Peterson DE. Oral toxicity of chemotherapeutic agents. Semin Oncol 1992;19:478–491.

305. Nieweg R, van Tinteren H, Poelhuis EK, Abraham-Inpijn L. Nursing care for oral complications associated with chemotherapy: A survey among members of the Dutch Oncology Nursing Society. Cancer Nurs 1992;15:313–321.

306. Lockhart PB, Clark JR. Oral complications following neoadjuvant chemotherapy in patients with head and neck cancer. NCI Monograph 1990;9:99–101.

307. Sica S, Pagano L, Salutari P, et al. Acute parotitis during induction therapy including L-asparaginase in acute lymphoblastic leukemia. Ann Hematol 1994;68:91–92.

308. Pan CV, Quintela AG. Doxycycline-induced parotitis [letter]. Postgrad Med J 1991;67:313.

309. Wolf M, Leventon G. Acute iodine-induced enlargement of the salivary glands. J Oral Maxillofac Surg 1990;48:71–72.

310. Thompson DF. Drug-induced parotitis. J Clin Pharm Ther 1993;18:255–258.

311. Robb ND, Smith BGH. Prevalence of pathological tooth wear in patients with chronic alcoholism. Br Dent J 1990;169:367–369.

312. Freidlander AH, Gorelick DA. Dental management of the cocaine addict. Oral Surg Oral Med Oral Pathol 1988;65:45–48.

313. Martin SD. Drug-induced parotid swelling [letter]. Br J Hosp Pharm 1993;50:496.

314. Burgeois JA, Drexler KG, Hall MJ. Hypersalivation and clozapine [letter]. Hosp Community Psychiatry 1991;42:1174.

315. Grabowski J. Clonidine treatment of clozapine-induced hypersalivation. J Clin Psychopharmacol 1992;12:69–70.

316. Screeby LM, Schwartz S. A reference guide to drugs and dry mouth. Gerodontology 1986;5:75–99.

317. Screeby LM, Valdini A. Xerostomia: A neglected symptom. Arch Int Med 1987;147:1333–1337.

318. Navazesh M. Xerostomia in the aged. Dent Clin North Am 1989;33:75–79.

319. Lewis IK, Hanlon JT, Hobbins MJ, Beck JD. Use of medications with potential oral adverse drug reactions in community-dwelling elderly people. Spec Care Dent 1993;13:171–176.

320. Atkinson JC, Wu AJ. Salivary gland dysfunction: Causes, symptoms, treatment. J Am Dent Assoc 1994;125:409–416.

321. Handelman SL, Baric JM, Saunders RH, Espeland MA. Hyposalivatory drug use, whole stimulated salivary flow, and mouth dryness in older, long-term care residents. Spec Care Dent 1989;9:12–18.

322. Navazesh M. Salivary gland hypofunction in elderly patients. J Calif Dent Assoc 1994;22:62–68.

323. Pallasch TJ. Anesthetic management of the chemically dependent patient. Anesth Prog 1992;39:157–161.

324. Pallasch TJ, Joseph CE. Oral manifestations of drug abuse. J Psychoactive Drugs 1987;19:375–377.

325. Baddour HM, Audemorte TB, Layman FD. The occurrence of diffuse gingival hyperplasia in a patient using marijuana. J Tenn Dent Assoc 1983;64:39–43.

326. Darling MR, Arendorf TM, Coldrey NA. Effect of cannabis use on oral candidiasis carriage. J Oral Pathol Med 1990;19:319–321.

327. Lee CYS, Mohammadi H, Dixon RA. Medical and dental implications of cocaine abuse. J Oral Maxillofac Surg 1991;49:290–293.

328. Yukna RA. Cocaine periodontitis. Int J Periodontics Restorative Dent 1991;11:73–79.

329. Krutchkoff DJ, Eisenberg E, O'Brien JE, Ponzillo JJ. Cocaine-induced dental erosions. N Engl J Med 1990;322:408.

330. Dello Russo NM, Temple HV. Cocaine effects on gingiva. J Am Dent Assoc 1982;104:13.

331. Gargiulo AV Jr, Toto PD, Gargiulo AW. Cocaine-induced gingival necrosis. Periodontal Case Rep 1985;7:44–45.

332. Quart AM, Small CB, Klein RS. The cocaine connection: Users imperil their gingiva. J Am Dent Assoc 1991;122:85–87.

333. Pallasch TJ, McCarthy FM, Jastak ET. Cocaine and sudden cardiac death. J Oral Maxillofac Surg 1989;47:1188–1191.

Systemic Effects of Periodontal Diseases

Steven Offenbacher, Catherine C.M.E. Champagne, and James D. Beck

- What Systemic Diseases Are Linked with Periodontal Disease?
- Who Is at Risk?
- How Can Oral Infection Affect Overall Health?
- How Do Periodontal Pathogens Get into the Bloodstream?
- How Do Periodontal Pathogens Cause Systemic Inflammation?
- What Is the Evidence Linking Periodontal Disease to Heart Disease?
- What Is the Threat of Periodontal Infection During Pregnancy?
- What Is the Relationship Among Periodontitis, Pneumonia, and Osteoporosis?
- What Risk Does Periodontal Disease Pose for Diabetics?
- Other Data from Animal Models
- Potential Impact on Dentistry

Systemic conditions, such as diabetes mellitus, have long been known to have an impact on oral tissues. Dental students are taught that the state of a patient's oral health is a window to, or reflection of, his or her systemic health. Indeed, many observant practitioners have correctly identified systemic conditions in patients, ranging from systemic lupus erythematosus to pregnancy, based simply on oral signs and symptoms. The discipline of oral medicine has traditionally focused on the diagnosis and treatment of these oral manifestations of systemic diseases.

In recent years, however, it has been recognized that many systemic conditions are multifactorial, and researchers do not know all the causes of these conditions. This is especially true for major chronic debilitating illnesses and for illnesses that involve inflammatory processes. For example, approximately one third of all myocardial infarctions occur in people who have none of the traditional risk factors like high blood pressure or high cholesterol levels. In other words, there are many behaviors, exposures, or

genetic traits that interact over time along the causal path to ultimately control the expression of disease, and studies have not identified all these separate causes or the interactions that may occur. Large longitudinal, epidemiological studies examining disease patterns in populations have been conducted to identify potential risk factors for certain common chronic illnesses, such as cardiovascular disease. These studies have been remarkably enlightening; for example, they have demonstrated not only the severely damaging effect that smoking has on cardiovascular health but also the more insidious damage caused by second-hand, or passive-exposure, smoking.

Scientists have also begun to analyze the dental measurements of periodontal disease and caries that were added to these studies a couple of decades ago. The results that have emerged from these long-term studies have come as a surprise to dental scientists and educators. For example, findings show that severe oral infections, especially periodontal disease, in otherwise healthy individuals appear to place these individuals at significant increased risk for developing certain health problems, including stroke and myocardial infarction. These effects cannot be explained by other traditional risk factors for heart disease, such as smoking, age, gender, cholesterol levels, exercise, blood pressure, socioeconomic status, or education. New research findings raise the possibility that periodontal disease may increase the risk of dying from a myocardial infarction almost twofold, and the risk of having a stroke almost threefold. The effect of periodontal disease on systemic well-being has been termed *periodontal medicine* to describe the potential injurious effects of periodontal disease on systemic health.[1] What is perhaps even more surprising is that the magnitude of the deleterious effects of periodontal disease on cardiovascular fitness may be as harmful as smoking or high cholesterol.

These early findings require confirmation by additional prospective and intervention studies. Many years of clinical and basic research will be needed to determine whether the association between these cardiovascular conditions and periodontal disease is actually causative. However, these associations provide the impetus to move the profession of dentistry and the discipline of periodontology further from a mechanical/surgical discipline and closer to a medical model of diagnosis, prevention, and therapy. Thus, the impact of new research and the emergence of periodontal medicine as a new discipline has the potential to revolutionize dentistry in a manner that has not been seen since the days of G. V. Black.

What Systemic Diseases Are Linked with Periodontal Disease?

Several conditions appear to be associated with patients who have more periodontal disease. The association with heart disease has been demonstrated by at least four cross-sectional[2–5] and five longitudinal studies,[6–10] beginning with studies by the Finnish physician Matilla.[2,3] Early studies include associations of periodontal or oral infections (as determined by total dental index scores that included caries, periodontal lesions, and endodontic lesions) with various forms of cardiovascular disease, including stroke and myocardial infarction. More recent studies demonstrate a relationship between periodontal disease (as measured by attachment loss and bone loss) and both incident (new cases) and progressing cardiovascular disease. Periodontal disease seems to be associated with the chronic atherosclerotic process that leads to atheroma formation[11] and impaired perfusion and vasospasm, as well

as with the acute thromboembolic events such as myocardial infarction and stroke.[7,10,12,13]

Not all reports, however, have found an association between periodontal disease and cardiovascular disease.[14–16] It has been suggested that the association between these diseases is due to the overwhelming effect and interaction with smoking, a common behavioral risk factor for both conditions.[15] Alternatively, the failure to show a positive relationship may reflect the shortcomings of analyzing preexisting data from studies that were not adequately designed to provide detailed assessments of periodontal status or the fact that the magnitude of the effect of periodontal disease on cardiovascular disease appears to be only mild to moderate (odds ratios of 1.5 to 2.5) rather than severe (odds ratios higher than 3.0).[17]

Three issues surrounding the apparent conflicting data appear worthy of comment. First, in one series of studies, the same data set was analyzed by three independent research groups,[6,10,15] and two of the three groups found significant associations.[6,10] Second, newer studies that have adequate periodontal measures establish a link of periodontal disease with early subclinical changes in cardiovascular status, such as increased carotid artery thickening (an index of early atherosclerotic disease as measured by ultrasonography).[11] These investigations, published in the cardiology journals, have been well controlled for potential confounders, such as smoking. Finally, experiments in cell and animal models have demonstrated the biologic feasibility of periodontal pathogens enhancing atherogenesis and thromboembolic events.[12,13,18–20] Studies have suggested that periodontal disease may worsen diabetes by worsening glycemic control.[21–28] This effect is presumably a consequence of the metabolic stress induced by infection, which would increase blood lipid and blood glucose levels and induce a state of insulin resistance.[29,30] Thus, the chronic infection may predispose an individual to increased risk for developing states of metabolic dysregulation, leading to type 2 diabetes. Within people with diabetes mellitus, the metabolic stress of periodontal infection would worsen glycemic control and increase the need for hypoglycemic agents.

During pregnancy, the presence of periodontal disease in the mother appears to be associated with an increased risk for premature delivery and low birth weight for gestational age.[31–38] In a pregnant mother with periodontal infection, the transient bacteremias associated with periodontitis and periodontal progression appear to represent a special risk.[36] Evidence analyzing fetal cord blood obtained at delivery indicates that maternal oral pathogens or bacterial products become blood-borne and target the placenta and fetus.[39]

The threat of periodontitis to overall health extends across the lifetime of an individual. Several studies [40–43] indicate that the oral flora can harbor respiratory pathogens, especially in older institutionalized disabled individuals, and this reservoir appears to enhance the risk of aspiration pneumonia. Periodontal pathogens have also been associated with aspiration pneumonia[44,45] and appear to present a special risk in dysphagic individuals.[46] Although it remains to be proven, these associations are consistent with the concept that oral infection actually worsens an existent systemic condition or places the individual at greater risk along a causal path.

The importance of these associations should not be exaggerated, however. The links may simply be a reflection of a currently unidentified, underlying trait that places an individual at risk for all of these conditions in a nonspecific manner. Many of these conditions share a "common soil." For example, periodontitis, cardiovascular disease, and diabetes mellitus all tend to be more common in individuals who are older, male, smokers, and less educated. The common soil concept does not negate the potential importance of oral health, however. For example, the links among poverty, low socioeconomic status, low education level, and increased risk of disease all require a biologic rationale. Perhaps periodontal disease is one of the underlying components of higher risk among these individuals. Certainly, the surgeon general's report[47] emphasizes that poor oral health is one potential cause of, or contributor to, health disparities among different populations. It is important to realize, however, that periodontal disease is associated with these systemic conditions even after adjustments for education and poverty index. Thus, periodontal disease is not simply a surrogate marker for other social factors.

Who Is at Risk?

The most severe forms of periodontal disease do not affect everyone. Population studies in the United States demonstrate that only 7% to 15% of the adult population has severe forms of periodontal disease.[48] It is interesting to note that the prevalence of periodontitis in rural China is comparable to that in the United States. This population has no access to dental care, does not practice toothbrushing, and has very poor oral hygiene.[49] Clearly, periodontal pathogens are necessary, but not sufficient, for disease.[50,51] Studies conducted in twins suggest that approximately half the expression of periodontal disease that affects the population appears to be due to genetic factors.[52] In other words, periodontitis has a large genetic component, and much of the susceptibility to disease is inherited. Smoking and diabetes, not plaque accumulation, appear to be the major risk factors for periodontal disease. Thus, it is certainly reasonable to suggest that eventually re-

searchers will identify genetic traits that make individuals susceptible to periodontal disease, and some of these genes may also make someone susceptible to other conditions, such as heart disease. Thus, it will be important to do more research to determine whether these associations are actually causally related.

The search for new risk factors and causes of these systemic conditions is far from complete. As has been discussed, approximately one third of all myocardial infarctions occur in people with no known risk factors such as high blood pressure or elevated blood lipid levels. Furthermore, it is a generally accepted medical fact that acute infections, such as pneumonia, are causally related to more severe acute events like myocardial infarction, acute-onset diabetes mellitus, and premature delivery. What remains to be clarified is exactly how a long-standing, low-grade infection like periodontal disease is manifested systemically.

How Can Oral Infection Affect Overall Health?

On the surface, the biologic feasibility of an oral infection's having an influence on systemic conditions such as heart disease seems obtuse. However, the data are now compelling that certain periodontal pathogens have a domain or "territory" that far exceeds the periodontal pocket. Three key organisms have been identified as causative of periodontal diseases: *Porphyromonas gingivalis*, *Treponema denticola*, and *Bacteroides forsythus*. These organisms have been defined as the "red cluster" of pathogens[53] associated with periodontal disease (see Fig 5-4), the major subgingival inhabitants that emerge late in maturing plaque. They do not colonize easily and require a lush biofilm ecosystem to support adherence, growth, and emergence. In contrast to supragingival organisms that largely rely on salivary components and dietary nutrients for growth, organisms of the red cluster rely mainly on host serum proteins and blood components for sustenance. The organisms of the red cluster have special enzymes and proteins that enable them to trigger mild host inflammation and enhanced gingival crevicular flow to ensure an adequate food and nutrient supply from the serum. These organisms are analogous to predatory animals like tigers or sharks, and they are at the top of their food chain within the subgingival ecosystem. These organisms have evolved with human beings over the eons and have no other known habitat or transmission vectors. As organisms evolve and move up the food chain, the size of the territory or domain also increases. These organisms have acquired unique stealthlike properties that enable them to evade neutrophil defenses, invade tissues, and get into the bloodstream.

In patients with periodontitis, recurrent, albeit transient, bacteremias occur and initiate a systemic antibody response to these pathogens. This antibody response is clearly protective and serves as a selective pressure that helps limit the infection. In addition, however, there is evidence that these organisms disseminate and target the liver to induce activation of the hepatic acute-phase response. This response is characterized by elevations of serum inflammatory mediators and hepatic secretion of acute-phase proteins, such as C-reactive protein (CRP) and haptoglobin. Inflammation and bacteria at a systemic level—even a low systemic level—when repeated acutely and aggravated chronically over many years, theoretically can provide severe cumulative damage to systemic health. Thus, it is the direct systemic action of blood-borne oral bacteria or bacterial products and the chronic inflammation caused by this hematogenous exposure that are currently thought to provide a risk to health.

How Do Periodontal Pathogens Get into the Bloodstream?

Levels of periodontal pathogens of the red cluster (*P gingivalis*, *B forsythus*, and *T denticola*) are elevated in the subgingival plaque of patients with chronic periodontitis.[53,54] *P gingivalis* is the best-characterized pathogen, and its ability to invade the host is most impressive. For example, *P gingivalis* is capable of evading neutrophil clearance (phagocytosis and killing), invading through the epithelium to the tissues, secreting enzymes that digest host tissues to enable penetration and spreading, and triggering vasopermeability to facilitate hematogenous dissemination. The organisms have been identified at many distant sites, such as within atheromatous plaques,[55,56] where they do not necessarily cause a large localized inflammatory reaction, abscess, or localized tissue destruction. Fetal cord blood also contains antibodies against *P gingivalis*, indicating that fetal exposure can occur in utero in mothers with periodontal disease.[39] The mechanisms by which *P gingivalis* avoids activating the acquired immune response and evades immune surveillance are not fully understood. Certain proteins secreted by this species mimic those of the host and serve to "naturally" suppress the immune response. Thus, the organism evades host clearance and detection and is stealthlike. This property may enable these organisms to persist in the body for extended periods.

Other periodontal pathogens also appear to gain systemic egress and become blood-borne. The pocket epithelium surface area has been suggested to approximate a wounded area for microbial penetration.[57] The clinical sign of bleeding on probing reflects ulceration of the epithelium and represents a sizable periodontal lesion surface area, or "wound," that may serve as a significant portal of entry for many periodontal organisms.[8,17,58] The organisms also create a toxic reservoir of bacterial lipopolysaccharide (LPS) that is highly inflammatory and represents approximately one third the weight of the gram-negative bacterial plaque mass. The LPS is released within the pocket and penetrates into the tissues. Within the tissues, LPS interacts with cells of the macrophage lineage to stimulate the release of inflammatory mediators. These inflammatory mediators include prostaglandin E_2 (PGE_2), interleukin 1β (IL-1β), and tumor necrosis factor α (TNF-α). These molecules activate other cells, including fibroblasts and osteoclasts, to cause connective tissue destruction and bone resorption. Thus, these host-produced mediators of inflammation cause vasodilation and destruction of the periodontal ligament, the gingival connective tissues, and the alveolar bone.[59] The magnitude and quality of this inflammatory response seems to be an important determinant of periodontal disease severity. That is, patients who secrete more PGE_2, IL-1β, and TNF-α simply have more inflammation and more periodontal disease.

As discussed above, not everyone gets periodontal disease, but we are all exposed to similar oral pathogens. Some patients seem to never get periodontal disease, no matter how poor their oral hygiene habits.[49,60,61] It now appears that the genetic and behavioral differences that influence our individual inflammatory response are a key determinant of who will get severe periodontal disease. Certain genes associated with an excess production of IL-1β have been associated with severe forms of periodontal disease.[62,63] Exposures and behaviors can also modify inflammatory states and periodontal disease expression. For example, diabetes mellitus and smoking both enhance the inflammatory response to bacterial LPS while simultaneously impairing the ability to fight infection by compromising neutrophil function. Thus, an exaggerated inflammatory response results in more tissue destruction and what is seen clinically as more severe pocketing and bone loss in patients with diabetes and smokers.

The concept of an underlying exaggerated inflammatory trait characterizing patients with the most severe forms of periodontitis needs to be considered in the context of the observed associations between periodontitis and systemic disease. If a patient responds to the oral flora with a severe, tissue-damaging inflammatory response, might that same individual also respond poorly to other types of inflammatory challenges? Perhaps there is an underlying hyperinflammatory trait that places an individual at risk for not only periodontitis but many other conditions, including cardiovascular disease. This does not necessarily negate the potential importance of oral infection as a contributor to these systemic maladies, but it points out that there may be underlying mechanisms or causes yet to be identified that may better explain the observed associations between periodontal disease and other systemic conditions such as cardiovascular disease. Additional research in this area is needed.

How Do Periodontal Pathogens Cause Systemic Inflammation?

Periodontitis elicits a systemic inflammatory response that reflects the activation of the hepatic acute-phase response. The liver can be activated by bacteria; bacterial products such as LPS; cytokines like IL-1β, TNFα, and IL-6; and oxidized lipids produced as a consequence of oxidative stress. This activation results in the synthesis of acute-phase proteins such as CRP and haptoglobin. Ebersole et al[64] were the first to report that patients with periodontitis had slight elevations in both CRP and haptoglobin. Studies by Slade et al[65] using data from a national survey of almost 14,000 people confirm that periodontitis is associated with small increases in CRP, even after adjusting for other potential activators of the acute-phase response. Studies by Loos et al[66] also demonstrate that periodontitis patients have elevations in levels of serum IL-6, CRP, and white blood cells, even after adjusting for other stressors such as other sources of infection, diabetes, and smoking.

It is important to point out that the increases in CRP seen in patients with periodontitis in these studies are modest (twofold to threefold higher) compared with the increases seen in acute infection. Acute systemic infections like pneumonia can increase the CRP level 100-fold to 1,000-fold—the kind of elevation that is considered typical of severe acute pathology, such as pneumonia, encephalitis, or acute arthritis. Increases in laboratory values of only twofold or threefold are not considered by physicians to be "abnormal." It is interesting to note that the data from the study of Slade et al[65] would suggest that the normal laboratory values of CRP have been derived using people who were systemically healthy, but many probably had periodontal disease. Unfortunately, it would appear that many laboratory "normal ranges" of serum blood chemistry values probably did not take into account whether the "healthy" persons used to define *normal ranges* had periodontal disease or not. For this reason, the

CRP values associated with periodontal disease would be considered high normal. Recently, however, studies by Ridker and colleagues have shown that "high normal" levels of CRP in "apparently healthy males" were predictive of future myocardial infarctions and peripheral artery disease.[67] Indeed, Ridker reports that for diagnosing cardiovascular risk, serum CRP levels, in addition to cholesterol levels, provide the best diagnostic indicators of risk for future myocardial infarction.[68–70]

Thus, in light of these recent data suggesting that even mild increases in CRP enhance cardiac risk, the small elevations in CRP elicited by periodontal disease might be considered potential warning flags among cardiologists. Preliminary data[71] have been reported on the relationship between periodontal status, blood CRP levels, and the severity of subclinical atherosclerosis using B-mode ultrasonography to measure the wall thickness of the carotid vessels. These findings suggest that some (approximately half) of the linkage between high CRP levels and increased carotid wall thickness appears to be attributable to periodontal disease. Much work needs to be done to clarify what is triggering the acute-phase response and whether blood levels of CRP can be used for diagnosing systemic dissemination, assessing cardiovascular risk, and monitoring the systemic effects of periodontal treatment. Reports by Ebersole and others[64] and Elter and colleagues (personal communication, 2002) suggest that periodontal therapy may reduce levels of CRP. Thus, it appears likely that the future of periodontal medicine will probably include monitoring hepatic activation using blood tests similar to CRP tests, and practitioners will need to work with physicians to diagnose, monitor, and control CRP levels that are attributable to oral infection.

What Is the Evidence Linking Periodontal Disease to Heart Disease?

The evidence linking periodontal disease to cardiovascular disease has been summarized. Five longitudinal studies have shown that preexistent periodontal disease, as determined by direct oral examination, independently conferred excess risk for increased morbidity or mortality due to cardiovascular disease.[6–10] The increased risk ranges from a modest 20% (odds ratio of 1.2) to 180% (odds ratio of 2.8). A study by Beck and colleagues demonstrated a dose response; that is, with increasing periodontal disease, there is an incremental increase in risk for death due to myocardial infarction and stroke.[8] A study by Genco and colleagues demonstrates an association between coronary heart disease and periodontitis in a population that is largely nonsmoking.[72] Some studies include more than 1,000 subjects, and others more than 10,000 subjects. Some extend over decades. Most of these studies began as cardiovascular disease studies and have controlled for traditional risk factors such as gender, smoking, body mass, serum lipid levels, exercise, familial history, socioeconomic status, education, and other cardiovascular risk factors. Thus, several criteria appear to be satisfied for establishing an association: multiple studies, large numbers of subjects, prospective cohort design, valid cardiovascular and oral examination data, and specificity by controlling for confounders and covariables.

However, the magnitude of the risk is variable and appears modest in many studies. Modest degrees of excess risk, such as odds ratios less than 2, may potentially be due to what epidemiologists refer to as *residual confounding*, or the potential existence of other underlying risk factors that were not fully considered, adjusted for, or even measured. This issue, however, is always a potential problem, as there is always one more parameter that could be considered in any study design. The report by Arbes et al[73] analyzing the National Health and Nutrition Examination Survey (NHANES) III data shows a strong association between a history of myocardial infarction (a very robust and valid measure of cardiovascular disease) and increasing periodontal disease severity in a dose-response manner. The greater the periodontal disease, the greater the risk with odds ratios greater than 5 for the most severe periodontal disease groups. This was present after adjusting for age; race; gender; levels of serum cholesterol, low-density lipoprotein, and high-density lipoprotein; smoking; body mass index; physical activity; familial history; hypertension; diabetes mellitus; socioeconomic status; and education. With odds ratios of this magnitude, the likelihood is lower that residual confounding is responsible for a spurious finding. Thus, the epidemiological association data are fairly strong.

What Is the Threat of Periodontal Infection During Pregnancy?

Case-control and prospective human studies[31–38] suggest that periodontal disease in the mother is a potential risk factor for premature birth and low birth weight. Studies have indicated that after considering other traditional obstetric risk factors such as smoking, alcohol, age, race, level of prenatal care, and other infections, periodontal disease remains an independent contributor for an increase in prematurity,[31,32,36,37] preeclampsia,[36] and low birth weight.[31,32,34,36,37] The numbers of human studies

conducted are not as extensive as those supportive of a cardiovascular disease linkage, and there are negative reports,[33,35] but there are supportive data from animal models.[74,75] These data have been recently summarized.[36,37,39] Preliminary reports of interim findings from larger prospective studies, such as the Oral Conditions and Pregnancy Study at the University of North Carolina and Duke University,[36,39] as well as studies at University of Alabama Birmingham,[37] continue to show a significant association between more severe periodontal disease and increased incidence of premature delivery. The risk of preterm delivery increases to threefold among mothers with mild periodontal disease and increases to tenfold among mothers with moderate to severe disease.[36] There is also a significant effect of maternal periodontal disease on fetal growth restriction resulting in smaller babies for gestational age.[36] As stated before, these findings are controlled for other potential obstetric risk factors, including level of prenatal care, education, other infections, smoking, weight gain, and previous history of preterm delivery.

Overall, these data suggest that periodontal disease may have as large an impact on the prevalence of prematurity as smoking or alcohol consumption.[36] There are estimates that suggest that as many as 18% of all premature births may be prevented by providing periodontal treatment, assuming periodontal disease is truly associated with the causal pathway and can be eliminated by treatment. Preliminary reports by Mitchell-Lewis and colleagues[35] on convenience populations suggest that periodontal treatments may reduce the risk of prematurity. Reports by Lopez et al[38] of a randomized, no-treatment-controlled trial among pregnant women with periodontal disease suggest that periodontal therapy may reduce the rate of preterm delivery approximately fivefold. These promising reports of early findings need to be confirmed in multicenter, randomized, placebo-controlled clinical trials.

What Is the Relationship Among Periodontitis, Pneumonia, and Osteoporosis?

The oral cavity can serve as a reservoir for the dissemination of pathogens, especially in the medically compromised individual. This topic has been the subject of recent reviews.[44,76,77] Scannapieco and colleagues[40] have led this line of investigation, linking periodontal status to increased risk for chronic obstructive pulmonary disease (COPD) and aspiration pneumonia. The data suggest that periodontal pathogens shed into the saliva can be aspirated via the bronchia to the lung and thereby serve as one of the potential causes of pneumonia, especially in people who are debilitated, infirm, and aged.[44,45] The more severe the periodontal disease status of the patient, the greater the apparent risk for aspiration pneumonia. Furthermore, the mature periodontal flora can serve as a habitat for respiratory tract pathogens, especially in hospitalized individuals with dysphagia secondary to stroke[40–43] and during prolonged intubation. This oral colonization of respiratory pathogens in these compromised individuals appears to increase the risk for pulmonary involvement.[42,76] An association between periodontal disease and COPD has been reported, based on the NHANES III data set of more than 10,000 individuals.[78] Although the data from case-control studies and population surveys appear to demonstrate a possible association, few prospective data demonstrate that preexistent periodontal disease enhances the likelihood of developing pneumonia or COPD. Clearly, this area merits further study.

Some reports have associated osteoporosis with more severe periodontal disease.[79] However, it should be pointed out that osteoporosis is a systemic metabolic bone disease that has widespread effects on the skeleton. The alveolar bone is not a privileged site, and in osteoporosis it also suffers from a lack of bone mineral density and a marked decrease in trabecular cortication. Thus, it is not surprising that the osteolytic effects of periodontitis on the alveolar crestal bone result in greater clinical bone loss in patients with osteoporosis. There are no longitudinal data suggesting that more severe periodontal disease results in more severe osteoporosis. Although the systemic load of inflammatory mediators could at least theoretically have an effect on skeletal mass, the data to date suggest that osteoporosis modifies the expression of periodontal disease rather than the converse.

What Risk Does Periodontal Disease Pose for Diabetics?

Many epidemiological studies have confirmed that diabetes is strongly associated with periodontitis, with odds ratios in the range of 2 to 3. More recent investigations lead by Grossi et al,[26] Taylor et al,[25] and others (for a review, see Taylor[28]) have clearly demonstrated that periodontal disease is associated with impaired fasting glucose levels and an increased demand for insulin, apparently a consequence of insulin resistance (insulin tolerance). The metabolic stress of infection would tend to shift a person with normal glucose tolerance (euglycemic) toward a prediabetic state of type 2 diabetes mellitus. It has been suggested that this metabolic effect is a consequence of systemic LPS, TNF-α, IL-1β, and IL-6—all of which enhance insulin resistance.[29,30] Perhaps the best example is the effects of acute infection in a prediabetic individual. It is well appreciated by the medical community that hospitalized prediabetic individuals with acute infections, such as pelvic inflammatory disease, pneumonia, encephalitis, nephritis, bacterial endocarditis, and appendicitis, have the potential for the induction of a temporary state of diabetes mellitus that requires short-term insulin therapy. The same basic metabolic stressor mechanisms have been suggested to be involved in periodontitis as a greatly attenuated, but chronic, challenge. Experiments are under way to definitively determine whether periodontal therapy reduces the need for insulin use in people with diabetes and reduces the risk for the onset of type 2 diabetes. Taylor et al have published longitudinal data supporting the idea that periodontal disease is associated with an increased risk (nearly sixfold) of having poor glycemic control at follow-up.[25] Much of their data suggest that periodontal disease is a metabolic stressor associated with insulin tolerance and that periodontal therapy can reduce the level of glycosylated hemoglobin, a marker of glycemic control.

Other Data from Animal Models

Animal models of infections with periodontal pathogens and experimental periodontitis have demonstrated the deleterious effect of infection on atherosclerosis,[20] diabetes,[80,81] and fetal growth.[74,75] These data not only help establish biologic plausibility but also provide important clues regarding the potential mechanisms of cellular and molecular pathogenesis. There is an increasing body of evidence in support of the biology of the local-to-systemic pathological pathways, from cellular mechanisms to animal models of disease; human clinical data, however, will require more time and research. For example, it has been known for decades in the veterinary field that dogs with periodontal problems are at much greater risk for cardiovascular disease.[82,83] Periodic scaling and oral prophylaxis are a standard of veterinary canine care, not just to save teeth or prevent bad breath but also to save hearts. Unfortunately, parallel experiments in humans have lagged behind. It will require at least 5 to 15 years of clinical research and the completion of multicentered, randomized, placebo-controlled clinical trials to gain an adequate body of evidence to affect the standard of care. The potential benefits of oral therapy in pregnant women may represent a more accessible end point because of the definitive and timely nature of the clinical end point.

Thus, although the association data and biologic rationale contribute evidence quickly, the final clinical studies that change the standard of care are just beginning and will require more support for clinical research and more time for scrutiny and assimilation. Nonetheless, with each published study, the likelihood of these associations being spurious observations becomes less probable. It appears more likely that some or most of these associations contain a component of risk that is attributable to, or a consequence of, periodontal infection and that the chronic systemic burden of oral microbes and attendant inflammation plays a role in systemic disease. Thus, it would appear likely that practitioners of the future will have to consider how periodontal infection affects multiple organ systems.

Potential Impact on Dentistry

Periodontal medicine appears to be garnering additional evidence on the systemic effects of periodontal disease, with new reports and publications appearing at an increasing rate. Although there are a few negative findings[14–16] and appropriate cautionary editorial assessments,[84–88] to cite just a few, the evidence in support of the concept that periodontal infection has an effect on systemic health continues to mount. Without intervention studies demonstrating a systemic therapeutic benefit of periodontal therapy, there is no concrete evidence to justify a change in oral health care policy or the current standards of care. However, studies in progress have the potential to alter this position in a rapid and dramatic manner. Thus, it is prudent to be conservative, but prepared for the future.

At this moment one can say that a healthy mouth is part of a healthy lifestyle and that evidence suggests that poor oral health may be as detrimental to general health as other risk factors, such as smoking or high cholesterol levels. Although the beneficial systemic effects of oral therapy have not been demonstrated, the oral benefits clearly have a positive impact on the quality of life.

If periodontal disease is demonstrated by multicentered, randomized, controlled clinical trials to be causally related to some of the key systemic conditions described above, dental professionals will have to rapidly confront several issues. There will be a sudden appreciation by the public and by physicians that dentistry can no longer be considered solely as a luxury and as elective health care. Recent polls indicate that 85% of the US public is aware that poor oral health can worsen general health. Thus, the larger problem is the perception of the separation of oral health and systemic health among health care professionals, the nature of health care and the system by which it is delivered, and issues centering on access and utilization. The recognition of the medical necessity for periodontal care will increase the perceived importance of dental

services, and the demand for dental services will increase. In contrast to many diseases, such as mental illness, most cancers, and arthritis, periodontitis represents a modifiable risk factor that can be prevented and treated. Consider, for example, the nationwide maternal prenatal care programs that seek to reduce the rate of prematurity. These programs face the formidable task of reducing substance abuse among pregnant women, including the use of alcohol, tobacco, and other drugs. By comparison, oral prevention programs and services have been shown to be highly efficient and effective against periodontal diseases (and caries). Thus, research findings that clearly demonstrate the medical necessity for periodontal care among pregnant women would undoubtedly lead to a rapid and profound increase in the priority of dental services in such high-risk populations.

Dentistry will move far beyond saving teeth and smiles, and practitioners will be given the opportunity, and be expected, to assume a greater responsibility and obligation for patients' overall health. Although it may take a decade for this to unfold, dentistry will be profoundly affected in many ways, from education to the practice of dentistry and health care policy.

References

1. Williams RC, Offenbacher S. Periodontal medicine: The emergence of a new branch of periodontology. Periodontol 2000 2000;23:9–12.
2. Mattila KJ, Nieminen MS, Valtonen VV, et al. Association between dental health and acute myocardial infarction. Br Med J 1989;298:779–781.
3. Mattila KJ, Valle MS, Nieminen MS, et al. Dental infections and coronary atherosclerosis. Atherosclerosis 1993;103:205–211.
4. Grau AJ, Buggle F, Ziegler C, et al. Association between acute cerebrovascular ischemia and chronic and recurrent infection. Stroke 1997;28:1724–1729.
5. Loesche WJ, Schork A, Terpenning MS, et al. The relationship between dental disease and cerebral vascular accident in elderly United States veterans. Ann Periodontol 1998;3:161–174.
6. DeStefano F, Anda RF, Kahn HS, et al. Dental disease and risk of coronary heart disease and mortality. Br Med J 1993;306:688–691.
7. Mattila KJ, Valtonen VV, Nieminen M, Huttunen JK. Dental infection and the risk of new coronary events: Prospective study of patients with documented coronary artery disease. Clin Infect Dis 1995;20:588–592.
8. Beck J, Garcia R, Heiss G, et al. Periodontal disease and cardiovascular disease. J Periodontol 1996;67(suppl):1123–1137.
9. Morrison HI, Ellison LF, Taylor GW. Periodontal disease and risk of fatal coronary heart and cerebrovascular diseases. J Cardiovasc Risk 1999;6:7–11.
10. Wu T, Trevisan M, Genco RJ, et al. Periodontal disease and risk of cerebrovascular disease: The first national health and nutrition examination survey and its follow-up study. Arch Intern Med 2000;160:2749–2755.

11. Beck JD, Elter JR, Heiss G, et al. Relationship of periodontal disease to carotid artery intima-media wall thickness: The atherosclerosis risk in communities (ARIC) study. Arterioscler Thromb Vasc Biol 2001;21:1816–1822.

12. Herzberg MC, Meyer MW. Effects of oral flora on platelets: Possible consequences in cardiovascular disease. J Periodontol 1996;67(suppl):1138–1142.

13. Meyer MW, Gong K, Herzberg MC. *Streptococcus sanguis*–induced platelet clotting in rabbits and hemodynamic and cardiopulmonary consequences. Infect Immun 1998;66:5906–5914.

14. Joshipura KJ, Rimm EB, Douglass CW, et al. Poor oral health and coronary heart disease. J Dent Res 1996;75:1631–1636.

15. Hujoel PP, Drangsholt MT, Spiekerman C, DeRouen TA. Periodontal disease and coronary heart disease risk. JAMA 2000;284:1406–1410.

16. Howell TH, Ridker PM, Ajani UA, et al. Periodontal disease and risk of subsequent cardiovascular disease in U.S. male physicians. J Am Coll Cardiol 2001;37:445–450.

17. Beck JD, Offenbacher S. The association between periodontal diseases and cardiovascular diseases: A state-of-the-science review. Ann Periodontol 2001;6:9–15.

18. Deshpande RG, Khan MB, Genco CA. Invasion of aortic and heart endothelial cells by *Porphyromonas gingivalis.* Infect Immun 1998;66:5337–5343.

19. Dorn BR, Dunn WA Jr, Progulske-Fox A. Invasion of human coronary artery cells by periodontal pathogens. Infect Immun 1999;67:5792–5798.

20. Li L, Messas E, Batista EL Jr, et al. *Porphyromonas gingivalis* infection accelerates the progression of atherosclerosis in a heterozygous apolipoprotein E-deficient murine model. Circulation 2002;105:861–867.

21. Williams RC Jr, Mahan CJ. Periodontal disease and diabetes in young adults. JAMA 1960;172:776–778.

22. Wolf J. Dental and periodontal conditions in diabetes mellitus. A clinical and radiographic study. Proc Finn Dent Soc 1977;73(suppl):1–56.

23. Miller LS, Manwell MA, Newbold D, et al. The relationship between reduction in periodontal inflammation and diabetes control: A report of 9 cases. J Periodontol 1992;63:843–848.

24. Seppälä B, Seppälä M, Ainamo J. A longitudinal study on insulin-dependent diabetes mellitus and periodontal disease. J Clin Periodontol 1993;20:161–165.

25. Taylor GW, Burt BA, Becker MP, et al. Severe periodontitis and risk for poor glycemic control in patients with non–insulin-dependent diabetes mellitus. J Periodontol 1996;67(suppl):1085–1093.

26. Grossi SG, Skrepcinski FB, DeCaro T, et al. Treatment of periodontal disease in diabetics reduces glycated hemoglobin. J Periodontol 1997;68:713–719.

27. Collin HL, Uusitupa M, Niskanen L, et al. Periodontal findings in elderly patients with non–insulin-dependent diabetes mellitus. J Periodontol 1998;69:962–966.

28. Taylor GW. Bidirectional interrelationships between diabetes and periodontal diseases: An epidemiologic perspective. Ann Periodontol 2001;6:99–112.

29. Mizock BA. Alterations in carbohydrate metabolism during stress: A review of the literature. Am J Med 1995;98:75–84.

30. Michie HR. Metabolism of sepsis and multiple organ failure. World J Surg 1996;20:460–464.

31. Offenbacher S, Katz V, Fertik G, et al. Periodontal infection as a possible risk factor for preterm low birth weight. J Periodontol 1996;67(suppl):1103–1113.

32. Dasanayake AP. Poor periodontal health of the pregnant woman as a risk factor for low birth weight. Ann Periodontol 1998;3:206–212.

33. Davenport ES, Williams CE, Sterne JA, et al. The East London study of maternal chronic periodontal disease and preterm low birth weight infants: Study design and prevalence data. Ann Periodontol 1998;3:213–221.

34. Offenbacher S, Jared HL, O'Reilly PG, et al. Potential pathogenic mechanisms of periodontitis-associated pregnancy complications. Ann Periodontol 1998;3:233–250.

35. Mitchell-Lewis D, Engebretson SP, Chen J, et al. Periodontal infections and pre-term birth: Early findings from a cohort of young minority women in New York. Eur J Oral Sci 2001;109:34–39.

36. Offenbacher S, Lieff S, Boggess KA, et al. Maternal periodontitis and prematurity. Part I: Obstetric outcome of prematurity and growth restriction. Ann Periodontol 2001;6:164–174.

37. Jeffcoat MK, Geurs NC, Reddy MS, et al. Current evidence regarding periodontal disease as a risk factor in preterm birth. Ann Periodontol 2001;6:183–188.

38. Lopez NJ, Smith PC, Gutierrez J. Higher risk of preterm birth and low birth weight in women with periodontal disease. J Dent Res 2002;81:58–63.

39. Madianos PN, Lieff S, Murtha AP, et al. Maternal periodontitis and prematurity. Part II: Maternal infection and fetal exposure. Ann Periodontol 2001;6:175–182.

40. Scannapieco FA, Stewart EM, Mylotte JM. Colonization of dental plaque by respiratory pathogens in medical intensive care patients. Crit Care Med 1992;20:740–745.

41. Terpenning M, Bretz W, Lopatin D, et al. Bacterial colonization of saliva and plaque in the elderly. Clin Infect Dis 1993;16(suppl):S314–S316.

42. Fourrier F, Duvivier B, Boutigny H, et al. Colonization of dental plaque: A source of nosocomial infections in intensive care unit patients. Crit Care Med 1998;26:301–308.

43. Russell SL, Boylan RJ, Kaslick RS, et al. Respiratory pathogen colonization of the dental plaque of institutionalized elders. Spec Care Dentist 1999;19:128–134.

44. Scannapieco FA. Role of oral bacteria in respiratory infection. J Periodontol 1999;70:793–802.

45. Terpenning MS, Taylor GW, Lopatin DE, et al. Aspiration pneumonia: Dental and oral risk factors in an older veteran population. J Am Geriatr Soc 2001;49:557–563.

46. Kurihara M, Nishimura F, Hashimoto T, et al. Immunopathological diagnosis of cicatricial pemphigoid with desquamative gingivitis. A case report. J Periodontol 2001;72:243–249.

47. U.S. Department of Health and Human Services. Oral Health in America: A Report of the Surgeon General. Rockville, MD: U.S. Dept of Health and Human Services, National Institute of Dental and Craniofacial Research, 2000.

48. Papapanou PN. Periodontal diseases: Epidemiology. Ann Periodontol 1996;1:1–36.

49. Baelum V, Wen-Min L, Fejerskov O, Xia C. Tooth mortality and periodontal conditions in 60–80-year-old Chinese. Scand J Dent Res 1988;96:99–107.

50. Beck JD, Koch GG, Zambon JJ, et al. Evaluation of oral bacteria as risk indicators for periodontitis in older adults. J Periodontol 1992;63:93–99.

51. Socransky SS, Haffajee AD. The bacterial etiology of destructive periodontal disease: Current concepts. J Periodontol 1992;63:322–331.

52. Michalowicz BS. Genetic and heritable risk factors in periodontal disease. J Periodontol 1994;65(suppl):479–488.

53. Socransky SS, Haffajee AD, Cugini MA, et al. Microbial complexes in subgingival plaque. J Clin Periodontol 1998;25:134–144.

54. Ximenez-Fyvie LA, Haffajee AD, Socransky SS. Comparison of the microbiota of supra- and subgingival plaque in health and periodontitis. J Clin Periodontol 2000;27:648–657.

55. Chiu B. Multiple infections in carotid atherosclerotic plaques. Am Heart J 1999;138:S534–S536.

56. Haraszthy VI, Zambon JJ, Trevisan M, et al. Identification of periodontal pathogens in atheromatous plaques. J Periodontol 2000;71:1554–1560.

57. Page RC, Offenbacher S, Schroeder HE, et al. Advances in the pathogenesis of periodontitis: Summary of developments, clinical implications and future directions. Periodontology 2000 1997;14:216–248.

58. Offenbacher S, Madianos PN, Champagne CM, et al. Periodontitis-atherosclerosis syndrome: An expanded model of pathogenesis. J Periodontal Res 1999;34:346–352.

59. Offenbacher S. Periodontal diseases: Pathogenesis. Ann Periodontol 1996;1:821–878.

60. Papapanou PN, Baelum V, Luan WM, et al. Subgingival microbiota in adult Chinese: Prevalence and relation to periodontal disease progression. J Periodontol 1997;68:651–666.

61. Baelum V, Luan WM, Chen X, Fejerskov O. A 10-year study of the progression of destructive periodontal disease in adult and elderly Chinese. J Periodontol 1997;68:1033–1042.

62. Engebretson SP, Lamster IB, Herrera-Abreu M, et al. The influence of interleukin gene polymorphism on expression of interleukin-1beta and tumor necrosis factor-alpha in periodontal tissue and gingival crevicular fluid. J Periodontol 1999;70:567–573.

63. Shirodaria S, Smith J, McKay IJ, et al. Polymorphisms in the IL-1A gene are correlated with levels of interleukin-1alpha protein in gingival crevicular fluid of teeth with severe periodontal disease. J Dent Res 2000;79:1864–1869.

64. Ebersole JL, Machen RL, Steffen MJ, Willmann DE. Systemic acute-phase reactants, C-reactive protein and haptoglobin, in adult periodontitis. Clin Exp Immunol 1997;107:347–352.

65. Slade GD, Offenbacher S, Beck JD, et al. Acute-phase inflammatory response to periodontal disease in the US population. J Dent Res 2000;79:49–57.

66. Loos BG, Craandijk J, Hoek FJ, et al. Elevation of systemic markers related to cardiovascular diseases in the peripheral blood of periodontitis patients. J Periodontol 2000;71:1528–1534.

67. Ridker PM, Cushman M, Stampfer MJ, et al. Inflammation, aspirin, and the risk of cardiovascular disease in apparently healthy men. N Engl J Med 1997;336:973–979.

68. Ridker PM, Glynn RJ, Hennekens CH. C-reactive protein adds to the predictive value of total and HDL cholesterol in determining risk of first myocardial infarction. Circulation 1998;97:2007–2011.

69. Ridker PM, Buring JE, Shih J, et al. Prospective study of C-reactive protein and the risk of future cardiovascular events among apparently healthy women. Circulation 1998;98:731–733.

70. Ridker PM, Stampfer MJ, Rifai N. Novel risk factors for systemic atherosclerosis: A comparison of C-reactive protein, fibrinogen, homocysteine, lipoprotein(a), and standard cholesterol screening as predictors of peripheral arterial disease. JAMA 2001;285:2481–2485.

71. Slade GS, Ghezzi E, Heiss G, et al. Relationship between periodontal disease and C-reactive protein among adults in the Atherosclerosis Risk in Communities study. Ann Intern Med 2002 (accepted).

72. Genco RG, Wu TJ, Grossi S, et al. Periodontal microflora related to the risk for myocardial infarction: A case control study [abstract 2811]. J Dent Res 1999;78(spec. issue):457.

73. Arbes SJ Jr, Slade GD, Beck JD. Association between extent of periodontal attachment loss and self-reported history of heart attack: An analysis of NHANES III data. J Dent Res 1999;78:1777–1782.

74. Collins JG, Windley HW III, Arnold RR, Offenbacher S. Effects of a Porphyromonas gingivalis infection on inflammatory mediator response and pregnancy outcome in hamsters. Infect Immun 1994;62:4356–4361.

75. Collins JG, Smith MA, Arnold RR, Offenbacher S. Effects of Escherichia coli and Porphyromonas gingivalis lipopolysaccharide on pregnancy outcome in the golden hamster. Infect Immun 1994;62:4652–4655.

76. Terpenning MS. The relationship between infections and chronic respiratory diseases: An overview. Ann Periodontol 2001;6:66–70.

77. Garcia RI, Nunn ME, Vokonas PS. Epidemiologic associations between periodontal disease and chronic obstructive pulmonary disease. Ann Periodontol 2001;6:71–77.

78. Scannapieco FA, Ho AW. Potential associations between chronic respiratory disease and periodontal disease: Analysis of National Health and Nutrition Examination Survey III. J Periodontol 2001;72:50–56.

79. Wactawski-Wende J. Periodontal diseases and osteoporosis: Association and mechanisms. Ann Periodontol 2001;6:197–208.

80. Lalla E, Lamster IB, Feit M, et al. A murine model of accelerated periodontal disease in diabetes. J Periodontal Res 1998;33:387–399.

81. Lalla E, Lamster IB, Feit M, et al. Blockade of RAGE suppresses periodontitis-associated bone loss in diabetic mice. J Clin Invest 2000;105:1117–1124.

82. Wilkinson GT. Myocarditis in puppies, unidentified feline illness and gingivitis in cats. Vet Rec 1979;104:149–150.

83. DeBowes LJ. The effects of dental disease on systemic disease. Vet Clin North Am Small Anim Pract 1998;28:1057–1062.

84. Joshipura K, Ritchie C, Douglass C. Strength of evidence linking oral conditions and systemic disease. Compend Contin Educ Dent Suppl 2000;21:12–23.

85. Genco RJ, Trevisan M, Wu T, Beck JD. Periodontal disease and risk of coronary heart disease. JAMA 2001;285:40–41.

86. Di Napoli M, Papa F, Bocola V. Periodontal disease, C-reactive protein, and ischemic stroke. Arch Intern Med 2001;161:1234–1235.

87. Wehrmacher WH. Periodontal disease and risk of myocardial infarction. J Am Coll Cardiol 2001;38:1273–1274.

88. Katz J, Marc H, Porter S, Ruskin J. Inflammation, periodontitis, and coronary heart disease. Lancet 2001;358:1998.

Infection Control and Personnel Safety

John A. Molinari

- Historical Perspective
- Principles of Microbial Transmission
- Rationale for Infection Control and Safety Guidelines
- Aseptic Technique
- Practical Barrier Techniques
- Hepatitis B Vaccination and Other Immunizations
- Postexposure Evaluation and Follow-up
- Instrument Recirculation, Sterilization, and Monitoring
- Environmental Surface and Equipment Asepsis
- Water Quality
- Waste Management

Historical Perspective

Progress in controlling the transmission of infectious diseases has been steady and highlighted by extraordinary individual achievements. The development and refinement of new principles, procedures, and products to meet the increasingly complex demands of patient care have created a safer environment for patients and health professionals alike. The implementation of appropriate practices, devices, and procedures to attain the current level of infection control initially required the recognition of science-based infectious disease risks, as well as determined cooperation among numerous professional groups. Routine application of effective infection control strategies continues to require a major commitment by medical and dental care providers, along with their willingness to respond to documented and emerging biomedical and clinical science–based information.

The fields of microbiology, patient care, and infection control have benefited from the advancement of scientific knowledge elucidating the etiologies of many infectious diseases, their modes of transmission to susceptible hosts, and strategies designed to control their spread.

Table 16-1 is a representative list of achievements that have provided a foundation for many of today's routine infection control practices. One of these milestones was the successful development and introduction in the 1790s of a smallpox vaccine by Edward Jenner, an English physician. He astutely observed that dairy milkmaids who had developed vesicles associated with cowpox were immune to smallpox. Jenner later induced this protective immunity in other townspeople by injecting extracted vesicular fluid from the hands of those affected women into the arms of susceptible individuals. By 1800, approximately 6,000 people had been vaccinated and protected in this manner, ushering in the era of vaccination and a new philosophy of preventive medicine.

Although it may be difficult for current clinicians to relate to many of the early problems and perceptions confronted by scientists and clinicians 100 to 300 years ago, one need go back only a relatively short time to find important 20th-century dental infection control challenges and successes (Box 16-1).

Dental medicine has come a long way in achieving the current level of infection control success. Many dental professionals may not be aware of all the protective aspects of routinely applied precautions, in part because

Table 16-1 Representative Milestones in Infectious Diseases and Their Control

Year	Researcher	Contributions
1546	Fracastoro	Reported concept of contagion and modes of disease transmission
1675	van Leeuwenhoek	First described bacteria and protozoa ("animalcules") under microscope; built the first simple microscope
1750	Pringle	Observed relationship of putrefaction to disease; performed studies with agents he called "antiseptics"
1796	Jenner	Introduced smallpox vaccination as an effective preventive method against disease outbreaks
1827	Alcock	Emphasized disinfectant properties of hypochlorite
1840s to 1870s	Nightingale	Emphasized importance of sanitation; used statistics, surveillance, and data collection
1843	Holmes	Applied epidemiology to demonstrate direct transmission of infection by health care personnel; demonstrated contagiousness of childbed fever (puerperal sepsis) from doctors and nurses
1861	Semmelweis	Instituted hospital procedures to reduce mortality from puerperal septicemia; emphasized role of hand hygiene in prevention of cross-infection
1860s and 1870s	Lister	The "father of clean and decent surgery"; introduced aseptic technique for surgery and care of wounds; introduced phenols (carbolic acid)
1860s to 1880s	Pasteur	Established microbiology as a science; developed process of pasteurization
1870s and 1880s	Koch	Isolated and demonstrated infectivity of anthrax bacillus; discovered *Mycobacterium tuberculosis*; formulated Koch's postulates for infectious disease investigation; examined effects of numerous disinfectants against bacteria

From Molinari.[1] Copyright © 1999 American Dental Association. Adapted (2002) with permission of ADA Publishing, a Division of ADA Business Enterprises, Inc.

Box 16-1 20th-Century Accomplishments in Infection Control

- Recognition of relationship between microbial pathogens and risk of occupational transmission of infectious disease: blood-borne, airborne, wound, acute, chronic
- Development and refinement of efficient aseptic techniques: hand-washing procedures, classes of antiseptics, infection control cleaning procedures
- Conversion from chemical immersion to heat sterilization procedures for instrument reprocessing
- Adaptation to use of personal protective barriers during patient care: gloves, face masks, eyewear, clinic coats and gowns
- Receipt of hepatitis B vaccine and other vaccines recommended for health professionals
- Application of universal precautions against blood-borne disease as infection control standard for patient treatment

- Adaptation of safer procedures to minimize accidental exposures to contaminated sharp items
- Development and use of newer technologies to prevent microbial cross-contamination and facilitate better infection control: sterilizers; personal and equipment barriers; automated instrument cleaning equipment; reusable, heat-stable dental instrumentation; single-use disposable needles; technical advancements in promoting dental unit water asepsis
- Provision of routine care to patients with increasing variety of immune system compromise
- Discovery and development of antimicrobial antibiotics to treat clinical infections

From Molinari.[1] Copyright © 1999 American Dental Association. Adapted (2002) with permission of ADA Publishing, a Division of ADA Business Enterprises, Inc.

---

certain occupational infections now occur only infrequently in schools, clinics, and practices. As a consequence of this trend, a decreasing percentage of students and practitioners are able to directly relate to certain repercussions of asepsis failures.

Current infection control and personnel safety practices were initially developed in the 1960s to limit the potential transmission of blood-borne pathogens in clinical settings.

The primary target of these precautions was hepatitis B virus (HBV).[2,3] This virus remains the most infectious microbial organism targeted for universal or standard infection control precautions in health care. A large volume of accumulated evidence documented HBV as the major occupational microbial challenge for health care workers, but widespread implementation of infection control principles and procedures became integrated into many dental

Table 16-2 Representative Infectious Diseases Encountered in Dentistry

Condition	Habitat	Route
Respiratory diseases		
Common cold	Upper respiratory tract	Aerosols, contact
Sinusitis	Upper respiratory tract	Aerosols, droplet
Pharyngitis	Upper respiratory tract	Aerosols, droplet
Pneumonia	Respiratory tract	Aerosols, droplet
Tuberculosis	Respiratory tract, oral cavity	Aerosols, droplet
Childhood diseases		
Chicken pox	Oral cavity, skin	Droplet, contact
Herpangina	Oral cavity, oropharynx	Droplet, contact
Hand-foot-and-mouth disease	Oral cavity, hands, feet	Droplet, ingestion, contact
Rubella and rubeola	Respiratory tract, oral cavity, skin	Droplet, contact with saliva/blood/exudate
Mumps	Parotids, pancreas, testes, central nervous system	Droplet, contact with saliva
Cytomegalovirus infection	Salivary glands	Droplet, contact with saliva and blood
Sexually transmitted diseases		
Herpetic infections	Oral cavity, pharynx, genitals, skin, viscera	Contact with lesion, saliva, blood, other body fluids
Acute herpetic gingivostomatitis	Oral cavity, gingiva, pharynx	Contact with lesion, saliva, blood, other body fluids
Herpetic whitlow	Fingers, hands	Contact with oral lesion, saliva, exudate, blood
Gonococcal infections	Oral cavity, pharynx	Contact with blood, lesion exudate, nasopharyngeal secretions
Chlamydial infections	Genitals, eyes, oropharynx	Contact with lesion exudate, genital secretions, secretions from eyes
Trichomonal infections	Genitals, oropharynx, oral cavity, gastrointestinal tract	Contact with mucosa, lesion exudate, saliva, body fluids, blood
Condyloma acuminatum	Anogenital skin, oral cavity, other mucosal areas	Contact with lesion, mucosa, blood, autoinoculation
Syphilis	Genitals, skin, oral mucosa, oropharynx	Contact with mucosa, blood, body fluids, congenital
Infectious mononucleosis	Skin, oral mucosa, genitals, parotids, saliva	Contact with mucosa, saliva, lesion exudate
Hepatitis A	Liver, gastrointestinal tract	Ingestion, rarely by blood
Hepatitis B	Liver, blood, body fluids	Contact with blood, saliva, body fluids
Hepatitis C	Liver, blood	Contact with blood
Hepatitis D	Liver, blood	Contact with blood
Hepatitis E	Liver	Possible contact with blood
HIV infection	Blood, oral cavity, mucosa, skin	Contact with blood, semen, nonintact skin

practices only after the emergence and recognition of the well-publicized acquired immunodeficiency syndrome (AIDS) pandemic in the early 1980s.[4,5] The same recommended protocols and procedures for minimizing HBV infection were subsequently applied to both human immunodeficiency virus (HIV, the etiologic agent of AIDS) and, more recently, hepatitis C virus (formerly associated with blood-borne non-A, non-B hepatitis).[5–15] Statements in published regulations, guidelines, and recommendations from numerous health professional organizations have reinforced the position that infection control procedures should be used routinely to minimize cross-infection of all occupational infectious diseases.[16–22] Representative examples are listed in Table 16-2.

Dentistry has confronted many occupational challenges since the publication of the initial American Dental Association infection control recommendations in 1978.[3] Despite documentation of transmission of other infectious diseases in the dental environment, it was the impact of HBV and HIV infections in the 1980s that forever changed the way dentistry was practiced. The recognition that many persons infected with these and other microbial pathogens neither show symptoms for extended periods nor give positive histories of prior infection led the Centers for Disease Control (CDC) to recommend the practice of treating all patients as though they are infected with HBV or HIV.[5] This approach to patient care is termed *universal infection control precautions*. The term has been modified in recent years to *standard infection control precautions*, and protection against the hepatitis C virus has also been included under this infection control umbrella.[14,15]

Today, governmental regulations from federal agencies, such as the Occupational Safety and Health Administration (OSHA), and state and local health departments require dental practitioners to be trained in appropriate infection control and other safety precautions. Dental health care workers are required to routinely follow these measures during patient care to reduce potential risks of disease transmission to both patients and themselves. Mandated standards and recommendations from public health agencies also call for a reduction of potential risks from occupational exposures through a series of other practice controls. This chapter discusses state-of-the-art infection control and safety components, as well as their implications for the practice of periodontics.

Principles of Microbial Transmission

Initial recognition of the potential for microbial cross-transmission is essential prior to applying appropriate infection control precautions during the provision of dental care. Dental health care workers and patients can be exposed to a wide variety of microorganisms via blood and other oral/respiratory secretions. There are multiple potential sources for microbial cross-contamination and infection during treatment, including blood; saliva; nasal discharge; hands; instruments; aerosolized spatter from waterlines, ultrasonic scaler units, and the patient's mouth; and other contaminated used items. When considering routes of microbial transmission in clinical settings, two different, yet compatible, approaches can be cited. The first approach describes three general routes of transmission:

1. *Direct contact with a lesion, organisms, or potentially infectious secretions when performing intraoral procedures.* The earlier practice of treating patients without wearing gloves (ie, "wet-fingered" dentistry) is an example.

2. *Indirect contact via contaminated instruments, equipment, or disposable items.* Accidental percutaneous exposures from used needles or other sharps are placed in this category and remain a major concern for dental health care workers and advisory agencies.

3. *Aerosolization of microorganisms from patients' blood or saliva while using devices that can generate droplet spatter.* Exposure to aerosols created by equipment such as dental handpieces, air-water devices, and ultrasonic scaling units can lead to a variety of mild to severe respiratory infections, including influenza and bacterial pneumonia.[2,4,16,17,23]

A second system of exposure designation describes information similar to the above, while using dental health care workers and patients as modes of microbial and disease transmission during patient care:

1. *Patient–to–dental health care worker passage of potentially infectious microbes.* This transmission can occur through breaks in the skin, from accidental sharps exposure, or through exposed mucous membranes (from airborne microorganisms in sprays or spatter particles).

2. *Dental health care worker–to–patient exposure to potentially infectious microbes.* This transmission represents a microbial challenge as a result of accidental bleeding into a patient's mouth following an accidental sharps exposure or through respiratory droplets passed from the care provider to the patient.

3. *Patient-to-patient transmission of infectious microorganisms.* This kind of transmission has a much lower chance of occurring, although it has been noted, primarily in medicine, from the use of improperly reprocessed instruments or improper hand washing and/or glove wearing by health care workers.

4. *Dental practice–to–community transmission of infectious microorganisms.* This form of transmission may take place as a result of improper waste management or improper decontamination of dental impressions and appliances.[19,21]

The most common risks of exposure are those from patient to health care professional. Minimizing the potential for this mode of transmission, therefore, is a primary focus for a comprehensive infection control program. The potential for risk of microbial transmission can vary, depending on the number of microbial pathogens present during exposure, host susceptibility to infection, and pathway of exposure (see Table 16-2).[16] It is therefore necessary to understand the nuances of these different transmission modes to be able to implement appropriate control measures. In addition, recognition of infection control challenges should be supplemented by the application of a few general guidelines regarding standard precautions for patient care:

1. Reduce the concentration of pathogens so that normal host resistance mechanisms can prevent infections.
2. Break the cycle of infection by reducing cross-contamination as much as possible.
3. Treat every patient and instrument as if potentially infectious for a life-threatening blood-borne disease.
4. Protect patients and personnel from occupational exposure and possible infection.[17,23,24]

Rationale for Infection Control and Safety Guidelines

Because dental health care workers are at potential risk of exposure and possible infection from a variety of microbial diseases (see Table 16-2), it is essential that they protect themselves and their patients from cross-infection. A number of individual, rational approaches used in concert can accomplish effective infection control. Practices aimed at reducing occupational risks include, among others, routine use of aseptic techniques, immunization of care providers with available vaccines, use of protective barriers to physically reduce tissue exposure to pathogenic microorganisms, use of appropriate engineering controls and other safety measures, and use of effective sterilization and disinfection procedures.

Infection control and safety guidelines for dentistry have been published by a number of agencies and associations. The American Dental Association (ADA) focused on HBV prevention in dental settings when it released its initial report in 1978, suggesting procedures for reducing contamination and cross-contamination.[3] In addition to the recognized health care risks for HBV, the description of the first cases of AIDS in 1981 and 1982 stimulated the CDC to publish occupational infection control guidelines for health care workers, which included recommendations for the use of gloves, gowns, and extraordinary steps to avoid injury.[5] Subsequent ADA recommendations in 1988[6] and 1992[7] expanded the scope of certain practices and protocols, including more routine application of gloves, masks, and eyewear and sterilization procedures. In May 1993 the CDC, renamed the Centers for Disease Control and Prevention, published updated guidelines replacing the 1986 recommendations.[9] The CDC and ADA guidelines are directed toward protecting both dental care providers and their patients from potential infections and hazards during provision of care. To protect dental health care workers from occupational exposures, the federal government passed into law and published the blood-borne pathogens rule in December 1991.[10] The rationale and specific components of this OSHA law are designed to protect employees in workplaces, including dental staff personnel, practitioners who are associates, and practitioners in the employ of their own corporations. The latest series of ADA infection control recommendations, released in 1996, reinforced the tenets and practices found in the earlier CDC and OSHA documents.[11]

Aseptic Technique

A fundamental principle that runs through all aspects of infection control practices is the routine application of aseptic technique. This refers to the use of procedures that break the cycle of infection and reduce the potential for cross-contamination. At the heart of all applications of this principle is the requirement for cleaning. Patient care providers are constantly reminded to wash and clean hands routinely before and after patient care (in many instances, washing hands at certain times during treatment is also necessary); to clean instruments before employing sterilization procedures; to clean surfaces before application of disinfectants; and to clean dentures before spraying them with, or immersing them in, chemical agents. Appropriate cleaning accomplishes a number of infection control goals: (1) reduction in the number of contaminating microorganisms, (2) removal of organic matter and debris that can interfere with sterilization and disinfection procedures, and (3) assistance in keeping work areas clean.[16–21]

One component singled out for special mention in the "clean it first" category is the washing of hands. The clinical impact of this practice cannot be overstated. Hand washing is the single most important infection control procedure for minimizing the potential for the development of nosocomial infections.[9,25–28] Its primary purpose is to reduce the microbial population on the hands by removing the accumulated macroscopic and microscopic bioburden. The most frequently used classes of antimicrobial antiseptics available are chlorhexidine gluconate, parachlorometaxylenol, and triclosan. Each agent is capable of providing substantivity, a residual antimicrobial effect, following each succeeding hand-washing procedure during the day.

With regard to routine, nonsurgical dental procedures, hand washing is mandatory before treatment, between patient appointments, after glove removal, and before leaving treatment areas. In addition to general considera-

Box 16-2 Hand Washing

General Considerations
- Be aware of skin sensitivities of personnel.
- Perform a thorough surgical scrub at the beginning of the day.
- Jewelry and long nails should not be permitted.

Hand-Washing Procedure
1. Wet hands and wrists under cool, running water.
2. Dispense a sufficient amount of a hand-washing agent to cover the hands and wrists.
3. Rub the agent into all areas, paying particular attention to thumbs, fingertips, and areas between fingers.
4. Clean thoroughly under nails.
5. Rinse hands with cool water.
6. Use disposable towels to dry hands.
7. Dry hands completely before donning gloves.
8. Keep epithelial integrity intact and prevent dry skin, use water-based lotions.

care workers and their patients. Dental care providers must wear protective attire such as disposable gloves, eyewear, face masks or chin-length shields, and other protective clothing when performing treatment procedures capable of causing splash, spatter, or contact with body fluids or mucous membranes, or when touching items or surfaces that may be contaminated with these fluids (Box 16-3). These treatment procedures include the use of high- or low-speed handpieces, manipulation with sharp cutting instruments during periodontal and prophylaxis treatments, spraying water and air into a patient's mouth, intraoral surgical procedures, cleanup of the treatment area, and instrument reprocessing.

Disposable materials must be discarded after a single use. Reusable materials must be reprocessed in an acceptable manner (either by sanitization, disinfection, or sterilization) based on the level of contamination and the inherent ability of the material to withstand the level of reprocessing. If the materials are damaged or become permeable during use, they must be replaced with fresh items to prevent contamination and maintain barrier efficacy. The practitioner should choose either sterile or clean barriers (eg, gloves), as dictated by the procedures.[9,20]

Gloves

Properly fitting gloves protect health care providers from direct exposure through cuts and abrasions, which often can be visually undetected on the hands. Gloves used during the provision of patient care are single-use items and must not be used on another patient or be washed with a detergent. The ADA initially approached the issue of practitioners wearing disposable gloves in an important 1976 publication aimed at protecting dental health care workers from occupational HBV infection. At that time, the ADA Council of Dental Therapeutics wrote: "The use of gloves in a practice should be encouraged through dental school training for those procedures in which there is bleeding."[29] The language was strengthened and expanded in later series of ADA and CDC statements and recommendations. In today's health professional activities, the routine use of disposable gloves constitutes the single most important aspect of personal protective equipment.[1]

The most common type of glove worn during patient treatment is made of latex. This material can be manufactured in a number of sizes and specifications (ambidextrous, right or left hand, low powder, powder-free, or low protein), can provide a comfortable fit and tactility for most users, and provides an effective barrier during the time needed for most routine procedures. Other types of disposable gloves include medical vinyl, nitrile, and neoprene. The use of sterile latex or other treatment glove materials is indicated when surgical procedures are

tions that apply to all forms of hand-washing procedures (Box 16-2), application of a thorough 1-minute wash at the beginning of the work day, followed by 15-second washes for the remainder of the day, except at the end of the day, is recommended.

Surgical procedures require more rigorous hand washing. This involves a scrub technique to clean nails, hands, and forearms with a surgical antiseptic and a soft sterile brush or sponge. Lather for 5 to 7 minutes using multiple scrub-and-rinse cycles, and dry with sterile towels.

Routine hand washing, a fundamental application of aseptic technique, is a frequent source of dermatitis or exudative problems, which can have either immunologic or nonspecific irritant etiologies. Dental care providers who have exudative lesions or weeping dermatitis should refrain from direct patient contact until the condition is resolved. They can also take steps to return damaged skin to epithelial integrity by ceasing to use antiseptics that remove skin oils and replacing them with a nonantiseptic, mechanical cleansing agent, such as liquid soap and water.

Practical Barrier Techniques

Physical barriers play an important role in reducing tissue contact with potential pathogens and thus reduce cross-contamination and cross-infection between dental health

---

Box 16-3 Criteria for Protective Barriers

Face Mask

1. It must fit the face well to minimize open spaces on the side of the face.
2. It should be able to prevent penetration of aerosolized particles generated during the procedure for which the mask is worn.
3. It should not rest against the mouth, as the wearer's breath can condense and wet the fabric.[20]

Eyewear

1. It should have solid side shields to afford peripheral protection.
2. It must meet the American National Standards Institute Occupational and Educational Eye and Face Protection Standard for impact resistance.
3. It should be able to withstand cleaning and disinfection between patient procedures.
4. It should not distort the operator's vision.

Outer Clothing

1. The outer occupational garment should be fluid resistant and not fluid proof.
2. Appropriate garment material should not permit blood or other potentially infectious fluids to pass through or reach the health care worker's clothes or epithelial/mucosal tissues.
3. For routine dental procedures, cotton or cotton/polyester laboratory coats or clinic jackets are usually satisfactory.
4. Protective garments must be changed at least when visibly soiled.
5. Protective garments must be removed before leaving the workplace.

---

performed. These are found as right- and left-handed fitted items, and they offer clinicians excellent tactility, comfort, and dexterity.

As an alternative to the repeated glove changes that may be required during temporary interruptions in treatment, less expensive plastic or food handler gloves may be worn over contaminated gloves (overgloving) to prevent cross-contamination to other clean items. The use of these loose-fitting, mostly copolymer overgloves is not intended for patient care without a more effective barrier underneath, and they should be removed and discarded when treatment is to resume. Another type of nontreatment glove used routinely is worn when handling and cleaning contaminated instruments, cleaning up the operatory area, surface cleaning, and carrying out disinfection procedures. By necessity for the tasks undertaken, these are puncture resistant, resistant to chemical toxicity, and able to withstand multiple cleaning and disinfection exposures. These utility gloves are usually made of nitrile or neoprene, and some types can even withstand repeated heat sterilization in an autoclave.

The increasing use of natural rubber latex (NRL) in a wide assortment of health care and personal products has led to an increase in the incidence of allergic reactions to latex. In addition to latex gloves used in health care environments, a number of other devices can contain latex, including blood pressure cuffs, dental dams, elastic bands on masks, adhesive bandages, vascular catheters, nitrous oxide nose cones, prophylaxis cups, and intubation tubes. Allergic reactions to items such as latex gloves, rubber dams, and mask elastic bands occur as one of two types: type I (immediate, or immunoglobulin E) and type IV (delayed hypersensitivity).

Type I hypersensitivity is the result of a humoral immunoglobulin E response against certain latex proteins.[30–34] The clinical reaction usually occurs as a localized urticaria, or cutaneous anaphylaxis, within minutes after a sensitized person comes in contact with latex allergens. Donning latex gloves or placing a rubber dam are common stimuli. The individual can rapidly develop this "wheal and flare reaction" and develop itching, hives, and possibly local edema. In some instances when these individuals are challenged via the airborne route from aerosolized allergens, more serious respiratory symptoms, such as wheezing, coughing, shortness of breath, and respiratory distress can occur. Perspiration of the hands can induce sensitization by leaching water-soluble protein allergens from the latex glove material. Natural rubber latex proteins can also adhere to glove powder particles and remain suspended in the air during removal of such items from boxes. Clinicians are addressing the risk of allergic reaction to airborne latex through an increased use of nonpowdered gloves.

In contrast, type IV hypersensitivity develops from the infiltration of sensitized CD4+ lymphocytes and other leukocytes.[30,32,33] Development of this contact dermatitis is much slower, often taking 12 to 24 hours after the challenge. The resultant chronic inflammation presents with characteristic epithelial lesions from induration and walling off of affected sites, leading to necrosis, scabbing, and epithelial sloughing within 72 to 96 hours. The specific immune response in this instance is directed against certain water-soluble chemicals added during the manufacturing process, including chemical accelerators, vulcanizers, and antioxidants.

A number of governmental, manufacturing, and health care organization initiatives have been undertaken to protect health care workers and their patients from these types of adverse reactions.[35,36] Among the initiatives are the following:

- Nitrile, vinyl, neoprene, and other nonlatex gloves may be worn by sensitive dental care providers during patient treatment, in addition to an expanding list of other nonlatex items and materials. For example, many brands of prophylaxis cups and orthodontic elastic bands are now latex-free.
- Dental health care workers should be aware of developing technologies concerning the manufacture of nonlatex gloves and be able to devise special precautions for patients with latex allergies. For example, they can be scheduled as the first patients of the day to minimize exposure to aerosolized latex particles. In addition, specific treatment areas with minimal presence of items containing latex can be set up. Food and Drug Administration (FDA) regulations in effect as of September 1998 disallowed the use of the misleading term *hypoallergenic* to describe latex gloves and required all medical devices containing NRL to be labeled as such, including a cautionary statement warning of the potential of NRL to cause allergic reactions.

Masks

Dental health care providers are routinely exposed to high concentrations of aerosols and spatter during various treatment procedures involving the use of a handpiece, ultrasonic scaler, or air/water spray, as well as while grinding items contaminated with saliva or even cleaning contaminated instruments. Airborne microorganisms that can be infectious via this route of exposure include staphylococci, streptococci, tubercle bacilli, herpesviruses, influenza viruses, and gonococci. The routine use of an approved face mask will protect dental personnel from microbe-laden droplets.

The personal barriers are considered medical devices and are therefore reviewed by the FDA for approval. Masks that filter at least 95% of particles 3.0 to 3.2 µm provide effective protection, with many types now able to filter out 1-µm particles.[37] These masks should be changed at least

between each patient appointment, and more frequently when they are exposed to heavy spatter or aerosols during treatment or when they become moist or wet. This is an important consideration, as wet fabric may serve as a vehicle for microbial passage through the mask.

Protective Eyewear

The eyes and surrounding tissues of dental health care personnel can be exposed to a variety of macroscopic and microscopic particles that can cause mechanical trauma (eg, tooth fragments, amalgam, surgical tissue debris), chemical injury from splashing, or infection (eg, conjunctivitis caused by staphylococci, gonococci, or herpes simplex viruses). HBV was also shown years ago to be infectious through the conjunctiva in susceptible primates. Protective eyewear such as goggles, glasses with side shields, or face shields should be used during procedures in which aerosol generation or splash/spatter is anticipated.[9,11,20] One should choose an appropriate device based on the level of protection indicated.

A face mask should be used in conjunction with an eye protection device, even if the device is a face shield, to reduce bacterial contamination through the nasal and oral portals of entry.

Rubber Dam

In many restorative and endodontic dental procedures, the routine use of a rubber dam provides an effective intraoral barrier affording protection for both the dental health care provider and the patient.[38] When the use of a rubber dam is indicated in any dental procedure, a high-volume evacuator must be used if splash or spatter is generated. When used together, the dental dam and high-volume evacuator minimize both the potential for spatter during treatment and care provider contact with the patient's oral mucosa and secretions.

Furthermore, the ventilation systems and air flow should remove suspended aerosols from the operatory. Prior to construction of a new operatory, one must consider incorporation of an office design that reduces retention of aerosols. In established offices, portable or fixed devices that remove aerosols and decontaminate the air using high-volume suction, ultraviolet radiation, and filtration may be an option.

Protective Clothing

The following portion of the December 6, 1991, federal OSHA *Bloodborne Pathogens Standard* mandated employers to address employee protective clothing:[10] "Gowns, Aprons, and Other Protective Body Clothing:

Appropriate protective clothing such as, but not limited to, gowns, aprons, lab coats, clinic jackets, or similar garments shall be worn in occupational exposure situations. The type and characteristics will depend upon the task and degree of exposure anticipated."

Although most of the discussion in drafting language for the regulations centered on concern for reducing potential exposure of health care workers' skin to patients' blood, the basic premise for the final wording was related to a perception of cleanliness.

Hepatitis B Vaccination and Other Immunizations

The hepatitis B vaccine is provided free to any employee who may have occupational exposure to blood-borne pathogens,[10] including the practitioner, dental assistant, dental hygienist, and lab technician, and it applies to full-time, part-time, temporary, and probationary employees. Employers must provide vaccination within 10 working days of initial assignment. New employees can continue to provide patient care during the period required to complete the vaccination series. The employee, along with a copy of the standard, is sent to a designated medical health care professional for evaluation. This professional evaluates the employee for contraindications to vaccination and then either vaccinates the employee or discusses the contraindications. The health care professional sends the employer a written opinion on whether the vaccine is indicated and whether it was received. The employer then provides a copy of the written opinion to the employee within 15 days. The time sequence for receipt of the vaccine is 0, 1, and 6 months for the 3-injection regimen.

Employees may refuse to be vaccinated, but they must sign the "Informed Refusal for Hepatitis B Vaccination" form, currently found in appendix A at the end of the *Bloodborne Pathogens Standard.* The US Public Health Service guidelines do not recommend booster doses, but if a booster is recommended in the future, it must be provided at no cost to the employee. Documentation of the hepatitis B vaccination should be placed in the employee's medical record.

The perception that vaccination of health care workers involves only hepatitis B protection is now clearly outdated. The trend away from widespread dependency on, and use of, antimicrobial chemotherapy has been gaining momentum since the early 1990s. A new phase of immunization practices to prevent disease has already been initiated to protect at-risk health care workers from nosoco-

mial transmission of vaccine-preventable infections such as influenza, measles, mumps, rubella, varicella (chicken pox), and *Streptococcus pneumoniae* pneumonia.[39–41]

Postexposure Evaluation and Follow-up

The *Bloodborne Pathogens Standard* requires that any employee who has an exposure incidence be offered immediately a free, confidential medical evaluation and follow-up.[10,15] An exposure incident may be defined as a needle stick or puncture wound from a contaminated object, a splash of blood or body fluid onto mucous membranes, or a splash of blood or body fluids onto nonintact skin.

An employee exposure incident should be reported to the safety and health manager or the employer. The employee should see a health care professional as soon as possible for medical evaluation. If the source individual (usually the patient) can be identified, he or she should be sent to the health care professional for blood testing along with the employee. Documents that should accompany the employee include a copy of the *Bloodborne Pathogens Standard*, the employee's job description, an incident report describing the circumstances, and the employee's hepatitis B vaccine status and other relevant medical information.

The medical consulting professional will evaluate the exposure incident, arrange for blood testing of the employee and source individual, notify the employee of the results of all testing, provide counseling, provide postexposure prophylaxis, and evaluate any reported illnesses.[12,14,42–44]

The medical consultant should then send the employer documentation that the employee was informed of the evaluation results and the need for any follow-up, and provide a recommendation on whether hepatitis B vaccine was indicated and if the vaccine was received. The employer should also provide a copy of this written opinion to the employee within 15 days of the completed evaluation.

Any exposure incident should be evaluated to determine how it could be prevented in the future. This evaluation should be documented and may be accomplished with specific information in the following categories: type of exposure incident; measures taken to prevent recurrence; evaluation of policies, engineering controls, work practices, and personal protective equipment used at the time of the exposure incident; and any other areas with similar patterns of occurrence.

Table 16-3 Major Methods of Heat Sterilization[46]

Method	Temperature	Pressure	Cycle time	Advantages	Disadvantages
Steam autoclave	121°C/250°F 134°C/273°F	15 psi 30 psi	15–20 min 3–5 min	Rapid turnaround time, low cost per cycle, no toxic/hazardous chemicals.	May corrode instruments, cannot be used with many plastics.
Dry-heat oven	160°C/320°F 170°C/340°F		2 h 1 h	Does not corrode instruments, no toxic/hazardous chemicals, low cost per cycle.	Long cycle time; cannot be used with plastics; paper products may char.
Rapid heat transfer	190°C/375°F		12 min for wrapped items; 6 min for unwrapped items	Short cycle, items are dry after cycle.	Cannot sterilize liquids, may damage plastic and rubber items; door cannot be opened before end of cycle; small capacity per cost; unwrapped items are quickly contaminated after cycle.
Unsaturated chemical vapor	131°C/270°F	20 psi	30 min	Good turnaround time, less corrosive to instruments.	Uses toxic/hazardous chemicals; requires fume ventilation; cannot be used with many plastics.
Ethylene oxide	Room temperature		10–16 h (depends on material)	Can be used with almost all materials, including dental appliances, and instruments.	Very long cycle time; uses toxic/hazardous chemical; requires special ventilation.

Instrument Recirculation, Sterilization, and Monitoring

A basic principle for effective infection control is as follows: *Do not disinfect when you can sterilize.* In fact, sterilization of contaminated instruments is the most important component of an asepsis program. An initial distinction must therefore be made between the antimicrobial outcomes of sterilization and disinfection. *Sterilization* is defined as the destruction of all forms of life, with particular reference to microbial forms. The limiting requirement and basic criterion for accomplishment of sterilization is the destruction of high numbers of bacterial and mycotic spores, the most heat-resistant microbial forms. In contrast, *disinfection* refers only to the inhibition or destruction of pathogens. Spores are not killed during disinfection.[16–18,20,21,23]

The use of heat has long been recognized as the most efficient, reliable method of sterilization. The standard of care in this area has evolved to the level where all reusable heat-stable instruments; high-speed handpieces; low-speed handpiece components used intraorally; ultrasonic tips; reusable prophylaxis angles; and other contaminated items that come in contact with patients' blood, saliva, or mucous membranes must be sterilized in an FDA 510K cleared-heat sterilizer before use.[9,11,45] Multiple appropriate meth-

ods of heat sterilization are available and effective in dental care settings. These include steam under pressure (autoclave), dry heat, and unsaturated chemical vapor units. Exposure to ethylene oxide gas at room temperature is also useful in limited circumstances in large facilities for heat-labile reusable items.[17,18,46,47] Major features, conditions of use, and characteristics of these sterilization modalities are presented in Table 16-3.[46] While a practitioner may prefer one type of heat sterilizer over another, it is important to remember that no single method of sterilization may be suitable for the range of items used in dental care. It must also be mentioned that the ongoing data collection by the Environmental Protection Agency (EPA), FDA, and OSHA led to the development of increasingly stringent standards for ethylene oxide emissions, residue limits, and allowable exposure limits for workplace personnel.

The historical practice of using liquid chemical sterilants in dentistry (ie, cold sterilization), including agents such as glutaraldehyde or chlorine dioxide, is no longer necessary or appropriate, since most reusable instruments and devices used in dentistry can withstand sterilization by one of the common processes mentioned above.[48] If certain devices cannot be sterilized, single-use disposable items should be considered.

With regard to cleaning and reprocessing contaminated instruments between patient treatment procedures,

Table 16-4 Common Causes of Sterilization Failure

Improper instrument cleaning	
Poor cleaning	Debris and bioburden can insulate organisms from contact with the sterilizing agent
Improper packaging	
Wrong packaging material	Prevents penetration of sterilizing agent; packaging material may melt
Excessive packaging material	Retards penetration of the sterilizing agent
Cloth wrap in a chemical vapor sterilizer	Can absorb chemicals, preventing sufficient vaporization for sterilization
Closed container in steam or chemical vapor sterilizers	Prevents direct contact with the sterilizing agent
Improper loading of the sterilizer	
Overloading	Increases heating time and retards penetration of the sterilizing agent to the center of the sterilizer load
Packages or cassettes loaded too close together, even without overloading	May prevent or delay contact of sterilizing agent with all items in the chamber
Improper timing	
Incorrect operation of the sterilizer	Does not allow sufficient time at proper temperature to achieve microbial kill
Timing for sterilization begun before proper temperature is reached (for units with non-automatic timers)	Does not allow sufficient time at proper temperature to achieve microbial kill
Dry-heat sterilizer door opened during sterilizing cycle	Does not allow sufficient time at proper temperature to achieve microbial kill
Sterilizer timer malfunction	Timer does not accurately reflect chamber conditions, resulting in insufficient time at proper temperature to achieve microbial kill
Improper temperature	
Incorrect operation of the sterilizer	Does not allow sufficient heat for proper time interval to achieve microbial kill
Sterilizer malfunction	Gauges do not accurately reflect chamber conditions, resulting in insufficient heat for proper time interval to achieve microbial kill
Improper method of sterilization	
Solutions or water processed in a chemical vapor sterilizer	Sterilizing agent does not penetrate the solution
Solutions or water processed in a dry-heat sterilizer	Liquids boil over and evaporate
Processing heat-sensitive items	Items melt or distort

Compiled from Miller and Palenik[49] and Cottone et al.[17]

the instrument recirculation system should be logical and organized to *(1)* most efficiently accomplish reprocessing and sterilization and *(2)* minimize procedures that can place employees at risk for percutaneous sharps exposures or other hazards. An instrument recirculation system may be divided into several subsections or areas: receiving, cleaning, packaging, sterilization, storage, and dispensing.[17,18] Many choices for implementation are available for practitioners, each of which can be effective when used appropriately.

Receiving area. Instruments and other contaminated materials arrive at the receiving area and undergo early preparation, such as immersion in a holding solution and disposal of waste. The initial use of a holding solution (usually a detergent and/or enzymatic cleaner in water) is not required, but it may be useful in keeping the biobur-

den moist when instrument cleaning cannot occur for extended intervals.

Cleaning area. Precleaning contaminated instruments is the most important preparatory step, since bioburden can act as a barrier to subsequent sterilization. Instruments are most commonly placed in an ultrasonic cleaner for the prescribed period and then inspected visually for any residual bioburden. The residual bioburden may then be removed by an additional cycle of cleaning in an ultrasonic cleaner or by scrubbing with a long-handled brush and then rinsed.

Packaging area. In the packaging area, sufficient counter space is needed to carry out several different procedures to prepare instruments for sterilization. These procedures include organization of supplies into unit doses and grouping of dried instruments into appropriate cassettes, pouches, bags, or wraps suitable for heat sterilization methods.

Sterilization area. The sterilization area needs sufficient space for sterilizers as required by the size of the practice and the number of treatment operatories, as well as appropriate ventilation required to vent fumes and sterilizer odors. Additional space is necessary to allow cooling of cassettes, trays, and packages after removal from sterilizers.

Storage area. The storage area of the system calls for sufficient space to store sterilized packages before they are needed in patient treatment.

Dispensing area. An organized location for the preparation of instrument setups and their distribution to operatories brings all the other steps together prior to the provision of patient care.

Quality control. The application of effective quality control measures is essential in instrument reprocessing. How does one know that the most important piece of infection control equipment is functioning properly? Unfortunately, numerous equipment malfunction and human factors can adversely affect a sterilizer's performance (Table 16-4). It is therefore imperative that sterilizer effectiveness be routinely monitored and verified using specific chemical and biologic indicators. In 1993, the CDC updated earlier dental infection control recommendations, stating that "proper functioning of sterilization cycles should be verified by the periodic use (at least weekly) of biologic indicators (ie, spore tests)."[9] Heat-sensitive chemical indicators, such as those that change color after exposure to heat, are useful in detecting major unit malfunctions or human errors during sterilization procedures, yet they do not ensure adequacy of the sterilization cycle. These chemical process monitors can be used with each load of processed instruments to detect major problems.

Biologic indicators containing heat-resistant *Bacillus* spores provide the best challenge for sterilization cycles. Two species are used: *Bacillus stearothermophilus* and *Bacillus subtilis*. It is important to note that a spore vehicle designed for one sterilization method is not necessarily the proper modality to use for other methods. Calibrated *B stearothermophilus* spore–impregnated paper strips or glass vials are the appropriate biologic monitors for autoclaves and unsaturated chemical vapor sterilizers, while *B subtilis* preparations provide an effective challenge for conditions in dry-heat sterilizers and ethylene oxide units. Proof of destruction of these resistant microbial forms is used to infer that all microorganisms exposed to the same conditions have been destroyed, thereby representing the most sensitive check of sterilizer efficiency.[9,11,16–18,20,50]

Environmental Surface and Equipment Asepsis

A number of operatory surfaces become contaminated with patient blood, saliva, and other materials during dental treatment. The decontamination of these operatory treatment surfaces between patient appointments is an important component of an effective infectious disease control program.[51,52] The routine use of chemical disinfectants and/or disposable covers is warranted in certain instances because it is not possible, or necessary, to sterilize all contaminated items or surfaces.

A standard system of classification for chemical sterilants and disinfectants was first proposed by Spaulding in 1972.[48] This system was originally devised for classifying hospital instruments according to their use and degree of contamination, but it was adapted to include dental instrument and equipment asepsis. A modification of the original scheme was first published in 1991 and is presented in Table 16-5.[48] Patient care items and equipment are placed into one of three categories (critical, semicritical, and noncritical) and treated according to the type of tissue exposure, bioburden contamination, and relative risk of microbial transmission and disease. In addition, representative classes for chemical germicide use are included for their sterilization or disinfection capabilities. Different classes of disinfectants are defined based on their effectiveness against vegetative bacteria, tubercle bacilli, fungal spores, lipid-containing and non-lipid–containing viruses, and bacterial endospores.[48,51] To assist in determining which surfaces may be covered with disposable barriers, the Organization for Safety and Asepsis Procedures developed a classification that distinguishes among touch, transfer, and splash, spatter, and aerosol surfaces[18] (Box 16-4).

When selecting the type of chemical to be used as a cleaner and/or disinfectant, a number of factors should be considered[4,48,53,54]:

1. Cleaning of object. Precleaning contaminated surfaces is a necessary first step before disinfection; all commercial disinfectants require a clean surface to be effective. Directions for use that appear on manufacturers' labels must be approved by the EPA prior to release of the product. Certain classes of disinfectants, such as aqueous agents that also contain surfactants, may be used as both cleaner and disinfectant.
2. Presence of organic load (bioburden) on the surface.
3. Type and level of contamination.
4. Chemical concentration of the disinfectant and required effective exposure time.
5. Nature of the contaminated object.

Table 16-5 Modified CDC/Spaulding Classification of Contaminated Environmental Surfaces[48*]

Classification	Description	Dental clinic/lab examples	Relative risk of disease	Surface recycling processes
Critical surfaces	Penetrates tissue; contacts open tissue	• Hand instruments • Cutting instruments • Burs, files, and needles • Handpieces and scaler tips	High	• Heat sterilization • Sterile, single-use disposables
Semicritical surfaces	Contacts mucosa	• Hand instruments • Mouth props • Plastic prophylaxis angles • Rubber dam frames	Intermediate	• Heat sterilization • Single-use disposables • Chemical sterilization*
Noncritical surfaces (intraoral contact)	May contact skin and/or mucous membranes of dental personnel; contact patient after fabrication, handling, or repair	• Impressions • Prostheses • Splints • Other appliances	Low	• Thorough rinsing followed by intermediate-level disinfection[†‡]
Noncritical surfaces (no intraoral contact)	Contacts unbroken skin	• Blood pressure cuffs • Face masks (eg, nitrogen dioxide)	Low	• Sanitize with detergent (no blood or saliva) • Intermediate-level disinfection[†] • Removable covers
Environmental surfaces (patient care)	Usually contacts dental personnel, but not patients	• Dental unit surfaces • Laboratory equipment • X-ray equipment	Very low	• Sanitize with detergent (no blood or saliva) • Intermediate-level disinfection[†] • Removable covers
Environmental surfaces (housekeeping)	Rarely contacts dental personnel or patients	• Floors • Walls • Countertops	Minimal	• If no obvious blood, sanitize with detergent • When blood is present, use intermediate-level disinfection[†]

* To be used only on items that are destroyed by heat.
† Some examples include iodophors, combination synthetic phenolics, bromides, and sodium hypochlorite.
‡ Process is repeated if item is returned to the patient.

6. Temperature and pH of the disinfection process and effects on treated surfaces.

Environmental surfaces must be disinfected with an EPA-registered intermediate-level hospital disinfectant (capable of killing *Mycobacterium tuberculosis, Pseudomonas aeruginosa, Salmonella typhimurium, Escherichia coli*, hydrophilic viruses, and lipophilic viruses). The disinfection may be carried out at the beginning of a morning session before seating the first patient and at the end of the day. A spray-wipe-spray technique should be followed to sanitize (spray-wipe) and disinfect (spray) the surfaces. To reduce waiting time between patients, disposable barriers may be used where appropriate. Disinfection should be performed between patients if contamination (blood, saliva, or bioburden) is visible; otherwise, a change of barriers is sufficient between patients.

High-touch areas can be designated and barrier wrapped with a disposable barrier. Electrical switches and nonsealed controls of equipment must not be sprayed directly with a disinfectant; they must be barrier wrapped. Areas that are not designated as high touch should not be touched, and only those with barriers may be handled. Antiseptic formulations may not be used as surface disinfectants. Surface disinfectants such as sodium hypochlorite preparations, iodophors, complex or synthetic phenolics, and bromides that are water-based sprays are better cleaners and disinfectants than alcohol-based foams and aerosols, as the latter tend to evaporate faster, and the alcohol may hinder removal of bioburden.[54] Commercially prepared cloth wipes are also available; they contain a range of alcohol concentrations in addition to other disinfectant agents. Wipes with high concentrations of alcohol may not be suitable as initial surface cleaners, and their inability to keep contact surfaces wet for required disinfection intervals should also be considered before use. The time of contact of the disinfectant with the surface is very important, as is the room temperature. The user must follow the manufacturer's instructions with regard to the material compatibility, time, and temperature when using any chemical germicide.[48,51]

Box 16-4 Classification and Management of Environmental Surfaces

Touch surfaces Surfaces that are usually touched and contaminated during dental procedures (eg, dental light handles, dental unit handle and controls, headrest adjustment mechanisms, dental chair switches). Touch surfaces should be kept to a minimum. If a surface must or might be touched, it should be cleaned and disinfected or covered with a barrier that is impervious to liquid. Barriers must be single-use and replaced between patients. Surfaces should be cleaned and disinfected at the end of each clinic day. Place new barriers before the first patient of the next clinic day.

Transfer surfaces Surfaces that are not touched but are usually contacted by contaminated instruments (eg, instrument trays, dental unit handpiece holders). To maintain asepsis, transfer surfaces should be treated in the same manner as touch surfaces.

Splash, spatter, and aerosol surfaces All surfaces in the operatory other than touch or transfer surfaces. Splash and spatter surfaces need not be disinfected but should be cleaned at least daily.

Barrier choices range from inexpensive plastic food wrap to commercially available custom-made covers. Plastic food wraps that are 1.5 feet wide by 2,000 feet long are available in dispenser rolls that may be mounted on a bracket on the wall or on a cart. Areas that may be covered are equipment controls, chair switches, light handles, headrests, hand-handled soap dispensers, coupling areas of the air and water tubings for the air/water syringe, and handpieces. Controls that are operated by foot need not be wrapped but may be sanitized. For surgical procedures it is necessary to follow the institution protocols on surgical asepsis, which may require additional steps as prescribed by individual institutional guidelines that conform to CDC recommendations. It is necessary to maintain and service equipment and replace consumables as prescribed by the manufacturers. The suction lines should be cleaned with a disinfectant or with enzymatic cleaners using protocols designated by the manufacturers. Patients should be instructed to avoid closing their mouths around the saliva ejector, as it could cause a reverse/negative pressure, leading to sucking back of contaminants from the suction lines. Hollow-bore instruments such as air/water syringe tips are difficult to clean and can retain bioburden inside the lumen. It is best to use single-use disposable tips, because they are inexpensive and easy to change.

Water Quality

For approximately 40 years practitioners have known that dental unit water systems are contaminated by both non-pathogenic and pathogenic organisms that colonize the system and waterlines and soon form biofilms inside the lumens of the waterlines.[55] Although the water coming into the system from an external source is potable (< 500 CFU/mL bacteria and < 1 CFU/mL coliform bacteria), water coming out of the units may have as many as 1 million CFU/mL. To date, there is no published evidence of serious health problems for either patients or dental care providers from contact with dental water. However, exposing patients or dental professionals to water of poor microbiologic quality is inconsistent with both universally accepted infection control principles and the high level of asepsis standards routinely exhibited in most dental facilities.[56]

Investigators have identified multiple classes of organisms in dental unit water samples, ranging from nonpathogenic to pathogenic microbes.[56–59] Types of microbes commonly associated with water from the dental unit water systems include *Bacterionema* species; *Corynebacterium* species; gram-negative bacilli and cocci; *Klebsiella* species; *Neisseria catarrhalis*; *Pseudomonas* species, including *P aeruginosa*, *P pyogenes*, and *P cepacia*; *Staphylococcus epidermidis*; *Streptococcus* species, including *S mutans*, *S salivarius*, and *S mitis*; *Actinomyces* species; enterococci; α-hemolytic streptococci; *Staphylococcus aureus*; *B subtilis*; *E coli*; *Flavobacterium* species; nonhemolytic streptococci; *Legionella pneumophila*; *Mycobacterium* species; *Aspergillus niger*; *Cladosporium* species; *Achromobacter*; and *Alcaligenes faecalis*.

It is necessary to understand the potential of water contamination on the outcome of care if the dental unit water is used. There are two levels of care in dentistry based on the extent of surgery and exposure of underlying bone. For treatment that does not expose bone, and where extensive surgery is not performed, the water can be of potable quality and not sterile. For surgery that exposes the underlying bone, sterile water or saline should be used to avoid postoperative infection. Furthermore, the water delivery system must be sterile to avoid contaminating the water and/or saline used in surgery. Filtered and bacteria-free water are not necessarily sterile water, so filtered water should not be used in this instance.[56]

Dental units with water systems capable of being sanitized and disinfected and that have a fixture for an alternative water system (separate reservoir) should be used. If ultrasonic scalers are being used, a system with a device to attach sterile surgical solution (water/saline) can be used. Devices that have an external peristaltic pump around which the water/saline lines are wrapped are better than those that pump fluid through the unit, because the solution in the former case will not come in contact with the external environment or the inner surfaces of a contaminated unit. Devices (electronic pumps) that are autoclavable, with attachments for saline bottles and bags, are also available.

In September 1995, the ADA issued a draft statement on the quality of water used in dental treatment.[60] The statement proposed that by the year 2000, water used during nonsurgical dental procedures contain no more than 200 CFU/mL mesophilic heterotrophic bacteria. (Similar standards are in effect for dialysate used in hemodialysis units.) The statement further encouraged industry and researchers to improve the design of dental equipment, and it suggested that all dental units being manufactured or marketed in the United States be equipped or retrofitted with a separate water reservoir independent of the public water supply.

Successful engineering and manufacturing of these and other options for improving water quality continue to provide dental practitioners with multiple choices for exerting better control over the quality of source water used in patient care. These choices include the following:

1. An alternate water supply that bypasses community and dental unit water by providing sterile and/or distilled water directly into waterline attachments
2. Filtration involving in-line filters to remove bacteria immediately before dental unit water enters instrument attachment
3. Chemical disinfection involving periodic flushing of lines with a disinfectant followed by appropriate rinsing of lines with water
4. Thermal inactivation of facility water at a centralized source
5. Ozonation using units designed for either single-chair or entire-practice waterlines
6. Ultraviolet irradiation of water prior to entrance into individual unit waterlines

Waste Management

Dental facilities routinely must deal with a variety of waste materials, which may range from noninfectious to infectious, hazardous, or even toxic. The implementation and application of logical procedures in safely handling, storing, and disposing of waste items further minimize occupational risks to practice professionals.[61,62]

A number of sometimes-confusing terms have been developed to describe different waste categories (Box 16-5).[18] Adding to practitioners' questions about this area is the fact that many areas of the United States have local and

---

Box 16-5 Glossary of Waste Management Terms

Contaminated waste Items that have had contact with blood or other body secretions.
Hazardous waste Waste posing a risk or peril to humans or the environment.
Infectious waste Waste capable of causing an infectious disease.
Medical waste Any solid waste* that is generated in the diagnosis, treatment, or immunization of human beings or animals in research pertaining thereto, or the production or testing of biologicals. The term does not include hazardous waste or household waste. Only a small percentage of medical waste is infectious and needs to be regulated.
Regulated waste Infectious medical waste that requires special handling, neutralization, and disposal.
Toxic waste Waste capable of having a poisonous effect.

From Miller and Palenik.[18p233]
* Solid waste includes discarded solid, liquid, semiliquid, or contained gaseous materials.

---

municipal regulations. The following suggestions may assist personnel in implementing appropriate regulations:

1. All waste must be discarded in accordance with applicable federal, state, and local regulations.
2. In general, blood- and saliva-stained items are not considered regulated waste.
3. Items saturated with blood and/or saliva (ie, fluid can be expelled with squeezing) are considered regulated medical waste.
4. With regard to biohazard communication, containers regulated for medical waste must be labeled with the appropriate biohazard symbol. Included in this category are sharps containers, contaminated pans used for cleaning bioburden-laden instruments, bags of contaminated laundry, and specimen containers.
5. Used needles and other contaminated sharps are to be placed in a puncture-resistant, leak-proof container that is closable and either contains a biohazard label or is red.
6. Unfixed tissue, teeth, items saturated with blood or saliva, and items caked with blood or saliva must be discarded in containers or bags that are closable and leak-proof and that contain a biohazard label or are red.
7. Liquid blood collected in a cannister must have a biohazard label.

Summary

Effective infection control must be a routine activity of dental professionals. Much has been accomplished over the years. The implementation and routine application of a vast array of logical, effective techniques and procedures have protected both health care workers and patients, who expect safe care. The provision of dental treatment continues to be guided by appropriate recommendations of dental professionals, health professional organizations, and regulatory governmental agencies. It is important always to respond to emerging challenges in infectious disease control with new information and technologies.

References

1. Molinari JA. Dental infection control at the year 2000. Accomplishment recognized. J Am Dent Assoc 1999;130:1291–1298.
2. Crawford JJ. State-of-the-art: Practical infection control in dentistry. J Am Dent Assoc 1985;110:629–633.
3. Infection control in the dental office. American Dental Association Council on Dental Materials and Devices Council on Dental Therapeutics. J Am Dent Assoc 1978;97:673–677.
4. Runnells RR. Infection Control in the Former Wet Finger Environment. Salt Lake City: Publishers Press, 1984.
5. Recommended infection control practices for dentistry. MMWR Morb Mortal Wkly Rep 1986;35:237–242.
6. Infection control recommendations for the dental office and dental laboratory. Councils on Dental Materials, Instruments and Equipment, Dental Practice, and Dental Therapeutics. J Am Dent Assoc 1988;116:241–248.
7. Infection control recommendations for the dental office and the dental laboratory. J Am Dent Assoc 1992;123:1–8.
8. Guidelines for prevention of transmission of HIV and HBV to health care and public safety workers. MMWR Morb Mortal Wkly Rep 1989;38:1–37.
9. Recommended infection control practices for dentistry. MMWR Morb Mortal Wkly Rep 1993;41(RR-8):1–12.
10. Department of Labor, Occupational Safety and Health Administration. Occupational exposure to bloodborne pathogens: Final rule (29 CFR Part 1910.1030). Fed Regist 1991;56: 64004–64182.
11. Infection control recommendations for the dental office and the dental laboratory. Councils on Scientific Affairs and Dental Practice. J Am Dent Assoc 1996;127:672–680.
12. Recommendations for preventing transmission of the human immunodeficiency virus and the hepatitis B virus during exposure-prone invasive procedures. MMWR Morb Mortal Wkly Rep 1991;40(RR-8):1–9.
13. Public Health Service statement on management of occupational exposure to human immunodeficiency virus, including considerations regarding zidovudine postexposure use. MMWR Morb Mortal Wkly Rep 1990;39(RR-1):1–14.
14. Recommendations for prevention and control of hepatitis C virus (HCV) infection and HCV-related chronic disease. MMWR Morb Mortal Wkly Rep 1998;47(RR-19):1–39.
15. Occupational Safety and Health Administration. Occupational exposure to bloodborne pathogens, needlestick and other sharps injuries: Final rule (29 CFR Part 1910, docket no. H370A). Fed Regist 2001;66(12):5318–5325.
16. Centers for Disease Control and Prevention. Practical infection control in the dental office. Washington, DC: U.S. Department of Health and Human Services, October 1993.
17. Cottone JA, Terezhalmy GT, Molinari JA. Practical Infection Control in Dentistry, ed 2. Baltimore: Williams & Wilkins, 1996.
18. Miller CH, Palenik CJ. Infection Control and Management of Hazardous Materials for the Dental Team, ed 2. St Louis: Mosby, 1998.
19. Miller CH. Infection control strategies for the dental office. In: Ciancio SG (ed). ADA Guide to Dental Therapeutics, ed 1. Chicago: American Dental Association, 1998:489–504.
20. Organization for Safety and Asepsis Procedures (OSAP) Research Foundation. Infection Control in Dentistry Guidelines. Annapolis: Organization for Safety and Asepsis Procedures, 1999.
21. Miller CH, Palenik CJ. Sterilization, disinfection and asepsis in dentistry. In: Block SS (ed). Disinfection, Sterilization and Preservation. Philadelphia: Lippincott Williams & Wilkins, 2001: 1049–1068.
22. NIOSH Alert. Preventing needlestick injuries in health care settings. DHHS (NIOSH) Publication No. 2000-108. Cincinnati: National Institute for Occupational Safety and Health, 1999.
23. Cottone JA, Molinari JA. State-of-the-art infection control in dentistry. J Am Dent Assoc 1991;123:33–40.
24. Molinari JA. Practical infection control for the 1990's: Applying science to government regulations. J Am Dent Assoc 1994;125: 1189–1197.
25. Larson E. A causal link between handwashing and risk of infection? Examination of the evidence. Infect Control Hosp Epidemiol 1988;9:28–36.
26. Garner JS, Favero MS. CDC guideline for handwashing and hospital environmental control, 1985. Infect Control 1986;7:231–235.
27. Larson EL. APIC guideline for handwashing and hand antisepsis in health care settings. Am J Infect Control 1995;23:251–269.
28. Widmer AF. Replace hand washing with use of a waterless alcohol rub? Clin Infect Dis 2000;31:136–143.
29. Type B (serum) hepatitis and dental practice. Council on Dental Therapeutics. J Am Dent Assoc 1976;92:153–159.
30. Hamann CP. Natural rubber latex protein sensitivity in review. Am J Contact Dermat 1993;28:94–100.
31. Sussman G, Tarlo S, Dolovich J. The spectrum of IgE-mediated responses to latex. JAMA 1991;265:2844–2847.
32. Hamann CP, Kick SA, Sullivan K. Taking up the gauntlet: Accepting the challenge of glove evaluation. J Healthc Mater Manage 1993;11:24–37.
33. Burton AD. Latex allergy in health care workers. Occup Med 1997;12:609–626.
34. Hamann CP, Turjanmaa K, Reitschel R, et al. Natural rubber latex hypersensitivity: Incidence and prevalence of type I allergy in the dental professional. J Am Dent Assoc 1998;129:43–54.
35. US Food and Drug Administration. Natural rubber-containing medical devices; user labeling (21 CFE Part 801). Fed Regist 1997;62(189):51021–51030.
36. National Institute for Occupational Safety and Health (NIOSH). Preventing allergic reactions to natural rubber latex in the workplace. US Dept Health and Human Services publication 97-135. Government Printing Office, 1997.

37. National Institute for Occupational Safety and Health (NIOSH), Centers for Disease Control and Prevention, US Public Health Service. Respiratory protective devices: Final rule and notice. Fed Regist 1995;60(110):30335–30398.

38. Cochran MA, Miller CH, Sheldrake MA. The efficacy of the rubber dam as a barrier to the spread of microorganisms during dental treatment. J Am Dent Assoc 1989;119:141–144.

39. Hepatitis B virus: A comprehensive strategy for eliminating transmission in the United States through universal childhood vaccination. MMWR Morb Mortal Wkly Rep 1991;40(RR-13):1–25.

40. General recommendations of immunization. MMWR Morb Mortal Wkly Rep 1994;43(RR-1):1–38.

41. Immunization of health-care workers. MMWR Morb Mortal Wkly Rep 1997;46(RR-18):1–42.

42. Molinari JA. HIV, health care workers and patients: How to ensure safety in the dental office. J Am Dent Assoc 1993;124: 51–56.

43. Gerberding JL. Management of occupational exposures to blood-borne viruses. N Engl J Med 1995;332:444–451.

44. Update: Provisional Public Health Service recommendations for chemoprophylaxis after occupational exposure to HIV. MMWR Morb Mortal Wkly Rep 1996;45:468–472.

45. Young JM. Dental air-powered handpieces: Selection, use and sterilization. Compend Contin Educ Dent 1993;14:358–368.

46. Miller CH. Sterilization and disinfection: What every dentist needs to know. J Am Dent Assoc 1992;123:46–54.

47. Runnells RR. Countering the concerns: How to reinforce dental practice safety. J Am Dent Assoc 1993;124:65–73.

48. Favero MS, Bond WW. Chemical disinfection of medical and surgical materials. In: Block SS (ed). Disinfection, Sterilization, and Preservation. Philadelphia: Lippincott Williams & Wilkins, 2001:881–917.

49. Miller CH, Palenik CJ. Infection Control and Management of Hazardous Materials for the Dental Team, ed 1. St Louis: Mosby, 1994:132–170.

50. Biological indicators for verifying sterilization. Council on Dental Therapeutics. J Am Dent Assoc 1988;117:653–654.

51. Rutala WA. Guideline for selection and use of disinfectants. Am J Infect Control 1996;24:313–342.

52. Rutala WA, Cole EC. Ineffectiveness of hospital disinfectants against bacteria: A collaborative study. Infect Control 1987;8: 501–506.

53. Molinari JA. Surface disinfection and disinfectants. Calif Dent Assoc J 1985;110:73–78.

54. Molinari JA, Gleason MJ, Cottone JA, et al. Cleaning and disinfectant properties of dental surface disinfectants. J Am Dent Assoc 1988;117:179–182.

55. Blake GC. The incidence and control of bacterial infection of dental units and ultrasonic scalers. Br Med J 1963;115: 413–416.

56. Mills SE. The dental unit waterline controversy: Defusing the myths, defining the solutions. J Am Dent Assoc 2000;131: 1427–1441.

57. Abel LC, Miller RL, Micik RE, et al. Studies on dental aerobiology. IV. Bacterial contamination of water delivered by dental units. J Dent Res 1971;50:1567–1569.

58. Gross A, Devine MJ, Cutright DE. Microbial contamination of dental units and ultrasonic scalers. J Periodontol 1976;47: 670–673.

59. Bagga BSR, Murphy RA, Anderson AW, et al. Contamination of dental unit cooling water with oral microorganisms and its prevention. J Am Dent Assoc 1984;109:712–716.

60. American Dental Association. Statement on Dental Unit Waterlines (adopted December 13, 1995). Chicago: American Dental Association, 1995.

61. Infectious Waste Disposal in the Dental Office, Questions and Answers. Chicago: American Dental Association, 1989.

62. Rutala WA, Weber DJ. Infectious waste: Mismatch between science and policy. N Engl J Med 1991;325:578–582.

CHAPTER 7

Examination of Patients to Detect Periodontal Diseases

Thomas G. Wilson, Jr, and Ingvar Magnusson

- Examination of Soft Tissues for Clinical Trials
- Evaluation of Oral Hygiene for Clinical Trials
- Periodontal Probing Technology
- Suggested Clinical Approach
- Clinical Charting
- Periodontal Screening and Recording

Descriptive indices of oral health and oral hygiene are used to evaluate the need for periodontal therapy and the effect of different therapeutic regimens. The individual response to periodontal therapy is evaluated by recording and documenting differences in these indices and measurements. Such documentation helps improve the accuracy of the diagnosis and reduces the risk of too little or too much therapy. Before any data are collected, it is important to understand what the data indicate and the validity of that information. This chapter first describes the indices used for clinical trials and then presents information on data collection appropriate for daily practice.

Examination of Soft Tissues for Clinical Trials

The index system most commonly used to evaluate gingival status in clinical trials is the system (or modifications thereof) devised by Löe and Silness,[1] in which the gingival units are scored as follows: 0 = healthy gingiva; 1 = slight inflammation; 2 = moderate inflammation with bleeding

on pressure; and 3 = severe inflammation with spontaneous bleeding. Later, Löe[2] modified the system by changing the score of 2 from bleeding on pressure to bleeding on probing. The index was modified further by Gordon et al,[3] who used a noninvasive scoring system ranging from 0 to 4. The Löe-Silness score of 1 was divided into two categories: mild inflammation of any portion of the gingival unit, and mild inflammation of the whole gingival unit. This modified index was recommended by Lobene[4] for use in clinical trials. Lobene et al[5] showed that this modified gingival index had a high correlation with the Löe-Silness index; these authors listed the advantages of this system as follows:

1. It is noninvasive, thereby eliminating concerns about the disruption of soft tissue or plaque in the gingival region, as well as obviating infection control practices that would be required if sulcular probing were done.
2. It is logistically simpler. Decision making is simplified if bleeding considerations do not have to be superimposed on visual determinations.
3. There is less variability in its implementation if bleeding on pressure or probing is eliminated. This feature,

Table 17-1 Loesche Papillary Bleeding Score (PBS) Compared with Löe-Silness Gingival Index (GI)

PBS	GI	Comparison
0	0	Healthy gingiva; no bleeding on insertion of Stimudent interproximally
1	1	Edematous, reddened gingiva; no bleeding on insertion of Stimudent interproximally
2	2	Bleeding without flow on insertion of Stimudent interproximally
3	2	Bleeding with flow along gingival margin on insertion of Stimudent interproximally
4	2	Copious bleeding on insertion of Stimudent interproximally
5	3	Severe inflammation, marked redness, and edema; tendency for spontaneous bleeding

in combination with item 2, can result in greater accuracy in interexaminer calibration.

4. It affords greater sensitivity in detecting therapeutic efficacy. The expansion of the scale at its low end makes this index more sensitive to improvements in gingival health following treatment.

No one index should be recommended for general use; different indices may suit different examiners. Most important is that the examiner be consistent. Although visual assessment provides information on marginal inflammation, bleeding on probing provides information about the status of the bottom of the pocket (ie, the epithelium–connective tissue interface).

Often, gingival inflammation is defined as bleeding only. Lang et al[6] studied bleeding on probing as a predictor for the progression of periodontal disease and found that bleeding was a limited but useful indicator in clinical diagnosis for patients in the periodontal maintenance phase. Different methods to record bleeding have been described, the most simple being just the presence or absence of bleeding on probing at a particular site. The percentage of bleeding sites can then be calculated. Saxer and Mühlemann[7] described a papilla bleeding index (PBI) in which the sulcus is swept with a blunt periodontal probe and the amount of papillary bleeding is recorded 20 to 30 seconds after each quadrant has been probed. The amount of bleeding is scored from 1 (minimal) to 4 (profuse), and the PBI is calculated by adding all the bleeding scores and dividing by the number of papillae examined.

Histologically, it has been shown that an increase in the inflammatory infiltrate parallels an increase in the PBI. Loesche[8] introduced a papillary bleeding score in which bleeding was rated from 0 to 5 after a Stimudent interdental cleaner (Johnson & Johnson) was inserted interproxi-mally. This scoring system, which was related to the Löe-Silness gingival index (Table 17-1), was simplified by Caton and Polson[9] in the Eastman interdental bleeding index, in which the presence or absence of bleeding was recorded after a Stimudent interdental cleaner had been inserted and removed four times. Caton et al[10] reported that the Eastman interdental bleeding index was a more reliable clinical indicator for detecting interdental inflammatory lesions than was the PBI.

In a calibration study, Magnusson et al[11] assessed the intraexaminer and interexaminer variability of 11 previously calibrated examiners with regard to a noninvasive gingival index (Gordon et al[3]) and the papillary bleeding score (Loesche[8]). The results are illustrated in Fig 17-1. The intraexaminer correlation coefficient between two examination visits was 0.94 for the papillary bleeding score and 0.68 for the gingival index. The interexaminer correlation coefficient was 0.96 for the papillary bleeding score and 0.64 for the gingival index. It can thus be concluded that the papillary bleeding score is highly reproducible and suitable for use in the evaluation of periodontal therapy.

Earlier, a classification system for the appearance of gingival inflammation was described by Schour and Massler.[12] In 1956, Russell[13] described a periodontal index of the occurrence and severity of periodontal disease, which has been widely used in descriptive studies. This periodontal index consists of both qualitative and quantitative criteria. Qualitatively, the presence of gingival inflammation is recorded. Quantitatively, the tooth is scored as 1 if the inflammation is present only in localized areas and 2 if inflammation is present around the circumference of the tooth. A score of 6 is given if the tooth has deepened pockets and a score of 8 if it has lost its function.

All the index systems previously described are reversible, and the scores can return to 0 after successful periodontal

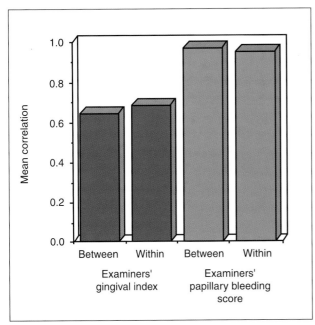

Fig 17-1 Pearson correlation coefficient between and within examiners for the papillary bleeding score and the gingival index.

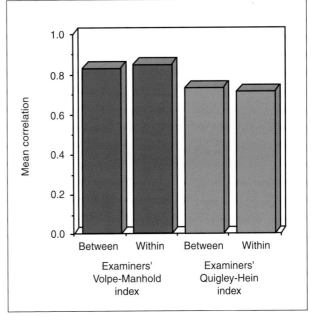

Fig 17-2 Pearson correlation coefficient between and within examiners for the Volpe-Manhold index and the Quigley-Hein index.

therapy. To get an indication of the amount of lost attachment, Ramfjord[14] recommended that it be measured in millimeters from the cementoenamel junction to the bottom of the pocket and be used in a periodontal disease index. This type of index is irreversible, because lost attachment is rarely regained completely after periodontal therapy.

Evaluation of Oral Hygiene for Clinical Trials

Ramfjord[14] suggested the use of an index to evaluate oral hygiene status, and Greene and Vermillion[15] devised an oral hygiene index to relate oral hygiene status to the presence of disease. This index consists of both a debris index, scored 0 to 3 (eg, a score of 1 would indicate that one third of the surface was covered), and a calculus index, also scored 0 to 3. It was shown that 90% of periodontal disease could be related to the amount of plaque and calculus present and to the subject's age.[16] The increase in the oral hygiene index with age was explained mainly by an increase of calculus.

Quigley and Hein[17] modified the oral hygiene index to develop an index for the evaluation of different oral hygiene measures. This modified index used a scoring range from 0 to 5 by inserting two low values between scores 0 and 1 in the oral hygiene index system. The extended score permits a more sensitive assessment of therapeutic efficacy.

Silness and Löe[18] developed a plaque index system that has been widely used in epidemiological studies. This system evaluates the thickness of the plaque at the gingival margin as follows: 0 = no plaque; 1 = nonvisible plaque that can be scraped from the tooth surface with a probe; 2 = visible plaque; and 3 = abundant plaque. To evaluate calculus formed during shorter clinical trials, Ennever et al[19] developed a calculus surface index to be used on the lingual surface of the four mandibular incisors. The tooth surface was divided into four fields by two intersecting diagonal lines, and the presence (1) or absence (0) of calculus was then registered in each field. Volpe and Manhold,[20] in studying the development of calculus over longer periods, measured the amount of calculus along two intersecting diagonal lines on the lingual surfaces of mandibular incisors and canines and added the resultant 12 numbers.

Magnusson et al[11] studied the reproducibility of the Volpe-Manhold index and the Quigley-Hein index. The intraexaminer and interexaminer correlations were calculated for 11 calibrated examiners (Fig 17-2). The intraexaminer correlation coefficient was 0.85 for the Volpe-Manhold index and 0.72 for the Quigley-Hein index. The interexaminer correlation coefficient was 0.84 for the Volpe-Manhold index and 0.73 for the Quigley-Hein index, indicating that these indices are acceptably reproducible.

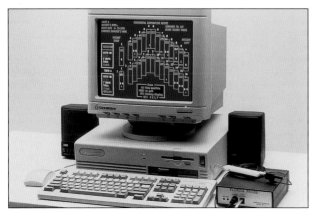

Fig 17-3 Florida Probe system. The probe handpiece is connected to the computer and a foot switch.

Periodontal Probing Technology

Probing-depth measurements yield important information regarding periodontal status and response to therapy. In clinical research, however, the gold standard for active disease at a site is a measurable loss of attachment. A number of studies have attempted to correlate attachment level with other clinical parameters. For example, Badersten et al[21] tried to relate probing level changes in treated subjects to other clinical characteristics in an attempt to determine if any other clinical parameter could be used to predict disease activity (ie, loss of attachment). Sites with a shallower initial probing depth demonstrated a higher incidence of attachment gain and a lower incidence of attachment loss than did deeper sites. All other investigated characteristics, including plaque, bleeding, suppuration, tooth surface, and tooth position, showed either weak association or no association with probing attachment change following therapy.

Currently, then, it appears that the only reliable clinical method for assessing progression or remission of periodontal disease is to monitor longitudinal changes in probing attachment level measurements recorded from a fixed reference point. The aim of probing attachment level measurements is to determine the most coronal connective-tissue fibers of the periodontal ligament. Several studies evaluating the location of the probe tip in both healthy and diseased conditions[22-26] have shown that in a healthy periodontium, the probe tip usually stops short of the connective tissue attachment, whereas when gingival inflammation is present, the probe tip penetrates the apical termination of the junctional epithelium and goes into the connective tissue.

Studies have also shown that the penetration of the probe is positively correlated with probing forces,[27-29] indicating that to obtain reproducible measurements, it is important to probe with a standardized force. Badersten et al[30] studied the reproducibility of probing attachment level measurements using a manual probe and found that approximately 90% of the recordings could be repeated within ±1 mm difference. This was found for intraexaminer and interexaminer comparisons of two calibrated examiners. The level of reproducibility varied notably between patients and was improved following nonsurgical periodontal therapy.

Automatic Constant-Force Probes

Following a workshop titled "Quantitative Evaluation of Periodontal Diseases by Physical Measurement Techniques," the National Institute for Dental Research requested proposals to develop and clinically evaluate an improved periodontal probing-depth attachment level measurement system.[31] The new periodontal probe system was to meet the following criteria:

1. A precision of approximately 0.1 mm
2. A range of 10 mm
3. Constant probing force
4. Noninvasive; lightweight for comfortable use over an extended period; easy to learn
5. Ability to access any location around all teeth
6. A guidance system to ensure that measurements are taken from the same part of the sulcus each time (desirable but not mandatory)
7. Complete sterilization of all portions entering or nearing the mouth (cold sterilization not acceptable)
8. No biohazard from material or electric shock
9. Digital output

These criteria were more or less met by Gibbs et al,[32] who developed the Florida Probe system (Florida Probe Corporation), which combined the advantages of constant probing force with precise electronic measurement and computer storage of the data. Consisting of a probe handpiece, a digital readout, a foot switch, a computer interface, and a computer, the Florida Probe (Fig 17-3) eliminates the potential errors associated with visual reading. The system was studied by Magnusson et al[33] and correlated to standard probe measurements. They concluded that the reproducibility of probing-depth measurements obtained with the electronic probe was significantly superior to the reproducibility of the measurements obtained with a standard probe. There was no difference in time consumption between the two methods; however, data from the electronic probe are entered into the computer automatically, thereby eliminating the need for an assistant to record the measurements. At present, these devices are primarily indicated for clinical trials when appropriate.

Suggested Clinical Approach

Periodontal diseases are found in all patient groups, regardless of age or socioeconomic status; therefore, a periodontal examination should be performed for every patient who has teeth.[34] It is important for dental professionals to record the findings of these examinations.

Comprehensive Periodontal Examination for Daily Practice

The concepts detailed in this chapter are changing rapidly. Continued updating of knowledge on the subject is of utmost importance.

To judge the efficacy of active therapy and periodontal maintenance, the clinician must have adequate and accurate baseline data; without this baseline, it is difficult to define success. With accurate baseline data, gathered before treatment begins, selection of appropriate treatment is easier. Careful examination of patients with periodontal diseases is critical, and adequate time should be allowed during all phases of therapy for this procedure. Data gathered before active therapy will lead to an initial

diagnosis that will guide the patient's initial therapy and can prevent both undertreatment of inflammatory lesions (which is common) and their overtreatment. Re-evaluations will guide later therapy (see chapter 26).

Health History

The initial periodontal examination starts with a questionnaire completed by the patient. It should contain vital statistics (eg, age and weight), address, employment and marital status, a review of medical and dental histories, and the patient's chief complaint (see box). Questions concerning present and past compliance with oral hygiene procedures and periodontal maintenance are included.

The practitioner should review the health history with the patient. The initial visit is an appropriate time to determine both the patient's goals for therapy and motivation to seek care. In many cases, these goals will be unfocused, and patients will need the assistance of the dental professional in formalizing their desired end points in therapy. Setting goals serves several purposes, including ameliorating concerns about the proposed care, helping the patient develop realistic expectations, and identifying and then overcoming barriers to therapy. Both parties sign and date the health history, which should be updated periodically. (See appendix 1 for more information on the health history and a sample form.)

Health History Items

1. Basic information (name, address, patient height, weight, etc)
2. What most concerns the patient about his or her mouth (chief complaint)
3. Medical history
   - Information on past and present illnesses
   - Medications presently taken
   - Any allergies
   - Possible need for premedication before dental visits (certain cardiovascular conditions, such as mitral valve prolapse, artificial heart valves, certain prosthetic vein or artery replacements, and others; certain prosthetic devices, such as prosthetic hips or prosthetic knees) When there is a question, the patient's physician should be contacted. (See appendix 2 for specific information on medicating these patients.)

- Any present problems that may affect dental treatment (eg, pregnancy; transmissible diseases such as HIV infection, hepatitis, tuberculosis; tobacco use)
4. Dental history
   - Current oral hygiene practices
   - Previous dental or periodontal problems
   - History of temporomandibular joint problems
   - History of parafunctional habits (bruxing or clenching)
   - History of negative experiences with dentistry
   - Degree of compliance to suggestions by dental professionals (to suggested oral hygiene procedures or to suggested maintenance visits)
5. Family history
   - History of periodontal problems
   - History of heart disease or hypertension
   - History of diabetes

Positive answers to health history questions can affect parts of the examination. For example, a patient may have a type of heart murmur that requires premedication before dental procedures that cause bleeding (see appendix 2). Information of this type can be obtained in a telephone interview or by having the patient mail in the completed health history form before the first visit. Appropriate medications can then be prescribed or other modifications made before the visit.

Gathering Data on Risk Factors

Identifying and then reducing or eliminating risk factors known to be involved in the etiology or progression of periodontal diseases will improve the chances for halting or reversing the disease process. The more of these factors that can be eliminated or ameliorated, the better the prognosis (see chapter 20).

Primary local risk factors
1. Bacteria
   • Number and percentage of species (determined, if appropriate, by bacterial sampling and antibiotic specificity testing)
   • Retentive areas
     — Periodontal pockets
     — Poorly fitting dental restorations
     — Poor tooth alignment
     — Tongue
2. Compliance
   • To suggested oral hygiene
   • To suggested periodontal maintenance

Primary systemic risk factors
1. Smoking
2. Diabetes
3. Interleukin 1 genotype

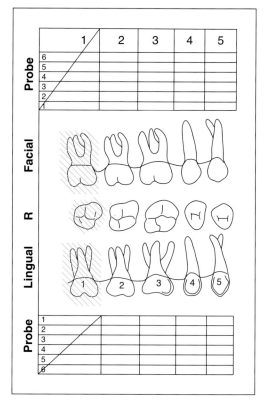

Fig 17-4 Clinical charting: Recording missing teeth

• Missing teeth are marked with a slash.
• Unerupted teeth are circled.
• Dental caries can be recorded at this time.

Radiographic Examination and Radiographic History

A set of appropriate radiographs is essential for making a proper diagnosis (see chapter 18). Each patient is unique, but most adults with teeth require a full-mouth series of periapical radiographs accompanied by posterior vertical bitewing radiographs. At present, these are best exposed using a parallel (right-angle) technique. The combination of panoramic and bitewing radiographs rarely provides enough information to make a correct diagnosis.

Radiographs should be kept to a minimum, but for patients with ongoing periodontal disease, a full set of radiographs may need to be obtained often. A set of seven vertical bitewing radiographs is preferred over four horizontal posterior radiographs in adults because they provide an increased view of the coronal portion of the alveolar bone in both the maxilla and mandible. Mounts are available that allow placement of several series of bitewing radiographs in the same holder, thus permitting the clinician to follow bone patterns over time.

A practitioner can gain perspective on a patient's condition by comparing the patient's old radiographs and periodontal probing charts to get an indication of the relative stability of the periodontium. This is important in making a correct diagnosis, since patients with slow progressive deterioration will fit into different diagnostic categories and receive therapy different from patients in whom rapid bone loss has been documented.

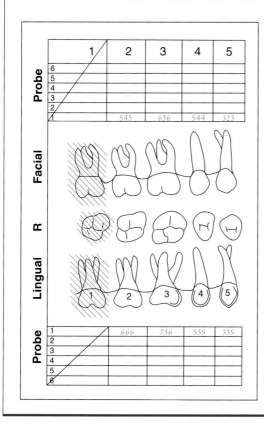

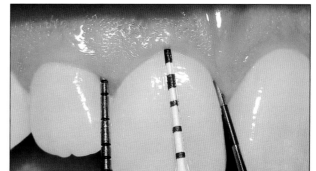

Fig 17-5 Clinical charting: Record probing depths

To obtain the most accurate manual readings, use a thin probe positioned as parallel to the long axis of the tooth as possible, and drag it through the sulcus (pocket). Pictured here are thin probes (0.4- to 0.5-mm diameters) with Williams markings (1, 2, 3, 5, 7, 8, 9, and 10 mm) *(left)*; a variation of the Community Periodontal Index of Treatment Needs (CPITN) markings (PSR, or periodontal screening and recording) (0.5, 3.5, 5.5, 8.5, and 11.5 mm) *(center)*; and 3-, 6-, 9-, and 12-mm markings *(right)*.

Clinical Charting

The patient's teeth are counted, and missing or impacted teeth are indicated on the chart (Fig 17-4).

Probing Depths

The manual periodontal probe is the clinician's most important diagnostic tool. It is used to obtain information on the health of the soft tissues, bone loss, tissue tone, subgingival calculus deposits, bone loss in furcations, and variations in root anatomy. However, it does have limitations. Probing depths found with these devices can vary greatly, depending on probe angulation, pressure applied, health of the tissue, diameter of the probe, and operator variables. In inflamed tissue, the probe passes through the junctional epithelium (epithelial attachment) and into the connective tissue.[35] This means that the true histologic depth of the pocket is not being measured. Consequently, the term *probing depth* often replaces the more traditional term *pocket depth*. Probing depth has been described as

the distance between the gingival margin and the apical depth of the periodontal probe tip penetration.[36] Manual probing remains an art, and great diligence is needed to standardize one's technique and thereby ensure reproducible readings (Figs 17-5).[27]

Probing tells the informed clinician more about the status of the periodontium than does any other clinical diagnostic test. As the operator gains experience, the information obtained from the use of this tool increases. A step-by-step approach to developing a standardized probing technique is described. A set of accurate full-mouth radiographs on the viewbox will improve the operator's chance of obtaining accurate readings.

1. *Selecting a probe with accurate standardized markings.* Reproducibility is the key to proper probing. Each periodontal probe should have accurate, well-defined, permanent, and easily readable markings. The probe should be thin (no more than 0.5 mm in diameter) and made from metal (plastic for implants) (Figs 17-6 to 17-8). It is suggested that a manual, standardized, thin metal probe be used around teeth, because these probes have the greatest

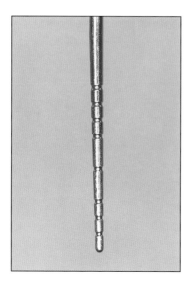
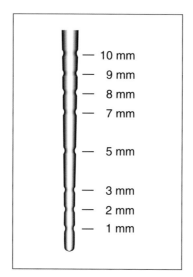

Fig 17-6 Michigan-O probe. This thin (0.5 mm in diameter) metal probe has Williams markings outlined in black (Hu-Friedy, Chicago). With Williams markings there are no marks for the 4- and 6-mm depths. It is suggested that the rings be in black to make the markings easier to read.

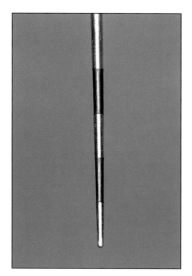
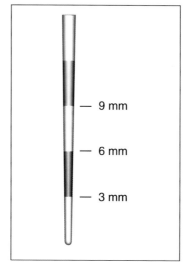

Fig 17-7 Marquis 2× probe. This thin metal probe is 0.5 mm in diameter and is marked in alternating black and silver 3-mm segments.

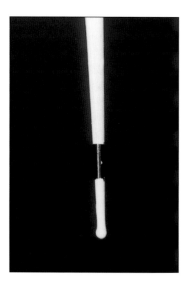
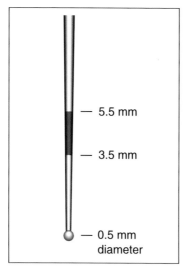

Fig 17-8 Community Periodontal Index of Treatment Needs Type E probe (Pro-Dentec, Batesville, AR). This thin plastic probe is 0.5 mm in diameter at the tip and has a 2-mm colored band from 3.5 to 5.5 mm. It can also be used with the periodontal screening and recording examination discussed later in this chapter.

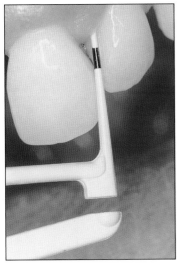
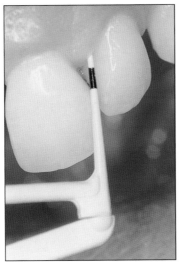
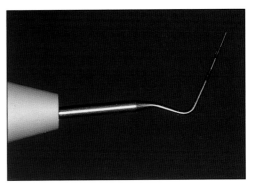

Fig 17-9 This probe is said to deliver a known force of 20 g. The force is delivered when the two parts of the probe meet *(right)* (Pro-Dentec).

Fig 17-10 Electronic probe that beeps after a force of 20 g has been applied (Laboratoire Peridental, Chateauneuf-Du-Faou). (For another example, see Fig 17-3; also see Mombelli et al.[37])

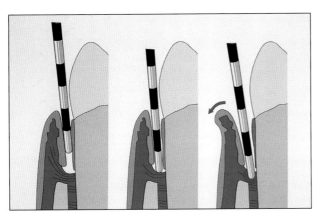
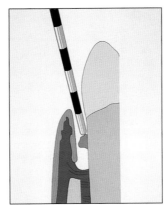

Fig 17-11 The health of the gingival tissue can directly affect the depth of penetration of the probe tip. With very tight tissue, the probe may not penetrate to the base of the pocket *(left)*. In flaccid tissue, the tip may go far into the connective tissue *(right)*. *(center)* The desired relation between probe tip and soft tissue.

Fig 17-12 Deposits of subgingival calculus may keep the probe tip from penetrating to the depth of the pocket. It is usually possible to work around this obstacle.

reproducibility of markings. A probe that delivers standardized force is helpful, but most are too expensive, or the markings are not standardized sufficiently to allow reproducible readings.

2. Standardizing probing pressure. The harder one pushes, the more the probe penetrates into the soft tissues of the periodontium.[26] The tip also travels further apically in inflamed than it does in healthy tissue.[22] This means that all probing depths are relative. To standardize the depth of penetration to the greatest degree possible, a standardized probing force should be used. This standardization can take many forms. A known force is best achieved by using a probe with a reproducible force (Figs 17-9 and 17-10). A variety of new probes designed to deliver a standardized force are entering the market. Forces from 25 g[38] to 50 g[39] have been suggested as appropriate. Many patients find a 50-g force uncomfortable; forces in the range of 20 to 25 g seem to be more comfortable and are still useful. At these lower forces, care must be taken to properly evaluate pockets with tight gingival tissue, very deep pockets, and large subgingival calculus deposits, since significant errors in readings can occur (Figs 17-11 and 17-12). In the end, the best that can be hoped for is accuracy within 1 mm. However, this often complicates clinical decisions[40] (see chapter 20).

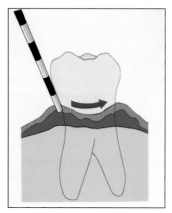

Fig 17-13 The probe is placed into the sulcus at the distal (or mesial) aspect of the tooth.

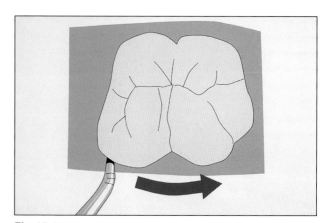

Fig 17-14 The probe is dragged through the sulcus.

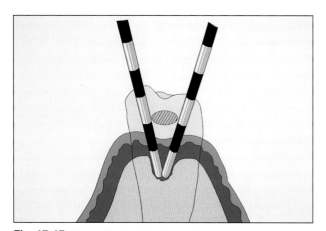

Fig 17-15 The probe is placed touching the contact area and kept as close to parallel to the long axis of the tooth root as possible.

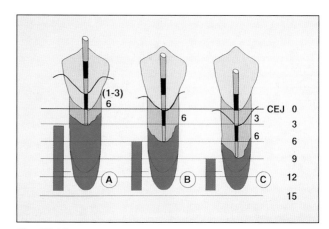

Fig 17-16 The clinical attachment level can be determined by adding the probing depth to the amount of gingival recession (or, subtracting from the probing depth if the patient has hyperplastic tissue). (A) A 6-mm probing depth that results from a normal attachment level and 3 mm of hyperplastic tissue. (B) A 6-mm pocket that results from 3 mm of attachment loss. (C) A 6-mm pocket with 9 mm of attachment loss. (CEJ) Cementoenamel junction.

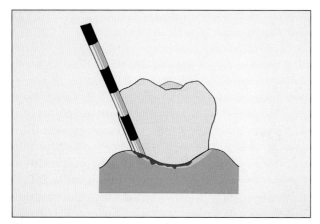

Fig 17-17 Bleeding (and sometimes suppuration) can be found during the probing procedure.

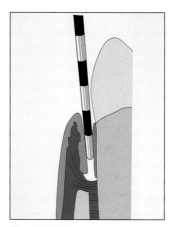

Fig 17-18 Root roughness and calculus can sometimes be felt during probing.

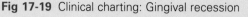

Fig 17-19 Clinical charting: Gingival recession

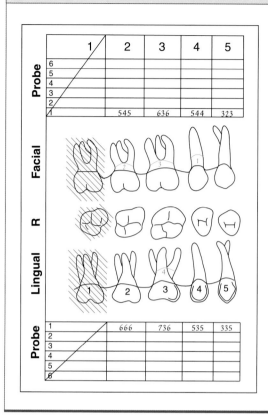

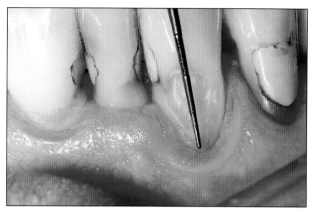

In this example, the pocket probing depth is 3 mm. If the amount of recession were not recorded, the fact that approximately 7 mm of attachment had been lost (equal to a 10-mm probing depth) would have been overlooked when the chart was read.

3. *Learning to properly position the probe.* An important part of the art of probing is position. The probe is positioned as close as possible to parallel to the long axis of the tooth and then dragged through the sulcus. In interproximal areas, the probe tip is placed at the deepest part of the pocket (on that side) and rested on the contact area[41] (Figs 17-13 to 17-15).

4. *Assessments made with a probe.* Despite its limitations, the manual probe is suggested for use in daily clinical practice. When it is used along with the measure of gingival recession, the clinical attachment can be determined (Fig 17-16). One can also measure the presence or absence of bleeding on probing. Suppuration can frequently be seen but is more often found following finger pressure on the buccal or lingual gingiva. Deposits of subgingival calculus can also be detected, as can the character of the soft tissue (Figs 17-17 and 17-18).

Clinicians must remember that probing depths can be misleading in the presence of excessively tight or flaccid tissue, when there are large deposits of calculus, or when visibility or placement of the probe is hindered. Even though these problems make it difficult to standardize probing-depth readings, the information obtained makes it well worth the effort. Despite its limitations, at present probing is the best clinical indicator of disease state.

An excellent time to collect probing charts from the patient's previous clinicians is before the initial examination. Although probe readings can vary from office to office, the perspective they provide (especially when combined with previous radiographs) is of great value when establishing a diagnosis.

Gingival Recession or Hyperplasia

Gingival recession or hyperplasia is measured from a set point on the tooth, usually the cementoenamel junction, the margin of a restoration, or the occlusal (incisal) edge. It provides perspective for pocket probing depth (Fig 17-19). In most cases, midbuccal and midlingual (palatal) recessions are recorded, but interproximal recession can add information and is often used in clinical trials.

Fig 17-20 Clinical charting: Bleeding on probing, suppuration, and bacterial plaque

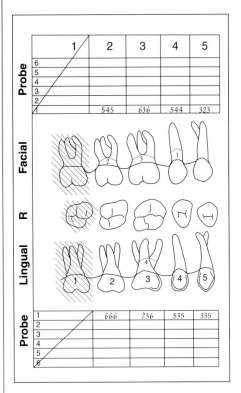

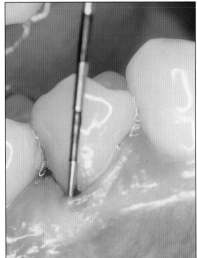

In clinical practice, the following parameters are recorded as either present or absent:

- Bleeding on probing, as noted in the clinical photograph, can be recorded as a dot above the pocket probing depth or on a modified O'Leary chart.[42]
- Suppuration is found by pressing the gingival tissues or is seen when pocket probing depths are recorded. It is recorded as a circle with a dot in the center.
- Supragingival bacterial plaque can be recorded on the chart if desired.

Bleeding on Probing, Bacterial Plaque, and Suppuration

Bleeding on probing can be found in two ways: (1) as an independent process, by dragging the tip of a thin periodontal probe through the gingival sulcus, using a pressure of 20 to 25 g,[38] or (2) by recording any bleeding seen up to 30 seconds after the probing-depth reading of a particular site has been taken. The importance of this index may be found in its absence rather than its presence, because absence of bleeding almost always indicates gingival health (Fig 17-20).

At the same time the clinician detects bleeding on probing, any visible supragingival dental plaque also can be recorded. Remember that bleeding on probing gives more information concerning tissue health than does the accumulation of plaque.

Suppuration can be found when using the periodontal probe or by exerting pressure on the gingival tissues near the gingival margin.

Tooth Mobility

Tooth mobility can be measured in daily clinical practice in two ways: when pressure is placed on individual teeth while the jaws are apart (bidigital mobility) (Fig 17-21) and when the teeth are in function (fremitus) (Fig 17-22). Registration of tooth mobility is an important part of a periodontal examination because it represents a combination of the height of the alveolar bone and the width of the periodontal ligament. Inflammation will affect the coronal part of the periodontal ligament by increasing mobility. The inflammatory status has to be considered in the evaluation of mobility. However, because tooth mobility may be attributable to causes other than periodontal disease (such as periapical lesions and trauma), it is essential to determine its cause. Increased mobility often occurs in a reduced but healthy periodontium. To determine if changes in mobility have occurred as a result of either therapy or disease, it is important to document and record both initial and posttherapy data.

Fig 17-21 Clinical charting: Tooth mobility (bidigital)

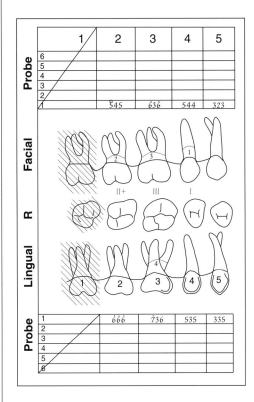

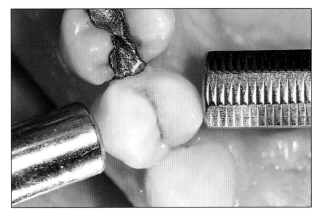

At present there is no simple, inexpensive, reproducible system for documenting bidigital mobility. This measurement is performed by alternately pressing on the buccal and lingual surfaces of the teeth with the nonworking ends of two instrument handles. The clinician can then use a modification of the Lindhe scale, as recommended by Fleszar et al[43]:

Class 0: Physiologic mobility; firm tooth
Class I: Slightly increased mobility
Class II: Definite to considerable increase in mobility, but no impairment of function
Class III: Extreme mobility; a loose tooth that would be uncomfortable in function (a plus sign can be used for intermediate values, eg, I+). This approach obviously leads to a great deal of individual variation. However, some degree of reproducibility is possible within one's own office.

Lindhe developed the following method for recording tooth mobility[45]:

Degree 1. The crown of the tooth moves 0.2 to 1 mm in a horizontal direction.
Degree 2. The crown of the tooth moves more than 1 mm in a horizontal direction.
Degree 3. The crown of the tooth moves in a vertical direction.

Fleszar et al[43] devised a similar system, as follows[46]:

Class I. The tooth has slightly increased mobility.
Class II. The tooth has definite to considerable increase in mobility, but no impairment of function.

Class III. The tooth has extreme mobility; it would be uncomfortable in function.

Measuring tooth mobility manually as described is the simplest and most practical method in a clinical setting. For research purposes, however, there are more sophisticated and more precise methods that use various mechanical devices.[47,48]

Furcations

Bone loss in furcations can be clinically assessed in two ways. The first method uses a Nabers probe. The second uses a traditional probe placed horizontally and describes it in millimeters (Fig 17-23).

Fig 17-22 Clinical charting: Tooth mobility (fremitus)

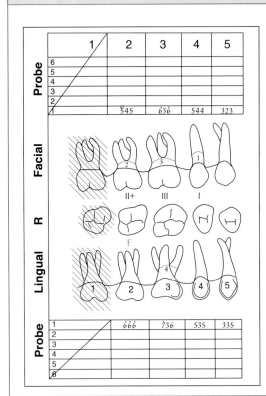

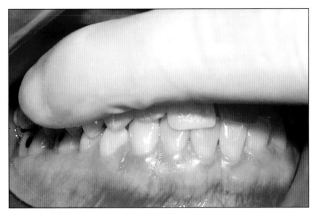

Fremitus (functional mobility) is the movement of teeth during function or parafunction. Fremitus can often be detected earlier than bidigital tooth mobility and has been associated, in the presence of inflammation, with increased bone and attachment loss (pocket formation) when compared with teeth without fremitus.[44] The photograph shows testing for fremitus. The index finger is placed on the buccal surface of the maxillary teeth, and the patient is asked to grind in lateral and protrusive movements. Any movement seen or felt is termed fremitus.

Fig 17-23 Clinical charting: Furcations

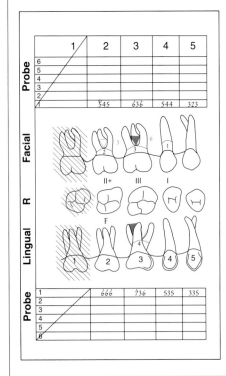

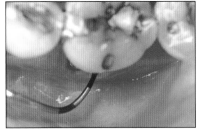

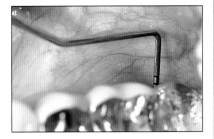

Nabers probes are useful for mesial and distal furcae of maxillary molars and interproximal furcae of maxillary premolars. The furcae can be classified in one of the following manners:

Approach 1

Class I: A depression that does not catch a curette or probe

Class II: A furca deep enough to catch a curette or probe but not contiguous with other furcae on the same tooth

Class III: Through-and-through bone loss

Standard probes can be used horizontally in buccal and lingual furcae. When combined with the determination of vertical probing depths, this approach is an accurate way to quantify bone loss, but this form of analysis is usually feasible only in buccal furcations in the maxilla and in buccal and lingual furcations in the mandible.

Approach 2

The horizontal measurement (in millimeters) is taken using a standard periodontal probe.

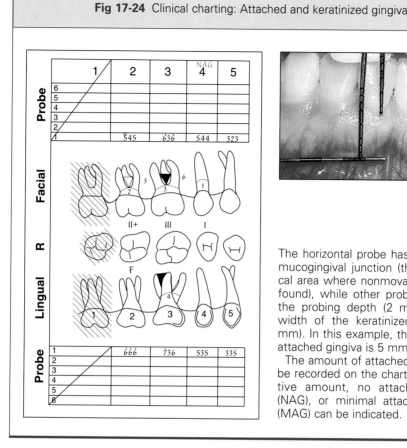
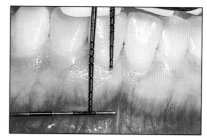

Fig 17-24 Clinical charting: Attached and keratinized gingiva

The horizontal probe has located the mucogingival junction (the most apical area where nonmovable tissue is found), while other probes measure the probing depth (2 mm) and the width of the keratinized gingiva (7 mm). In this example, the amount of attached gingiva is 5 mm.

The amount of attached gingiva can be recorded on the chart, or the relative amount, no attached gingiva (NAG), or minimal attached gingiva (MAG) can be indicated.

Attached and Keratinized Gingiva

The keratinized tissue of the gingiva extends from the mucogingival junction to the most coronal aspect of the midfacial or midlingual surface of the free gingival margin. The amount of attached gingiva is found by subtracting the midfacial or midlingual pocket probing depth from the width of keratinized gingiva (Fig 17-24). For additional information, see chapter 32.

Periodontal Screening and Recording

The screening tool described in this section is a variation of the Community Periodontal Index of Treatment Needs (CPITN Alternative II),[49] which has been endorsed by the World Health Organization. This index was modified by the American Academy of Periodontology as the periodontal screening and recording (PSR).[50] In almost every instance, a full examination is preferred over the use of this approach.

The PSR is designed for patients at least 18 years old and assays every surface of every tooth. It involves the use of a thin periodontal probe with a colored strip (running from 3.5 to 5.5 mm) with a 0.5-mm ball at the tip (see Fig 17-8). During this examination, the entire sulcus (pocket) of each tooth or implant is probed. Readings are taken at the mesiofacial, midfacial, and distofacial areas, as well as corresponding lingual/palatal areas. The probe is inserted into the crevice until resistance is met, at which point a reading is taken. The highest reading for each sextant is then recorded in a box specific for that sextant (Fig 17-25). Each sextant is rated according to the PSR scale of criteria (Table 17-2). The code then guides the need for a more comprehensive examination and suggests broad outlines for therapy.

An asterisk (*) placed in the box indicates a clinical abnormality found in that sextant. These abnormalities include, but are not limited to, bone loss in a furcation, tooth mobility, and mucogingival problems or gingival recession that extends from the cementoenamel junction apically for 3.5 mm (into the colored area of the probe). If an abnormality (asterisk) appears in codes 0 to 2, notation and/or treatment of that condition is warranted (Figs 17-26

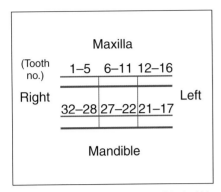

	Maxilla			
(Tooth no.)	1–5	6–11	12–16	
Right	32–28	27–22	21–17	Left
	Mandible			

Fig 17-25 Chart for use with PSR. An X is used to indicate any sextant with no teeth and no dental implants, and the severity of the disease is indicated by a set of numbers ranging from 0 to 4 (see Table 17-2).

Table 17-2 Scale Used with PSR

PSR code	Probing depth	Calculus/defective margins	Bleeding on probing
0	Colored area visible	No	No
1	Colored area visible	No	Yes
2	Colored area visible	Yes	May be present
3	Colored area partially visible	May be present	May be present
4	Colored area not visible	May be present	May be present

Fig 17-26 PSR code 0: Health	**Fig 17-27** PSR code 1: Gingivitis	**Fig 17-28** PSR code 2: Gingivitis
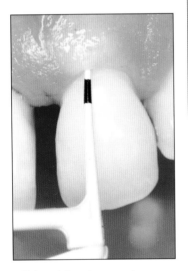	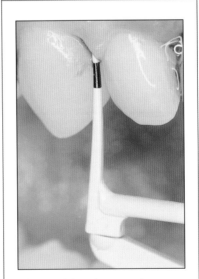	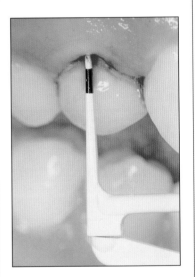
• Colored band on probe completely visible • No bleeding on probing • No calculus or defective margins	• Colored band on probe completely visible • Signs of gingivitis (eg, bleeding on probing) • No calculus or defective margins found	• Colored band on probe completely visible • Supragingival or subgingival calculus present • Defective margins detected

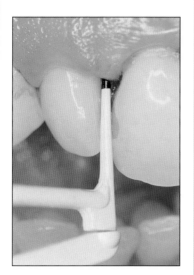

Fig 17-29 PSR code 3: Chronic periodontitis with early or moderate attachment loss

- Colored band on probe only partially visible
- Perform a comprehensive examination in that quadrant

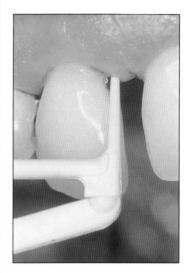

Fig 17-30 PSR code 4: Chronic periodontitis with moderate attachment loss or a form of aggressive periodontitis

- Colored band on probe not visible
- Perform a comprehensive examination

to 17-28). If a code 3 or 4 is found, comprehensive examination and treatment are necessary (Figs 17-29 and 17-30). For code 3 situations, the entire sextant is probed and recorded. If a code 4 is recorded, the entire mouth is examined using the approaches described in this chapter. This system does not distinguish among the various types of gingivitis or periodontitis.

References

1. Löe H, Silness J. Periodontal disease in pregnancy, I. Prevalence and severity. Acta Odontol Scand 1963;21:532–551.
2. Löe H. The gingival index, the plaque index and the retention index systems. J Periodontol 1967;38(suppl):610–616.
3. Gordon JM, Lamster IB, Seiger MC. Efficacy of Listerine antiseptic in inhibiting the development of plaque and gingivitis. J Clin Periodontol 1985;12:697–704.
4. Lobene RR. Discussion: Current status of indices for measuring gingivitis. J Clin Periodontol 1986;13:381–382.
5. Lobene RR, Mankodi SM, Ciancio SG, et al. Correlations among gingival indices: A methodological study. J Periodontol 1989; 60:159–162.
6. Lang NP, Joss A, Orsanic T, et al. Bleeding on probing: A predictor for the progression of periodontal disease? J Clin Periodontol 1986;13:590–596.
7. Saxer UP, Mühlemann HR. Motivation und Aufklarung. Schweiz Monatsschr Zahnheilkd 1975;85:905–919.
8. Loesche WJ. Clinical and microbiological aspects of chemotherapeutic agents used according to the specific plaque hypothesis. J Dent Res 1979;58:2404–2412.
9. Caton JG, Polson AM. The interdental bleeding index: A simplified procedure for monitoring gingival health. Compend Contin Educ Dent 1985;6:90–92.
10. Caton J, Polson A, Bouwsma O, et al. Associations between bleeding and visual signs of interdental gingival inflammation. J Periodontol 1988;59:722–727.
11. Magnusson I, Marks RG, Taylor M, et al. Intra- and interexaminer correlation of some oral indices [abstract 1970]. J Dent Res 1990;69:355.
12. Schour I, Massler M. Gingival disease in postwar Italy (1945): Prevalence of gingivitis in various age groups. J Am Dent Assoc 1947;35:475–482.
13. Russell AL. System of classification and scoring for prevalence surveys of periodontal disease. J Dent Res 1956;35:350–359.
14. Ramfjord SP. Indices for prevalence and incidence of periodontal disease. J Periodontol 1959;30:51–59.

15. Greene JC, Vermillion JR. Oral hygiene index: A method for classifying oral hygiene status. J Am Dent Assoc 1960;61:172–179.

16. Russell AL. International nutrition surveys: A summary of preliminary dental findings. J Dent Res 1963;42(suppl):233–244.

17. Quigley GA, Hein JW. Comparative cleansing efficiency of manual and power brushing. J Am Dent Assoc 1962;65:26–29.

18. Silness J, Löe H. Periodontal disease in pregnancy, II. Correlation between oral hygiene and periodontal condition. Acta Odontol Scand 1964;22:121–135.

19. Ennever J, Sturzenberger OP, Radike AW. The calculus surface index method for scoring clinical calculus studies. J Periodontol 1961;32:54–57.

20. Volpe AR, Manhold JH Jr. A method of evaluating the effectiveness of potential calculus inhibiting agents. NY State Dent J 1962;28:289–290.

21. Badersten A, Nilveus R, Egelberg J. Effect of nonsurgical periodontal therapy, VIII. Probing attachment changes related to clinical characteristics. J Clin Periodontol 1987;14:425–432.

22. Armitage GC, Svanberg GK, Löe H. Microscopic evaluation of clinical measurements of connective tissue attachment levels. J Clin Periodontol 1977;4:173–190.

23. Magnusson I, Listgarten MA. Histological evaluation of probing depth following periodontal treatment. J Clin Periodontol 1980;7:26–31.

24. Polson AM, Caton JG, Yeaple RN, Zander HA. Histological determination of probe tip penetration into gingival sulcus of humans using an electronic pressure-sensitive probe. J Clin Periodontol 1980;7:479–488.

25. Jansen J, Pilot R, Corba N. Histologic evaluation of probe penetration during clinical assessment of periodontal attachment levels: An investigation of experimentally induced periodontal lesions in beagle dogs. J Clin Periodontol 1981;8:98–106.

26. Fowler C, Garrett S, Crigger M, Egelberg J. Histological probe position in treated and untreated human periodontal tissues. J Clin Periodontol 1982;9:373–385.

27. Hassell TM, Germann MA, Saxer UP. Periodontal probing: Interinvestigator discrepancies and correlations between probing force and recorded depth. Helv Odontol Acta 1973;17:38–42.

28. Van der Velden U, de Vries JH. Introduction of a new periodontal probe: The pressure probe. J Clin Periodontol 1978;5:188–197.

29. Van der Velden U. Probing force and the relationship of the probe tip to the periodontal tissues. J Clin Periodontol 1979;6:106–114.

30. Badersten A, Nilvéus R, Egelberg J. Reproducibility of probing attachment level measurements. J Clin Periodontol 1984;11:475–485.

31. Parakkal PF. Proceedings of the workshop on quantitative evaluation of periodontal diseases by physical measurement techniques. J Dent Res 1979;58:547–553.

32. Gibbs CH, Hirschfeld JW, Lee JG, et al. Description and clinical evaluation of a new computerized periodontal probe—The Florida Probe. J Clin Periodontol 1988;15:137–144.

33. Magnusson I, Fuller WW, Heins PJ, et al. Correlation between electronic and visual readings of pocket depths with a newly developed constant force probe. J Clin Periodontol 1988;15:180–184.

34. American Dental Association. Diagnosing and Managing the Periodontal Patient. American Dental Association Risk Management Series. Chicago: American Dental Association, 1986.

35. Caton J. Periodontal diagnosis and diagnostic aids. In: Proceedings of the World Workshop in Clinical Periodontics. Princeton, NJ: American Academy of Periodontology, 1989:1–22.

36. Proye M, Caton J, Polson A. Initial healing of periodontal pockets after a single episode of root planing monitored by controlled probing forces. J Periodontol 1982;53:296–301.

37. Mombelli A, Mühle T, Frigg R. Depth-force patterns of periodontal probing. Attachment-gain in relation to probing force. J Clin Periodontol 1992;19:295–300.

38. Magnusson I, Clark WB, Marks RG, et al. Attachment level measurements with a constant force electronic probe. J Clin Periodontol 1988;15:185–188.

39. Hugoson A. Gingival inflammation and female sex hormones: A clinical investigation of pregnant women and experimental studies in dogs. J Periodontal Res 1970;5(suppl):1–18.

40. Haffajee AD, Socransky SS, Goodson JM. Comparison of different data analysis for detecting changes in attachment level. J Clin Periodontol 1983;10:298–310.

41. Watts TL. Probing site configuration in patients with untreated periodontitis: A study of horizontal positioned error. J Clin Periodontol 1989;16:529–533.

42. O'Leary TJ, Drake RB, Naylor JE. The plaque control record. J Periodontol 1972;43:38.

43. Fleszar TJ, Knowles JW, Morrison EC, et al. Tooth mobility and periodontal therapy. J Clin Periodontol 1980;7:495–505.

44. Pihlstrom BL, Anderson KA, Aeppoli D, Schaffer EM. Association between signs of trauma from occlusion and periodontitis. J Periodontol 1986;57:1–6.

45. Lindhe J. Textbook of Clinical Periodontology. Copenhagen: Munksgaard, 1983.

46. Lindhe J. Textbook of Clinical Periodontology, ed 2. Copenhagen: Munksgaard, 1989.

47. Muhlemann HR. Periodontometry, a method for measuring tooth mobility. Oral Surg Oral Med Oral Pathol 1951;4:1220–1233.

48. Robertson G. The multiple impulse method of tooth mobility assessment: An evaluation of the Periotest. Third North Sea Conference on Periodontology. Maastricht, The Netherlands: British, Dutch and Scandinavian Society on Periodontics, 1990:62.

49. Ainamo J, Barmes D, Beagrie G, et al. Development of the World Health Organization Community Periodontal Index of Treatment Needs CPITN. Int Dent J 1982;32:281–291.

50. Lo Frisco C, Cutler R, Bramson JB. Periodontal screening and recording: Perceptions and effects on practice. J Am Dent Assoc 1993;124:226–229, 231–232.

Radiography in Periodontal Assessments

Samuel J. Zeichner
- Indications for Radiographic Examination
- Optimal Radiographic Techniques
- Optimizing Radiographic Interpretation
- Documenting Radiographic Findings
- Radiographic Anatomy of the Periodontium
- Radiographic Findings of Various Conditions
- Radiographic Correlations with Disease

Marjorie Jeffcoat
- Subtraction Radiography

Recent epidemiological studies and demographic trends suggest that in ensuing decades there will be substantial numbers of adults in the United States who need periodontal therapy.[1] Because radiologic evaluation is an integral part of periodontal assessment, techniques for obtaining and interpreting radiographs merit special attention. This chapter presents a clinically relevant approach for optimizing the acquisition and interpretation of radiographic examinations. Specifically, this chapter addresses the capacities and limitations of conventional radiographic techniques, including panoramic, periapical, and bitewing radiography. Geometric and technical considerations, such as paralleling versus bisecting-the-angle techniques and kilovolt (peak), are discussed.

Methods for optimizing radiographic interpretation include an organized, systematic, sequential approach to radiologic analysis of the periodontium and related structures. Also discussed are normal radiographic anatomy and its variants, the radiographic appearance of periodontal diseases, methods for documentation of radiographic findings, and systemic diseases that affect the periodontium. Helpful interpretive hints are presented. The overall goal of this chapter is to provide the reader with the skills needed to comprehensively evaluate a radiographic examination.

Indications for Radiographic Examination

Radiographic examination is based on each patient's unique needs. The concept that radiographic examination is need based rather than time based is fundamental and well accepted in modern dental medicine.[2] Thus, radiographs are not prescribed merely because a patient has not had a recent examination or to rule out occult disease of the jaws.[3] In some cases, only after the practitioner obtains a thorough history and performs a physical examination can he or she determine which radiographs should be ordered for the patient. For example, consider a healthy 22-year-old patient who presents with gingival bleeding on periodontal probing and recurrent caries associated with a molar. A comprehensive radiographic examination for this patient might consist simply of two posterior bitewing radiographs and one periapical view of the affected molar. In

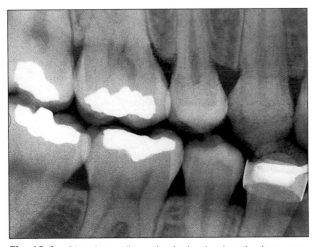

Fig 18-1a Bitewing radiograph obtained using the long-cone-paralleling technique accurately demonstrates the mandibular alveolar crest to be situated 1 mm apical to the CEJs.

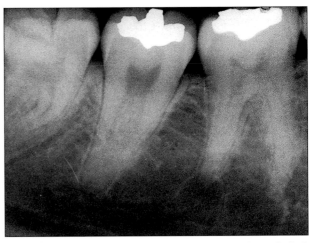

Fig 18-1b Same region as in Fig 18-1a, but the radiograph deviates from parallelism. The improperly angulated radiograph underestimates alveolar bone height. The alveolar crest misleadingly appears to be slightly coronal to the CEJs. Moreover, the crestal cortication disappears.

contrast, a comprehensive examination for a patient who presents with multiple missing, carious, tilted, and mobile teeth might consist of selected periapical views and vertical bitewing radiographs.

In essence, each radiographic examination is tailored to suit the unique diagnostic needs of individual patients. No radiographs may be required, or more than 20 intraoral radiographs may be needed. The necessity for radiographs and their quantity depend solely on the patient's clinical status, dental history, and oral anatomy, as well as the practitioner's treatment planning goals.

Optimal Radiographic Techniques

Selection of appropriate radiographic methods optimizes the diagnostic yield from intraoral radiography. For some diagnostic tasks, such as evaluating alveolar bone heights and assessing the cortication of the alveolar crest, bitewing radiographs are more reliable than periapical radiographs. For other tasks, such as determining crown-to-root ratios or visualizing the periodontal ligament spaces, periapical views are the more appropriate radiographic option. For obtaining periapical views, the long-cone-paralleling technique is preferred to the bisecting-the-angle technique because the paralleling technique produces less distortion. The principles of the long-cone-paralleling technique have been presented elsewhere.[4]

Figures 18-1a and 18-1b illustrate a common misleading radiographic observation caused by lack of parallelism. Figure 18-1a correctly demonstrates the alveolar crest to be situated approximately 1 mm subjacent to the cementoenamel junctions (CEJs) of the mandibular molars. This radiograph was obtained with the surface of the film positioned parallel to the long axis of the teeth and parallel to the central grooves of the occlusal surfaces. Concurrently, the x-ray beam was positioned approximately parallel to the occlusal plane and perpendicular to the contact points. In contrast, in Fig 18-1b (a radiograph of the same region), the alveolar crest appears to be situated coronal to the CEJs. Anatomically this is not possible. In this obvious example, the inaccurate position of the alveolar crest resulted from deviations from parallel technique. Moreover, the crestal cortication appears to be absent. This is explained diagrammatically in Fig 18-2. As illustrated here, when the x-ray beam traverses parallel to the alveolar crest and CEJs, the correct anatomic relationship is depicted on the resultant radiograph. However, when the x-ray beam is angulated with respect to the crests (which more likely occurs with maxillary posterior

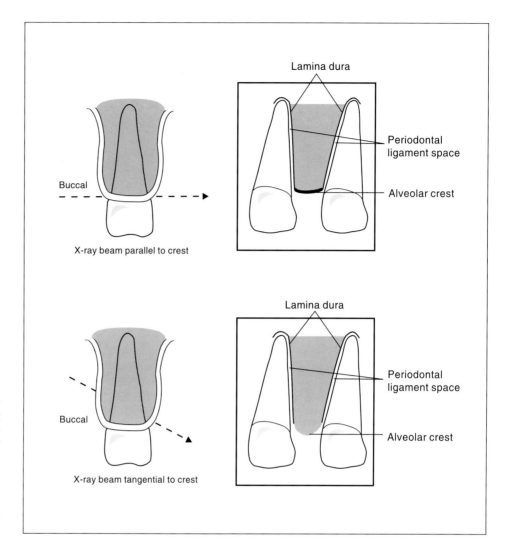

Fig 18-2 When the x-ray beam traverses parallel to the alveolar crest and CEJs, the correct anatomic relationships are depicted on the resultant radiograph. When the x-ray beam is angulated with respect to the crest and traverses the crest tangentially, the image of the crest is projected coronally, and the cortical bone of the crest appears indistinct or absent.

periapical radiographs), the image of the crest is projected coronally. Thus, it is not uncommon for improperly angulated radiographs to underestimate alveolar bone levels.

When the x-ray beam passes parallel to the crest, the entire buccolingual dimension of the crest is projected on the radiograph, and the image of the crest shows as a distinct radiopaque line. In contrast, when the beam traverses the crest tangentially, passing through a short distance of cortical bone, the radiograph is not likely to display a discernible line. Figures 18-3a and 18-3b depict bone heights on a correctly positioned bitewing radiograph and a corresponding periapical radiograph that deviates moderately from parallelism. The periapical film underestimates the level of the alveolar bone in relation to the CEJs. The clinical importance of recognizing these artifacts is discussed later in this chapter.

Another technical factor to consider is x-ray beam quality (ie, energy of the x-ray photons that make up the beam). Beam quality is largely influenced by kilovolt (peak), or kVp. X-ray machines operating at high-kVp levels (80 kVp or greater) generate an x-ray beam with a higher average photon energy. A photon beam with a high kVp can better delineate the subtle changes in mineralization of the alveolar crest than can low-kVp techniques. In short, conventional radiographic examination of the periodontium is best accomplished using periapical and bitewing views with the long-cone-paralleling method and an x-ray beam of high kVp.

Panoramic radiography has limited utility in evaluating the periodontium.[5] This may be attributed to inherently low resolution and geometric distortion that poorly define the presence and relative location of the alveolar crest.

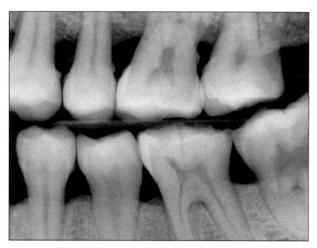
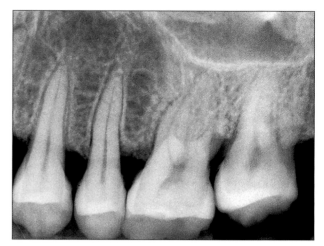

Figs 18-3a and 18-3b Comparison of alveolar bone heights as depicted on a correctly positioned bitewing radiograph *(left)* and a corresponding periapical radiograph *(right)* that deviates from parallelism. The periapical radiograph underestimates the level of alveolar bone in relation to the CEJs.

Optimizing Radiographic Interpretation

Just as good-quality radiographs are fundamental to diagnosis and treatment planning, an organized, systematic, sequential method of radiographic interpretation is equally important. Because the untrained eye tends to dart from radiograph to radiograph and skip randomly from region to region, the clinician must deliberately compensate for this natural tendency by using a systematic approach. The systematic interpretive method is a structured, repetitive process. Each radiograph is viewed repeatedly and in an invariable sequence. Each repetition focuses on a separate clinically relevant anatomic region. Consequently, a comprehensive interpretation can require more than 15 minutes to evaluate 15 to 20 intraoral radiographs.

An organized, systematic radiographic analysis begins by placing the properly mounted radiographs on a suitable light box and confirming the patient's identity and date of exposure. (If previous radiographic examinations are available, these should be on hand for comparison.) Next, the clinician should briefly view the set of radiographs in their entirety, making certain that *(1)* there are no distortions caused by improper radiograph placement or excessive vertical angulation of the x-ray beam (this can be ascertained by comparing buccal and lingual cusp tips of posterior teeth; if cusp tips superimpose, then the radiographs were obtained with adequate parallelism), *(2)* the bitewing and periapical radiographs show each interproximal area without significant overlap, *(3)* the periapical views include the root apices plus at least 3 mm of adja-

cent bone, and *(4)* the radiographs demonstrate the alveolar crest.

With a confirmation of the diagnostic adequacy of the radiographic examination, a detailed study of the radiographs can begin. A helpful hint that facilitates reproducible, comprehensive, sequential interpretation is to imagine the set of radiographs as a road map. Visualize an origin. Visualize a destination, and consistently follow the intervening route without variation. For the intraoral radiographic examination, the central origin is the occlusal plane. The destination is bidirectional: *(1)* the most cephalad structures displayed on the radiographs (usually the maxillary sinus in the maxilla) and *(2)* the most caudad structures (usually the inferior border of the mandible). The intermediate structures that should be viewed en route are (in sequence) *(1)* the crowns of the teeth, *(2)* the pulp chambers and root canals, *(3)* the alveolar crests and overlying gingiva, *(4)* the laminae dura and periodontal ligament spaces, *(5)* the interdental and inter-radicular bone, *(6)* the alveolar bone apical to the roots of the teeth, and *(7)* the maxillary sinus and inferior mandibular border.

To illustrate, given a complete mouth survey, the right molar bitewing radiograph is viewed, and the surface of the crowns is traced. Is the enamel intact, or are there defects, adherent calculus, or malcontoured restorations? Are there missing, malposed, or nonerupted teeth? More anteriorly, this process is repeated with the premolar bitewing radiograph. Next, observations are reconfirmed by visually tracing the crowns on the maxillary and mandibular right posterior periapical views. Continuing around the dental arches, the crowns depicted on the anterior periapical views are inspected. Then the left bitewing and posterior periapical radiographs are examined, focusing solely on the dental crowns.

After analysis of the crowns, the pulp chambers and (where visible) the root canals are analyzed in the right molar bitewing view. Internal resorption or other pulpal abnormalities are noted. Root canal fillings, root fractures, or root perforations are evaluated, and the remaining radiographs are sequentially inspected, with attention to the pulp chambers and root canals. When every radiograph has been viewed, the right posterior bitewing radiograph is reconsidered.

The alveolar crest and overlying gingiva are observed. Is the gingiva hyperplastic? Are foreign bodies evident? The presence or absence of crestal cortication is ascertained. The level of the alveolar crest in relation to the CEJs of adjacent teeth is noted. The contour of the crestal bone, including the presence of osseous abnormalities (described later in this chapter), is assessed. As before, observations are repeated for every radiograph. (Bitewing radiographs tend to be more reliable than periapical views for evaluating the alveolar crest. Discrepancies are reconciled in favor of the bitewing findings.)

The next step of the interpretation addresses the periodontal ligament spaces and laminae dura. The right posterior radiographs are examined: Are the laminae dura intact or interrupted? Are they well defined or indistinct? Are the periodontal ligament spaces of uniform dimension or notably widened? Each remaining radiograph is inspected in sequence.

The interdental and inter-radicular bones on each radiograph are evaluated. Are there atypical areas of increased or diminished radiodensity? Is there an absence of furcational bone? The size, shape, and location of discernible lesions are noted. Are the borders well circumscribed or ill defined? Is the internal architecture heterogeneous or homogeneous? Abnormal findings in the bone apical to the roots of teeth are noted.

Finally, the most peripheral structures visible on the radiographs are inspected: Are the maxillary sinuses and nasal cavity well aerated, or are they opacified? Are their bony boundaries intact? Is there thickening of the mucosal lining? Is the inferior mandibular border intact or interrupted, thinned, expanded, or eroded?

Documenting Radiographic Findings

Even the most meticulous radiographic interpretation is deficient if it is inadequately documented. Proper documentation facilitates communication among caregivers, simplifies transactions with third-party payers, and cir-

cumvents potential medicolegal problems. For these and other reasons, accrediting agencies have issued standardized guidelines for reporting radiographic findings.[6] Accordingly, an appropriate radiologic report should include the patient's name, the date of the radiographic examination, the number and type of radiographs making up the examination, a description of the findings in objective terms, and the signature of the licensed practitioner. Additionally, the radiographic record may include a summary of the findings (ie, radiologic impression); a notation of technical inadequacies that might impair the diagnostic quality of the examination; a statement explaining why, in the judgment of the clinician, additional views were deferred or not obtained; and recommendations for further radiographic evaluation.

The radiologic report is generally written narratively in the patient's chart. Some clinicians prefer to note the radiographic findings on a separate page, form, or diagram in the patient's record. When a patient is referred to a radiologist for radiographic examination, the radiologist sends the referring doctor a consultation letter that describes the radiographic findings. An example of a comprehensive radiologic report is illustrated in Fig 18-4.

Radiographic Anatomy of the Periodontium

The normal radiographic appearance of the alveolar crest is characterized by the presence of cortical bone. This crestal cortication appears as a thin but distinct radiopaque line contiguous with the laminae dura of adjacent teeth. In the posterior regions, the junction of the alveolar crest with the laminae dura is boxlike, forming a sharp, distinct angle (Fig 18-5). In the mandibular anterior region, the alveolar crest between adjacent teeth is normally spear shaped or knifelike (Fig 18-6). In the maxillary anterior region, the alveolar crest may be rounded (Fig 18-7). In all regions, the normal alveolar crest lies 1 to 2 mm subjacent to the CEJ of adjacent teeth and parallels adjacent CEJs.

Radiographic Findings of Various Conditions

Chronic Periodontitis with Early or Moderate Attachment Loss

The subtle inflammatory changes associated with early periodontitis are not easily discerned radiographically. Both good-quality radiographs and close examination are

The Maxillofacial Radiology Center
at
LENOX HILL RADIOLOGY & MEDICAL IMAGING ASSOCIATES
Samuel J. Zeichner, D.M.D.

New York, NY 10021

61 EAST 77TH STREET
(212) 650-0442

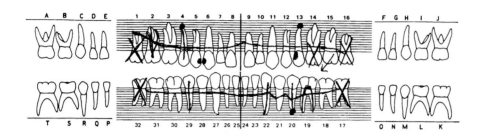

January 3, 2002

Dr. Robert L. Stevenson
4321 Park Avenue, Suite 2201
New York, New York 10021

Re: William Shakespeare
Hx: missing and mobile teeth, left facial swelling
Exam: complete mouth survey
Date: January 2, 2002

Dear Dr. Stevenson:

The examination consists of 14 periapical and 2 bitewing radiographs.

Caries, missing, tilted, and endodontically treated teeth are diagrammed above along with approximate alveolar bone levels.

Calculus is present. There is generalized loss of crestal cortication with evidence of horizontal alveolar bone loss in the right posterior maxilla. Blunting of the mandibular interdental bone is noted and vertical bony defects are seen adjacent to teeth #s 8, 20, and 21. There is an absence of furcational bone associated with tooth # 2.

The periodontal ligament spaces associated with teeth #s 4 and 20 are notably widened. The laminae dura are indistinct or absent. A punctate radiopacity is noted apical to # 20 and most likely represents ectopic endodontic filling material. The lamina dura apical to # 13 is absent. An elliptical area of lytic bone measuring 5 mm in widest dimension adjoins the root apex.

IMPRESSION:
    1) rarefying osteitis tooth # 13
    2) furcational periodontitis tooth # 2
    3) marginal periodontitis and osseous defects #s 8, 20, and 21
    4) apical periodontitis (or healing apical periodontitis) #s 4 and 20
    5) caries, missing, tilted, and endodontically treated teeth

Sincerely,

Samuel J. Zeichner, D.M.D., M.A., M.S.

Fig 18-4 A comprehensive report documents radiographic findings.

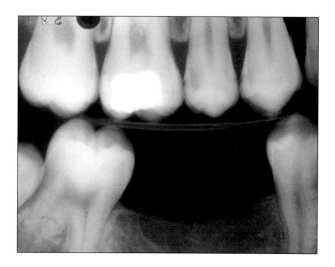

Fig 18-5 Radiographic appearance of normal periodontium in the posterior region of the mandible and maxilla.

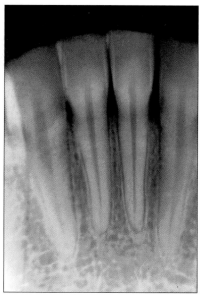

Fig 18-6 Radiographic appearance of normal periodontium in the anterior region of the mandible.

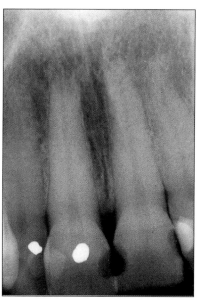

Fig 18-7 Radiographic appearance of normal periodontium in the anterior region of the maxilla.

required. Early radiographic changes associated with periodontitis include localized thinning or loss of the crestal cortication (Fig 18-8a) and/or blunting of mandibular anterior interdental bone (Fig 18-8b). The absence of crestal cortication is a noteworthy sign of disease, because at no site in the healthy body can medullary bone be observed adjacent to soft tissue without an intervening layer of cortical bone. It also should be noted that radiography inherently lacks sensitivity. Thus, clinical disease invariably precedes the ability to detect abnormalities radiographi-

cally. Moreover, as previously described, artifacts may simulate the absence of an intact alveolar crest.

As the inflammatory process progresses, not only does the cortical bone of the alveolar crest demineralize but the underlying bone of the marginal periodontium resorbs as well. With this resorption, patterns of osseous abnormalities are observed radiographically. For example, the alveolar crest may appear to lie more than 2 mm subjacent to CEJs yet still parallel to the occlusal plane (Fig 18-9). This is commonly termed *horizontal bone loss*. Other osseous

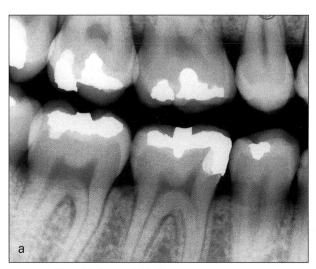
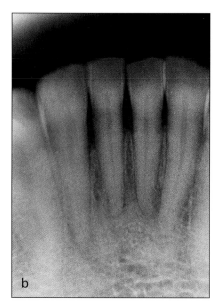

Figs 18-8a and 18-8b Radiographic findings associated with chronic periodontitis with early attachment loss. *(a)* There is loss of crestal cortication in the maxilla and mandible. *(b)* There is blunting of the mandibular anterior interdental bone.

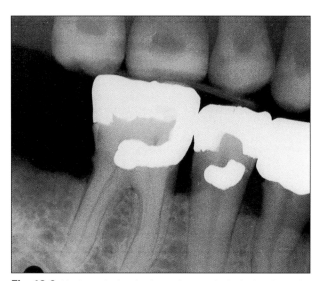

Fig 18-9 Horizontal alveolar bone loss typical of chronic periodontitis with mild to moderate attachment loss.

defects associated with chronic periodontitis with early or moderate attachment loss include interproximal crater formation (cupping defect), disparate buccal and lingual bone margins, angular bony defects (vertical bony defect), and resorption of furcational bone (furcation involvement). The interproximal crater is the most common osseous abnormality[7] and manifests as a cup-shaped depression in the alveolar crest. The apical margin of the defect is generally poorly defined and may appear to blend with the underlying bone (Fig 18-10). Another radio-

graphic finding typical of this form of periodontitis is two separate and distinct interproximal bone levels (Fig 18-11). This occurs when there has been disproportionate resorption of the buccal and lingual cortices. Consequently, the radiograph delineates the crestal margin of each individual cortical plate.

Angular bony defects are yet another radiographic manifestation of periodontitis with early or moderate attachment loss. Unlike the normal crestal contour in which the interproximal alveolar crest parallels adjacent CEJs, angular bony defects are characterized radiographically by oblique orientation of the alveolar crest. As a result, when the pattern of bone destruction progresses vertically along the root of a tooth, the radiographs may demonstrate a V-shaped crevice, with the root of the tooth making up one side of the defect (Fig 18-12). This osseous abnormality is termed a *vertical defect, angular defect,* or *triangular defect* (terminology derived from the three sides that make up its borders). Some or all of these osseous abnormalities may be found on radiographic examination of patients with chronic periodontitis with early or moderate attachment loss. With advancing periodontitis, there is destruction of bone in the furcations of multirooted teeth. Radiographically, this appears as furcational radiolucencies. The absence of furcational bone when accompanied by signs of inflammation is indicative of a more substantial attachment loss.

Aggressive Forms of Periodontitis

Aggressive periodontitis may demonstrate some or all of the radiographic findings associated with the previously

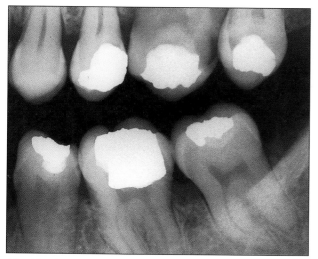

Fig 18-10 Interproximal crater in the mandibular molar region.

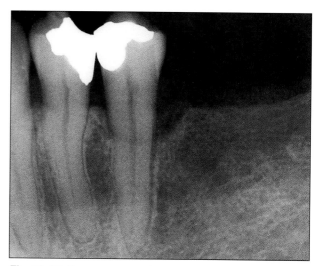

Fig 18-11 Two separate and distinct interproximal bone levels associated with the mandibular second premolar. This is a consequence of disproportionate resorption of the buccal and lingual cortices.

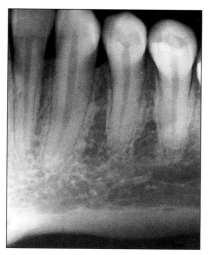

Fig 18-12 A vertical bony defect is seen between the canine and first premolar.

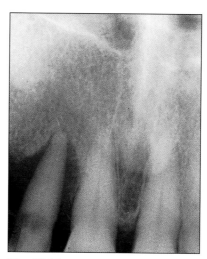

Fig 18-13 A vertical (angular) bony defect involving the root apex of the right lateral incisor.

mentioned forms of periodontitis. Additionally, there may be substantial horizontal bone loss such that the alveolar crest appears at or below the level of the apical third of roots. Moreover, vertical (angular) bony defects may involve the root apices (Fig 18-13). The periodontal ligament spaces may be notably widened and the laminae dura conspicuously absent. In such cases, it is common to find radiographic evidence of concurrent marginal periodontitis, bone loss in the furcations, and apical periodontitis.

Radiographic Correlations with Disease

Findings Suggestive of Periodontal Disease

Certain radiographic findings demonstrate a strong correlation with periodontal disease. It is helpful to recognize these so-called red flags. For example, open contacts,

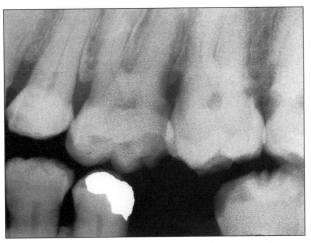

Fig 18-14 Calculus telegraphs underlying inflammatory changes.

malcontoured dental restorations, open restorative margins, or tilted, rotated, or otherwise malposed teeth predispose to the accumulation of bacteria. Inflammatory periodontal disease frequently is seen in conjunction with such radiographic observations. Similarly, the radiographic appearance of calculus often telegraphs underlying inflammatory changes (Fig 18-14). In addition, hypererupted teeth may call attention to the radiographic signs of occlusal trauma, such as widened periodontal ligament spaces and atypical laminae dura.

Findings Suggestive of Systemic Disease

A few systemic conditions may intensify the severity of periodontitis or cause radiographically observable changes in the periodontium. Endocrinopathies, hematologic disorders, hereditary disturbances, and immunodeficiencies have been associated with radiographic findings indicative of rapidly progressing periodontitis with severe bone destruction.

Most notable of the endocrinopathies is uncontrolled diabetes mellitus. Patients with diabetes mellitus are more prone to develop severe and rapid alveolar bone loss than are patients with normal glucose metabolism.[8]

Of the hematologic disorders, acute forms of monocytic, myelogenous, and lymphoid leukemia have been reported occasionally to mimic destructive periodontitis.

Hereditary disturbances affecting the periodontium are similarly rare. Chediak-Higashi syndrome (characterized by oculocutaneous albinism, photophobia, nystagmus, and recurrent infection) may be accompanied by destruction of the periodontium.[9] Papillon-Lefèvre syndrome (characterized by hyperkeratosis of the palms and soles)

may include extensive generalized horizontal alveolar bone loss.[10]

In the immunocompromised patient, the ability to resist infection is diminished. Individuals taking immunosuppressive agents or patients with AIDS may manifest particularly rapid alveolar bone destruction.[11]

Periodontal manifestations of systemic disease are uncommon. Nonetheless, rapid loss of alveolar bone, in the absence of the usual causative agents, should prompt the clinician to consider underlying systemic abnormalities.

Subtraction Radiography

Most assessment of progressive alveolar bone loss in clinical practice today is achieved by interpretation, ie, visual comparison of radiographs taken over time. Unfortunately, it is difficult to detect small changes in bone that occur between examinations using interpretation because the radiograph contains a superimposed background of teeth, cortical bone, and trabecular bone. Unchanging superimposed structures often make it difficult to see small changes in alveolar bone that have occurred between examinations in spite of the fact that these changes have been registered in the film itself.

Digital subtraction radiography was introduced to dentistry in the 1980s.[12–16] This technique is used to detect small changes in hard tissues that occur between examinations. In brief, digital subtraction radiography uses specialized computer programs to remove all structures that have not changed from a set of two x-ray films taken at different examinations. This image-processing procedure subtracts unchanging teeth, cortical bone, and trabecular pattern, leaving only the bone gain or loss standing out against a neutral gray background on the subtraction image. The area of change may be superimposed on the original radiograph to improve the ability of the clinician to interpret the subtraction image (Fig 18-15). Additional software can determine the size, mass, or density of the region of change. These techniques have been shown to be more than 90% sensitive and specific in detecting small bony changes. More recently, this quantitative method has been shown to correlate highly with techniques used to measure bone mass in medicine (such as dual-energy x-ray absorptiometry).[17]

Summary

Radiologic evaluation is an integral part of periodontal assessment. Radiographic examination is based on each patient's unique situation and the practitioner's treatment planning goals. Conventional radiographic examination

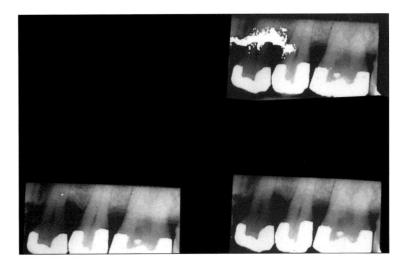

Fig 18-15 The lower right and left panels represent radiographs taken 6 months apart. Although bone loss on the first premolar is evident in both radiographs, it is difficult to determine whether or not progressive bone loss has occurred between examinations. The upper panel shows the area of change detected by subtraction radiography superimposed on the original radiograph. On the computer monitor, this area appears in shades of red, indicating bone loss. In this black-and-white figure, the area of bone loss is shown in white to facilitate visualization.

of the periodontium is best accomplished with selected periapical and bitewing views employing the long-cone-paralleling method and a high-kVp x-ray beam. Assessment of progressive alveolar bone loss may be enhanced by using image-processing techniques such as digital subtraction radiography. Radiographic interpretation can be optimized by using a structured, repetitive viewing process such as that illustrated in this chapter.

Normal radiographic anatomy of the periodontium is characterized by crestal cortication. The alveolar crest may be boxlike, spear shaped, or rounded, depending on the anatomic region. In all regions, the normal alveolar crest lies 1 to 2 mm subjacent to the CEJ of adjacent teeth and parallels adjacent CEJs. Radiographic findings associated with chronic periodontitis include loss of crestal cortication, horizontal alveolar bone loss, interproximal crater formation, disparate buccal and lingual cortical bone margins, vertical bony defects, and resorption of furcational and periapical bone. Periodontal manifestations of systemic disease are uncommon. Nonetheless, rapidly progressing attachment loss, in the absence of the usual causative agents, should prompt the clinician to consider underlying systemic abnormalities.

References

1. Douglass C, Fox C. Cross-sectional studies in periodontal disease: Current status and implications for dental practice. Adv Dent Res 1993;7(1):25–31.
2. American Dental Association Council on Dental Materials, and Equipment. Recommendations in radiographic practices: An update. J Am Dent Assoc 1989;118:115–117.
3. Zeichner S, Ruttimann E, Webber R. Dental radiography: Efficacy in the assessment of intraosseous lesions of the face and jaws in asymptomatic patients. Radiology 1987;162:691–695.
4. Goaz P, White S. Oral Radiology Principles and Interpretation, ed 3. St. Louis: Mosby, 1992:151–218.
5. Muhammed A, Manson-Hing L. A comparison of panoramic and intraoral radiographic surveys in evaluating a dental clinic population. Oral Surg Oral Med Oral Pathol 1982;54:108–117.
6. ACR Commission on Standards and Accreditation. ACR standard for communication-diagnostic radiology. Resolution 5-1991. Reston, VA: American College of Radiology, 1991.
7. Prichard JF. Advanced Periodontal Disease, Surgical and Prosthetic Management, ed 2. Philadelphia: WB Saunders, 1965:116.
8. Emrich L, Shlossman M, Genco R. Periodontal disease in non-insulin dependent diabetes mellitus. J Periodontol 1991;62:123–130.
9. Hamilton RE Jr, Giasanti JS. The Chediak-Higashi syndrome: Report of a case and review of the literature. Oral Surg Oral Med Oral Pathol 1974;37:754–761.
10. Farzim I, Edalat M. Periodontosis with hyperkeratosis palmaris and plantaris: A case report. J Periodontol 1974;45:316–318.
11. Winkler JR, Grassi M, Murray PA. Clinical description and etiology of HIV-associated periodontal disease. In: Robertson PB, Greenspan JS (eds). Perspectives on Oral Manifestations of AIDS. Littleton, MA: PSG Publishing, 1988.
12. Webber RL, Ruttimann UE, Grondhal HG. X-ray image subtraction as a basis for assessment of periodontal changes. J Periodontal Res 1982;17:509–511.
13. Hausmann E, Christersson L, Dunford R, et al. Usefulness of subtraction radiography in the evaluation of periodontal therapy. J Periodontol 1985;56:4–7.
14. Braegger U, Pasquali L, Weber H, Kornman KS. Computer-assisted densitometric image analysis (CADIA) for the assessment of alveolar bone density change in furcations. J Clin Periodontol 1989;16:46–52.
15. Jeffcoat M. Radiographic methods for the detection of progressive alveolar bone loss. J Periodontol 1992;63(suppl):367–372.
16. Webber RL. Oral imaging as a diagnostic tool for assessing osseous changes. J Bone Miner Res 1993;8:S543–S548.
17. Jeffcoat MK, Lewis CE, Reddy MS, et al. Post-menopausal bone loss and its relationships to oral bone loss. Periodontol 2000 2000;23:94–102.

Supplemental Diagnostics for the Assessment of Periodontal Diseases

Gary C. Armitage
- Current Concepts of Periodontitis Progression
- Supplemental Diagnostic Tests
- Detection of Putative Bacterial Pathogens
- Host-Derived Products in Gingival Crevicular Fluid

Chester W. Douglass
- Interpretation of Diagnostic Tests in Clinical Practice
- Efficacy of Diagnostic Tests
- Threshold for Disease
- A Diagnostic Test Checklist

In the past two decades, there has been extensive interest in the development, testing, and refinement of diagnostic aids for early detection of the presence and progression of periodontitis. With traditional techniques, such as periodontal probing and inspection of conventional radiographs, it is relatively easy, even for the novice clinician, to detect the presence of moderate to severe periodontitis. The challenge is to detect the earliest changes associated with the progression of periodontitis. If one can detect the disease earlier, treatment becomes less complicated and frequently more effective.

Current Concepts of Periodontitis Progression

Periodontitis was once viewed as a single, plaque-induced, nonspecific infection that progressed at a slow, more or less constant rate. Almost every case of untreated gingivitis was believed to progress to chronic periodontitis. In the past, most individuals were believed to be equally susceptible to developing periodontitis.

It is now known that these concepts were overly simplistic and partially wrong. Based on extensive clinical research, it is clear that (1) not all cases of untreated gingivitis lead to periodontitis; (2) there are several forms of periodontitis, which progress at widely varying rates; (3) relatively specific qualitative changes in the subgingival flora are associated with disease progression; and (4) susceptibility to periodontal infections is highly variable and appears to be related to genetically determined specific host responses to periodontal pathogens. These newer views of the natural history of periodontal diseases have encouraged researchers to develop diagnostic aids for the identification of factors associated with the progression of periodontitis.

Supplemental Diagnostic Tests

Traditional methods for determining the progression of periodontitis assess the degree of damage that has occurred to the periodontal tissues over time. These techniques include the use of calibrated periodontal probes and radiographs. In recent years, automation and computer technology have been applied to the use of both periodontal probes and radiographs to improve sensitivity and ease of use. These technologies are discussed in chapters 17 and 18.

Supplemental diagnostic tests can be used to perform two basic tasks. The first is screening to separate patients with and without disease. The second is to detect sites or patients at high risk for progressive disease. This task is more demanding than the first. It is also more important, since the clinician can usually distinguish healthy tissue from diseased tissue based on customary clinical criteria.

The clinical value of fully validated diagnostic tests is considerable, because they are potentially useful in (1) identifying the presence of therapeutic targets (ie, periodontal pathogens), (2) monitoring the response to therapy, (3) identifying sites at high risk for progression, and (4) assisting the clinician in determining a patient-specific recall interval during the maintenance phase of periodontal therapy. Some supplemental diagnostic tests are currently available and others are under development. Most of them are designed to provide information presumably associated with progressing periodontal lesions.

Supplemental diagnostic tests fall into four general categories and can be used to detect the presence of putative pathogens, host-derived enzymes, tissue-breakdown products, or inflammatory mediators.

Detection of Putative Bacterial Pathogens

Although more than 300 different bacteria have been isolated from periodontal pockets, a relatively small subset has been implicated as playing a role in the etiology of periodontal infections.[1] At the 1996 World Workshop in Periodontics in which an evidence-based approach was used to come to conclusions, it was agreed that there are sufficient data to consider the following three microorganisms as etiologic agents for certain forms of periodontitis: *Actinobacillus actinomycetemcomitans, Porphyromonas gingivalis,* and *Bacteroides forsythus. A actinomycetemcomitans* is most often found in aggressive forms of periodontitis, whereas *P gingivalis* and *B forsythus* are found more frequently in chronic periodontitis.[2] In addition to these three bacteria, there is some evidence for an etiologic role for *Campylobacter rectus, Eubacterium nodatum, Fusobacterium nucleatum, Prevotella intermedia, Peptostreptococcus micros, Streptococcus intermedius, Treponema denticola,* and the spirochetes associated with necrotizing ulcerative gingivitis.[2] Finally, some initial data suggest that in certain patients *Eikenella corrodens,* enteric rods, *Pseudomonas, Selenomonas, Staphylococcus,* and yeasts may have an etiologic role.[2]

Since most of these microorganisms are part of the resident (normal) flora in many people without periodontitis, merely demonstrating their presence is insufficient to conclude that they are of etiologic importance in an individual patient.[3] Therefore, in making the decision to perform a microbial analysis of the patient's periodontal flora, the clinician must be reasonably certain that some information useful for the management of the patient's infection might be obtained. For example, compliant patients who have been treated for periodontitis and still have a clinically evident periodontal infection might be good candidates for microbial testing. Results of such testing may shed some light on the nature of the patient's periodontal infection and provide the clinician with some guidance on what type of antimicrobial intervention might be appropriate.

Several strategies have been developed to detect periodontal pathogens. They include culture, microscopic examination, nucleic acid analyses, detection of specific bacterial antigens, detection of specific bacterial enzymes, and molecular analysis of 16S ribosomal RNA (rRNA) genes of bacteria.

Cultural Analysis of Subgingival Flora

Cultural analysis involves properly collecting a subgingival plaque sample, placing it immediately in reduced transport fluid, and sending it to a licensed clinical laboratory that is set up to cultivate and identify oral anaerobes and other microorganisms present in the subgingival environment. Once received by the laboratory, the sample is dispersed, diluted, and then plated on selective and nonselective media. Putative pathogens are identified, and sensitivity to various antibiotics is determined. The clinician is then sent a laboratory report of the findings, which can be used as a guide in treating the periodontitis. This process is obviously too involved and costly for use with every patient, but it can be very important for a small subset of individuals who continue to experience disease progression despite excellent compliance and well-executed conventional therapy (eg, those with refractory chronic periodontitis). Microbial testing might also be appropriate for young patients with highly destructive forms of periodontitis or those with an unusual clinical presentation. In such patients, particularly if systemic antibiotic therapy is being planned as part of the treatment, cultural analysis of the flora is highly desirable.

In many cases, cultural analysis of the subgingival flora allows the clinician to select an antibiotic that has a beneficial effect on resolving the patient's periodontal infection. This, however, is not always the case. In some instances, cultural testing does not reveal any useful information on the nature of the infection (ie, no putative pathogens are detected). In other cases, *P gingivalis* and other pathogens may be found at low levels, but administration of the antibiotics based on the laboratory report has no discernible clinical effect. It should be remembered that even with microbiologic testing, clinicians cannot be absolutely certain that the bacteria cultured from a given periodontal pocket are the pathogens responsible for the patient's periodontal disease.[3] In addition, it should be emphasized that not all periodontal bacteria can be cultured. Indeed, it has been estimated that approximately 50% of the oral flora cannot be grown in the laboratory.[4]

Microscopic Examination of Subgingival Flora

In the 1970s and early 1980s, it became popular to examine the subgingival flora with phase-contrast or dark-field microscopes. Such analyses of the subgingival flora can only distinguish between motile and nonmotile bacteria and categorize them into general morphotypes (eg, cocci or rods). Determination of genus, species, and antibiotic susceptibilities is not possible in microscopic analysis.

Information obtained with microscopic analysis was believed by some to be useful in the diagnosis and monitoring of periodontal disease.[5] It is true that motile forms such as spirochetes increase dramatically during periodontitis,[6–10] but there is considerable doubt that this observation is of any value in monitoring periodontal disease.[3,11–13]

Nucleic Acid Probes

Nucleic acid probes can be used to identify complementary nucleic acid sequences in specific bacteria.[3] The probes use DNA, RNA, or synthetic oligonucleotide sequences that hybridize with nucleic acids of bacteria present in periodontal pockets. They can detect specific plaque microorganisms at levels as low as 10^2. One of the main advantages of nucleic acid probes is that obtaining plaque samples is uncomplicated and requires minimal chairtime. Plaque samples can be collected quickly by inserting a sterile paper point to the base of a given pocket. The paper point is then placed in an empty vial and mailed to a licensed commercial laboratory for analysis. No special transport or media are necessary since living bacteria are not required and the bacterial nucleic acid (eg, DNA) is largely stable. Most commercial laboratories routinely provide a report on the presence and approximate amounts of *P gingivalis, A actinomycetemcomitans, B forsythus, P intermedia, C rectus, E corrodens, F nucleatum,* and *T denticola.* In addition, a rapid (40-minute) chairside DNA probe assay for *B forsythus* and *P gingivalis* has been developed.[14]

Although nucleic acid probes can reliably detect putative periodontal pathogens, their usefulness in clinical situations has not been established.[3] The major problem with these assays is that they provide no information regarding the antibiotic susceptibilities of the detected pathogens. Currently the only way to obtain this information is by growing the bacteria in culture and then testing their sensitivity to a battery of antibiotics. Some licensed clinical laboratories use nucleic acid (primarily DNA) probes to supplement the findings of cultural analysis of the flora. In most situations, when periodontal pathogens are cultured from a plaque sample, they are also detected by DNA probe assays. However, in many instances plaque samples are negative for the pathogens when tested in culture but are positive when subjected to DNA probe assays. This is especially true when the pathogen is difficult to grow, such as is the case with *B forsythus.*

Detection of Antigens of Suspected Pathogens

Another strategy for the detection of subgingival pathogens is the rapid chairside detection of antigens specific to them. This approach uses monoclonal or polyclonal antibodies directed against antigens that are unique to a given bacterium. Of the two general systems that have reached the prototype stage, the first uses latex beads coated with antibody specific for *A actinomycetemcomitans, P gingivalis,* and *P intermedia.*[15] The antibody-coated beads are simply mixed with suspensions of subgingival plaque; if the target bacteria are present, the beads clump together, which allows visual evaluation. The second system uses monoclonal antibodies labeled with a fluorescent marker. Antigen-antibody complexes formed on addition of plaque suspensions can be read with a fluorimeter.[16] Neither of these chairside systems are commercially available, and it is unlikely that they will be marketed since their clinical utility is uncertain. The basic problem is that knowledge of the presence or absence of a few putative pathogens is usually of no particular value to clinicians in diagnostic or treatment-planning procedures.

Detection of Enzymatic Activity of Suspected Pathogens

A limited number of periodontal pathogens produce a trypsinlike enzyme capable of hydrolyzing β-naphthylamide derivatives, mainly N-alpha-benzoyl-DL-arginine-2-naphthylamide (BANA). BANA is colorless, but upon hydrolysis, β-naphthylamide is released and reacts with a variety of dyes to form colored products. The solid-phase test for BANA activity in plaque samples uses Evans black dye as the indicator.[17] It has been estimated that approximately 95% of the BANA hydrolysis by a subgingival plaque sample is from its combined content of *P gingivalis, T denticola,* and *B forsythus.*[18]

A BANA-hydrolysis chairside test (eg, PerioScan, Oral-B Laboratories) has been used in a number of epidemiological studies as a screening method for identifying people who harbor putative periodontal pathogens.[19–22] In these studies, plaques from approximately 64% of adult subjects[20] and 66% of the sites[21] examined were BANA positive. It has also been reported that approximately 56% of children and adolescents (ages 2 to 18 years) without periodontitis have BANA-positive dental plaques.[19] In this young population approximately 21% of sampled sites were BANA positive. Since a high percentage of patients and sites without periodontitis are carriers of putative periodontal pathogens as detected by the BANA hydrolysis test, there is no diagnostic significance to the mere presence or absence of BANA-positive organisms on an individual patient basis.

Evaluation of the BANA hydrolysis test as a risk factor for the progression of periodontitis has been examined in a large longitudinal epidemiologic study of older adults.[23] In this study, a positive BANA hydrolysis test was found to be a significant risk factor for periodontitis in white subjects, but not in black subjects. Therefore, the data suggest that the test might only be a valid method of risk assessment in some populations.

Based on the results of randomized clinical trials, one group of investigators has suggested that microbiologic testing for anaerobic bacteria, using either darkfield spirochete counts or BANA hydrolysis, is useful in deciding if an antibiotic (eg, metronidazole) that is bactericidal for obligate anaerobes should be administered.[24–27] Although these studies suggest that, compared to mechanical treatment alone, the use of metronidazole in conjunction with scaling and root planing (S/RP) has certain beneficial effects, such as reducing the need for periodontal surgery and tooth extraction,[26,27] it is less clear if the microbiologic testing was actually of any value in the antibiotic selection process. For example, in one of these double-blind studies only patients with BANA-positive sites were enrolled.[26] Presumably, if the BANA hydrolysis test is of value in identifying a therapeutic target (ie, the anaerobes *T denticola, P gingivalis,* and *B forsythus*), then metronidazole treatment should result in significant reductions in these putative pathogens compared to controls (S/RP + placebo). However, results from this 2-year study indicate that at all time periods, there were no significant differences between the metronidazole and control groups with regard to the subgingival content of the bacteria targeted by the BANA hydrolysis test (ie, *P gingivalis* and one member of the *Treponema* species).[26] In the control group, the diagnostic information provided by the BANA hydro-

lysis test was, in a sense, ignored since the subjects did not receive any antibiotics. Use or nonuse of the BANA hydrolysis test did not have a significant impact on the microbiologic targets of therapy.

In this same study statistically significant reductions in the darkfield spirochete counts (presumably including some BANA-negative treponemes) were observed in both the metronidazole and control groups 4 to 6 weeks after treatment.[26] For the scaling and root planing plus metronidazole group, the mean proportions ± standard deviations of spirochetes were 59 ± 18% at baseline versus 22 ± 17% 4 to 6 weeks posttreatment. For the control group, which received scaling and root planing plus placebo, the values were 60 ± 13% at baseline versus 35 ± 20% posttreatment. The spirochete counts 4 to 6 weeks after treatment were not significantly different between the metronidazole and control groups ($P = .06$). If a positive BANA hydrolysis test was the correct basis on which to select metronidazole as the antibiotic of choice (ie, because of an "anaerobic infection"), it would seem that a more powerful effect on the target flora would have been observed. Indeed, this result was unexpected since metronidazole should have had a more potent suppressive effect on the spirochete populations. One possible explanation for this result might be that subjects assigned to the metronidazole group did not take all of their medication, and this was evident when compliance was checked.[28]

It has been known for a long time that anaerobic bacteria are of probable etiologic importance in the development of chronic periodontitis.[1] However, bacteria that are not obligate anaerobes are also considered to be putative periodontal pathogens.[1] Nearly all patients with chronic periodontitis are heavily colonized by anaerobes. This does not mean, however, that anaerobic bacteria are the principal cause of all cases of chronic periodontitis. Proponents of the BANA hydrolysis test imply that a positive assay is synonymous with the presence of an "anaerobic infection" and therefore administration of metronidazole is justified.[24–27] However, the data do not unequivocally support this view.

Diagnostic tests for monitoring the results of periodontal treatment can be of considerable value at two different stages of therapy: *(1)* at the end of active therapy when the clinician is faced with the decision as to whether treatment is really completed (ie, therapeutic endpoint monitoring), and *(2)* at the maintenance phase of periodontal therapy when the clinician must decide if the initial therapeutic result has had long-term stability.[3] The BANA hydrolysis test has been proposed for both of these purposes.[29–33] Cross-sectional comparisons of BANA hydrolysis have been made using subgingival plaques from treated and untreated patients.[30–32] Not surprisingly in all of these studies, plaques from treated and maintained patients consistently gave lower percentages of BANA-positive reactions than did plaques from untreated patients. For example, in one of these studies only 7.5% (3 of 40) of the plaques from sites clinically judged as healthy or responsive to treatment were BANA positive, whereas 80.4% (37 of 46) of the diseased untreated sites gave positive reactions.[32] In addition, 60% (6 of 10) of the treated sites clinically judged to be unresponsive to therapy were BANA positive.[32] Although these data point to the possible usefulness of the BANA hydrolysis test in a clinical setting, results from cross-sectional studies cannot be used to establish the clinical utility of a diagnostic test for monitoring therapeutic outcomes. Longitudinal studies are needed for this purpose.

Use of the BANA hydrolysis test for purposes of therapeutic endpoint monitoring has been evaluated in two short-term studies in which the effects of scaling and root planing on BANA scores were determined.[34,35] In the first study, the effects of subgingival instrumentation on BANA scores in periodontitis patients was determined 3 months after scaling and root planing.[34] Sites with either gingivitis or periodontitis were monitored. For the gingivitis sites 64.3% (9 of 14) were BANA positive prior to treatment, and 28.6% (4 of 14) were positive 3 months after treatment. For the periodontitis sites 85.7% (12 of 14) were BANA positive prior to treatment, and 78.6% (11 of 14) were positive after treatment. The treatment-induced reductions in BANA reactions were not significantly different between the gingivitis and periodontitis sites ($P = .08$).[34] Obviously, the results of this study should be viewed with caution since only a small number of sites were monitored.

In the second study, sites in periodontitis patients were judged to be clinically "healthy" (absence of bleeding and color change; probing depth 3 mm or less) or "diseased" (presence of bleeding and color change; probing depth 5 mm or greater).[35] BANA hydrolysis scores were then taken, and the sites were treated with scaling and root planing. After 4 to 6 weeks the sites were again clinically evaluated and tested for BANA hydrolysis. Response to treatment was judged as "better," "no change," or "worse." An improvement or deterioration was recorded if a change in bleeding or color scores was noted and if there was a 2-mm or greater change in probing depth or clinical attachment level. Prior to treatment 83.3% (105 of 126) of the sites were BANA positive. Of the BANA-positive sites, 15.2% (16 of 105) were judged to be clinically healthy. Following treatment 60% of the sites were judged to have improved ("better" category), 36% exhibited no change, and 4% were worse. There was only a 52% agreement between clinical judgment of response to treatment and BANA scores. The authors concluded that the BANA hydrolysis test did not reliably reflect the clinically judged outcome following treatment.[35]

Based on available data, no firm conclusions can be drawn regarding the clinical usefulness of BANA hydrolysis as a stand-alone test for monitoring the results of periodontal therapy. The clinical utility of the test has never been longitudinally evaluated in a treated and well-maintained population over a prolonged period of time. For a time the test was available to clinicians in Europe and Canada, but questions about its value in day-to-day clinical practice never resulted in its widespread use.

Molecular Analysis of 16S Ribosomal RNA Genes of Bacteria

Most of our understanding of the oral flora comes from cultural studies in which clinical specimens are collected and then bacteria in the sample are grown on artificial media in the laboratory. Unfortunately, approximately 50% of the oral flora cannot be cultured, and therefore current knowledge of the flora is incomplete.[4] Indeed, knowledge of the microbial community is fragmentary at best. It has been estimated that greater than 99% of microorganisms observable in nature cannot be cultivated using standard techniques.[36] In the past two decades a quiet revolution in bacterial taxonomy and classification has been underway. Microbiologists have been using similarities and differences in well-conserved 16S rRNA gene sequences to determine the relation of one bacterium to another.[37] The method is culture-independent and therefore permits the detection of previously unknown microorganisms.[38]

Application of 16S rRNA gene technology to characterization of the oral flora is just beginning. In almost all cases where this method has been applied to the oral flora, unexpected microbial diversity has been found, including the discovery of new genera of bacteria.[39–47] For example, in one study a single plaque sample from a 9-mm periodontal pocket in a patient with severe periodontitis was analyzed using 16S rRNA technology.[40] If 98% or greater sequence similarities were used, 23 species of spirochetes were detected. If 92% or greater sequence similarities were used, there were 8 major groups (each containing multiple species) and only 2 of the groups contained named species (eg, *T denticola* and *T vincentii*). Other oral spirochetes such as *T pectinovorum* and *T socranskii* were not represented in any cluster.[40] Therefore, a large number of phylogenetically different spirochetes were isolated from a single pocket. Analysis of the subgingival flora using the 16S rRNA gene technology in a group of 15 patients who were either periodontally healthy or had a variety of periodontal infections revealed at least 57 different *Treponema* species.[47] Clearly, as this method is more widely applied to characterization of the periodontal flora in health and disease, our current view

Table 19-1 Host-Derived Components of GCF That Have Been Preliminarily Studied as Possible Markers for the Progression of Periodontitis*

Enzymes and inhibitors	Tissue-breakdown products	Inflammatory mediators

• Aspartate aminotransferase
• Alkaline phosphatase
• β-glucuronidase
• Elastase
• Elastase inhibitors
  —α_2-macroglobulin
  —α_1-proteinase inhibitor
• Cathepsins
  —cysteine proteinases (B, H, L)
  —serine proteinase (G)
• Trypsinlike enzymes
• Immunoglobulin-degrading enzymes
• Glycosidases
• Dipeptidyl peptidases
• Nonspecific neutral proteinases
• Collagenases
  —matrix metalloproteinase-1
  —matrix metalloproteinase-3
  —matrix metalloproteinase-8
• Gelatinases
  —matrix metalloproteinase-2
  —matrix metalloproteinase-9
• Stromyelysins
• Myeloperoxidases
• Lactate dehydrogenase
• Carboxypeptidase
• Creatinine kinase
	• Glycosaminoglycans
	  —hyaluronic acid
	  —chondroitin-4-sulfate
	  —chondroitin-6-sulfate
	  —dermatan sulfate
	• Hydroxyproline
	• Fibronectin fragments
	• Connective tissue proteins
	  —osteonectin
	  —osteocalcin
	  —type I collagen peptides
	• Keratin
	• Laminin
	• Calprotectin
	• Hemoglobin β-chain peptides
	• Pyridinoline crosslinks
		• Cytokines
		  —interleukin 1α
		  —interleukin 1β
		  —interleukin 1ra
		  —interleukin 6
		  —interleukin 8
		  —tumor necrosis factor α
		  —interferon α
		• Prostaglandin E$_2$
		• Acute-phase proteins
		  —lactoferrin
		  —transferrin
		  —α_2-macroglobulin
		  —α_1-proteinase inhibitor
		  —C-reactive protein
		• Autoantibodies
		  —anticollagen antibody
		  —antidesmosomal antibody
		• Antibacterial antibodies
		  —immunoglobulin G$_1$ to G$_4$
		  —immunoglobulin M
		  —immunoglobulin A
		  —secretory immunoglobulin A
		• Plasminogen activator (PA)
		• PA inhibitor-2
		• Substance P
		• Neurokinin A

*For review, see Armitage.[3]

of the nature of the disease-producing periodontal flora will change.

First-generation DNA microarray systems are already in widespread use in research laboratories throughout the world. Advanced semiautomated DNA microarray systems that are under development will eventually allow clinicians to completely characterize the microbial flora from a single site or pocket. In addition, as the technology is developed further it should be possible to determine the presence of plasmids in the resident flora. This information could potentially be useful in determining the sensitivity of the flora to antibiotics without first culturing the bacteria. Although these statements are far-reaching and speculative, in the next few decades it is likely that this technology will have a significant impact on the clinical management of periodontal infections.

Host-Derived Products in Gingival Crevicular Fluid

An array of enzymes, tissue-breakdown products, and inflammatory mediators are released from host cells and tissues during the development and progression of periodontal infections. Some of these substances have been suggested as possible markers for the detection of progressing periodontal lesions. A large number of studies of gingival crevicular fluid (GCF) have been conducted with the general goal of devising rapid chairside assays for markers of disease progression. More than 50 components of GCF have been preliminarily evaluated for this purpose (Table 19-1). The strategy used by most investigators is to first establish in cross-sectional studies that a potential marker is present in the GCF from periodontitis sites and is absent or at low levels at healthy and gingivitis sites. If a marker can be shown to be strongly related to the severity of periodontitis, the next step is to longitudinally demonstrate that it accurately identifies sites at a high risk of progressing.

For a marker to be clinically useful it must be able to distinguish between sites with high and low risks of progression. This is a very difficult task since both nonprogressing and progressing sites are frequently inflamed, and the vast majority of the potential markers examined so far are strongly associated with periodontal inflammation. A marker may be a reliable indicator of the severity of inflammation, but it might be unable to distinguish sites with stable gingivitis from those with gingivitis on the verge of progressing to periodontitis. It is equally difficult for a marker to distinguish between progressing and nonprogressing sites with periodontitis. Finally, for a marker to have the maximum utility in clinical practice, it should be able to identify progressing sites in patients who have been treated and are in the maintenance phase of periodontal care. Therefore, longitudinal studies of treated and maintained patients are needed to fully validate any GCF assays designed to detect sites at high risk for future attachment loss.

Host-Derived Enzymes

Since many enzyme assays depend on colorimetric reactions, they are relatively easy to adapt to rapid chairside tests. For this reason, a great deal of work has been done on developing tests for enzymes in GCF that may be related to the progression of periodontitis. Among the host-derived enzymes present in GCF that have received the most attention are aspartate aminotransferase (AST),[3,48–55] matrix metalloproteinases (MMPs)[3,56–63] and related neutral proteases,[3,35,64–66] β-glucuronidase,[3,66–70] elastase,[3,61,71–75] alkaline phosphatase,[3,76,77] dipeptidyl peptidases,[3,79–81] and cathepsins.[3,82–85] Some of these enzymes are released from dead and dying cells of the periodontium; some come from polymorphonuclear neutrophils (PMNs); and others are produced by inflammatory, epithelial, and connective tissue cells at affected sites.[3]

Aspartate Aminotransferase

Aspartate aminotransferase is released by dead and dying host cells. In medicine, it is a useful marker for the cell death that occurs in cardiac muscle after a myocardial infarction or in the liver during hepatic disease. In fact, it is released from the dead cells of virtually all tissues of the body. Results from several longitudinal studies of patients with progressive periodontitis, in which increased clinical attachment loss was used as the criterion for progression,

suggest that AST levels in GCF might serve as a marker for disease progression on a site-by-site basis.[48–52] A rapid chairside test for the enzyme in GCF has been developed.[50] Since AST is also elevated at sites with gingivitis and nonprogressing periodontitis, it remains to be established if its levels in GCF can help distinguish between inflamed sites that are breaking down and those that are not.[3] The GCF assay for AST was marketed under the brand name of PocketWatch (Steri-Oss).

Matrix Metalloproteinases

Matrix metalloproteinases are a family of collagenases produced by a wide variety of cells such as neutrophils, macrophages, fibroblasts, keratinocytes, and osteoclasts. They characteristically function best at neutral pH and contain a Zn^{++} binding site within the catalytic domain of the molecule. There are small differences in the molecular forms of MMPs depending on their cellular source (eg, MMP-1 is produced by fibroblasts and epithelial cells; MMP-8 primarily comes from neutrophils). Gelatinases MMP-2 and MMP-9 are closely related enzymes that degrade similar collagen substrates.[3] In a 12-month longitudinal study of a treated, but not maintained, population of periodontitis patients, progressing sites had elevated GCF levels of active collagenase compared to nonprogressing sites.[58] In another study, when full-mouth GCF gelatinase levels were longitudinally monitored over a 2-year period using a mouthrinsing technique, samples from patients with recurrent periodontitis had significantly higher levels of neutrophil-derived gelatinase (MMP-9) than successfully treated patients.[57] The mouthrinsing technique to obtain clinical samples has also been applied to a population of stable (nonprogressing/maintained) periodontitis patients and untreated individuals with severe periodontitis.[61] In this study, levels of neutrophil-derived collagenase (MMP-8) were approximately 18 times higher in mouthrinse samples from severe periodontitis patients than in those obtained from stable periodontitis patients. A chairside immunofluorometric test for GCF levels of MMP-8 on a site-specific basis has been developed and has undergone preliminary clinical testing.[62]

Polymorphonuclear Neutrophilic Leukocytes

Polymorphonuclear neutrophilic leukocytes are prominent inflammatory cells found in GCF from sites with gingivitis or periodontitis. They are the first line of defense against bacteria that colonize periodontal pockets. PMNs release a wide range of lysosomal enzymes when challenged by bacteria. The logic behind the idea that some of these enzymes might serve as markers for the progression of periodontitis is simple. When periodontitis progresses, subgingival bacteria overwhelm local host defenses (including PMNs), and lysosomal enzymes from dead neutrophils are released into the GCF in abundance. A rapid (less than 15 minutes) chairside test for some of these lysosomal enzymes (ie, nonspecific neutral proteinases) has been developed (Periocheck, ACTech).[64–66] These proteinases have been shown to be elevated in GCF from sites with advanced periodontitis.[65] However, this test has not been longitudinally evaluated to determine if it can identify sites that are at an increased risk for progression.

Preliminary work from two longitudinal studies has shown that GCF levels of another lysosomal enzyme, β-glucuronidase, were elevated in patients in whom increased clinical attachment loss was detected over 6- and 12-month observation periods.[67–69] Lower levels of the enzyme were found in patients with nonprogressing disease. However, since the data were analyzed on a full-mouth or subject basis, it is unclear if the GCF content of β-glucuronidase would have any predictive value for the identification of sites at high risk of losing additional attachment. It remains to be determined if a rapid chairside GCF test for β-glucuronidase can be developed into a useful method for detecting the progression of periodontitis on a site-by-site basis.

Elastase

Elastase is a prominent neutral proteinase released into GCF by PMNs. Data from multiple cross-sectional studies indicate that GCF samples taken from sites with periodontitis have significantly higher total elastase activity than GCF from healthy or gingivitis sites.[3] A prototype of a chairside test for GCF elastase was developed and tested in two 6-month longitudinal studies of patients with untreated periodontitis.[72,73] In both studies, the progression of periodontitis was assessed by subtraction radiography (see chapter 18). Although elastase levels were somewhat predictive of disease progression, a false-positive result (ie, a positive test at nonprogressing sites) occurred approximately 50% of the time. This finding raises serious questions about the clinical usefulness of GCF elastase levels in identifying sites at high risk of progressing.

Alkaline Phosphatase

Alkaline phosphatase is an enzyme produced by many cells of the periodontium, including osteoblasts, fibroblasts, and neutrophils.[3] A new ultrasensitive assay for the enzyme has made it possible to accurately determine its levels in small amounts of GCF.[77,78] In a 3-month longitudinal study of treated periodontitis patients, the diagnostic accuracy for GCF alkaline phosphatase (at a threshold of 1,300 μIU/30 s) as a predictor of future attachment loss was 77% with a 77% positive predictive value and a 76% negative predictive value.[78] These results are promising, but longer-term longitudinal studies in a treated and maintained population are needed.

Dipeptidyl Peptidases

Dipeptidyl peptidases (DPPs) are a group of proteinases produced by a variety of host cells and are found in serum.[79] Bacterial dipeptidyl peptidases differ from the host-derived enzymes in that the bacterial forms are more sensitive to inactivation by heat.[80] However, bacterial and host DPPs have similar substrates.[79,80] In a 2-year longitudinal study of treated and maintained chronic periodontitis patients, a strong relationship was found between GCF levels of host DPPs (DPP II and DPP IV) and the progression of periodontitis.[79] In a similar study, an even stronger relationship was found between disease progression and bacterial DPPs on a site-specific basis.[81] This relationship might be related to the fact that *P gingivalis*, a known periodontal pathogen, is a major source of bacterial DPPs.[80] The available data suggest that development of a cost-effective and rapid chairside test for bacterial DPPs in GCF is justified.

Cathepsins

Cathepsins B, H, and L are cysteine proteinases that play an important role in intracellular protein degradation.[3] In a cross-sectional study of patients with chronic periodontitis, highly significant correlations were found between GCF cathepsin B/L activity and gingival bleeding, probing depth, and clinical attachment loss.[82] In addition, significant decreases in cathepsin B/L activity have been noted after scaling and root planing.[83,84] In a 2-year longitudinal study of treated and maintained chronic periodontitis patients, a strong relationship was found between GCF levels of host cathepsin B and the progression of periodontitis.[85] A rapid chairside test for cathepsin B should be developed so that its utility in clinical practice can be fully evaluated.

Tissue-Breakdown Products

One of the major features of periodontitis is the destruction of connective tissue and bone. Abundant amounts of breakdown products from these tissues are released during the disease. It would therefore seem logical that the GCF levels of these products would increase during the progression of periodontitis. Among the tissue components and breakdown products that have been preliminarily examined as possible markers for progressing periodontitis are glycosaminoglycans,[3,86–92] hydroxyproline,[3,93] fibronectin fragments,[3] various connective tissue proteins,[3] keratin,[3] laminin,[94] calprotectin,[95–97] hemoglobin β-chain oligopeptides,[98] and pyridinoline crosslinks.[99]

Glycosaminoglycans

Glycosaminoglycans (GAGs) are polysaccharides linked to protein cores of proteoglycans and are important components of the ground substance of connective tissues. Some of the GAGs that are released into the surrounding environment during connective tissue destruction include hyaluronic acid, chondroitin-4-sulfate, and chondroitin-6-sulfate. All of them can be found in GCF at inflamed sites.[3] As a potential marker for the progression of periodontitis, chondroitin-4-sulfate (C-4-S) is perhaps the most interesting since it makes up approximately 94% of the GAG content of bone.[86] Therefore, it has been suggested that the appearance of large amounts of C-4-S in GCF might be a marker for ongoing destruction of alveolar bone.[90,91] Indeed, there is a surge in the GCF content of C-4-S during the active phase of orthodontic tooth movement when bone resorption is at its peak.[88,89] GCF from sites that responded poorly to scaling and root planing have been reported to contain elevated levels of C-4-S.[90] In addition, findings from a pilot study of a small group of progressing periodontitis sites indicated that sulfated GAGs are elevated compared with nonprogressing control sites.[91] A simple assay for C-4-S suitable for chairside testing has not yet been developed, but these preliminary results suggest that some effort should be made to develop one since it appears to be a promising marker for periodontal bone destruction.

Hydroxyproline

Hydroxyproline, an amino acid, is found in high levels in collagen. Therefore, its content in GCF has been preliminarily evaluated as a possible marker for connective tissue destruction.[3] Unfortunately, data from a cross-sectional study indicate that the hydroxyproline content of GCF cannot distinguish between sites with gingivitis or periodontitis.[93] Other products released on the destruction of periodontal connective tissue and bone such as collagen telopeptides,[3] osteocalcin,[3] osteonectin,[3] and laminin,[94] have only been examined in preliminary studies. Of particular interest for future investigations is the pyridinoline cross-linked carboxyterminal telopeptide of type I collagen, which is bone-specific.[99]

Calprotectin

Calprotectin is a cytoplasmic calcium-binding protein of many cells, including keratinocytes, monocytes, macrophages, and neutrophils.[95] It makes up 50% to 60% of the total cytoplasmic protein of neutrophils. Although it is normally present in serum, saliva, and some other body fluids, it is released in abundance at sites of inflammation where lysis of cells is a common event. Because of this, it is considered a possible systemic marker of inflammatory diseases. Results from several studies have shown that the levels of calprotectin in GCF are positively correlated with biochemical markers of periodontal inflammation including interleukin 1β (IL-1β),[96] prostaglandin E$_2$ (PGE$_2$),[96] as-

partate aminotransferase,[97] and collagenase.[97] There are, however, no studies directly linking GCF levels of calprotectin with an increased risk of the progression of periodontitis.

Inflammatory Mediators

Numerous inflammatory mediators are produced by tissues with gingivitis or periodontitis. Some of these mediators play a central role in the destructive processes observed in periodontitis, which has led some investigators to examine the possibility that certain inflammatory mediators may be used as markers for progressive lesions.[3] Inflammatory products and mediators that have received the most attention include prostaglandin E$_2$,[3,100–105] proinflammatory cytokines,[3,105–110] acute-phase proteins,[3,111] immunoglobulin (Ig) types and subclasses,[106,112–115] and various nonspecific indicators or modifiers of the inflammatory response.[116–120]

Prostaglandin E$_2$

Prostaglandin E$_2$ is a metabolite of arachidonic acid that can increase vascular permeability and induce bone resorption. GCF from sites with periodontitis have elevated levels of PGE$_2$ compared with crevicular fluids collected from healthy or gingivitis sites.[100] However, there is extensive variability in GCF levels of PGE$_2$ obtained from sites with similar clinical characteristics.[101,102] In untreated periodontitis patients, GCF levels of PGE$_2$ do not appear to be able to distinguish between progressing and nonprogressing sites.[103] In addition, reductions in PGE$_2$ levels have been reported to occur in some patients after nonsurgical therapy,[104] but no changes have been detected up to 3 months after periodontal surgery.[102,105] Collectively, these findings cast doubt on the usefulness of PGE$_2$ as a marker for detecting sites at an increased risk for disease progression.

Proinflammatory Cytokines

Proinflammatory cytokines that have been preliminarily investigated as possible markers for the progression of periodontitis include interleukin 1α (IL-1α),[3,106] IL-1β,[3,105,107–108] interleukin 1 receptor antagonist (IL-1ra),[109] interleukin 6 (IL-6),[3] interleukin 8 (IL-8),[3,106,110] tumor necrosis factor α (TNF-α),[3] and interferon α (IFN-α).[106] GCF levels of most of these cytokines nonspecifically increase at sites of gingival inflammation irrespective of whether the sites have gingivitis or periodontitis. Therefore, their utility as diagnostic markers is questionable. However, IL-1β, which has been associated with bone resorption, has been reported to be elevated at progressing sites, compared with nonprogressing sites, in patients with refractory chronic periodontitis.[106]

Acute-Phase Proteins

Acute-phase proteins or reactants are a group of products whose levels increase in serum and tissue fluids during episodes of acute inflammation and tissue destruction.[3] Among the acute-phase proteins in GCF that have been studied as possible markers for the progression of periodontitis are α_2-macroglobulin, α_1-proteinase inhibitor, C-reactive protein, transferrin, and lactoferrin.[3] Although acute-phase proteins play important roles in combating bacterial infections, their levels in GCF do not appear to be able to distinguish between sites with gingivitis and those with periodontitis.[3] In addition, no difference in their levels has been detected in GCF from nonprogressing and progressing sites in treated periodontitis patients on a periodontal maintenance therapy program.[111]

Other Indicators

Data from a large number of studies indicate that extensive variation exists on a site and patient basis with regard to local and systemic antibody production against putative periodontal pathogens.[3] GCF contains locally produced specific antibody types and subclasses that have been suggested as potential markers for the progression of periodontitis.[3,112–115] It has been reported that an elevation of GCF IgA from treated but not maintained[70,114] and treated/maintained[115] periodontitis patients lowers the risk of disease progression, suggesting that this immunoglobulin has a "protective" role. If confirmed, this observation has the potential to be adapted into a risk assessment test for the progression of periodontitis.

Although some GCF-based tests have the potential to be clinically useful, much more work has to be done to fully validate their value in clinical situations. In addition, no GCF-based tests have been approved by the Food and Drug Administration for use in clinical practice as tests for the progression of periodontitis. Currently, there are no completely validated diagnostic or prognostic tests that can help identify progressing cases of periodontitis other than longitudinal assessments of clinical attachment levels as measured with calibrated periodontal probes or documentation of additional bone loss as determined with radiographs. Before purchasing any new tests or devices, it is important to make sure that data from well-controlled longitudinal studies justify their use in clinical practice.

Interpretation of Diagnostic Tests in Clinical Practice

To efficiently use diagnostic tests, dental care providers need to use a set of decision rules known collectively as *clinical decision analysis*.[121] These rules consist of a series of comparison methods that can be used by general practitioners, periodontists, and dental hygienists for weighing the benefits and disadvantages of using alternative periodontal diagnostic tests. As discussed throughout this text, scientific advances are leading to the development of a wide variety of specific diagnostic tests, which are providing practitioners with the ability to detect periodontal disease activity where previously only crude measurement methods were available. Decision analysis concepts, combined with clinical selection criteria as outlined in chapters 17, 18, and 20, can then be used to differentiate patients who are more likely to benefit from certain diagnostic tests from patients who would probably not benefit.

The crucial question is, Are the diagnostic decisions made by practitioners more accurate when they are based on a new diagnostic test for periodontal disease than when they are based on clinical measurement methods alone? Since periodontal disease is primarily a chronic condition, it is the risk of disease progression into subsequent stages of more serious tissue destruction that the practitioner is trying to predict more accurately. If a new biologically based test can identify patients at high risk for further attachment loss, the efficacy of the test warrants its use.

Efficacy of Diagnostic Tests

There are a few principal concepts that must be understood by practitioners when they use diagnostic tests. The most basic of these concepts are *(1)* the gold standard, *(2)* accuracy, *(3)* sensitivity, *(4)* specificity, *(5)* positive predictive value, and *(6)* negative predictive value.

The most difficult concept to grasp is that of the gold standard, which is supposed to be the truth about whether disease is present or absent. A gold standard measure is obtained from an independent definitive diagnosis of disease presence or absence, which is usually provided by histopathological examination of the tissues. Clearly, a true gold standard measure is impractical when evaluating many diagnostic tests, because biopsies of the periodontal attachment apparatus cannot usually be readily obtained without sacrificing the tooth. It is this gold standard (or truth about whether periodontal disease is present or absent) against which a new diagnostic test is evaluated. This comparison between a new test and the gold standard will determine if the test can accurately differentiate patients who have periodontal disease from those who do not. However, in situations where the gold standard is perhaps not quite so gold, the best available independent assessment is made. After all, truth is only a matter of degree or acceptability[122]; or to put it another way, Newhauser and Yin say the gold standard is "the best there is."[123]

Table 19-2 Decision Matrix

Test result	Gold standard		
	Disease present (D+)	Disease absent (D–)	Total
Positive (T+)	TP	FP	TP + FP
Negative (T–)	FN	TN	FN + TN
Total	TP + FN	FP + TN	

TP = true positive; FP = false positive; FN = false negative; TN = true negative.

A diagnostic test can still be valuable when there is reason to doubt the gold standard against which it was tested, if test results consistently converge with other measures of the pathological condition under question. In situations where there are already-accepted diagnostic tests as previously outlined, a new diagnostic test could improve the diagnostic process by being less costly, more effective, less risky, or easier to conduct. Hence it is worth the effort to understand the efficacy of a particular diagnostic test and to be familiar with the gold standard against which it was compared.

The basic method used to compare a diagnostic test with the gold standard is the decision matrix shown in Table 19-2. Here, test results (test positive and test negative) in the left-hand column are cross-tabulated with the independent gold standard, which tells whether disease is truly present or absent. This 2 × 2 comparison shows four kinds of test results. Positive test results on patients with disease are true-positive (TP) results; positive test results on patients without disease are false-positive (FP) results; negative test results on patients with disease are false-negative (FN) results; and negative test results on patients without disease are true-negative (TN) results. Ideally, all tests would produce either true-positive or true-negative results. This is called the *accuracy* of a test and is calculated as TP + TN/all tests conducted, ie, the proportion or percentage of times that the test gives accurate results. With these definitions, the four basic measurements of diagnostic efficacy can be calculated. Sensitivity and specificity characterize the effectiveness of a test in identifying patients who do (sensitivity) and patients who do not (specificity) have disease. These two measurements are calculated vertically in Table 19-2.

Sensitivity (the true-positive ratio) is calculated as TP/TP + FN. This measurement indicates the proportion of patients with periodontal disease that has been correctly identified with the test results. Sensitivity signifies the probability of obtaining a positive test result given that the patient, in fact, has periodontal disease; hence, sensitivity represents the proportion or percentage of times that the test results help correctly identify patients with disease.

Specificity (the true-negative ratio) is calculated as TN/FP + TN. This measurement indicates the proportion of patients who do not have periodontal disease that has been correctly identified with the test results. Specificity signifies the probability of obtaining a negative test result given that the patient, in fact, does not have periodontal disease. Hence, specificity represents the proportion or percentage of times that the test results help correctly identify patients who do not have disease.

In dental practice settings, practitioners are faced with one patient at a time, and they do not know a priori whether the patient has disease; they only know whether diagnostic test results are positive or negative. They do not know for sure if the test results are true positive or true negative. The chance of false-positive and false-negative results must be considered. Hence, the question is, What percentage of positive test results are true-positive results versus false-positive results; or conversely, what percentage of negative test results are true-negative versus false-negative results? To answer these questions, return to Table 19-2; consider the decision matrix in a horizontal dimension, and calculate two types of predictive values.

Positive predictive value is calculated as TP/TP + FP, which indicates the proportion or percentage of true-positive results of all positive results. That is, what percentage of all positive test results are, in fact, true-positive results according to the gold standard? In other words, when the test result is positive, what is the probability that the patient (or site) really has disease?

Negative predictive value is calculated as TN/FN + TN, which indicates the number of true-negative test results of all negative test results. That is, what percent of all negative test results are, in fact, true-negative test results according to the gold standard?

It is important to understand that both the positive predictive value and the negative predictive value are affected by disease prevalence in the population being tested. If the prevalence of the disease is high, there will be many true-positive test results, and if the specificity of the test is good, there will be relatively few false-positive results. Hence, a large number of true-positive test results and few false-positive test results yield a high positive predictive value. That is, the vast majority of positive test results will be correct.

However, if the prevalence of disease is low, there will surely be fewer true-positive test results. But since no test is perfect, there will also be at least a few false-positive results. The actual number of false-positive results could be almost as many as the few true-positive results. Hence, the proportion or percentage of true-positive results out of all positive (TP + FP) test results might not be high. Such is the

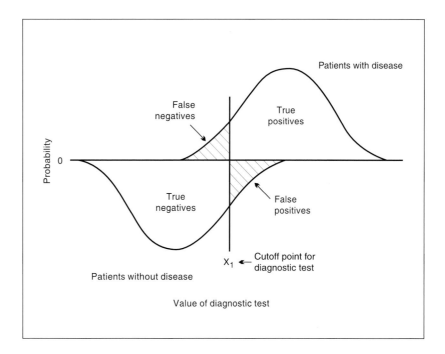

Fig 19-1 Relationship between sensitivity and specificity.

case for screening for HIV. With such a low disease prevalence within the population, a diagnostic test would have to be nearly perfect to avoid a substantial percentage of false-positive results for HIV.

Most new diagnostic tests are evaluated in specific populations to obtain sufficient positive and negative test results to adequately evaluate them. The sensitivity and specificity results from such evaluations are valuable, because these measurements of diagnostic test efficacy are not affected by variations in the prevalence of the disease. However, the positive and negative predictive values of a diagnostic test will vary across most dental practice patient populations because the proportion of patients with moderate or severe periodontal disease (ie, the prevalence of periodontal disease) varies across different types of dental practices.

Threshold for Disease

When using a diagnostic test as part of a patient examination, at what stage of progression does one actually label the process being observed as periodontal disease? Unfortunately, in many patients there is no clear demarcation between disease and no disease. Periodontal disease presents throughout a range from incipient to severe. Hence it may be reasonable for practitioners to consider more than one threshold of disease at which the test result is determined to be positive to get a sense of the magnitude of risk taken when making this decision one way or the other.

Figure 19-1 shows the distribution of patients without active periodontal disease below the horizontal line (or x-axis) and patients with active periodontal disease above the line. Both show a normal (bell-shaped) distribution, which may not be the case in a particular practitioner's office. The diagnostic test results lie on a continuum (the horizontal line) of test values representing increasing levels of risk factors or risk indicators,[124] such as periodontal pathogens or enzyme activity, from low on the left to high on the right. The two curves usually overlap as shown. Thus, for any diagnostic cutoff point that identifies most of the diseased cases correctly, some normal cases will be falsely identified as positive (false-positive results). Similarly, some of the patients who do have periodontal disease will be falsely identified as negative (false-negative results). Which is worse: not treating a patient who has periodontal disease because of a false-negative test result, or treating a patient who does not have periodontal disease because of a false-positive test result?

Figure 19-1 demonstrates that there is a trade-off between sensitivity, which includes false-negative results, and specificity, which includes false-positive results. The practitioner must know the cutoff point at which the result becomes positive and then think about which way to lean for each patient. A false-positive result may be the situation to avoid, particularly if the recommended treatment for a particular patient is an invasive surgical procedure. Hence, the practitioner will want to be conservative in interpreting positive test results. With such dramatic nonreversible therapy, caution should be taken to have no false-positive results; ie, the clinician should correctly identify

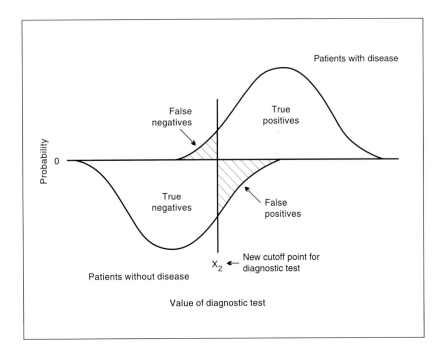

Fig 19-2 Relationship between sensitivity and specificity, with a lower cutoff point for the diagnostic test than shown in Fig 19-1.

those who do not have severe disease and so choose a higher cutoff point that yields high specificity and few, if any, false-positive results.

Conversely, when missing the disease is considered the worst outcome, the cutoff point or clinician's judgment should err on the side of high sensitivity (fewer false-negative results). The diagnostic cutoff point (identified as x_2) would be shifted to the left (Fig 19-2). Choosing a lower cutoff value will result in more true-positive and fewer false-negative results, as desired, but there will also be more false-positive results because specificity is lowered as sensitivity is raised. In contrast, if the test itself is risky or expensive and a false-negative could be tolerated at the disease level being considered, then the diagnostic cutoff should be shifted to the right, where test results will be more specific, so that false-positive results are reduced while false-negative results increase. The treating clinician should go through this thought process every time a diagnostic test is used. Diagnostic testing should be considered an aid to the diagnostic process rather than a device or procedure that provides the diagnosis. The practitioner must provide the diagnosis using all the available data.

The value of a particular diagnostic test may differ dramatically between patients. The practitioner must consider the added value of the test over existing diagnostic information for a particular patient, along with the specific preferences of that patient.[125] Information costs money and time, so capturing additional information is of value only if it changes what the doctor or patient knows or would do. For example, in a patient with a history of periodontitis and a family and medical history suggestive of

an increased risk of disease progression, an additional diagnostic test may provide little added value, because the probability of future disease is so high already. Likewise, some patients may have such strong feelings about treatment outcomes, costs, and side effects that they will only choose among a limited set of treatment options. A diagnostic test that suggests a therapy that is generally unacceptable to a particular patient will be of low practical value to that patient.

A Diagnostic Test Checklist

Before adopting a test for routine clinical practice, the following six questions need to be answered:

1. Does the scientific theory or biologic logic of the test fit with the current body of knowledge about diagnosing periodontal disease?
2. Has the technical merit of the test been evaluated and compared with the technical merit of other tests?
3. Has the efficacy of the test been evaluated in terms of sensitivity, specificity, and positive and negative predictive values?
4. Has the effect of the test on a practitioner's diagnostic and treatment decisions been evaluated?
5. Has the influence of the test on oral health outcomes been assessed?
6. Has the cost-effectiveness of the test been evaluated? Is the added expense justified by increased effectiveness or by avoiding other expenses?

To better understand and effectively use diagnostic tests, clinicians must become familiar with, and comfortable in using, clinical decision analysis concepts. Mastery of these basic concepts[126] will lead to the provision of clinical services that are based on scientific principles, thus improving patient care. Diagnostic tests are intended to increase the probability of correct diagnoses, but they are not substitutes for the practitioner's judgment. Diagnostic tests provide data that must be weighed along with the clinician's assessment of the patient's medical and dental history and clinical examination. While not a substitute for the clinician's judgment, diagnostic tests can be very useful if the six questions previously listed can be answered, giving the clinician a basis for knowledgeable interpretation of test results.

References

1. Haffajee AD, Socransky SS. Microbial etiological agents of destructive periodontal diseases. Periodontol 2000 1994;5:78–111.
2. Consensus Report. Periodontal diseases: Pathogenesis and microbial factors. Ann Periodontol 1996;1:927–930.
3. Armitage GC. Periodontal diseases: Diagnosis. Ann Periodontol 1996;1:37–215.
4. Wilson MJ, Weightman AJ, Wade WG. Applications of molecular ecology in the characterisation of uncultured microorganisms associated with human disease. Rev Med Microbiol 1997;8:91–101.
5. Keyes PH, Rams TE. A rationale for management of periodontal diseases: Rapid identification of microbial "therapeutic targets" with phase-contrast microscopy. J Am Dent Assoc 1983;106:803–812.
6. Listgarten MA, Helldén L. Relative distribution of bacteria at clinically healthy and periodontally diseased sites in humans. J Clin Periodontol 1978;5:115–132.
7. Armitage GC, Dickinson WR, Jenderseck RS, et al. Relationship between the percentage of subgingival spirochetes and the severity of periodontal disease. J Periodontol 1982;53:550–556.
8. Savitt ED, Socransky SS. Distribution of certain subgingival microbial species in selected periodontal conditions. J Periodontal Res 1984;19:111–123.
9. Omar AA, Newman HN, Bulman J, Osborn J. Associations between subgingival plaque bacterial morphotypes and clinical indices? J Clin Periodontol 1991;18:555–566.
10. Ojima M, Tamagawa H, Nagata H, et al. Relation of motility of subgingival microflora as a clinical parameter to periodontal status in human subjects. J Clin Periodontol 2000;27:405–410.
11. Greenstein G, Polson A. Microscopic monitoring of pathogens associated with periodontal diseases. A review. J Periodontol 1985;56:740–747.
12. Listgarten MA, Schifter CC, Sullivan P, et al. Failure of a microbial assay to reliably predict disease recurrence in a treated periodontitis population receiving regularly scheduled prophylaxes. J Clin Periodontol 1986;13:768–773.
13. Lembariti BS, Mikx FHM, van Palenstein Helderman WH. Microscopic spirochete counts in untreated subjects with and without periodontal tissue destruction. J Clin Periodontol 1995;22:235–239.
14. Tanner ACR, Maiden MFJ, Zambon JJ, et al. Rapid chair-side DNA probe assay of Bacteroides forsythus and Porphyromonas gingivalis. J Periodontal Res 1998;33:105–117.
15. Nisengard RJ, Mikulski L, McDuffie D, Bronson P. Development of a rapid latex agglutination test for periodontal pathogens. J Periodontol 1992;63:611–617.
16. Wolff LF, Anderson L, Sandberg GP, et al. Bacterial concentration fluorescence immunoassay (BCFIA) for the detection of periodontopathogens in plaque. J Periodontol 1992;63:1093–1101.
17. Loesche WJ, Bretz WA, Lopatin D, et al. Multi-center clinical evaluation of a chairside method for detecting certain periodontopathic bacteria in periodontal disease. J Periodontol 1990;61:189–196.
18. Loesche WJ, Lopatin DE, Giordano J, et al. Comparison of the benzoyl-DL-arginine-naphthylamide (BANA) test, DNA probes, and immunological reagents for ability to detect anaerobic periodontal infections due to Porphyromonas gingivalis, Treponema denticola, and Bacteroides forsythus. J Clin Microbiol 1992;30:427–433.
19. Watson M-R, Lopatin DE, Bretz WA, et al. Detection of two anaerobic periodontopathogens in children by means of the BANA and ELISA assays. J Dent Res 1991;70:1052–1056.
20. Drake CW, Hunt RJ, Beck JD, Zambon JJ. The distribution and interrelationship of Actinobacillus actinomycetemcomitans, Porphyromonas gingivalis, Prevotella intermedia, and BANA scores among older adults. J Periodontol 1993;64:89–94.
21. Bretz WA, Eklund SA, Radicchi R, et al. The use of a rapid enzymatic assay in the field for the detection of infections associated with adult periodontitis. J Public Health Dent 1993;53:235–240.
22. Watson MR, Bretz WA, Loesche WJ. Presence of Treponema denticola and Porphyromonas gingivalis in children correlated with periodontal disease of their parents. J Dent Res 1994;73:1636–1640.
23. Beck JD. Methods of assessing risk for periodontitis and developing multifactorial models. J Periodontol 1994;65:468–478.
24. Loesche WJ, Syed SA, Morrison EC, et al. Metronidazole in periodontitis. I. Clinical and bacteriological results after 15 to 30 weeks. J Periodontol 1984;55:325–335.
25. Loesche WJ, Schmidt E, Smith BA, et al. Effects of metronidazole on periodontal treatment needs. J Periodontol 1991;62:247–257.
26. Loesche WJ, Giordano JR, Hujoel P, et al. Metronidazole in periodontitis: Reduced need for surgery. J Clin Periodontol 1992;19:103–112.
27. Loesche WJ, Giordano J, Soehren S, et al. Nonsurgical treatment of patients with periodontal disease. Oral Surg Oral Med Oral Pathol Oral Radiol Endod 1996;81:533–543.
28. Loesche WJ, Grossman N, Giordano J. Metronidazole in periodontitis (IV). The effect of patient compliance on treatment parameters. J Clin Periodontol 1993;20:96–104.
29. Loesche WJ. The identification of bacteria associated with periodontal disease and caries by enzymatic methods. Oral Microbiol Immunol 1986;1:65–70.
30. Gusberti FA, Syed SA, Hoffman T, Lang NP. Diagnostic methods for the assessment of potential periodontal disease activity: Enzymatic activities of bacterial plaque and their relationship to clinical parameters. In: Lehner T, Cimasoni G (eds). The Borderland Between Caries and Periodontal Disease III. Geneva, Switzerland: Médecine et Hygiène, 1986:165–174.
31. Loesche WJ, Syed SA, Stoll J. Trypsin-like activity in subgingival plaque. A diagnostic marker for spirochetes and periodontal disease? J Periodontol 1987;58:266–273.

32. Schmidt EF, Bretz WA, Hutchinson RA, Loesche WJ. Correlation of the hydrolysis of benzoyl-arginine naphthylamide (BANA) by plaque with clinical parameters and subgingival levels of spirochetes in periodontal patients. J Dent Res 1988;67:1505–1509.

33. Loesche WJ, Giordano J, Hujoel PP. The utility of the BANA test for monitoring anaerobic infections due to spirochetes (*Treponema denticola*) in periodontal disease. J Dent Res 1990;69:1696–1702.

34. Smith AJ, Wade WG, Greenman J, Addy M. Analysis of cultivable *Porphyromonas gingivalis* with trypsin-like protease enzyme activity and serum antibodies in chronic adult periodontitis. Oral Diseases 1995;1:70–76.

35. Hemmings KW, Griffiths GS, Bulman JS. Detection of neutral protease (Periocheck) and BANA hydrolase (Perioscan) compared with traditional clinical methods of diagnosis and monitoring of chronic inflammatory periodontal disease. J Clin Periodontol 1997;24:110–114.

36. Amann RI, Ludwig W, Schleifer K-H. Phylogenetic identification and in situ detection of individual microbial cells without cultivation. Microbiol Rev 1995;59:143–164.

37. Tanner A, Maiden MFJ, Paster BJ, Dewhirst FE. The impact of 16S ribosomal RNA-based phylogeny on the taxonomy of oral bacteria. Periodontol 2000 1994;5:26–51.

38. Hugenholtz P, Goebel BM, Pace NR. Impact of culture-independent studies on the emerging phylogenetic view of bacterial diversity. J Bacteriol 1998;180:4765–4774.

39. Paster BJ, Dewhirst FE, Olsen I, Fraser GJ. Phylogeny of *Bacteroides, Prevotella*, and *Porphyromonas* spp. and related bacteria. J Bacteriol 1994;176:725–732.

40. Choi BK, Paster BJ, Dewhirst FE, Göbel UB. Diversity of cultivable and uncultivable oral spirochetes from a patient with severe destructive periodontitis. Infect Immun 1994;62:1889–1895.

41. Choi BK, Wyss C, Göbel UB. Phylogenetic analysis of pathogen-related oral spirochetes. J Clin Microbiol 1996;34:1922–1925.

42. Spratt DA, Weightman AJ, Wade WG. Diversity of oral asaccharolytic *Eubacterium* species in periodontitis – identification of novel phylotypes representing uncultivated taxa. Oral Microbiol Immunol 1999;14:56–59.

43. Dymock D, Weightman AJ, Scully C, Wade WG. Molecular analysis of microflora associated with dentoalveolar abscesses. J Clin Microbiol 1996;34:537–542.

44. Moter A, Hoenig C, Choi BK, et al. Molecular epidemiology of oral treponemes associated with periodontal disease. J Clin Microbiol 1998;36:1399–1403.

45. Kroes I, Lepp PW, Relman DA. Bacterial diversity within the human subgingival crevice. Proc Natl Acad Sci USA 1999;96:14547–14552.

46. Willis SG, Smith KS, Dunn VL, et al. Identification of seven *Treponema* species in health and disease-associated dental plaque by nested PCR. J Clin Microbiol 1999;37:867–869.

47. Dewhirst FE, Tamer MA, Ericson RE, et al. The diversity of periodontal spirochetes by 16S rRNA analysis. Oral Microbiol Immunol 2000;15:196–202.

48. Persson GR, DeRouen TA, Page RC. Relationship between gingival crevicular fluid levels of aspartate aminotransferase and active tissue destruction in treated chronic periodontitis patients. J Periodontal Res 1990;25:81–87.

49. Persson GR, Page RC. Diagnostic characteristics of crevicular fluid aspartate aminotransferase (AST) levels associated with periodontal disease activity. J Clin Periodontol 1992;19:43–48.

50. Chambers DA, Imrey PB, Cohen RL, et al. A longitudinal study of aspartate aminotransferase in human gingival crevicular fluid. J Periodontal Res 1991;26:65–74.

51. Persson GR, Alves MEAF, Chambers DA, et al. A multicenter clinical trial of PerioGard in distinguishing between diseased and healthy periodontal sites. I. Study design, methodology and therapeutic outcome. J Clin Periodontol 1995;22:794–803.

52. Magnusson I, Persson RG, Page RC, et al. A multi-center clinical trial of a new chairside test in distinguishing between diseased and healthy periodontal sites. II. Association between site type and test outcome before and after treatment. J Periodontol 1996;67:589–596.

53. Atici K, Yamalik N, Eratalay K, Etikan I. Analysis of gingival crevicular fluid intracytoplasmic enzyme activity in patients with adult periodontitis and rapidly progressive periodontitis. A longitudinal study model with periodontal treatment. J Periodontol 1998;69:1155–1163.

54. Kuru B, Yilmaz S, Noyan Ü, et al. Microbiological features and crevicular fluid aspartate aminotransferase enzyme activity in early onset periodontitis patients. J Clin Periodontol 1999;26:19–25.

55. Wong MY, Lu CL, Liu CM, et al. Relationship of the subgingival microbiota to a chairside test for aspartate aminotransferase in gingival crevicular fluid. J Periodontol 1999;70:57–62.

56. Lee W, Aitken S, Kulkarni G, et al. Collagenase activity in recurrent periodontitis: Relationship to disease progression and doxycycline therapy. J Periodontal Res 1991;26:479–485.

57. Teng YT, Sodek J, McCulloch CAG. Gingival crevicular fluid gelatinase and its relationship to periodontal disease in human subjects. J Periodontal Res 1992;27:544–552.

58. Lee W, Aitken S, Sodek J, McCulloch CAG. Evidence of a direct relationship between neutrophil collagenase activity and periodontal tissue destruction in vivo: Role of active enzyme in human periodontitis. J Periodontal Res 1995;30:23–33.

59. Halinen S, Sorsa T, Ding Y, et al. Characterization of matrix metalloproteinase (MMP-8 and -9) activities in the saliva and in gingival crevicular fluid of children with Down's syndrome. J Periodontol 1996;67:748–754.

60. Mohd H, Said S, Sander L, et al. GCF levels of MMP-3 and MMP-8 following placement of bioresorbable membranes. J Clin Periodontol 1999;26:757–763.

61. Mancini S, Romanell R, Laschinger CA, et al. Assessment of a novel screening test for neutrophil collagenase activity in the diagnosis of periodontal diseases. J Periodontol 1999;70:1292–1302.

62. Chen HY, Cox SW, Eley BM, et al. Matrix metalloproteinase-8 levels and elastase activities in gingival crevicular fluid from chronic adult periodontitis patients. J Clin Periodontol 2000;27:366–369.

63. Bhide VM, Smith L, Overall CM, et al. Use of a fluorogenic septapeptide matrix metalloproteinase assay to assess responses to periodontal treatment. J Periodontol 2000;71:690–700.

64. Bowers JE, Zahradnik RT. Evaluation of a chairside gingival protease test for use in periodontal diagnosis. J Clin Dent 1989;1:106–109.

65. Bowers JE, Hawley CE, Romberg E. A clinical test for proteolytic enzymes in gingival crevicular fluid: Comparison with periodontal probing depth and bleeding on probing. Int J Periodontics Restorative Dent 1991;11:411–422.

66. Bader HI, Boyd RL. Long-term monitoring of adult periodontitis patients in supportive periodontal therapy: Correlation of gingival crevicular fluid proteases with probing attachment loss. J Clin Periodontol 1999;26:99–105.

67. Lamster IB, Oshrain RL, Harper DS, et al. Enzyme activity in crevicular fluid for detection and prediction of clinical attachment loss in patients with chronic adult periodontitis. Six month results. J Periodontol 1988;59:516–523.

68. Lamster IB, Oshrain RL, Celenti RS, et al. Indicators of the acute inflammatory and humoral immune responses in gingival crevicular fluid: Relationship to active periodontal disease. J Periodontal Res 1991;26:261–263.

69. Lamster IB, Holmes LG, Gross KBW, et al. The relationship of β-glucuronidase activity in crevicular fluid to probing attachment loss in patients with adult periodontitis. Findings from a multicenter study. J Clin Periodontol 1995;22:36–44.

70. Grbic JT, Singer RE, Jans HH, et al. Immunoglobulin isotypes in gingival crevicular fluid: Possible protective role of IgA. J Periodontol 1995;66:55–61.

71. Layik M, Yamalik N, Çaglayan F, et al. Analysis of human gingival tissue and gingival crevicular fluid β-glucuronidase activity in specific periodontal diseases. J Periodontol 2000;71:618–624.

72. Palcanis KG, Larjava IK, Wells BR, et al. Elastase as an indicator of periodontal disease progression. J Periodontol 1992;63: 237–242.

73. Armitage GC, Jeffcoat MK, Chadwick DE, et al. Longitudinal evaluation of elastase as a marker for the progression of periodontitis. J Periodontol 1994;65:120–128.

74. Jin LJ, Söder PÖ, Leung WK, et al. Granulocyte elastase activity and PGE_2 levels in gingival crevicular fluid in relation to the presence of subgingival periodontopathogens in subjects with untreated adult periodontitis. J Clin Periodontol 1999;26: 531–540.

75. Yamalik N, Çaglayan F, Kilinç K, et al. The importance of data presentation regarding gingival crevicular fluid myeloperoxidase and elastase-like activity in periodontal disease and health status. J Periodontol 2000;71:460–467.

76. Jin L, Söder B, Corbet EF. Interleukin-8 and granulocyte elastase in gingival crevicular fluid in relation to periodontopathogens in untreated adult periodontitis. J Periodontol 2000;71:929–939.

77. Chapple ILC, Matthews JB, Thorpe GH, et al. A new ultrasensitive chemiluminescent assay for the site-specific quantification of alkaline phosphatase in gingival crevicular fluid. J Periodontal Res 1993;28:266–273.

78. Chapple IL, Garner I, Saxby MS, et al. Prediction and diagnosis of attachment loss by enhanced chemiluminescent assay of crevicular fluid alkaline phosphatase levels. J Clin Periodontol 1999;26:190–198.

79. Eley BM, Cox SW. Correlation between gingival crevicular fluid dipeptidyl peptidase II and IV activity and periodontal attachment loss. A 2-year longitudinal study in chronic periodontitis patients. Oral Dis 1995;1:201–213.

80. Suido H, Neiders ME, Barua PK, et al. Characterization of N-CBz-glycyl-glycyl-arginyl peptidase and glycyl-prolyl peptidase of Bacteroides gingivalis. J Periodontal Res 1987;22:412–418.

81. Eley BM, Cox SW. Correlation between gingivain/gingipain and bacterial dipeptidyl peptidase activity in crevicular fluid and periodontal attachment loss in chronic periodontitis patients. A 2-year longitudinal study. J Periodontol 1996;67:703–716.

82. Eley BM, Cox SW. Cathepsin B/L-, elastase-, tryptase-, trypsin-, and dipeptidyl peptidase IV-like activities in gingival crevicular fluid: Correlation with clinical parameters in untreated chronic periodontitis patients. J Periodontal Res 1992;27:62–69.

83. Eley BM, Cox SW. Cathepsin B/L-, elastase-, tryptase-, trypsin-, and dipeptidyl peptidase IV-like activities in gingival crevicular fluid: A comparison of levels before and after periodontal surgery in chronic periodontitis patients. J Periodontol 1992;63: 412–417.

84. Eley BM, Cox SW. Cathepsin B/L-, elastase-, tryptase-, trypsin-, and dipeptidyl peptidase IV-like activities in gingival crevicular fluid. A comparison of levels before and after basic periodontal treatment of chronic periodontitis patients. J Clin Periodontol 1992;19:333–339.

85. Eley BM, Cox SW. The relationship between gingival crevicular fluid cathepsin B activity and periodontal attachment loss in chronic periodontitis patients: A 2-year longitudinal study. J Periodontal Res 1996;31:381–392.

86. Waddington RJ, Embery G, Last KS. Glycosaminoglycans of human alveolar bone. Arch Oral Biol 1989;34:587–589.

87. Giannobile WV, Riviere GR, Gorski JP, et al. Glycosaminoglycans and periodontal disease: Analysis of GCF by safranin O. J Periodontol 1993;64:186–190.

88. Samuels RHA, Pender N, Last KS. The effects of orthodontic tooth movement on the glycosaminoglycan component of gingival crevicular fluid. J Clin Periodontol 1993;20:371–377.

89. Waddington RJ, Embery G, Samuels RHA. Characterization of proteoglycan metabolites in human gingival crevicular fluid during orthodontic tooth movement. Arch Oral Biol 1994;39: 361–368.

90. Smith AJ, Addy M, Embery G. Gingival crevicular fluid glycosaminoglycan levels in patients with chronic adult periodontitis. J Clin Periodontol 1995;22:355–361.

91. Waddington RJ, Langley MS, Guida L, et al. Relationship of sulphated glycosaminoglycans in human gingival crevicular fluid with active periodontal disease. J Periodontal Res 1996;31: 168–170.

92. Yan F, Marshall R, Wynne S, et al. Glycosaminoglycans in gingival crevicular fluid of patients with periodontal class II furcation involvement before and after guided tissue regeneration. A pilot study. J Periodontol 2000;71:1–7.

93. Akalin FA, Sengün D, Eratalay K, et al. Hydroxyproline and total protein levels in gingiva and gingival crevicular fluid in patients with juvenile, rapidly progressive, and adult periodontitis. J Periodontol 1993;64:323–329.

94. Figueredo CMS, Gustafsson A. Increased amounts of laminin in GCF from untreated patients with periodontitis. J Clin Periodontol 2000;27:313–318.

95. Kido J, Nakamura T, Kido R, et al. Calprotectin, a leukocyte protein related to inflammation, in gingival crevicular fluid. J Periodontal Res 1998;33:434–437.

96. Kido J, Nakamura T, Kido R, et al. Calprotectin in gingival crevicular fluid correlates with clinical and biochemical markers of periodontal disease. J Clin Periodontol 1999;26:653–657.

97. Nakamura T, Kido J, Kido R, et al. The association of calprotectin level in gingival crevicular fluid with gingival index and the activities of collagenase and aspartate aminotransferase in adult periodontitis patients. J Periodontol 2000;71:361–367.

98. Mäkinen KK, Sewón L, Mäkinen PL. Analysis in gingival crevicular fluid of two oligopeptides derived from human hemoglobin β-chain. J Periodontal Res 1996;31:43–46.

99. Giannobile WV, Lynch SE, Denmark RG, et al. Crevicular fluid osteocalcin and pyridinoline cross-linked carboxyterminal telopeptide of type I collagen (ICTP) as markers of rapid bone turnover in periodontitis. A pilot study in beagle dogs. J Clin Periodontol 1995;22:903–910.

100. Nakashima K, Roehrich N, Cimasoni G. Osteoclacin, prostaglandin E_2 and alkaline phosphatase in gingival crevicular fluid: Their relations to periodontal status. J Clin Periodontol 1994;21:327–333.

101. Offenbacher S, Collins JG, Yalda B, Haradon G. Role of prostaglandins in high-risk periodontitis patients. In: Genco R, Hamada S, Lehner T, et al (eds). Molecular Pathogenesis of Periodontal Disease. Washington, DC: ASM Press, 1994:203–213.

102. Needleman IG, Moles DR, Collins AM. Periodontal flap surgery with 25% metronidazole gel. (2). Effect on gingival crevicular fluid PGE_2. J Clin Periodontol 2000;27:193–197.

103. Nakashima K, Giannopoulou C, Anderson E, et al. A longitudinal study of various crevicular fluid components as markers of periodontal disease activity. J Clin Periodontol 1996; 23:832–838.

104. Sengupta S, Fine J, Wu-Yang CY, et al. The relationship of prostaglandins to cAMP, IgG, IgM and α-2-macroglobulin in gingival crevicular fluid in chronic adult periodontitis. Arch Oral Biol 1990;35:593–596.

105. Alexander DCC, Martin JC, King PJ, et al. Interleukin-1 beta, prostaglandin E_2, immunoglobulin G subclasses in gingival crevicular fluid in patients undergoing periodontal therapy. J Periodontol 1996;67:755–762.

106. Mathur A, Michalowicz B, Castillo M, Aeppli D. Interleukin-1 alpha, interleukin-8 and interferon-alpha levels in gingival crevicular fluid. J Periodontal Res 1996;31:489–495.

107. Lee HJ, Kang IK, Chung CP, Choi SM. The subgingival microflora and gingival crevicular fluid cytokines in refractory periodontitis. J Clin Periodontol 1995;22:885–890.

108. Figueredo CMS, Ribeiro MSM, Fischer RG, Gustafsson A. Increased interleukin-1β concentration in gingival crevicular fluid as a characteristic of periodontitis. J Periodontol 1999; 70:1457–1463.

109. Ishihara Y, Nishihara T, Kuroyanagi T, et al. Gingival crevicular interleukin-1 and interleukin-1 receptor antagonist levels in periodontally healthy and diseased sites. J Periodontal Res 1997;32:524–529.

110. Özmeriç N, Bal B, Balos K, et al. The correlation of gingival crevicular fluid interleukin-8 levels and periodontal status in localized juvenile periodontitis. J Periodontol 1998;69: 1299–1304.

111. Adonogianaki E, Mooney J, Kinane DF. Detection of stable and active periodontitis sites by clinical assessment and gingival crevicular acute-phase protein levels. J Periodontal Res 1996; 31:135–143.

112. Reinhardt RA, McDonald TL, Bolton RW, et al. IgG subclasses in gingival crevicular fluid from active versus stable periodontal sites. J Periodontol 1989;60:44–50.

113. Kinane DF, Takahashi K, Mooney J. Crevicular fluid and serum IgG subclasses and corresponding mRNA expressing plasma cells in periodontitis lesions. J Periodontal Res 1997;32:176–178.

114. Lamster IB, Smith QT, Celenti RS, et al. Development of a risk profile for periodontal disease: Microbial and host response factors. J Periodontol 1994;65:511–520.

115. Grbic JT, Lamster IB, Fine JB, et al. Changes in gingival crevicular fluid levels of immunoglobulin A following therapy: Association with attachment loss. J Periodontol 1999;70:1221–1227.

116. Kinnby B, Matsson L, Åstedt B. Aggravation of gingival inflammatory symptoms during pregnancy associated with the concentration of plasminogen activator inhibitor type 2 (PAI-2) in gingival fluid. J Periodontal Res 1996;31:271–277.

117. Xiao Y, Bunn CL, Bartold PM. Detection of tissue plasminogen activator (t-PA) and plasminogen activator inhibitor 2 (PAI-2) in gingival crevicular fluid from healthy, gingivitis and periodontitis patients. J Clin Periodontol 2000;27:149–156.

118. Linden GJ, McKinnell J, Shaw C, Lundy FT. Substance P and neurokinin A in gingival crevicular fluid in periodontal health and disease. J Clin Periodontol 1997;24:799–803.

119. Hanioka T, Takaya K, Matsumori Y, et al. Relationship of the substance P to indicators of host response in human crevicular fluid. J Clin Periodontol 2000;27:262–266.

120. Lundy FT, Mullally BH, Burden DJ, et al. Changes in substance P and neurokinin A in gingival crevicular fluid in response to periodontal treatment. J Clin Periodontol 2000;27:526–530.

121. Weinstein M, Feinberg H. Clinical Decision Analysis. Philadelphia: Saunders, 1980.

122. Browner W, Newman T, Cummings S. Designing a new study: Diagnostic tests. In: Hulley S, Cummings S (eds). Designing Clinical Research. Baltimore: Williams and Wilkins, 1988.

123. Newhauser D, Yin X. Deciding whether a new test measure is useful. Med Care 1991;29:685–689.

124. Beck JD. Identification of risk factors. In: Beck JD (ed). Risk Assessment in Dentistry. [Proceedings of a conference, June 2–3, 1989, Chapel Hill, North Carolina.] Chapel Hill: University of North Carolina, 1989:8–13.

125. Holtzman S, Kornman K. Decision analysis for periodontal therapy. J Dent Educ 1992;56:844–862.

126. Douglass C, McNeil B. Clinical decision analysis methods applied to diagnostic tests in dentistry. J Dent Educ 1983;47: 708–712.

Part II

Clinical Management of the Periodontal Patient in Health and Disease

Conditions of the Periodontium

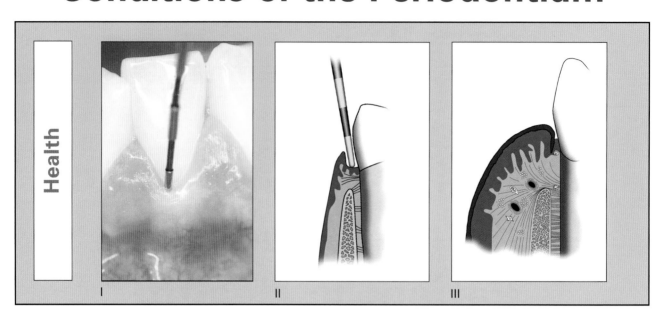

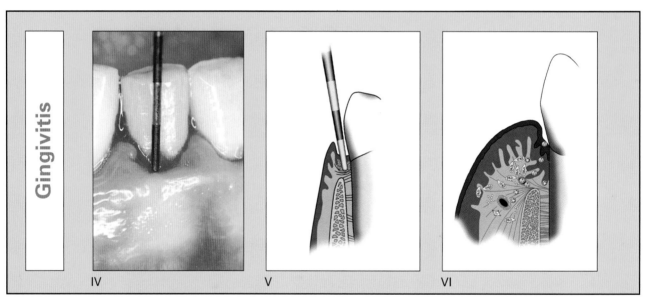

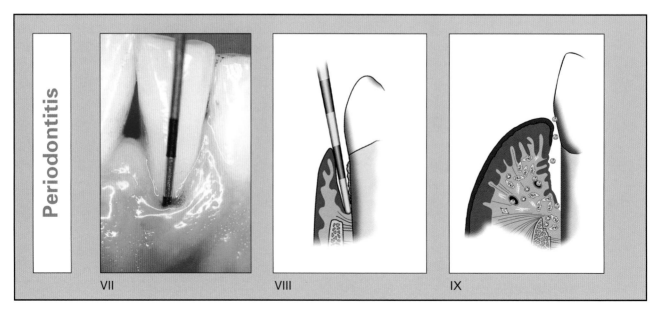

The Periodontium in Health and Disease

There are three primary conditions of the periodontal tissues: health, gingivitis, and periodontitis. These stages of periodontal health and disease will be highlighted in several places in this text. They are represented on the clinical, light-microscopic, and electron-microscopic levels (the latter two schematically) on the facing page.

Health

In health, the soft tissue has the following clinical characteristics (Fig I):

1. The gingival tissue is pink and stippled (it may appear darker in individuals with darker skin coloration).
2. It shows no signs of inflammation (eg, bleeding on probing).
3. The coronal margin of the soft tissue is located at or slightly coronal to the cementoenamel junction.
4. The probing depth ranges from 1 to 3 mm.

A light-microscopic view of healthy tissue, with a periodontal probe in place, shows the following (Fig II):

1. The tip of the probe rests (ideally) at the bottom of the clinical sulcus.
2. Very few inflammatory cells are found in the connective tissues at the base of the sulcus.
3. The alveolar bone is located 2 to 3 mm apical to the base of the junctional epithelium.

The same healthy tissue, viewed with an electron microscope, reveals deeper structures (Fig III):

1. The junctional epithelium is intact and is in close contact with the tooth surface at or just apical to the cementoenamel junction.
2. There are no (or few) inflammatory cells located apical to the junctional epithelium.
3. The connective tissue fibers of the gingiva that support the junctional epithelium are intact.

Gingivitis

In gingivitis, the clinical picture of the soft tissues presents as follows (Fig IV):

1. The gingival tissue is often red or red-blue in color.
2. The tissue shows other signs of inflammation, including bleeding on probing.
3. The coronal margin of the soft tissues is located at or slightly coronal to the cementoenamel junction.
4. In cases where the most coronal extent of the soft tissue is at or slightly coronal to the cementoenamel junction, probing depths range from 1 to 3 mm. In cases with swelling (or hyperplasia) of the tissues, there may be deeper probing depths.

A light-microscopic view of gingivitis, with a periodontal probe in place, shows added detail (Fig V):

1. The tip of the probe often rests within the connective tissue.
2. Large numbers of inflammatory cells are found in the connective tissues at the base of the junctional epithelium.
3. The alveolar bone is located 2 to 3 mm apical to the base of the junctional epithelium and is not affected to any great extent by the inflammatory lesion.

If the same tissue with gingivitis is viewed with an electron microscope, more is evident (Fig VI):

1. The junctional epithelium has been converted into a pocket epithelium. Cells of the junctional epithelium have proliferated into the area formerly occupied by connective tissue.
2. Large numbers of plasma cells are present in this lesion.
3. The connective tissues of the gingiva that supported the junctional epithelium have been destroyed.

Periodontitis

In periodontitis, the soft tissues present the following clinical signs (Fig VII):

1. The gingival tissue is often red or red-blue in color, but may appear normal.
2. On probing, the tissue shows other signs of inflammation, including bleeding and, possibly, suppuration.
3. The coronal margin of the soft tissues can be located at any level relative to the cementoenamel junction.
4. Probing depths in the range of 4 mm or more are seen.

A light-microscopic view of periodontitis provides additional data (Fig VIII):

1. The tip of the probe often rests within the connective tissue.
2. Large numbers of inflammatory cells are found in the connective tissues at the base of the pocket.
3. Bone loss is evident.

The same tissue shows even more detail when viewed with an electron microscope (Fig IX):

1. The junctional epithelium has further degenerated. Junctional epithelial cells have proliferated into the area formally occupied by connective tissue, and a space (the periodontal pocket) filled with inflammatory cells and debris is evident.
2. Plasma cells and lymphocytes are the predominate inflammatory cells in this lesion.
3. The connective tissues of the gingiva have been destroyed and in some areas replaced by masses of inflammatory cells or unorganized scarlike fibrous tissue.
4. Alveolar bone has been destroyed and is located more than 2 to 3 mm apical to the base of the cementoenamel junction. Osteoclastic bone resorption may be evident.

Making a Clinical Diagnosis and Treatment Plan

Kenneth S. Kornman and Thomas G. Wilson, Jr
- Diagnostic Categories
- General Approach to Periodontal Care
- Evaluation of Risk Factors
- Establishing a Prognosis
- Developing a Treatment Plan

Diagnostic Categories

There are many different classifications and names for periodontal diseases. Early classification schemes were based on histologic observations that were interpreted from the perspective of disease-causation concepts at the time.[1–8] During the 1970s and 1980s, clinical practice was based on the concept that all periodontal disease in adults was simply a function of the degree of plaque exposure. Therapy was therefore focused on the removal of subgingival plaque and calculus and the establishment of a gingival anatomy that was compatible with easy plaque removal by the patient and the clinician. A diagnostic system emerged that rated the severity of past destruction, because the amount and configuration of bone destruction and connective tissue attachment helped to determine the complexity of the therapy required to remove subgingival deposits.[9–11]

In the 1980s, several clinically distinct conditions were identified and described, and they became the basis for terminology.[12] When those descriptions were first presented, it was hoped that new microbial and immunologic technology would allow investigators to demonstrate distinct biologic patterns that matched the clinical patterns.

This goal was achieved for some forms of periodontal disease that affect children and young adults (see chapters 5 and 8), but in adult patients there were multiple biologic patterns within each clinical pattern.[3,10,11,13–23] Although the use of objective biologic markers as a guide to periodontal diagnosis is an important goal to pursue, biologic parameters do not currently add value to clinical assessments in the diagnosis of most cases of periodontitis (see chapter 19).

The diagnostic categories presented below attempt to provide a practical classification system that could be used to guide therapy for each patient. The categories largely reflect the system formulated by the International Workshop for a Classification of Periodontal Diseases and Conditions.[24]

Modified Diagnostic Categories for Use in Daily Practice

Most of the periodontal problems seen in daily practice are chronic. General guidelines on the clinical management of these chronic problems are outlined in this chapter. More specific information on treatment can be found in subsequent chapters.

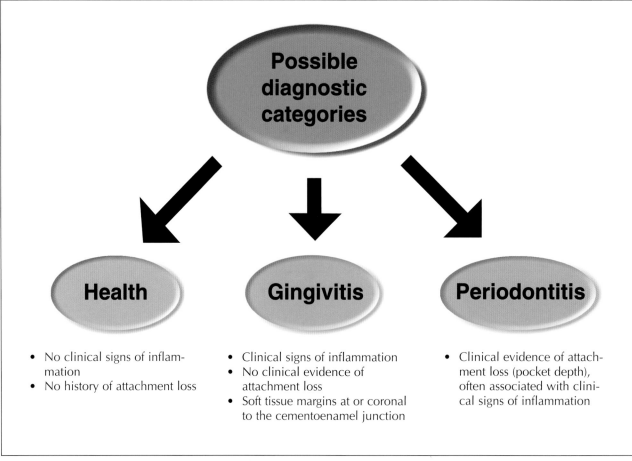

Fig 20-1 The diagnostic categories used to make a diagnosis and treatment plan.

Developing treatment plans for patients with inflammatory periodontal disease is simplified when patients are separated into three general groups—health, gingivitis, and periodontitis—based on clinical and radiographic evidence gathered during the examination (Fig 20-1). Treatment will be guided by the most severe of these categories found in each individual patient.

Health

This group consists of healthy patients who have no current disease and no history of attachment loss. This is in contrast to patients who have had previous attachment loss but show no manifestations of current disease. The distinction between patients who have never had attachment loss and those who have had attachment loss is important, because patients, especially adults, with no disease history are less likely to develop disease than those who have had attachment loss.

Gingivitis

Dental plaque–induced gingivitis. Gingivitis is most often a response of the gingival tissues to bacterial plaque and its by-products. Most patients will have a form of gingival inflammation that is reversible following the removal of plaque, calculus, and other plaque-retaining features and with the patient's regular oral hygiene measures. Dental plaque–induced gingivitis is characterized by probing depths of 3 mm or less and bleeding on probing. The soft tissues will usually be located at or coronal to the cementoenamel junction and are often reddened and edematous (Fig 20-2).

Other forms of gingivitis. There are several forms of gingivitis that are seen less frequently than plaque-induced gingivitis (Figs 20-3 to 20-8). These forms are often difficult to diagnose and treat, and they may involve systemic disorders; these conditions are best managed by someone with substantial experience in the area. This chapter concentrates on plaque-induced gingivitis.

Fig 20-2 Dental plaque–induced gingivitis

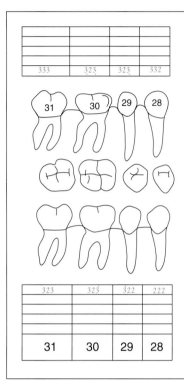

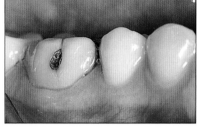

Clinical signs of inflammation such as bleeding on probing are seen.

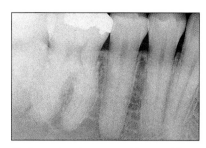

Radiographs show no evidence of bone loss.

Probing depths are 3 mm or less.

Clinical presentation

- Most common form of periodontal disease
- Probing depths ranging from 1 to 3 mm
- Clinical signs of inflammation such as bleeding on probing or gingival redness and edema
- Plaque usually present; calculus often seen
- Precedes periodontitis but does not always lead to periodontitis
- Reversible with plaque and calculus removal

Radiographic presentation

- No bone loss seen

Fig 20-3 Non–plaque-induced linear gingival erythema

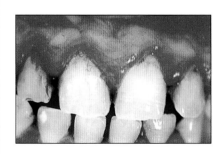

- Sometimes associated with HIV disease
- Erythema of the free and attached gingiva
- Extends into the alveolar mucosa
- Spontaneous gingival bleeding
- Usually does not respond to plaque-control therapy
- Possibly a *Candida* species infection

(Courtesy Dr Terry Rees.)

Fig 20-4 Necrotizing ulcerative gingivitis (NUG)

Other commonly used names: Trench mouth, Vincent's angina, Vincent's disease

Clinical presentation

- Accompanied by pain, gingival bleeding, and halitosis

- *Prevetolla intermedia*, fusiform bacteria, and spirochetes have been associated

- Repeated episodes may lead to bone loss

- Patient may be systemically stressed, immunocompromised, or malnourished

- Some patients may present with systemic signs, including fever and leukocytosis. In severe cases, systemic antibiotics may be appropriate

- Ulcerative and necrotic ("punched out") destruction of one or more dental papillae

Radiographic presentation

- No bone loss evident radiographically unless *(1)* patient has had repeated episodes or *(2)* NUG has developed in a patient who has previously had periodontitis.

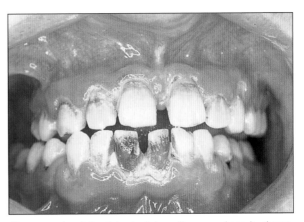

The necrosis of the interdental papillae seen here is characteristic of NUG.

Therapy consists of gentle debridement by the dental professional on several consecutive days while encouraging the patient to practice improved personal oral hygiene. (For more information on treatment, see chapter 29.)

Fig 20-5 Plaque-induced gingivitis modified by endocrine factors

- Presents during natural or induced hormonal change.

- Has been reported in pregnancy, a few days prior to menstruation, during puberty, and in some women taking oral contraceptives for extended periods of time.

- Has been associated with an increase in specific bacteria (eg, *Prevotella intermedia*) and immunoregulatory changes.

- Although hormone-influenced gingivitis is reversible, hormonal changes in a patient with untreated or unstable periodontitis may induce substantial loss of attachment.

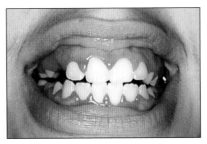

Puberty-associated gingivitis.

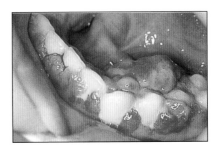

Pregnancy-associated gingivitis with pyogenic granuloma.

- Treatment in most instances consists of local debridement, scaling and root planing, and improved plaque control techniques. Surgical correction is sometimes necessary in severe cases.

(Courtesy Dr Terry Rees.)

Fig 20-6 Plaque-induced gingival enlargements associated with medications

The condition appears to represent an exaggerated tissue response to plaque modified by the presence of certain medications.

There are three commonly used medications that cause most of these overgrowths. They are phenytoin (Dilantin, Parke-Davis and other manufacturers), cyclosporine (Sandimmune, Sandoz), and nifedipine (Adalat, Miles; Procardia, Pfizer). In general, the better the patient's oral hygiene, the less the problem. For an excellent review, see Butler et al.[25]

Treatment can include changing medications (if appropriate), scaling and root planing (see chapter 22), or surgery (see chapter 23).

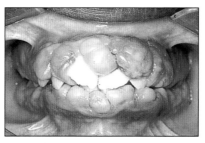

Phenytoin-induced overgrowth.

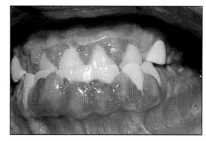

Cyclosporine-induced overgrowth.

Clinical presentation

- Overgrowth often interproximal
- Oral hygiene difficult once tissue is enlarged

Fig 20-7 Non–plaque-induced gingival manifestations of systemic conditions

- Mucocutaneous disorders: erosive lichen planus, pemphigoid; pemphigus
- Allergic reactions

After diagnosis, treatment of a mucocutaneous disease must often be coordinated with the patient's physician. Topical and/or systemic corticosteroids are frequently administered. Allergic reactions are treated primarily by discontinuing use of the causative material.

(Courtesy of Dr Terry Rees.)

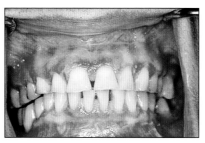

Localized atrophic and erosive gingival lesions in erosive lichen planus.

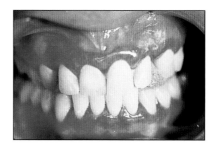

Generalized atrophic gingivitis common in benign mucous membrane pemphigoid.

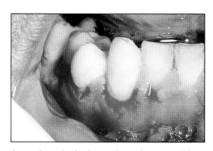

Irregular gingival erosions in pemphigus vulgaris.

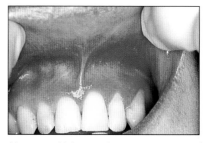

Hypersensitivity reaction to a tartar-control toothpaste.

Fig 20-8 Other causes of gingivitis

- Blood disorders
- Nutritional deficiencies
- Tumors
- Mouth breathing
- Bacterial and viral infection

Oral treatment is often palliative while underlying systemic disorders are being managed. Oral debridement and meticulous oral hygiene are initiated when possible. Surgical correction is usually necessary for tumors or hyperplastic gingival enlargements.

(Courtesy of Dr Terry Rees.)

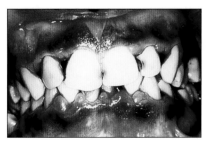

Spontaneous gingival bleeding in a patient suffering from idiopathic thrombocytopenic purpura.

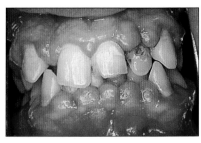

Gingival hyperplasia resulting from inadequate plaque control in a patient who is a chronic mouth breather.

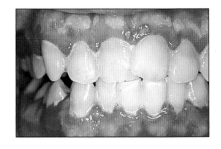

Generalized gingivitis and vesiculation associated with primary herpetic gingivostomatitis.

Fig 20-9 Recurrent gingivitis superimposed on previous attachment loss

- Results from a failure of the patient to clean correctly
- Clinical signs of gingival inflammation seen in areas of previous attachment loss
- No new attachment loss

This condition should be treated and monitored aggressively to prevent further attachment loss. Patients with previous attachment loss are more likely than those without previous attachment loss to have additional loss in the future. This disease state should be viewed with more alarm than plaque-associated gingivitis without previous attachment loss.

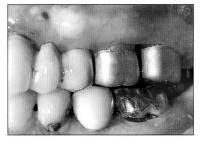

Before treatment for chronic periodontitis with moderate attachment loss.

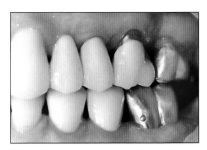

The patient was treated surgically, then restored. For 20 years, the patient's periodontal status was stable and classified as treated chronic periodontitis.

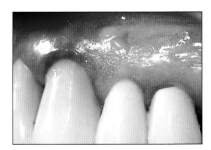

When gingivitis occurred, it was treated aggressively because of the patient's history of attachment loss.

Fig 20-10 Generalized chronic periodontitis with early or moderate attachment loss (untreated)

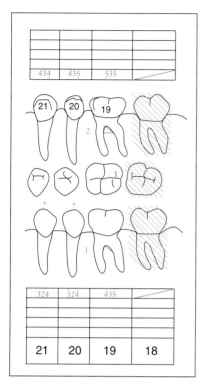

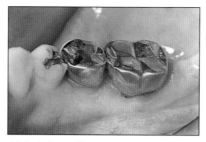

Clinical signs of inflammation are present.

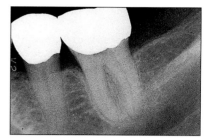

No bone loss is apparent on the radiograph of the same area.

Clinical presentation

- 4- to 6-mm pocket probing depths
- No furcation invasion (no bone loss in the furca) (early)
- Bone loss in furcae (moderate)
- Bleeding on probing and/or suppuration usually present

- May see fremitus or bidigital tooth mobility

Assuming systemic risk factors are absent or controllable, there should be a predictably positive response to therapies directed at cleaning bacterial deposits from the root surface and controlling supragingival plaque.

Probing depths range up to 6 mm. Because of bone loss in furcations, this patient would have a diagnosis of moderate generalized chronic periodontitis.

Periodontitis

Periodontitis is marked by attachment loss and clinical signs of inflammation. In this text, periodontitis is separated into two major divisions, chronic and aggressive forms, which can be either generalized or localized.

Chronic periodontitis with early or moderate attachment loss. By definition, patients with *early* or *moderate* periodontitis have probing depths of 4 to 6 mm, with the gingival margin at or near the cementoenamel junction. Bleeding on probing, suppuration, or other signs of clinical inflammation are found in untreated cases. The designation *early* is reserved for those patients who have no bone loss in the furcations. Those with furcation invasion are said to be in the *moderate* category, because bone loss in furcations makes the patient harder to treat and the long-term prognosis more guarded. The patient with no previous history of professional therapy for periodontal disease will be classified as *untreated*.

Untreated chronic periodontitis with early or moderate attachment loss is the type most commonly encountered in clinical practice (Fig 20-10). Clinically detectable progression is usually slow, but other studies suggest that progression may occur in bursts of attachment loss.[26] Untreated chronic periodontitis is usually associated with accumulation of supragingival and subgingival bacteria that collect where the patient does not (or cannot) clean. Calculus is present in varying degrees but is usually a clinical feature.

Cases previously treated but with new signs and symptoms of disease are termed *recurrent*. These cases fall into two divisions: recurrent gingivitis with previous attachment loss (Fig 20-9) and recurrent periodontitis (also called *relapsing periodontitis*) (Fig 20-11), where additional attachment loss is seen in localized areas. Both types of recurrent periodontitis are attributable to lack of proper oral hygiene by the patient, inadequate treatment of the disease by the therapist, or a combination of these factors. Recurrent periodontitis is to be distinguished from the case in which attachment loss continues and is more generalized throughout the mouth, despite the best efforts of the therapist and the patient. This is an aggressive form termed *refractory periodontitis*.

Fig 20-11 Recurrent periodontitis (also called *relapsing periodontitis*)

- Results from a failure of the patient or the therapist (or both) to control the local bacterial factors that cause the disease (as opposed to refractory periodontitis in which breakdown continues despite the best efforts of both dentist and patient).

- New attachment loss is evident in many areas following therapy.

This condition should be treated and monitored aggressively to prevent further attachment loss. Patients with previous attachment loss are more likely

than those without previous attachment loss to have additional loss in the future. Most specialists distinguish these cases from refractory periodontitis.

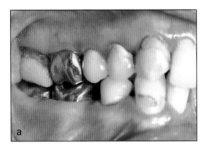
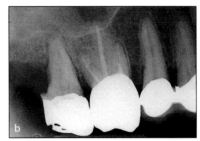
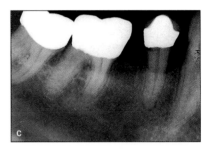
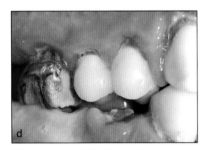
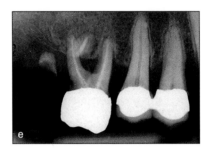
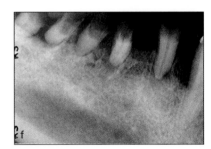

The patient in 1978 (a–c). She was treated (nonsurgically) for periodontitis and active dental caries. Her compliance to suggested personal oral hygiene was never adequate to control her disease. She was given a diagnosis of recurrent periodontitis and the results of her inaction are seen in 1986 (d–f).

Aggressive forms of periodontitis. Lesions of the aggressive forms of periodontitis are often characterized by rapid loss of attachment (Figs 20-12 to 20-18). This group includes a large number of diseases that are differentiated from early and moderate chronic periodontitis because their response to therapy directed at cleaning the root surface and controlling supragingival plaque is less predictable. These cases may be detected clinically by the rapidity or severity of bone loss or generalized progression after treatment. These problems seem to be due in part to systemic conditions. These diseases are considered as a group because of their less predictable response to traditional periodontal therapy.

Chronic periodontitis with generalized severe attachment loss is considered an aggressive form of periodontitis

(see Fig 20-12). Severe attachment loss is usually associated with probing depths of 7 mm or more, advanced bone loss in furcations, or radiographic bone loss of 50% or more seen with multiple teeth. All of these definitions assume that the gingival tissues approximate the cementoenamel junction and that root length is normal.

Periodontitis associated with systemic diseases and conditions. A number of systemic problems have been implicated in periodontal breakdown (Figs 20-19 and 20-20). They include human immunodeficiency virus (HIV) disease, type 1 diabetes mellitus, nutrition deficiencies such as scurvy, stress, Papillon-Lefèvre syndrome, Down syndrome, and others (see chapters 13 and 14).

Fig 20-12 Generalized chronic periodontitis with severe attachment loss

Clinical presentation

- 7-mm or deeper probing depths
- Furcation invasion ranging from early to through-and-through
- Bleeding on probing and/or suppuration usually present
- Fremitus and bidigital tooth mobility usually seen

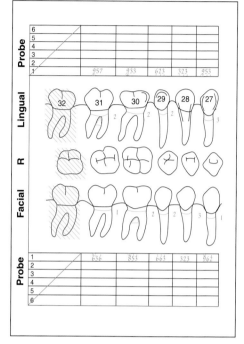

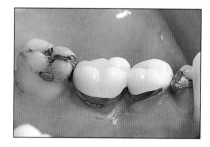

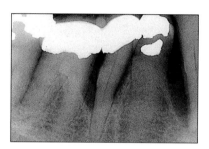

Severe bone loss is seen radiographically.

Probing depths are 7 mm or greater.

Fig 20-13 Localized aggressive periodontitis (previously termed *localized prepubertal periodontitis*) or periodontitis as a manifestation of systemic disease

Clinical presentation

- Little or no inflammation of gingiva
- Usually amenable to standard periodontal therapy with appropriate antibiotics
- Seen after eruption of primary teeth

Radiographic presentation

A radiograph of the area seen clinically shows bone loss localized to the distal of the deciduous first molar.

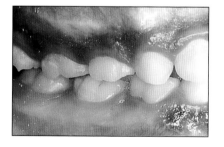

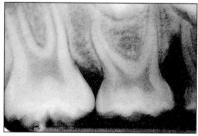

(Courtesy of Dr Jayne Delaney.)

Fig 20-14 Generalized aggressive periodontitis (previously termed *generalized prepubertal periodontitis*) or periodontitis as a manifestation of a systemic disease

Clinical presentation

- Extreme gingival inflammation

- Rapid bony destruction

- Often accompanied by severe functional defects of neutrophils and monocytes

- Recurrent otitis media and upper respiratory infections or recurrent skin infections may be found

- In some cases the more severe lesions are refractory to antibiotics[18]

(Courtesy of Dr Jayne Delaney.)

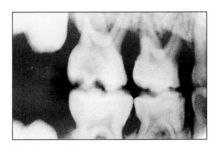

Radiographic presentation

- Generalized bone loss is evident.

Fig 20-15 Localized juvenile aggressive periodontitis (previously termed *localized juvenile periodontitis*)

Clinical presentation

- Occurs around puberty

- No demonstrable systemic modifying factors

- Usually localized to molars and incisors

- Minimal inflammation and plaque apparent

- Often associated with a systemic host defense defect, although usually no evidence of overt systemic disease

- Associated with a specific bacterial species

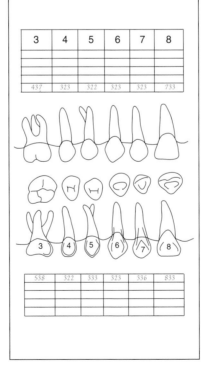

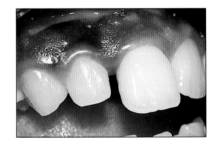

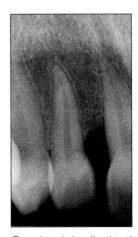

Bone loss is localized to the distal of the maxillary central incisor and maxillary first molar.

Fig 20-16 Generalized juvenile aggressive periodontitis as a manifestation of systemic disease (previously termed *generalized juvenile periodontitis*)

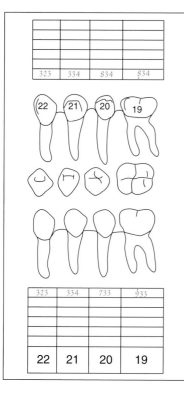

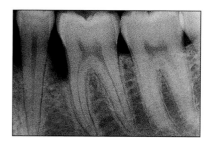

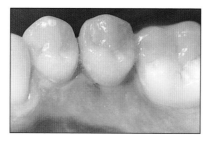

Clinical presentation

- Occurs around puberty to young adulthood
- Rapid bone destruction
- Usually accompanied by minimal inflammation and minimal visible plaque
- Often associated with a systemic host defense defect
- Lesions often refractory to antibiotics or other therapy

Radiographic presentation

Despite the clinically healthy appearance of the gingiva, severe bony destruction around premolars and molars can be seen radiographically.

Fig 20-17 Generalized aggressive periodontitis in an adult (previously termed *rapidly progressive periodontitis*)

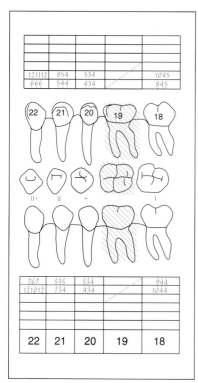

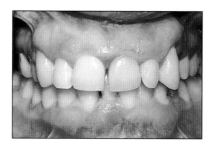

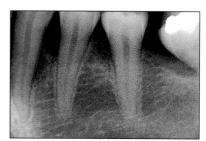

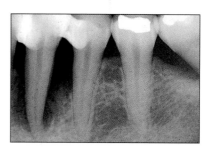

Clinical presentation

- Seen in young adults and some older patients
- Characterized by periods of severe gingival inflammation, edema, and rapid bone loss
- Malaise, depression, and lowered immune competency have been reported

This radiograph, taken 6 months after the one above, reveals rapid bony deterioration.

The progressive increase in probing depths is seen over a 6-month period.

Fig 20-18 Refractory periodontitis

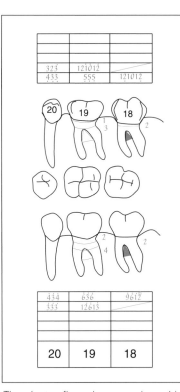

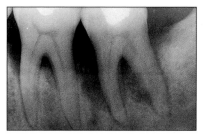

Initial radiograph of a 45-year-old woman with no known systemic diseases.

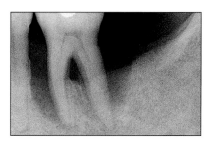

This radiograph was taken 9 months after the initial radiograph.

The chart reflects increases in probing depths over a 9-month period.

Clinical presentation

Refractory periodontitis has multiple clinical presentations.

- Attachment loss: May be seen after an initial period of stability following traditional therapy, or may be seen with no evidence of stability.
- Pattern of disease progression: Multiple teeth are affected; progression occurs even in sites with minimal or no initial loss of attachment or bone loss.
- Oral hygiene: May be better than the typical adult periodontitis case; highly variable between patients.
- General: May be a collection of different diseases with multiple biologic problems that produce similar clinical presentations.

Fig 20-19 Necrotizing ulcerative periodontitis (NUP)

Clinical presentation

- Usually observed in individuals with HIV infection, immunosuppression, or severe malnutrition
- General or localized rapid soft and hard tissue destruction
- Bone sequestration may be present
- Teeth may become mobile
- Spontaneous, usually nocturnal, gingival bleeding
- Fetid breath
- Intense, deep-seated pain
- May be preceded by necrotizing ulcerative gingivitis

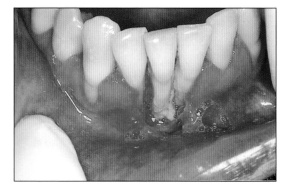

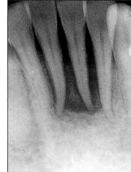

For treatment, see chapter 29.

Fig 20-20 Necrotizing stomatitis

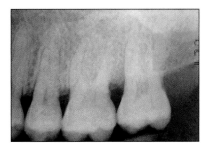

Initial radiograph.

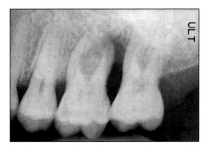

Radiograph taken 7 weeks after the initial radiograph.

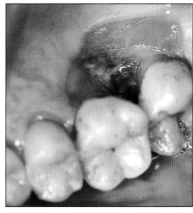

Clinical presentation at the time the second radiograph was taken.

- Many of the features of necrotizing ulcerative periodontitis
- Localized acute necrotic area of the oral mucosa usually overlying bone
- Exposure and sequestration of bone are common

(Courtesy of Dr Michael Glick. Reprinted from Muzyka and Glick,[27] with permission.)

Fig 20-21 Gingival recession

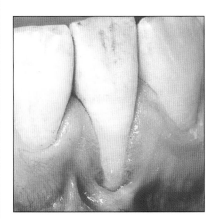

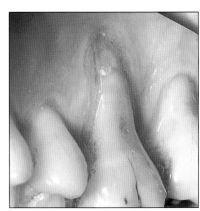

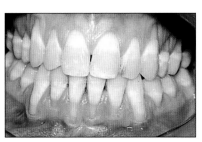

- May be localized or generalized, facial (buccal) or lingual (palatal)
- True periodontal pockets not always present
- Often associated with local anatomic variations, including bony fenestrations or dehiscences and inadequate bands of attached gingiva

---

Fig 20-22 Peri-implant mucositis (also called *peri-implant gingivitis*)

- Seen around dental implants.
- The soft tissues surrounding the implant exhibit the same manifestations of inflammation as those seen around teeth with gingivitis.

For treatment, see chapter 38.

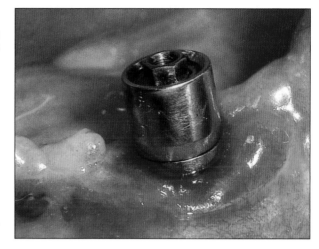

The tissue around this implant has the same clinical manifestations found with dental plaque–induced gingivitis.

Fig 20-23 Peri-implantitis

Clinical presentation

- Often accompanied by bleeding on probing
- Probing depths increased from baseline

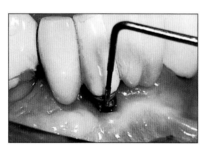

Bone loss seen clinically and radiographically around a fibro-osseous implant.

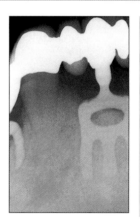

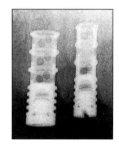

Bone loss seen around osseointegrated implants.

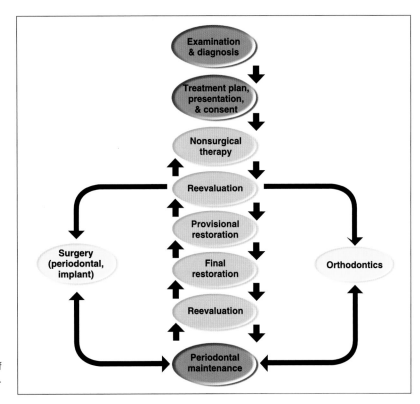

Fig 20-24 The relationship of various aspects of therapy for patients with periodontal diseases. (Modified from Corn and Marks.[30])

Gingival Recession

Gingival recession can occur secondary to an anatomic problem or as a result of a disease process (Fig 20-21).

Peri-implantitis

The soft and hard tissues surrounding implants can be affected by inflammatory lesions (Figs 20-22 and 20-23). In general, inflammation is more prevalent around fibro-osseous implants than around osseointegrated implants. Early evidence suggests that the microflora around failing implants mimics that around teeth with periodontitis.[28–30]

General Approach to Periodontal Care

The basic approach to all patients who may have periodontal disease is the same: perform an examination, make an initial clinical diagnosis (see Fig 20-1), identify the risk factors for future progression of the disease, establish a prognosis, present treatment alternatives to the patient, obtain informed consent, and then treat the patient. In most cases, this involves initial nonsurgical therapy; reevaluation; and when the disease is clinically stable, placing the patient into periodontal maintenance care (formerly called *supportive periodontal treatment*) (Fig 20-24).

As a general rule, clinical signs of inflammation should be reduced or eliminated before adjunctive care is started. The exceptions are patients in pain or who have caries or endodontic lesions that need immediate care. Provisional restorations, orthodontic therapy, and periodontal and implant surgery usually follow initial nonsurgical periodontal therapy performed to reduce inflammation. A series of reevaluations throughout therapy guides further care. The therapy outlined later in this chapter will deal primarily with the most common periodontal diseases and conditions.

Evaluation of Risk Factors

The sine qua non for the initiation and continuation of inflammatory periodontal diseases is bacteria; if there are no bacteria, there is no disease (see chapters 1 and 5). While a limited number of bacteria are associated with disease progression, most of the risk for disease progression can be explained simply by the presence of plaque deposits in general; in other words, the persistent presence of plaque constitutes a significant risk for disease.

In aggressive periodontitis cases, however, the clinical level of plaque may be misleading relative to the risk for disease. This is often due to the presence of a specific pathogenic bacteria that may not form large plaque deposits but may be very destructive. In addition, due to genetic or acquired factors that change the body's response, patients with aggressive periodontitis may be hyper-responsive to small bacterial challenges. In chronic forms of these diseases, the bacterial ecosystem varies from patient to patient and from tooth surface to tooth surface.

To improve the prognosis, periodontopathic bacteria need to be eliminated or controlled. The dental professional can eliminate retentive areas that shelter bacteria and can routinely disturb the ecosystem of any remaining pathogens during active and maintenance care. Once this occurs, it is primarily the patient's responsibility to disrupt bacterial organization on a daily basis (personal oral hygiene) and to present for periodontal maintenance as suggested by the dental team. The importance of patient compliance cannot be overemphasized.

Within the last few years, a number of systemic risk factors have been found to modify the course of disease. If these risk factors are identified and eliminated or ameliorated, then the patient's prognosis improves.

Research and clinical experience indicate that the individual local and systemic risk factors discussed below significantly increase the risk for more severe disease, disease progression, and a less favorable response to therapy. These factors do not guarantee periodontal disease but rather change the patient's individual response. It is assumed that these factors, at a minimum, add to the risk of periodontal disease; some studies suggest that two risk factors found together may multiply the risk. This discussion is only meant to point out common risk factors. More detailed information can be found elsewhere in this text.

Local Risk Factors

Specific Bacterial Pathogens

Studies for many years have shown that the failure to eliminate specific bacterial pathogens is associated with an increased risk of future disease progression. The bacteria that have been studied include *Actinobacillus actinomycetemcomitans*, *Porphyromonas gingivalis*, *Bacteroides forsythus*, and spirochetes.

Compliance

In general, individuals who follow suggested oral hygiene and maintenance schedules experience less disease, better healing, and less tooth loss compared with individuals who do not comply.

Past History of Severe Generalized Disease

The majority of individuals will develop only mild to localized moderate disease in response to moderate plaque levels. Severe generalized destruction suggests a problem with the patient's host response. The causative factor may or may not be discovered, and the problem may be transient. However, several studies indicate that past severe disease is one of the best predictors of future problems (see chapter 1).

Poor Clinical Response to Initial Therapy

After the removal of subgingival bacterial accumulations and regular plaque control, sites that are accessible for cleaning should demonstrate a predictable clinical response. For instance, sites with initial probing depths of 4 to 5 mm on single-rooted teeth should have no bleeding after probing, and probing depths should have decreased by at least 1 mm. If the majority of such sites do not respond as described, it may indicate either something of concern in the biologic response or in the patient's compliance with home care. It should be emphasized that sites with pocket depths 6 mm or greater and diseased sites on multirooted teeth are not used to evaluate the patient's response to initial therapy, because those sites are rarely accessible for adequate cleaning during the initial, nonsurgical phase of therapy.

Systemic Risk Factors

Diabetes Mellitus

Individuals with diabetes mellitus who do not adhere to medical regimens tend to have more severe disease and a less predictable response to the initial phase of therapy (see chapter 13).

Smoking

Studies have consistently shown that individuals who smoke more than 10 cigarettes per day have an increased risk of more severe disease, have a less predictable clinical and microbial response to initial therapy, and have a more complicated therapeutic response (see chapter 12).

Interleukin 1 Genotype

Individuals who carry a specific variation in the interleukin 1 (IL-1) genes tend to have higher levels of bacterial pathogens, tend to overproduce inflammatory mediators, are at increased risk for severe generalized disease, and have less favorable long-term responses to certain therapies (see chapter 11).

IL-1 Genotype–Positive Smokers

Evidence is accumulating that individuals who smoke and are positive for the IL-1 genotype are at greater risk for tooth loss due to chronic periodontitis than are individuals with only one of these risk factors (see chapter 11).

Menopause

Data indicate that the skeletal bone loss that leads to osteoporosis in postmenopausal women who are not receiving hormonal replacement therapy will also affect bone metabolism in the maxilla and mandible and thereby influence disease patterns (see chapter 13).

Establishing a Prognosis

A prognosis is determined by the number of risk factors that can be reduced or eliminated; the greater the reduction in risk factors, the better the prognosis. Some risk factors, such as smoking and noncompliance with professional suggestions, can be eliminated. Others, like diabetes mellitus, can be reduced, while genetic factors are unchangeable. A patient with diabetes mellitus who smokes and is IL-1 positive should stop smoking and reduce or eliminate other risk factors to avoid exacerbation of the disease. Just as the patient with a family history of heart disease must refrain from smoking and monitor diet and exercise, individuals at high risk for tooth loss due to periodontal disease must eliminate other potential risk factors that could contribute to inflammatory periodontal disease.

Developing a Treatment Plan

Treatment planning decisions should be based on *(1)* the extent and pattern of past destruction of bone and connective tissues and *(2)* the expected risk for future disease progression.

Past patterns of destruction influence the treatment options that should be considered. For example, if horizontal loss of bone and connective tissue is minimal, guided tissue regeneration would not be the optimal treatment option.

Expected risk for future disease progression also influences treatment options. For example, if two males at age 40 had similar past destruction but one smoked 20 cigarettes each day, one would expect the future disease progression and, more important, the response to treatment to differ between the two patients. Based on the prediction of a different course of disease, different treatment approaches would be considered for the two patients. This information would then be used to educate the patients about the level of individual risk.

There are, of course, no facts about the future, but only estimates of probability. We all make probability estimates, usually unconsciously, about many aspects of our lives. For example, we awaken one day in March and must select clothes to wear. Without looking outside or turning on the weather report, our experience tells us that

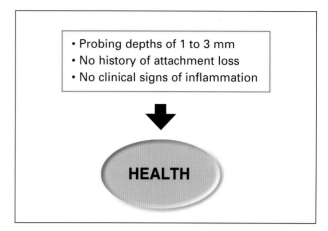

- Probing depths of 1 to 3 mm
- No history of attachment loss
- No clinical signs of inflammation

HEALTH

Fig 20-25 Initial diagnosis of health.

a certain range of weather is likely. We then look outside, access the weather report, and make a final decision. The decision on what clothes are appropriate for the weather that day is based on both experience and information. Information improves accuracy in decision making. However, predictions are probability estimates, not facts. If the weather report calls for a 60% chance of showers, we know that it may not rain; but given our information and experience, we make a decision.

Clinical decision making is very similar. Clinical decisions, which have substantial costs and risks, must be made with incomplete information. You have clinical data on a new case and experience about how similar cases have responded to your treatment. You gather additional information to improve your estimate of risk for a particular patient: Is he a smoker? Does he have diabetes? Is he genetically predisposed to more severe disease? Finally, during treatment, you continuously observe the patient's response to therapy and revise your estimates about the risk for future disease—for this specific patient.

Any amount of information is valuable in estimating a patient's risk for future disease, with and without therapy. This estimate is a critical part of the treatment plan and of the discussion with the patient. Through reevaluation at various stages of therapy, you can redetermine the patient's risk based on how the patient has complied with, and responded to, therapy.

Health

If the patient has no history of attachment loss and no clinical signs of inflammation, the periodontal diagnosis is health (Fig 20-25). Treatment for these patients involves therapy for any dental complaints or problems and counseling on the need to modify any risk factors. These patients are reevaluated after 1 year.

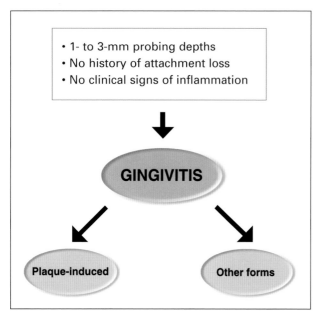

Fig 20-26 Initial diagnosis of gingivitis.

Gingivitis

There are two major subcategories of gingivitis: dental plaque–induced and non–plaque-induced gingivitis. A diagnostic overview for dental plaque–induced gingivitis is given in Fig 20-26. For greater detail, see chapter 22. Treatments for non–plaque-induced gingivitis are discussed elsewhere in this book.

Initial Diagnosis: Dental Plaque–Induced Gingivitis

Dental plaque–induced gingivitis is the most common inflammatory periodontal disease. It is characterized by clinical signs of inflammation that may include color changes of the gingiva, swelling of the soft tissues, and bleeding on probing. Bacterial plaque, as well as supragingival and subgingival calculus, is often a major clinical feature of this disease.

Treatment or Referral. Cases with an initial diagnosis of dental plaque–induced gingivitis should be handled by the general practitioner in the following manner:

1. Evaluate the patient's oral hygiene.
2. Take steps to improve the patient's oral hygiene, if necessary.
3. Remove calculus and bacterial products from the teeth (see chapter 22 for more details).
4. Eliminate or ameliorate risk factors.

Reevaluation. The case is reevaluated 30 to 60 days after initial treatment by redetermining the clinical indices gathered at the initial visit. The current status is then compared with the baseline.

Making a Final Diagnosis. The final diagnosis is based on the response of periodontal tissues to removal of dental plaque and its products. There are three possible final diagnoses:

1. *Dental plaque–induced gingivitis that has been arrested.* In this case, the clinical signs of inflammation have been eliminated, and the patient is placed in periodontal maintenance.
2. *Dental plaque–induced gingivitis that has not been arrested.* This diagnosis is made when the reason for continued signs of clinical inflammation is the failure of the therapist or the patient to remove sufficient bacteria and their products, not when the inflammation has a systemic or non–plaque-related component. The local factors should be identified and eliminated. A second re-evaluation is performed, and if inflammation has been resolved, a final diagnosis of arrested dental plaque–induced gingivitis is made, and the patient enters maintenance.
3. *Non–plaque-induced gingivitis.* If the patient performs oral hygiene measures effectively, the therapist has removed the local factors, and clinical signs of inflammation still exist, a final diagnosis of non–plaque-induced gingivitis is made. It should be noted that some patients may exhibit good oral hygiene at the reevaluation appointment but may have been inconsistent in their oral hygiene practices over time. These patients may have little plaque but will still have gingival inflammation. It is important to look for signs of tissue trauma and isolated areas of plaque accumulation that may suggest inconsistent plaque removal.

Initial Diagnosis: Non–Plaque-Induced Gingivitis

Many factors, ranging from hormonal factors to HIV infection, may contribute to gingivitis. Because treatment varies with etiology, therapy is discussed in other sections of this text.

Periodontitis

There are two subgroups of periodontitis: chronic and aggressive periodontitis.

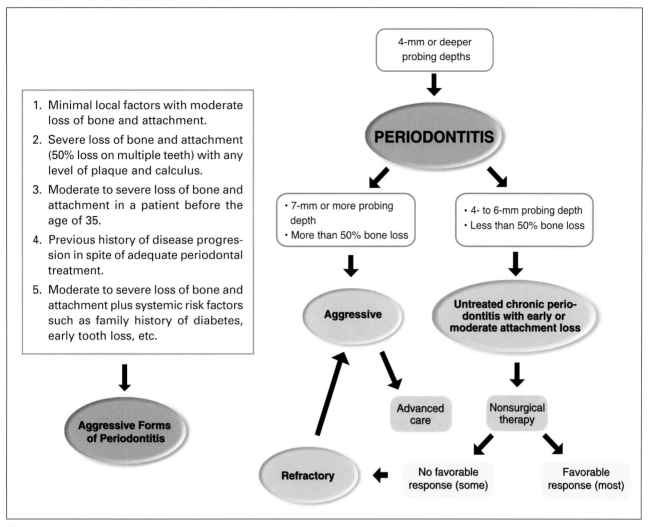

1. Minimal local factors with moderate loss of bone and attachment.
2. Severe loss of bone and attachment (50% loss on multiple teeth) with any level of plaque and calculus.
3. Moderate to severe loss of bone and attachment in a patient before the age of 35.
4. Previous history of disease progression in spite of adequate periodontal treatment.
5. Moderate to severe loss of bone and attachment plus systemic risk factors such as family history of diabetes, early tooth loss, etc.

Aggressive Forms of Periodontitis

4-mm or deeper probing depths

PERIODONTITIS

- 7-mm or more probing depth
- More than 50% bone loss

- 4- to 6-mm probing depth
- Less than 50% bone loss

Aggressive

Untreated chronic periodontitis with early or moderate attachment loss

Advanced care

Nonsurgical therapy

Refractory

No favorable response (some)

Favorable response (most)

Fig 20-27 A decision diagram to aid in making an initial diagnosis for patients with periodontitis.

Initial Diagnosis: Chronic Periodontitis

Chronic forms of periodontitis are the most common. They are characterized by bone loss (probing depth of 4 mm or greater) and soft tissue margins at the cementoenamel junction with signs of clinical inflammation.

This category is further subdivided according to whether or not bone has been lost in the furcations. This distinction is important because once bone has been lost between the roots of a tooth, it becomes much harder for the patient and the clinician to clean these areas, thus leading in many cases to further attachment loss. For the purposes of this text, *chronic periodontitis* with early attachment loss refers to cases that have 4- to 6-mm probing depths and no bone loss in the furcations. *Chronic periodontitis with moderate attachment loss* (4- to 6-mm probing depth) involves bone loss in the interfurcal areas up to Class II, but not including through-and-through (Class III) furcation defects (Fig 20-27). *Severe periodonti-*

tis is defined here as having probing depths of 7 mm or greater.

The approach outlined in this section can be used to treat patients with an initial diagnosis of early to moderate chronic periodontitis or patients who were first diagnosed with an aggressive form of periodontitis that has been converted to a chronic state. With patients in the latter group, the traditional approaches described here can be used once the microorganisms and/or other risk factors associated with the more aggressive problems have been reduced or eliminated.

The treatment of chronic periodontitis is divided into two stages: active therapy and periodontal maintenance (formerly called *supportive periodontal therapy*). Active therapy is subdivided into initial and surgical therapy. The outline of therapy used in this chapter for these chronic problems was introduced in the late 1950s,[31] but with certain modifications it is still relevant (see Fig 20-24).

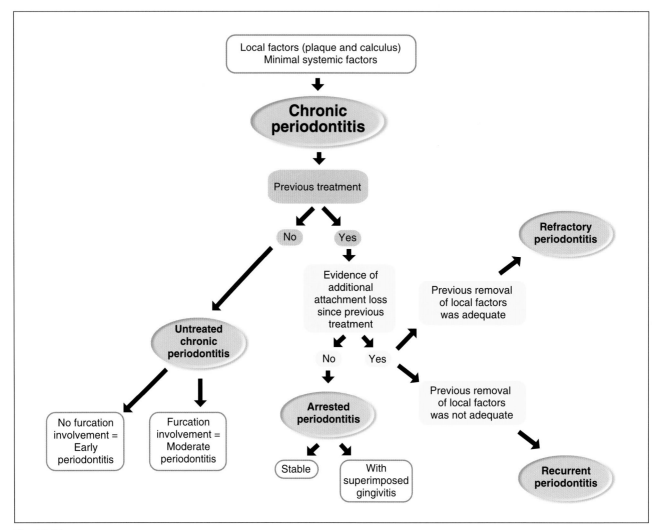

Fig 20-28 A decision diagram to aid in making a treatment plan for patients with chronic periodontitis.

Treatment/referral and initial therapy. Initial therapy for patients with early to moderate localized or generalized periodontitis should be performed by the general practitioner (Figs 20-28 and 20-29). It begins after the first examination has been completed, an initial diagnosis has been made, risk factors have been identified, and the patient has accepted a treatment plan.

The first step in initial therapy should be a review of the patient's oral hygiene and a discussion of risk factors. Scaling and root planing usually follow. In most cases of early attachment loss, these procedures eliminate the local factors well enough to be the only form of periodontal therapy needed prior to maintenance. Surgery is rarely needed in early cases, but it is occasionally used to correct some gingival deformity that inhibits plaque removal.

The goal of initial therapy is to remove enough local irritants to stop the progression of attachment loss and to encourage the patient to comply with suggested oral hygiene and periodontal maintenance so that the stability achieved by the active therapy can be maintained. In many cases with moderate attachment loss (bone loss in the furcations), the goal of removing all of the tooth-borne subgingival accretions will not be met using traditional closed scaling and root planing.[32–35] These studies cited show that in pockets deeper than 5 mm, it is likely that some subgingival bacterial plaque and calculus will remain despite as much as 30 minutes of subgingival scaling and root planing on a single tooth using traditional approaches. Even after scaling and root planing have been performed with surgical access, some bacterial deposits may remain on the roots. Endoscopy (discussed later in

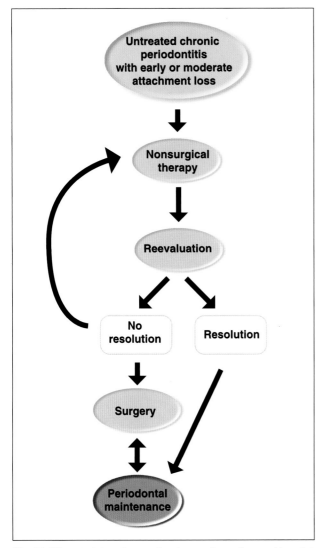

Fig 20-29 A decision diagram for therapy for patients with an initial diagnosis of chronic periodontitis.

perienced following surgery. When hypermobility, increasing tooth mobility, or fremitus still exists after occlusal adjustment, habit appliances, splinting of teeth, or both are often warranted. In cases of advanced mobility, procedures designed to reduce this parameter can be performed at the same time that closed subgingival scaling and root planing are done.

The initial stage of therapy for periodontitis is often an ideal time to place dental implants. For example, if the treatment plan calls for two-stage implants, then stage 1 surgery (placement) can be performed at the same time that closed subgingival scaling and root planing are done. If periodontal surgery is subsequently indicated, it can be performed when the implants are uncovered. One-stage implants can be placed during either the initial or surgical phase.

Reevaluation. The initial phase of therapy is intended to begin to achieve the therapeutic objectives of reducing and controlling the bacterial challenge and inflammation. Reevaluation allows the practitioner to assess how the patient has responded to the therapy and to identify additional therapeutic needs. Although experienced practitioners often identify areas requiring surgical intervention at the initial examination, in most cases the reevaluation is essential to the recognition of atypical response patterns and should be performed prior to embarking on a therapeutic approach that could produce a less-than-optimal outcome, such as surgery or restorative dentistry. In the treatment planning process described in this chapter, reevaluation is the means of confirming or modifying the presumptive diagnosis. Until more specific diagnostic tools are available, clinical response to scaling, root planing, and plaque control provide a practical approach of grouping patients and selecting therapy for the most predictable clinical outcomes.

Results of reevaluation and establishing a final diagnosis

1. The following are common findings seen after initial therapy at sites on single-rooted teeth that initially had 4- to 6-mm probing depths:
   a. A decrease in probing depths of 1 to 2 mm
   b. Elimination or substantial reduction of the clinical signs of inflammation, especially on probing
2. Rationale: Single-rooted teeth with shallow to moderate probing depths are accessible for scaling and root planing and plaque control. It is therefore possible to accurately assess the quality of therapy and the patient's response to therapy with minimal complicating factors. Such assessments cannot be made in sites with furcation involvement or deeper pocket probing depths. Accessible sites in a patient with chronic periodontitis will show a good response to local therapy.

this chapter) or surgery allow a more efficient removal of bacterial deposits in deep pockets.[34] In general, the deeper the probing depths, the less chance of removing these deposits.

After a short healing period (usually 30 to 60 days), data are again collected, and a reevaluation is performed. If inflammation is still found around a tooth with fremitus or a tooth mobility of one and a half (I+) is found, then occlusal therapy should be considered for that tooth. The adjustment often removes occlusal interferences such as fremitus and nonworking and working interferences on periodontally involved teeth. In addition, it often eliminates or ameliorates thermal sensitivity and discomfort ex-

3. A failure to get the expected response in accessible sites may indicate:
   a. Inadequate scaling and root planing
   b. Inadequate home care
   c. Failure to reduce or ameliorate systemic risk factors
   d. A more aggressive disease pattern (an aggressive form of periodontitis)
4. If the expected response in accessible sites is not achieved, rule out:
   a. Inadequate scaling and root planing
   b. Inadequate home care
   c. Failure to control systemic risk factors
5. Assign a final diagnosis of an aggressive form of periodontitis if the expected response is not achieved in accessible sites despite adequate scaling and root planing and home care.
6. If the expected response in accessible sites is achieved:
   a. Assign a final diagnosis of chronic periodontitis.
   b. Plan further treatment as necessary for remaining sites with evidence of disease.

Possible outcomes at reevaluation

1. *No sites with evidence of disease remain.* In this case, the soft tissues appear clinically normal, and the probing depths are 3 mm or less in all sites. The final diagnosis is arrested chronic periodontitis. This case is now transferred to periodontal maintenance.
2. *Periodontitis has not been arrested.* The presence of sites with clinical inflammation and probing depths greater than normal can mean one of two things: either the initial diagnosis of chronic periodontitis was incorrect, or the pockets were too deep or tortuous to allow adequate removal of bacteria and their products. Therefore, the clinical signs and symptoms of disease could not be controlled.
   a. If areas accessible to closed subgingival scaling and root planing (usually single-rooted, nonfurcated teeth with initial probing depths of 4 to 6 mm) have shown resolution of clinical signs of inflammation, but inaccessible areas (usually furcations) still have clinical signs of inflammation, the final diagnosis is chronic periodontitis that has not been arrested. Further professional therapy is needed to manage individual sites in the mouth. This therapy can consist of additional closed subgingival scaling and root planing, possibly with the dental endoscope or surgical therapy (see the following section).
   b. If areas accessible to closed subgingival scaling and root planing still show signs of clinical inflammation and/or attachment loss, and the patient and clinician have done an adequate job of removing tooth-borne accretions, a final diagnosis of an aggressive form of periodontitis is made. At this point, one

should consider referral to a clinician with advanced experience in the management of such cases (see chapter 27).

- The presence of sites with clinical inflammation but probing depths reduced to 3 mm or less usually indicates that the professional therapy was successful, but the patient is not doing an adequate job with oral hygiene. The patient should be reinstructed, reevaluated, and when appropriate, placed in periodontal maintenance with a final diagnosis of arrested chronic periodontitis.
- The presence of sites with no clinical inflammation but with probing depths greater than 3 mm presents a diagnostic and clinical challenge, because without scrupulous oral hygiene measures by the patient and frequent periodontal maintenance, these cases tend to relapse. It is best to inform the patient of the potential problem and then schedule periodontal maintenance in 3 months. At each periodontal maintenance visit, the case must be carefully evaluated for signs of clinical inflammation or attachment loss. The final diagnosis will most likely be chronic periodontitis, depending on the patient's responses during periodontal maintenance. These patients may require surgical care if attachment loss progresses.

Therapy for deeper probing depths found following initial therapy. **Surgical therapy.** Some deeper lesions can be controlled with traditional closed scaling and root planing. However, other cases with a final diagnosis of moderate (and occasionally early) chronic periodontitis that still have deepened pockets with clinical signs of inflammation often benefit from surgery. Surgical approaches in chronic periodontitis cases may differ greatly, depending on the severity of previous destruction and the objectives of therapy. Surgery in early to moderate cases of chronic periodontitis offers the following advantages:

1. Less treatment time for the patient than with closed subgingival scaling and root planing
2. Increased visualization of the root surface for more effective scaling and root planing (compared with traditional methods of closed subgingival scaling and root planing)
3. The chance to perform pocket reduction surgery, which allows the following:
   a. The ability to predictably reduce probing depths with concomitant diminution of periodontopathic bacteria
   b. Improved access for oral hygiene by the patient
   c. Easier access for root planing during periodontal maintenance

In such cases, surgery may have the following disadvantages:

1. Increased root sensitivity to thermal insult
2. Esthetic changes in anterior areas

Surgical candidates should be carefully selected. To be a candidate, the patient should be in good enough physical health to undergo surgery; the teeth must be stable enough to allow a comfortable healing period; and the patient optimally is an adequate complier to suggested oral hygiene measures, periodontal maintenance, or both. In most cases, patients also should have had adequate closed subgingival scaling and root planing to prevent unneeded surgery or to prepare the tissues for surgery and should have probing depths of 5 mm or greater, and clinical signs of inflammation. The decision to perform surgery is made by both the therapist and the patient after informed consent.

At present, because of a lack of accuracy in deciding when the disease process is active, both overtreatment and undertreatment probably occur. Once clinicians are better able to establish when true disease activity is occurring, it will be possible to treat more accurately and more selectively.

Once the decision is made to proceed with surgery, the therapist must decide—again with the patient's consent—which form (or forms) of surgery will be best. Following therapy, the case is reevaluated, and the patient is directed for further care, usually periodontal maintenance.

There is much debate concerning the most effective means to reduce pocket probing depths associated with shallow interdental osseous craters. These craters are the most commonly found bony defect associated with periodontitis[36] and usually are manifested clinically as interproximal probing depths ranging from 5 to 6 mm. In cases where other surgical criteria are met and where the gingival tissues are close to the cementoenamel junction on posterior teeth with normal root lengths, pocket reduction is most predictably performed using positive architecture osseous surgery.[37–39] The same procedure can be used to lengthen clinical crowns to enhance restorative procedures or esthetics.

The Dental Endoscope. The dental endoscope allows visualization of the subgingival environment at a magnification of up to 50×. This device allows removal of toothborne accretions to levels heretofore impossible. The cleaner root surface produced has resulted in clinical responses not routinely produced using traditional blind approaches.[40]

Compliance and its effect on treatment planning. Chronic inflammatory diseases are not currently curable.

Evidence is provided by the recent finding that the greatest single predictor of future disease activity is history of periodontitis. Patients with these problems require continuous monitoring of their periodontal status and oral hygiene and often need frequent periodontal maintenance visits to maintain attachment levels. Thus, patient compliance with professional suggestions is of utmost importance in containing these diseases. Unfortunately, most patients have been shown not to comply with either suggested oral hygiene measures[41] or periodontal maintenance, thus leading to the need for re-treatment or to loss of teeth.[42] Patients who do not meet their clinicians' requirements for oral hygiene often experience additional attachment loss after surgery.

Initial Diagnosis: Severe Generalized Chronic Periodontitis and Aggressive Periodontitis

Patients in whom disease is severe or in whom disease progression is rapid are not "managing" the bacterial challenge as well as patients with early or moderate chronic periodontitis. The use of the term *aggressive* indicates that the disease most likely progressed more rapidly than is normally seen in early or moderate adult periodontitis. Such situations are most likely the result of inadequate host defenses, but occasionally they are caused by an unusual bacterial challenge. The relationship between disease and plaque accumulation in these cases is less clear. Therefore, the approach to therapy differs from the approaches used in chronic periodontitis (Fig 20-30).

Treatment/referral. These cases are often difficult to control, and relapses occur frequently. Since they represent a very small percentage of total cases seen in the average general dental office and since they require advanced diagnostics and therapy, these cases may be best managed in a specialist office.

Several general principles apply to these cases. First, because severe chronic periodontitis and generalized aggressive periodontitis are often associated with alterations in host defenses, the therapy should begin by exploring the risk factors that may contribute to changes in the defense systems. Increasing evidence in recent years has implicated genetic influences on periodontal disease severity. Although the genetic factors cannot currently be altered, it is often valuable to test for these defects, especially in smokers. Nongenetic factors, including smoking, diabetes mellitus, viral infections, and prolonged stress, have been shown to produce substantial alterations in host defenses. Smoking and diabetes mellitus have been strongly associated with severe chronic periodontitis, and clinicians have long believed that there is a link between stress and periodontitis. Since these factors are modifiable,

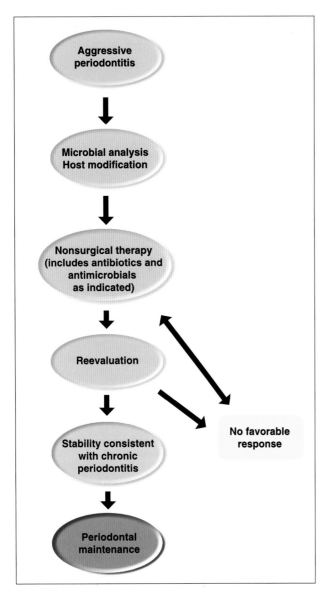

Aggressive periodontitis

↓

Microbial analysis Host modification

↓

Nonsurgical therapy (includes antibiotics and antimicrobials as indicated)

↓

Reevaluation

↓

Stability consistent with chronic periodontitis

↓

Periodontal maintenance

No favorable response

Fig 20-30 A decision diagram for therapy for patients with an initial diagnosis of aggressive periodontitis or severe chronic periodontitis.

may be necessary. Bacterial sampling and antibiotic specificity testing may be helpful in these cases. Future therapies directed at strengthening the host response may provide new opportunities for managing these diseases.

Third, surgery may not be advisable in aggressive forms of periodontitis until the infection is under control. Localized aggressive periodontitis in young patients (previously termed *localized juvenile periodontitis*) appears to be an exception to this principle. In most cases of severe and rapidly progressing disease, an altered host defense may make the response to surgery unpredictable. This is very different from the situation in early to moderate chronic periodontitis.

Accepted diagnostic categories for the aggressive forms are not well defined. The goal of therapy in aggressive cases is to halt the bacterial process and to achieve a more favorable balance between the bacteria and the host so that conventional therapy may be more predictably applied.

Initial therapy is modified in these cases to attempt to control systemic factors that may influence treatment response and to achieve more definitive control of the bacterial challenge. The guidelines for therapy in aggressive forms of periodontitis are very different from those in chronic periodontitis. Therapy for aggressive periodontitis is outlined in chapter 24.

References

1. Bernier JL. Report of the committee on classification and nomenclature. J Periodontol 1957;28:56.
2. Box HK. Periodontal studies. Dent Items Interest 1940;62:915.
3. Carranza FA Sr, Carranza FA Jr. A suggested classification of common periodontal diseases. J Periodontol 1959;30:140.
4. Carranza FA Jr. Classification of periodontal disease. In: Carranza FA Jr (ed). Glickman's Clinical Periodontology. Philadelphia: Saunders, 1984:193–194.
5. Fish EW. Paradontal Disease. London: Eyre and Spottiswoode, 1944.
6. Orban B. Classification of periodontal disease. Paradentologie 1949;3:159.
7. Thoma KH, Goldman HM. Classification and histopathology of paradontal disease. J Am Dent Assoc 1937;24:1915.
8. Weski O. Paradentopathia and parodentosis. Paradentium 1937;8:169.
9. Diagnosis of Periodontal Diseases. Chicago: American Academy of Periodontology, 1992:1.
10. Genco RJ, Goldman HM, Cohen W (eds). Contemporary Periodontics. St. Louis: Mosby, 1990:65.
11. Grant D, Stern I, Listgarten M. Periodontics. St. Louis: Mosby, 1988.
12. Current Procedural Terminology for Periodontics. Chicago: American Academy of Periodontology, 1989.
13. Kornman KS, Newman MG, Alvarado R, et al. Clinical and microbiological patterns of adults with periodontitis. J Periodontol 1991;62:634–642.

they should be assessed and managed to the extent possible as part of the therapy.

Second, the lack of a strong association between plaque accumulations and disease severity in the aggressive forms of periodontitis and the host alterations noted above often mean that these patients are less responsive to conventional periodontal therapy, which is focused on plaque removal from the root surfaces. This does not mean that plaque control is unimportant, but rather that more specific approaches to controlling the bacterial challenge

14. Nevins M, Becker W, Kornman K. Consensus report discussion. In: Proceedings of the World Workshop in Clinical Periodontics. Chicago: American Academy of Periodontology 1989: I23–I24.

15. Baer P, Benjamin S. Periodontal Diseases in Children and Adolescents. Philadelphia: Lippincott, 1974.

16. Baer PN. The case for periodontosis as a clinical entity. J Periodontol 1971;42:516–520.

17. Saxen L. Juvenile periodontitis. J Clin Periodontol 1980;7:1–19.

18. Page RC, Bowen T, Altman L, et al. Prepubertal periodontitis. I. Definition of a clinical disease entity. J Periodontol 1983;54: 257–271.

19. Page RC, Beatty P, Waldrop TC. Molecular basis for the functional abnormality in neutrophils from patients with generalized prepubertal periodontitis. J Periodontal Res 1987;22:182–183.

20. Delaney JE, Kornman KS. Microbiology of subgingival plaque from children with localized prepubertal periodontitis. Oral Microbiol Immunol 1987;2:71–76.

21. Page RC, Altman LC, Ebersole JL, et al. Rapidly progressive periodontitis: A distinct clinical condition. J Periodontol 1983;54: 197–209.

22. Haffajee AD, Socransky SS, Dzink JL, et al. Clinical, microbiological and immunological features of subjects with refractory periodontal diseases. J Clin Periodontol 1988;15:390–398.

23. Glossary of Periodontal Terms, ed 3. Chicago: American Academy of Periodontology, 1992.

24. Armitage GC. Development of a classification system for periodontal diseases and conditions. Ann Periodontol 1999;4(1):1–6.

25. Butler RT, Kalkwarf KL, Kaldahl WB. Drug-induced gingival hyperplasia: Phenytoin, cyclosporine, and nifedipine. J Am Dent Assoc 1987;114(1):56–60.

26. Goodson JM, Tanner ACR, Haffajee AD, et al. Patterns of progression and regression of advanced destructive periodontal disease. J Clin Periodontol 1982;9:472–481.

27. Muzyka BC, Glick M. HIV infection and necrotizing stomatitis. Gen Dent 1994;42:66–68.

28. Lekholm U, Ericsson I, Adell R, Slots J. The condition of the soft tissues at tooth and fixture abutments supporting fixed bridges: A microbiological and histological study. J Clin Periodontol 1986;13:558–562.

29. Mombelli A, Van Oosten MA, Schurch E Jr, Lang NP. The microbiota associated with successful or failing osseointegrated titanium implants. Oral Microbiol Immunol 1987;2:145–151.

30. Becker W, Becker BE, Newman MG, Nyman S. Clinical and microbiologic findings that may contribute to dental implant failure. Int J Oral Maxillofac Implants 1990;5:31–38.

31. Corn H, Marks MH. Strategic extraction in periodontal therapy. Dent Clin North Am 1969;13:817–843.

32. Stambaugh RV, Dragoo M, Smith DM, Carasal L. The limits of subgingival scaling. Int J Periodontics Restorative Dent 1981; 1(5):30–41.

33. Waerhaug J. Healing of the dento-epithelial junction following subgingival plaque control. II. As observed on extracted teeth. J Periodontol 1978;49(3):119–134.

34. Caffesse RG, Sweeney PL, Smith BA. Scaling and root planing with and without periodontal flap surgery. J Clin Periodontol 1986;13:205–210.

35. Brayer WK, Mellonig JT, Dunlap RM, et al. Scaling and root planing effectiveness: The effect of root surface access and operator experience. J Periodontol 1989;60(1):67–72.

36. Saari JT, Hurt WC, Biggs NL. Periodontal bony defects on the dry skull. J Periodontol 1968;39:278–283.

37. Everett FG, Waerhaug J, Widman A. Leonard Widman: Surgical treatment of pyorrhea alveolaris. J Periodontol 1971;42:571–579.

38. Schluger S. Osseous resection—A basic principle in periodontal surgery. Oral Surg Oral Med Oral Pathol 1949;2:316–325.

39. Ochsenbein C, Ross S. A reevaluation of osseous surgery. Dent Clin North Am 1969;13:87–102.

40. Stambaugh RV, Myers G, Ebling KL, et al. Endoscopic visualization of the submarginal gingiva dental sulcus and tooth root surfaces. J Periodontol 2002;73:374–382.

41. Johansson LA, Oster B, Hamp SE. Evaluation of cause-related periodontal therapy and compliance with maintenance care recommendations. J Clin Periodontol 1984;11(10):689–699.

42. Wilson TG, Glover ME, Schoen J, et al. Compliance with maintenance therapy in a private periodontal practice. J Periodontol 1984;55:468–473.

The Healthy Patient

Thomas G. Wilson, Jr, and Kenneth S. Kornman

- Collecting the Clinical and Radiographic Evidence
- Interpreting the Evidence
- Making a Clinical Diagnosis
- Determining Risk Factors
- Estimating the Prognosis
- Formulating a Treatment Plan and Treating the Patient

R ecent advances allow the clinician to determine a patient's prognosis more reliably and thereby develop a treatment plan better tailored for that individual. The clinician uses an approach based on the analysis of local and systemic risk factors for developing inflammatory periodontal disease. The clinician gathers information about the patient's oral condition as outlined in chapter 17. Local risk factors, such as bacterial status and the presence of pockets or rough subgingival margins that may shelter the bacteria, can be gleaned from these data. In some cases of aggressive disease, the identification of specific bacteria and their antibiotic susceptibility may be helpful. Clinicians now understand that certain systemic risk factors also can have a significant effect on the clinical course of periodontal disease. Among the strongest systemic factors are smoking, diabetes mellitus, and certain genetic modifications. The prognosis can be determined by the extent to which the local and systemic risk factors can be eliminated or ameliorated.

The order of therapy is to *(1)* collect the clinical and radiographic evidence, *(2)* interpret the evidence, *(3)* make a clinical diagnosis, *(4)* determine risk factors, *(5)* determine the prognosis, *(6)* formulate a treatment plan, and *(7)* treat the patient.

There are three basic clinical conditions of the periodontium: health, gingivitis, and periodontitis. These conditions may be seen separately or in combination. The details of an actual case will be used to illustrate how to approach clinical and radiographic examinations, diagnosis, and treatment systematically. This sequence is the same one used in daily practice, and it will be followed in the chapters on

gingivitis, chronic periodontitis, and aggressive forms of periodontitis. The reader will be given an outline and then referred to other sections of this text for further information on individual subjects. Case histories are used to demonstrate how an experienced practitioner sifts through the available data to focus on what is important in each case.

Collecting the Clinical and Radiographic Evidence

John Brooks presents to your practice, having just moved from another city. His main concern (chief complaint) is to continue his regular dental therapy. Like all patients, he fills out a health history form, which you review with him (see appendix 1). He brings with him a letter from his previous practitioner summarizing his dental history and a complete set of radiographs taken within the past year. In the initial telephone conversation it was learned that the patient had a heart murmur. His physician was contacted, and appropriate antibiotic prophylaxis was suggested. The patient took the medication as prescribed before his appointment. (See appendix 2 for more details.)

In your initial interview with the patient, you find him to be a well-nourished, well-oriented man who is 36 years old. He has a family history of heart disease. He works as an architect for a well-known local firm. His goals for his stomatognathic system include keeping his teeth for as long as possible in a healthy and comfortable state.

THE EVIDENCE

Health History

1. Medical
   - Mr Brooks' health history reveals nothing that would influence his oral health, but he does have a heart murmur.
2. Dental
   - The patient sees his practitioner for examination and appropriate treatment as often as suggested.
   - He knows a great deal about his dental condition.
   - He reports no history of periodontal disease.
   - He reports that he brushes his teeth and uses dental floss twice daily and has done so for many years.

Extraoral Examination

1. The head and neck are inspected visually for asymmetries and abnormal features. Any deviations from normal are recorded.
   - None are found.
2. The temporomandibular joints are inspected by palpation during range-of-motion movements, and any noise or tenderness is recorded.
   - Mr Brooks' joints elicit no sounds during movement and are not tender to palpation.
3. The lips are examined and any abnormalities (including location and size) noted, since a large percentage of oral neoplasms are found here.
   - Mr Brooks' lip tissues show no signs of abnormalities.

Intraoral Examination

1. Any discoloration (usually white, red, or black) of the oral mucosal tissues is recorded, including location and size.
2. The tongue is grasped at the tip with cotton gauze and gently moved anteriorly to inspect the lateral borders, since this is the most frequent site for intraoral neoplasms and changes associated with certain chronic conditions.
   - No abnormalities are found.

Clinical Examination (see chapter 17)

1. Dental (Figs 21-1a to 21-1c)
   - All teeth are present and in good alignment.
   - No dental caries, periapical lesions, or other dental abnormalities are noted.
   - The teeth are not mobile.
   - The patient has only one dental restoration, an amalgam on the mandibular right first molar.
2. Periodontal: The periodontal findings are compatible with the clinical definition of health (Fig 21-2).
   - Probing depths are 1 to 3 mm, with the gingival margins at or slightly coronal to the cementoenamel junctions (CEJs).
   - No bleeding on probing is found. No redness, change of color, swelling, or other signs of gingival inflammation are noted.

   These findings are associated with clinical health of the gingival tissues.

Radiographic Examination

The normal radiographic appearance of the alveolar crest is characterized by the presence of cortical bone. This crestal cortication appears as a thin but distinct radiopaque line contiguous with the laminae dura of adjacent teeth. In the posterior regions, the junction of the alveolar crest with the laminae dura is boxlike, forming a sharp, distinct angle. In all regions, the normal alveolar crest lies 1 to 2 mm subjacent to the CEJ of adjacent teeth and parallels adjacent CEJs. (See chapter 18 for more information.)
- Radiographic examination is normal (Figs 21-3 and 21-4).

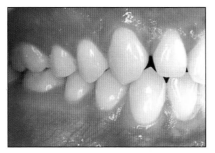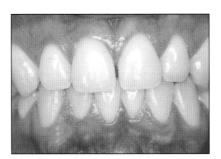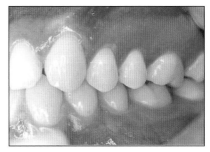

Figs 21-1a to 21-1c This patient exhibits no clinical signs of gingival inflammation and has no history of attachment loss.

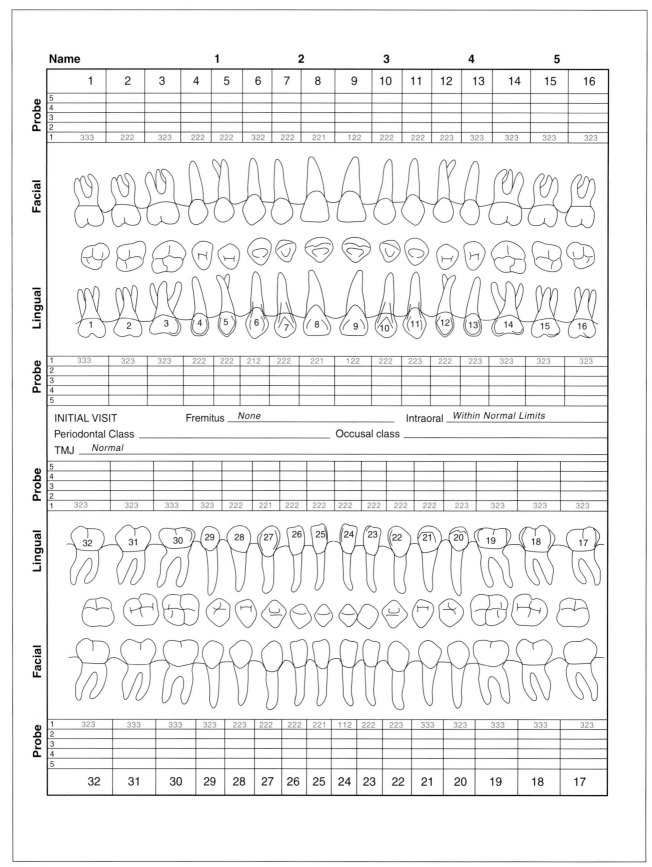

Fig 21-2 Periodontal charting for this patient.

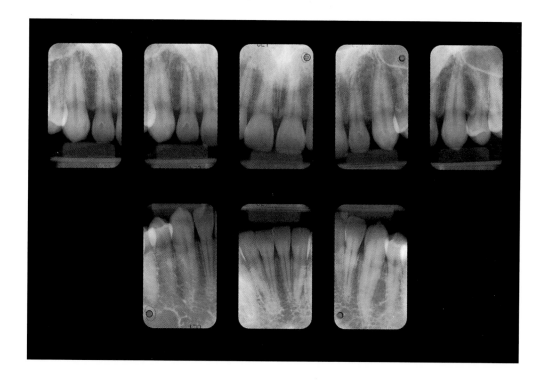

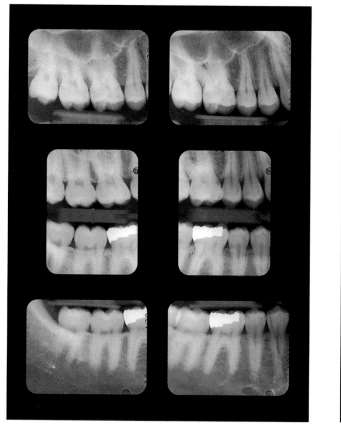

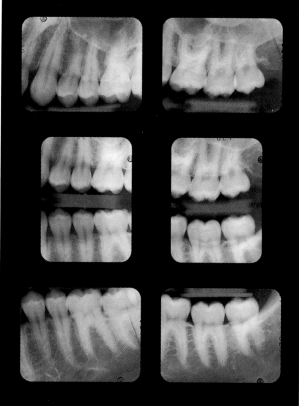

Fig 21-3 Full-mouth series of radiographs from this healthy patient.

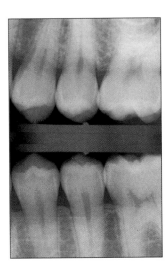

Fig 21-4 Posterior vertical bitewing radiograph from the patient. The alveolar crests are 1 to 2 mm apical to the CEJs of the teeth.

Interpreting the Evidence

After reading this section you should have a basic understanding of the clinical and radiographic signs found in the healthy patient. In the following sections you will be able to review the knowledge that you need to make a differential diagnosis. The most likely disease or condition will be selected as the initial diagnosis, and this will be the driving force behind the initial treatment of this patient.

1. Make sure that the patient has no extraoral or intraoral problems that should be dealt with first. In Mr Brooks' case, none of these problems is evident.
2. Look for a systemic component to the disease process. Since all these findings are normal (except the heart murmur, which has already been dealt with), attention can be focused on the dental and periodontal findings.
3. Review the clinical sign and symptoms.
4. Review the radiographic signs.

The remainder of this section will focus on the third and fourth steps.

Clinical Signs and Symptoms

Gingival Inflammation

➤ *Gingival tissues are pale pink with no signs of inflammation.*

Healthy attached gingiva is pale pink and frequently stippled. Mr Brooks' tissues show no edema or redness as the result of inflammation, and the gingival margin has a regular, scalloped outline slightly coronal to the CEJ. The mucogingival line is usually clearly visible because of the

difference in color between the noninflamed pale pink attached gingiva and the deeply red alveolar mucosa.

The texture of the healthy attached gingiva and the interproximal gingival tissue is firm, in contrast to the edematous, swollen tissue in gingivitis, and the interdental papillae fill most of the interproximal spaces. The depth of the gingival sulcus, or pocket, in health does not exceed 3 mm, because there is no apical migration of the junctional epithelial attachment or loss of the periodontal ligament fibers, as seen in periodontitis (see chapter 3).

With minimal accumulation of bacteria at the gingival margin and in the sulcus, normal structures are intact, with minimal loss or modification of the gingival epithelium and connective tissue. Histologic evaluation of tissue from Mr Brooks would most likely show an occasional lymphocyte or plasma cell in the connective tissue. The number of neutrophils within the sulcular epithelium and gingival crevice would be minimal (see chapter 8).

When gingival health is observed in the presence of good oral hygiene, the supragingival plaque is immature and thinly covers the enamel surface at the gingival margin. The plaque is dominated by early colonizers such as streptococci, *Veillonella* species, and *Actinomyces* species, because good oral hygiene frequently disrupts the ecology. These bacteria produce small-molecular-weight compounds that are capable of inducing some tissue inflammation, but they are probably at low levels in the healthy patient (see chapter 5).

Examination of immunologic responses in periodontal health can focus on both systemic reactivities and local responses associated with the transudate in the gingival sulcus. Specific peripheral T-cell responses to suspected periodontopathic bacteria are generally very low in periodontally healthy subjects. Serum antibody levels to these bacteria are also generally low; however, healthy subjects do exhibit antibodies to various proposed pathogens, including *Actinobacillus actinomycetemcomitans, Porphyromonas gingivalis, Prevotella intermedia, Eubacterium corrodens,* and *Campylobacter rectus.* The healthy population exhibits a range of antibody levels to these types of bacteria, and specificity studies combined with microbiologic data suggest that the antibodies are directed to cross-reacting antigenic epitopes that may be expressed by microorganisms in the commensal microbiota. The local transudate contains a variety of serumlike proteins, glycoproteins, and lipoproteins, the concentration of which appears to depend on the molecular size and represents a filtering through the tissues into the sulcus. Finally, the presence of subgingival plaque, even in the healthiest sulcus, is the basis for the host inflammatory response to these bacteria. Thus, although clinical inflammation is absent, low levels of certain inflammatory mediators (prostaglandins and leukotrienes), as well as some cytokines, can be detected. How these molecules contribute to the maintenance of health in conjunction with normal treatment modalities is unknown (see chapters 8 and 9).

Probing Depths

➤ *Probing depths are 3 mm or less.*

The periodontal probe stops at different levels in the epithelium or connective tissue subjacent to the junctional epithelium, depending on the amount of inflammation present.

The periodontal attachment apparatus that connects the gingiva and periodontal ligament to the tooth is composed of connective tissue fibers that insert into the root surface and an epithelial attachment (the junctional epithelium) that involves epithelial cells from the gingiva attaching to the tooth surface by means of hemidesmosomes. In health and gingivitis, the normal level of the connective tissue attachment is approximately at the CEJ. In patients with periodontitis, the coronal portion of the connective tissue is at a more apical position. The clinically measured level of attachment is an indication of the severity of the previous periodontal destruction. Probing depth is measured with a periodontal probe as the distance from the gingival margin to where the probe stops at the most apical part of the sulcus or pocket. If there is no recession, one then measures the distance from the gingival margin to the CEJ and subtracts this distance from the probing depth to determine the clinical attachment level—ie, the amount of attachment loss apical to the CEJ. If there is recession, the distance from the CEJ to the free gingival margin is added to determine clinical attachment level. (See chapter 17 for specific information on how to probe.) Although the primary determinant of probing depth and clinical attachment level is the location of the connective tissue attachment, the actual measurement is a function of not only the connective tissue attachment location but also the amount of inflammation in the area, the pressure applied to the probe, and the diameter of the probe.

When there is minimal or no inflammation, the connective tissue fibers are intact, and the gingival epithelium is attached to the tooth via an epithelial attachment. The probe stops somewhere within the epithelial attachment and is somewhat coronal to the connective tissue attachment. When inflammation is present, the basal epithelial cells turn over more rapidly, preventing cell maturation and reducing the integrity of the epithelial attachment. In addition, the collagen fibers that make up the connective tissue attachment undergo some destruction. The net result is that with inflammation, the periodontal probe passes completely through the epithelial attachment and usually stops apical to the most coronal part of the connective tissue attachment.

With the increasing pressure on the periodontal probe, the apical penetration is increased (a higher probing-depth reading is found). With minimal inflammation the probe may stop within the epithelium or penetrate just into the underlying connective tissue, but with greater inflammation an increase in pressure results in more apical penetration of the probe into the connective tissue (again resulting in a higher probing-depth reading).

Relationship of Gingival Margin to CEJ

➤ *The gingival margin is located at or slightly coronal to the CEJ.*

The relationship of the gingival margin to the CEJ is important in establishing how much clinical attachment has been lost (and therefore to help make a correct diagnosis). In a healthy patient, the gingival margin will be located at or slightly coronal to the CEJ, as it was in Mr Brooks' case. The location of the free gingival margin is taken into account in a measurement called the *clinical attachment level (CAL)* (see chapter 17 for more details). The CAL is the sum of the number of millimeters of gingival recession and the probing depth. It is a good reflection of the amount of supporting tissue that has been destroyed by disease. If the probing depth alone is used, then one will not correctly assess the amount of destruction that has occurred. For example, deep pseudopockets reflect sites with hyperplasia or altered passive eruption without CAL. These conditions are often found on the lingual and distal aspects of second molars. As another example, one should be more concerned about a probing depth of 3 mm with 9 mm of recession than the same probing depth with no recession. This is because the 3-mm probing depth with no recession has no attachment loss, while the 3-mm probing depth with 9 mm of recession represents 12 mm of attachment loss and a great deal of destruction of the support for that tooth.

Radiographic Signs

The normal radiographic appearance of the alveolar crest is characterized by the presence of cortical bone. This crestal cortication appears as a thin but distinct radiopaque line contiguous with the laminae dura of adjacent teeth. In the posterior regions, the junction of the alveolar crest with the laminae dura is boxlike, forming a sharp, distinct angle. In the mandibular anterior region, the alveolar crest between the adjacent teeth is normally spear shaped or knifelike. In the maxillary anterior region, the alveolar crest may be rounded. In all regions, the normal alveolar crest lies 1 to 2 mm subjacent to the CEJ of adjacent teeth and parallels adjacent CEJs. (See chapter 18 for more information.)

Making a Clinical Diagnosis

1. Is the periodontium clinically healthy? *Yes, because there are no signs of inflammation and no previous attachment loss has occurred.*

The absence of visual signs of inflammation indicates gingival health. Measurements of the subgingival sulcus depths are 3 mm or less, and the gingival tissues are located in their normal position. This means that the coronal portion of the free gingival margin is located at or slightly coronal to the CEJ. Mr Brooks has no clinically detectable loss of periodontal support. The absence of gingival bleeding from the probed areas is also an important sign. It has been demonstrated that gingival tissues that do not bleed following gentle probing are healthy and that minimal or no periodontal attachment loss can be anticipated in these patients within the next 3 to 4 months.

2. Is this plaque-associated gingivitis? *No, because there are no signs of gingival inflammation.*
3. Is this chronic periodontitis? *No, because there are no radiographic signs of bone loss, and probing depths are 3 mm or less, with the soft tissues at the level of the CEJ.*
4. Is this an aggressive form of periodontitis? *No (for the same reasons it is not chronic periodontitis).*
5. So what is the presumptive diagnosis? *Health.*

Determining Risk Factors

Several factors, both local and systemic, can affect disease progression. Local factors include bacteria and any niches that protect them from daily disruption by the patient, as well as the degree to which the patient complies with the practitioner's suggestions. As previously discussed, if bacteria are allowed to remain undisturbed, they initiate and sustain an inflammatory reaction in the periodontal tissues, which will lead to tooth loss in some patients if untreated. As bacterial plaque matures, it can allow colonization of more pathogenic organisms. Where probing depths are shallow (3 mm or less) and the patient disrupts the plaque with daily oral hygiene, the clinical signs of gingivitis (such as bleeding on probing and color changes) can be reversed. If those patients have routine periodontal maintenance visits, they generally keep their teeth longer than those who do not. Unfortunately, many patients do not clean their teeth as suggested and do not schedule maintenance visits as often as recommended. This lack of compliance is a major risk factor of disease progression.

Systemic risk factors for progression of gingivitis to periodontitis include smoking, diabetes mellitus, and genetic factors. Patients who smoke develop periodontal disease more rapidly, heal more poorly, and lose teeth more rapidly compared with nonsmokers (see chapter 12). Individuals with diabetes mellitus experience more tooth loss from periodontal disease than do those who do not have the disease (see chapter 13). In general, the less severe the diabetes and the better its control, the better the prognosis for the patient's periodontal problem. A genetic change in the genes responsible for one of the inflammatory mediators in periodontal disease (interleukin 1) can result in increased levels of attachment loss and tooth loss compared with patients without the change (see chapter 11). In addition, patients who smoke and are positive for the interleukin 1 genotype are at greater risk than those without this combination of factors.

The following is a summary of the risk factors for Mr Brooks:

Local risk factors
1. There is no inflammation; therefore, whatever bacteria this patient harbors are not causing clinical signs of disease.
2. The patient's compliance to suggested oral hygiene has been good.

Systemic risk factors
1. The patient does not and has not smoked.
2. The patient has no family history of diabetes mellitus and does not currently have the disease.
3. The patient was not tested for the interleukin 1 genotype because there are no clinical signs of disease and he does not smoke.

Estimating the Prognosis

The prognosis depends on the degree to which local and systemic risk factors can be controlled. In Mr Brooks' case, there are no known risk factors; therefore, his prognosis is very good.

Formulating a Treatment Plan and Treating the Patient

At present Mr Brooks needs no periodontal treatment, so any needed dental therapy (eg, restorative dentistry or orthodontics) can be started. He is scheduled for a re-evaluation and cleaning (if needed) in 1 year. The patient is told of his diagnosis. He is informed that periodontal disease can have negative systemic effects, therefore it is important that he maintain his dental health (see chapter 15).

Treating Dental Plaque– Induced Gingivitis

Thomas G. Wilson, Jr, and Kenneth S. Kornman
- Collecting the Clinical and Radiographic Evidence
- Interpreting the Evidence
- Making a Clinical Diagnosis
- Determining Risk Factors for Disease Progression
- Determining the Prognosis
- Formulating a Treatment Plan

Bjorn Steffensen and John S. Sottosanti
- Defining Plaque-Induced Gingivitis
- Progression of Plaque-Induced Gingivitis to Periodontitis
- Prevention and Treatment Methods for Plaque-Induced Gingivitis
- Treatment Goals
- Patient Examination
- Informing the Patient
- Patient Factors in Plaque Control
- Treating Plaque-Induced Gingivitis
- Managing Appointments

Recent advances allow the clinician to determine a patient's prognosis more successfully and thereby develop a treatment plan tailored for that individual. The clinician uses an approach based on the analysis of local and systemic risk factors for developing periodontitis. The clinician gathers the same information about the patient's oral condition outlined in chapter 17. Local risk factors are gleaned from these data. These risk factors include deep pockets, rough subgingival margins, and other areas that may shelter microbes. In some cases, identification of specific bacteria and determination of antibiotic susceptibility may be helpful (see chapter 5). This is most commonly recommended for cases in which (1) the clinical severity of destruction exceeds expectations, given the level of bacterial plaque, or (2) systemic risk factors are present that suggest that the patient's host response may not adequately control the bacterial challenge. Among the strongest systemic risk factors are smoking, diabetes mellitus, and a genetic modification that puts the patient at increased risk. The prognosis for the case can be determined by the extent to which the bacterial and systemic risk factors can be eliminated or ameliorated.

The order of therapy is to (1) collect the clinical and radiographic evidence; (2) interpret the evidence; (3) make a clinical diagnosis, (4) determine risk factors for disease progression, (5) determine the prognosis using risk factor analysis, (6) formulate a treatment plan, and (7) treat the patient.

There are three basic clinical conditions of the periodontium: health, gingivitis, and periodontitis. These may be seen separately or in combination. Gingivitis connotes inflammation of the gingival tissues, which is presumed to precede periodontitis. This section details the findings of a patient with plaque-induced gingivitis.

THE EVIDENCE

Health history

1. Medical
   - Ms Padgett's health history reveals nothing that would negatively influence her oral health. She does not smoke, have diabetes mellitus, or have a family history of diabetes mellitus. Because of her prosthetic knee, her oral health could affect her general health. Her physician is contacted and suggests that she receive antibiotics before dental work.
2. Dental
   - The patient has seen a dental practitioner in the past only when she has been in pain.
   - She is an intelligent person who does not understand much about dentistry.
   - She brushes twice daily but does not use dental floss.

Extraoral Examination

1. The head and neck are inspected visually for asymmetries and abnormal features.
   - ➤ No deviations from normal are noted.
2. The temporomandibular joints are inspected by palpation during range-of-motion movements, and any noise or tenderness is recorded.
   - ➤ The joints move well, and there is no noise or pain on palpation.
3. The lips are examined and any abnormalities (including location and size) are noted, since a large percentage of oral lesions are found here.
   - ➤ No abnormalities are found. This is recorded.

Intraoral Examination

1. Any discoloration (usually white, red, or black) of the oral mucosal tissues is recorded, including location and size.
   - ➤ No abnormalities are found.
2. The tongue is grasped at the tip with cotton gauze and gently moved anteriorly to inspect the lateral borders since this is the most frequent site for intraoral tumors and changes associated with certain chronic conditions.
   - ➤ No abnormalities are found.

Risk Factors

1. Local
   - Bacteria are present, but there are no niches that would prevent their removal by the patient.
   - Compliance to suggestions on oral hygiene (flossing) and periodic maintenance visits is not and has not been good.
2. Systemic
   - She does not smoke.
   - She has no family history of diabetes mellitus and does not currently have the disease.
   - There are two possible approaches to the use of genetic testing in patients with gingivitis: to test before therapy begins or to test following initial therapy when generalized signs of inflammation (eg, bleeding on probing) are seen in patients with adequate oral hygiene. Testing becomes more important in patients who smoke.

Clinical Examination (see chapter 17)

1. Dental (Fig 22-1)
   - ➤ All teeth are present except the third molars, which were extracted 4 years ago at the suggestion of her previous practitioner.
   - ➤ There is bacterial plaque at the gingival margins of a number of teeth.
   - ➤ Calculus is present on the lingual aspect of the mandibular anterior teeth.
   - ➤ The teeth are not mobile.
   - ➤ No clinical evidence of dental caries is found.
2. Periodontal (Figs 22-2 and 22-3)
   - ➤ Probing depths are 3 mm or less.
   - ➤ There is bleeding found after probing in a number of areas.
   - ➤ Some interproximal gingival tissues are red and slightly swollen.
   - ➤ No gingival recession has occurred.

Radiographic Examination (Fig 22-4)

- ➤ Radiographic findings are within normal limits.

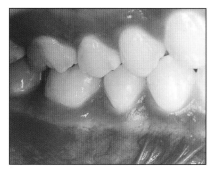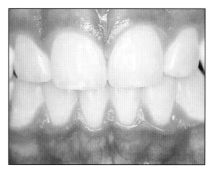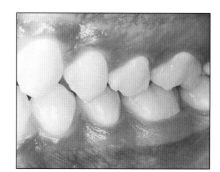

Figs 22-1a to 22-1c The patient's dental and periodontal condition at the initial visit.

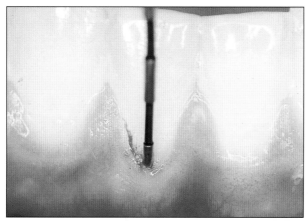

Fig 22-2 Facial view of the mandibular anterior teeth at the initial visit. Note the bacterial plaque and bleeding seen on probing.

Collecting the Clinical and Radiographic Evidence

Penny Padgett presents to your office. Her reason for coming (chief complaint) is that she has not had a dental checkup in the past few years.

Like all patients, she fills out a health history (see appendix 1). Because it has been a number of years since a full-mouth series of radiographs was obtained, you suggest a complete set of right-angle and bitewing radiographs (see chapter 18).

In your initial interview with the patient, you find a well-nourished, well-oriented woman who is 42 years old. She has just graduated from college and started her own business. Her goals for her stomatognathic system include keeping her teeth for as long as possible in a healthy and comfortable state. In the initial telephone interview, she said she has had a prosthetic knee replacement, and her physician suggests premedication.

Interpreting the Evidence

After reading this section you should understand the clinical, microbiologic, and radiographic signs associated with this patient's disease. You should also understand how bacteria can collect in the interproximal regions of the teeth of patients who do not remove these microbes on a daily basis (which will be true of most of your patients). In the following sections, you will be able to review the knowledge that you will use to make a differential diagnosis. The most likely disease will be selected as the clinical diagnosis. This diagnosis, along with elimination or moderation of systemic risk factors, will be the driving force behind the initial treatment of this patient. The following steps are important for determining a diagnosis:

1. Make sure the patient has no extraoral or intraoral problems that should be dealt with first. *In this case,*

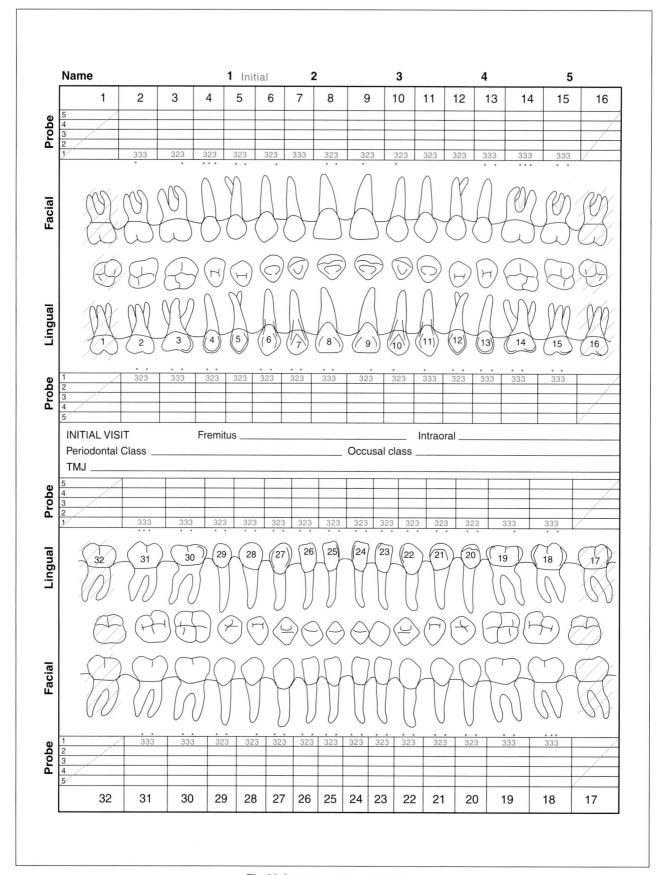

Fig 22-3 Initial periodontal charting.

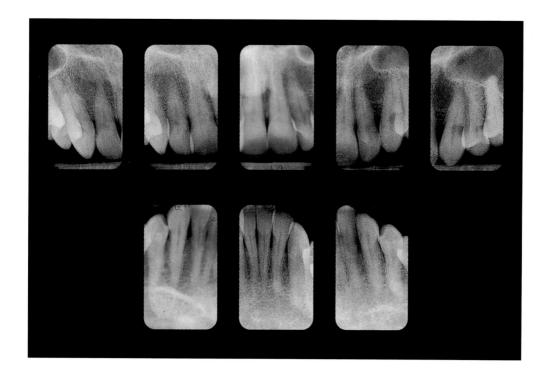

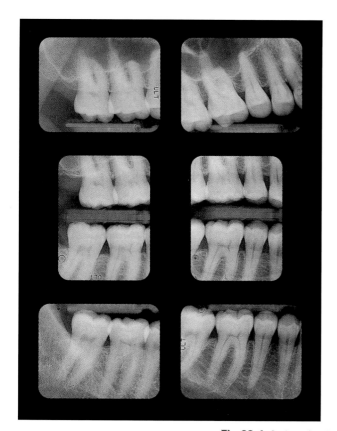

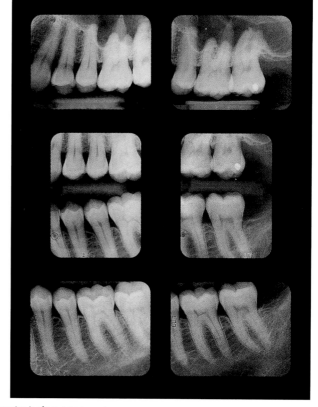

Fig 22-4 Series of radiographs before treatment.

the patient should be premedicated with antibiotics because her physician believes it will protect her knee prosthesis. It is often prudent to have the patient's physician suggest appropriate antibiotics and to verify that the recommendation is consistent with current guidelines for preventing infection of the prosthesis.

2. Look for a systemic component to the disease's process. *No systemic component is evident in this case.*
3. Review the patient's clinical signs and symptoms.
4. Review the patient's radiographic signs.

Clinical Signs and Symptoms

Gingival Inflammation

➤ *The gingival tissues are inflamed.*

Role of plaque. The gingival inflammation seen is the result of plaque accumulation. This will be manifested as redness, swelling, and contour changes of the gingival tissues, as well as bleeding seen after probing.

Supragingival calcifications called *calculus* (primarily mineralized plaque) form on enamel surfaces and are most common adjacent to the parotid and sublingual salivary gland ducts. Supragingival calculus formation is primarily the result of calcium and salivary proteins, which combine to form a calcified matrix. Supragingival calculus may be prevented by careful and regular cleaning and plaque removal. It generally may be removed easily by a professional, since the supragingival calculus crystals do not bind tightly to the enamel crystals.

Subgingival calculus forms primarily as the result of calcifications in the bacterial cell walls of the subgingival plaque. In chronic periodontitis the anaerobic bacteria that form the majority of subgingival plaque bacteria produce alkaline products that are conducive to calculus formation. In some forms of periodontitis (eg, aggressive periodontitis), the predominant bacteria are acid forming, and calculus is less extensive.

Subgingival calculus forms a mechanical union with the roughened porous cemental surface, making its complete removal difficult without removing superficial cementum layers. Although subgingival calculus has a rough surface, there is no evidence that direct physical irritation is involved in the initiation of periodontitis. However, the calculus surface is always covered with bacterial plaque, and as the calculus mass increases, the bacterial covering is moved more and more apically into a position of greater threat to the periodontal tissues.

If plaque is not removed or substantially disrupted on a regular basis, bacterial changes occur that result in the clinical signs of gingivitis. In the mid-1960s, there were many theories about the cause of gingivitis and periodontitis. Studies in Denmark[1] demonstrated that plaque accumulation was the primary factor in the initiation of gingival inflammation, and clinical signs of inflammation were preceded by specific microbial changes in these bacteria. These studies used the experimental gingivitis model in which dental students received professional cleanings and oral hygiene instruction until they achieved essentially perfect gingival health. The dental students then abstained from all oral hygiene practices for 3 weeks. During that time, plaque accumulated rapidly and went through a predictable series of bacterial changes. These changes were characterized by a shift from gram-positive cocci to gram-negative rods, filaments, and spirochetes. Dramatic microbial changes were evident after 3 to 5 days of no cleaning and preceded clinical signs of inflammation. It is now known that many of the gram-negative bacterial species observed in the experimental gingivitis study depend on nutrition and physical environmental changes produced by the mature growth of gram-positive bacteria. Gram-negative microorganisms, which are usually microaerophilic or anaerobic, cannot attach, grow, and survive without substantial colonization by gram-positive bacteria.

As a result of this observation, it was demonstrated that careful and clinically complete plaque removal once every 48 hours is sufficient to prevent gingivitis development. If the plaque removal is incomplete or if the time between cleanings is greater than 48 hours, gingivitis gradually develops on a histologic level. This is seen clinically a few days later.

Bacterial changes. In gingivitis, the plaque is composed primarily of gram-positive microorganisms. As the plaque matures, it changes in composition to include more gram-negative anaerobic organisms.

Bacterial accumulation on the teeth, forming dental plaque, follows a predictable and reproducible process. In adults, after the teeth are cleaned, salivary proteins selectively attach to tooth surfaces and form a salivary pellicle. Gram-positive cocci and rods, predominantly *Streptococcus* and *Actinomyces* species, attach to teeth within hours of cleaning and form the first layers of plaque. In supragingival areas, if plaque is removed once or twice daily, microbial samples will show almost entirely *Streptococcus* and *Actinomyces* species. With less frequent cleaning, the plaque ecology in supragingival niches such as interproximal areas will resemble the plaque ecology of marginal and subgingival plaque.

At the gingival margin, if plaque is not removed on a regular basis, gram-negative rods such as *Fusobacterium* and *Prevotella* species usually start to enter the ecosystem after 1 or 2 weeks of no cleaning. This is usually seen interproximally in patients who do not floss. Subsequent to this, motile gram-negative rods and filaments such as spirochetes, *Eikenella corrodens*, and *Campylobacter* species appear. All the gram-negative species are either anaerobic (ie, they are killed in the presence of oxygen or air) or microaerophilic (ie, they prefer small amounts of air or oxygen, but not too much). The gram-negative species are ecologically favored by the preceding accumulation of *Streptococcus* and *Actinomyces* species. The gram-negative species do not attach well to the tooth surface but do attach very nicely to *Actinomyces* cells. In addition, many of the gram-negative anaerobes have nutrition requirements that are met either by gram-positive microorganisms or by the increased products from the crevicular fluid flow that result from the early deposition of plaque.

The net result is that when undisturbed, a sequential acquisition of microbial species occurs on the tooth surface beginning with *Streptococci* species and culminating in gram-negative bacteria. Some of these bacteria come in proximity to the gingival tissue or are capable of attaching to it and generate various products capable of destroying the tissue. In health, gingivitis, and most forms of periodontitis, bacterial accumulation and by-products are present at high amounts in the gingival sulcus. Although it is uncertain to what extent the bacterial toxins and products penetrate the sulcular lining, they do induce the inflammatory reactions that result in the clinical signs of gingivitis.

If the teeth are cleaned and plaque is allowed to accumulate undisturbed over a 21-day period (the experimental gingivitis model), plaque accumulates predictably and gingivitis develops. The development of clinically detectable gingivitis appears to coincide with the acquisition of gram-negative rods and filaments. Although early studies in this area suggested that gram-negative bacteria may be responsible for gingivitis, well-defined studies using antimicrobial agents that selectively inhibited either gram-positive or gram-negative microorganisms demonstrated that gingivitis would develop in the absence of gram-negative bacteria if sufficient levels of gram-positive microorganisms accumulated. The only successful means of preventing gingivitis development involved either mechanical or chemical methods that kept bacterial levels uniformly low. These studies suggest that although gingivitis requires bacteria, it is most likely a natural result of nonspecific accumulations of plaque in the dentogingival region. Different individuals exhibit very different degrees of inflammation with the same amount of plaque accumulation. Studies have indicated that a substantial part of the gingival inflammatory response may be a genetically determined response of an individual to bacterial challenge (see chapter 11).

Inflammatory changes. In gingivitis, the inflammatory process spreads through the connective tissue subjacent to the junctional epithelium. As bacterial plaque accumulates in the gingival sulcus area, low-molecular-weight products from the bacteria enter the gingival tissue and initiate early signs of inflammation, including vascular dilation and attraction (chemotaxis) of polymorphonuclear neutrophils (PMNs). At the same time, various acute-phase inflammatory mediators are activated in the serum that leaks into the tissue from the dilated vessels. At this point, histologic changes are evident and include dilated blood vessels and an increase in PMNs in the tissue. These biochemical changes cause early clinical signs of gingivitis such as redness and edema from vascular dilation and proliferation and efflux of serum proteins.

As the inflammation becomes more chronic, high-molecular-weight bacterial products, including both antigens and endotoxin (lipopolysaccharide), enter the tissue, activate a more extensive inflammatory mechanism, and initiate a specific and nonspecific immune response. Histologically one sees an increase in lymphocytes, and with special staining one may see that substantial amounts of collagen fiber have been at least partially destroyed just apical to the junctional epithelium. Clinically, the tissue has less integrity and appears more edematous, and the periodontal probe now penetrates the epithelial attachment and superficial layers of the connective tissue attachment.

Probing Depths

➤ *Probing depths are 3 mm or less.*

The periodontal probe penetrates to different levels, depending on the amount of inflammation present. The periodontal attachment apparatus that connects the gingiva and periodontal ligament to the tooth is composed of connective tissue fibers that insert into the root surface and an epithelial attachment that involves epithelial cells from the gingiva attaching to the tooth surface by means of hemidesmosomes. In health and gingivitis, the connective tissue attachment is approximately at the cementoenamel junction (CEJ). In periodontitis, the coronal portion of the connective tissue is at a more apical position. The clinically measured level of attachment (probing depths are also often used) is an indication of the severity of periodontal destruction. This clinical measurement is made with a periodontal probe that is held gently but firmly in the hand and used to measure the distance from the most apical part of the sulcus, or pocket, to the gingival margin (probing depth) or to the CEJ (clinical attachment level, or CAL). Although the aim of clinical probing is to locate the bottom of the pocket and the connective tissue attachment, the actual measurement is a function of not only the connective tissue attachment location but also the amount of inflammation in the area, the pressure applied to the probe, and the diameter of the probe (Fig 22-5).

With minimal or no inflammation, the connective tissue fibers are intact, and the gingival epithelium is attached to

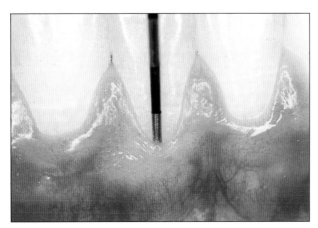

Fig 22-5 View of the mandibular anterior region following initial nonsurgical therapy.

the tooth by an epithelial attachment. The probe stops somewhere within the epithelial attachment and is somewhat coronal to the connective tissue attachment. With inflammation in the area, the basal epithelial cells turn over more rapidly, preventing cell maturation and reducing the integrity of the epithelial attachment. In addition, the collagen fibers that make up the connective tissue attachment undergo some destruction. The net result is that with inflammation, the periodontal probe passes completely through the epithelial attachment and usually stops just apical to the most coronal part of the connective tissue attachment.

With increasing pressure on the periodontal probe, the apical penetration is increased. With minimal inflammation, this may result in complete penetration of the epithelial attachment, but with greater inflammation an increase in pressure results in more apical penetration of connective tissue.

Clinical Attachment Level
➤ *The coronal border of the junctional epithelium is located at or slightly coronal to the CEJ.*

The relation of the gingival margin to the CEJ and to the coronal portion of the junctional epithelium is important to know in establishing a proper diagnosis. The location of the free gingival margin is taken into account in measuring the CAL. The CAL is the sum of the number of millimeters of gingival recession and the probing depth. If the probing depth alone is used, errors can be made in reading a chart. One should be more concerned about a probing depth of 3 mm with 9 mm of recession than the same probing depth with no recession because the former situation represents 12 mm of attachment loss, while the lat-

ter represents no attachment loss. Many clinicians choose to use probing depths alone. Some record facial and lingual gingival recessions, while a few record six areas of recession per tooth.

Radiographic Signs

In gingivitis with no loss of attachment, the level of the interproximal bone seen on the radiographs should be the same level as that seen in health (see Fig 22-4). The radiographic appearance of the alveolar crest is characterized by the presence of cortical bone. This crestal cortication appears as a thin but distinct radiopaque line contiguous with the laminae dura of adjacent teeth. In the posterior regions, the junction of the alveolar crest with the laminae dura is boxlike, forming a sharp, distinct angle. In the mandibular anterior region, the alveolar crest between adjacent teeth is normally spear shaped or knifelike (see Fig 22-4). In the maxillary anterior region, the alveolar crest may be rounded. In all regions, the normal alveolar crest lies 1 to 2 mm subjacent to the CEJ of adjacent teeth and parallels adjacent CEJs.

Making a Clinical Diagnosis

1. Is this periodontal health? *No, there are signs of inflammation.*
2. Is this gingivitis? *Yes, because there are signs of gingival inflammation.*
3. Is this periodontitis? *No, because there has been no attachment loss, and there is no bone loss seen on radiographs.*
4. What type of gingivitis is this? *It is dental plaque–induced gingivitis, because there are no identifiable systemic findings that would suggest that it is another form of gingivitis.*
5. What is the periodontal diagnosis? *Dental plaque–induced gingivitis.*
6. What is the dental diagnosis? *Health.*

Determining Risk Factors for Disease Progression

Several factors, both local and systemic, can affect disease progression. Local factors include bacteria and any niches that protect them from daily disruption of the plaque by the patient, along with the degree to which the patient complies with the dental therapist's suggestions. As previously discussed, if allowed to remain undisturbed, bacteria initiate and sustain an inflammatory reaction in the periodontal tissues, which if untreated will lead to tooth loss in some patients. As bacterial plaque matures, it can allow colonization of more pathogenic organisms. Where probing depths are shallow (3 mm or less) and the patient disrupts the plaque with daily oral hygiene measures, the clinical signs of gingivitis (such as bleeding on probing and color changes) can be reversed. If those patients have routine periodontal maintenance visits, they generally will keep their teeth longer than those who do not. Unfortunately, many patients do not clean their teeth as suggested and do not schedule maintenance visits as often as needed. This lack of compliance is a major risk factor of disease progression.

Systemic risk factors for progression of gingivitis to periodontitis include smoking, diabetes mellitus, and a specific genetic change. Patients who smoke develop periodontal disease more rapidly, heal more poorly, and lose teeth more rapidly than those who do not (see chapter 12). Individuals with diabetes mellitus experience more tooth loss from periodontal disease than do those who do not have diabetes mellitus (see chapter 13). In general, the less severe the diabetes mellitus and the better its control, the better the prognosis for the patient's periodontal problem. A genetic change in those genes responsible for one of the inflammatory mediators in periodontal disease (interleukin 1, or IL-1) results in increased levels of attachment and tooth loss compared with patients without the change (see chapter 11). In addition, patients who smoke and are also positive for the IL-1 genotype have many times greater risk than those without this combination of factors.

Determining the Prognosis

An assessment of Ms Padgett's risk factors reveals the following:

Local risk factors
1. The patient has bacteria that are associated with disease, but there are no physical barriers to disturbing those bacteria (no probing depth greater than 3 mm, no overhanging dental restorations, etc).
2. The patient is not complying with past recommendations for personal oral hygiene and maintenance care.

Systemic risk factors
1. The patient does not and has not smoked.
2. The patient has no family history of diabetes mellitus and does not currently have the disease.
3. The patient has not been tested for the IL-1 genotype.

We know that the patient is at risk for disease progression if she continues to ignore suggestions concerning oral

hygiene and maintenance. Therefore, it would be advisable to instruct the patient in oral hygiene practices, clean her teeth, and evaluate her response 30 to 45 days after the cleaning. If improved oral hygiene, along with the professional removal of calculus and plaque, results in clinical signs of health (normal tissue color and size and no bleeding on probing), then the patient is placed on periodontal maintenance. If on reevaluation the patient has multiple areas of bleeding on probing, then her oral hygiene is reassessed, and she is seen again. If bleeding persists despite good oral hygiene, genetic testing and a consultation with her physician to rule out systemic factors are prudent.

The number of risk factors present and the number that can be controlled or eliminated determine the prognosis. In this case, the prognosis depends to a great degree on how well the patient complies with the recommendations. If she maintains good oral hygiene and comes back for suggested maintenance care, the prognosis is good. If she does not comply with the recommendations, her periodontal outlook is more guarded.

Formulating a Treatment Plan

The following is a standard treatment plan for patients with dental plaque–induced gingivitis.

1. *Initial therapy to control the inflammatory periodontal disease.*
   a. Oral hygiene instructions, including the use of dental floss.
   b. Removal of tooth-borne dental plaque and calculus. This may require as little as the use of a rubber cup polisher or as much as supragingival scaling with local anesthesia, depending on the amount and tenacity of the deposits, as well as the patient's tolerance of the procedures.
2. *Reevaluation of therapy 30 days after completion of initial therapy.* There are three possible final diagnoses at that time:
   a. Dental plaque–induced gingivitis that has been arrested (Fig 22-6). In this case, the clinical signs of inflammation have been eliminated, and the patient is placed on periodontal maintenance (see chapter 28).
   b. Dental plaque–induced gingivitis that has not been arrested. The reason for continued signs of clinical inflammation can be the failure of the therapist or the patient to remove sufficient bacteria and their products, or the inflammation may have a systemic component. This is most commonly the result of inconsistent plaque control by the patient. If oral hygiene is good and the test for the IL-1 genotype has

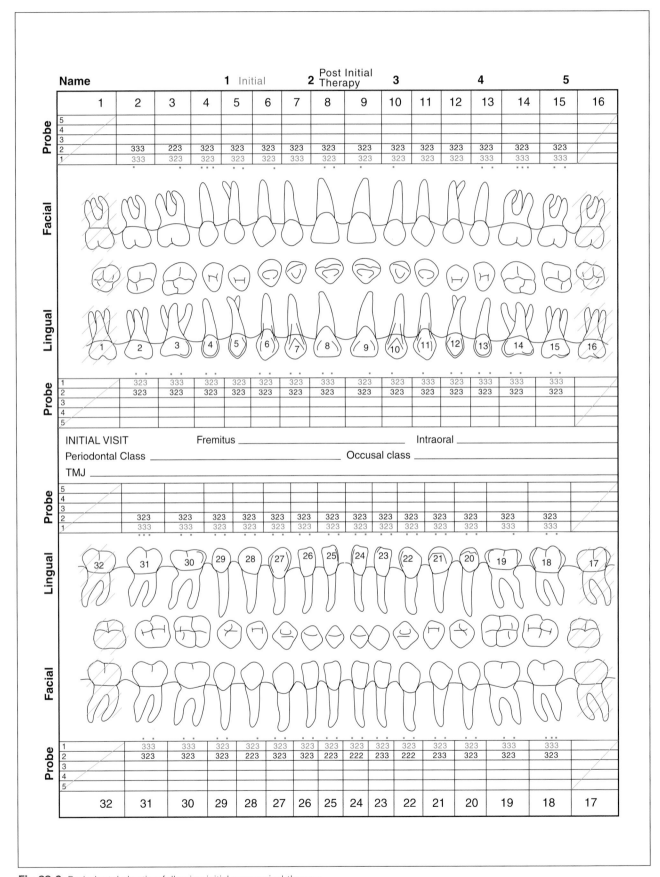

Fig 22-6 Periodontal charting following initial nonsurgical therapy.

not been performed, testing is suggested. A second reevaluation is performed, and if the inflammation has resolved, the patient enters the maintenance phase. If the therapist and the patient have performed properly but signs of inflammation are still present, one of the other forms of gingivitis may be present.

c. Another form of gingivitis. When the patient performs appropriate oral hygiene measures, the therapist has eliminated local factors, and clinical signs of inflammation still exist, then a final diagnosis of some other form of gingivitis may be made. Those patients normally need further evaluation. Some patients may exhibit good oral hygiene at the reevaluation appointment but may have been inconsistent in their oral hygiene practices over time. These patients may have little plaque but still have gingival inflammation. It is important to look for signs of tissue trauma and isolated areas of plaque accumulation that may suggest inconsistent plaque removal.

3. *Periodontal maintenance.* On average, patients with dental plaque–induced gingivitis do well if seen twice a year by the professional. At this visit the disease process is monitored; oral hygiene is evaluated; and any appropriate maintenance therapy, including cleaning the teeth, is performed. See chapter 28 for more information on this aspect of therapy.

Defining Plaque-Induced Gingivitis

The term *gingivitis* has been defined as inflammation of the marginal gingiva.[2] Dental plaque–induced gingivitis is the most prevalent inflammatory condition of the gingiva. However, the identification of several specific etiological factors that modify the level of gingival inflammation has led to the development of an extended classification system for gingival inflammation and lesions.[3] In addition to dental plaque, it is recognized that systemic factors associated with the endocrine system (eg, in puberty-associated gingivitis; menstrual cycle–associated gingivitis; pregnancy-associated gingivitis, including pyogenic granuloma; and diabetes mellitus–associated gingivitis), blood dyscrasias (eg, in leukemia-associated gingivitis), medications (eg, in drug-influenced gingival enlargements and oral contraceptive–associated gingivitis), and malnutrition (eg, in ascorbic acid–deficiency gingivitis) may contribute to the development of unique forms of gingivitis. In addition, certain gingival conditions are the primary results of specific bacterial (eg, *Neisseria gonorrhea*, *Treponema pallidum*, and streptococci) or viral (eg, herpes simplex or varicella zoster) infections. This chapter will primarily focus on dental plaque–induced gingivitis and also briefly discuss how some of the most common systemic modifiers alter the clinical picture and patient management.

The clinical signs of inflammation in the gingival tissues reflect the classic signs of all inflammation: rubor (redness), tumor (swelling), calor (warmth), and dolor (pain). These signs may be readily apparent to the practitioner or dental hygienist, but the threshold for discomfort is commonly not reached by patients with plaque-induced gingivitis. This chronic inflammation is therefore often not apparent to the individual and is tolerated well over an extended period.

Gingivitis is ubiquitous in most populations from early childhood to older age, reaching prevalences of around 90%. However, inflammatory conditions in the gingival tissues (such as plaque-induced gingivitis) reflect a disease state and are not compatible with oral health. For this reason it is of concern that plaque-induced gingivitis is widespread in the general population.

It is generally accepted that the main causative factor in the development of plaque-induced gingivitis is undisturbed accumulation of plaque in the dentogingival area.[1,4] (See chapter 5 for details.) However, the use of plaque-removing measures ensures the reversal of gingival inflammation and return to gingival health.[5]

To present strategies for the management of plaque-induced gingivitis, this chapter discusses the risk of progression of gingivitis to periodontitis and rationales for treatment. Current knowledge about treatment approaches and their validity are addressed. Finally, this chapter contains a thorough etiology-based treatment approach that further details aspects of clinical examination pertinent to chronic gingivitis, available treatment options, and recommendations for patient treatment.

Progression of Plaque-Induced Gingivitis to Periodontitis

In the past it was widely accepted that gingivitis left untreated over time would lead to destructive periodontitis.[6] The periodontal destruction was also believed to progress at a relatively constant rate over the years. However, studies have radically altered this perception of the periodontal disease process. Current evidence strongly indicates that the probability of periodontal destruction developing in a site with gingival inflammation is less than previously believed, and that at least some of the destructive disease events occur in short episodes, or "bursts," at individual sites.[7,8] Although the theory of disease progression in bursts has been questioned,[9] the great difference in the prevalence of gingivitis versus destructive periodontitis in the adult population supports a site-specific nature of periodontal disease progression. As mentioned, the prevalence of gingivitis in some studies has approached 90% of the examined persons, but only about 10% of the individuals exhibited signs of advanced periodontitis.[10–12] Such results have been shown in populations with poor oral hygiene, severe gingivitis, and very limited access to oral health care,[12,13] as well as in populations with a better level of oral hygiene and access to dental services.[10,14] The risk of developing early or moderate periodontitis is higher. This is illustrated by surveys in the United States that found the prevalence of persons with at least one site of attachment loss of at least 4 mm to be 24%.[11]

In clinical studies, periodontal changes can be monitored over time in greater detail than in epidemiologic surveys. When a group of 61 adults with varying severity of gingivitis but no periodontitis was observed during 3 years with no treatment, the incidence of conversions of plaque-induced gingivitis to periodontitis was low.[15] This study illustrates that over a relatively short time, compared with lifelong exposure, only a few sites of gingivitis will have a clinically measurable loss of periodontium with conventional diagnostic methods.

The principle that periodontitis does not always develop at sites of gingivitis has been supported by results from long-term experimental studies of dogs.[16,17] As a result of plaque accumulation by having been fed a soft diet, in the absence of oral hygiene measures, local periodontal lesions and bone loss were provoked experimentally. However, from the results of these investigations it became clear that there were great variations in disease susceptibility among the animals. Some of the dogs did not develop periodontitis at any sites of gingivitis. In other studies of dogs in the age range of 8 to 14 years and characterized by large amounts of plaque deposits, calculus, and plaque-induced gingivitis, approximately 20% presented no signs of periodontal breakdown during examination.[16]

Histologically, there is evidence from such animal models that in a periodontium with long-standing gingivitis, there will be episodes of acute inflammation in localized areas. At these sites there is ulceration of the junctional epithelium and infiltration by neutrophils, as well as increased osteoclast activity. The active periods are then followed by longer quiescent periods.[18,19]

The results of clinical studies in humans also have demonstrated that attachment loss at individual sites tends to occur in episodic bursts of disease activity.[7,8,20] It was determined that a low frequency of recorded sites (2% to 6%) showed clinical breakdown during a 1-year period. These data were derived from a combination of gingivitis and periodontitis sites in patients with past episodes of periodontitis and may therefore overestimate the risk of pro-

gression for patients with gingivitis only. However, the results are in agreement with the previously described studies of disease progression patterns in other models and, therefore, clearly point to the relationship between gingival inflammation and progression to destructive periodontal disease.

In summary, current knowledge indicates that although gingivitis is widespread, only a small number of gingivitis sites in a limited number of susceptible persons will develop into periodontitis with loss of attachment. The mechanism of attachment loss is probably episodic bursts of acute inflammatory activity at select sites. Such localized disease activity may be determined by unbalanced alterations in the pathogenicity of the plaque, the host response, and local factors.

Prevention and Treatment Methods for Plaque-Induced Gingivitis

When considering the need for prevention and treatment of plaque-induced gingivitis, an important factor is the cost-benefit ratio as it relates to the economic, functional, and personal well-being of the individual, as well as to the population as a whole. For the professional who is confronted daily with plaque-induced gingivitis in the individual patient, two questions arise: (1) Can plaque-induced gingivitis be prevented and treated effectively? and (2) What are the benefits of such efforts?

Several studies have evaluated the effects of various periodontal procedures over time in controlling periodontal health status. In a unique approach, the effects of prophylactic measures were evaluated among large groups of Swedish persons.[21,22] Groups of 209 schoolchildren aged 7 to 14 years and 375 adults received individualized oral hygiene instructions and regular frequent prophylactic treatments by dental hygienists. After 2 years for the children and 3 years for the adults, the periodontal status was carefully reevaluated. The children generally had very limited plaque accumulation on their teeth and only negligible signs of gingivitis. The adults who followed the program adopted improved oral hygiene habits and had only negligible signs of gingivitis and no new periodontal attachment loss. This status was clearly better than that of a control group, which, in spite of regular dental care, had gingivitis, continued loss of periodontium, and new caries lesions.

Comparable results of preventive periodontal approaches have been shown among such differing groups as factory workers in Norway, young Californian employees, and US Air Force students during study periods of 3 to 5 years.[23–25]

On the basis of these reports, it may be concluded that the combination of regular and thorough self-care by individuals and preventive professional therapy does lead to improved gingival health, decreased attachment loss, and maintenance of the natural dentition. From an economic aspect, over time the initial expense of preventive programs may well be converted to substantial gains from savings on complex treatment procedures such as tooth replacements. Based on existing data, a US governmental task force strongly emphasized the value of preventive measures in managing gingivitis and periodontitis.[26]

In the context of a population approach and the previously described limited risk of disease progression, if frequent dental visits for periodontal management were prescribed for all persons, clinicians would be overtreating for a proportion of the population that is at low risk. But whereas it might therefore be best to direct efforts only toward persons at risk, at this time risk profiles for identifying this population are only in the developmental stages. Moreover, it is known from closely monitored patients with histories of mild to moderate periodontitis as an indicator of susceptibility that the periodontal disease process will progress if left untreated.[20]

Today it remains a major problem that there is no easy, reliable method of differentiating periodontal sites with disease activity from stable sites. One very interesting line of research has correlated bleeding on probing with the risk for progressing periodontal attachment loss. Although the presence of bleeding on probing is not accurate in predicting progression of periodontal attachment loss, the absence of bleeding, in contrast, is closely correlated with stability of a site over time during maintenance therapy.[27,28] Therefore, there is considerable promise in this method of treating patients with periodontitis.

Once a patient has been identified as susceptible, has undergone quality care, and is under careful maintenance, the prognosis for long-term periodontal health is good. It is known from longitudinal studies of posttreatment maintenance therapy that repeated prophylaxis to control gingival inflammation at regular intervals will greatly delay or prevent reemergence of active disease in the patient.[29]

In conclusion, on a population basis, clinicians should make it a top priority to develop diagnostics that identify persons at risk for periodontal disease or sites of disease activity. Currently, with limited availability of reliable diagnostic indicators, treatment for chronic gingivitis should be based on a preventive approach. Controlled oral hygiene, in combination with professional prophylaxis at regular intervals, generally is effective in preventing the transition from gingivitis to periodontitis. In persons with chronic gingivitis, care should focus on behavioral modification, motivation of the patient, and elimination of local factors important to plaque retention.

Oral Hygiene Control

In spite of a better understanding of the role of microorganisms in plaque-induced gingivitis, a scientific basis for intercepting the development of gingival inflammation by targeting specific microorganisms has not yet emerged. Therefore, in preventing and treating plaque-induced gingivitis in the majority of patients, one currently has to rely on a nonspecific model aiming for regular plaque removal and elimination of plaque-retaining factors. Motivating children to remove plaque not only reduces gingivitis but also lowers the caries incidence rate.[30]

As described previously, gingival inflammation can be controlled in both adults and children who follow intensive recall programs provided by dental hygienists.[21,22] The challenge, however, is to achieve the level of patient motivation for optimal oral health at which the responsibility for thorough oral hygiene can be transferred successfully from the practitioner to the patient.

Methods for motivation and patient instruction have been researched: scientifically based theories that are now available should be integrated into daily practice.[31,32] Individualized oral hygiene interventions may be required to improve oral hygiene behavior, skills, and attitudes. For example, some people may accept and respond well to repeated instructions, but others may react with resistance to this approach and demand greater personal responsibility.[23,24,33]

To involve the patient in a process leading to greater self-interest and personal responsibility, self-instruction programs have yielded encouraging long-term improvements in achieving oral cleanliness and gingival health.[21,34,35] Success in such patient motivation and instruction also relies on active feedback mechanisms, which may be built into self-instructional programs.[35] The oral hygiene therapist should be available to the patient for counseling and demonstrations, develop a good understanding of personality characteristics, and develop an individualized schedule for reevaluation and feedback.[31,36]

Researchers have found that improvements in oral hygiene levels do not depend so much on toothbrush designs or specific methods as they do on the performance and motivation of the person using any of the methods.[36] Although no specific toothbrush design appears to be universally superior in plaque removal, it has been recognized that soft, rounded-end bristles may be less damaging to the gingival tissues.[37]

Toothbrushing may be effective in removing plaque on buccal and lingual surfaces, but it will not reach interdental plaque. To accomplish this a number of other oral hygiene devices have been made available. These include dental floss or tape, interdental brushes, and toothpicks.[36] The oral hygiene therapist should carefully analyze the needs and manual dexterity of each patient and then develop an optimal oral hygiene regimen with the patient.

Plaque and Plaque-Retaining Factors

Three local contributing factors that are central to the accumulation of plaque and the subsequent development of gingival inflammation are (1) tooth anatomic factors; (2) dental restorations and appliances; and (3) root fractures, cemental tears, and root resorptions.

Although tooth position does influence plaque accumulation, it took several attempts to define the precise role of malalignment on plaque accumulation. It has become clear that malaligned teeth have little effect on the oral hygiene level of teeth with either excellent or very poor plaque control levels; however, in patients with medium degrees of plaque control, malalignment could be isolated as an important contributory factor to local plaque accumulation and gingival inflammation.[38] In general, it has been difficult to correlate specific morphologic dental shape or form with gingival inflammation. However, surface irregularities such as dental grooves do constitute local plaque traps. The grooves, which display a variety of forms and shapes, may originate on enamel and have various extensions on the root. Palatogingival grooves have been detected with a prevalence of 8.5% on maxillary anterior teeth, most commonly in the lateral incisors.[39] There is increased plaque accumulation and gingival inflammation associated with the grooves,[39] and there is a potential for periodontal disease progression at such sites. Enamel projections and pearls are developmental aberrations. It is controversial to what extent these integral parts of the tooth structures modify the periodontal disease process. An interdental exposed enamel pearl on the root surface may promote plaque accumulation as well as the local disease process.

It is now clear that fixed restorations with margin discrepancies or poor design, which interfere with optimal plaque control, contribute to the development of gingivitis. As an example, if restoration margins extend subgingivally, they allow for accumulation and development of a pathogenic microbiota and permit induction of gingival inflammation.[40] Because optimal margins reduce the detrimental effects on the periodontium, all restoration margins should be well adapted and corrected if there is a discrepancy. Like fixed restorations, the design of removable prosthetics should take into consideration the access for plaque removal. This would include avoiding direct coverage of, or contact between, the dentogingival zone and connecting elements, connectors, or clasps. Also, the patient may benefit from the creation of open spaces between frameworks and abutment teeth, which allow for

cleaning with various tools such as interdental brushes. Meticulous plaque control around implants is an important component of preventing peri-implantitis and will be discussed in more detail in chapter 38.

Tooth fractures may provide niches for plaque accumulation and result in gingival inflammation that may extend deeply into the periodontium. This is dependent on the extent of the tooth fracture, which may be coronal only or may involve both the crown and root structure. The practitioner should carefully examine teeth that display localized inflammation for tooth fractures, using careful history taking, clinical examination, and radiographic examination.[41] Tears of the cementum from the tooth surface may occur during aging. In most cases, such cemental tears apparently remain asymptomatic. However, in cases where cemental tears are exposed in the pocket, they may enhance the localized inflammatory process, probably through added bacterial accumulation and reduced access for plaque removal. Diagnosis of cemental tears involves both clinical probing and radiographic examination. If the localized inflammation remains clinically unresolved, cemental tears may be detected during exploratory flap surgery that enables direct visualization of the area.[42] An additional, but rather uncommon, diagnosis to consider if localized gingival inflammation is encountered is external root resorption. This root defect may be detected on radiographs and by careful probing of the root surface.

The professional who is responsible for the care of a patient should ensure that all plaque traps, including insufficient restoration contours or margins, are eliminated (see chapter 30 for details on the effects on the periodontium of restorative procedures). Also, in the treatment-planning phase, prosthetic devices that in their designs interfere with optimal plaque control by infringing on the dentogingival region should be evaluated and, whenever possible, avoided or replaced. This is important to prevent gingival inflammation that on a longer-term basis can create permanent loss of periodontal support.[43–45]

To establish optimal conditions for oral hygiene control and patient motivation, all calculus deposits should be removed. This may be done manually with hand instruments, such as scalers and curettes, or with ultrasonic devices. The procedure may be time-consuming with both approaches. Ultrasonic devices tend to leave rougher surfaces following instrumentation, but comparisons of the two methods have not shown any significant differences in the clinical response.[46]

Traditionally, prophylaxis has included the removal of extrinsic tooth stains. This part of treatment may not have any significant effect in preventing periodontal breakdown, but from cultural and societal expectations, and possibly motivational benefits, it appears that polishing can hardly be avoided.[47] Surface-abrasive pumice for polishing should contain fluorides to compensate for the abrasive effects on the enamel.[48] Rather than polishing all tooth surfaces at each appointment, it is appropriate to selectively polish only those surfaces that have plaque or staining.

Despite prior concerns, there now appears to be sufficient evidence that air-powered abrasive devices are acceptable methods of stain removal. The injuries to gingival tissues are minor and reversible, and the systemic introduction of salts is not significant.[49,50] When working in the vicinity of exposed root surfaces, however, the practitioner should take care to prevent loss of tooth structure.[51]

Chemotherapeutics

The use of chemotherapeutic products for controlling gingivitis in patients with no history of periodontal disease has not been widely accepted, with the exception of special patient groups who are unable to maintain oral plaque control. These may include persons with impaired manual dexterity, systemically compromised individuals, or postoperative patients.[52–55] In these cases, antimicrobial products have been used as adjuncts to regular plaque-control procedures.

Although the general attitude toward plaque- and gingivitis-controlling agents in the past has been one of skepticism, a number of new antimicrobial products are emerging for use in the general population. Several commercially available products do not lead to bacterial resistance or have severe adverse effects. Therefore, the use of such agents may change the general approach to oral plaque control.

The main interest has been in antiseptics with broad spectra of antimicrobial activity. Other agents, which function through enzymatic dispersion of the plaque matrix or interference with bacterial aggregation or attachment to the tooth surface, have received less attention. However, it is likely that such products will appear on the market at any time.[56]

Of concern is the high alcohol content—as high as 25%—of several marketed antiseptic products. Thus, a National Cancer Institute publication,[57] based on a large population-based case-control study, expressed concern that regular use of mouthrinses with high alcohol content could contribute to oral and pharyngeal cancer. It appears that the concentrations of alcohol used have little, if any, antimicrobial effect, but traditionally alcohol has been included to aid in solubilization of the active ingredients. It is hoped that innovative approaches may produce preparations that eliminate the high alcohol content. Patients encouraged to avoid alcohol intake for medical or other reasons should carefully determine the alcohol content of mouthrinses prior to using them.

Chlorhexidine

Among the antimicrobial products available today, those based on chlorhexidine digluconate have superior antimicrobial efficacy.[52,53,58] This ingredient has been effective in supragingival plaque control and in reducing gingival inflammation when used in mouthrinses and gels, or when delivered with irrigation devices.[59–62] Although the use of chlorhexidine rinses may result in a beneficial change in the microbial composition, this change is temporary. Once the rinse is discontinued, the microbial profile will revert to one similar to the original.[63] In addition, the reduction in sensitivity to chlorhexidine among certain bacterial species was temporary and diminished after cessation of the rinses.[64]

Beneficial results have been obtained in both short-term clinical studies and after long-term use of chlorhexidine. Reductions in plaque and gingivitis scores, as well as reduced gingival bleeding, were demonstrated after 2 years of use of oral rinses among medical and dental students,[65] and after 6 months of use of rinses among schoolchildren[66] or adults.[59] Medical parameters, including blood counts, urinalysis, and sedimentation rate, were not affected after such extended periods of use.[67] Thus, long-term use of chlorhexidine can be considered safe and efficacious, and therefore useful for patient groups characterized by less resistance to bacterial plaque accumulation. These include patients with systemic conditions, the physically or mentally handicapped, and others with increased susceptibility to periodontal disease.[61]

Realization of the apparent benefits that would be gained by delivery of chlorhexidine during brushing with the dentifrice as the vehicle has been hampered by the chemical characteristics of chlorhexidine. Interactions with other components of the dentifrice have inactivated chlorhexidine.[68] New dentifrice formulations that are compatible with chlorhexidine are being developed and hold promise based on their demonstrated plaque-reducing effects.[69,70]

Distinct adverse effects associated with chlorhexidine products have limited their use. These effects include individually varying degrees of brownish staining of the teeth, tongue, and restorations.[55] Also, increased calculus deposition has been observed, and some patients have reported mucosal irritation and changes in taste sensation.[61,71] A reduction in the concentration of the rinse might provide less staining but carries with it the risk of lower efficacy.

Chlorhexidine has become an integral part of dental practice for use over limited periods when regular oral hygiene measures do not suffice for effective plaque control.[72]

Triclosan

The adverse effects of chlorhexidine have stimulated the search for other products that inhibit plaque formation and gingival inflammation. A nonionic antimicrobial agent with broad-spectrum activity against gram-positive and gram-negative bacteria,[73,74] triclosan (2,4,4'-trichloro-2' hydroxydiphenyl ether) has attracted interest. Although less effective than chlorhexidine in mouthrinses, it does not have major adverse effects and can be included in dentifrices without loss of activity (eg, Colgate Total, Colgate-Palmolive).

Effective formulations of triclosan (0.3%) in dentifrices, in combination with sodium fluoride (0.24%) and a copolymer (2%) or a zinc salt, have been tested for periods ranging from 7 days to 7 and 12 months. When patients used the dentifrice containing triclosan, significantly less new supragingival plaque developed.[75–78] Moreover, the triclosan dentifrice of this composition not only prevented new plaque formation but also had an effect on established plaque and gingivitis. Thus, after 3 and 6 months, users of the experimental dentifrice showed a reduction in preexisting plaque and gingivitis levels compared with a traditional dentifrice containing fluoride but no triclosan.[79]

Initial studies did not show alterations in the composition of the plaque. Whereas the total cultivable flora was reduced significantly after 6 months' use of the triclosan dentifrice, the normal microflora composition was not disrupted, colonization with periodontal or opportunistic pathogens was not promoted, and bacterial resistance was not acquired.[80]

It is noteworthy that triclosan inhibits a specific bacterial enzyme involved in fatty acid synthesis[81] that is also the target for isoniazid, which is a primary medication for treatment of tuberculosis. Although not identified as a clinical problem at this time, the widespread use of triclosan in soaps and general household cleaning products combined with the potential for development of bacterial resistance has been raised as a concern.[82]

Triclosan, at a lower concentration (0.15%) in combination with a zinc salt (0.4%), has shown some encouraging initial results when used as a component of mouthrinse; there was a significant reduction in plaque and gingivitis levels during a 21-day experimental period when compared with a placebo rinse.[83] In light of these results, triclosan may hold promise as an antimicrobial agent for long-term use.

Other Antimicrobial Products

Some oral chemotherapeutic rinses and dentifrices are based on essential oils (eg, Listerine, Pfizer). One should be aware, however, that the alcohol content is substantial for solubility. Another active ingredient is sanguinarine, which is an extract from the plant *Sanguinaria canadensis* (eg, Viadent). It is noteworthy that extended use of Viadent products has been associated with development of oral mucosal leukoplakic changes.[84] A third interesting agent is hexetidine (ie, Oraldene, Warner Wellcome), a hexahydropyrimidine derivative, which in combination with Zn^{2+} ions exhibits considerable antibacterial and antifungal properties.[85] Clinically, this preparation has been found to inhibit plaque accumulation and gingivitis well compared with chlorhexidine.[86] All three of these agents have been shown to be associated with some reduction in plaque accumulation and gingival inflammation and have fewer adverse effects than chlorhexidine-based products for use over extended periods.[52,87] Comparative studies, however, have generally shown that the effects of such other products are less pronounced than those of chlorhexidine.[52,58,87]

Baking Soda and Hydrogen Peroxide

Introduced as part of the Keyes technique, the use of baking soda and hydrogen peroxide has maintained a user group over a number of years. It has been proposed that these ingredients reduce gingival inflammation. However, extensive short- and long-term studies of baking soda and hydrogen peroxide as adjuncts to regular oral hygiene procedures have failed to demonstrate clinical or antimicrobial benefits of the combined treatment over conventional oral hygiene methods alone.[88–92] When delivered with an irrigator, hydrogen peroxide did not provide added benefits compared with regular plaque control measures.[93]

A combination product of hydrogen peroxide and povidone-iodine has shown promising reduction in gingivitis over water, as assessed by bleeding on probing during a 2- to 3-week period of supervised daily mouthrinsing.[94,95]

Calculus-Controlling Dentifrices

Oral hygiene products are now available for the control of calculus formation. These are the anticalculus or tartar-controlling dentifrices. Most prominent among the active compounds used are the soluble pyrophosphates, which act by interfering with crystal growth in the forming calculus.[96–98] Clinical studies have demonstrated convincingly that a large proportion of people benefit from using the pyrophosphate-containing dentifrices. One third of the examined persons had no calculus formation after 6 months, and approximately two thirds had fewer surfaces with calculus formation compared with a group using a regular dentifrice.[99–102] A significant but lower anticalculus effect has been observed with the use of zinc salt (0.5%) in combination with triclosan in a dentifrice.[103]

These results certainly point to beneficial effects of calculus-controlling dentifrices not only for individual patients but for the broader population as well. In some patients pyrophosphates may be irritating to oral mucous membranes and contribute to hypersensitivity reactions.[104] Furthermore, it should be clearly understood that reduction of supragingival calculus formation has little or no effect on the progression of periodontal disease.

Treatment Goals

Presented in the following sections is an approach to managing plaque-induced gingivitis. This clinical approach relies on a review of the literature and on experience from treating patients with plaque-induced gingivitis in practice. The aims of treatment are to address etiologic factors, including plaque-related factors, as well as to pay careful attention to the individual patient's behavior and uniqueness.

The rationale for treating a patient with plaque-induced gingivitis is based not solely on an assessment of the risk for progression to periodontitis in susceptible patient groups,[7,8,11,15,20] but also on other aspects of importance to the patient. These include the general social and physical well-being and function of the patient. A preventive approach in the absence of manifest periodontitis changes may be beneficial in preventing the occurrence of attachment loss, as well as caries.[21,22]

In the absence of special circumstances, such as systemic conditions, the approach to treatment would apply measures founded on the nonspecific plaque hypothesis.[2,4,5] Thus, the aims of treatment for plaque-induced gingivitis are to establish patient understanding and behaviors that, in conjunction with professional treatment, will lead to the establishment and maintenance of a plaque-free dentition, physiologic gingival contour, gingival health with absence of gingival inflammation, and oral comfort.

Patient Examination

Patients with plaque-induced gingivitis deserve the same careful examination as patients with more advanced forms of periodontal deterioration. A number of the components of the examination are of particular importance during the initial visits of new patients. However, as a general rule, at each periodontal maintenance visit, the patient with plaque-induced gingivitis should not be treated or dismissed without assessing periodontal health and entering the findings in the patient record.

Medical, Dental, and Family History

A thorough review of the patient's medical condition should precede treatment at each visit. This is important not only to prevent medically derived complications during the treatment session but also because several common physiologic or medical conditions—such as pregnancy, uncontrolled diabetes mellitus, and puberty—are known to influence gingival health[105–107] (Figs 22-7 to 22-9) (see also chapters 12 to 14). Based on evidence that tobacco is a contributing causative factor in periodontal diseases,[108–112] the dental visit provides an opportunity to advise patients about the risks of tobacco use and to assist in smoking cessation. Reviewing the dental history of the patient, as well as determining the dental status of family members, may also provide the practitioner with important clues.

Understanding the Patient

There are great variations in attitude, ability, and life circumstances that affect a patient's response to the services and advice offered by the dental team. These include personality type, previous dental experiences, age, and general life conditions, among others. It is important to understand how to interact with individual patients. Examination of the teeth, gingival tissues, and deposits (food debris [Fig 22-10], calcified and noncalcified plaque [Figs 22-11 and 22-12], and inflammatory changes) may provide important information about the patient, pointing to factors such as level of oral hygiene skills, dental knowledge, manual dexterity, motivation, and self-esteem. The section describing plaque control discusses these patient characteristics in more detail.

Clinical Examination

Patients with plaque-induced gingivitis do not exhibit loss of attachment, but edema and hyperplasia often occur (see Figs 22-8 and 22-9), causing an increase in probing depth. Probing depths should be measured at each visit to assess the results of therapy and also to provide baseline data should a progressive condition develop. It is not acceptable practice to assume that plaque-induced gingivitis is a stable condition without risk of progression to periodontitis.

The recording should include notation of bleeding (dots) and exudation (circled dots) placed above or below the corresponding probing-depth score. Supragingival plaque and calculus may be categorized by presence/absence from individual surfaces (O'Leary index) after staining with disclosing solution. The circles include markings indicating the surfaces where plaque has been left to accumulate (Fig 22-13).

The placement of restorations and other dental procedures can cause changes in conditions that promote gingival inflammation.[113,114] Possible iatrogenic problems include

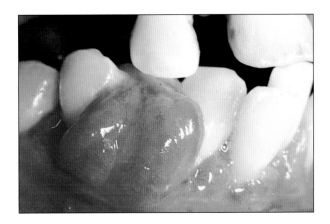

Fig 22-7 Pregnancy. An increase in inflammation and even tumor-like growths are common in pregnant women. This may begin in the second month and continue to increase until the eighth month. Pregnancy is a time when intensive plaque-control measures should be instituted, particularly because antibiotics and other medications should be minimized. Scaling, when necessary, should also be performed. In this patient, the tumor grew to be very large; scaling, combined with improved plaque control, caused it to shrink. It was excised after delivery of the baby.

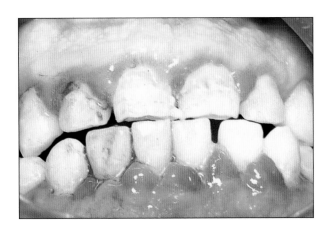

Fig 22-8 Uncontrolled diabetes mellitus. Patients suspected of having diabetes should be referred immediately to their physicians for appropriate testing. Patients with controlled diabetes can have a normal tissue response and should be treated in the same way as persons without the disease, with the exception that the clinician should make sure that the usual dosages of insulin have been taken and the appropriate meals have been eaten. Morning appointments after breakfast are ideal. In this patient, the maxillary arch was scaled weeks earlier. Note the persistent inflammation of the maxillary gingiva and the violent tissue reaction of the unscaled mandibular arch.

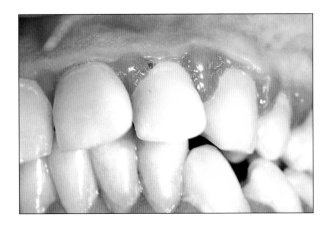

Fig 22-9 Puberty. Gingival tissues that are very inflamed, bleed easily, and are often hyperplastic may characterize the onset of puberty in some individuals with poor oral hygiene. Excellent oral hygiene may reduce or negate the hormonal influence in most of these individuals. The hyperplastic tissue response shown here is a reaction to local irritants. Shrinkage of the papillae and reduction of pocket depth is expected after plaque control and scaling.

insufficient fixed partial denture contours, overhanging or deficient margins, inappropriate width of embrasure spaces, and open contacts between neighboring restorations. Also, prosthetic devices may be designed in ways that promote plaque retention and gingival inflammation.

Such iatrogenic factors can be assessed with the aid of explorers, radiographs, and mouth mirrors and be recorded to better understand the effects of local factors in causing the gingival inflammatory changes. Corrective actions to eliminate these factors may then be undertaken.

Fig 22-10 Food debris. Most often this minor problem that can be corrected easily, but it indicates a potentially serious situation. The patient may simply be ignorant of proper oral hygiene measures or may be unaware of proper etiquette regarding visits to a health care practitioner. Occasionally this lack of basic oral hygiene will alert the clinician to mental disturbances such as depression or senility. Often the condition may be related to physical impairments such as Parkinson disease, severe arthritis, or disability caused by a stroke. In this patient, food debris is present upon initial examination. This patient has been receiving psychiatric treatment.

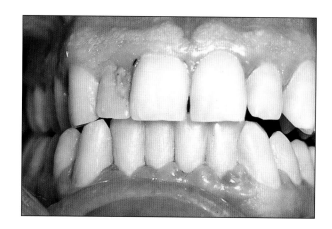

Fig 22-11 Noncalcified plaque. Heavy plaque deposits will usually be visible to the naked eye. They may be heavy in all areas, indicating an absence of knowledge or motivation regarding plaque control. Alternatively, they may be simply in localized areas, very often in difficult-to-reach places such as the lingual surfaces of mandibular molars and the distal surfaces of maxillary second molars. Heavy plaque associated with subjacent bleeding gingival tissues usually indicates long-standing accumulation. In this patient, heavy plaque without bleeding might indicate more food debris than actual bacterial accumulation, and the duration of its existence might be several days or less. Heavy plaque accumulation was responsible for an intense inflammatory response, as evidenced by the dramatic color change.

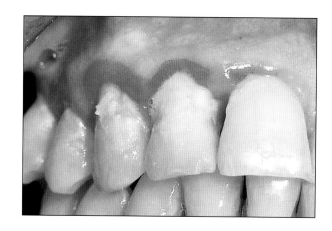

Fig 22-12 Calcified plaque (calculus). Heavy supragingival deposits may be the result of a long span of time since the patient's last dental scaling, poor plaque-removal techniques, or a rapid calcification rate. A rapid calcification rate plus an overextended recall period resulted in the heavy accumulation of calculus in this patient. The gingival tissue may be either red or magenta, indicating an inflammatory response related to a local irritant. When there is much color change and little or no visible plaque and calculus, one must be concerned about a possible systemic condition that is weakening the patient's immune response. Determine whether the number of local irritants is commensurate with the amount of inflammation. Increased levels of inflammation with little plaque and calculus may mean a more aggressive periodontal problem or may necessitate a medical consultation, whereas increased levels of plaque and calculus with moderate to severe inflammation may require no more than plaque-control instruction and calculus removal.

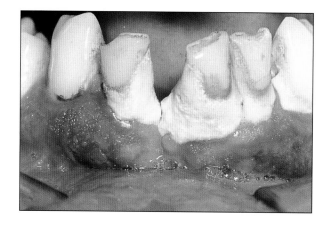

Tobacco use affects the appearance of the gingiva in a way that is significant during the clinical examination of patients with plaque-induced gingivitis. Comparisons of twins revealed fewer signs of gingival inflammation such as gingival bleeding among smokers compared with nonsmokers.[115,116] Thus, when examining patients who smoke, one should remember that smokers commonly will not show the same degree of gingival inflammation as nonsmoking patients despite a similar degree of disease involvement.[115–118] Although the general clinical impres-

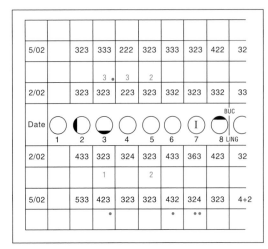

Fig 22-13 These are pocket chartings on the maxillary right quadrant recorded 3 months apart. The red dots represent pockets that bled on probing; no exudate was present. The red numbers above or below the pocket recordings represent millimeters of recession. The black markings within the circles represent tooth surfaces that retain plaque. The center of the circle can be used to record tooth mobility if it is present (see tooth 7).

sion among smokers is one of recurrent and greater staining and accumulation of deposits, strict study conditions have indicated that the rate of plaque accumulation and the bacterial composition is similar between patients with or without the habit.[119,120] However, patients who use tobacco show a less beneficial response to periodontal treatment[121] and have a higher risk for periodontal attachment loss[109,112] and tooth loss.[109]

Other causative factors, such as crowding and tooth malalignment, mouth breathing, allergies, orthodontic appliances, and ill-fitting removable partial dentures may contribute to the severity of the gingivitis (see chapters 12 to 14, 20, and 21 for details). Each situation must be reviewed individually and the causative factors eliminated to the extent possible.

Informing the Patient

After the data from the examination have been compiled, it is important to inform the patient about the results. This should include the diagnosis, expected treatment required, and prognosis. Also, the expected long-term measures required to maintain a healthy periodontium should be explained to the patient. Such a conversation should be in language that is appropriate for the individual patient so that the message is clear and complex terms and specialty expressions are avoided.

The patient is informed that he or she has a gingival infection that needs to be treated and that treatment consists of four parts:

1. One or more visits related to the control of the bacterial plaque that is infecting the gingivae
2. A dental scaling and polishing appointment
3. A reevaluation appointment to determine the level of disease control

4. A regular periodontal maintenance program to maintain the teeth and gingiva in a state of health

Some patients are reluctant to schedule a plaque-control appointment if they believe they will simply be shown how to brush their teeth. They may think that it is an insult to their intelligence and a waste of their time. However, it is essential that patients understand the critical role they play in maintaining their own oral health. Plaque deposition is a continual process, and within days of cessation of its removal, the signs of gingival inflammation will occur.[1] Biannual appointments with the dental hygienist will do little to alleviate the disease condition without full cooperation from the patient. To promote patients' understanding of their role in the comprehensive treatment, the following points may be stated:

1. The anatomy of their teeth and gingiva makes it difficult for them to remove the bacterial plaque and may necessitate individual instruction.
2. They will be shown new techniques that will allow them to brush further under the gums and to clean better between the teeth. The word *new* must be emphasized.
3. If appropriate for their condition, mechanical appliances and mouthrinses may be helpful. This will be determined after the type and location of their plaque have been analyzed.
4. It is important to reduce the infection first so that during scaling there will be less bleeding and tenderness.

Patient Factors in Plaque Control

Following treatment planning and consent by the patient, an initial and particularly important aspect of the treatment will be to convey to the patient the importance of oral hygiene. This will include cooperation between the dental team and the patient, but ultimately it relies on the efforts of the patient. It is important, therefore, that the practitioner and oral hygiene therapist gain an in-depth understanding of the patient. The following sections present important personal factors to consider and adjust for in treatment planning.

Degree of Dental Phobia

Unfortunately, many patients are not relaxed in the dental environment because of a previous traumatic experience. Anxiety may hinder successful achievement of the treatment aims. Therefore, it is important to let these patients know that treatment will not be painful for them and that they are free to express concerns at any time. The following questions are helpful in determining whether or not dental phobia will be a factor in the patient's receptiveness to treatment and can be included in the dental history:

1. *Have you ever had a bad dental experience?* Follow this question on the history form with the words *yes* and *no*, with a notation to circle one answer.
2. *Do you have any concerns about dental treatment?* Again, this question should be followed by *yes* and *no*, and there should be a place for comments.

If one or both of these questions is answered in the affirmative, patients should be invited to share whatever information they would like. They can then be reassured that their treatment should be a pleasant experience and given the reasons why.

Oral sedation can be used during scaling if the degree of dental fear is unusually high. The benefits of psychologically treated dental phobia last much longer than the benefits of medicinal sedation, however.[122]

Degree of Unfilled Dental Needs

It is important to determine whether patients are embarrassed about the poor condition of their oral cavity. The clinical examination should note untreated caries lesions, fractured teeth, unreplaced missing teeth, and lost restorations. It is also wise to determine the cause of such findings, whether dental phobia, financial problems, stress, depression, or fatigue. The clinician's approach should be one of compassion, empathy, and understanding.

Age

Teenagers and young adults may be very difficult to motivate, because oral hygiene is often not a priority. Special

approaches to communicate with and motivate these patients may be applied. For example, because this age group is usually very concerned about relationships with the opposite sex, it can be very helpful to discuss how materia alba, plaque, and gingivitis contribute to bad breath.

Dental Knowledge

Many people come from cultural, ethnic, or social backgrounds where little value is placed on the preservation of the natural dentition. Such patients may assume that complete dentures are inevitable. Explaining alternative routes of treatment, showing them dentures, and discussing their potentially negative aspects may help the patient choose preventive dental care approaches.

Physical or Mental Disabilities

The patient's dexterity, deformity, or malfunction will need to be assessed. In some instances, mechanical devices can help overcome the problem. In other cases, a spouse or caretaker may need to perform the functions for the patient, and he or she should be present at the plaque-control appointment.

Personality Types

A skilled plaque-control therapist can recognize that different personalities respond best to different approaches. When teaching plaque control, it may be useful to recognize four distinct personality types. Obviously, there will be some overlap of traits in many individuals.

1. *The people type*—pleasant, wants to be liked, informal. The therapist should be friendly, patient, and open, and minimize details unless asked.
2. *The analytical type*—formal, conservative, needs to understand the process, wants to do a thorough job. The best approach is to be organized and detailed.
3. *The in-charge type*—businesslike, wants control. The therapist should provide definite answers and allow the patient options.
4. *The socialite type*—friendly, concerned with image, wants attention and approval. The best approach is to emphasize how skills can promote image and to praise the patient.

Level of Unfulfilled Needs

Psychologist Abraham Maslow, in his theory of self-actualization,[123,124] described peoples' necessity to have basic needs met before being concerned about higher needs. For instance, a man feeling intense pain must have it relieved

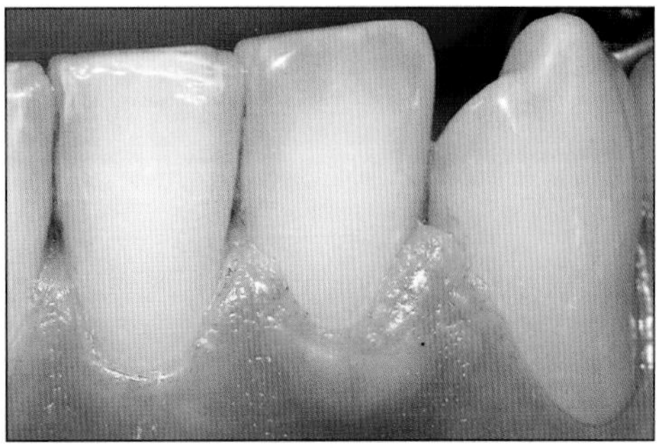

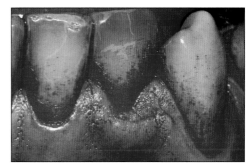

Fig 22-14 A patient with no evidence of gingival inflammation. Note the pink color, the flat, pointed papillae, and the presence of stippling.

Fig 22-15 Disclosing solution has stained difficult-to-see plaque. Patients with reasonably good oral hygiene will stain mostly in the interproximal areas and, sometimes, adjacent to the marginal tissues. Check the lingual surfaces of the mandibular molars carefully, since it is a very common place for residual plaque.

before he will be concerned about his appearance. Other basic needs are for food and shelter. People who are hungry and have nowhere to sleep are likely to be unconcerned about bleeding gingiva. The therapist must determine whether basic needs are being met for a specific patient and interpret how this will affect his or her ability to receive dental treatment. Once basic needs are met and patients have reasonably high self-esteem, they will be concerned about the function and esthetics of their dentition.

Treating Plaque-Induced Gingivitis

Patient Motivation

It is important for patients with plaque-induced gingivitis to understand that their condition is a bacterial infection that is harmful to delicate tissues. If they showed the same amount of infection on the surface of their skin as they do in the oral cavity, they would most likely seek the help of a physician. Photographs, drawings, or models of teeth and plaque deposits may be shown to the patient to help explain the disease. Some clinicians use a microscope or video monitor to show patients plaque samples from their mouth. This tool, however, is not accurate for prediction of disease progression.[125,126]

Another approach that has recently gained some recognition is the measurement of subgingival temperature, which is increased during plaque-induced gingivitis.[127,128] A commercial instrument can measure the subgingival temperature, assist in recording hot spots, and provide a printed record of their location. Patient motivation may be

enhanced as the patients improve their home care between office visits in an attempt to improve upon the previous score. In the context of disease progression from gingivitis to periodontitis, there is initial evidence to suggest that increased temperatures may precede subsequent attachment loss and thus may identify sites at risk.[89]

The concept of subgingival plaque and the need for its removal should be explained. A drawing done by the therapist or a pamphlet with printed depictions of plaque often suffice. It may be helpful to compare subgingival plaque and its need for removal to dirt under the fingernail and how that needs to be scraped away. Demonstrating the presence of plaque on a tooth with a periodontal probe helps the patient visualize it.

Once the patient understands what plaque is and where it resides, the next issue is to describe the changes it can cause in the oral cavity. Bleeding, color changes, edema, bad taste, and bad breath can be discussed in general before relating them to conditions in the patient's own oral cavity. Wherever possible, the disease condition is compared with the normal situation, using the healthy areas of the patient's oral cavity or photographs of normal tissues (Fig 22-14). The possible progression of gingivitis to periodontitis should be discussed using a visual aid.

Teaching Manual Oral Hygiene

Teaching oral hygiene may be approached in different ways, including instruction or self-instruction. It is important that the patient be integrally involved in order to promote greater self-interest and personal responsibility.[34,35,129] The approaches may need substantial adjustment based on factors such as age and manual dexterity.[130] However, the oral hygiene instruction is a fundamental part of success in the management of plaque-induced gingivitis and in preventing recurrence, and it should receive careful attention. The following describes an approach to oral hygiene instruction in a clinical setting and provides examples of the use of different oral hygiene tools:

1. Seat the patient in a dental chair, and review his or her oral condition.
2. Demonstrate color changes, bleeding, and edematous papillae.
3. Scrape visible plaque using a probe until it can easily be seen as a white mass at the end of the probe. When necessary, use a disclosing solution (Fig 22-15). Note that it is important to obtain the patient's permission before using a dye, because patients might have important engagements after their dental appointments. Minimize residual stain by coating the patient's lips with petroleum jelly and applying the disclosing solution to the marginal and interproximal areas with a soaked cotton tip before having the patient rinse lightly.
4. Show the patient the stained plaque and let him or her know that it extends under the gingiva and between the teeth further than can be seen.
5. Explain that brushing under the gums and contoured dental flossing are the most important techniques to master.

Brushing

Toothbrushes are available in a variety of shapes and should have a relatively small head (1 to 1¼ inches for adults; smaller for children) (Fig 22-16). Many come with oversized handles for better gripping. The bristles should be of soft nylon and multitufted, with polished ends.

Give patients a suitable new brush, and ask them to demonstrate their technique first. Some will need only minor corrections. Others will need extensive counseling, with considerable detail.

Interdental Cleaning

No one type of dental floss is superior to other types in all situations. If the rules regarding the use of floss are too stringent, patients will be reluctant to floss at all. A lightly waxed, mint-flavored floss is tolerated well by most patients. It is important that the floss slip easily between the teeth and past restorative margins without tearing and becoming lodged in the interproximal spaces.

Most people who do not floss believe that it is too time-consuming and too difficult a skill for them to master. Many people who floss do it incorrectly and simply use it to remove food particles lodged between the teeth.

For patients who say they do floss, hand them a container of floss, and ask them to show you their technique.

Many will tear off a short piece, often about 6 to 12 inches in length, wrap it around their index fingers, and attempt to floss. Explain to them that there is an easier way, and show them how to take a longer piece of floss (at least 18 inches) and wrap it several times around each middle finger. Demonstrate how to use the thumbs and index fingers of each hand to guide the floss to the mesial and distal portion of each interdental papilla. Floss should be contoured sufficiently by these fingers to extend it past the line angles of the teeth out onto the facial and lingual surfaces. An up-and-down motion of the floss on each proximal surface is then required to sufficiently remove the subgingival plaque.

Tell patients who are not flossing that there have been improvements in the techniques that will make it easier for them to do. These patients also need to understand that flossing is essential to cleaning under the gingiva between the teeth, where most disease occurs. Toothpicks or rubber tips do not do the same thing.

Children may find flossing easier if they start with a shorter piece of floss (about 12 inches); tie the ends together with a square knot to form a loop; grasp the loop with the third, fourth, and fifth fingers of each hand; and use the thumb and index fingers to guide the floss.

Besides the basic brush and dental floss, many other useful aids are available (Fig 22-17). Some adult patients will need to use a floss holder because of dexterity problems, arthritis, or other reasons. Defer to this device only when absolutely necessary, however, because these holders usually stretch the floss very tightly, preventing it from being wrapped around proximal tooth surfaces or being slipped subgingivally.

When teeth are spaced apart or the gingiva has receded to allow sufficient room, interdental brushes may be preferred for their ease of use and their ability to penetrate into concave root surfaces.

End-tuft brushes are brushes that have bristles only at the very end of the head (see Fig 22-17). Special areas, such as the distal surfaces of second molars, may require an end-tuft brush. They are also good for reaching difficult-access areas when teeth are crowded.

Toothpicks can be broken and the pointed ends attached to plastic handles, creating a wooden dental instrument excellent for penetrating into the deep grooves of teeth, as well as for cleaning at the gingival margin and slightly subgingivally on the facial and lingual surfaces (Fig 22-18). Before the patient uses the toothpick, have him or her blunt the sharp tip by running it under warm water and then tapping it on a hard surface.

Wooden interdental cleaners (eg, Stim-U-Dent) can be useful for dislodging retained food particles from between the teeth. Because of their small size and packaging, they can be carried in purses and pockets and are useful when eating away from home. The wooden tip should be thor-

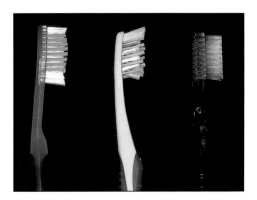

Fig 22-16 Three styles of brushes effective for the removal of plaque. *Left to right:* Blue brush with a wave design for better access; white brush with a criss-cross pattern for improved plaque control; and a rose brush with a standard head small enough for hard-to-reach areas in smaller mouths.

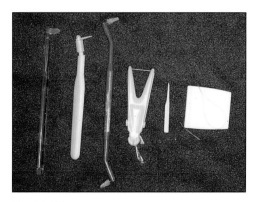

Fig 22-17 Additional useful plaque-control aids include (left to right) an end-tuft brush, toothpick in holder, double-ended interdental brush, floss holder, plastic interdental cleaner, and dental floss with loop threader.

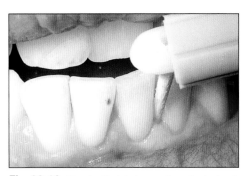

Fig 22-18 The toothpick traces the gingival sulcus of a mandibular anterior tooth.

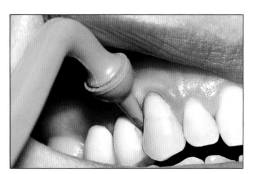

Fig 22-19 The rubber tip is used to apply pressure to an inflamed papilla. Note blanching of the tissue and the angle at which the tip is applied.

oughly moistened in the mouth to soften it. The pointed end is inserted between the teeth and gently moved in and out.

Plastic interdental cleaners are similar to wooden ones and are made by a variety of manufacturers. Since they are usually thin, they have a better chance of some subgingival penetration. However, because they are constructed of harder material, they are not as comfortable to use as the wooden instruments.

Rubber-tip stimulators were once considered essential in the reduction of interproximal inflammation. It is now known, however, that plaque removal is the primary method of controlling gingivitis. Stimulators are sometimes used to aid in plaque removal by applying contouring pressure to hyperplastic interdental papillae (Fig 22-19).

When teeth are in tight proximity and the papilla fills the interdental area, no interdental brush, pick, or stimulator will penetrate the interproximal subgingival area as well as properly contoured dental floss. For this reason,

proper brushing and flossing techniques are essential in the control of gingivitis.

Powered Appliances

Powered brushes, combined with updated information on pulsating irrigation devices, provide further ammunition in the war against plaque and gingivitis. Patients who have been poor manual brushers may quickly improve their ability to remove plaque with a powered brush and thus improve their gingival health.[131] However, powered devices eventually stop working. Patients should be made aware of this and be counseled in manual techniques so that plaque levels will not increase while a brush is being repaired or replaced.

Multiple rotating tuft brushes with direction reversal consist of separate tufts of soft bristles that can rotate very rapidly (a reported 4,200 times per minute, reversing direction 46 times per minute), causing the bristles to extend outward toward the interproximal spaces and into the subgingival areas. Some dentifrices, such as tartar-control types, can damage the delicate gears in the head. Controlled studies have demonstrated improved plaque reduction scores[132] and significantly reduced gingival bleeding[133] for these brushes compared with manual brushing.

Multiple rotating tuft brushes are indicated for (1) patients with persistent marginal plaque; (2) handicapped patients; (3) patients with poor manual dexterity; (4) patients with Parkinson disease; and (5) orthodontic patients.

Disadvantages of multiple rotating tuft brushes
1. The head is large.
2. A recharging stand must be carried when traveling (a battery model is also available).
3. Abrasive grit clogs the gears; the manufacturer recommends a proprietary dentifrice.
4. Claims of interproximal cleansing often discourage patients from using dental floss.

Multiple rotating tuft brushes with oscillation, containing 29 stationary tufts, are available. Instead of the bristle tufts rotating, the head of the brush has a counter-rotational and simultaneous oscillating action. When compared with the use of a popular manual brush in a population of 70 healthy adults, this brush scored significantly better for reduction in gingivitis for both the whole mouth or just interproximal areas.[134] Another version has a three-dimensional head action in addition to the rotation and oscillation movements. It has been shown to significantly reduce both bleeding on probing and plaque when compared with a manual brush.[135]

Advantages of multiple rotating tuft brushes with oscillation:
1. The medium-sized head is effective in most areas.
2. It is easy to use.
3. It can be used with all types of dentifrice.
4. One charge lasts a long time.
5. Handle size is comfortable for adults and children.

Disadvantages
1. Head will not reach into tight areas.
2. Tightness of bristles retain dentifrice during rinsing.
3. Interproximal areas must be flossed.

Single rotating tuft brushes are based on the cleansing principles long used by the dental hygienist when performing prophylactic procedures with contra-angle handpieces and rubber polishing cups. The brushes come in several shapes and sizes, and one is narrow and pointed for better penetration into interproximal areas and other tight spaces. The head is small and can reach virtually any area in the oral cavity. The small head size and the availability of a variety of brushes may make it comparable to using a variety of traditional manual aids.[136]

Advantages of the single rotating tuft brush
1. Soft bristles are kind to both hard and soft dental tissues.
2. The small head can reach into tight areas.
3. The brush can be used with dentifrice for stain removal.
4. Patients with orthodontic appliances, fixed partial dentures, and implants find it easy to use.
5. It is convenient for travel, because the charge lasts a long time.

Disadvantages
1. Subtle changes in angles and directions may be difficult for patients with poor coordination or mental retardation.
2. Considerable instructional time is necessary.
3. Some patients are unable to tolerate the tickling.
4. Success can depend on flossing as an adjunctive procedure.

Sonic brushes can vibrate at 31,000 brush strokes per minute. They have a rectangular, medium-sized head containing hundreds of soft-rippled bristles. Used with dentifrice, the sonic brush can produce a foam that penetrates subgingival areas. The brush combines acoustic vibrations and dynamic fluid activity with direct mechanical scrubbing of tooth surfaces. Its plaque reduction has been shown to be as much as three times greater than manual brushing. The sonic brush causes no soft tissue abnormalities after 6 months' use, and there is significant reduction in gingivitis and sulcular bleeding scores.[137]

Advantages of the sonic brush
1. Plaque removal is excellent.
2. It may adversely affect bacteria beyond the reach of the bristles by decreasing their aggregation tendencies.[138]
3. Stain removal is very effective.
4. It has a 2-minute timer to prolong brushing time.
5. It appeals to technically trained individuals.

Disadvantages
1. The sound is disturbing to some.
2. In vivo studies supporting subgingival antibacterial claims are needed.
3. The technique for cleansing is considerably different from manual techniques.

Ultrasonic brushes include a traditional manual-style toothbrush head and bristles combined with a piezoelectric emitter in the brush head, which delivers 16 million cycles of ultrasonic energy per second. Patients with moderate gingivitis see a clinically significant improvement after 1 month.[139]

Advantages of ultrasonic brushes
1. There is a long history of ultrasonic energy as an aid in cleansing dental instruments.
2. The patient can use traditional brushing techniques, such as the modified Bass technique.

Concern
Few studies support the claims of this brush type.

Pulsating Irrigation

When pulsating water irrigation was introduced more than 25 years ago, it was intended to dislodge plaque and food particles, particularly around fixed partial dentures. The procedure never became popular as a plaque-control device, however, because plaque was not totally removed from tooth surfaces and occasionally abscesses developed. This was because root planing with concomitant calculus removal was not performed before the irrigation procedures were started. The literature shows that patients who have less than optimal plaque control can improve their effectiveness by using supragingival irrigation.[140]

A greater understanding of the microbiology and pathogenesis of gingivitis has brought renewed interest in the ability of pulsating irrigation to reduce not only plaque accumulations but also gingival inflammation. Irrigation is now believed to qualitatively alter dental plaque toward less pathogeneity,[141,142] thereby reducing plaque-induced gingivitis even when performed with plain water.[143] As previously reviewed, the addition of antimicrobial agents may further increase the effect of irrigation. When used around dental implants, irrigation with a subgingival irrigation tip and chlorhexidine (0.06%) has been shown to improve plaque, gingival, and stain indices when compared with a chlorhexidine (0.12%) oral rinse.[144]

Pulsating irrigation, used in addition to brushing and flossing, is recommended for *(1)* patients with special food-retentive areas (eg, pontics, diastemata, and orthodontic appliances); *(2)* patients with persistent gingivitis even after manual plaque control has been mastered to the extent of the patient's ability; and *(3)* patients who enjoy the feeling of cleanliness they derive from the irrigation.

Chemical Plaque Control

Patients are intrigued by the possibility that application of topical agents can aid them in plaque control. Because plaque buildup is constant and relentless, patients are often willing to spend considerable sums of money, en-

dure strong tastes, and to a lesser degree, tolerate stains on the teeth caused by the agents. These antimicrobial agents are particularly effective in patients with plaque-induced gingivitis and no deep pockets. When delivered by mouth-rinsing and even by irrigation, there is very limited effect on the microbial flora of deeper pockets.

Chlorhexidine is a potent antiplaque agent available in Europe in a 0.2% concentration and in the United States in a 0.12% concentration (with a prescription) under the brand names of Peridex or PerioGard. Unfortunately, the adverse effects limit its use over extended periods. Dilution of chlorhexidine to half concentration reduces the therapeutic benefit but also cuts cost, staining, taste alteration, and calculus formation.

Chlorhexidine may be indicated:

1. As treatment for gingivitis when conventional manual and mechanical techniques are insufficient
2. As the initial method of plaque control when plaque-induced gingivitis has resulted in extreme gingival sensitivity to touch
3. For longer control of gingivitis, if only minimal adverse effects are observed

Potential side effects include:

1. Varying degrees of brown stain on the teeth, tongue, and silicate and resin restorations. We recommend that patients avoid concurrent use of tobacco, coffee, tea, and red wine; also, chlorhexidine should be used very cautiously by patients with bonded restorations or cracked or pitted enamel.
2. Prolonged alteration or transient impairment of taste perception. Patients should be informed in advance that this adverse effect will occur and lasts for a few days.
3. Excessive supragingival calculus formation (from accumulation of calcifying dead bacterial organisms). One solution is to use a tartar-control dentifrice[145] and to brush more frequently.

Alternatives to chlorhexidine for long-term use include essential oil–based mouthrinses (eg, Listerine or Viadent). The effects are generally less than those of chlorhexidine.[58,146] Listerine has been approved by the American Dental Association for control of plaque and gingivitis. It is recommended that patients rinse with it for 30 seconds in the morning and evening. It is contraindicated for patients who cannot tolerate the taste, who experience a burning sensation, or who avoid alcohol (alcohol content is 26.9%).

Managing Appointments

Oral Hygiene

For patients who need minimal improvement in plaque control, one visit of 30 to 60 minutes should be sufficient. Important feedback as to the patient's progress can be delivered at the scaling appointment. All dental needs, such as manual toothbrushes, floss, disclosing solution, and a plastic dental mirror, should be provided for the patient to take home and begin using immediately.

It is very difficult for most patients to master more than two new oral hygiene techniques in one treatment session. For patients with very poor oral hygiene who need to begin with education about basic brushing and flossing techniques, it is best to schedule two sessions approximately 1 week apart. The second session can begin with an evaluation of what has been accomplished since the last appointment, along with what further improvements can be made. Subsequently, new aids such as the end-tuft brush or the toothpick holder might be introduced. The second appointment might include a determination that the patient's manual brushing technique is not adequate and that a battery-powered mechanical brush is needed. Above all else, one should be flexible in teaching and motivating patients to attain higher levels of oral hygiene.

Calculus Removal

Calcified aggregates of dead bacteria and other debris are termed *calculus*. Such deposits are plaque retentive, just as overhanging restoration margins are, and their removal is required to provide the patient with the easiest access for keeping the dentogingival area free of plaque. The calculus may attach to the tooth by mechanically locking into cracks, resorptions, carious lesions, and other defects of the tooth surface.[147] Calculus deposits require careful instrumentation, either with hand instruments or mechanical devices for removal.

Calculus removal may be technically challenging in patients with gingivitis. These patients commonly have no significant attachment loss; the gingival tissues are near normal levels, with the interdental papillae filling the interdental spaces. However, to prevent future attachment loss, the subgingival calculus must be completely removed.

There is substantial variation within and among individuals in the extent of calculus deposition.[148–150] Even after complete professional calculus removal, those who initially had the most calculus re-form new deposits most rapidly.[151] It has been observed among heavy calculus formers that the calculus buildup occurs most rapidly during the first 4 weeks after scaling and polishing. Thereafter, the calculus deposition is substantially slower.[152] This phenomenon has been confirmed in a tube-fed patient with poor oral hygiene.[153]

Clinically, it is evident that calculus removal leads to less bleeding, less discomfort, and less edema. To convey to patients the primary significance of home plaque control, consider starting the calculus removal 2 weeks after the individualized instruction in procedures for plaque removal. Most patients with plaque-induced gingivitis can undergo scaling in one session of 45 to 60 minutes. Occasionally, two or more sessions are needed, depending on the amount and tenacity of the calculus and the degree of stain. Once scaling is complete, the patient should return for a reevaluation session in 2 to 4 weeks, the amount of time needed for maximum healing to take place.

As described previously, pyrophosphate-containing dentifrices are available for over-the-counter purchase. The recommendation of this adjunct to home oral hygiene procedures and regular professional cleaning may be valuable for patients who tend to form heavy calculus deposits.

Posttreatment Evaluation

At the reevaluation session, the response to treatment is assessed, and pretreatment and posttreatment chartings are compared. Plaque control and tissue response (probing depths and signs of inflammation, including bleeding on probing, color, and consistency) are evaluated, and the patient is encouraged to continue the high level of achievement or to strive for improved levels of excellence. When necessary, additional instruction is given.

A determination is then made regarding periodontal maintenance. An individualized recall schedule for periodontal maintenance appointments should depend on the response of the patient and commonly consists of visits in intervals of 3 to 12 months. In more severe cases with less than satisfactory response to treatment, periodontal maintenance appointments should be made every 3 to 4 months. If a chemical agent such as chlorhexidine is being used, the therapist should make a decision to (1) stop use of the agent and not replace it with another, (2) replace it with an agent that has fewer adverse effects for that individual or is less costly if finances are a problem, or (3) continue the agent but vary the mode of delivery (eg, use irrigation).

If the patient has not responded to treatment as expected, every attempt should be made to determine the cause. Some reasons might be patient noncompliance in controlling plaque, an underlying systemic problem, or the presence of subgingival calculus. Patient noncompliance might require one or more additional sessions of instruction and motivation, or the addition of different aids, such as a mechanical toothbrush and/or a floss holder. Suspected systemic complications may necessitate a medical consultation. It may also be determined that additional scaling or root planing is necessary.

References

1. Löe H, Theilade E, Jensen SB. Experimental gingivitis in man. J Periodontol 1965;36:177–187.

2. Glossary of Periodontal Terms, ed 4. Chicago: American Academy of Periodontology, 2001.

3. Armitage GC. Development of a classification system for periodontal diseases and conditions. Ann Periodontol 1999;4:1–6.

4. Theilade E, Wright WH, Jensen SB, Löe H. Experimental gingivitis in man. A longitudinal clinical and bacteriological investigation. J Periodontal Res 1966;1:1–13.

5. Löe H, Schiott CR. The effect of mouthrinses and topical application of chlorhexidine on the development of dental plaque and gingivitis in man. J Periodontal Res 1970;5:79–83.

6. Greene JC. Oral hygiene and periodontal disease. Am J Public Health 1963;53:913–922.

7. Socransky SS, Haffajee AD, Goodson JM, Lindhe J. New concepts of destructive periodontal disease. J Clin Periodontol 1984;11:21–32.

8. Goodson JM, Tanner ACR, Haffajee AD, et al. Patterns of progression and regression of advanced destructive periodontal disease. J Clin Periodontol 1982;9:472–481.

9. Jeffcoat M, Reddy M. Progression of probing attachment loss in adult periodontitis. J Periodontol 1991;62:185–189.

10. Hugoson A, Jordon T. Frequency distribution of individuals aged 20–70 years according to severity of periodontal disease. Community Dent Oral Epidemiol 1982;10:187–192.

11. National Institute of Dental Research. Oral Health of United States Adults: National Findings. Washington DC: National Institute of Dental Research, 1987.

12. Löe H, Anerud A, Boysen H, Morrison E. Natural history of periodontal disease in man. Rapid, moderate, and no loss of attachment in Sri Lankan laborers 14 to 46 years of age. J Clin Periodontol 1986;13:431–445.

13. Ismail AI, Eklund SA, Burt BA, Calderone JJ. Prevalence of deep periodontal pockets in New Mexico adults age 27 to 74 years. J Public Health Dent 1986;46:199–206.

14. Beck JD, Lainson PA, Field HM, Hawkins BF. Risk factors for various levels of periodontal disease and treatment needs in Iowa. Community Dent Oral Epidemiol 1984;12:17–22.

15. Listgarten MA, Schifter CC, Laster L. 3-year longitudinal study of the periodontal status of an adult population with gingivitis. J Clin Periodontol 1985;12:225–238.

16. Page RC, Schroeder HE. Periodontitis in Man and Other Animals: A Comparative Review. New York: Karger, 1982.

17. Lindhe J, Hamp SE, Löe H. Experimental periodontitis in the beagle dog. J Periodontal Res 1973;23:432–437.

18. Garant PR, Cho MI. Histopathogenesis of spontaneous periodontal disease in conventional rats. I. Histometric and histologic study. J Periodontal Res 1979;14:297–309.

19. Garant P. An electron microscopic observation of osteoclastic alveolar bone resorption in rats mono-infected by *Actinomyces naeslundii*. J Periodontol 1976;47:717–723.

20. Lindhe J, Haffajee AD, Socransky SS. Progression of periodontal disease in adult subjects in the absence of periodontal therapy. J Clin Periodontol 1983;10:433–442.

21. Axelsson P, Lindhe J. Effect of controlled oral hygiene procedures on caries and periodontal disease in adults. J Clin Periodontol 1978;5:133–151.

22. Lindhe J, Axelsson P. The effect of controlled oral hygiene and topical fluoride application on caries and gingivitis in Swedish school children. Community Dent Oral Epidemiol 1973;1:9–16.

23. Suomi JD, Greene JC, Vermillion JR, et al. The effect of controlled oral hygiene procedures on the progression of periodontal disease in adults: Results after third and final year. J Periodontol 1971;42:152–160.

24. Lightner LM, O'Leary TJ, Drake RB, et al. Preventive periodontic treatment procedures: Results over 46 months. J Periodontol 1971;42:555–561.

25. Lövdal A, Arno A, Schei O, Waerhaug J. Combined effect of subgingival scaling and controlled oral hygiene on the incidence of gingivitis. Acta Odontol Scand 1961;19:537–555.

26. U.S. Preventive Services Task Force. Guide to clinical preventive services: An assessment of the effectiveness of 169 interventions. Report of the U.S. Preventive Services Task Force (prepublication copy). Baltimore: Williams & Wilkins, 1989.

27. Lang NP, Joss A, Orsanic T, et al. Bleeding on probing. A predictor for the progression of periodontal disease? J Clin Periodontol 1986;13:590–596.

28. Chaves ES, Caffesse RG, Morrison EG, Stults DL. Diagnostic discrimination of bleeding on probing during maintenance periodontal therapy. Am J Dent 1990;3:167–170.

29. Knowles JW, Burgett FG, Nissle RR, et al. Results of periodontal treatment related to pocket depth and attachment level. Eight years. J Periodontol 1979;50:225–233.

30. Okada M, Kuwahara S, Kaihara Y, et al. Relationship between gingival health and dental caries in children aged 7–12 years. J Oral Sci 2000;42:151–155.

31. Glavind L. Means and methods in oral hygiene instruction of adults. A review. Tandlaegebladet 1990;94:213–246.

32. Kiyak HA, Mulligan K. Behavioral research related to oral hygiene practices. In: Löe H, Kleinman DV (eds). Dental Plaque Control Measures and Oral Hygiene Practices. Oxford: IRL Press, 1986.

33. Glavind L. Effect of monthly professional mechanical tooth cleaning on periodontal health in adults. J Clin Periodontol 1977;4:100–106.

34. Glavind L, Zeuner E, Attstrom R. Oral cleanliness and gingival health following oral hygiene instruction by self-educational programs. J Clin Periodontol 1984;11:262–273.

35. Glavind L, Attstrom R. Oral hygiene instruction of adults by means of a self-instructional manual. J Clin Periodontol 1981;8:165–176.

36. Frandsen A. Mechanical oral hygiene practices. In: Löe H, Kleinman DV (eds). Dental Plaque Control Measures and Oral Hygiene Practices. Oxford: IRL Press, 1986.

37. Breitenmoser J, Morman W, Mühlemann H. Damaging effects of tooth brush bristle end form on gingiva. J Periodontol 1979;70:212–216.

38. Ainamo J. Relationship between malalignment of teeth and periodontal disease. Scand J Dent Res 1972;80:104–110.

39. Withers JA, Brunsvold MA, Killoy WJ, Rahe AJ. The relationship of palato-gingival grooves to localized periodontal disease. J Periodontol 1981;52:41–44.

40. Lang NP, Kiel RA, Anderhalden K. Clinical and microbiological effects of subgingival restorations with overhanging or clinically perfect margins. J Clin Periodontol 1983;10:563–578.

41. Schetritt A, Steffensen B. Diagnosis and management of vertical root fractures. J Can Dent Assoc 1995;61:607–613.

42. Ishikawa I, Oda S, Hayashi J, Arakawa SJ. Cervical cemental tears in older patients with adult periodontitis. Case reports. J Periodontol 1996;67:15–20.

43. Lang NP, Kaarup-Hansen D, Joss A, et al. The significance of overhanging filling margins for the health status of interdental periodontal tissues of young adults. Schweiz Monatsschr Zahnmed 1988;98:725–730.

44. Ramfjord SP, Ash MM Jr. Periodontology and Periodontics. Philadelphia: WB Saunders, 1979.

45. Valderhaug J, Birkeland JM. Periodontal conditions in patients 5 years following insertion of fixed prostheses. Pocket depth and loss of attachment. J Oral Rehab 1976;3:237–243.

46. Badersten A, Nilvéus R, Egelberg J. Effect of nonsurgical periodontal therapy. I. Moderately advanced periodontitis. J Clin Periodontol 1981;8:57–72.

47. Sheiham A. The prevention and control of periodontal disease. In: International Conference on Research in the Biology of Periodontal Disease. Chicago: University Press, 1977:309–376.

48. Tinanoff N, Wei SH, Parkins FM. Effect of a pumice prophylaxis on fluoride uptake in tooth enamel. J Am Dent Assoc 1974;88:384–389.

49. Snyder JA, McVay JT, Brown FH, et al. The effect of air abrasive polishing on blood pH and electrolyte concentrations in healthy mongrel dogs. J Periodontol 1990;61:81–86.

50. Mishkin DJ, Engler WO, Javed T, et al. A clinical comparison of the effect on the gingiva of the Prophy-Jet and the rubber cup and paste techniques. J Periodontol 1986;57:151–154.

51. Galloway SE, Pashley DH. Rate of removal of root structure by the use of the Prophy-Jet device. J Periodontol 1987;58:464–469.

52. Bral M, Brownstein CN. Antimicrobial agents in the prevention and treatment of periodontal disease. Dent Clin North Am 1988;32:217–241.

53. Lindhe J (ed). Mouthrinses in the treatment and prevention of gingivitis [proceedings of a symposium, 11 Dec 1987]. J Clin Periodontol 1987;15:485–530.

54. Kornman KS. Antimicrobial agents. In: Löe H, Kleinman DV (eds). Dental Plaque Control Measures and Oral Hygiene Practices. Oxford: IRL Press, 1986.

55. Greenstein G, Berman C, Jaffin R. Chlorhexidine. An adjunct to periodontal therapy. J Periodontol 1986;57:370–377.

56. American Academy of Periodontology Committee on Research Science and Therapy. Chemical Agents for Control of Plaque and Gingivitis. Chicago: American Academy of Periodontology, 1994.

57. Winn D, Blott W, McLaughlin J, et al. Mouthwash use and oral conditions in the risk of oral and pharyngeal cancer. Cancer Res 1991;51:3044.

58. Siegrist BE, Gusberti FA, Brecx MC, et al. Efficacy of supervised rinsing with chlorhexidine digluconate in comparison to phenolic and plant alkaloid compounds. J Periodontal Res 1986;21 (suppl 16):60–73.

59. Grossman E, Reiter G, Sturzenberger OP, et al. Six-month study of the effects of a chlorhexidine mouthrinse on gingivitis in adults. J Periodontal Res 1986;21(suppl 16):33–43.

60. Lie T, Enersen M. Effects of chlorhexidine gel in a group of maintenance-care patients with poor oral hygiene. J Periodontol 1986;57(6):364–369.

61. Lang NP, Brecx MC. Chlorhexidine digluconate: An agent for chemical plaque control and prevention of gingival inflammation. J Periodontal Res 1986;21(suppl 16):74–89.

62. Löe H, Schiott C. The effect of suppression of the oral microflora upon the development of dental plaque and gingivitis. In: McHugh WD (ed). Dental Plaque. Edinburgh: E & S Livingstone, 1970.

63. Briner WW, Grossman E, Buckner RY, et al. Effect of chlorhexidine gluconate mouthrinse on plaque bacteria. J Periodontal Res 1986;21(suppl 16):44–52.

64. Briner WW, Grossman E, Buckner RY, et al. Assessment of susceptibility of plaque bacteria to chlorhexidine after six months' oral use. J Periodontal Res 1986;21(suppl 16):53–56.

65. Löe H, Schiott CR, Glavind L, Karring T. Two years' oral use of chlorhexidine in man. I. General design and clinical effects. J Periodontal Res 1976;11:135–144.

66. Lang NP, Hotz P, Graf H, et al. Effects of supervised chlorhexidine mouthrinses in children. A longitudinal clinical trial. J Periodontal Res 1982;17:101–111.

67. Schiott CR, Löe H, Briner WH. Two years' oral use of chlorhexidine in man. IV. Effect on various medical parameters. J Periodontal Res 1976;11:158–164.

68. Barkvoll P, Rolla G, Svendsen A. Interaction between chlorhexidine digluconate and sodium lauryl sulphate in vivo. J Clin Periodontol 1989;16:593–595.

69. Jenkins S, Addy M, Newcombe R. The effects of a chlorhexidine toothpaste on the development of plaque, gingivitis and tooth staining. J Clin Periodontol 1993;20:59–62.

70. Yates R, Jenkins S, Newcombe R, et al. A 6-month home usage trial of a 1% chlorhexidine toothpaste. I. Effects on plaque, gingivitis, calculus and toothstaining. J Clin Periodontol 1993;20:130–138.

71. Flotra L, Gjermo P, Rolla G, Waerhaug J. Side effects of chlorhexidine mouth washes. Scand J Dent Res 1971;79:119–125.

72. Albandar J, Gjermo P, Preus H. Chlorhexidine use after two decades of over-the-counter availability. J Periodontol 1994;65:109–112.

73. Furia J, Schenkel A. New broad spectrum bacteriostat. Soap Chem Spec 1968;44:47–122.

74. Regos J, Zak O, Solf R, et al. Antimicrobial spectrum of triclosan, a broad-spectrum antimicrobial agent for topical application. III. Comparison with some other antimicrobial agents. Dermatol 1979;158:72–79.

75. Mankodi S, Walker C, Conforti N, et al. The clinical effect of a triclosan-containing dentifrice on plaque accumulation and the development of gingivitis. A 6-month study. Clin Prev Dent 1992;14:4–10.

76. Saxton C, Lane R, Van der Ouderaa F. The effects of a dentifrice containing a zinc salt and non-cationic agent on plaque and gingivitis. J Clin Periodontol 1987;14:144–148.

77. Garcia-Godoy F, DeVizio W, Volpe A, et al. Effect of triclosan copolymer/fluoride dentifrice on plaque formation and gingivitis: A 7-month clinical study. Am J Dent 1994;3:S15–S26.

78. Svatun B, Saxton C, Rolla G, Ouderaa V. A one-year study on the maintenance of gingival health by a dentifrice containing a zinc salt and non-ionic antimicrobial agent. J Clin Periodontol 1989;16:75–82.

79. Lindhe J, Rosling B, Socransky S, Volpe A. The effect of a triclosan-containing dentifrice on established plaque and gingivitis. J Clin Periodontol 1993;20:327–334.

80. Walker C, Borden L, Zambon J, et al. The effects of a 0.3% triclosan-containing dentifrice on the microbial composition of supragingival plaque. J Clin Periodontol 1994;21:334–341.

81. Heath RJ, Rock CO. A triclosan-resistant bacterial enzyme. Nature 2000;406:145–146.

82. Travis J. Popularity of germ fighter raises concern. Sci News 2000;157:342.

83. Schaeken M, van der Hoeven J, Saxton C, Cummins D. The effect of mouthrinses containing zinc and triclosan on plaque accumulation and development of gingivitis in a 3-week clinical test. J Clin Periodontol 1994;21:360–364.

84. Damm DD, Curran A, White DK, Drummond JF. Leukoplakia of the maxillary vestibule—An association with Viadent? Oral Surg Oral Med Oral Path Oral Radiol Endod 1999;87:61–66.

85. Giertsen E, Svatun B, Saxton A. Inhibition by hexetidine and zinc. Scand J Dent Res 1987;95:49–54.

86. Hefti AF, Huber BJ. The effect on early plaque formation, gingivitis and salivary bacterial counts of mouthwashes hexetidine/zinc, aminefluoride/tin or chlorhexidine. J Clin Periodontol 1987;14:515–518.

87. Brecx M, Brownstone E, MacDonald L,et al. Efficacy of Listerine, Meridol and chlorhexidine mouthrinses as supplements to regular toothcleaning measures. J Clin Periodontol 1992;19: 202–207.

88. Wolff L, Pihlstrom B, Bakdash M, et al. Salt and peroxide compared with conventional oral hygiene. II. Microbial results. J Periodontol 1987;58:301–307.

89. Haffajee A, Socransky S, Goodson J. Subgingival temperature. II. Relation to future periodontal attachment loss. J Clin Periodontol 1992;19:409–416.

90. Bakdash M, Wolff L, Pihlstrom B,et al. Salt and peroxide compared with conventional oral hygiene. III. Patient compliance and acceptance. J Periodontol 1987;58:308–313.

91. Cerra M, Killoy W. The effect of sodium bicarbonate and hydrogen peroxide on the microbial flora of periodontal pockets. J Periodontol 1982;53:599.

92. Wolff L, Pihlstrom B, Bakdash M, et al. Four-year investigation of salt and peroxide regimen compared with conventional oral hygiene. J Am Dent Assoc 1989;118:67.

93. Jones C, Blinkhorn A, White E. Hydrogen peroxide, the effect on plaque and gingivitis when used in an oral irrigator. Clin Prev Dent 1990;12:15.

94. Clark W, Magnusson I, Walker C, et al. Efficacy of Perimed antibacterial system on established gingivitis. J Clin Periodontol 1989;16:630.

95. Marvniak J, Clark W, Walker C, et al. The effect of three mouthrinses on plaque and gingivitis development. J Clin Periodontol 1992;19:19.

96. Gaengler P, Kurbad A, Weinert W. Evaluation of anti-calculus efficacy. An SEM method of evaluating the effectiveness of pyrophosphate dentifrice on calculus formation. J Clin Periodontol 1993;20:144–146.

97. Addy M, Koltai R. Control of supragingival calculus. Scaling and polishing and anticalculus toothpastes: An opinion. J Clin Periodontol 1994;21:342–346.

98. Stookey G, Jackson R, Beiswanger B. Clinical efficacy of chemicals for calculus prevention. In: Ten Cate JM (ed). Recent Advances in the Study of Dental Calculus. Oxford: IRL Press, 1989:235–258.

99. Lobene R. A clinical study of the anticalculus effect of a dentifrice containing soluble pyrophosphates and sodium fluoride. Clin Prev Dent 1986;8:5–7.

100. Lobene R. Anticalculus effect of a dentifrice containing pyrophosphate salts and sodium fluoride. Compend Contin Educ Dent 1987;8:175–178.

101. Lobene R. A clinical comparison of the anticalculus effect of two commercial dentifrices. Clin Prev Dent 1987;9:3–8.

102. Rosling B, Lindhe J. The anticalculus efficacy of two commercially available anticalculus dentifrices. Compend Contin Educ Dent 1987;8:278–282.

103. Stephen K, Saxton C, Ritchie C, Morrison T. Control of gingivitis and calculus by a dentifrice containing a zinc salt and triclosan. J Periodontol 1990;61:674–679.

104. DeLattre VF. Factors contributing to adverse soft tissue reactions due to the use of tartar control dentifrice: A report of a case and literature review. J Periodontol 1999;70:803–807.

105. Ervasti T, Knuuttila M, Pohjamo L, Haukipuro K. Relation between control of diabetes and gingival bleeding. J Periodontol 1985;56(3):154–157.

106. Setia A. Severe bleeding from a pregnancy tumor. Oral Surg 1973;36:192.

107. Sutcliffe P. A longitudinal study of gingivitis and puberty. J Periodontal Res 1972;7:52–58.

108. Holm G. Smoking as an additional risk for tooth loss. J Periodontol 1994;65:996–1001.

109. Grossi SG, Zambon JJ, Ho AW, et al. Assessment of risk for periodontal disease. I. Risk indicators for attachment loss. J Periodontol 1994;65:260–267.

110. American Academy of Periodontology. The Etiology and Pathogenesis of Periodontal Diseases. Chicago: The American Academy of Periodontology, 1992.

111. Robertson PB, Walsh M, Greene J, et al. Periodontal effects associated with the use of smokeless tobacco. J Periodontol 1990;61:438–443.

112. Christen A, McDonald J, Christen J. The Impact of Tobacco Use and Cessation on Nonmalignant and Precancerous Oral and Dental Diseases and Conditions. Indianapolis: Indiana University School of Dentistry, 1991.

113. Pennell BM, Keagle JG. Predisposing factors in the etiology of chronic inflammatory periodontal disease. J Periodontol 1977; 48(9):517–532.

114. Lang NP, Kiel RA, Anderhalden K. Clinical and microbiological effects of subgingival restorations with overhanging and clinically perfect margins. J Clin Periodontol 1983;10(6): 563–578.

115. Preber H, Bergstrom J. Occurrence of gingival bleeding in smoker and nonsmoker patients. I. Acta Odontol Scand 1985; 43:315–320.

116. Bergstrom J, Floderus-Myrhed B. Co-twin control study of the relationship between smoking and some periodontal disease factors. Community Dent Oral Epidemiol 1983;11:113–116.

117. Bergstrom J, Preber H. Tobacco use as a risk factor. J Periodontol 1994;65:545–550.

118. Lang NP, Tonetti MS, Suter J, et al. Effect of interleukin-1 gene polymorphisms on gingival inflammation assessed by bleeding on probing in a periodontal maintenance population. J Periodontal Res 2000;35:102–107.

119. Swenson H. The effects of cigarette smoking on plaque formation. J Periodontol 1979;50:146–147.

120. Kenney EB, Saxe SR, Bowles RD. The effect of cigarette smoking on anaerobiosis in the oral cavity. J Periodontol 1975;46: 82.

121. Ah MKB, Johnson GK, Kaldahl WB, et al. The effect of smoking on the response to periodontal therapy. J Clin Periodontol 1994;21:91–97.

122. Johren P, Jackowski J, Gangler P, et al. Fear reduction in patients with dental treatment phobia. Br J Oral Maxillofac Surg 2000;38:612–616.

123. Maslow A. Toward a Psychology of Being. New York: D. Van Nostrand, 1968.

124. Harris N, Christen A. Primary Preventive Dentistry. Norwalk: Appleton and Lange, 1987.

125. Keyes P, Rams T. A rationale for management of periodontal disease: Rapid identification of microbial "therapeutic targets" with phase contrast microscopy. J Am Dent Assoc 1983;106:803.

126. Caton J. Periodontal diagnosis and diagnostic aids. In: Proceedings of the World Workshop in Clinical Periodontics. Chicago: American Academy of Periodontology, 1989:1–22.

127. Isogai E, Isogai H, Hirose K, et al. Subgingival temperature is elevated when gingivitis is present. J Periodontol 1994;65:710–712.

128. Holthuis A, Gelskey S, Chebih F. The relationship between gingival tissue temperature and various indicators of gingival inflammation. J Periodontol 1981;52:187–189.

129. DeBiase C. Dental Health Education Theory and Practice. Philadelphia: Lea and Febiger, 1991:7–18.

130. DeBiase C. Dental Health Education Theory and Practice. Philadelphia: Lea and Febiger, 1991:243–264.

131. Barnes CM, Russell CM, Weatherford TW III. A comparison of the efficacy of 2 powered toothbrushes in affecting plaque accumulation, gingivitis, and gingival bleeding. J Periodontol 1999;70:840–847.

132. Soparkar P, Newman M, DePaolo P. The efficacy of a novel toothbrush design. J Clin Dent 1991;2(4):107–110.

133. Killoy WJ, Love JW, Love J, et al. The effectiveness of a counter-rotary action powered toothbrush and conventional toothbrush on plaque removal and gingival bleeding. A short term study. J Periodontol 1989;60(8):473–477.

134. Barnes C, Weatherford T, Menaker L, et al. A comparison of the Braun, Oral-B Plaque Remover (D5) electric and a manual toothbrush in affecting gingivitis. J Clin Dent 1993;4:48–51.

135. van der Weijden FA, Timmerman MF, Piscaer M, et al. A comparison of the efficacy of a novel electric toothbrush and a manual toothbrush in the treatment of gingivitis. Am J Dent 1998;11(Spec Issue):S23–28.

136. Boyd R, Murray P, Robertson P. Effect on periodontal status of rotary electric toothbrushes vs. manual toothbrushes during periodontal maintenance. I. Clinical results. J Periodontol 1989;60:390–395.

137. Johnson B, McInnes C. Clinical evaluation of the efficacy and safety of a new sonic toothbrush. J Periodontol 1994;65:692–697.

138. MacNeill S, Walters DM, Dey A, et al. Sonic and mechanical toothbrushes: An in vitro study showing altered microbial surface structures but lack of effect on viability. J Clin Periodontol 1998;25:988–993.

139. Terezhalmy G, Gagliardi V, Rybicki L, et al. Clinical evaluation of the efficacy and safety of the Ultrasonex ultrasonic toothbrush. Compend Contin Educ Dent 1994;15:866–874.

140. Greenstein G. Nonsurgical periodontal therapy in 2000: A literature review. J Am Dent Assoc 2000;131:1580–1592.

141. Flemmig TF, Newman MG, Doherty FM, et al. Supragingival irrigation with 0.06% chlorhexidine in naturally occurring gingivitis. I. 6 month clinical observations. J Periodontol 1990;61(2):112–117.

142. Newman MG, Flemmig TF, Nachnani S, et al. Irrigation with 0.06% chlorhexidine in naturally occurring gingivitis. II. 6-month microbiological observations. J Periodontol 1990;61:427–433.

143. Chaves E, Kornman K, Manwell M, et al. Mechanism of irrigation effects on gingivitis. J Periodontol 1994;65:1016–1021.

144. Felo A, Shibly O, Ciancio SG, et al. Effects of subgingival chlorhexidine irrigation on peri-implant maintenance. Am J Dent 1997;10:107–110.

145. McFall WT Jr. Supportive treatment. In: Nevins M, Becker W, Kornman K (eds). Proceedings of the World Workshop in Clinical Periodontics, July 23–27, 1989. Chicago, American Academy of Periodontology, 1989.

146. Page RC, Schroeder HE. Pathogenesis of inflammatory periodontal disease. A summary of current work. Lab Invest 1976;34(3):235–249.

147. Selvig K. Attachment of plaque and calculus to tooth surfaces. J Periodontal Res 1970;5:8–18.

148. Muhler J, Ennever J. The occurrence of dental calculus through several successive periods in a selected group of subjects. J Periodontol 1962;33:22–25.

149. Statistics NCH. Oral hygiene in adults. Vital and health statistics. US Public Health Service. Washington, DC: Government Printing Office, 1966.

150. Suomi J, Smith L, McClendon B, et al. Oral calculus in children. J Periodontol 1971;42:341–345.

151. Blank L, Rule J, Colangelo G, et al. The relationship between first presentation and subsequent observations in heavy calculus formers. J Periodontol 1994;65:750–754.

152. Conroy C, Sturzenberger O. The rate of calculus formation in adults. J Periodontol 1968;39:20–22.

153. Klein F, Dicks J. Evaluation of accumulation of calculus in tube-fed, mentally handicapped patients. J Am Dent Assoc 1984;108:352–354.

Treating Chronic Periodontitis with Early or Moderate Attachment Loss

Thomas G. Wilson, Jr, and Kenneth S. Kornman
- Collecting the Clinical and Radiographic Evidence
- Interpreting the Evidence
- Making a Clinical Diagnosis
- Determining Risk Factors for Disease Progression
- Determining the Prognosis
- Formulating a Treatment Plan

Michael K. McGuire, Bengt G. Rosling, and Thomas G. Wilson, Jr.
- Nonsurgical Therapy for Early and Moderate Periodontitis

Dan M. Loughlin, Kenneth L. Kalkwarf, and Erwin P. Barrington
- Surgical Therapy for Periodontitis with Moderate Attachment Loss

Dan M. Loughlin, Mark E. Glover, and Robert M. Loughlin
- Clinical Crown Lengthening
- Postoperative Care and Periodontal Maintenance

Janet M. Guthmiller
- Local Delivery of Antimicrobial Agents in the Treatment of Periodontitis

Recent advances allow the clinician to determine a patient's prognosis more successfully and thereby develop a treatment plan tailored for the individual. The clinician uses an approach based on the analysis of local and systemic risk factors for developing inflammatory periodontal disease. The clinician gathers the same information about the patient's oral condition outlined in chapter 17. Local risk factors are gleaned from these data. These bacterial factors include deep pockets and other areas, such as rough subgingival margins, that may shelter microbes. In some cases, identification of specific bacteria and determination of antibiotic susceptibility may be helpful (see chapter 5). This is most commonly recommended for cases in which (1) the clinical severity of destruction exceeds expectations, given the level of bacter-ial plaque or (2) systemic risk factors are present that suggest that the patient's host response may not adequately control the bacterial challenge. Among the strongest systemic factors are smoking, diabetes mellitus, and a genetic modification that puts the patient at increased risk. The prognosis for the case can be determined by the extent to which the risk factors can be eliminated or ameliorated.

The order of therapy is to (1) collect the clinical and radiographic evidence; (2) interpret the evidence; (3) make a clinical diagnosis; (4) determine risk factors; (5) estimate the prognosis; (6) formulate a treatment plan; and then (7) treat the patient.

There are three basic clinical conditions of the periodontium: health, gingivitis, and periodontitis. These may be seen separately or in combination. The following

THE EVIDENCE

Health History

1. Medical
   - Mr Wilson's health history reveals nothing that would influence his oral health, except that he has a heart murmur and takes several doses of a nonsteroidal anti-inflammatory drug daily.
   - He smokes one pack of cigarettes per day.
   - There is no current or family history of diabetes mellitus.
2. Dental
   - The patient saw a practitioner (his father) regularly until he was in college. Since then, his visits have been sporadic.
   - He is an intelligent person who does not take good care of his teeth.
   - His oral hygiene consists of brushing his teeth twice a day.
   - The patient says that he is under a great deal of stress, which will continue. When under stress, he frequently grinds his teeth (bruxism) at night.
   - His teeth are very sensitive to iced drinks.

Extraoral Examination

1. The head and neck are inspected visually for asymmetries and abnormal features.
   - ➤ The findings are within normal limits except for a small lesion on the left cheek that the patient has noticed within the last 6 months.
2. The temporomandibular joints are inspected by palpation during range-of-motion movements; any noise or tenderness is recorded.
   - ➤ The findings are within normal limits except for a slight pop in the left temporomandibular joint on opening. The patient says that this condition has not changed for years.
3. The lips are examined for any abnormalities (including location and size), since a large percentage of oral neoplasms are found here.
   - ➤ No abnormalities are found.

(continued)

case involves a patient with a form of chronic periodontitis. Included is an overview of the clinical, radiographic, and basic scientific principles associated with this class of disease.

Collecting the Clinical and Radiographic Evidence

Mr Wilson presents to your office. His reason for coming (chief complaint) is that his wife has complained lately that he has bad breath. He completes a health history and presents you with a full-mouth series of radiographs taken recently.

In your initial interview with the patient, you find a well-nourished, well-oriented man who is 52 years old. He is a manager of an international business firm. He has never thought about his goals for his teeth, but after discussing the subject with you, he says that his appearance is important and that he thinks healthy teeth and gums are an important part of his overall well-being.

Interpreting the Evidence

After reading this section, one should understand how to interpret the clinical, microbiologic, and radiographic signs associated with this patient's disease. One should also understand how bacteria can collect in the interproximal regions of the teeth of patients who do not remove these microbes daily (which is true of most patients). Later sections will review the knowledge used to make an expert diagnosis, which, along with elimination or modification of systemic risk factors, will become the driving force behind the initial treatment of the patient. Following the reevaluation of initial (nonsurgical) therapy, a final diagnosis will be made that will direct further active treatment. Once the disease has been arrested, the patient will be placed in periodontal maintenance. The following steps are important for determining a diagnosis:

1. Make sure the patient has no extraoral or intraoral problems that should be dealt with first.
2. Look for a systemic component to the disease process.
3. Review the patient's clinical signs and symptoms.
4. Review the patient's radiographic signs.

Intraoral Examination

1. Any discoloration (usually white, red, or black) of the oral mucosal tissues is recorded, including location and size.

   ➤ No abnormalities are found.

2. The tongue is grasped at the tip with cotton gauze and gently moved anteriorly to inspect the lateral borders, since this is the most frequent site for intraoral neoplasms and changes associated with certain chronic conditions.

   ➤ No abnormalities are found.

Risk Factors

1. Local
   - Bacteria are present, and in some areas the patient cannot remove them (eg, the cement around a single-unit fixed partial denture and probing depths greater than 3 mm). (See "Radiographic Examination" below.)
   - Compliance with suggested oral hygiene (flossing) measures and periodic maintenance is poor.

2. Systemic
   - The patient smokes.
   - He does not have diabetes, and there is no family history of the disease.
   - His genetic status is undetermined at his first visit, but testing is recommended. Because this patient smokes and has periodontitis (see "Clinical Examination" below), it is important to determine his genetic susceptibility to the disease. If he is positive for the interleukin 1 (IL-1) genotype, he has a greater risk for tooth loss; if he continues to smoke and is IL-1 positive, it increases his risk multiple times (see chapter 11). The patient is tested and is IL-1 positive.

Clinical Examination

1. Dental (Fig 23-1)

   ➤ All teeth are present except maxillary third molars.
   ➤ There are several dental restorations; some are serviceable, and some have poorly adapted margins.

   ➤ There is bacterial plaque at the gingival margins of most of the teeth, especially in the interproximal regions.
   ➤ The full-coverage restorations on the maxillary left lateral incisor and the maxillary left first molar have open margins.
   ➤ Supragingival calculus is present on the lingual aspect of the mandibular teeth.
   ➤ The teeth have bidigital mobility that ranges up to Class II on the Miller scale, and fremitus is present on several of the molars.

2. Periodontal (Fig 23-2)

   ➤ Probing depths range from 2 to 6 mm, with the deeper areas found in the interproximal regions of the posterior teeth; bone loss is found in the furcations of most of the molars.
   ➤ There is bleeding found after probing in all the posterior interproximal regions and on the facial and lingual aspects of several of the posterior teeth. When the clinician uses fingers to press the gingival tissues in an occlusal direction, suppuration is found in a few areas associated with deeper probing depths. The soft tissues around the maxillary left lateral incisor and the maxillary left first molar are very inflamed.
   ➤ Deposits of subgingival calculus are detected.
   ➤ Minimal gingival recession has occurred.

Radiographic Examination

Radiographic examination (Fig 23-3) is normal except for the following: In contrast to a healthy periodontium, early changes of periodontitis seen on radiography include thinning or loss of the crestal cortication, blunting of mandibular anterior interdental bone, alveolar crest greater than 2 mm subadjacent to cementoenamel junctions (CEJs), cupping, cratering, or vertical bony defects associated with the alveolar crest. A radiopaque area, possibly dental cement, is seen on the distal aspect of the maxillary left first molar associated with the single-unit fixed partial denture on that tooth.

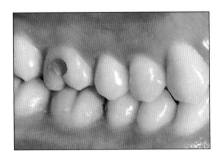 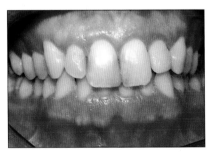 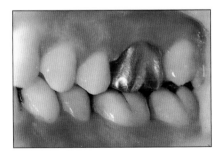

Figs 23-1a to 23-1c The patient's dental and periodontal condition at the initial examination.

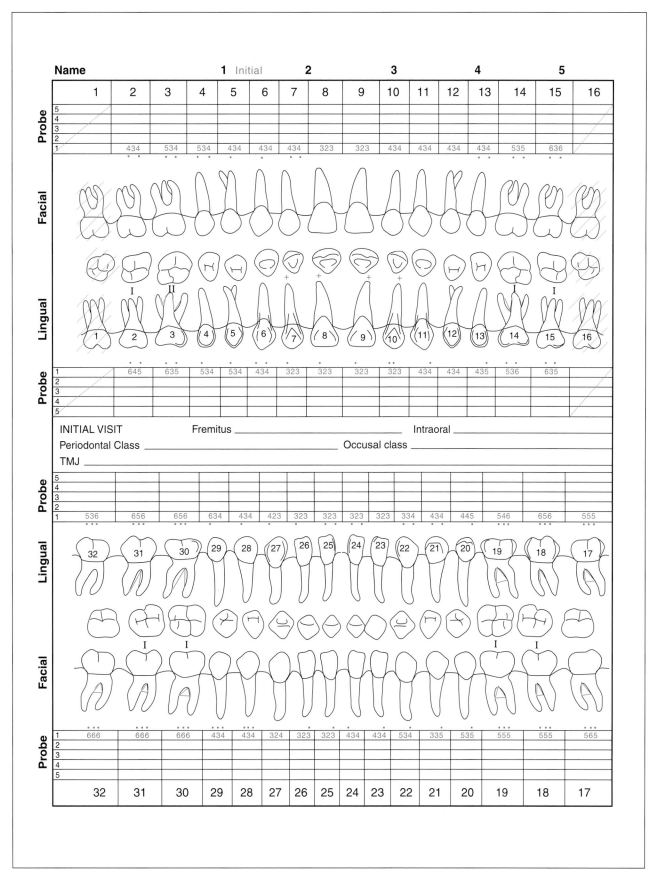

Fig 23-2 Charting taken at the initial visit.

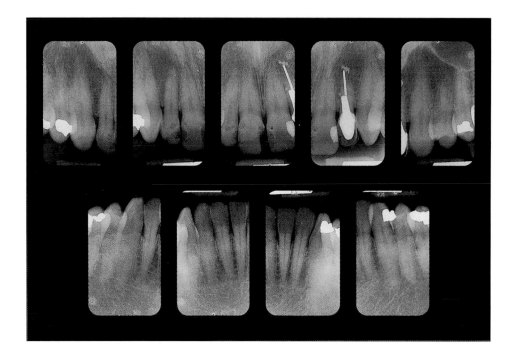

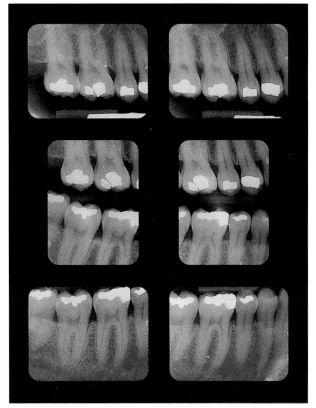 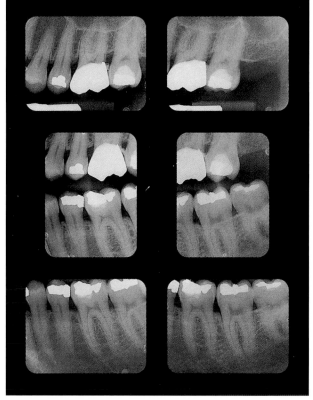

Fig 23-3 Initial radiographs.

Extraoral and Intraoral Problems

In Mr Wilson's case, no problems are evident except a slight pop in the left temporomandibular joint on opening and a lesion on his left cheek. The patient should be counseled on the potential problems associated with temporomandibular joint dysfunction and how to reduce them. A habit appliance will be recommended to ameliorate his joint noise, reduce his thermal sensitivity, and possibly reduce future problems. The patient is told to contact his physician if the lesion on his cheek persists.

Systemic Condition

Mr Wilson has a heart murmur. Patients with certain types of murmurs need to take antibiotics before invasive dental procedures (see appendix 2). Often patients are aware of this and will have taken their medication before the appointment. If not, check with the patient's physician about the need for antibiotic coverage.

The patient takes large doses of nonsteroidal anti-inflammatory drugs (NSAIDs) daily. NSAIDs have many influences on the clinical signs of periodontitis; they all inhibit the cyclooxygenase enzyme that is responsible for the synthesis of prostaglandins. All NSAIDs reduce clinical signs of inflammation, and some NSAIDs have been shown to reduce the progression of bone loss in periodontitis. Aspirin, unlike other NSAIDs, has an inhibition of cyclooxygenase that is irreversible. This irreversible effect is significant only in platelets, which cannot synthesize new enzymes. The net effect is a reduction in platelet aggregation and a prolonged bleeding time. Therapeutic doses of aspirin or NSAIDs may irritate gastric mucosa and increase blood loss, frequently without overt symptoms. This patient therefore may have periodontal and nonperiodontal effects of prolonged aspirin or NSAID therapy. The periodontal effects may involve some reduction in bone loss, but an increase in gingival bleeding tendency. The patient must also be watched for gastrointestinal adverse effects from the medication. Prolonged bleeding should be expected during scaling and root planing or surgical procedures.

There is accumulating evidence that chronic inflammatory diseases, such as periodontitis, may have negative effects in the cardiovascular system (see chapter 15). It may be appropriate to inform the patient of current information on this topic.

Clinical Signs and Symptoms

Excessive Occlusal Forces
Bidigital tooth mobilities range up to Class II, and there is fremitus on the molars. The patient's teeth hurt when he drinks cold fluids. When this information is combined with the fact that the patient is aware of bruxism (grinding his teeth) at night, one must suspect that most of these clinical findings are related to this habit. The clinician must decide whether these signs and symptoms warrant therapy. If any of these symptoms concern the patient or if the problems are getting worse (increasing tooth mobility, development of muscle pain, or increasing thermal sensitivity), then therapy is warranted. In this case, in the opinion of the therapist, clinical symptoms plus patient concerns warrant occlusal bruxism therapy.

Problems with Restorations
The patient has several amalgam restorations that are failing, and the fixed partial dentures on the maxillary left lateral incisor and first molar have open margins. The patient is informed that these restorations should be replaced following resolution of the clinical signs of inflammation.

Periodontal Tissue Inflammation
➤ *The gingival tissues are inflamed.*

Role of plaque. If supragingival plaque is left undisturbed for more than a few days, the bacterial ecology matures and produces both microbial changes and changes in the gingival tissues. Patients who do not clean well in interproximal sites usually have a mature plaque ecology. These ecological changes allow the establishment of a subgingival ecosystem in which the bacteria thrive. Although the supragingival plaque is essential for the formation of the subgingival plaque ecology, the two become somewhat independent as the subgingival plaque becomes well established. For example, once the subgingival plaque is established, removal of supragingival plaque will have only a limited effect on the subgingival bacteria. The deeper the probing depths, the more independent the two ecosystems become. Therefore, after periodontitis has produced a loss of attachment, removal of supragingival plaque alone will not be sufficient to stop the disease process. In that situation, one must also direct attention to the subgingival plaque.

Bacterial changes. Extensive research has been directed at determining which bacteria are responsible for the initiation of attachment loss and bone loss and therefore produce the conversion from gingivitis to periodontitis. Unfortunately, this question is still unresolved. In chronic periodontitis, however, there are distinct microbial findings that are not consistent with health and should therefore be eradicated as a goal of therapy. *Porphyromonas gingivalis* is frequently present in disease but not in health. Failure to eliminate *P gingivalis* has been associated with a clinical failure to control the disease. Although the data are less convincing, *Bacteroides forsythus* and certain types of *Prevotella intermedia* are increased in periodontitis (see chapter 5).

Inflammatory changes. Histologically, Mr Wilson's lesion appears similar to, but larger than, the lesion of chronic gingivitis, and loss of bone is evident at the coronal aspect of the alveolar bone. There is a heavy infiltrate of plasma cells and B lymphocytes, as well as T lymphocytes and macrophages within the lesion. The accumulation of inflammatory and immune cells may follow the course of larger blood vessels originating from the alveolar bone. At the time of the actual loss of bone, the zone of injury may extend closer to the surface of the underlying bone, thus bringing the inflammatory infiltrate closer to the surface of the alveolar bone. The gingival crevicular fluid from these patients contains appreciable amounts of neutrophil-derived enzymes (ie, β-glucuronidase and neutrophil elastase), cytokines (IL-1), and eicosanoids (prostaglandin E_2 [PGE_2]) (see chapter 9).

Immune findings. Chronic periodontitis associated with breakdown of the barrier function of the epithelia in the sulcus, loss of connective tissue integrity, and bone resorption involves local and systemic immunologic responses. While polymorphonuclear leukocytes (PMNs) remain a significant component of the cellular infiltrate in the tissues and predominate in the gingival sulcus, increases in the mononuclear cell population are noted, including T cells, B cells, and macrophage/monocytes. The distribution of T-cell phenotypes (and presumably functions) in this infiltrate has been shown to be altered, with a prevalence of $T_{C/S}$ (CD8$^+$) cells. The changes in local T cells result in a dysregulation of host responses to the plaque antigens and contribute to the additional influx of B cells, with some differentiation into plasma cells. There is a dramatic increase in local mediators and cytokines, including molecules associated with cell disruption (PGE_2) and cell stress (IL-1, IL-6, and tumor necrosis factor α), as well as more sophisticated mechanisms for recruitment of host defenses (IL-8, monocyte chemotactic peptide-1 [MCP-1], and C' activation). Immunoglobulins in the gingivocrevicular fluid (GCF) generally reflect the plasma cell infiltrate, with immunoglobulin G (IgG) predominating; however, local increases in specific antibody are not as prevalent as in the more aggressive forms of periodontitis. Systemic immune reactions may reflect or contribute to the local changes with alterations in inflammatory mediators, altered T-cell functions, and elevations in serum antibody levels. In particular, the literature demonstrates elevations in serum antibody to *P gingivalis* in a majority of these patients, although individual subjects may show significant responses to other proposed pathogens (ie, *Campylobac-*

ter rectus or *P intermedia*). While these inflammatory and immune responses characterize this disease to some extent, the functions and importance of these responses to maintaining homeostasis of the periodontium or contributing to tissue destruction remain enigmatic.

Probing Depths

➤ *The probing depths are greater than 3 mm.*

The periodontal probe stops at different levels, depending on the amount of inflammation present. The periodontal attachment apparatus, which connects the gingiva and periodontal ligament to the tooth, is composed of both connective tissue fibers that insert into the root surface and an epithelial attachment that involves epithelial cells from the gingiva attaching to the tooth surface by means of hemidesmosomes. In health and gingivitis, the connective tissue attachment is approximately at the CEJ. In periodontitis, the coronal portion of the connective tissue is at a more apical position. The clinically measured level of attachment is an indication of the severity of periodontal destruction. This clinical measurement is made with a periodontal probe, which is held gently but firmly in the hand and used to measure the distance from the most apical part of the sulcus or pocket to the gingival margin (probing depth) or to the CEJ (clinical attachment level) (see chapter 17 for specific information on how to probe). Although the primary determinant of probing depth and clinical attachment level is the location of the connective tissue attachment, the actual measurement is a function of not only the connective tissue attachment location but also the amount of inflammation in the area, the pressure applied to the probe, and the diameter of the probe.

With minimal or no inflammation, the connective tissue fibers are intact, and the gingival epithelium is attached to the tooth via an epithelial attachment. The probe stops within the epithelial attachment, somewhat coronal to the connective tissue attachment. With inflammation in the area, the basal epithelial cells turn over more rapidly, preventing cell maturation and reducing the integrity of the epithelial attachment. In addition, the collagen fibers that make up the connective tissue attachment undergo some destruction. The net result is that in the presence of inflammation, the periodontal probe passes completely through the epithelial attachment and usually stops just apical to the most coronal part of the connective tissue attachment.

With increasing pressure on the periodontal probe, the apical penetration is increased. With minimal inflammation, this may result in complete penetration of the epithelial attachment. With greater inflammation, however, an increase in pressure results in more apical penetration of connective tissue.

Connective tissues. The biochemical events occurring in the connective tissues of a patient with mild chronic periodontitis will be closely associated with the inflammatory infiltrate. With the accumulation of inflammatory cells, numerous cytokines, interleukins, and bioactive molecules are released; they amplify the inflammatory reaction, as well as act directly and indirectly on the resident fibroblasts. A principal response of fibroblasts to the inflammatory process is release of the matrix-degrading metalloproteinases. These enzymes lead to significant degradation of matrix collagens and proteoglycans. Excessive release of reactive oxygen species (eg, oxygen-derived free radicals) is possible, which can further add to the tissue destruction. At the same time that tissue destruction is occurring, the cells at the periphery of the inflammatory lesion are stimulated to increase their matrix synthesis in an attempt to wall off the inflammatory lesion.

An important feature of any destructive lesion is the disruption of the delicate balance between matrix formation and matrix degradation. In the case of destructive periodontal inflammation, the balance is tipped toward degradation so that the rate of formation is insufficient to accommodate for the loss of matrix structure associated with the degradative processes.

The inflammatory process leads to the release of numerous breakdown products of the extracellular matrix, which may be detected in the gingival crevicular fluid. These products include breakdown products of collagens, proteoglycans, and hyaluronic acid. In addition, in inflamed tissues the levels of detectable tissue collagenase increase and appear to correlate with the level of tissue destruction (see chapter 6).

Bone changes. In patients with 4- to 6-mm probing depths where the gingival margins are located approximately at the CEJ (chronic periodontitis), the supporting bone appears similar to that found in healthy patients. In both types of patients, bone is under constant turnover. Osteoclasts resorb bone and set the stage for osteoblast recruitment, attachment, and new bone formation. In patients with chronic periodontitis, bacterial products and factors produced as part of the host response affect both the resorptive stages (ie, osteoclast-mediated events) and synthetic stages (ie, osteoblast-mediated events) of the process. In disease, there is an increase in the rate of bone resorption compared with new bone formation, resulting in net bone loss. Nothing is abnormal about the bone during this process. It is simply responding to the local factors produced by the bacteria and immune system. During treatment, bacteria are eliminated from the local environment, and therefore the host response to the bacteria (ie, local factor production) is greatly reduced. Bone physiol-

ogy and turnover return to normal, and the progression of the disease is halted (see chapter 7).

Periodontal pathology. Clinically, periodontitis is associated with loss of gingival tissue attachment and firmness. This is due to the inflammatory infiltration with extended loss of collagen fibers, including periodontal ligament fibers and edema of the connective tissue. The attached gingiva is erythematous as a result of the inflammation with increased amounts of vessels and vasodilation. The mucogingival line, therefore, often is not clearly visible in periodontitis. Due to the loss of periodontal ligament fibers and apical migration of junctional epithelium, the probing depth is more than 3 mm in the posterior interproximal regions. The pocket epithelium has increased permeability and is ulcerated in some areas. This situation, combined with vascular exudation of serum as part of the inflammatory process, facilitates an increased flow of pocket fluid—the crevicular exudate, which is also increased in gingivitis. The inflammatory process in periodontitis is associated with increased plasma-cell infiltration.

Clinical Attachment Level
➤ *The free gingival margins are at, or slightly coronal to, the CEJ in most areas.*

The relation of the margin of the gingival tissues to the CEJ is important in establishing a proper diagnosis. The location of the free gingival margin is taken into account in a measurement called the clinical attachment level (CAL). The CAL is the sum of the number of millimeters of gingival recession and the probing depth. If the probing depth alone is used, errors can be made in reading a chart. One should be more concerned about a probing depth of 3 mm with 9 mm of recession than the same probing depth with no recession. The first example represents 12 mm of attachment loss, while the second example represents no attachment loss.

Radiographic Signs

Radiographs reveal signs of early changes associated with periodontitis including loss of crestal cortication and alveolar crests that are more than 2 mm subadjacent to the CEJs.

Making a Clinical Diagnosis

1. Is this periodontal health? *No, because there are clinical signs of inflammation and radiographic evidence of bony changes.*

2. Is this gingivitis? *There is gingivitis, but because there has been attachment loss, gingivitis is not the most severe disease finding.*

3. Is this periodontitis? *Yes, because there has been attachment loss (pocket formation) and bone loss.*

4. What subgroup of periodontitis is this?

   a. Is this chronic periodontitis? *Yes, because of the following: (1) The patient has not been previously treated for periodontitis and is 52 years old. (2) There are abundant local factors (plaque and calculus) associated with the clinical signs of inflammation. This would indicate slowly progressing (chronic) disease.*

   b. Is this aggressive periodontitis? *No, for the reasons stated above.*

5. Therefore, what is the initial periodontal diagnosis? *Chronic periodontitis.* There are three subclassifications of the disease:

   a. Early chronic periodontitis: Probing depths of 4 to 6 mm; no furcation invasion

   b. Moderate chronic periodontitis: Probing depths of 6 mm or greater; furcation involvement

   c. Severe chronic periodontitis: Probing depths of 7 mm or greater. This type of periodontitis is now classified as an aggressive form.

There has been bone loss in the furcations in this untreated patient, with 4- to 6-mm probing depths. The coronal margins of the soft tissues are at or close to the CEJs, and there are clinical signs of inflammation. *The initial diagnosis is chronic periodontitis with moderate attachment loss.*

Determining Risk Factors for Disease Progression

Several risk factors, both local and systemic, can affect disease progression. Local factors include bacteria and any niches that protect them from daily disruption of the plaque by the patient, as well as the degree to which the patient complies with the dental therapist's suggestions. As previously discussed, if allowed to remain undisturbed, bacteria initiate and sustain an inflammatory reaction in the periodontal tissues, which if untreated will lead to tooth loss in some patients. As bacterial plaque matures, it can allow colonization of more pathogenic organisms. Where probing depths are shallow (in the range of 3 mm or less) and the patient disrupts the plaque with daily oral hygiene, the clinical signs of gingivitis (eg, bleeding on probing and color changes) can be reversed. Patients who visit the dental office for routine periodontal maintenance generally keep their teeth longer than those who do not.

Unfortunately, many patients do not clean their teeth as suggested and do not schedule maintenance visits as often as recommended. This lack of compliance is a major risk factor in disease progression.

Systemic risk factors for the progression of gingivitis to periodontitis include smoking, diabetes mellitus, and a specific genetic change that predisposes the patient to attachment loss. Patients who smoke develop periodontal disease more rapidly, heal more poorly, and lose teeth more rapidly compared with those who do not (see chapter 12). For diabetics, the less severe the diabetes and the better its control, the better the prognosis for the patient's periodontal problem. An anomaly in the genes responsible for one of the inflammatory mediators in periodontal disease (IL-1) results in increased levels of attachment loss and tooth loss compared with patients without the change (see chapter 11). In addition, patients who smoke and are also positive for the IL-1 genotype have many times greater risk of tooth loss than individuals without this combination of risk factors.

The following is a summary of Mr Wilson's risk factors:

Local risk factors

1. The patient has bacteria that are associated with disease, and there are physical barriers to disturbing these bacteria (probing depths greater than 3 mm and improperly adapted dental restorations).

2. The patient is not complying with recommendations for personal oral hygiene and maintenance care.

Systemic risk factors

1. The patient smokes.

2. The patient has no family history of diabetes and does not currently have the disease.

3. The patient is positive for the IL-1 genotype.

Determining the Prognosis

The prognosis depends on the degree to which local and systemic risk factors can be controlled. In this case, a number of long-term behavioral changes (eg, improved compliance and smoking cessation) will be needed to improve the probability that the disease process will be arrested. The probability that the average patient will make significant long-term behavioral changes is not high. Active periodontal therapy usually results in short-term clinical improvement, but most patients initially improve compliance and then return to old habits.

The number of risk factors present and the number that can be controlled or eliminated determine the prognosis. This patient is at a high risk because he does not comply with professional suggestions about oral hygiene and maintenance. This means that he carries large numbers of periodontal pathogens, and his bone loss shows him to be susceptible to periodontal disease. The fact that he smokes and is IL-1 positive significantly increases his risk of tooth loss. Therefore, the short-term prognosis for this case is good, whereas it is guarded for the long term unless the patient complies with good dental practices and stops smoking.

Formulating a Treatment Plan

The fact that this patient has never had periodontal therapy more complex than occasional periodontal maintenance care would argue that he should first have traditional closed subgingival scaling and root planing (probably with local anesthesia). The fact that he is genotype positive indicates that he should be reevaluated early (30 to 45 days after scaling) and seen frequently for maintenance, regardless of what other therapy is performed. If his oral hygiene is good but he still has signs of inflammation in areas accessible for removal of subgingival deposits, more closed subgingival scaling and root planing may be appropriate. Advanced procedures, such as closed subgingival scaling and root planing using the dental endoscope or pocket reduction surgery, can be helpful in reducing probing depths that are greater than 5 mm after closed subgingival scaling and root planing and show signs of inflammation, such as bleeding on probing or continued attachment loss. In general, the less the patient smokes, the better the prognosis.

The following specific treatment plan was followed for Mr Wilson:

1. *Begin initial therapy to control inflammatory periodontal disease* (for details, see chapter 22). There is universal agreement that higher levels of oral hygiene are associated with longer tooth retention.
   a. Give the patient oral hygiene instructions, including instructions on the use of dental floss.
   b. Fabricate and deliver a maxillary hard acrylic habit appliance to help reduce the thermal sensitivity of the teeth and possibly reduce their clinical mobility. Some practitioners feel that it is beneficial to adjust the occlusion after the patient has worn the bite guard and experienced a reduction in tooth mobility and thermal sensitivity; others disagree. (See chapter 31 for a discussion on this topic.) The patient is instructed to wear the appliance while sleeping.
   c. Remove tooth-borne plaque and calculus. This patient has interproximal probing depths up to 6 mm in the posterior teeth. A number of studies have shown that complete removal of tooth-borne plaque and calculus in pockets this deep rarely occurs using tra-

ditional methods of closed subgingival scaling and root planing. The clinician is then presented with three treatment options: *(1)* traditional closed subgingival scaling and root planing; *(2)* closed subgingival scaling and root planing using the dental endoscope; or *(3)* periodontal surgery. In this case, closed subgingival scaling and root planing with the endoscope, under local anesthesia, is preferred.
   d. Advise the patient to stop smoking. The patient agreed to quit smoking.
2. *Reevaluate initial therapy 30 to 45 days after its completion.*
   a. If soft and hard tissues have returned to health (3-mm probing depths with no signs of clinical inflammation), then the patient is given a final diagnosis of arrested chronic periodontitis and will be placed on periodontal maintenance.
   b. If the soft tissues in the areas accessible to oral hygiene and subgingival scaling and root planing have not returned to health, the following guidelines should be followed:
      • If the therapist has failed to eliminate local factors, or if the patient is not removing plaque, then the problem should be rectified.
      • If the therapist and the patient have done an adequate job of eliminating local factors and there are no visible signs of inflammation but inflammation is found in deeper pockets, then surgery is a good option.
      • If signs of inflammation persist in areas well cleaned by both therapist and patient, then a final diagnosis of aggressive periodontitis is assigned.
3. *Assess the teeth* for the presence or absence of fremitus, as well as to see if the bidigital mobility has decreased and if the other symptoms caused by the patient's bruxism have diminished. If indicated, occlusal adjustment can be performed at this time. In this case, the patient still had bidigital tooth mobility and thermal sensitivity. He received an occlusal adjustment, followed by provisional restorations on the maxillary left lateral incisor and first molar (Figs 23-4 and 23-5).
4. *Perform additional therapy as needed for areas with inflammation.* Further therapy was indicated for Mr Wilson (Fig 23-6). Although the soft tissues in the areas easily accessible to oral hygiene and subgingival scaling and root planing returned to health, the deeper interproximal areas of molars and premolars still showed signs of inflammation (Figs 23-7a to 23-7c). Treatment options again include traditional or endoscopic scaling and root planing or periodontal surgery. Areas without root abnormalities and furcations (the anterior teeth) had responded well to closed subgingival scaling and root planing because these areas are easier for the pa-

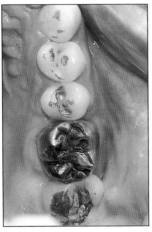

Fig 23-4 A number of occlusal interferences were found on the teeth, along with bidigital mobility, fremitus, and thermal sensitivity. These interferences were eliminated when they were still present after nonsurgical reduction of inflammation and the patient's wearing an occlusal habit appliance.

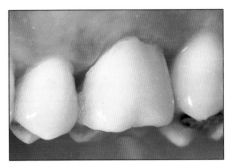

Fig 23-5 Provisional restorations were placed on the maxillary left lateral incisor and first molar following nonsurgical therapy because areas of active dental caries were found when the tissues receded.

tient to clean and more accessible for the therapist removing subgingival calculus. This time, surgery was chosen:

   a. To give the therapist better access to remove calculus and bacteria from the roots.

   b. To quickly reduce the probing depths and thus give the patient and the professional better access to remove bacteria and their products during the maintenance phase of care.

5. *Perform periodontal surgery.* At the patient's request, the mandibular third molars were removed during surgery.

6. *Perform a second reevaluation 90 days after surgical treatment.* Any clinical signs of disease that remain are treated until the disease is controlled or the teeth are lost. The patient will be reevaluated again at the conclusion of all active treatment.

7. *Determine final diagnosis.* The clinical signs of disease in this case had been arrested. The patient was given a final diagnosis of arrested chronic periodontitis and was placed on periodontal maintenance.

A patient with chronic periodontitis has a chronic, low-grade infection of the attachment apparatus of the teeth. To control this disease, the clinician must reduce the bacterial mass to one that allows maintenance of a steady state. As noted above, to do this, the professional should remove bacteria and their products in any areas that promote bacterial accumulation, such as overhanging restorative margins. This process is simple compared with the next step, which is motivating the patient to maintain the steady state created by active therapy. The patient must clean the teeth daily and return routinely for professional monitoring of the disease process and removal of the bacteria and their products, if necessary. This step is called *periodontal maintenance.* Maintenance allows the practitioner to find any disease recurrence in its early stages and to take steps to stabilize the patient's condition.

The case described here has been an exception so far in that the patient has complied with suggestions concerning smoking cessation, oral hygiene, and the frequency of periodontal maintenance. This approach has been successful in keeping his periodontal disease under control (Figs 23-8 to 23-10). Most patients do not comply with suggested oral hygiene measures or frequency of maintenance, and most continue to smoke; therefore, most patients experience recurrence of their problems. These patients require re-treatment, though usually in selected sites, and often experience tooth loss. Maintaining the steady state created in active care requires positive behavioral changes by the patient, which are often difficult to sustain (see chapter 28).

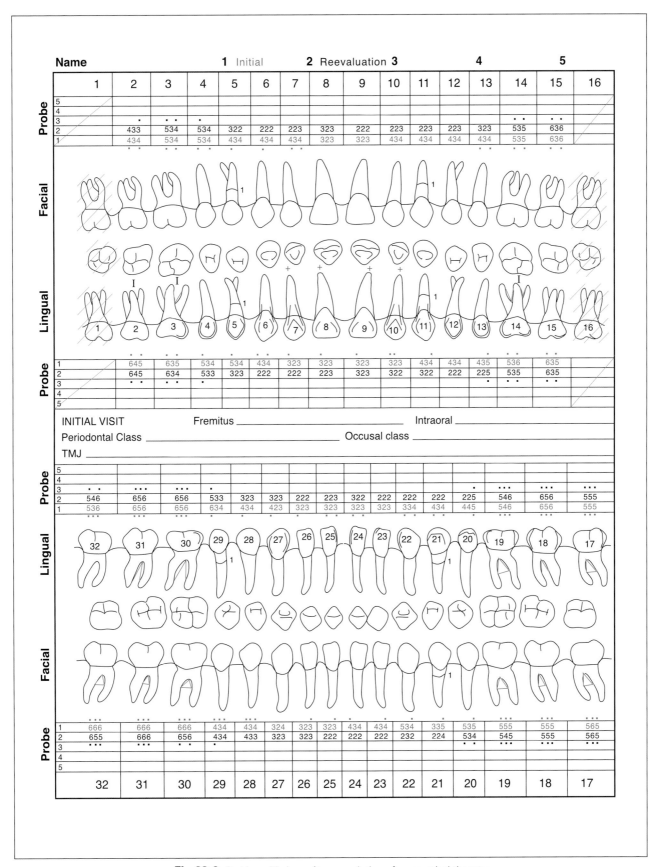

Fig 23-6 Probings 90 days after completion of nonsurgical therapy.

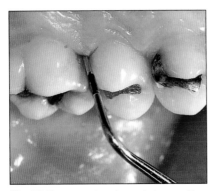

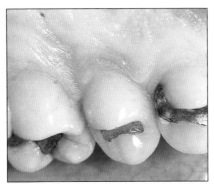

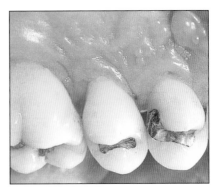

Fig 23-7a Palatal surface of the maxillary right posterior sextant at the initial examination.

Fig 23-7b Palatal surface of the maxillary right posterior sextant at the second reevaluation. Deepened probing depths associated with clinical signs of inflammation were still present 3 months after initial nonsurgical therapy.

Fig 23-7c Palatal surface of the maxillary right posterior sextant 5 years after surgery; note interproximal gingival recession.

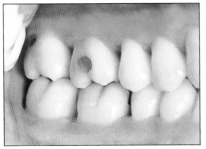

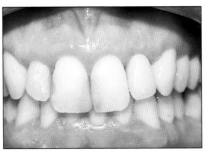

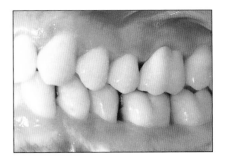

Figs 23-8a to 23-8c Patient's clinical presentation 5 years after surgery.

Nonsurgical Therapy for Early and Moderate Periodontitis

Convincing evidence of the central role of microorganisms in the etiology of gingivitis and periodontitis has been presented.[1–3] Early diagnosis and cause-related therapy are considered the main principles in treatment and may well be the key to successful results in the overall clinical management of periodontal diseases.

Although the reduction or elimination of systemic risk factors can help control periodontal diseases, the elimination of bacterial dental plaque and/or bacterial retention factors may be the only practical way to arrest progressive breakdown of the periodontal tissues in the vast majority of patients.[4–11]

The effectiveness of mechanical supragingival plaque control to prevent and resolve existing gingival inflammation (see chapter 22) was documented by Löe et al,[12] Nyman et al,[13] and Axelsson and Lindhe.[14] In contrast, supragingival plaque control alone has been demonstrated to have only limited effect in arresting the progressive course of periodontitis.[15–17] Thus, optimal periodontal therapy must always consist of a combination of supragingival and subgingival plaque control procedures.

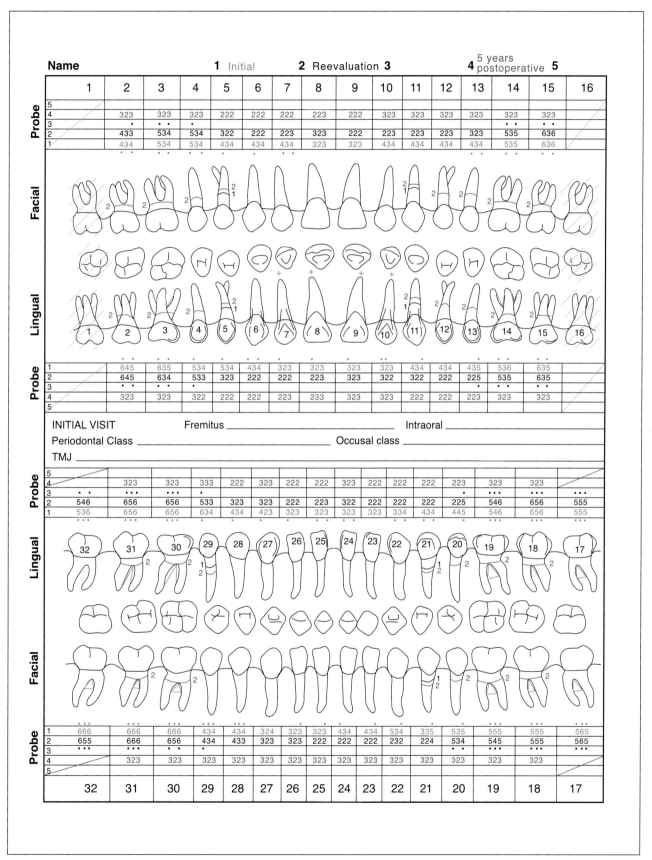

Fig 23-9 Probing chart for the area seen in Figs 23-8a to 23-8c. The probing depths closest to the teeth *(red)* are pretreatment, the middle ones *(black)* are from the second reevaluation, and the last ones *(blue)* are 5 years postsurgery.

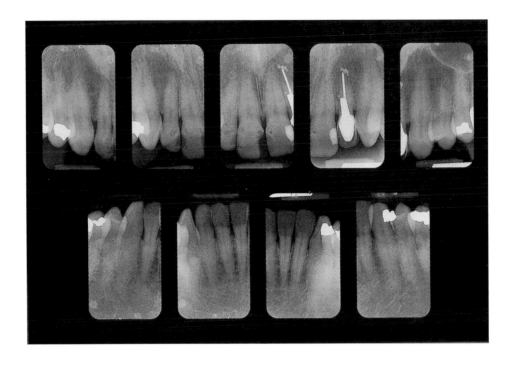

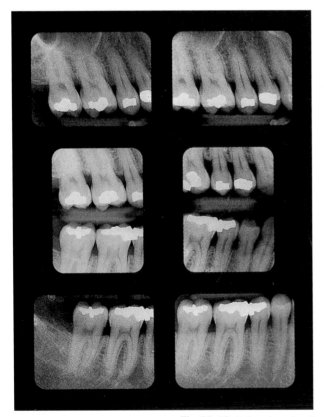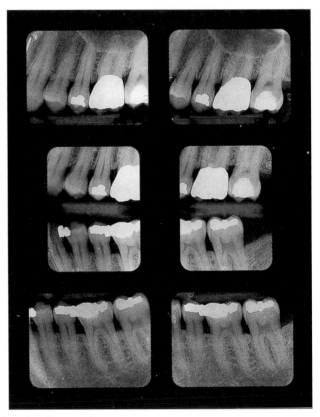

Fig 23-10 Full series of radiographs taken 5 years after surgery.

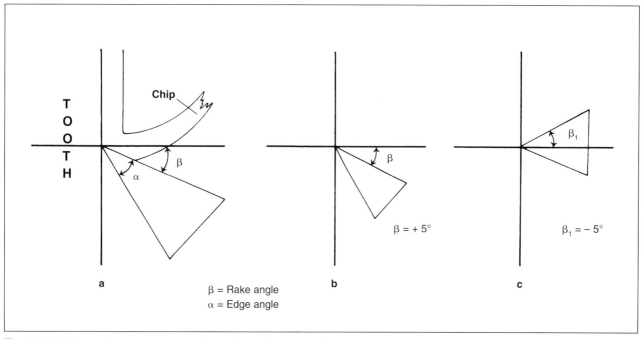

Fig 23-11 *(a)* The scaling procedure should result in the formation of chips. To facilitate the scaling procedure, the edge of the instrument should be applied with a rake angle of approximately ±5 degrees. A working angle of this magnitude will result in optimal cutting, even with low pressure on the instrument. *(b)* Increased angulation of the instrument will increase the risk for "chopping" strokes, resulting in nicks and/or scratches on the root surface. *(c)* An increasingly negative cutting angle will reduce the cutting effect of the instrument at a constant force. A sharp edge facilitates an optimal result.

General Considerations

The periodontal literature is replete with studies demonstrating that scaling and root planing are generally effective in controlling periodontal disease when probing depths do not exceed 4 mm.[18–20] These data would suggest that scaling and root planing with effective plaque control should be the treatment of choice for patients with early chronic periodontitis (Fig 23-11). The literature demonstrates that scaling and root planing, combined with effective plaque control, usually treats early periodontitis successfully (Figs 23-12a and 23-12b).[21–23]

The goal of treatment should be to render the roots biologically compatible with soft tissue by eliminating calculus and altered cementum and by reducing periodontal pathogenic microorganisms. Therapy should also address environmental factors affecting bacterial colonization, such as root surface irregularities, defective restorations, tooth malposition, and occlusion, as well as the patient's ability to perform effective oral hygiene. These efforts combined should resolve the inflammation, decrease probing depth, and increase attachment level.

The general practitioner or the dental hygienist under the supervision of the practitioner (depending on the hy-

gienist's skills and interests) can perform the treatment discussed in this chapter.

The sequence of treatment for patients with slight or moderate chronic periodontitis can and should be adapted to their individual needs. The first part of any evaluation should begin with a review of the patient's medical history to ascertain contraindications to dental treatment or the need for premedication prior to therapy.

Oral Hygiene Instructions, Education, and Motivation

It is best to begin patient education and oral hygiene instructions before scaling and root planing (see chapter 22). The initial examination should have been an educational experience for the patient; if it was not, the patient should explore the mouth with a mirror as the practitioner points out signs of the disease, such as edema, bleeding, purulence, and recession. It is also helpful if the practitioner has discovered what has motivated the patient to seek treatment and connect those wants to the dental needs demonstrated in the examination. The clinician should also try to discover what fears, real or imagined, the patient brings to treatment. These fears are best confronted

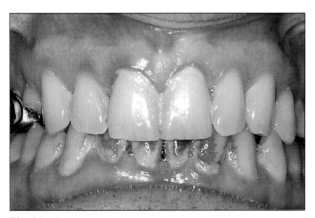

Fig 23-12a Patient with large amounts of plaque and calculus that have resulted in early chronic periodontitis.

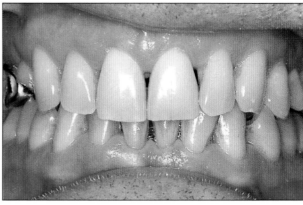

Fig 23-12b Same patient following scaling, root planing, and oral hygiene instruction. Note the resolution of the inflammation.

and resolved before starting therapy. The patient's expectations of the therapy should also be explored to make sure they are realistic.

The importance of effective personal oral hygiene and its relationship to the success of treatment should also be discussed before therapy. Even though the central role of dental plaque in the etiology and pathogenesis of periodontal disease is unquestionable, the effect of supragingival plaque control alone on the healing response of periodontal tissues in established periodontitis is limited.[15,17,24,25] Thus, it is important to stress that supragingival plaque control per se cannot prevent disease progression in already established periodontitis. However, it is possible to achieve a limited decrease in probing depth principally as a result of reduction in inflammatory edema. It is also important to stress that it is possible to achieve a low plaque score independent of the level of initial probing depth. The decisive role of supragingival plaque control for the long-term result of periodontal therapy is unquestionable.[5,6,13,26]

An oral hygiene instructional visit may be best scheduled as a separate appointment prior to any scaling and root planing. During this visit, the patient can be introduced to disclosing tablets and proper brushing and flossing techniques. Plaque and its relationship to the disease can be discussed, but the clinician must remember that motivation is more important than information. At the next appointment, before beginning scaling and root planing, one should ask the patient what differences he or she has seen in the mouth following implementation of the new oral hygiene techniques. For example, does the patient notice less bleeding and swelling or better breath? The patient must establish what he or she can do and take responsibility for the disease. If oral hygiene instructions are given for the first time as part of the scaling and root planing appointment, it is likely that the patient will assume that all of the changes noted after the appointment are due to the scaling and not to any personal efforts. This line of

thought breeds dependency and over the long run is counterproductive. An acceptable and realistic level of plaque control may be visible plaque not exceeding 15% to 20% of the tooth surfaces.

Patient and Operator Protection

To protect both the operator and the patient, proper aseptic technique should be followed (see chapter 16). Instruments should be sterilized and appropriate barrier techniques used. The clinician should wear eye protection, a mask, and gloves. Having the patient rinse with chlorhexidine for 30 seconds prior to treatment reduces the spread of microorganisms by atomization during therapy.[27] The clinician should explain to the patient what the scaling and root planing appointment will include, answer any questions, and secure informed consent. In general, there is very little patient risk associated with this treatment, and the benefits are many. By eliminating the inflammation associated with periodontitis, the patient should notice less bleeding and swelling of the gingiva and improvement in both taste and breath odor.

Scheduling the Appointment

Insufficient time is frequently allocated for scaling and root planing. It is not uncommon in a research setting for an operator to spend up to 15 minutes instrumenting one surface of one tooth, but in clinical practice one could easily take 45 minutes to an hour to scale and root plane an average quadrant. Whenever possible, all periodontally involved teeth should be treated at one visit to minimize the probability of reinfection from untreated pockets. The procedure should be performed systematically (not skipping around) to ensure that all areas are instrumented. Systematic use of individual instruments is also important. Using one instrument on all surfaces where it is applicable before moving on to the next instrument minimizes instrument transfer and makes efficient use of time.

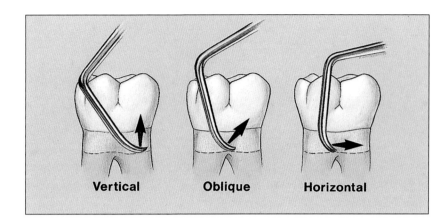

Fig 23-13 Exploration of the root surface is usually accomplished with a vertical, oblique, or horizontal motion.

Vertical   **Oblique**   **Horizontal**

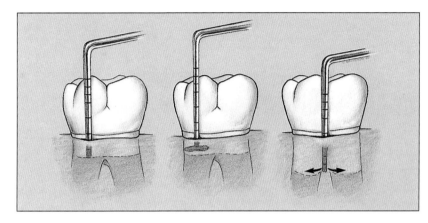

Fig 23-14 Subgingival exploration with a periodontal probe. The probe is capable of determining probing depth, as well as detecting root surface deposits and root topography.

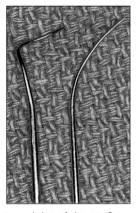

Fig 23-15 The curved tips of the no. 2 explorer and EXS-3A explorer allow exploration of difficult-to-reach areas.

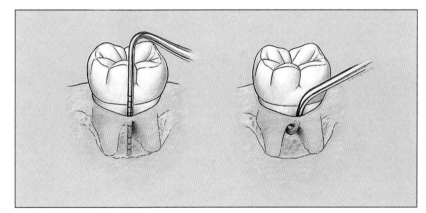

Fig 23-16 The periodontal probe can provide useful information on root surface topography, but the furcation probe is necessary to totally explore a furcation.

Basic Strokes in Root Instrumentation

Exploratory Strokes

Two basic strokes are used during root instrumentation: exploratory and working. Exploratory strokes provide information regarding the root surface. The information is usually gained by the use of an explorer, but scalers and curettes can also be used with light strokes to identify areas that require further work. Exploratory strokes are the only strokes in which the same amount of pressure is used on both the push and pull aspects. This light pressure is usually directed in a vertical, oblique, or horizontal fashion (Fig 23-13). The periodontal probe is typically not thought of as an explorer, but with experience one can use it to explore the root surface for deposits and surface irregularities, as well as to ascertain pocket depths (Fig 23-14). There are limitations, however, to the straight periodontal probe. Explorers with a curved tip provide better access into root depressions and furcations (Figs 23-15 and 23-16).

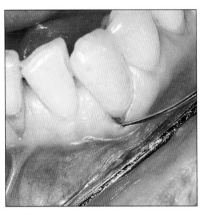

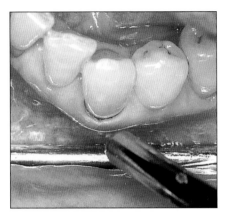

Fig 23-17a A large piece of calculus can be seen on the root surface of the canine through the translucent gingiva, and its presence is confirmed by an explorer.

Fig 23-17b The deposit can be visualized by directing a stream of air from the air-water syringe directly into the sulcus.

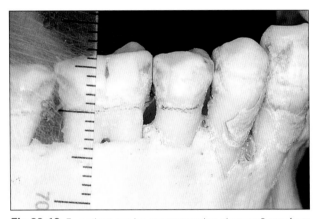

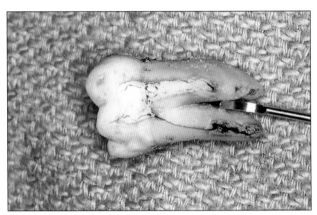

Fig 23-18 Furcations can be encountered as close as 3 mm from the CEJ. This photograph of a dry skull demonstrates a grade II furcation involvement approximately 3 mm from the CEJ.

Fig 23-19 Note the relationship between the size of the furcation opening and the blade of a Gracey curette.

Prior to beginning treatment, a fine explorer is used to examine the periodontal pockets to be instrumented. A long-standing periodontal lesion contains dental plaque and subgingival calculus in close contact with the tooth substance. Small irregularities caused by resorption of the root cementum are constantly found; they result in firm retention of plaque and calculus to the root surface, which constitutes the main reason for the root planing procedure. The information gained from this exploration, combined with a review of the periodontal chart and radiographs, will allow the operator to establish the topography of the pockets, root morphology, tissue tone, root surface deposits, and patient sensitivity. This exploration will assist in determining which areas will require more time for scaling and root planing, help in instrument selection, and determine the need for local anesthesia. Local anesthesia will often be necessary, but its use will depend on the skill of the operator and patient tolerance.

Studies evaluating the effectiveness of scaling and root planing consistently demonstrate that the most difficult areas to instrument effectively are furcations, grooves, abnormalities, concavities, and the CEJ.[18,20,28] Because of the difficulty in debriding these areas adequately, they should be explored carefully before moving on to another area. These explorations require a keenly developed tactile sensitivity. Figures 23-17a and 23-17b show commonly used methods to evaluate the root surface prior to instrumentation.

Furcation involvement can be a problem even in the patient with moderate chronic periodontitis with attachment loss of only 2 to 4 mm (probing depths of 4 to 6 mm). Gher and Vernino[29] demonstrated that furcations frequently occur as close as 3 mm to the CEJ (Fig 23-18). Bower[30] reported that 58% of the furcation openings he examined were smaller than the smallest curette blade available (Fig 23-19). This means that even when there is

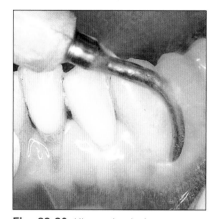

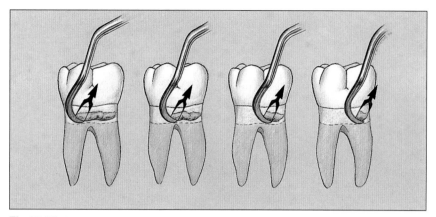

Fig 23-20 Ultrasonic devices are extremely effective for gross debridement. Here the tip of the ultrasonic device can be seen removing the large deposits of calculus discovered facial to the canine (see Figs 23-17a and 23-17b).

Fig 23-21 It is inefficient and sometimes impossible to remove large root-surface deposits with a single stroke. In gross scaling it is best to engage only a portion of the deposit at a time. This type of sectional scaling ensures that the entire deposit will be removed. Here four strokes are required.

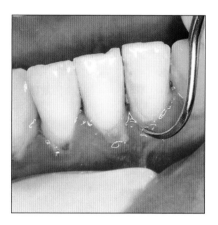

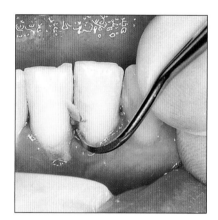

Fig 23-22 Proper use of a scaler during gross debridement. The entire portion of the calculus being instrumented is removed with a deliberate working stroke.

adequate access to the furcation, there may not be instruments available to adequately debride the furcation. These facts should encourage the practitioner to aggressively treat patients with early periodontitis before 5 mm or more of probing depth is found. At 5 mm or more, significant furcation involvement is often encountered, changing the prognosis dramatically.

Working Strokes

Once a plan of action has been established, one usually begins with gross scaling. Root surface debridement is usually accomplished with what is called a *working stroke*. This type of stroke provides constant lateral pressure of the instrument against the root surface. The lateral pressure is applied only on the pull strokes. The two types of working strokes used are the scaling stroke and the root planing stroke.

Scaling stroke. Scaling is the gross removal of plaque and calculus from the tooth surface. The literature is not clear as to whether hand instruments or ultrasonic devices are superior in terms of scaling.[31,32] Traditionally, both supragingival and subgingival gross debridement are accomplished by manual, ultrasonic, or combination techniques (Fig 23-20). Supragingival plaque and calculus removal is beneficial,[33] but one should limit the amount of supragingival root planing, because it does not contribute to the success of therapy and leads to root surface sensitivity. Gross scaling should be performed in a systematic fashion not only from tooth to tooth but also section by section on the actual root surface deposit (Fig 23-21). Each scaling stroke should overlap the previous one to ensure complete removal of deposits. Scaling should not be thought of as a shaving process in which layers are removed. Shaving often leaves a smooth layer of burnished calculus, difficult to distinguish from the root surface. Instead, all calculus should be removed with strong, deliberate working strokes (Fig 23-22). One should not hesitate, however, to repeat these strokes until the tooth surface has been adequately scaled.

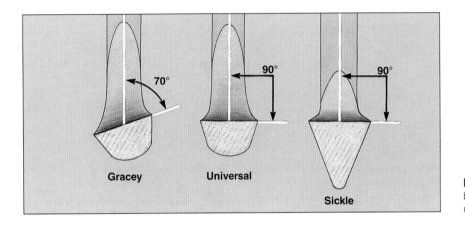

Fig 23-23 Note the relationship of the blade to the shank on the Gracey curette, universal curette, and sickle scaler.

Ultrasonic scalers have traditionally played an important role in gross scaling. Holbrook and Low[34] have suggested customizing the tip design of ultrasonic scalers to permit more efficient scaling. These tips are then used with ultrasonic instruments that can have their frequency, amplitude, and water flow manually adjusted to ensure that the tip energy is kept at the minimal level to accomplish a given clinical task. These customized inserts permit access to areas that are very difficult to instrument adequately. At least one study has shown ultrasonic instrumentation to be more effective than hand scaling in grade II and III furcations.[35]

Root planing stroke. Definitive removal of tooth-borne accretions, termed *root planing*, begins at the completion of scaling. Although it is academically beneficial to separate scaling from root planing, they are in reality tied one to the other. The two procedures fall along a continuum, with scaling at the beginning and root planing near the end. Many instruments have been developed to plane the root, including but not limited to curettes, chisels, hoes, and files.

Curettes are generally the instrument of choice for subgingival root planing, primarily because their shape and size promote tactile sensitivity and provide the best access to difficult areas. There are two broad categories of curettes: universal and limited utility. Universal curettes can be used on a number of surfaces of teeth and on different teeth. Examples of these curettes are the Columbia 4R4L or 13-14. Limited-utility curettes, such as the Gracey curette, can be used only on particular surfaces of specific teeth. The major difference between the two types of curettes is the angle that the blade makes with the shank of the instrument (Fig 23-23). Experience with the instrument and the specific area being instrumented will generally dictate which curette will be used. Once the curette has been chosen, the manner in which it is used will determine its effectiveness.

Typically, the curette is held so that the working edge of the blade forms a 60- to 80-degree angle with the root surface. Under light pressure the curette is worked under the gingival margin while the instrument is kept in light contact with the root or calculus. Often, to allow the curette to pass over the calculus, the blade must be closed toward the tooth surface at or near an angle of 0 degrees. The instrument continues along the root surface until soft tissue resistance is felt, indicating the depth of the pocket. Once at the base of the defect, the angle of the blade is reestablished, and the deposit is removed through a deliberate working or power stroke (Fig 23-24). During instrumentation with a curette, it is often useful to vary the force of the stroke from the power stroke to exploratory strokes. The lighter exploratory strokes allow the clinician to determine where more work is needed.

Just as in scaling, root planing strokes should be overlapped. Root surfaces are generally concave or convex, and it is important to try to remove all deposits and altered root cementum. The direction of the stroke will vary depending on the tooth anatomy, design of the instrument, topography of the defect, and access. Most strokes are directed apicocoronally (vertically), but often it is necessary to make oblique, horizontal, and circumferential strokes to engage the interproximal concavities, incipient furcation involvements, and CEJs (Fig 23-25).

Definitive root planing begins once all detectable subgingival deposits have been removed (Fig 23-26). A more delicate stroke is generally used for smoothing and planing the root surface. The curettes must be exquisitely sharp for root planing, and it is not uncommon to use a completely different set of curettes for root planing than were used for subgingival scaling or to resharpen curettes during treatment. As before, it is important to use overlapping strokes to ensure that the entire pathologically exposed root surface has been instrumented. It may take many strokes to render the root glassy smooth and hard, prior to moving on to another area.

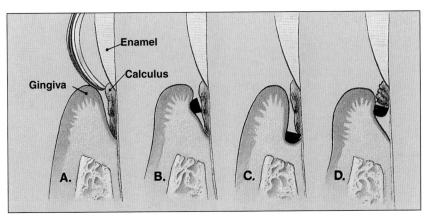

Fig 23-24 Subgingival scaling. (A) The curette is inserted under the free gingival margin. (B) The curette is passed over the root surface and deposits by closing its angle to near 0 degrees. (C) The base of the pocket is felt, and the proper angulation of the blade is reestablished. (D) The deposit is removed through a deliberate working stroke.

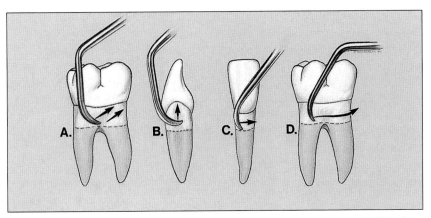

Fig 23-25 Subgingival scaling or root planing strokes: (A) oblique, (B) vertical, (C) horizontal, and (D) circumferential.

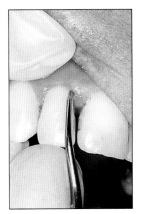

Fig 23-26 Once subgingival debridement is complete, definitive root planing is begun.

It is often difficult to determine when the root has been planed enough. It is best to dry the field, blow air into the sulcus for direct vision when possible, and explore the root surface with a fine explorer. Fiber optics may be useful, and transillumination of the root is sometimes productive. Surgical telescopic glasses are often beneficial, as they allow the operator to visually detect root surface imperfections not visible to the naked eye.

Determining the end point of scaling and root planing demonstrates the difficulty of translating the results of research to clinical practice. Research projects have clearly shown that it is possible to scale and root plane pathologically exposed root surfaces, removing the endotoxins and rendering the root surface biologically compatible with the soft tissue.[36] These studies are able to determine their end points by very sophisticated measurements, yet when using traditional methods in clinical practice one must continue to rely on crude and highly subjective methods such as exploring the root surfaces for roughness with an explorer. As crude as this measurement is, it has historically been effective. The ultimate test of the effectiveness of root instrumentation does not occur until 4 to 6 weeks after scaling, when the soft tissue response to therapy is reevaluated. (This reevaluation visit is covered later in the chapter.)

The importance of sharp instruments cannot be overemphasized. It is difficult to sharpen instruments effectively, and many resources are available to provide guidance. Instruments should be sharpened prior to use and while performing scaling and root planing. To make this possible, a sterile sharpening stone should be kept on the tray.

Closed Subgingival Scaling and Root Planing with a Dental Endoscope

As detailed above, traditional approaches to removing subgingival deposits require the clinician to use blind tactile methods to determine when the root surface is free of deposits. The dental endoscope allows the clinician to see in real time, as well as to watch the removal of these accretions. The use of this device can lead to removal of significantly more of the calculus and plaque attached to the root surface. This represents a quantum leap in the ability to remove subgingival deposits and has produced short-term results heretofore unseen in the average patient.

The device consists of a viewing screen, light source, and fiber-optic cable with a lens at one end. This lens is small enough to be contained in an explorer tip that will easily penetrate into the periodontal pocket. Magnification of 25× to 50× is provided and viewed in real time on a screen.

There are two ways to use this device for scaling and root planing. One is to look with the explorer (50× magnification), identify the position of the deposits, and then use traditional approaches for scaling and root planing. The ability to see deposits before their removal allows clinicians to accurately target their efforts and, more important, to see when the root surface is clean. The advantages are obvious. The second way is to use other attachments or devices to watch in real time as deposits are engaged and removed.

The results achieved thus far have surpassed those seen using traditional closed approaches. The use of the device, along with closed subgingival scaling and root planing, has resulted in clinically significant probing-depth reduction in almost every clinical situation, ranging from patients undergoing scaling and root planing for the first time to therapy for recalcitrant pockets in long-time periodontal maintenance patients. In nonresponsive areas or when bone regeneration is desired, this device can be used along with minimally invasive surgery techniques.

Training on the instrument and its use is necessary, and the initial learning curve is often steep. However, the results are well worth the effort.

Therapy is preceded and followed by explicit oral hygiene instructions, and the patient is placed on frequent periodontal maintenance therapy. A second visit is usually scheduled 1 week after the first session; at this visit, the areas are evaluated for signs of inflammation. Any inflammation, as manifested by bleeding on probing, has always been found to be associated with subgingival deposits. Most first visits involve the administration of a local anesthetic, while follow-up is usually done without it.

Curettage

Curettage is rarely part of the treatment for mild chronic periodontitis, because studies have demonstrated no advantage to soft tissue curettage as part of scaling and root planing.[37] Only sulci exhibiting disease should be instrumented. Scaling and root planing of healthy sulci is unnecessary and can actually promote attachment loss.[19,38]

Coronal Polishing and Postoperative Instructions

Once scaling and root planing is complete, the defect should be irrigated to remove fragments of calculus, shavings of cementum, and other debris. The supragingival portions of the tooth are generally polished with a handpiece and rubber cup or with an air-powder device. Oral hygiene instructions should be reviewed, and particular attention should be given to areas that will be difficult for the patient to maintain. Patients should be informed that they might experience some discomfort in the scaled areas. Over-the-counter analgesics are usually adequate for postoperative pain relief.

Postscaling Oral Hygiene Instructions

It is often useful to schedule patients for an oral hygiene instructional visit after completion of the scaling and root planing. Patients should be asked if they are experiencing difficulty in performing any of the oral hygiene procedures they have been asked to do. This oral hygiene appointment can be particularly effective in demonstrating where patients are having difficulty with home care. It can be explained to the patient that all plaque was removed at the previous visit and that therefore any plaque found today has accumulated since the last appointment. This demonstrates areas the patient finds difficult to clean.

Time should be spent developing effective ways to clean the areas patients finds difficult to maintain. Often, areas that patients say they have difficulty with may not be the same areas an examination reveals to be problematic. Positive reinforcement of properly performed home care is extremely important. One should point out as many areas as possible where the patient is effectively cleaning at home. Home care effectiveness or a plaque score should be recorded, and the types of home care devices given to the patient should be documented.

Reevaluation

The next appointment typically takes place 4 to 6 weeks after completion of the scaling and root planing.[39] Although the primary function of the reevaluation visit is to determine the effectiveness of the scaling and root planing, it is also appropriate to review home care proficiency. Areas that are not responding as expected can be reinstrumented. Sometimes residual root surface deposits will be apparent due to tissue resolution. Probing depths should be recharted, and bleeding on probing and purulence should be recorded. All inflammation, bleeding on probing, and purulence should be eliminated. Depending on the preoperative tissue response, a reduction of probing depth from 1 to 2 mm would be expected.

The reevaluation appointment may reveal other problems requiring special consideration. For example, gingival hyperplasia or interproximal cratering may require a gingivectomy or gingivoplasty to create an environment more conducive to maintenance care (see chapter 28). Plaque-retentive or biologically incompatible dental restorations should be replaced, and other local factors that could make supportive periodontal treatment difficult should be corrected.

One should expect to resolve mild chronic periodontitis with the procedures mentioned up to this point. If the expected results are not achieved (ie, bleeding on probing is not eliminated and probing depth is not reduced by 1 to 2 mm), one might consider referral of the patient to a periodontist for more advanced treatment. It is unlikely that performing more of the same procedures will improve the results. If the expected results are not achieved, the patient should be referred for more specialized care and not continue to be treated for mild chronic periodontitis.

The Role of Antimicrobial Therapy

Because most of the infecting organisms in periodontal diseases can be accessed through the orifice of the periodontal pocket, mechanical debridement of the plaque-infected root surfaces logically has been suggested as the first choice of therapy for early chronic periodontitis. Combining this treatment with the application of antimicrobial agents locally in the periodontal pocket may represent an adjunct for managing periodontopathic microflora to supplement mechanical debridement of the root surfaces in select cases (see "Local Delivery of Antimicrobial Agents," discussed later in this chapter). However, a certain risk for uncontrolled adverse reactions and bacterial drug resistance must be considered.[40]

The topical use of antimicrobial agents with low toxicity and a broad antimicrobial spectrum may be helpful in enhancing the effects of mechanical subgingival debride-

ment.[15,41,42] Furthermore, by applying chemical agents topically, a relatively low total dose can be administered while achieving high concentrations at the site of infection.

Although the use of antimicrobial agents in the treatment of periodontal diseases may be promising, it is important to stress that results from clinical studies seem to indicate that traditional subgingival scaling and supragingival plaque control procedures, when performed adequately, are sufficient treatments for most early lesions. Traditional periodontal scaling and root planing carried out without supplemental periodontal surgery has been demonstrated to be one practical way to arrest periodontal tissue breakdown.[26,43–45] Tagge et al[16] and Hughes and Caffesse[46] demonstrated clinical improvement in gingivitis and periodontal pocket depths following subgingival mechanical debridement of mild periodontitis lesions. Waerhaug[18] showed that optimal subgingival debridement might be difficult in periodontal pockets of depths exceeding 3 to 5 mm. Thus, mechanical debridement needs to be combined with surgical procedures to improve accessibility to the infected root surfaces in some moderate and many severe periodontitis lesions.[7,11,21,47] However, there is overwhelming documentation in the literature supporting the clinical value of supragingival and subgingival scaling as a powerful basic therapy in the treatment of early periodontitis and some cases of moderate periodontitis.

Based on the concept of specificity of bacterial infection in periodontal diseases, it should be possible to use appropriate systemic antimicrobial agents to supplement mechanical debridement in the management of periodontal disease. However, Listgarten et al[48] suggested that systemic tetracycline therapy had only a minor additional effect on the periodontal microflora and clinical healing as compared with scaling and root planing alone. Other studies, however, have indicated that systemic antimicrobial therapy may be useful in the treatment of chronic periodontitis.[40,49–51]

Topical application of antibacterial agents can also be an adjunct in the management of early chronic periodontitis to supplement mechanical debridement. Topical use of chlorhexidine digluconate as a mouthrinse will substantially diminish gingival inflammation.[52–56] Although the effect of chlorhexidine on established periodontitis appears limited when delivered supragingivally,[57] it has demonstrated promising results when delivered subgingivally.[58,59] Ultimately, however, Garrett[60] was unable to show any difference in clinical or microbiologic parameters between periodontal lesions scaled and root planed and those also irrigated with 0.2% chlorhexidine or tetracycline solutions.

Other agents with expected antimicrobial activity (including stannous fluoride,[61] hydrogen peroxide,[62] io-

---

Current Concepts of Chronic Periodontitis

- Therapy for early chronic periodontitis is aimed at reducing or altering the makeup of bacteria and their products and at reducing or eliminating areas that retain those bacteria.
- Early diagnosis and treatment are important to stop disease progression.

- Early intervention usually involves improved oral hygiene and closed subgingival scaling and root planing by the dental professional.
- The use of clinical parameters, not bacterial indicators, is the preferred method for judging success.
- For long-term success, active therapy must be followed by periodontal maintenance.

Overview of Scaling and Root Planing Treatment for Chronic Periodontitis

(Appropriate instrumentation is mentioned, but operators must develop their own techniques.)
1. Review the patient's medical history.
2. Undertake patient education and oral hygiene instruction. Using a hand mirror, demonstrate to the patient problems such as plaque deposits, inflammation, bleeding pus, and pockets, and explain their relationship to periodontal disease. Emphasize brushing and flossing techniques:
   - Brush at the dentogingival interface.
   - Floss as deeply as possible.
   - Inform the patient of an initial period of discomfort from this technique.
3. When patients return for the first scaling visit, ask if they can detect any improvement in the mouth from the new oral hygiene technique; it is important to establish what they can accomplish themselves. Discuss with patients their hopes, fears, and expectations regarding scaling and root planing. Explore periodontal pockets (Hu-Friedy EXD 11-12, EXS-3A, and CH3 and Nabers 2N furcation probes), review charting and radiographs, and determine the need for anesthetics. Then undertake gross scaling (ultrasonics TFI-10), as well as scaling and root planing:
   - Maxillary molars and premolars: Columbia 4R4L, Gracey 13-14 for typically apicocoronal strokes on distal surfaces (if tissue is very inflamed, this instrument is useful with the tip pointed into the sulcus with horizontal strokes); Gracey 11-12 for mesial surfaces; Gracey 1-2 or 5-6 for facial and lingual surfaces.
   - Maxillary anterior teeth: Gracey 1-2 good with horizontal strokes; SH 6/7 effective for burnished subgingival calculus at the CEJ.
   - Mandibular molars and premolars: Gracey 11-12 or 13-14, Columbia 4R4L, S 107/108 Sickle (effective for subgingival flinty calculus); Gracey 1-2 or 5-6 for facial or lingual surfaces.
   - Mandibular anterior teeth: SH 6/7; Gracey 13-14 (good angulation for access to lingual surfaces of mandibular anterior teeth); Gracey 1-2.
   - Polish according to patient's specific needs: prophy jet, rotary cup with pumice, and rotary cup with paste for resin composite or porcelain laminate veneers.
   - Give oral hygiene instructions, emphasizing problem areas.
4. In oral hygiene instructions after scaling and root planing, motivation is much more important than information.
5. Reevaluate to determine soft tissue response usually 4 to 6 weeks following scaling and root planing. The patient is placed on an appropriate maintenance schedule if therapy was successful or is referred for more specialized care if treatment was not effective.

---

dine,[15,63] and tetracycline[64]) have also been evaluated for topical use in periodontal treatment. Both positive and negative results have been reported with these agents. To minimize the risk of any adverse effects, antimicrobial agents with low toxicity and a broad antimicrobial spectrum should be used. Also, the optimal concentration, the duration of the drug exposure, and bacteriostatic or bactericidal properties are important pharmacologic properties to observe.[65]

Periodontal Maintenance

After treatment is complete and the patient is clinically stable, data (eg, probing depth, bleeding on probing, purulence, and mobility) are collected to serve as a baseline for further evaluation and to provide the therapist with information to determine the most appropriate periodontal maintenance schedule. Assuming appropriate response to therapy and adequate home care, one might initially place the average patient with early chronic periodontitis on a 3-month periodontal maintenance interval. The actual length of this interval, however, should be customized for the patient's particular problems (see chapter 28). Such factors as oral hygiene, anatomic considerations, restorative plans, and the patient's risk factors for periodontal disease will ultimately determine the appropriate recall interval. This periodontal maintenance interval is shortened or lengthened appropriately, of course, depending on how the patient responds.

The results of treatment of the patient with early chronic periodontitis and some patients with moderate periodontitis can be dramatic and often very gratifying. The therapist and patient working together can predictably eliminate bleeding gingiva, improve breath, and enhance esthetics by eliminating soft tissue inflammation. The end result is a patient who appreciates not only the important part periodontics plays in an overall health care program but also the role he or she must assume in maintenance.

Surgical Therapy for Periodontitis with Moderate Attachment Loss

Numerous research endeavors during the past few decades have supplied a wealth of information regarding therapy for chronic periodontitis. Some of the information presented is relatively straightforward and easily transferable to clinical practice. Other information appears to be contradictory and has led to confusion for the practicing dentist.

Prior to the 1970s, periodontal therapy was primarily aimed at surgical elimination of the defect created by the periodontitis and reduction of "pocket depth." Longitudinal clinical trials conducted during the 1960s and 1970s demonstrated that surgical reduction of pocket depth was not absolutely necessary to halt progressive loss of clinical periodontal attachment. These studies verified that surgical debridement (with or without osseous resection), coupled with supportive periodontal therapy, could maintain periodontal stability. Later studies demonstrated that

closed debridement accomplished by root instrumentation without surgical flap reflection was also capable of halting the progress of chronic periodontitis and stabilizing mean clinical attachment levels when coupled with appropriate supportive periodontal therapy. The primary criticism of these original clinical trials was related to data management. Each study presented conclusions based on the comparison of mean data, which tends to mask the response of sites that respond differently from the majority of sites.

It has been argued that surgical periodontal therapy provides a major advantage over nonsurgical approaches due to its ability to provide access and visualization for root instrumentation. This theory has been accentuated by a series of studies demonstrating the inability of scaling and root planing procedures to predictably remove all etiologic agents (plaque/calculus) from the root surface. Kepic and associates[66] confirmed the preliminary findings of others and substantiated that the complete removal of calculus from periodontally diseased root surfaces is rare, regardless of whether ultrasonic devices or hand instruments are used, and regardless of whether an open surgical or closed nonsurgical approach is used.

These data appear to conflict with results reported from the previously mentioned longitudinal trials. If it is impossible to remove the etiologic factors from the root surface, how is it possible to halt periodontitis? This dilemma was probably best explained by Robertson[67] when he stated, "While total elimination of etiologic factors is the appropriate treatment goal, reduction of plaque and calculus below the threshold level that is acceptable to the host appears to control the infection process and improve the clinical signs of inflammation."

The stability of mean clinical attachment levels, as shown in the longitudinal trials, indicates that root instrumentation by both surgical and nonsurgical approaches is capable of reducing the level of etiologic agents below threshold levels at most sites in most individuals. Sites that do not respond like the mean are indicative of failure to reduce the etiologic levels below the patient's threshold. Such failure may be a consequence of inadequate debridement due to anatomic limitations (root surface aberrations, grooves, or furcations, or the presence of pockets) or due to an abnormally low patient threshold secondary to systemic complications.

Based on this information, a rationale for the treatment of chronic periodontitis must be predicated on debridement of the root surface associated with the periodontal defect. The initial approach to therapy should be the type of debridement that can be rendered in the most expeditious and cost-effective manner. Following adequate time for a healing response, an assessment should be completed. Those individuals, or sites within individuals, that do not

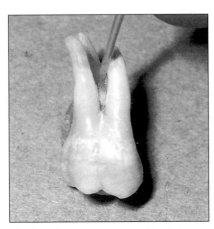

Fig 23-27 Note that the width of the furcation does not permit access with a hand curette of average width. A modified P10 ultrasonic scaler would fit better and potentially be more effective.

root surfaces, osseous defects, and the soft tissue wall of the periodontal defect.[68] Without direct visualization provided by a flap, it is rare that a clinician can effectively root plane beyond 5 mm of probing depth or into furcations of lesser depth.[18] The physical size of the curette is limiting in a narrow pocket. Root anatomy such as concavities, flutings, and grooves prevents intimate contact between the curette and root surface in combination with the overlying soft tissue. Furcations, even when shallow, present significant access problems.[18] In many cases they are too narrow to permit access with even the narrowest curettes (Fig 23-27).[69,70] Significant calculus can be readily missed when it is lodged under the ledge created at the CEJ. Smooth calculus is difficult to differentiate from a root surface by tactile sensation alone. With direct access and visualization, definitive root therapy is possible using mechanical therapy with hand curettes, ultrasonic curettes, or rotary instruments. This may be followed by chemical biomodification of the root surfaces with citric acid[71–73] or tetracycline[74] and the possible use of growth factors (see chapter 22). The potential for more definitive root therapy, mechanically and chemically, as well as the optional use of growth factors enhances the chances for regeneration of new attachment.

It is important that the granulomatous tissue be removed from the region of the periodontal defect due to the fact that it contains epithelium and the potential presence of bacterial infiltration.[75] Although unpredictable, a new connective tissue attachment may be formed following healing. More likely, healing will result in the creation of a long junctional epithelial attachment. Decreased probing depths may result, creating the significant clinical advantage of easier, more effective periodontal supportive therapy with less likelihood of future breakdown. The existing width or an adequate width of gingiva is preserved. Also, esthetic surgical procedures allow soft tissue morphology to be preserved or created, which has great benefit in the highly visible areas such as the maxillary anterior and premolar areas.

respond favorably to therapy should be reexamined, including appropriate evaluation of local or systemic complications that may be influencing their response. Decisions regarding additional treatment should factor in the results of such reexamination.

Diagnosis

Prior to making a determination of the surgical approach to use for maximum clinical effectiveness, an evaluation of attachment loss and relative oral anatomic structures is necessary. This requires the accurate use of a fine periodontal probe to evaluate attachment loss patterns, osseous defect morphology, and their relationship to the alveolus, teeth, and surrounding gingiva (see chapter 17).

Diagnostic radiographs are necessary to evaluate root morphology, root relationships, interdental and interradicular morphology, and a generalized pattern of alveolar crestal morphology, as well as to give some suggestion of osseous defect morphology (see chapter 18). Gingival width and thickness, tooth position in the alveolus, tooth-to-tooth relationships, and other anatomic considerations are observed via the oral examination. With this information one can then evaluate the disease status and determine the most appropriate therapy to use.

Rationale for Surgical Flap Approach to Treat Moderate Chronic Periodontitis

The primary objective and advantage of a surgical approach is visualization and access for debridement of the

Selection of Surgical Approach

All periodontal defects are not treated the same. In the selection of a therapeutic procedure, it is important that the clinician not make the patient fit a predetermined mode of therapy. Rather, the nature and extent of the patient's periodontal disease and the patient's other individual characteristics should be the determining factors in the choice of therapy. A skilled therapist will frequently use multiple procedures to treat a region affected by periodontal disease. These procedures could range from root planing, surgical flap access, and osseous resection to various regenerative procedures. The therapist must select those

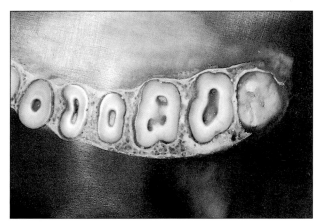

Fig 23-28a Note proximal root concavities on the molars and premolars in the maxillary posterior cross section, which make for difficult root instrumentation and decrease the chance for intimate flap-to-root surface adaptation.

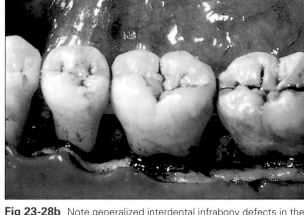

Fig 23-28b Note generalized interdental infrabony defects in the mandibular posterior area, and envision their continued presence following a repositioned flap procedure without osseous resection or regeneration.

procedures most appropriate for the given clinical circumstances and the esthetic, financial, and personal concerns of the patient. Surgical flap access therapy would be used for early to moderate defects not resolved by initial therapy. The repositioned flap without ostectomy would be the procedure of choice when esthetic concerns exist, such as in the maxillary anterior and premolar areas. In areas where esthetics are not a concern, such as most of the posterior areas, the apically positioned flap with or without ostectomy would be the procedure of choice, as there is usually greater probing depth reduction.

Repositioned Flap Without Ostectomy

The repositioned flap without ostectomy is suggested in areas of esthetic concern. A repositioned flap is essentially a flap that is replaced at or very near its presurgical position, as opposed to a flap that is apically positioned. Repositioned flaps have been known by a number of different names. They are all essentially open-flap debridement procedures with different names or perhaps entailing some slight technique modification. The most well known, and perhaps most commonly used, repositioned flap procedure is the modified Widman/Ramfjord flap procedure.

The primary objective of a flap procedure is access and visualization to allow appropriate root therapy and defect and flap wall debridement of granulomatous tissue and closure. The result is a healthy connective tissue flap wall adapted to a biologically clean tooth surface. This is felt to enhance the potential of creating a new connective tissue attachment. This circumferential intimate adaptation of the connective tissue wall of the flap to the root surface is much easier on facial and lingual surfaces, which perhaps partially accounts for the greater decrease in probing depths seen in these sites compared with interproximal

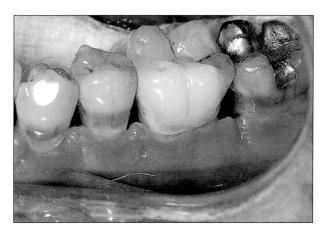

Fig 23-29 Note mandibular soft tissue craters following a repositioned flap procedure in the presence of infrabony craters. These craters present significant postoperative plaque control problems, supportive periodontal therapy concerns, and increased potential for progressive attachment loss.

areas following repositioned flap procedures. It is much easier to achieve good flap adaptation interproximally on convex or flat root surfaces that do not have concavities, flutings, grooves, or furcations or are associated with the presence of an infrabony defect. This procedure is particularly effective in the maxillary anterior region, where roots are essentially round and convex and the osseous defects are often suprabony. This procedure is not as effective in achieving pocket-depth reduction in the molar areas. In these areas, osseous defects are usually infrabony due to the osseous anatomy (Figs 23-28a and 23-28b).

A frequent problem with this procedure is the presence of postoperative interdental soft tissue craters, especially in the molar areas (Fig 23-29). Soft tissue crater formation is predisposed by the anatomic factors of proximal root

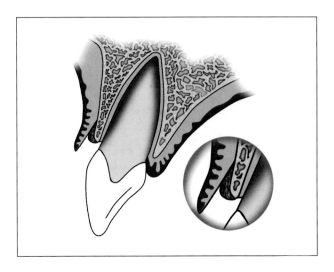

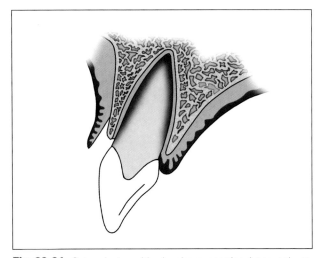

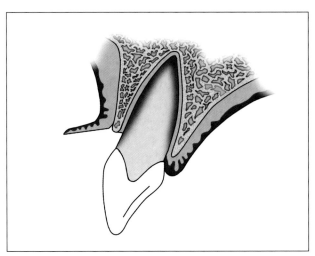

Fig 23-30 Exostosis requiring osteoplasty for smooth, intimate flap adaptation. Removal of the highlighted area is osteoplasty and does not involve any alveolar bone proper or attachment loss.

Fig 23-31 Osteoplasty, with alveolar supporting bone only removed. Note that there is no additional root exposure, and attachment remains the same.

Fig 23-32 Ostectomy, with alveolar bone proper removed. Note that there is additional root exposure and surgical removal of attachment.

concavities, infrabony defects, and narrow mesiodistal and wide faciolingual interdental widths. These factors inhibit intimate proximal flap-to-root surface adaptation, facial-lingual flap adaptation, and adequate flap nourishment from the underlying alveolus. The result is usually a soft tissue crater formation.

In the presence of thick bony margins and exostosis, good, intimate flap adaptation is not possible without some osteoplasty (Fig 23-30). This can be done judiciously without compromising esthetics or attachment levels. Osteoplasty involves removal of supporting alveolar bone, whereas ostectomy involves removal of alveolar bone proper. Alveolar bone proper consists of a thin lamella of bone that surrounds the root of the tooth and gives attachment to principal fibers of the periodontal lig-

ament. The supporting bone surrounds the alveolar bone proper and supports the sockets. The term *supporting bone* is frequently used incorrectly in the periodontal literature when the term *alveolar bone proper* should be used. Osteoplasty and ostectomy can be clinically differentiated in that increased root exposure occurs with ostectomy but not osteoplasty (Fig 23-31 vs Fig 23-32). Osteoplasty may reduce a thickened bony margin or marginal exostosis, but no additional root exposure or attachment loss occurs. Alveolar bone proper is removed during ostectomy, resulting in additional root exposure and clinical attachment loss at the site.

This procedure can be modified to achieve or preserve soft tissue esthetics. It may be very useful in visible sites such as the maxillary, anterior, and premolar regions.

Repositioned Flap Without Ostectomy

Advantages

- Access and visualization of the root surfaces and defects for debridement and root therapy
- Adaptation of healthy connective tissue to the root surfaces
- Less root hypersensitivity compared with an apically positioned flap
- Preservation of gingival width
- Preservation or creation of esthetic gingival morphology
- Relatively easy surgical procedure
- Relative postoperative comfort

Disadvantages

- Potential soft tissue crater formation postoperatively
- Residual probing depths in the presence of infrabony pockets
- Unpredictable attainment of new attachment
- Unstable long junctional epithelial attachment usually formed
- Intimate flap adaptation interproximally not always possible, especially in the posterior region

Periodontal Surgical Instrument List

- 2 mouth mirrors (one for chairside assistant's use for retraction and light reflection and one for the operator)
- Cotton pliers
- Periodontal probe
- 2 anesthetic syringes (one for block and one for infiltration)
- Minnesota retractor
- Prichard retractor PR 3
- Suture scissors
- La Grange soft tissue scissors
- Needle holder
- 2 scalpel blade holders (one for a 15c blade and one for a 12d blade)
- Tissue pickups
- Hemostat

- Molt curette 2/4 (used as a periosteal elevator)
- Curettes
  — Columbia 4R and 4L
  — McCall 13S/14S and 17/18
  — Prichard 1/2
  — Ultrasonic universal tip (P 10, fine)
- Osseous instruments
  — Ochsenbein chisels no. 1 and no. 2
  — Rhodes 36/37 back-action chisels
  — Loughlin 1/2 back-action chisels
  — Sugarman 1/2 bone files
  — Wedelstaedt chisel, narrow
- Surgical-length burrs, 7009 or an 8 round, 7004 or a 4 round and a 7903
- Sharpening stones for curettes and chisels
- Mixing spatula for the periodontal dressing

Proper flap design allows the entire gingiva to be preserved, or if indicated, it can be thinned or selectively sculpted to create a more esthetic morphology. Root hypersensitivity is not as great as with the apically positioned flap procedures, in which greater root exposure occurs.

With good surgical technique, postoperative discomfort is usually minimal following this procedure. There is minimal flap reflection, involvement of the osseous structures, and postoperative root exposure, and mature tissues cover the wound.

Technique

1. Primary incision. The location of the primary incision is based on the existing gingival width, thickness, and contour; surgical objectives; and esthetic considerations.

The incision should start at the point of the greatest scallop, which is usually mid-axis but is slightly distal to the mid-axis in the case of maxillary central incisors and canines (Figs 23-33 and 23-34). This incision is blended into the gingival crevice at approximately the line angle of the tooth (see Fig 23-33). Only a minimal amount of interdental tissue is removed, producing an exaggerated scallop to allow intimate adaptation of the flap to the entire root circumference during closure. With normal gingival anatomy, an internal bevel incision is directed to the alveolar crest and parallel to the long axis of the tooth starting 0.5 to 1 mm apical to the gingival margin (Fig 23-35). A crevicular incision may be used when esthetic concerns are primary or minimal gingival thickness is present (Fig 23-36). In the presence of thick, bulbous, or hyperplastic

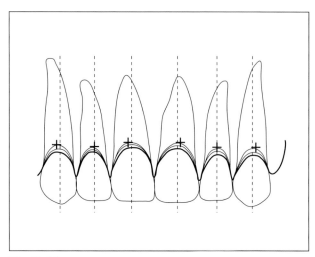

Fig 23-33 Primary incision outline, facial view. Note the location of the maximum scallop and then blending into the gingival crevice at the line angle area.

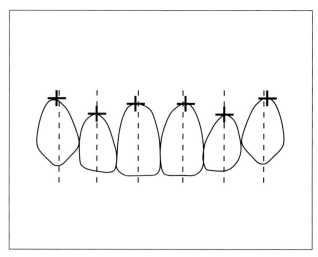

Fig 23-34 The maximum gingival scallop relative to the midline is slightly distal on the central incisors and canines and at the midline for the lateral incisors. This assumes normal tooth anatomy, position, and alignment.

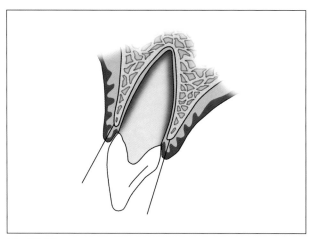

Fig 23-35 Primary incision with normal gingival width and thickness starting 0.5 to 1 mm apical to the free gingival margin.

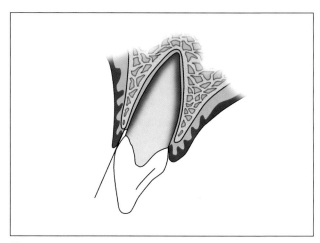

Fig 23-36 Sulcular incision with thin gingiva.

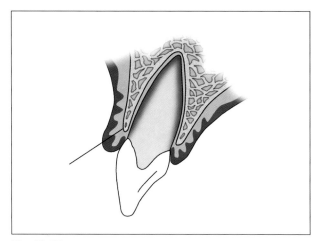

Fig 23-37 Thick gingiva with normal width. Remove excessive thickness.

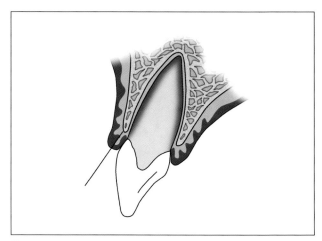

Fig 23-38 Thick gingiva with minimal width. Maintain the same width, but thin the tissue.

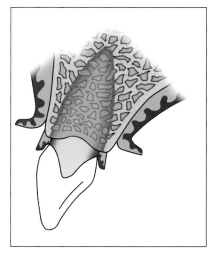

Fig 23-39 Flap elevation with minimal exposure of the alveolar crest.

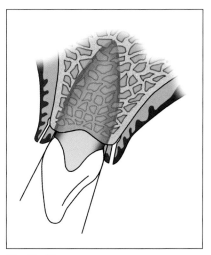

Fig 23-40 Second incision, from the base of the pocket to the alveolar crest.

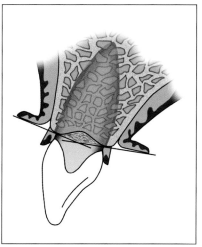

Fig 23-41 Third incision viewed from the proximal side with an Orban knife (1 and 2). Note granulomatous tissue left at the base of the infrabony crater.

tissue, a significantly greater amount of tissue is removed with the initial incision (Fig 23-37). With thick gingiva of minimal width, the gingiva is thinned, but the entire width is preserved (Fig 23-38). Most operators prefer to use a Bard-Parker 15c or 11 for the primary incision; however, in the posterior areas it may be necessary to use a 12d.

2. Flap elevation. A full-thickness flap is carefully elevated, exposing a minimum of 1 to 2 mm of alveolar bone for later access to the alveolar crest and root surfaces using a small periosteal elevator or Molt 2/4 curette (Fig 23-39).

3. Second incision. A second incision is made from the bottom of the pocket to the alveolar crest around the entire circumference of each tooth using a Bard-Parker 15c, 11, or 12d (Fig 23-40).

4. Third incision. Gently retracting the facial and lingual flaps with a Minnesota or Prichard retractor and using a small knife (Orban 1 and 2), a horizontal incision is made along the alveolar crest severing the supracrestal gingival fibers (Fig 23-41). Some operators believe they can remove a greater amount of the granulomatous tissue and leave significantly fewer tissue tags by peeling the tissue with a Molt 2 curette or using an Ochsenbein no. 2 chisel in a push-and-twist action.

5. Removal of granulomatous tissue and tissue tags. Remove the severed supracrestal gingival and granulomatous tissues and tissue tags with the sides and tips of sharp periodontal curettes (Fig 23-42).

6. Debridement and root planing. Thoroughly debride the osseous defects and root surfaces, and root plane all root surfaces exposed to the original pocket, with hand and ultrasonic curettes.

7. Inspection. After irrigation and aspiration, complete a thorough inspection of the root surfaces and osseous defects under good lighting to ensure that surgical objectives have been met (Fig 23-43).

8. Possible osteoplasty. In the presence of thick bony margins and exostosis, some judicious osteoplasty is frequently required to facilitate intimate flap adaptation.

9. Suturing. The most common method of suturing is by the use of routine interrupted sutures through the tips of the facial and lingual papillae, trying to achieve primary closure interproximally (Figs 23-44 and 23-45). This is the best method of suturing in areas without esthetic concerns and where maximum probing-depth reduction is desired. This approach, however, results in the facial papilla being

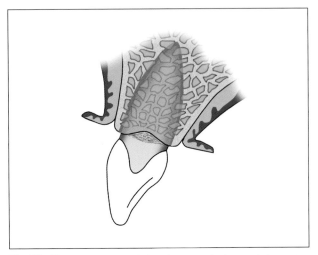

Fig 23-42 Note the granulation tissue at the base of the crater, which, along with tissue tags, is removed with the sides and tips of a curette.

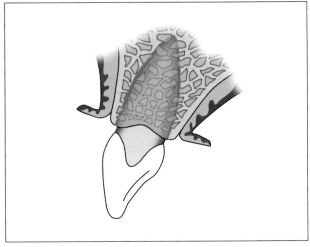

Fig 23-43 Thoroughly debride the defect and root surface, and root plane all diseased root surfaces. Then make a detailed inspection.

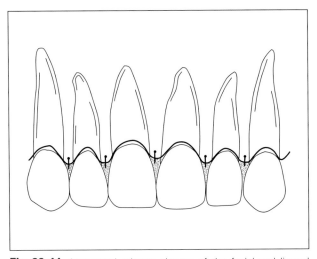

Fig 23-44 Attempted primary closure of the facial and lingual papillae, depressing the papillae apically to produce interdental dark triangles.

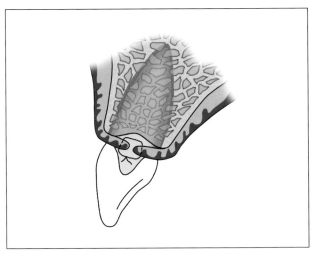

Fig 23-45 Proximal view of interrupted suture. Note depression of the facial papilla, which produces an open facial gingival embrasure and, when viewed from the facial aspect, a dark triangle.

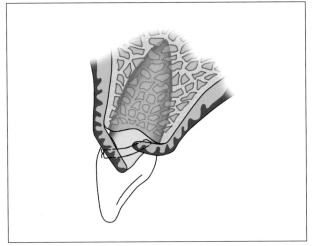

Fig 23-46 Vertical mattress suture of the facial papilla, elevating the facial papilla coronally and filling the facial gingival embrasure.

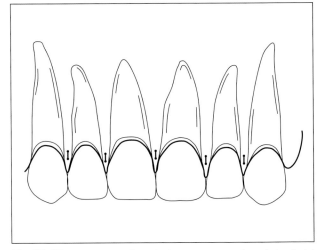

Fig 23-47 Facial view of vertical mattress suturing of the facial papillae. Note the significantly enhanced esthetics with the coronal positioning of the facial papillae.

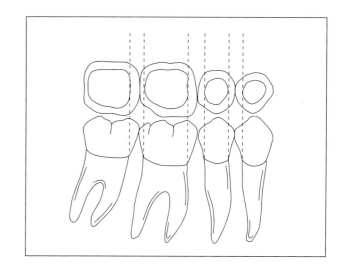

Fig 23-48 Note the much greater mesiodistal width at the CEJ area versus the contact region. The normal papillae are not wide enough to fill the space mesiodistally in the apical position without some alterations in incisions and/or suturing.

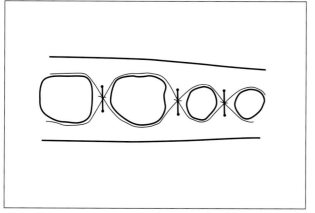

Fig 23-49 Note the open proximal root surfaces with traditional suturing with an apically positioned flap and widened interdental spaces.

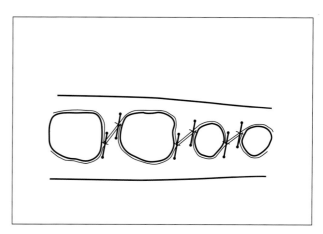

Fig 23-50 Note intimate flap adaptation on the proximal root surfaces with a modified suturing technique.

apically positioned, producing an open gingival embrasure that appears as a dark triangle (Fig 23-44). This is very unesthetic in the maxillary anterior region. This result can usually be prevented by the use of vertical mattress sutures for the facial papillae (Figs 23-46 and 23-47). Note in Fig 23-46 how, with the vertical mattress suture, the facial papilla is positioned more coronally, filling the gingival embrasure. A facial curtain effect is produced with enhanced esthetics from the facial aspect.

In the posterior areas, the mesiodistal interdental width becomes greater apically (Fig 23-48), and the normal papilla is not wide enough to contact both proximal tooth surfaces (Fig 23-49) without flap design and/or suturing modifications (Fig 23-50).

10. Flap adaptation. With moistened gauze, the primary flap is adapted around the necks of the teeth. Any excess blood is expressed to ensure intimate adaptation to the teeth and alveolus.

11. Application of periodontal surgical dressing (optional). If the flap is well adapted and there is no significant bleeding, a dressing is not required. The wound will be cleaner without a dressing, and faster soft tissue healing will occur. The use of a chlorhexidine mouthrinse effectively maintains supragingival plaque control during the postoperative period.

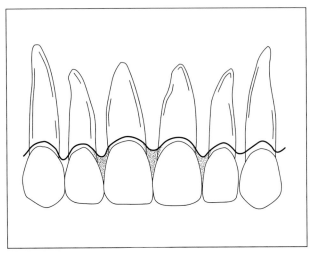

Fig 23-51 Facial view of apically positioned flap without osseous resection. Note the greater root exposure, lack of soft tissue to fill the facial gingival embrasures (producing the dark triangles), and generally unfavorable esthetics compared with Fig 23-47.

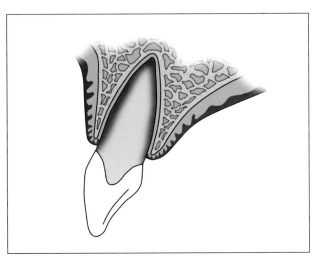

Fig 23-52 Proximal view of apically positioned flap without osseous resection. Note greater root exposure compared with Fig 23-46. There is less probing depth but also less favorable esthetics.

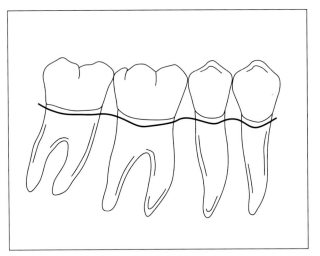

Fig 23-53 Facial view of apically positioned flap without ostectomy. Note increased root exposure.

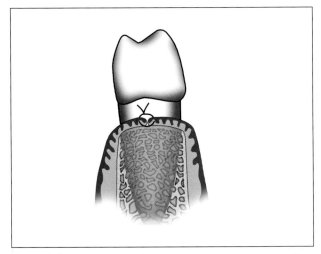

Fig 23-54 Proximal view of horizontal pattern of bone loss. Note the narrow faciolingual jaw width and thin radicular bone, anatomic features that predispose the patient to this pattern of bone loss. No residual probing depth remains with an apically positioned flap.

Apically Positioned Flap Without Ostectomy

The apically positioned flap without ostectomy is recommended in areas that do not have esthetic concerns and when greater probing-depth reduction is desired. This procedure is very similar to the repositioned flap procedure in most of its technique and objectives except for two essential differences: the marginal flap is initially reflected a greater distance, and following debridement of the osseous defects and root therapy, the flap is apically positioned and sutured at or slightly coronal to the alveolar crest (Figs 23-51 to 23-54). These differences result in both advantages and disadvantages compared with the repositioned flap procedure. There is greater probing-depth reduction when the gingival margin is apically positioned. This enhances the potential of effective periodontal maintenance and preservation of attachment levels. However, apical positioning can result in potentially unesthetic root exposure. More root exposure can potentially result in greater root hypersensitivity. Greater flap reflection and osseous exposure typically result in more postoperative pain. The interdental soft tissue area is usually slower to heal following apical positioning, since the interdental tissues are usually not coapted as closely as in the repositioned flap procedure.

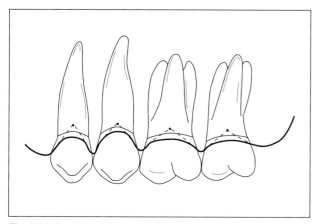

Fig 23-55 Apically positioned flap, palatal view of incision outline. Note the narrow radicular outline blending into the crevice at the line angle area, preserving maximal papilla width.

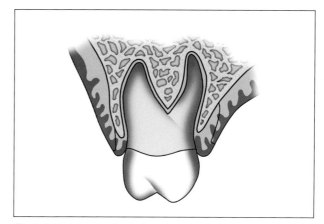

Fig 23-56 The proximal view of the apically positioned palatal flap demonstrates the site of the primary incision and the secondary thinning incision.

Apically Positioned Flap Without Ostectomy (compared with repositioned flap)

Advantages
- Potentially greater probing-depth reduction

Disadvantages
- Potentially unesthetic root exposure
- Potentially greater root hypersensitivity
- Potentially greater postoperative pain
- Usually slower interdental soft tissue healing
- Lack of flap adaptation in the presence of thick bony margins, exostosis, and tori without extensive osteoplasty

This surgical approach would not be the procedure of choice in areas of significant esthetic concern, such as the maxillary anterior and premolar areas. Generally, it is preferred in posterior regions without esthetic concern, since it usually results in greater pocket-depth reduction than the replaced flap procedure.

Total or near total pocket elimination may be possible in regions with thin radicular bone and narrow faciolingual jaw width with a horizontal pattern of bone loss and suprabony pockets (Fig 23-54). This occurs frequently in the mandibular incisor area but may occur in other areas with a very narrow facial-lingual jaw width and very thin radicular bone. This is one reason why it is so important that the therapist accurately evaluate preoperatively the osseous morphology and be able to predict morphologic results of the various surgical procedures.

Technique

The apically positioned flap procedure without ostectomy is very similar to the repositioned flap technique with the exceptions noted.

1. Primary incision. The primary incision design for the facial and lingual mandible and facial maxillary flaps is essentially the same as for the repositioned flap technique. Due to anatomic features of the palate that prevent its apical placement and its frequent need for thinning, its design is different. A surgical objective of the apically positioned flap procedure is the placement of the gingival margin just coronal to the alveolar crest. The postsurgical position and shape of the palatal gingival margin must be envisioned and that form placed with the initial incision (Fig 23-55). Some undermining and thinning of the palatal gingiva may also be required to allow the flap to freely adapt to the teeth and bone with a thin, tapering contour (Fig 23-56).

2. Flap elevation. The facial and lingual flaps are reflected to a greater extent, exposing additional alveolar marginal bone so that the mandibular and facial maxillary flaps can be apically positioned to the alveolar crestal level.

3. Second incision. Same as for the repositioned flap technique.

4. Third incision. Same as for the repositioned flap technique.

5. Removal of granulomatous tissue and tissue tags. Same as for the repositioned flap technique.

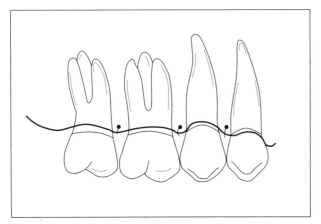

Fig 23-57 Apically positioned flap, facial view. Note root exposure.

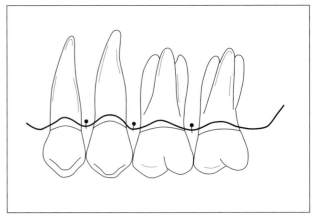

Fig 23-58 Apically positioned flap, palatal view of sutured flap in its resected apical position. Note root exposure.

6. Debridement and root planing. Same as for the repositioned flap technique.

7. Possible osteoplasty. Same as for the repositioned flap technique.

8. Apical positioning of the flap. The facial and lingual mandibular flaps and facial maxillary flaps are apically positioned to just cover the alveolar crests (Fig 23-57). The palatal flap is resected to conform to the shape and position of the palatal alveolar crest and local tooth form (Fig 23-58). Note the widened interdental mesiodistal width with apical positioning (see Fig 23-48). This results in the apically positioned papilla not being wide enough to fill the mesiodistal interdental space or provide intimate proximal root surface contact (see Fig 23-49).

9. Suturing. Use interrupted sutures or possibly continuous facial and lingual sling suturing, being careful not to draw the sutures so tight as to coronally displace the flaps. Sometimes modified suturing techniques may be used to enhance adaptation of the flap interproximally to the root surfaces (see Fig 23-50).

10. Flap adaptation. Same as for the repositioned flap technique.

11. Application of periodontal surgical dressing (optional). Same as for the repositioned flap technique.

Apically Positioned Flap with Ostectomy

Properly utilized in the presence of moderate osseous defects, the apically positioned flap procedure with ostectomy is the most effective surgical treatment available to predictably produce shallow probing depths. It is also required for surgical crown-lengthening procedures to establish biologic width for the epithelial and connective tissue attachment when caries, restorative margins, or root fractures extend near the alveolar crestal level. However, the procedure results in the sacrifice of some clinical attachment. Clinical expertise can minimize this occurrence and yet attain the clinical objectives. The procedure accentuates the potential for root hypersensitivity and, if used incorrectly, unesthetic root exposure.

Note the shallow interdental craters in Figs 23-59a and 23-59b. Following debridement and root therapy, flap closure with the interdental papillae bridges over the interdental craters; necrosis of the papillae tips and subsequent soft tissue crater formation are likely to occur (Figs 23-60a and 23-60b). Figures 23-61a and 23-61b demonstrate pocket elimination by osteoplasty and ostectomy. Figures 23-62a and 23-62b show the sutured interproximal papilla adapted to the underlying alveolus, which will provide some plasmatic circulation and less papilla necrosis. This, in combination with the lack of an underlying osseous crater, will result in positive gingival form and shallow probing depth. Proper application of this proce-

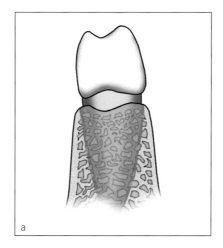
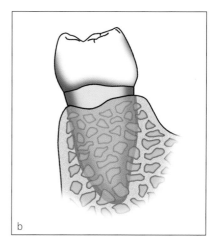

Fig 23-59a Proximal view of shallow interdental crater.

Fig 23-59b Proximal view of lingual shallow infrabony crater.

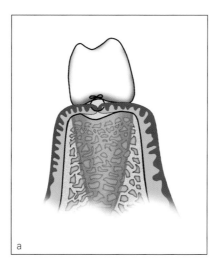
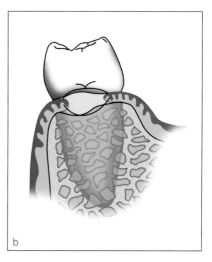

Fig 23-60a Even with primary apposition of papillae tips, necrosis of the papillae tips and a soft tissue crater will most likely result. The papillae tips are suspended in air and not contacting underlying bone for plasmatic circulation, and the flap vasculature is often not sufficient to maintain nourishment.

Fig 23-60b Apically positioned flap without ostectomy. Note the area where a soft tissue crater will develop, along with ultimate residual pocketing.

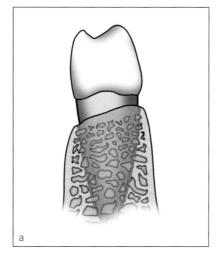
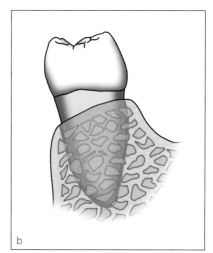

Fig 23-61a Ostectomy accomplished primarily from the lingual aspect. Note the absence of residual pocket depth.

Fig 23-61b Proximal view of ostectomy primarily accomplished from the lingual aspect.

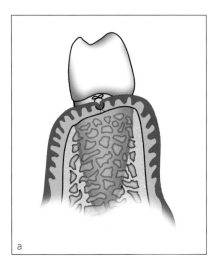 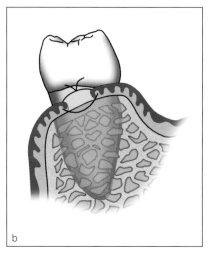

Fig 23-62a Ostectomy accomplished primarily from the lingual aspect. Note the absence of residual pocket depth. Primary closure as illustrated is not usually achieved.

Fig 23-62b Proximal view of a sutured flap following lingual ostectomy. Note the lack of primary closure; however, this area will heal nicely, without any residual pocketing.

Apically Positioned Flap with Ostectomy

Indications (infrabony defects)
- Adequate attachment remaining once physiologic osseous morphology has been established
- Esthetic limitations not present
- Anatomic limitations not present
- Root hypersensitivity concerns not present

Contraindications
- Alternative, more effective therapy
- Inadequate remaining attachment
- Anatomic limitations
- Esthetic limitations
- Root hypersensitivity concerns

Advantages
- Predictable reduction of probing depth if used appropriately
- Results relatively immediate; no prolonged waiting to determine outcome

Disadvantages (if used inappropriately)
- Clinical attachment removal
- Unesthetic root exposure
- Hypersensitive roots

dure requires advanced diagnostic knowledge, surgical training, and experience. A patient for whom this treatment is indicated is usually referred to a periodontist. For additional information on this procedure, the reader is referred to Kalkwarf et al.[76]

Clinical Crown Lengthening

If the margin of a restoration is placed subgingivally to gain retention because of a short clinical crown or because of caries, fractures, or perforations, periodontal health is frequently compromised. Gingivitis and attachment loss often result, leading to gingival recession or pocket formation. The restorative dentist is frequently faced with the task of simultaneously achieving mechanical, esthetic, and biologic goals. These goals must be

reached while achieving a retentive restoration. In addition, the restoration must maintain periodontal health while encompassing subgingival caries; fractures; areas of external or internal resorption; and perforations from endodontics, posts, and retentive pins. The anatomic and biologic guidelines and technical procedures that will permit the restorative practitioner to achieve an esthetic restoration that satisfies the restorative requirements and does not cause periodontal breakdown will be reviewed.

Biologic Width

The original concept of biologic width is based on histologic studies by Gargiulo et al[77] of the stages of passive eruption in normal cadaver periodontia. They noted that the average histologic width of the connective tissue attachment was 1.07 mm; of the epithelial attachment, 0.97

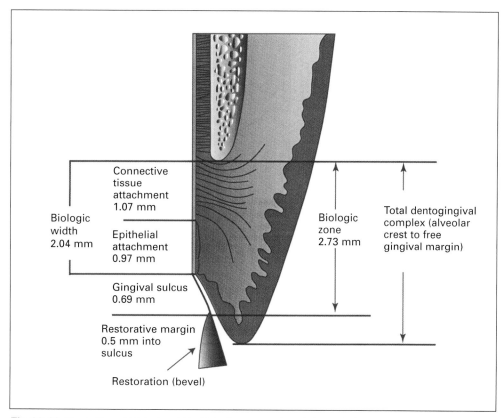

Connective
tissue
attachment
1.07 mm

Biologic
width
2.04 mm

Epithelial
attachment
0.97 mm

Biologic
zone
2.73 mm

Total dentogingival
complex (alveolar
crest to free
gingival margin)

Gingival sulcus
0.69 mm

Restorative margin
0.5 mm into
sulcus

Restoration (bevel)

Fig 23-63 Illustration of biologic width, biologic zone, and total dentogingival complex.

mm; and of the sulcus, 0.69 mm. The average combined width of the connective tissue attachment and the junctional epithelium of 2.04 mm has been referred to as the *biologic width* (Fig 23-63). Biologic width is believed to be very significant, because any violation of these anatomic structures by a restorative margin will lead to gingival inflammation and attachment loss.

The use of 2.04 mm as a universal biologic width may be questioned. First, the measurement for the biologic width is the average of the means of each of the four phases of passive eruption. There should always be some concern when an average is applied to all teeth—and especially in this case, when the use of the average of the means of each of the four phases pervades the literature. In the four stages of passive eruption, the individual range for the connective tissue attachment was 0.00 to 6.52 mm (mean, 1.07 mm); for the junctional epithelium, 0.08 to 3.72 mm (mean, 0.97 mm); and for the sulcus, 0.0 to 5.36 mm (mean, 0.69 mm). However, in this study the average width of the connective tissue attachment for each of the four stages was the most consistent, and the average for the junctional epithelium had the greatest variation as opposed to the individual measurements.

It has also been shown that there are variations in the biologic width when comparing individuals and when comparing anterior teeth versus molars. Vacek et al[78] have shown that the biologic width averages 0.33 mm greater for molars than for anterior teeth; the range was from 0.75 to 4.3 mm. The biologic width was consistent on the mesial, distal, facial, and lingual tooth surfaces of individual teeth. There are always some concerns with histologic anatomic interpretation. For example, sometimes it is difficult to determine the exact point where the periodontal ligament ends and the connective tissue attachment begins for measurement purposes. The formalin fixative causes some soft tissue shrinkage, which would primarily affect the free gingiva and sulcular depth. Also, anecdotal reports and comments from various clinicians note incidences of the margin of a restoration being 1 mm or less from the alveolar crest and the periodontium being in apparent health.

Restorative Margin Placement

For predictable and optimal periodontal health, the margin of the restoration unequivocally should be placed supragingivally. Obviously, this placement cannot always be achieved while satisfying the other restorative require-ments that are frequently present. Exceptions to supragin-gival placement could include areas of esthetic concern, subgingival caries, prior restoration, fracture, perforations from posts, root canals, retentive pins, external or internal resorption, extensive cervical erosion, short clinical crowns, and extreme root hypersensitivity. Frequently, the practitioner is faced with a dilemma of choosing between improved esthetics and less favorable periodontal health on the one hand and less favorable esthetics and better periodontal health on the other hand.

Maynard and Wilson[79,80] stated that if a restoration is to be placed apical to the gingival margin, it should be placed intracrevicularly and a minimum of 0.5 mm coronal to the junctional epithelium. *Intracrevicular restorations* were de-fined by Maynard and Wilson as being placed into, and confined within, the gingival crevice. *Intracrevicular* is a much more descriptive term than *subgingival*, which liter-ally could mean any place apical to the gingival margin. Subgingival placement of a restorative margin would per-mit violation of the junctional epithelium and connective tissue attachment, leading to gingival inflammation and attachment loss. It is significant to note that the term *intra-crevicular* limits not only the apical boundaries but the lateral boundaries as well. The apical extent of the restora-tive margin should be a minimum of 0.5 mm from the coronal aspect of the junctional epithelium. The lateral extent of the restoration should approximate that of the natural tooth. Maynard and Wilson also felt there should be a minimum of 1.5 to 2.0 mm sulcular depth to permit coverage of the restorative margin by the free gingiva.

Kois[81–83] believes the most important parameter for in-tracrevicular restorations is locating the base of the sulcus and the second most important parameter is locating the osseous crest. Precisely locating the base of the sulcus, the coronal extent of the junctional epithelium, is a problem. A healthy attachment has a histologic sulcus depth of ap-proximately 0.5 mm, yet clinically it measures 1.0 to 3.0 mm apical to the gingival margin. This discrepancy is due to the penetration of the periodontal probe into the junc-tional epithelium and possibly the connective tissue fibers. The degree and extent of penetration is variable, primarily based on probing depth pressure, diameter of the probe tip, and degree of gingival inflammation.

The therapist, therefore, is uncertain about the exact apical extent of the gingival sulcus, the coronal aspect of the junctional epithelium. To overcome this uncertainty, some authors have arbitrarily suggested placing the restorative margin a maximum of 0.5 to 1.0 mm apical to the gingival crest.[79,80] Kois,[81–83] however, advocates using the total gingival complex dimension to locate the apical base of the sulcus for intracrevicular margin location. He defines the total gingival complex dimension as the dis-tance from the free gingival margin to the alveolar crest (see Fig 23-63). This is measured under local anesthesia by probing carefully to the base of the sulcus, where some resistance should be felt if the periodontium is healthy. Then, while holding the probe tip against the root surface, advance the probe to the alveolar crest. This has also been referred to as *sounding to osseous crest* or *transgingival probing* (Figs 23-64a and 23-64b). This total measure-ment—gingival margin to alveolar crest—represents the dentogingival complex (see Fig 23-63). Kois uses the term *biologic zone* in referring to the combination of the con-nective tissue attachment, junctional epithelium, and sul-cus apical to the restored margin (see Fig 23-63).

Kois[82] demonstrated the dentogingival complex dimen-sion to be 3.0 mm on the midfacial aspect 85% to 90% of the time and 3.0 to 5.0 mm interproximally. This variation in measurement is noted by Kois to be the difference be-tween the gingival scallop and the osseous scallop. In general, the scallop is highly parabolic in the anterior re-gion and becomes nearly flat in the posterior region. If there has been no attachment loss, the alveolar crest par-allels the CEJ, as do the biologic width and biologic zone. The restorative margin then should parallel both the CEJ and the alveolar crest. The clinician must be especially cautious with preparations on the anterior teeth to follow this scallop, the CEJ, proximally. If the preparation is somewhat horizontal on the proximal surface, the bio-logic width and the biologic zone will be violated. The premolar CEJs are more horizontal and the molars nearly flat, as are their alveolar crests and biologic widths and zones. However, the alveolar crest and gingival margin may no longer be parallel to the CEJs once there has been alveolar crestal loss from periodontitis or gingival reces-sion, or following periodontal resective surgery. The ther-apist must then make adjustments to this alveolar crestal morphology and make the restoration margin parallel to the alveolar crest, not the CEJ. The apical extent of the restorative margin should then be a minimum of 2.5 mm from the alveolar crest: 1 mm of connective tissue attach-ment, 1 mm of junctional epithelium attachment, and 0.5 mm of sulcus apical to the restorative margin.

This concept is extremely important when considering tooth preparation after surgical crown-lengthening proce-dures before the gingival complex matures. Complete maturation of the periodontium following periodontal sur-gery can take up to 2 years. Seldom do patients or clini-cians wait for this complete healing to occur. Preparation of teeth after crown lengthening occurs at different inter-vals, ranging from 6 weeks to 2 years. The sooner a tooth is prepared after surgery, the more care one must use to prevent violating the biologic width.

Figure 23-65a shows the mesial aspect of a maxillary right canine 2 months after surgery with a probe sounding

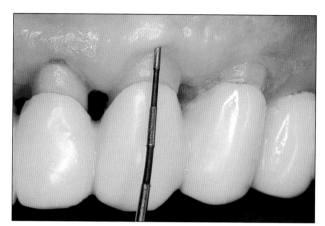

Fig 23-64a Measuring the dentogingival complex by sounding to bone.

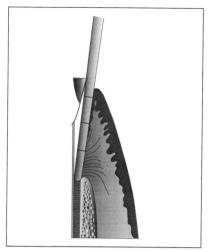

Fig 23-64b Illustration of measuring the dentogingival complex by sounding to bone.

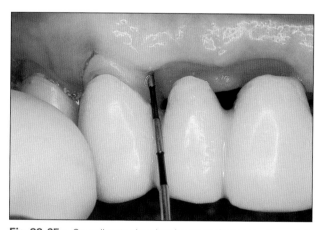

Fig 23-65a Sounding to the alveolar crest demonstrating a 1.5-mm total dentogingival complex 8 weeks after surgery.

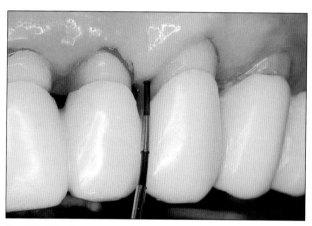

Fig 23-65b Sounding to the alveolar crest demonstrating a 3.0-mm total dentogingival complex 8 weeks after surgery.

to the osseous crest. The dentogingival complex measures only 1.5 mm at this stage of healing. The mesial surface is adjacent to an extraction site, where a soft tissue crater is still present. The mesial surface can easily be prepared too close to the bone. If the margin is placed 0.5 mm subgingivally, the margin will be 1 mm from the alveolar crest, thereby violating the biologic zone by 1.5 mm. The restorative margin should be placed 1 mm supragingival to this gingival margin to allow for the 2.5-mm minimum distance from the margin to the alveolar crest. However, the maxillary left canine (Fig 23-65b) shows a 3-mm dentogingival complex at the same stage of healing. A preparation margin placed 0.5 mm subgingivally will also be 2.5 mm from the alveolar crest, maintaining a minimal biologic zone.

It may be advisable to place the restorative margin farther than 2.5 mm from the alveolar crest during the early stages of healing, especially in the interproximal areas. As previously stated, the total dentogingival complex measures 3 to 5 mm interproximally. Following complete healing, a more definitive judgment can be made as to the exact placement of the margin. The use of provisional restorations will allow longer healing times before final restorations, permitting more accurate margin placement.

Predicting the position on the tooth where the gingival margin will heal is not an exact science, but with these guidelines one can more accurately place crown margins before the gingiva has completely matured. Experience will show that placing the margin of a final restoration 1

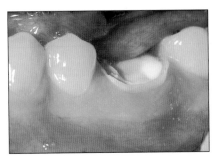

Fig 23-66a Inadequate clinical crown to achieve ferrule effect after post-and-core buildup.

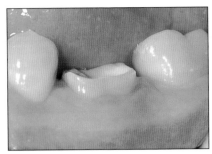

Fig 23-66b Postsurgical crown lengthening demonstrating tooth structure adequate to achieve the ferrule effect.

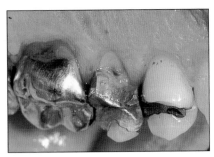

Fig 23-67 Palatal cusp fracture with a 1-mm palatal probing depth.

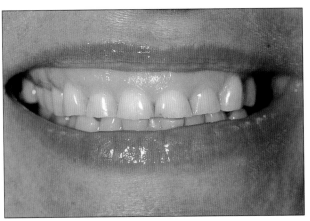

Fig 23-68a Incisal wear and uneven smile exposing excessive gingiva.

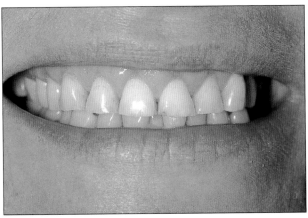

Fig 23-68b Postsurgical crown lengthening with improved esthetics prior to restoration.

mm or even 2 mm supragingivally at these early healing stages will result in complete coverage of the crown margin by the coronal growth of the gingiva. This coverage of root surfaces by the maturation of gingiva is predictable and reproducible.

Even placing the crown margins at the recommended 2.5-mm average distance from the alveolar crest can yield unsatisfactory results. If the periodontium consists of thin or narrow gingiva, or if the facial or lingual radicular bone is very thin or has fenestrations or dehiscences, gingival recession will be likely with any type of physical or bacterial stress.

The crown margins may remain exposed in some patients with biologic widths that are less than average. The gingiva can become red and inflamed when an individual's biologic width is violated. How does the practitioner know whether the patient undergoing treatment will have an average biologic width? Spear[84] has shown that the variation from the mean can be individually determined.

When possible, measuring the dentogingival complex on a contralateral unrestored and nonsurgically treated tooth gives the best measure of that individual patient's biologic width. When a contralateral tooth is not present, a premolar can be measured, because it has been shown by Spear to be an excellent measure of a patient's biologic width. Also, taking a presurgical measurement of the dentogingival complex of the teeth to be restored will help immensely in estimating the future healed gingival margin for that individual after surgery.

Other considerations in locating the restorative gingival margin include the length the preparation must be for retention, which is approximately 3.5 mm with a 6-degree taper. If a post-and-core buildup is involved, there should be at least 1.5 to 2 mm[85,86] of sound tooth structure between the post-and-core buildups and the restorative margin for the ferrule effect. The preservation of 1.5 to 2 mm of sound tooth structure will help avoid the common recurrent decay and root fractures seen when the margins of restorations are not extended adequately beyond the post-and-core buildups. Figure 23-66a shows a tooth with inadequate clinical crown remaining. A buildup could give adequate retention but will leave less than 2 mm of tooth structure for the ferrule effect without violating the biologic width. Figure 23-66b, which shows postsurgical healing following crown lengthening, demonstrates tooth structure adequate for placing the restoration margin 2 mm from the proposed buildup, achieving the ferrule effect.

Indications for Crown Lengthening

Essentially, crown lengthening is indicated when the biologic width or biologic zone has been violated or will be violated, as well as for areas of esthetic compromise. Crown lengthening is indicated when caries, fractures, perforations, or root resorption extends subgingivally so that the biologic zone will be violated with restorative correction (Fig 23-67). Short clinical crowns, either from delayed passive eruption or wear, will require added crown length to provide for retentive preparations. Patients whose teeth have delayed passive eruption and who have a gummy smile affecting overall esthetics can benefit from crown lengthening that surgically exposes the anatomic crown (Figs 23-68a and 23-68b).

Procedures in Crown Lengthening

Surgical crown lengthening should be considered in the overall treatment plan. This decision is made following a thorough periodontal, restorative, and prosthetic evaluation via a clinical and radiographic examination and a careful case analysis. Only after a thorough evaluation can it be determined whether crown lengthening is indicated, whether the posttreatment results will be desirable, and how best to achieve the desired results.

Clinically, the gingival and periodontal health must be evaluated, gingival width and thickness noted, and probing sulcular depths recorded. Is the facial and/or lingual radicular bone thick or thin? Are there fenestrations or dehiscences? This requires careful evaluation. It may be necessary to determine the width of the dentogingival complex and alveolar crestal bone level for the specific teeth of concern.

Radiographically, the generalized interdental crestal levels, interdental and inter-radicular widths, root lengths, root morphology, molar furcation levels, and root trunk lengths all must be noted. This information, in addition to probing depths, will determine the quantity of attachment present. Are there clinical or radiographic signs of pulpal involvement? What is the apical extent of the defect, such as caries, fracture, root perforation, or root resorption?

When the length of the root, level of the furcation, mesiodistal interdental width, and apical extent of the defect are known, one can determine whether crown lengthening is indicated, whether it is possible, and how best to accomplish it. Is the tooth critical to the overall treatment plan? If required, can the tooth be successfully treated endodontically? Will the surgical crown lengthening create an unesthetic result for the tooth in question and possibly the adjacent teeth? Will the tooth in question end up with an unfavorable ratio of clinical crown to clinical root or an inadequate amount of attachment? Will there be too great a sacrifice of attachment from the adjacent teeth to justify the procedure? Will a therapeutic furcation be created? How should the crown lengthening be done: gingivectomy, flap without osseous surgery, flap with osseous surgery, orthodontic extrusion?

Is there a more effective alternative treatment? Dental implants may be an alternative, because of their predictability. A fixed partial denture or removable partial denture may be a proper choice. Implants and partial dentures have the advantage that attachment from the adjacent teeth is not sacrificed. However, they each have their own deficiencies. The overall economics of the treatment must be considered. Is there a more cost-effective treatment for this patient? The cost of surgical crown lengthening and perhaps endodontic treatment, a buildup, a post and core, and crown could be significant.

Gingivectomy

Gingivectomy may be the treatment of choice in the case of delayed passive eruption, hyperplastic gingiva, or pseudopocketing associated with a gummy smile. Esthetics can be dramatically improved by exposing the anatomic crowns around the maxillary incisors, canines, and premolars and decreasing the amount of visible gingival tissue. Excess gingiva seems to be more common in teenage females and following orthodontic treatment.

Prior to selecting gingivectomy as the treatment of choice, one must determine the length of the anatomic crown versus the clinical crown to correctly diagnose the cause of the short clinical crown. Will adequate gingiva remain? There will need to be 3 to 5 mm of gingiva remaining[79,80]; 3 mm is generally thought to be the minimal amount of gingiva required to maintain health and resist the normal physical and bacterial stresses. If an intracrevicular restoration is to be placed, there should be 5 mm of gingiva[79,80] to withstand the added physical stress and the bacterial irritation associated with restorative margins. The gingiva should also be thick enough to prevent the restorative margin from showing through the gingiva, or it may need augmentation with a subepithelial graft. Where is the alveolar crest? Will there be enough width

411

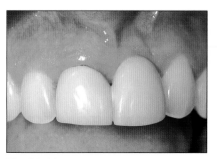

Fig 23-69a Grossly uneven gingival margins on right central incisor and left central incisor pontic.

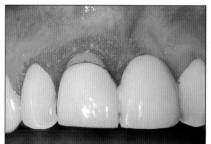

Fig 23-69b Gingivectomy and gingivoplasty of the right incisor.

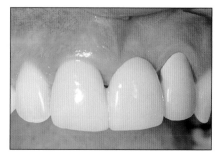

Fig 23-69c Final healing demonstrating even gingival margins on the right central incisor and left central pontic and greatly improved esthetics.

Diagnostic Criteria for Determining Which Crown-Lengthening Procedure Is Indicated

Clinical examination
- Periodontal health
- Gingival width and thickness
- Thickness of radicular bone
- Probing sulcular depth
- Sounding to marginal bony crest
- Esthetic evaluation, including smile line, gingival margin, incisal edge of teeth

Radiographic examination
- Interdental crestal margins
- Distance from contact points to interdental bone
- Root length
- Root morphology
- Furcation location or root trunk length
- Interdental width
- Apical extent of caries, prior restoration, fracture, root perforation, etc
- Pulpal involvement

---

between the alveolar crest and the CEJ to ensure stability for the connective attachment? If not, a flap and osseous procedure will be indicated. Is there any marginal exostosis that may require thinning? If so, a flap procedure will be required (Figs 23-69a to 23-69c).

Flap Without Osseous Resection

A flap-only procedure may be indicated where a narrow and thin band of gingiva is present and minimal crown lengthening is required. This could be treated by making a sulcular incision and apically positioning the flap. A flap without osseous resection may be indicated when there is excessive gingiva and the practitioner does not feel a gingivectomy is indicated or if less than 3 to 5 mm of gingiva would remain following resection. A flap approach may be used if the therapist is uncertain whether osseous surgery may be required. The need for osseous resection can be determined following flap reflection.

Flap With Osseous Resection

A flap with osseous resection is indicated in many clinical circumstances and is the most common crown-lengthening procedure. It is indicated when there is 3 mm of gingiva or less, where there would be less than 3 to 5 mm of gingiva remaining after a gingivectomy, or if osteoplasty or ostectomy would be required. Following the procedure, the flap can be repositioned or apically positioned as required.

When crown lengthening is performed for a single crown with a subgingival fracture or caries, a routine inverse bevel incision is used. It is extended to minimally include each adjacent tooth and occasionally more to facilitate flap reflection. The osteoplasty and ostectomy are carried out on the involved tooth and blended into the adjacent teeth to create a gradual rise and fall to the osseous architecture that the posthealing gingiva can assume (Figs 23-70a to 23-70e).

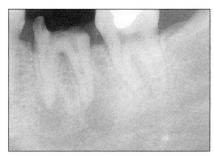

Fig 23-70a Radiograph showing a mandibular left first molar with an endodontic lesion and inadequate crown length.

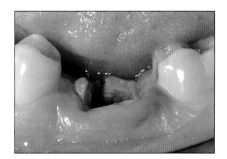

Fig 23-70b Mandibular left first molar with inadequate crown length.

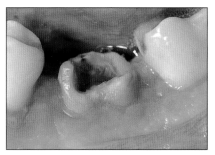

Fig 23-70c Postoperative crown lengthening of the mandibular left first molar with adequate tooth exposed for post-and-core buildup and crown preparation.

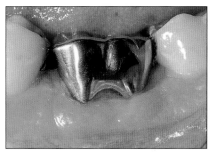

Fig 23-70d Completed restoration.

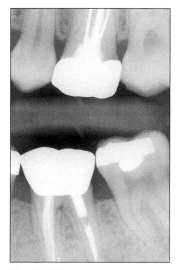

Fig 23-70e Twelve-year postoperative bitewing radiograph.

The amount of tooth exposure will vary from an absolute minimum of 3 mm[81,83] to as much as 5.5 mm.[87] There must be 1 mm for the connective tissue attachment, 1 mm for the junctional epithelial attachment, and 1 mm of sulcus depth (0.5 mm for the restorative margin and 0.5 mm between the restorative margin and the junctional epithelium). Additional root exposure will be required if there is a post and core, which requires an additional 1.5 to 2 mm (total of 4.5 to 5 mm) of sound tooth structure between the buildup and the crown margin for the ferrule effect.[85,86] Patients with thin, delicate gingiva, very thin radicular bone, or fenestrations and dehiscences are subject to recession and will need to have the margin placed farther than 2.5 mm from the alveolar crest. This also applies to patients who may be susceptible to periodontal disease.

The handling of the flap in areas of esthetic concern, such as the maxillary anterior and premolar regions, requires special considerations and modifications. If apical positioning of the gingival margin is anticipated, esthetics may be compromised. To allow papillary regeneration following flap reflection, the distance between the alveolar crest and the apical contact area should be no more than 5 mm.[88] This assumes a normal or narrow interdental width (Fig 23-71). If the interdental width is wide, less than 5 mm of interdental papilla will regenerate, leaving a dark triangle. The interdental width, general root taper, root alignment, and height from the alveolar crest to the apical aspect of the contact must be carefully noted and evaluated. If the interdental embrasures are wide or there is more than 5 mm between the alveolar crest and contact area, the design of the typical mucoperiosteal flap must be altered to preserve the interdental papilla. The incision outline then would include only the facial portion of the papilla (Fig 23-72). If the remaining papillary tissue is too thick, it can be carefully thinned with scissors or high-speed gingivoplasty diamonds, preserving the interdental papilla tissue.

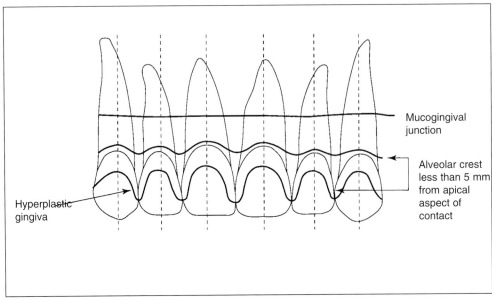

Fig 23-71 Hyperplastic gingiva and short clinical crowns; alveolar crest to apical aspect of contact is 5 mm or less, and inter-radicular width is normal.

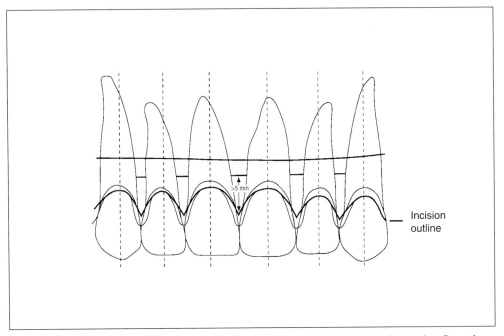

Fig 23-72 Situation requiring osseous surgery with wide inter-radicular spaces and more than 5 mm from alveolar crest to apical aspect of contact, with flap design to preserve interdental papilla.

Orthodontic Extrusion

Orthodontic extrusion of teeth with short clinical crowns, subgingival caries, defective restorations, fractures, perforations, and periodontal defects was advocated initially by Ingber.[89] It has the advantages of not having to sacrifice attachment from adjacent teeth and possibly a more esthetic overall result. However, a disadvantage is that the coronal gingiva and alveolar crest move coronally. This may require a flap and osseous surgical procedure to achieve functional and esthetic architecture. Kozlovsky et al[90] demonstrated that the coronal movement of the alveolar crest and gingiva could be prevented by a circumferential supracrestal fiberotomy and root planing to the alveolar crest every 2 weeks during the orthodontic extrusion (Figs 23-73a to 23-73d). Other disadvantages of orthodontic extrusion include added costs, longer treatment time, and

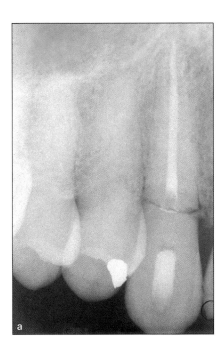

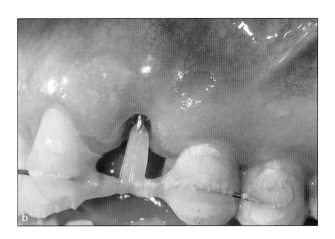

Fig 23-73a Radiograph of a horizontal fracture at the level of the alveolar crest.

Fig 23-73b Simple orthodontic extrusion of the root using an elastic and J-hook to extrude the tooth 4 mm.

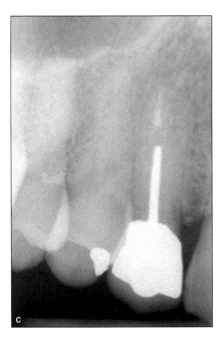

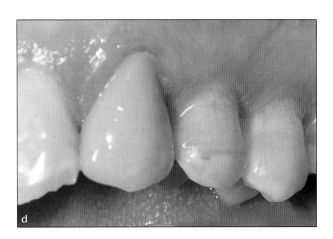

Fig 23-73c Two-year postoperative view of the radiograph.

Fig 23-73d Two-year postoperative view of the final restoration.

possibly unfavorable esthetic results. A root that is significantly narrower mesiodistally will create esthetic problems because the restored crown will be narrower in the cervical area than will the contralateral tooth. Also, the adjacent gingival embrasures may become wider, possibly creating recession of the gingival papilla and subsequent dark triangles.

The root trunk length of a molar must be carefully evaluated prior to extrusion. Orthodontic extrusion of a molar with a short root trunk could create a therapeutic furcation. If a significant furcation were created, it would not be a candidate for crown lengthening by orthodontic extrusion unless a root resection or hemisection could be performed to allow for such extrusion.

Postsurgical Periodontal Maintenance Procedures

General notes
- Follow the patient closely for 2 months postoperatively.
- Schedule weekly postoperative visits for the first 4 to 6 weeks.
- Prescribe chlorhexidine mouthrinse.

First week
- Remove periodontal surgical dressing if placed.
- Debride the wound with hydrogen peroxide and cotton-tipped swabs.
- Remove sutures if nonresorbable sutures were placed.
- Give the patient detailed plaque control instructions.

Subsequent weeks
- Evaluate healing and tissue morphology.
- Evaluate plaque control and give instructions as indicated.
- Desensitize roots as indicated.
- Determine the frequency of further appointments by the quality of plaque control and healing.

At 2-month intervals
- Perform postsurgical reevaluation, charting, and periodontal maintenance therapy.
- Establish periodontal maintenance frequency, and note any special concerns, such as areas of poor plaque control, unfavorable soft tissue morphology, significant residual probing depths, tooth hypermobility, or root hypersensitivity.

Postoperative Care and Periodontal Maintenance

The prophylactic use of systemic antibiotic coverage for routine surgical periodontal therapy is controversial. Little, if any, clinical benefit has been demonstrated with the routine use of antibiotics in these cases. With the widespread development of organisms resistant to many antibiotics, antibiotic use warrants careful consideration.

Postoperative pain is usually well controlled with the various narcotic pain medications available. Due to some of the undesirable effects of narcotics on the central nervous system, many clinicians have recently switched to nonsteroidal anti-inflammatory medications. These drugs also must be used with caution because severe gastrointestinal problems, ulceration, and bleeding have been reported, even with limited use.

It is very important that the patient be followed closely during the period immediately after surgical therapy until there is a reasonable level of tissue maturation, normal gingival morphology, and effective plaque control. Poor plaque control during healing could negate much of the anticipated benefits of the surgical procedure. Effective mechanical plaque control is difficult due to postoperative discomfort, altered gingival morphology, and sutures retaining plaque. Also, healing gingival tissues are highly vulnerable to injury from bacterial plaque by-products. Chemical plaque control with chlorhexidine mouthrinse has proved to be very beneficial in the early healing stages

following surgical therapy. It is routinely prescribed by most therapists for 2 to 3 weeks postoperatively until adequate comfort permits effective mechanical plaque control. The primary disadvantage of prolonged chlorhexidine use is the tooth staining that can occur and is difficult to remove. Chlorhexidine also tastes bad and can alter some patients' taste sensation.

The reader is referred to chapter 28 for additional information on periodontal maintenance.

Local Delivery of Antimicrobial Agents in the Treatment of Periodontitis

The primary etiology of periodontal disease is bacterial plaque. Although environmental,[91] behavioral,[92,93] and genetic[94] risk factors influence host response and disease progression, most, if not all, forms of periodontal disease should be considered infectious diseases. Recent advances aimed at altering the host's response to the bacterial infection appear to have promise[95,96]; however, most periodontal therapy remains focused on eradication of bacterial plaque and modifications of risk factors.

Between 1965 and 1970, the nonspecific plaque hypothesis suggested that the key factor in the initiation of tissue destruction was subgingival accumulation of microorganisms.[97] This theory did not stress the significance of any single bacterial species. Based on this theory, treatment of periodontal disease was primarily mechanical: root debridement performed either with or without surgical access to reduce the overall plaque mass.

It is estimated that more than 300 different bacteria reside in subgingival plaque.[98] Most of these organisms, however, are indigenous and are not considered pathogenic. Numerous studies have demonstrated a positive correlation between the presence of specific organisms and the occurrence of periodontitis.[1,99–101] These and other studies support the fact that a relatively small number of bacteria play a pivotal role in the initiation and progression of periodontitis.[102–104] In health, the indigenous flora and the host exist in a dynamic equilibrium. Perturbation of this equilibrium caused by colonization with a particular bacterium (or combination of bacteria) and/or an ineffective host response may result in the onset of disease. This finding has led to increased interest in chemical antimicrobial agents, which have the ability not only to suppress but also to eradicate the pathogenic players. Both systemic antimicrobial agents as well as locally delivered agents administered directly into the periodontal pockets have been used in the treatment of periodontal diseases. Local delivery alleviates many concerns associated with systemic antibiotic therapy, such as bacterial resistance, adverse effects (including superinfections and gastrointestinal irritation), lack of compliance, and the fact that periodontal destruction is often localized to a few teeth. This chapter discusses the current role of professionally administered subgingival antimicrobial agents used in the treatment of periodontitis. Other forms of antimicrobial therapy (eg, rinses and irrigation) have been used in the treatment of plaque and gingivitis, but they are not reviewed in this chapter.

The role of local delivery of antimicrobials is first reviewed and discussed relative to the more traditional mechanical treatment of periodontitis and to systemic antibiotics. Next, the agents most commonly used and currently available are presented, along with individual drug properties. The use of different agents is compared with the use of mechanical therapy, other agents, and systemic antibiotics. Specific recommendations for clinical use and contraindications follow. Finally, potential future studies to help determine the role of local delivery for treatment of periodontal disease are discussed.

Mechanical Plaque Removal Versus Local Delivery

Local delivery can be defined as the introduction of materials into the periodontal pocket designed to positively affect the treatment of inflammatory periodontal diseases.

Local delivery of any antimicrobial agent is not a replacement for good mechanical therapy. It may serve as

an adjunct to scaling and root planing in very specific situations, as will be discussed in following sections.

Although specific microbial species are believed to play a role in the disease process, periodontal therapy remains targeted toward removal of the plaque mass, as opposed to specific pathogens. However, in the process of mechanical root debridement, specific subgingival pathogenic species are removed or reduced to levels that result in improved clinical health and/or stabilization in periodontal maintenance patients.[105–107] Other benefits of mechanical debridement, whether performed as a part of initial therapy, surgical therapy, or periodontal maintenance, include the removal of calculus and endotoxin, disruption of the biofilm complex, induction of potentially protective antibody responses to certain pathogens,[108] and increased numbers of beneficial bacteria, such as streptococci.[109] Most benefits are in direct response to the mechanical action of scaling and root planing and cannot be achieved with local delivery of antimicrobial agents. Locally delivered antimicrobial agents can reduce the subgingival flora, but their effectiveness against plaque as a part of a biofilm is not known.

Potential advantages of local delivery include the fact that it can be easy to perform; takes little time; does not remove cementum, which often results in sensitivity; and is usually well tolerated by the patient.

Scaling and root planing have routinely been shown to be effective in the treatment of chronic periodontitis without the concomitant use of systemic or local antimicrobial agents.[110] When scaling and root planing are performed as a part of routine periodontal maintenance, periodontal pathogens are suppressed to a level that does not result in progressive disease in most patients.[111,112] There is no long-term evidence that the use of local delivery can reduce the interval for periodontal maintenance visits.

Many studies have shown that local delivery has the same clinical results as scaling and root planing in chronic periodontitis. Therefore, there is no clear advantage for using antimicrobial agents, either systemic or local, in these patients when good clinical results are obtained with scaling and root planing.

Systemic Delivery Versus Local Delivery

Not all periodontal pathogens are equally susceptible to mechanical debridement. Several bacteria, such as *A actinomycetemcomitans* and *P gingivalis*, can invade the epithelium[113,114] and therefore require supplemental antibiotics and/or surgery for eradication.

There are many advantages of using systemic delivery of antibiotics as opposed to local delivery in the treatment of periodontal diseases. The advantages include *(1)* treatment of multiple sites and potential microbial reservoirs (tongue, tonsils, and buccal mucosa); (2) treatment of organisms at the base of the pocket and in the tissue because of systemic absorption and delivery into oral tissues, gingival crevicular fluid, and saliva[115]; (3) availability of a variety of drugs and specific combinations of drugs to choose from; (4) shorter time to administer; and (5) lower cost.

Systemic antibiotics have been proven to be effective and are specifically recommended in the treatment of aggressive forms of periodontal disease.[116,117] In addition, they are effective in conjunction with scaling and root planing in deep periodontal pockets that are nonresponsive.[115,118,119]

In contrast, aggressive forms of periodontal disease that are associated with A actinomycetemcomitans infections are not routinely successfully treated with local delivery. In one study, the numbers of A actinomycetemcomitans actually increased with localized tetracycline delivery, and in another study A actinomycetemcomitans was resistant to localized metronidazole application.[120,121] This could be due to a reduction of antagonistic bacteria, the invasiveness of A actinomycetemcomitans, or the limited penetration of the medicament.

Local delivery does have the advantage of highly concentrated drug delivery without the adverse effects of systemic antibiotics. It also is accompanied by improved compliance and less propensity for development of bacterial resistance, which is the biggest concern with the use of systemic antibiotics.

Although transient increases in bacterial resistance have been shown for locally delivered tetracycline, minocycline, and metronidazole,[122–125] the high concentrations at a specific site decrease the overall chances of resistance due to ineffective drug dosing seen with systemic antibiotics. However, repeated use of locally delivered antimicrobial agents may result in leakage of low concentrations and an increased chance for developing resistant organisms. For example, there are limited data to suggest the development of resistance with the use of tetracycline.[126,127]

Local delivery of any antimicrobial agent is not a substitute for systemic antibiotics when they are indicated in specific periodontal diseases. When choosing local delivery, antibiotic selection is empirical; therefore, in cases where one needs to know the specific bacteria and antimicrobial susceptibility, microbiologic and antibiotic sensitivity testing are recommended.

Periodontitis is a mixed infection. There are drugs available today that target groups of microorganisms. However, broad-spectrum antibiotics are still widely used, even though they have the disadvantage of killing antagonistic bacteria as well. Practitioners must adhere to the judicious use of all antibiotics in light of this problem and increasing concerns about bacterial resistance.

The Agents

Local drug delivery offers the ability to reach bacteria at the base of a pocket and retains activity long enough to have bactericidal or bacteriostatic effects on offending pathogens. Depending on the duration of drug release, the agents are considered either sustained (less than 24 hours) or controlled (more than 24 hours).[128,129] Considering that the gingival crevicular fluid is capable of being replaced 40 times in 1 hour,[130] the drug should ideally be substantive (retained on root surfaces) or be delivered in a slow-release or controlled-release formulation. Local delivery results in a substantially higher drug concentration in the pocket compared with the equivalent systemic agent.

There are primarily six different antimicrobial agents in use for local delivery, and they are commercially available in various formulations (Table 23-1). The agents are discussed individually below. Properties of the locally delivered antimicrobial agents are compared in Table 23-2, and considerations for clinical use are reviewed in Table 23-3.

Tetracycline Fibers

Tetracycline fibers are 9-inch (23-cm) flexible ethylene vinyl acetate fibers loaded with 25% tetracycline hydrochloride. The fiber is layered back and forth, filling the periodontal pocket; it is then secured in place with a cyanoacrylate adhesive and covered with a periodontal dressing. After 10 days the fiber is removed.

Tetracycline is bacteriostatic in systemic forms, but it is bactericidal in the high concentrations delivered in the gingival sulcus. It is a substantive, broad-spectrum antimicrobial agent, which means it kills the antagonistic or beneficial bacteria, as well as the pathogens. Finally, resistance to tetracycline has been shown for 12% of normal oral flora,[132] and individuals can develop resistance to certain microorganisms after systemic administration of this antibiotic.[133]

Minocycline Gel

A lipid gel into which 2% minocycline hydrochloride has been incorporated is expressed into the periodontal pocket using a syringe until the pocket is overfilled. The gel resorbs within 1 day, and subsequent applications are recommended at 2 weeks and 4 weeks after the first application.

Minocycline is one of the tetracyclines, and therefore it is substantive, broad spectrum, and bacteriostatic. Its ability to successfully reduce the subgingival flora has been questioned.[134,135]

Minocycline Microspheres

One milligram of minocycline hydrochloride is microencapsulated into a bioabsorable polymer and delivered

Table 23-1 Local Delivery Antimicrobial Agents

Antimicrobial agent	Product	Company	Location
Tetracycline fiber	Actisite*†‡	Alza	Palo Alto, CA
Minocycline gel	Dentomycin†	Blackwell Supplies	Gillingham, United Kingdom
Minocycline microspheres	Arestin*	OraPharma	Warminster, PA
Doxycycline polymer	Atridox*	Atrix Laboratories	Fort Collins, CO
Metronidazole gel	Elyzol†‡	Dumex	Copenhagen, Denmark
Chlorhexidine chip	PerioChip*†‡	Perio Products	Jerusalem, Israel

*Currently approved for use in the United States.
†Currently approved for use in Europe.
‡Currently approved for use in Israel.

Table 23-2 Properties of Local Delivery Antimicrobial Agents

Antimicrobial agent	Delivery	Resorption	Duration of antimicrobial activity	Organisms targeted	Plasma concentration	Bacterial resistance
Tetracycline fiber	Controlled	None	10 d	Broad spectrum	Minimal	Possible
Minocycline gel	Sustained	1 d	1 d	Broad spectrum	Minimal	Possible
Minocycline microspheres	Controlled	≥14 d	≥14 d	Broad spectrum	Minimal	Possible
Doxycycline polymer	Controlled	27 d	7 d	Broad spectrum	Minimal	Possible
Metronidazole gel	Sustained	12–24 h	12–24 h	Anaerobes	Minimal*	Possible
Chlorhexidine chip	Controlled	7–10 d	7 d	Broad spectrum	Not detected	Minimal possibility

*Seventy percent of total dose, but still less systemic absorption than one 200-mg metronidazole tablet.[131]

Table 23-3 Handling Characteristics of Local Delivery Antimicrobial Agents

Antimicrobial agent	Ease of delivery	No. of sites treated per unit of product	Treatment time	Storage/Shelf life
Tetracycline fiber	Moderate	1–2	Approximately 10 min*	Room temperature/1.5 y
Minocycline gel	Easy	Multiple	Few seconds	Refrigerate/4 y
Minocycline microspheres	Easy	1	Few seconds	Room temperature/2 y
Doxycycline polymer	Easy	12	Few seconds†	Refrigerate/20 mo
Metronidazole gel	Easy	Multiple	Few seconds	Room temperature/3 y
Chlorhexidine chip	Easy	1	Less than 1 min	Refrigerate/3–18 mo

*May take an additional 10 minutes or longer to remove fiber.
†Must be removed from refrigeration 10 minutes prior to mixing; mixing requires approximately 2 minutes.

subgingivally as a powder via a syringe. On contact with the gingival crevicular fluid, it hydrolyzes and releases minocycline with minimum inhibitory concentrations, exceeding that required for periodontal pathogens, for at least 14 days.[136]

Like the other tetracycline derivatives, it has broad-spectrum activity and is bacteriostatic; however changes in the composition of the subgingival microorganisms have not yet been reported.

Doxycycline Polymer

Doxycycline polymer is a controlled-release system that requires mixing a 10% doxycycline hyclate powder with a bioabsorbable polymer to form a viscous liquid. The liquid is delivered with a syringe and a blunt cannula into the periodontal pocket, where it solidifies when it contacts the crevicular fluid. Following administration, it is recommended that the area be covered with a periodontal dressing or adhesive. Drug delivery occurs over 7 days, and the polymer resorbs after 27 days.

Doxycycline, also a tetracycline, is substantive, broad spectrum, and bacteriostatic. It can successfully reduce the populations of a number of periodontal pathogens.

Metronidazole Gel

Metronidazole bioabsorbable gel contains 25% metronidazole benzoate in a sesame oil matrix. The gel is delivered with a syringe and a blunt cannula into the periodontal pocket until the pocket is overfilled. The gel changes into a semisolid state when it contacts the gingival fluid. The activity and resorption occur within 12 to 24 hours (sustained delivery). The application is repeated 7 days later.

Metronidazole is bactericidal primarily toward anaerobes.[137] However, as used in this delivery system, its ability to reduce total anaerobic colony-forming units has been questioned.[125] Facultative organisms are not affected by this agent, and the development of resistant organisms after metronidazole use is not clear.[137]

Chlorhexidine Chip

The chlorhexidine chip delivers 2.5 mg chlorhexidine gluconate in a bioabsorbable hydrolyzed gelatin. The chip (4 mm × 5 mm × 0.35 mm) is placed into the periodontal pocket with a forceps. Activity is seen for 1 week, and resorption occurs shortly thereafter.

Chlorhexidine gluconate is an antiseptic with broad-spectrum antimicrobial activity (including activity against putative periodontal pathogens) and adheres to organic matter.[138] Resistance to chlorhexidine gluconate is unlikely.[139]

The decision regarding which antimicrobial agent to use is not typically based on the agents' individual antimicrobial properties. Clinical selection usually revolves around the agents' handling characteristics (see Table 23-3), the number of sites to be treated, allergic potential, cost, commercial availability, and approval by drug regulatory agencies. In general, adverse reactions to the local delivery agents are minimal; however, adverse effects such as toothache, gum soreness, and abscesses have been reported.

Clinical Trials of Local Delivery Agents

Table 23-4 summarizes the results of clinical trials using local delivery of antimicrobial agents.

Tetracycline Fibers

Clinical studies employing the local delivery of tetracycline fibers have tested its efficacy in pocket reduction, gains in clinical attachment, reduction of bleeding on probing, and suppression/elimination of subgingival bacteria both as a monotherapy and an adjunct to scaling and root planing.[140–144] Most of these studies have been conducted with patients who have chronic periodontitis or patients on maintenance therapy with probing depths of at least 5 mm. The length of the studies varied from 2 months to 5 years, and almost all studies used a single application of the fiber.

In general, the studies show that tetracycline fibers are as effective as scaling and root planing in improving periodontal clinical parameters. When tetracycline is combined with scaling and root planing and compared with scaling and root planing alone, the results are equivocal. Some studies show these treatments to be equally effective, while other studies report that the adjunctive use of tetracycline results in a superior statistical result. Most published studies report outcomes of 1 year or less. It is interesting to note that in a recent study where an initial (6-month) report showed the combination to be superior in terms of probing depth and attachment level, a 5-year follow-up of a subset of these patients found no significant difference in scaling and root planing alone versus scaling and root planing along with the fiber.[144] This finding warrants additional long-term studies involving greater numbers of patients.

Minocycline Gel

The studies evaluating the effectiveness of minocycline gel primarily examined its adjunctive potential when combined with scaling and root planing. However, the results of the studies conflict. Most studies do not consistently report improvements for either clinical parameters or microbiologic parameters with adjunctive minocycline therapy.[134,135,145,146] In fact, the longest trial (18 months) showed no advantage to using minocycline with scaling and root planing in terms of improvements in pocket depth, attachment levels, or bacterial colonization.[135]

Minocycline Microspheres

One large-scale multicenter study has been published using the minocycline microspheres.[136] Probing depth was reduced significantly more in the group receiving the combined therapy of locally delivered minocycline microspheres with scaling and root planing after 1 month and was maintained throughout the 9-month study. Clinical attachment levels were measured, but the outcomes of these measurements for the different groups were not reported.

Doxycycline Polymer

Doxycycline has been tested as a monotherapy only in the treatment of chronic periodontitis or in periodontal maintenance patients. Most studies (ranging from 3 to 18 months

Table 23-4 Range of Clinical Improvements Reported for Clinical Trials of Local Delivery Antimicrobial Agents

Antimicrobial agent	Probing-depth reduction (mm)	Attachment gain (mm)	Duration of studies
Tetracycline fiber[140–144]			2 mo–5 y
Fiber	0.57–1.02	0.54–0.65	
Fiber + S/RP	0.93–1.96	0.66–1.56	
S/RP	0.54–1.61	0.50–1.09	
Minocycline gel[134,135,143]			3–18 mo
Gel	—	—	
Gel + S/RP	1.0–1.7	0.5–0.8	
Placebo + S/RP	0.95–1.4	0.3–0.8	
S/RP	0.71	0.54	
Minocycline microspheres[136]			9 mo
Microspheres	—	—	
Microspheres + S/RP	1.32	—	
S/RP + vehicle	1.00	—	
S/RP	1.08	—	
Doxycycline polymer[147,148,150]			3–18 mo
Polymer	1.1–1.3	0.7–0.9	
Polymer + S/RP	—	—	
Placebo	0.8–1.8	0.1–1.0	
S/RP	0.9–1.3	0.7–0.9	
Metronidazole gel[143,151]			3 mo–175 d
Gel	1.6	0.70	
Gel + S/RP	0.93	0.54	
S/RP	0.71–1.6	0.50–0.54	
Chlorhexidine chip[154,155]			6–9 mo
Chip	—	—	
Chip + S/RP	0.95–1.16	0.31–0.75	
Placebo	0.69	0.55	
S/RP	0.65–0.70	0.47–0.58	

S/RP = scaling and root planing.

Dash indicates not evaluated or not reported.

in length) found that doxycycline was as effective as scaling and root planing in pocket reduction and clinical attachment gains.[147–149] However, in one study, doxycycline appeared to have better results than scaling and root planing and showed maximum improvement prior to the final (9th) month of evaluation.[150] Doxycycline and the control of scaling and root planing were both administered at baseline and at 4 months. Long-term follow-up is necessary to see if the improvements in clinical parameters are maintained. The benefits of doxycycline in adjunctive therapy, if any, are not known.

Metronidazole Gel

In general, the efficacy of metronidazole as a monotherapy is similar to that seen with scaling and root planing in terms of pocket reduction and gains in attachment. Its use as an adjunctive agent has not shown a substantial benefit in the treatment of chronic periodontitis or patients in periodontal maintenance.[121,151–153] The studies vary in length from 3 to 6 months and vary in number of metronidazole applications from 1 to 5 in 10 days.[121] The additional applications appear to have no benefit.

Chlorhexidine Chip

Large, multicenter clinical trials have found favorable benefits of the chlorhexidine chip used in conjunction with scaling and root planing.[154–156] These studies report the statistical significance of greater pocket reduction and more attachment gain for the combination therapy. The clinical significance, however, may not be as pronounced. A concern of the studies' design was the lack of any additional scaling and root planing in control sites but repeated chip applications in test sites every 3 months. However, the fact that the combined therapy resulted in more sites with pockets reduced by 2 mm or more suggests that there may be site-specific usefulness for the chlorhexidine chip as an adjunct to scaling and root planing.

The great majority of studies have focused on the use of local delivery of antimicrobial agents in nonsurgical therapy. Recently, a few studies have reported their use in surgical therapy. The results, however, are mixed. Needleman et al[157] saw no benefit relative to attachment levels when using metronidazole with flap surgery. Sander et al,[158] in contrast, reported a gain in clinical attachment when topical metronidazole was combined with GTR. More studies are needed in this area.

The results obtained with the different agents cannot be directly compared from study to study to determine which agent is best. Furthermore, there are a limited number of short-term studies, which reported no differences when comparing the efficacy of one local delivery agent versus another.[143,159]

Comparisons of local delivery and systemic administration of antimicrobial agents are also limited. Available studies show no superiority of one route versus the other when either the same antibiotic was used or when two different antibiotics were compared.[160] Additionally, limited information is available evaluating the concurrent administration of systemic and locally delivered antimicrobial agents.

Finally, several aspects must be considered when interpreting the results of clinical studies using various local delivery agents: (1) The format of the study protocol may dictate treatment or lack of treatment that is not consistent with periodontal therapy in periodontal practices. For example, in some studies scaling and root planing are performed at the onset of the trial and on completion of the trial (some subjects do not receive any debridement for 12 months). (2) The length of time allowed for scaling and root planing may be short (15 minutes per quadrant), longer, or not specified. (3) The qualifying probing depths in most studies are at least 5 mm. Many studies do not differentiate the distribution of deeper pockets (at least 7 mm deep) from the 5- and 6-mm probing depths. One could expect that deep and moderate pockets might respond dif-

ferently.[39] (4) Measurements of attachment levels are critical. Without knowing actual changes in attachment, probing-depth improvements may primarily reflect recession and not true gains in clinical attachment. (5) Some studies exclude multirooted teeth. (6) Most studies are conducted for very short times (the minimum necessary for approval by the respective drug agencies). Results may be promising, but do they hold true in long-term assessments? (7) Results are usually presented as being statistically significant. Whether or not they are clinically significant is open for interpretation.

Indications for Local Delivery of Antimicrobial Agents

Based on the results of clinical studies, local delivery of antimicrobial agents has a defined, but limited, beneficial response in periodontal therapy.[161] Although antimicrobial treatment as a monotherapy has similar results to scaling and root planing, it should not replace scaling and root planing but rather should be used in conjunction with them when conventional therapy has failed.[162]

Local delivery of antimicrobial agents has potential usefulness in the following patients:

1. Patients with chronic periodontitis who are in periodontal maintenance and who are otherwise stable but exhibit limited localized persistent or recurrent deep probing depths (Fig 23-74)
2. Patients with chronic periodontitis who have completed initial therapy, with localized nonresponsive sites, and in whom surgery is ruled out (Fig 23-75)

The first scenario is the primary indication for the current use of local delivery in periodontal therapy. If patients in periodontal maintenance exhibit generalized deep probing depths or osseous defects, surgical therapy may be indicated.

In the second scenario, local delivery in combination with scaling and root planing may be attempted after reevaluation of initial therapy. If the lesion persists after the combined use of mechanical and chemical therapy, the patient should be referred to a periodontist for definitive treatment.

Before incorporating local delivery of antimicrobial agents into a treatment plan, the practitioner must assess the ultimate goal of therapy or the desired outcome. Clinical reports evaluating local delivery agents generate statistically significant data, but the magnitude of the differences seen or the clinical importance is often not assessed.[163] For example, statistically significant data may reflect a 0.5-mm improvement in probing depth or attachment level as a result of the use of a particular prod-

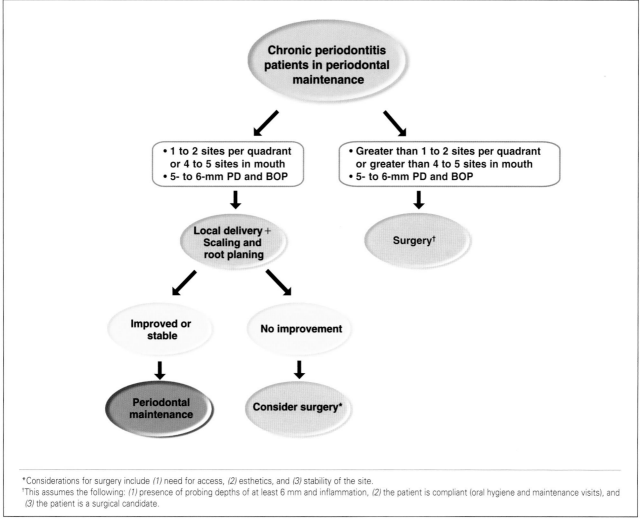

Fig 23-74 Therapy decisions for the use of local delivery during maintenance based on probing depths and nature of disease (localized versus generalized). PD = probing depth; BOP = bleeding on probing.

uct. One must consider if this is clinically justified, as well as the cost-benefit ratio for the patient. Clinically significant differences are the smallest changes that would convince one to choose an alternative therapy. Ultimately, this decision is determined by the individual practitioner.[163] If the goal of therapy is a stable periodontium, one must question whether this goal can be accomplished with scaling and root planing (with or without the use of antimicrobial agents) or whether surgery would be a better option.

Contraindications for Local Delivery of Antimicrobial Agents

Local delivery of antimicrobial agents should not be used alone, and it is not a replacement for traditional periodontal therapy. Additionally, local delivery is not suitable for certain periodontal patients. Local delivery should not be used in the following situations:

1. As a replacement for scaling and root planing in initial therapy or maintenance
2. As a replacement for surgical therapy
3. In patients with multiple areas requiring treatment
4. In patients with aggressive periodontitis (there are insufficient data to support the use of local delivery in aggressive forms of periodontitis)
5. As a substitute for systemic antibiotics (which are indicated for patients with aggressive periodontitis, certain periodontal diseases associated with systemic diseases, and patients with refractory disease or abscesses)

In terms of periodontal clinical parameters, there are no additional benefits for the use of local delivery of antimi-

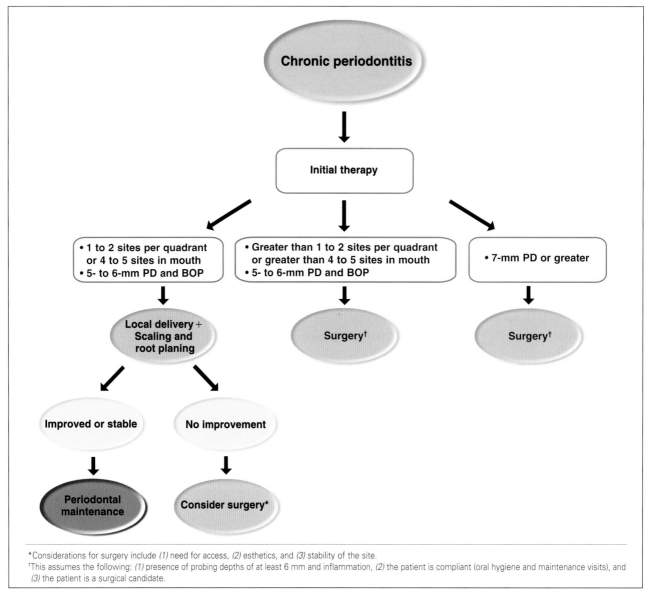

Fig 23-75 Therapy decisions for the use of local delivery after initial therapy based on probing depths and nature of disease (localized versus generalized). PD = probing depth; BOP = bleeding on probing.

crobial agents in place of scaling and root planing. One study proposed that local delivery reduced the need for periodontal surgery. However, this study examined local delivery in combination with systemic antibiotics.[164] Therefore, the effects of local delivery alone were not assessed. The patient with multiple deep periodontal defects is not a candidate for local delivery and is probably better treated with periodontal surgery.

Patients with aggressive periodontitis, periodontitis that is refractory, or periodontitis concomitant with certain systemic diseases have shown favorable response to systemic antibiotics.[165–167] Few data are available that compare the results achieved with local delivery to those of systemic

antibiotics in these patients.[160] While the results of studies of short-term local delivery appear equivalent to the results of systemic antibiotics in certain populations, the advantages and disadvantages of each (as discussed earlier in the chapter) must be considered. When multiple defects are present, systemic antibiotics are still recommended. Another consideration is the colonization of specific periodontal pathogens in special patient populations. For example, *A actinomycetemcomitans* is a frequent colonizer in localized aggressive periodontitis. The use of local delivery of tetracycline and metronidazole in *A actinomycetemcomitans* infections has not been shown to equivocally eliminate this pathogen.[120,121]

In summary, the primary application of local delivery at present is limited to localized sites in patients with chronic periodontitis. The effectiveness of local delivery is not clear in the treatment of specific defects, such as vertical bone loss, furcation involvement,[168] or around implants. If regenerative therapy is an option for vertical defects, it is the preferred treatment. Additionally, sufficient evidence does not exist to recommend the use of local delivery in specific probing depths, actively progressive sites, or specific periodontal procedures.

Future Studies

Many questions remain regarding the role of local delivery of antimicrobial agents in periodontal therapy. One of the most important is the long-term sequelae of these agents. There is limited information on the long-term outcome in terms of both clinical parameters and microbial resistance. Future studies should also address the potential of local delivery to reduce the need for periodontal surgery. Studies should also better define the role of locally delivered antimicrobial agents as adjuncts in specific periodontal procedures, as well as in treating different periodontal diseases, different lesions, and inflammation surrounding implants.

The benefits of specific local delivery agents used in combination, sequentially, or with systemic antibiotics also require further exploration. Also needed are studies evaluating their effectiveness in eradicating or suppressing potential pathogens, as well as beneficial species, in a biofilm environment.

Conclusions

Local antimicrobial delivery in the treatment of periodontal disease has a defined but limited usefulness. Meanwhile, the efficacy of traditional mechanical therapy targeted toward reduction of the plaque mass remains unquestioned. There is also substantial evidence in support of the use of systemic antimicrobial agents for specific pathogen infections and in certain forms of periodontitis. Clinicians must ask themselves if local delivery provides a benefit beyond currently accepted treatment modalities. Patients with generalized deep probing depths or vertical defects may be more appropriately treated with surgical therapy that may include regeneration.

The benefits of local delivery of antimicrobial agents and other medicaments are appealing, and future research should provide more information regarding the nature of the defects and the types of disease where it is indicated. While the advent of local delivery has not resulted in a treatment panacea, it has provided an additional mode of

therapy, primarily in the management of chronic periodontitis patients. Continued research will result in more clearly defined uses for these agents—for example, in the management of aggressive periodontitis and peri-implant disease. Ultimately, these agents may also have important treatment ramifications if the association of periodontal disease with systemic diseases holds true.

References

1. Slots J. Subgingival microflora in periodontal disease. J Clin Periodontol 1979;6(5):351–382.
2. Hamp SE. On the development and prevention of periodontal disease in the beagle dog [thesis]. Gothenburg: University of Gothenburg, 1973.
3. Lindhe J, Nyman S. The effect of plaque control and surgical pocket elimination on the establishment and maintenance of periodontal health. A longitudinal study of periodontal therapy in cases of advanced disease. J Clin Periodontol 1975;2(2):67–79.
4. Ramfjord SP, Knowles JW, Nissle RR, et al. Longitudinal study of periodontal therapy. J Periodontol 1973;44:66–77.
5. Rosling B, Nyman S, Lindhe J. The effect of systematic plaque control on bony regeneration in infrabony pockets. J Clin Periodontol 1976;3:38–53.
6. Rosling B, Nyman S, Lindhe J, Jern B. The healing potential of the periodontal tissues following different techniques of periodontal surgery in plaque-free dentitions. A 2-year clinical study. J Clin Periodontol 1976;3:233–250.
7. Lindhe J, Westfelt E, Nyman S, et al. Healing following surgical/non-surgical treatment of periodontal disease. A clinical study. J Clin Periodontol 1982;9:115–128.
8. Lövdal A, Arno A, Schei O, Waerhaug J. Combined effect of subgingival scaling and controlled oral hygiene on the incidence of gingivitis. Acta Odontol Scand 1961;19:537–555.
9. Suomi JD, Greene JC, Vermillion JR, et al. The effect of controlled oral hygiene procedures on the progression of periodontal disease in adults: Results after third and final year. J Periodontol 1971;42:152–160.
10. Waerhaug J. Plaque control in the treatment of juvenile periodontitis. J Clin Periodontol 1977;4:29–40.
11. Lindhe J, Socransky SS, Nyman S, et al. "Critical probing depths" in periodontal therapy. J Clin Periodontol 1982;9(4):323–336.
12. Löe H, Theilade E, Jensen SB. Experimental gingivitis in man. J Periodontol 1965;36:177–187.
13. Nyman S, Rosling B, Lindhe J. Effect of professional tooth cleaning on healing after periodontal surgery. J Clin Periodontol 1975;2:80–86.
14. Axelsson P, Lindhe J. Effect of controlled oral hygiene procedures on caries and periodontal disease in adults. J Clin Periodontol 1978;5:133–151.
15. Rosling B, Slots J, Webber RL, et al. Microbiological and clinical effects of topical subgingival antimicrobial treatment on human periodontal disease. J Clin Periodontol 1983;10:487–514.
16. Tagge DL, O'Leary TJ, El-Kafrawy AH. The clinical and histological response of periodontal pockets to root planing and oral hygiene. J Periodontol 1975;46:527–533.
17. Helldén LB, Listgarten MA, Lindhe J. The effect of tetracycline and/or scaling on human periodontal disease. J Clin Periodontol 1979;6:222–230.

18. Waerhaug J. Healing of the dento-epithelial junction following subgingival plaque control. II: As observed on extracted teeth. J Periodontol 1978;49:119–134.

19. Pihlström BL, McHugh RB, Oliphant TH, Ortiz-Campos C. Comparison of surgical and nonsurgical treatment of periodontal disease. A review of current studies and additional results after 6-1/2 years. J Clin Periodontol 1983;10:524–541.

20. Stambaugh RV, Dragoo M, Smith DM, Carasal L. The limits of subgingival scaling. Int J Periodontics Restorative Dent 1981;1(5):30–41.

21. Knowles J, Burgett F, Nissle R, et al. Results of periodontal treatment related to pocket depth and attachment level. Eight years. J Periodontol 1979;50:225–233.

22. Lindhe J, Westfelt E, Nyman S, et al. Long-term effect of surgical/non-surgical treatment of periodontal disease. J Clin Periodontol 1984;11:448–458.

23. Ramfjord SP, Knowles JW, Morrison EC, et al. Results of periodontal therapy related to tooth type. J Periodontol 1980;51:270–273.

24. Badersten A, Nilvéus R, Egelberg J. Effects of nonsurgical periodontal therapy. II. Severely advanced periodontitis. J Clin Periodontol 1984;11:63–76.

25. Badersten A, Nilvéus R, Egelberg J. Effect of nonsurgical periodontal therapy. III. Single versus repeated instrumentation. J Clin Periodontol 1984;11:114–124.

26. Badersten A, Nilvéus R, Egelberg J. Effect of nonsurgical periodontal therapy. I. Moderately advanced periodontitis. J Clin Periodontol 1981;8:57–72.

27. Guest GF, Cottone JA. Personal protection: The first line of defense. Tex Dent J 1987;104(9):16–18.

28. Rabbani GM, Ash MM Jr, Caffessee RG. The effectiveness of subgingival scaling and root planing in calculus removal. J Periodontol 1981;52:119–123.

29. Gher ME, Vernino AR. Root morphology: Clinical significance in pathogenesis and treatment of periodontal disease. J Am Dent Assoc 1980;101:627–633.

30. Bower RC. Furcation morphology relative to periodontal treatment. Furcation root surface anatomy. J Periodontol 1979;50:366–374.

31. American Academy of Periodontology. In: Nevins M, Becker W, Kornman K (eds). Proceedings of the World Workshop in Clinical Periodontics, July 23–27, 1989. Chicago: American Academy of Periodontology, 1989:II-1–II-20.

32. Walsh TF, Waite IM. A comparison of postsurgical healing following debridement by ultrasonic or hand instruments. J Periodontol 1978;49:201–205.

33. Ciancio SG, Genco RJ, Schallhorn RG, Goodsen JM. Non-surgical antibacterial approaches to periodontal treatment. J Am Dent Assoc 1988;116:22–32.

34. Holbrook TE, Low SB. Power-driven scaling and polishing instruments. In: Hardin J (ed). Clark's Clinical Dentistry. Philadelphia: JB Lippincott, 1989:1–24.

35. Leon LE, Vogel RI. A comparison of the effectiveness of hand scaling and ultrasonic debridement in furcations as evaluated by differential dark-field microscopy. J Periodontol 1987;58:86–94.

36. Jones WA, O'Leary TJ. The effectiveness of in vivo root planing in removing bacterial endotoxin from the roots of periodontally involved teeth. J Periodontol 1978;49:337–342.

37. Echeverria JJ, Caffesse RG. Effects of gingival curettage when performed one month after root instrumentation. A biometric evaluation. J Clin Periodontol 1983;10:277–286.

38. Ramfjord S, Caffesse R, Morrison E, et al. Four modalities of periodontal treatment compared over five years. J Periodontal Res 1987;22:222–223.

39. Morrison EC, Ramfjord SP, Hill RW. Short-term effects of initial, nonsurgical periodontal treatment (hygienic phase). J Clin Periodontol 1980;7:199–211.

40. Genco RJ. Antibiotics in the treatment of human periodontal diseases. J Periodontol 1981;52:545–558.

41. Goodson JM, Haffajee A, Socransky SS. Periodontal therapy by local delivery of tetracycline. J Clin Periodontol 1979;6:83–92.

42. Lindhe J, Heijl L, Goodson JM, Socransky SS. Local tetracycline delivery using hollow fiber devices in periodontal therapy. J Clin Periodontol 1979;6:141–149.

43. Hartzell TB. The practical surgery of the root surface in pyorrhea. Dental Cosmos 1911;53:513–521.

44. Black GV. A Work on Special Dental Pathology, ed 1. Chicago: Medico-Dental, 1915.

45. Waerhaug J, Arno A, Lövdal A. Dimension of instruments for removal of subgingival calculus. J Periodontol 1954;25:281–286.

46. Hughes TP, Caffesse RG. Gingival changes following scaling, root planing and oral hygiene. A biometric evaluation. J Periodontol 1978;49:245–252.

47. Pihlström B, Ortiz-Campos C, McHugh R. A randomized four-year study of periodontal therapy. J Periodontol 1981;52:227–242.

48. Listgarten MA, Lindhe J, Helldén L. Effect of tetracycline and/or scaling on human periodontal disease. Clinical, microbiological, and histological observations. J Clin Periodontol 1978;5:246–271.

49. Slots J, Mashimo P, Levine MJ, Genco RJ. Periodontal therapy in humans. I. Microbiological and clinical effects of a single course of periodontal scaling and root planing and of adjunctive tetracycline therapy. J Periodontol 1979;50:495–509.

50. Loesche WJ, Syed SA, Morrison EC, et al. Treatment of periodontal infections due to anaerobic bacteria with short-term treatment with metronidazole. J Clin Periodontol 1981;8:29–44.

51. Lindhe J, Liljenberg B, Adielson B, Borjesson I. The effect of metronidazole therapy on human periodontal disease. J Periodontal Res 1982;17:534–536.

52. Davies RM, Jensen SB, Schiott CR, Löe H. The effect of topical application of chlorhexidine on the bacterial colonization of the teeth and gingiva. J Periodontal Res 1970;5:96–101.

53. Löe H, Schiott C. The effect of suppression of the oral microflora upon the development of dental plaque and gingivitis. In: McHugh WD (ed). Dental Plaque. Edinburgh: E & S Livingstone, 1970.

54. Löe H, Schiott CR. The effect of mouth rinses and topical application of chlorhexidine on the development of dental plaque and gingivitis in man. J Periodontal Res 1970;5:79–83.

55. Löe H, Mandell M, Derry A, Schiott CR. The effect of mouth rinses and topical application of chlorhexidine on calculus formation in man. J Periodontol 1971;6:312–314.

56. Löe H, Schiott CR, Glavind L, Karring T. Two years oral use of chlorhexidine in man. I. General design and clinical effects. J Periodontal Res 1976;11:135–144.

57. Flötra L, Gjermo P, Rölla G, Waerhaug J. A 4-month study on the effect of chlorhexidine mouth washes on 50 soldiers. Scand J Dent Res 1972;80:10–17.

58. Cumming BR, Löe H. Optimal dosage and method of delivering chlorhexidine solutions for the inhibition of dental plaque. J Periodontal Res 1973;8:57–62.

59. Soh LL, Newman HN, Strahan JD. Effects of subgingival chlorhexidine irrigation on periodontal inflammation. J Clin Periodontol 1982;9:66–74.

60. Garrett JS. Effects of nonsurgical periodontal therapy on periodontitis in humans: A review. J Clin Periodontol 1983;10:515–523.

61. Mazza JE, Newman MG, Sims TN. Clinical and antimicrobial effect of stannous fluoride on periodontitis. J Clin Periodontol 1981;8:203–212.

62. Wennström J, Lindhe J. Effect of hydrogen peroxide on developing plaque and gingivitis in man. J Clin Periodontol 1970;6:115–130.

63. Talbot ES. The treatment of interstitial gingivitis and pyorrhea alveolaris. Dent Cosmos 1915;57:485–491.

64. MacAlpine R, Magnusson I, Kiger R, et al. Antimicrobial irrigation of deep pockets to supplement nonsurgical periodontal therapy. J Clin Periodontol 1983;10:568–575.

65. Davies BD, Dulbecco R, Eisen HN, Ginsberg HS. Microbiology, ed 3. New York: Harper & Row, 1980.

66. Kepic TJ, O'Leary TJ, Kafrawy AH. Total calculus removal: An attainable objective? J Periodontol 1990;61:16–20.

67. Robertson PB. The residual calculus paradox. J Periodontol 1990;61:65–66.

68. Caffesse RG, Sweeney PL, Smith BA. Scaling and root planing with and without periodontal flap surgery. J Clin Periodontol 1986;13:205–210.

69. Bower RC. Furcation morphology relative to periodontal treatment. Furcation root entrance architecture. J Periodontol 1979;50:23–27.

70. Bower RC. Furcation morphology relative to periodontal treatment. Furcation root surface anatomy. J Periodontol 1979;50:366–374.

71. Register A, Burdick F. Accelerated reattachment with cementogenesis to dentin, demineralized in situ. I. Optimum range. J Periodontol 1975;46:646–655.

72. Register A, Burdick F. Accelerated reattachment with cementogenesis to dentin, demineralized in situ. II. Defect repair. J Periodontol 1976;47:497–505.

73. Garrett J, Crigger M, Efelberg J. Effects of citric acid on diseased root surfaces. J Periodontal Res 1978;13:155–163.

74. Terranova V, Franzetti LC, Hic S, et al. A biochemical approach to periodontal regeneration: Tetracycline treatment of dentin promoting fibroblast adhesion and growth. J Periodontal Res 1986;21:330–337.

75. Saglie F, Carranza FA Jr, Newman MG, et al. Identification of tissue-invading bacteria in human periodontal disease. J Periodontal Res 1982;17:452–455.

76. Kalkwarf KL, Loughlin DM, Barrington EP. Moderate chronic adult periodontitis. In: Wilson TG Jr, Kornman KN, Newman MG (eds). Advances in Periodontics. Chicago: Quintessence, 1992:143–179.

77. Gargiulo WW, Wentz FM, Orban B. Dimensions of the dentogingival junction in humans. J Periodontol 1961;32:261–267.

78. Vacek J, Gher ME, Assad DA, et al. The dimensions of the human dentogingival junction. Int J Periodontics Restorative Dent 1994;14:155–165.

79. Maynard JG, Wilson RD. Physiologic dimensions of the periodontium significant to the restorative dentist. J Periodontol 1979;50:170–177.

80. Wilson RD, Maynard JG. Intracrevicular restorative dentistry. Int J Periodontics Restorative Dent 1981;1:34–49.

81. Kois JC. The restorative-periodontal interface: Biologic paramaters. Periodontol 2000 1996;11:29–38.

82. Kois JC. New paradigms for anterior tooth preparations: Rationale and technique. Contemp Esthet Dent 1996;2:1–9.

83. Kois JC. Altering gingival levels: The restorative connection. Part 1. Biological variables. J Esthet Dent 1994;6:3–9.

84. Spear F. Lecture at 1999 Annual Meeting of the American Academy of Periodontology. San Antonio, Texas.

85. Libman W, Nicholls J. Load fatigue of teeth restored with cast posts and cores and complete crowns. Int J Prosthodont 1995;8:155–161.

86. Barkhordar R, Tadke R, Abbasi J. Effect of metal collars on resistance of endodontically treated teeth to root fracture. J Prosthetic Dent 1989;61:676–678.

87. Wagenberg BD. Surgical tooth lengthening: Biological variables and esthetic concerns. J Esthet Dent 1998;10:30–36.

88. Tarnow DP, Magner AW, Fletcher P. The effect of the distance from the contact point to the crest of bone on the presence or absence of the interproximal dental papilla. J Periodontol 1992;63:995–996.

89. Ingber JS. Forced eruption. Part II. A method of treating nonrestorable teeth—Periodontal and restorative considerations. J Periodontol 1976;47:203–216.

90. Kozlovsky A, Tal H, Liebermann N. Forced eruption combined with gingival fiberotomy. A technique for clinical crown lengthening. J Clin Periodontol 1988;15:534–538.

91. Genco RJ. Current view of risk factors for periodontal diseases. J Periodontol 1996;67(suppl):1041–1049.

92. Grossi SG, Zambon JJ, Ho AW, et al. Assessment of risk for periodontal disease. I. Risk indicators for attachment loss. J Periodontol 1994;65:260–267.

93. Grossi SG, Genco RJ, Machtei EE, et al. Assessment of risk for periodontal disease. II. Risk indicators for alveolar bone loss. J Periodontol 1995;66:23–29.

94. Kornman KS, Crane A, Wang HY, et al. The interleukin-1 genotype as a severity factor in adult periodontal disease. J Clin Periodontol 1997;24:72–77.

95. Caton JG, Ciancio SG, Blieden TM, et al. Treatment with subantimicrobial dose doxycycline improves the efficacy of scaling and root planing in patients with adult periodontitis. J Periodontol 2000;71:521–532.

96. Howell TH, Williams RC. Nonsteroidal anti-inflammatory drugs as inhibitors of periodontal disease progression. Crit Rev Oral Biol Med 1993;4(2):177–196.

97. Theilade E. The non-specific theory in microbial etiology of inflammatory periodontal diseases. J Clin Periodontol 1986;13:905–911.

98. Moore WEC, Holdeman LV, Smibert RM, et al. Bacteriology of severe periodontitis in young adult humans. Infect Immun 1982;38:1137–1148.

99. Socransky SS. Microbiology of periodontal disease: Present status and future considerations. J Periodontol 1977;48:497–504.

100. Ranney RR, Debski BF, Tew JG. Pathogenesis of gingivitis and periodontal disease in children and young adults. Pediatr Dent 1981;3:89–100.

101. Slots J, Listgarten MA. *Bacteroides gingivalis, Bacteroides intermedius* and *Actinobacillus actinomycetemcomitans* in human periodontal diseases. J Clin Periodontol 1988;15:85–93.

102. Loesche WJ. Chemotherapy of dental plaque infections. Oral Sci Rev 1976;9:65–107.

103. Tanner ACR, Haffer C, Bratthall GT, et al. A study of the bacteria associated with advancing periodontitis in man. J Clin Periodontol 1979;6:278–307.

104. Slots J. Bacterial specificity in adult periodontitis. A summary of recent work. J Clin Periodontol 1986;13:912–917.

105. Rams TE, Listgarten MA, Slots J. Utility of 5 major putative periodontal pathogens and selected clinical parameters to predict periodontal breakdown in patients on maintenance care. J Clin Periodontol 1996;23:346–354.

106. Slots J, Emrich LJ, Genco RJ, Rosling BG. Relationship between some subgingival bacteria and periodontal pocket depth and gain or loss of periodontal attachment after treatment of adult periodontitis. J Clin Periodontol 1985;12:540–552.

107. Listgarten MA, Sullivan P, George C, et al. Comparative longitudinal study of 2 methods of scheduling maintenance visit: 4-year data. J Clin Periodontol 1989;16:105–115.

108. Ebersole JL, Taubman MA, Smith DJ, Haffajee AD. Effect of subgingival scaling on systemic antibody responses to oral microorganisms. Infect Immun 1985;48:534–539.

109. Axelsson P, Lindhe J. The significance of maintenance care in the treatment of periodontal disease. J Clin Periodontol 1981;8:281–294.

110. Mousques T, Listgarten MA, Phillips RW. Effect of scaling and root planing on the composition of human subgingival microflora. J Periodontal Res 1980;15:144–151.

111. Magnusson I, Lindhe J, Yoneyama T, Liljenberg B. Recolonization of a subgingival microbiota following scaling in deep pockets. J Clin Periodontol 1984;11:193–207.

112. Sbordone L, Ramaglia L, Gulletta E, Iacono V. Recolonization of the subgingival microflora after scaling and root planing in human periodontitis. J Periodontol 1990;61:579–584.

113. Sreenivasan PK, Meyer DH, Fives-Taylor PM. Requirements for invasion of epithelial cells by Actinobacillus actinomycetemcomitans. Infect Immun 1993;61:1239–1245.

114. Sandros J, Papapanou P, Dahlen G. Porphyromonas gingivalis invades oral epithelial cells in vitro. J Periodontal Res 1993;28:219–226.

115. Van Winkelhoff AJ, Rams TE, Slots J. Systemic antibiotic therapy in periodontics. Periodontol 2000 1996;10:45–78.

116. Van Winkelhoff AJ, Tijhof CJ, de Graaff J. Microbiological and clinical results of metronidazole plus amoxicillin therapy in Actinobacillus actinomycetemcomitans-associated periodontitis. J Periodontol 1992;63:52–57.

117. Kornman KS, Newman MG, Moore DJ, Singer RE. The influence of supragingival plaque control on clinical and microbial outcomes following the use of antibiotics for the treatment of periodontitis. J Periodontol 1994;65:848–854.

118. Loesche W, Giordano J, Soechren S, et al. Nonsurgical treatment of patients with periodontal disease. Oral Surg Oral Med Oral Pathol 1996;2:959–960.

119. Gordon JM, Walker CB, Lamster I, et al. Evaluation of clindamycin hydrochloride in refractory periodontitis: 12 month results. J Periodontol 1985;56(suppl):75–80.

120. Mandell R, Tripodi L, Savitt E, et al. The effect of treatment on Actinobacillus actinomycetemcomitans in localized juvenile periodontitis. J Periodontol 1986;57:94–97.

121. Riep B, Purucker P, Bernimoulin J-P. Repeated local metronidazole-therapy as adjunct to scaling and root planing in maintenance patients. J Clin Periodontol 1999;26:710–715.

122. Goodson JM, Tanner A. Antibiotic resistance of the subgingival microbiota following local tetracycline therapy. Oral Microbiol Immunol 1992;7:113–117.

123. Larsen T. Occurrence of doxycycline resistant bacteria in the oral cavity after local administration of doxycycline in patients with periodontal disease. Scand J Infect Dis 1991;23:89–95.

124. Preus HR, Lassen J, Aass AM, Ciancio SG. Bacterial resistance following subgingival and systemic administration of minocycline. J Clin Periodontol 1995;22:380–384.

125. Pedrazzoli V, Killian M, Karring T, et al. Comparative clinical and microbiological effects of topical subgingival application of metronidazole 25% dental gel and scaling in the treatment of adult periodontitis. J Clin Periodontol 1992;19:715–722.

126. Walker C. The acquisition of antibiotic resistance in the periodontal microflora. Periodontol 2000 1996;10:79–88.

127. Larsen T, Fiehn NE. Development of resistance to metronidazole and minocycline in vitro. J Clin Periodontol 1997;24:254–259.

128. Langer P, Peppas N. Present and future applications of biomaterials in controlled drug delivery systems. Biomaterials 1981;2:201–214.

129. Langer R. New methods of drug delivery. Science 1990;249:1527–1533.

130. Goodson JM. Pharmacokinetic principles controlling efficacy of oral therapy. J Dent Res 1989;68:1625–1632.

131. Stolze K, Stellfeid M. Systemic absorption of metronidazole after application of a metronidazole 25% dental gel. J Clin Periodontol 1992;19(suppl):693–697.

132. Lacroix JM, Walker CB. Detection and incidence of the tetracycline resistant determinant tet(M) in the microflora associated with adult periodontitis. J Periodontol 1995;66:102–108.

133. Olsvik B, Hansen BE, Tenover FC, Olsen I. Tetracycline-resistant microorganisms recovered from patients with refractory disease. J Clin Periodontol 1995;22:391–396.

134. Van Steenberghe D, Bercy P, Kohl J, et al. Subgingival minocycline hydrochloride ointment in moderate to severe chronic adult periodontitis: A randomized double blind, vehicle-controlled, multi-center study. J Periodontol 1993;64:637–644.

135. Timmerman M, van der Weljden G, van Steenbergen T, et al. Evaluation of the long-term efficacy and safety of locally applied minocycline in adult periodontitis patients. J Clin Periodontol 1996;23:707–716.

136. Williams RC, Paquette DW, Offenbacher S, et al. Treatment of periodontitis by local administration of minocycline microspheres: A controlled trial. J Periodontol 2001;72:1535–1544.

137. Greenstein G. The role of metronidazole in the treatment of periodontal diseases. J Periodontol 1993;64:1–15.

138. Stabbolz A, Kettering J, Aprecio R, et al. Retention of antimicrobial activity by human root surfaces after in situ subgingival irrigation with tetracycline HCl or chlorhexidene. J Periodontol 1993;64:137–141.

139. Greenstein G, Berman C, Jaffin R. Chlorhexidene: An adjunct to periodontal therapy. J Periodontol 1986;57:370–377.

140. Goodson J, Offenbacher S, Farr D, et al. Periodontal disease treatment by local drug delivery. J Periodontol 1985;56:265–272.

141. Goodson J, Cugini M, Kent R, et al. Multicenter evaluation of tetracycline fiber therapy: II. Clinical response. J Periodontal Res 1991;26:371–379.

142. Newman M, Kornman K, Doherty F. A 6-month multi-center evaluation of adjunctive tetracycline fiber therapy used in conjunction with scaling and root planing in maintenance patients: Clinical results. J Periodontol 1994;65:685–691.

143. Kinane DF, Radvar M. A 6-month comparison of 3 periodontal local antimicrobial therapies in persistent periodontal pockets. J Periodontol 1999;70:1–7.

144. Wilson TG, McGuire MK, Greenstein G, Nunn M. Tetracycline fibers plus scaling and root planing versus scaling and root planing alone: Similar results after 5 years. J Periodontol 1997;68:1029–1032.

145. Graca MA, Watts TLP, Wilson RE, Palmer RM. A randomized, controlled trial of a 2% minocycline gel as an adjunct to non-surgical periodontal treatment using a design with multiple matching criteria. J Clin Periodontol 1997;24:249–253.

146. Van Steenberghe D, Rosling B, Soder PO, et al. A 15-month evaluation of the effects of repeated subgingival minocycline in chronic adult periodontitis. J Periodontol 1999;70:657–667.

147. Garrett S, Johnson L, Drisko CH, et al. Two multicenter studies evaluating locally delivered doxycycline hyclate, placebo control, oral hygiene, and scaling and root planing in the treatment of periodontitis. J Periodontol 1999;70:490–503.

148. Garrett S, Adams, DF, Bogle G, et al. The effect of locally delivered controlled-release doxycycline or scaling and root planing on periodontal maintenance patients over 9 months. J Periodontol 2000;71:22–30.

149. Drisko CH. The use of locally delivered doxycycline in the treatment of periodontitis. Clinical results. J Clin Periodontol 1998;25:947–952.

150. Polson A, Garrett S, Stoller N, et al. Multi-center comparative evaluation of subgingivally delivered sanguinary and doxycycline in the treatment of periodontitis. II. Clinical results. J Periodontol 1997;68:119–126.

151. Rudhart A, Purucker P, Kage A, et al. Local metronidazole application in maintenance patients. Clinical and microbiological evaluation. J Periodontol 1998;69:1148–1154.

152. Stelzel M, Flores-de-Jacoby L. Topical metronidazole application compared with subgingival scaling. A clinical and microbiological study on recall patients. J Clin Periodontol 1996;23:24–29.

153. Stelzel M, Flores-de-Jacoby L. Topical metronidazole application in recall patients. Long-term results. J Clin Periodontol 1997;24:914–919.

154. Soskolne W, Heasman P, Stabholt A, et al. Sustained local delivery of chlorhexidene in the treatment of periodontitis: A multi-center study. J Periodontol 1997;68:32–38.

155. Jeffcoat M, Bray K, Ciancio S, et al. Adjunctive use of a subgingival controlled-release chlorhexidene chip reduces probing depths and improves attachment level compared with scaling and root planing alone. J Periodontol 1998;69:989–997.

156. Stabholz A, Shapira L, Mahler D, et al. Using the PerioChip in treating adult periodontitis: An interim report. Compend Contin Educ Dent 2000;21:325–328,330,332.

157. Needleman IG, Collins AM, Moles DR. Periodontal flap surgery with 25% metronidazole gel. (1). Clinical outcomes. J Clin Periodontol 2000;27:187–192.

158. Sander L, Frandsen EVG, Ambjerg D, et al. Effect of local metronidazole application on periodontal healing following guided tissue regeneration. Clinical findings. J Periodontol 1994;65:914–920.

159. Radvar M, Pourtaghi N, Kinane DE. Comparison of 3 periodontal local antibiotic therapies in persistent periodontal pockets. J Periodontol 1996;67:860–865.

160. Noyan O, Yilmaz S, Kuru B, et al. A clinical and microbiological evaluation of systemic and local metronidazole delivery in adult periodontitis patients. J Clin Periodontol 1997;24:158–165.

161. Greenstein G, Tonetti M. The role of controlled drug delivery for periodontitis. Position Paper. J Periodontol 2000;71:125–140.

162. Finkelman RD, Williams RC. Local delivery of chemotherapeutic agents in periodontal therapy: Has its time arrived? [discussion]. J Clin Periodontol 1998;25:978–979.

163. Greenstein G. Conceptualization vs. reality in the treatment of periodontal diseases. Compend Contin Educ Dent 1999;20:410–425.

164. Loesche WJ, Schmidt E, Smith A, et al. Effects of metronidazole on periodontal treatment needs. J Periodontol 1991;62:247–257.

165. Slots J, Rams TE. New views on periodontal microbiota in special patient categories. J Clin Periodontol 1991;18:411–420.

166. Schenkein HA, Van Dyke TE. Early-onset periodontitis: Systemic aspects of etiology and pathogenesis. Periodontol 2000 1994;1:7–25.

167. Special patient categories. Periodontol 2000 1994;6:1–124.

168. Tonetti M, Cortellini P, Carnevale G, et al. A controlled multicenter study of adjunctive use of tetracycline periodontal fibers in mandibular class II furcations with persistent bleeding. J Clin Periodontol 1998;25:737–745.

Treating Aggressive Forms of Periodontal Disease with Severe Bone Loss

Thomas G. Wilson, Jr, and Kenneth S. Kornman
- Defining Aggressive Periodontitis
- Collecting the Clinical and Radiographic Evidence
- Interpreting the Evidence
- Making a Clinical Diagnosis
- Determining Risk Factors for Disease Progression
- Determining the Prognosis
- Formulating a Treatment Plan
- Reevaluation and End Points in Therapy

James T. Mellonig and Michael A. Brunsvold
- Methods of Reconstruction of the Periodontium

There are the three basic clinical conditions of the periodontium: health, gingivitis, and periodontitis. These conditions may be seen separately or in combination. After reading this chapter, you should understand the clinical, microbiologic, and radiographic signs associated with aggressive periodontitis. You should also understand that the diseases in this category often do not respond to conventional periodontal therapy. The following sections review the knowledge needed to make a differential diagnosis and present an overview of treatment. Treatment for the individual diseases in this category is often difficult and unpredictable, so it is best handled by individuals with experience and formal advanced training in the field.

Defining Aggressive Periodontitis

The diagnosis of aggressive periodontitis is based on the observation that the patient's disease appears to be more severe or more progressive than one would expect given the level of bacterial challenge. The severity and pattern of periodontal destruction seen at the initial examination is, of course, the cumulative result of how well the patient has cleaned the teeth (ie, the bacterial challenge) and how well the patient's immunoinflammatory responses have protected against the bacterial challenge.

The vast majority of patients who brush their teeth once or twice each day and rarely use dental floss have early to localized moderate periodontitis by the age of 35. This level of disease results in spite of the robust protective immunoinflammatory responses that exist in most individuals. A person who has an excessive bacterial challenge or an altered immunoinflammatory response is likely to develop more severe disease. In some cases the altered immunoinflammatory response may allow severe destruction at an early age, even in the teenage years.

While *aggressive* refers to the patient's altered immunoinflammatory response, the term *severe* refers to the amount of destruction of the periodontal attachment apparatus. It generally means that at least one third of the periodontal support for a tooth has been destroyed. Severe disease may be seen with the following clinical presentations:

1. Generalized severe periodontal destruction in the primary dentition
2. Localized severe destruction limited to molars and incisors, with minimal to no destruction in other sites
3. Localized severe destruction at a few sites, with moderate disease affecting several other teeth
4. Generalized severe destruction in the permanent dentition

Generalized periodontal destruction in the primary dentition is very rare and is most commonly associated with a systemic defect such as neutrophil abnormalities or immune deficiencies (see chapter 14). This condition should be classified as a periodontal manifestation of a systemic disease. The management of such cases will not be considered in this text.

Localized severe destruction limited to molars and incisors with minimal to no destruction in other sites was previously classified as localized juvenile periodontitis or a form of early-onset periodontitis. Now classified as aggressive periodontitis, it has a prevalence of less than 1% and is seen first in the teenage years. Cases of localized aggressive periodontitis, in which destruction is limited to molars and incisors, often have deep vertical bone defects on the mesial surfaces of first molars and surprisingly low levels of supragingival plaque. This condition has different microbial patterns than does chronic disease in adults and is characterized by *Actinobacillus actinomycetemcomitans*, which may or may not be accompanied by *Porphyromonas gingivalis* (see chapter 5). This condition also has host defense characteristics that differ from both health and chronic periodontitis, including immunologic responses (see chapter 8), neutrophil responses (see chapter 14), and possibly gene variations involved in the immunoinflammatory responses (see chapter 11).

Localized aggressive periodontitis with severe bone loss is often not responsive to local mechanical therapy (ie, scaling and root planing) directed at reduction of bacterial accumulations on the teeth. This may be due to the pathogenic bacteria *A actinomycetemcomitans*, which attaches to and even invades the gingival tissues. The most effective therapies for such cases have been scaling and root planing combined with either antibiotics (such as combinations of metronidazole and amoxicillin) or surgery. When appropriate therapy is applied to localized aggressive cases with deep vertical defects, the healing response is often dramatic and may result in substantial regeneration. This chapter does not directly address the clinical management of localized severe destruction limited to molars and incisors, but the mechanical techniques needed are detailed in chapter 23.

Localized severe destruction at a few sites, with moderate disease affecting several other teeth, may result from one of two scenarios. The first is that the disease biology is consistent with chronic periodontitis with mild to moderate attachment loss, but the anatomy of a few sites leads to more severe localized destruction. The anatomic factors that can cause such a phenomenon include root fractures, root malformations or grooves, furcations that originate very close to the cementoenamel junction, among others. The second scenario is that the biology is consistent with generalized aggressive disease, but the case was identified before more generalized severe disease developed. Most cases of localized severe destruction at a few sites, with moderate disease affecting other teeth, are the result of the first scenario. It is therefore recommended that areas with moderate periodontitis be treated as described in chapter 23. Areas of severe bone loss will often respond (following initial therapy) to the surgical approaches described in that chapter. If the patient does not respond predictably to the therapy for chronic periodontitis, the therapist should consider reclassifying the disease as aggressive.

Generalized severe destruction in the permanent dentition is appropriately classified as aggressive periodontitis and is the primary focus of this chapter. Substantial data collected over many years support the concept that patients with severe generalized destruction are losing the host-bacteria battle more days than they are winning. Although such patients may be overtly healthy in terms of systemic disease, they most likely have subtle variations in host defense mechanisms that prevent adequate protection against the bacterial challenge. It is known that patients who smoke, are diabetic, have metabolic syndrome, or have certain common genetic variations, such as the proinflammatory interleukin 1 genotype, have altered host defense mechanisms and are at increased risk for severe disease and disease progression. The remainder of this chapter addresses the management of generalized aggressive periodontitis cases with severe bone loss.

Collecting the Clinical and Radiographic Evidence

P. A. Veazey presents to your office. His chief complaint is that his teeth "are getting loose." He was referred to a periodontist by his general practitioner.

He fills out a health history form and brings a complete set of right-angle and bitewing radiographs, which were obtained by his general practitioner.

In your initial interview with the patient, you find a well-nourished, well-oriented man who is 29 years old. He is a high school graduate who has a clerical job in a local munitions factory.

THE EVIDENCE

Health History

1. Medical
   - Mr Veazey's health history reveals nothing that would influence his oral health, except that he smokes an occasional cigarette and has a family history of diabetes mellitus.
2. Dental
   - The patient has only seen his practitioner every 6 months to have his teeth cleaned.
   - He is an intelligent person but has little understanding of dentistry.
   - He brushes his teeth twice daily and uses dental floss occasionally.
   - Both his parents experienced early tooth loss because of periodontal problems.
   - The patient reports that he grinds his teeth at night.

Extraoral Examination

1. The head and neck are inspected visually for asymmetries and abnormal features. Any deviations from normal are recorded.
   - ➤ No deviations from normal are found.
2. The temporomandibular joints are inspected by palpation during range-of-motion movements, and any noise or tenderness is recorded.
   - ➤ None is found in this patient.
3. The lips are examined and any abnormalities (including location and size) noted, since a large percentage of oral lesions are found here.
   - ➤ No abnormalities are found in this patient.

Intraoral Examination

1. Any discoloration (usually white, red, or black) of the oral mucosal tissues is recorded, including location and size.
   - ➤ None is found.
2. The tongue is grasped at the tip with cotton gauze and gently moved anteriorly to inspect the lateral borders, since this is the most frequent site for in-traoral neoplasms and changes associated with certain chronic conditions.
   - ➤ No abnormalities are found.

Risk Factors

1. Local
   - Bacteria are present and cannot be removed by the patient because of deepened probing sites.
   - Compliance with suggested oral hygiene and maintenance visits is average.
2. Systemic
   - The patient smokes.
   - He does not have diabetes mellitus but has a family history of the disease.
   - He is positive for the interleukin 1 genotype.

Clinical Examination

1. Dental (Figs 24-1a to 24-1d)
   - ➤ The patient has all of his teeth.
   - ➤ There are a number of mobile teeth.
   - ➤ The maxillary anterior teeth have drifted forward and become more crowded in the last few months, according to the patient.
2. Periodontal. The periodontal examination has the following positive findings (Fig 24-2):
   - ➤ Pocket probing depths range from 5 to 11 mm. Numerous pockets are 7 mm or deeper.
   - ➤ There are signs of gingival inflammation, including spontaneous bleeding, bleeding on probing, and suppuration.
   - ➤ There are no areas of gingival recession.

Radiographic Examination

The radiographic examination is normal except that there is severe bone loss around most of the remaining teeth (Fig 24-3). The loss is both horizontal and vertical (angular). The alveolar crest is more than 2 to 3 mm apical to the cementoenamel junction. The crown-to-root ratio is poor. There are widened periodontal ligament spaces around most of the teeth, and the laminae dura are absent in a number of areas. Calculus is not evident. In a number of areas, there is absence of bone in the furcae.

Interpreting the Evidence

The initial diagnosis of aggressive periodontitis will be the driving force behind the treatment of this patient. The following steps are important in making this diagnosis:

1. Make sure that the patient has no extraoral or intraoral problems that should be dealt with first.
2. Evaluate the local and systemic factors that might be contributing to the disease.
3. Review the patient's clinical signs and symptoms.
4. Review the patient's radiographic signs.

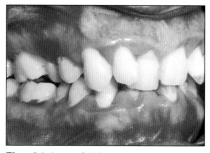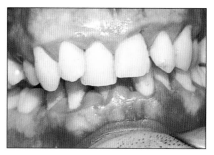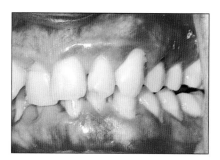

Figs 24-1a to 24-1c Patient's dental and periodontal condition at the initial presentation.

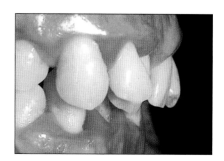

Fig 24-1d Patient's overbite/overjet in centric occlusion at the first visit.

Extraoral and Intraoral Problems

The patient does not exhibit any of these problems that might affect the outcome of therapy.

Systemic Condition

In Mr Veazey's case, three systemic factors should be taken into consideration. He has a family history of diabetes mellitus. He was screened for this disease, and the results were negative. The patient was counseled to stop smoking. This is especially important because he was found to be interleukin 1 (IL-1) positive, and individuals who smoke and who are positive for the IL-1 genotype have an increased probability of losing teeth as a result of periodontitis.

It should be noted that IL-1 genetic variations have been associated with more severe and more progressive periodontitis in adults (see chapter 11). Although studies indicate that IL-1 genetic variations are commonly found in aggressive periodontitis cases that previously would have been characterized as juvenile periodontitis, the variation associated with these cases is opposite the one associated with severe disease in adults. Adults with more severe disease have been found to have the less common variation, allele 2, which is generally classified as positive on the genetic test, whereas young patients with severe disease have been found to have the more common variation, allele 1.

Although the studies were well conducted, certain factors complicate the interpretation; for example, (1) most of the families or patients studied for aggressive periodontitis in juveniles were non-white, and (2) the clinical condition of aggressive periodontitis is very uncommon, yet the IL-1 gene variation that was implicated in the studies (allele 1) is found in the majority of the population.

In cases involving severe generalized periodontitis in the permanent dentition or localized severe destruction at a few sites with moderate disease affecting several other teeth, the IL-1 genetic variation may provide valuable information about the patient's risk for future disease progression. In cases of generalized severe periodontal destruction in the primary dentition or localized severe destruction limited to molars and incisors with minimal to no destruction in other sites, it is unclear how to interpret the IL-1 genetic variation.

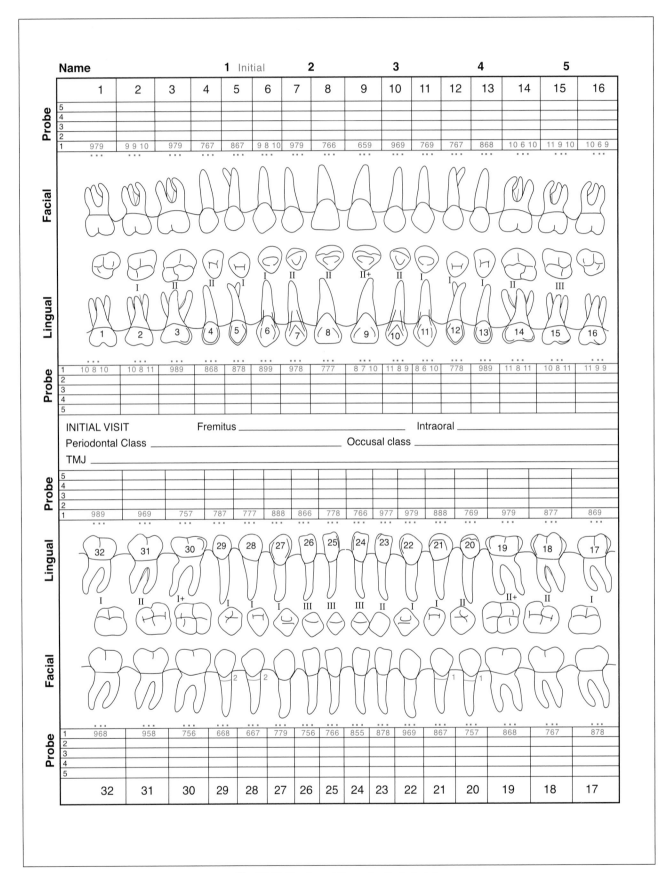

Fig 24-2 Charting at the patient's first visit.

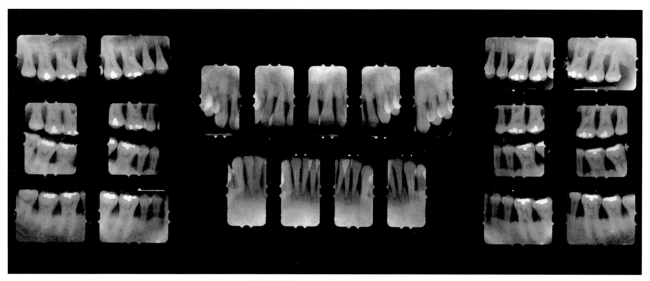

Fig 24-3 Original radiographs.

Clinical Signs and Symptoms

Periodontal Tissue Inflammation

➤ *Clinical signs of periodontal inflammation can be seen in aggressive forms of periodontal disease, but usually not to the degree seen in chronic periodontitis.*

Role of plaque. In the 1960s and 1970s, it was assumed that all inflammatory periodontal diseases were basically the same; the more plaque the patient had, the more disease that occurred. In the late 1970s and early 1980s, evidence began to accumulate that all patients did not respond the same to plaque accumulation and that severe bone loss occasionally occurred without clinically demonstrable plaque and calculus. Many of the patients with aggressive forms of periodontitis have minimal plaque levels. The low plaque levels are due to the different types of bacteria that are usually found in some of these diseases as compared with chronic periodontitis.

Patients with aggressive forms of inflammatory periodontal disease must have above-average compliance with suggested oral hygiene measures and suggested frequency of periodontal maintenance. Mr Veazey's oral hygiene measures, while adequate for some individuals, are not sufficient for patients in his disease category. He has scheduled regular cleanings when asked to do so by his practitioner (although the frequency of the cleanings should be increased to at least four times per year). In cases such as these, the therapist should consider the value of bacterial sampling and antibiotic specificity testing.

Bacterial changes. Chronic periodontitis results from plaque accumulations and the bacterial changes that accompany those accumulations. The primary problem in

aggressive forms of periodontitis appears to be an alteration in the normal inflammatory/immune processes. Some aggressive disease, notably that seen in teenagers, involves a defect in neutrophil function and also has a consistent bacterial pattern, with *Actinobacillus actinomycetemcomitans* dominating. Other forms of aggressive disease, including those that are refractory to conventional therapy, have more diverse inflammatory/immune alterations and a more diverse bacterial pattern. Although the patterns vary, the most frequent bacteria involved in aggressive forms of periodontitis are *A actinomycetemcomitans*, *Porphyromonas gingivalis*, and *Bacteroides forsythus*. An important goal in the treatment of these cases is to eliminate these bacterial species. Other species have also been reported in aggressive periodontitis, such as certain types of *Prevotella intermedia*, *Campylobacter rectus*, and *Eikenella corrodens*. The bacterial findings in refractory periodontitis are similar to those reported for some forms of aggressive periodontitis in adults. Some of these bacteria, such as *A actinomycetemcomitans, C rectus,* and *E corrodens*, if dominant in the plaque, would produce a clinical appearance of minimal plaque (see chapter 5).

Inflammatory changes. Periodontal lesions in patients with aggressive periodontitis appear similar to lesions in patients with chronic periodontitis, with a large tissue infiltrate of plasma cells, B lymphocytes, T lymphocytes, and macrophages. Bursts of active disease may occur frequently. Several studies have shown that in patients with chronic periodontitis and some forms of aggressive periodontitis, a decrease in the CD4 T-cell number occurs, leading to a decrease in the CD4-to-CD8 ratio (ratio of helper cells to suppressor cells) in gingival tissue (see chapter 9).

Immune findings. These pathological periodontal findings, which appear to be expressed in a subset of the general population, are manifested as rapid destructive lesions of the soft and hard tissues that are not always commensurate with local inciting factors and the level of inflammation. Minimal information is available concerning local and systemic immune responses in aggressive forms of periodontitis seen in prepubertal patients. In general, both the localized and generalized forms of this disease are associated with other medical conditions, which can be debilitating and life threatening. Frequently, decreases in neutrophil numbers and/or functions are intimately associated with these highly destructive diseases.

In contrast, localized aggressive periodontitis (formerly called *localized juvenile periodontitis*), which is seen in pubertal patients, has been extensively investigated and in some cases used as the paradigm for delineating host-parasite interactions in periodontal disease. As the categorization implies, this disease is manifested by severe, localized soft and hard tissue destruction, frequently in juxtaposition with extremely healthy sites. The localized diseased tissues demonstrate an increase in $T_{C/S}$ cells, potentially contributing to dysregulation of protective immune responses. These lesions have a significant increase in plasma cells predominated by immunoglobulin G and immunoglobulin A (IgG and IgA), with some evidence for an altered distribution of IgG subclasses when compared with the systemic cell population. A peculiar finding is that many of these patients exhibit minimal levels of local inciting factors and low levels of clinical inflammation accompanying severe destructive disease. Inflammatory mediators and cytokines are increased compared with healthy sites, but these levels may be more coincident with the extent of inflammation in the tissues. Levels of antibody to gingival crevicular fluid are often significantly increased in diseased sites; the most common is antibody reactive with *A actinomycetemcomitans*, the suspected pathogen in this disease. The local antibody elevations are often accompanied by colonization with the microorganism and appear to account for the local activation of both the alternative and classic complement pathways.

Systemic manifestations of this disease are noted by increases in circulating cytokines and stress proteins. Most pathognomonic of this disease is the high frequency of decreased neutrophil functions. Whether these alterations are genetically determined and contribute as a direct cause of the disease, or whether they reflect negative host-parasite interactions subjugating the neutrophil functions and provide a secondary susceptibility, remains to be determined.

In addition, circulating T cells may exhibit an increased sensitization to plaque antigens. Accompanying the characteristic *A actinomycetemcomitans* infection is a uniformly reported prevalence of elevated levels of serum antibody to this microorganism. The pathogen and antibody response are intimately associated and change with disease and treatment.

Generalized aggressive periodontitis may be seen in patients from the late teens through the mid-30s. This category contains a more heterogeneous group of diseases that included conditions formerly termed *rapidly progressive periodontitis* and *generalized juvenile periodontitis*. Many of the local and systemic immune characteristics of patients are virtually identical to those noted in younger subjects. These include altered neutrophil functions, elevations in gingival crevicular fluid mediators and cytokines and antibody to *A actinomycetemcomitans*, and systemic inflammatory and immune responses to this microorganism. Thus, these patients may have a decreased ability to manage the *A actinomycetemcomitans* infection, which progresses from a localized to a generalized disease. Alternatively, they may have altered host responses that progress rapidly to generalized disease on colonization with this pathogen.

A second subset of patients appears to reflect a disease associated with *P gingivalis* colonization similar to chronic periodontitis. Generally, patients with this type of disease are less associated with neutrophil dysfunctions. The patients exhibit extensive local immune responses specific for *P gingivalis*, as well as elevations in systemic antibody levels. Interestingly, this serum antibody has been suggested to be of low function and appears to increase in its effectiveness following treatment of the patients.

Finally, there appears to be a subset of generalized aggressive periodontitis patients that may overlap a subset seen in patients with disease refractory to conventional therapy. These patients may lack detectable putative pathogens in their subgingival plaque while presenting with elevations in levels of local and systemic antibodies to a battery of these microorganisms. These individuals may show alterations in systemic cellular immune functions, acute-phase reactants, and immunoglobulins, and they frequently smoke. Thus, the concept has been proposed that this patient subset is characterized by a complex of immune dysfunctions that result in increased susceptibility to colonization and/or tissue destruction initiated by many of the periodontopathogens.

As mentioned previously, this subset includes those patients who are refractory to conventional therapy. The immunologic and clinical characterizations of this group remain ill defined, but the patients' immune capacities may be altered such that standard treatment meets with limited success. Future studies will be required to more clearly delineate what, if any, immune abnormalities alter the susceptibility of these patients (see chapter 8).

Probing Depths

➤ *The probing depths are greater than 3 mm.*

With inflammation in the area, the basal epithelial cells turn over more rapidly, preventing cell maturation and reducing the integrity of the epithelial attachment. In addition, the collagen fibers that make up the connective tissue attachment undergo some destruction. The net result is that with inflammation, the periodontal probe passes completely through the epithelial attachment and usually stops just apical to the most coronal part of the connective tissue attachment.

With increasing pressure on the periodontal probe, the apical penetration is increased. With minimal inflammation this may result in complete penetration of the epithelial attachment, but with greater inflammation an increase in pressure results in more apical penetration of connective tissue.

Connective tissues. The biochemical events occurring in the connective tissues of a patient with aggressive periodontal disease are similar to those occurring in mild periodontitis, except that the magnitude and frequency of the destructive phases will be greater. In addition, the issue of whether some overriding systemic problems may exist should be investigated. For example, many diseases and systemic conditions are associated with defects in either the connective tissue matrices, their resident cells, or both (eg, rheumatoid arthritis, diabetes mellitus, medication intake, and dermatologic conditions).

The mechanism of matrix destruction will be closely related to the inflammatory response to bacterial plaque. Periodontal pathogens, through a variety of mechanisms, may stimulate cytokine production by circulating mononuclear phagocytes. These cytokines may activate release of metalloproteinases, which can initiate matrix destruction. The release of reactive oxygen species will also contribute to matrix disruption. In some instances, the level of enzymes has been found to be increased in patients suffering from aggressive forms of periodontitis. This may be due to the pathological state of the disease in which more rapid destruction of the periodontal tissues is seen compared with milder forms of periodontitis. Furthermore, if the disease progresses in intermittent bursts of activity, patients with aggressive periodontal destruction may be more likely to exhibit active disease at any given sampling time.

Due to the severity of the tissue destruction, the integrity of the tissues is likely to be severely compromised, which will have significant ramifications for the ability of the tissues to resolve the damage. For example, the diffusion of nutrients and cellular metabolic products will be compromised in tissues damaged by aggressive tissue destruction, which will have a profound effect on the resident cells and tissue as a whole.

The principal mechanism of tissue destruction is derived from the host response rather than being a direct effect of bacterial enzymes. This, however, does not alter treatment, which should be aimed at reducing the causative factor of the destructive phase—in this case, a variety of bacteria in the dental plaque (see chapter 6).

Bone changes. In aggressive forms of periodontitis, bone features are similar to those in moderate chronic periodontitis. However, because of a more aggressive host immune response caused by the presence of bacteria with higher virulence and increased local factor production, bone loss is greatly accelerated. No new factors have been discovered to account for the aggressive nature of this disease. It appears that there is simply an increase in quantity of the factors produced, resulting in more rapid bone loss. For this reason, some of these cases may have good regenerative potential, if the bacterial factors are successfully controlled. If treatment includes a regenerative phase, bone formation can be enhanced by inhibiting bone resorption, resulting in the formation of additional bone (see chapter 6).

Periodontal pathology. There are no distinct histopathological features that distinguish aggressive forms of periodontitis from chronic forms. However, the frequent lack of pronounced clinical signs of inflammation seen in chronic periodontitis is based on less prominent vascular changes (see chapter 4).

Clinical Attachment Level

➤ *The free gingival margin is at, or slightly coronal to, the cementoenamel junction (CEJ).*

The relation of the margin of the gingival tissues to the CEJ is important in establishing a proper diagnosis. The location of the free gingival margin is taken into account in a measurement called the *clinical attachment level*, which is the sum measurements of gingival recession and probing depth. If the probing depth alone is used, then errors can be made in reading a chart. As an example, one should be more concerned about a probing depth of 3 mm with 9 mm of recession than the same probing depth with no recession. The first situation represents 9 mm of attachment loss, while the second situation represents no attachment loss.

Radiographic Signs

Radiographic findings in these diseases include generalized loss of crestal cortication with evidence of substantial horizontal or vertical (or both) bone loss. In one or more areas, there may be an absence of furcational bone associated with multirooted teeth. Vertical bony defects are typical and may extend apically, involving root apices. The associated laminae dura may be absent and the periodontal ligament spaces considerably widened.

Other Areas for Consideration

Aggressive forms of periodontitis differ widely in treatment needs and response to therapy. Most of these cases will benefit to some degree from advanced diagnostics. These diagnostics often include selecting specific antibiotics to be used in conjunction with conventional therapy. Therapy can include surgical or nonsurgical care. These cases, as a rule, benefit from frequent periodontal maintenance following active care.

Parafunctional habits such as tooth grinding or clenching can contribute to the patient's problems. Clinical experience has shown that patients who clench or grind their teeth have increased thermal sensitivity and may experience more tooth mobility than patients without these habits. Most patients who have these habits are not aware of them, and some will strongly deny the habits. Many times the stronger the denial, the more pronounced the habit. While it should be clearly understood that trauma from the occlusion does not cause attachment loss, it seems that this process can exacerbate the destruction of a periodontium that is already inflamed.

Making a Clinical Diagnosis

1. Does the patient have any extraoral or intraoral problems that should be dealt with first? *In Mr Veazey's case, none are evident.*
2. An overview of the periodontal diagnostic process
   a. Signs and symptoms
      (1) Was there inflammation? *Yes.*
      (2) Was there loss of clinical attachment and/or bone? *Yes.*
   b. Making a differential diagnosis
      (1) Is there periodontal health? *No. There are signs of inflammation and bone loss.*
      (2) Is this gingivitis? *Gingivitis is present, but since there has been attachment loss, gingivitis is not the most severe disease present.*
      (3) Is this periodontitis? *Yes, because there has been attachment loss and bone loss.*
      (4) What subgroup of periodontitis is this?
          (a) Is this chronic periodontitis? *No, because there is generalized severe bone loss seen on radiographs.*

(b) Is this aggressive periodontitis? *Yes, because the patient is under age 35, there is more than 50% bone loss seen on radiographs, and the number of local factors present (plaque and calculus) does not match the amount of bone destruction. These findings suggest that this patient's host response is not adequately controlling the bacterial challenge or the patient is having an excessive destructive response to the bacterial challenge.*

Determining Risk Factors for Disease Progression

Several factors, both local and systemic, can affect disease progression. Local factors include bacteria and any niches that protect them from daily disruption of the plaque by the patient, as well as the degree to which the patient complies with the dental therapist's suggestions. As previously discussed, if allowed to remain undisturbed, bacteria initiate and sustain an inflammatory reaction in the periodontal tissues; if untreated, this condition will lead to tooth loss in some patients. As bacterial plaque matures, it can allow colonization of more pathogenic organisms. Where probing depths are shallow (3 mm or less) and the patient disrupts the plaque with daily oral hygiene, the clinical signs of gingivitis (eg, bleeding on probing and color changes) can be reversed. Patients who make routine periodontal maintenance visits generally keep their teeth longer than those who do not. Unfortunately, many patients do not clean their teeth as suggested and do not schedule maintenance visits as often as asked. This lack of compliance is a major risk factor for disease progression.

Systemic risk factors for progression of gingivitis to periodontitis include smoking, diabetes mellitus, and a specific genetic change that predisposes the patient to attachment loss. Patients who smoke develop periodontal disease more rapidly, heal poorly, and lose teeth more rapidly compared with those who do not smoke (see chapter 12). Individuals with diabetes mellitus experience more tooth loss from periodontal disease than do those who do not have the disease (see chapter 13). In general, the less severe the diabetes and the better its control, the better the prognosis for the patient's periodontal problem. An anomaly in the genes responsible for one of the inflammatory mediators in periodontal disease (IL-1) results in increased levels of attachment loss and tooth loss compared with patients without the change (see chapter 11). In addition, patients who smoke and are also positive for the IL-1 genotype have a much greater risk of tooth loss than patients without this combination of factors.

Mr Veazey has the following risk factors:

Local risk factors
1. The patient has bacteria that are associated with disease, and there are physical barriers to disturbing those bacteria (probing depths greater than 3 mm).
2. The patient is not complying with recommendations for personal oral hygiene.

Systemic risk factors
1. The patient smokes.
2. The patient has a family history of diabetes mellitus but does not currently have the disease.
3. The patient is positive for the IL-1 genotype.

Determining the Prognosis

A patient's prognosis depends on the degree to which it is possible to eliminate or ameliorate the risk factors. This patient's family history of diabetes mellitus and the fact that he is positive for the IL-1 genotype cannot be altered. Smoking is a very difficult habit to break, and risk is multiplied when the smoker is IL-1 positive. In addition, the patient's oral hygiene is not being maintained at a level needed for an individual with an aggressive form of periodontitis. Therefore, his overall prognosis is guarded. A guarded prognosis does not mean that the patient should not receive therapy but merely that he should understand the risks and benefits before proceeding.

Formulating a Treatment Plan

Aggressive periodontal diseases are often more difficult to control than their chronic counterparts. The ideal goal is to eliminate these diseases. More realistically, one would like to convert aggressive disease to a chronic problem. The following treatment was proposed:

1. *Sophisticated monitoring and advanced diagnostic and decision-making techniques.* These cases are best managed by an experienced periodontal therapist. Due to the aggressive nature of these diseases and the potential lack of response to conventional periodontal therapy, substantial loss of clinical attachment can occur rapidly, so frequent monitoring is required.
2. *Initial therapy to control inflammatory periodontal disease, combined with antibiotics.*
    a. The patient, who was already brushing with adequate frequency, was encouraged to continue this habit but to add interproximal cleaning with dental floss and an interproximal brush and to have his efficacy in plaque removal checked periodically.
    b. Counseling and other appropriate therapy for cessation of smoking was given, and the patient initially stopped the habit.
    c. Closed subgingival scaling and root planing were performed using nonspecific antibiotics. Therapy for this patient started before antibiotic specificity testing for periodontal pathogenic bacteria was available, but today bacterial sampling and antibiotic specificity testing would be used. It took a total of 16 hours of closed subgingival scaling and root planing by the periodontist on multiple visits to achieve the desired result.
3. *Reevaluation of therapy 30 days later.*
    a. Since the tissues showed clinical signs of health, therapy went to step 4.
    b. If the soft tissues had not returned to health, then the following guidelines would be followed:
        (1) If the therapist failed to remove local factors, this problem should be rectified.
        (2) If the therapist and the patient did an adequate job of removing local factors, then the bacteria would once again be sampled and therapy repeated until the disease was under control or the teeth lost.
4. *Placing provisional restorations.* Nonemergency restorative dentistry was postponed until the clinical signs of inflammation of the periodontal tissues were controlled. In this case, posterior fixed provisional restorations were placed to serve as anchorage units for fixed orthodontic appliances. Individual provisional crowns were joined to provide the needed stability. This was necessary because of the extreme mobility of the patient's posterior teeth and the concern that the posterior teeth might drift forward as much as the anterior teeth were retracted.
5. *Orthodontics* (Figs 24-4 to 24-6). If teeth are moved in the presence of inflammation, increased bone loss can occur compared with cases where inflammation was controlled (see chapter 33). This may be a special problem in aggressive forms of periodontitis. Clinical signs of inflammation must be controlled before orthodontic therapy begins, and inflammation and trauma from the occlusion should be kept under control during tooth movement. In this case, inflammation was kept under control by improving the patient's oral hygiene and by using closed subgingival scaling and root planing every 2 weeks during orthodontic therapy. New provisional fixed partial dentures were placed following completion of orthodontic care to act as orthodontic retention.

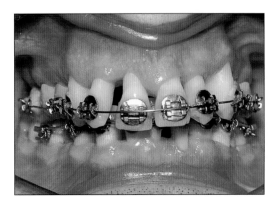

Figs 24-4a to 24-4c After resolution of clinical signs of inflammation and the placement of provisional fixed partial dentures in the posterior sextants, fixed orthodontic appliances were placed. The maxillary first premolars had been removed to allow space to retract the maxillary anterior teeth. (Orthodontics by Dr Gene Lambreth.)

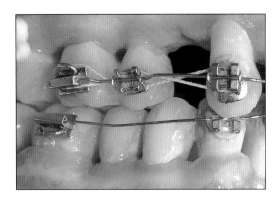

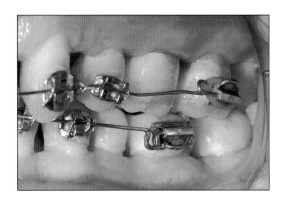

6. *Reevaluation of continued therapy.* At the conclusion of orthodontic treatment, a reevaluation of therapy was performed.
    a. If disease had remained active, it would have been treated until it was controlled or the teeth were lost.
    b. The clinical signs of the disease in this case were within normal limits following orthodontic therapy. Once orthodontic movement had been completed and the teeth stabilized, the occlusion was adjusted. In cases like this one, it is important that the therapist be sure that the disease process is arrested before final restorative dentistry is started. Therefore, the patient kept the provisional restorations for a year to give the therapist time to find and treat any disease recurrence. During this time, a hard acrylic maxillary habit device was constructed for the patient to wear at night to help ameliorate the damage caused by bruxism. The patient was placed on periodontal maintenance and seen every 2 months.
7. *Fixed restorative dentistry* (Figs 24-7a to 24-7c). Final restorative dentistry was performed approximately 1 year later.
8. *Reevaluation of active therapy.* At the conclusion of all of the treatment described, a reevaluation of therapy was performed.
    a. If disease had remained, it would have been treated until it was controlled or the teeth were lost.

b. Since the disease processes were arrested clinically, the patient was placed back into periodontal maintenance. In this case there was an initial arrest of the clinical and radiographic signs of disease.
9. *Periodontal maintenance.* Patients with aggressive periodontitis often require more frequent periodontal maintenance than patients with chronic periodontitis, so initially this patient was seen every 2 months for periodontal maintenance. A reevaluation of therapy is part of every periodontal maintenance visit.
10. *Moving the patient between periodontal maintenance and active therapy.* This patient stayed stable periodontally for approximately 6 years. Shortly after this, the patient dropped out of suggested treatment and was seen periodically over the next few years. Seventeen years after the start of therapy, the patient returned for an examination. He had good oral hygiene but little or no professional care for the preceding 10 years, and he had resumed his tobacco habit. Bone levels had drastically eroded in both arches (Figs 24-8 to 24-10). In general, the better these patients clean their teeth and the better their compliance to suggested periodontal maintenance, the more stable their conditions remain. This patient began a downhill spiral soon after leaving professional care. This is typical of aggressive forms of periodontitis.

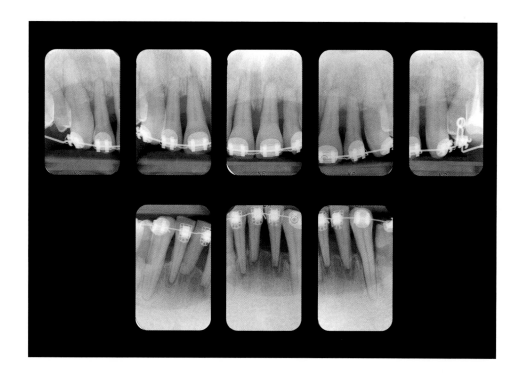

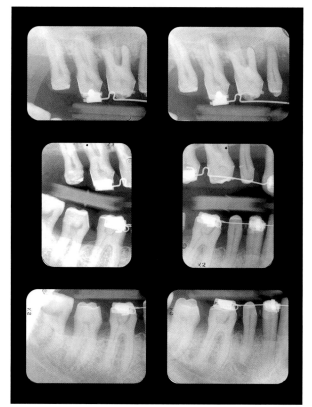

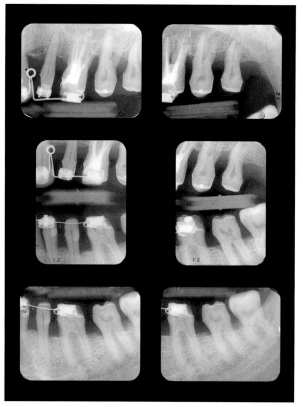

Fig 24-5 Radiographs taken during tooth movement.

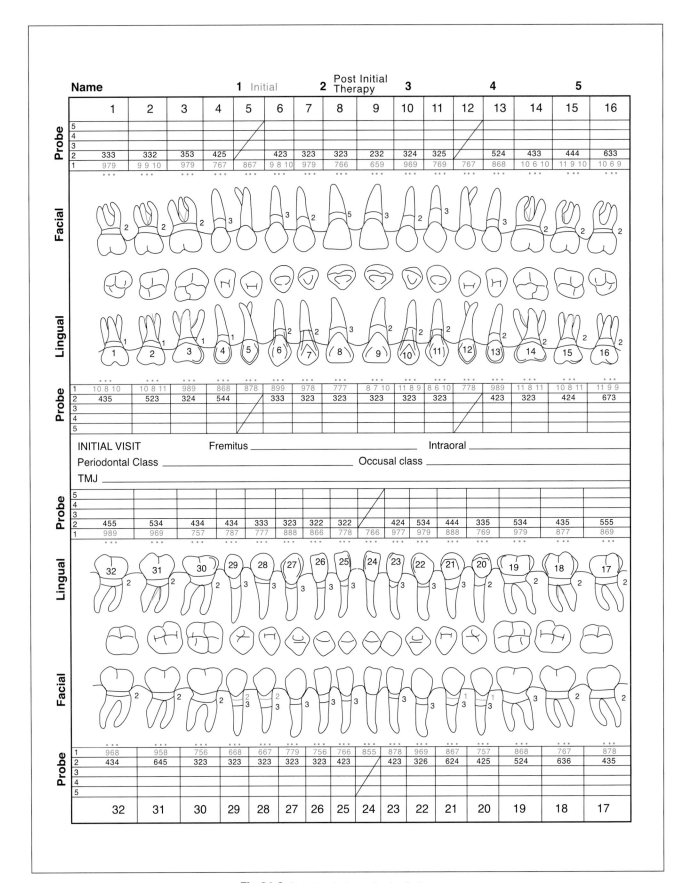

Fig 24-6 Charting during orthodontic therapy.

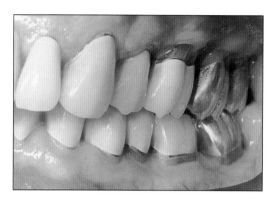

Figs 24-7a to 24-7c Final restorative dentistry was performed about 1 year after completion of orthodontic movement. (Restorative dentistry by Dr Frank Higginbottom.)

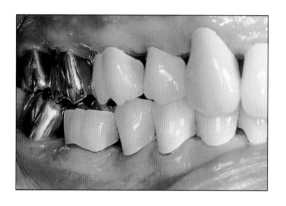

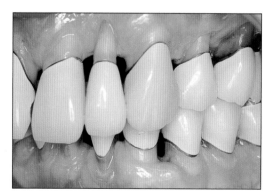

Figs 24-8a to 24-8c Patient 17 years after starting therapy. Notice the degree of gingival recession.

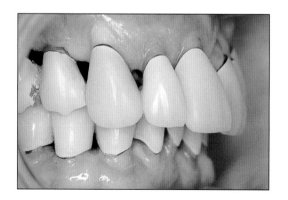

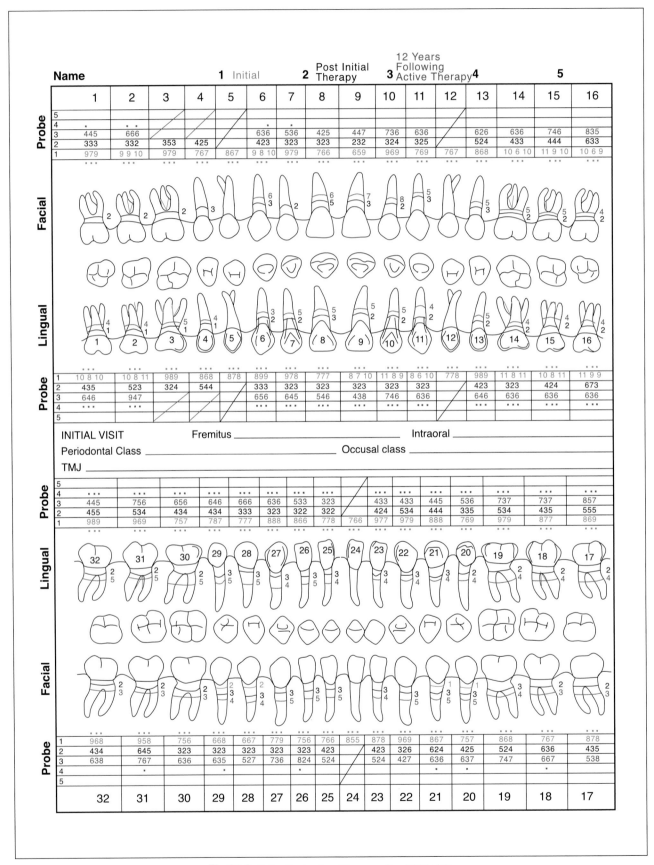

Fig 24-9 Patient's charting 17 years after initial visit.

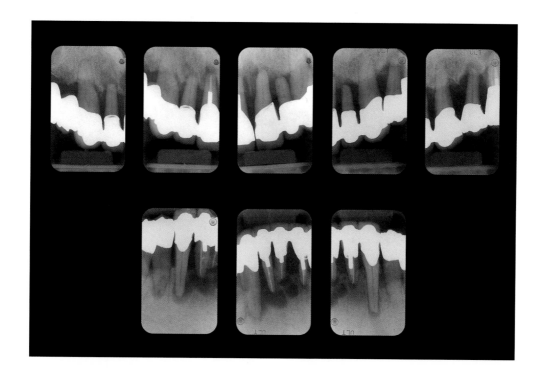

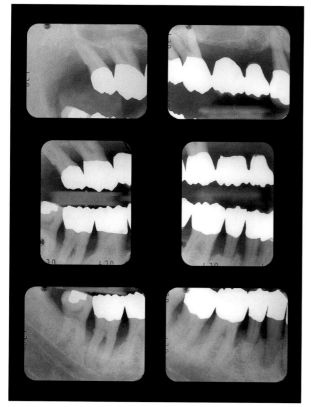

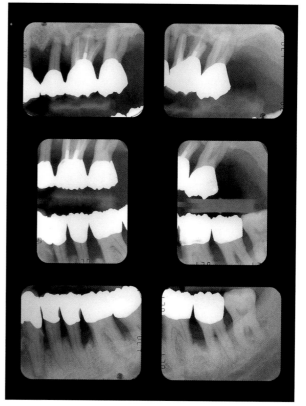

Fig 24-10 Radiographs 17 years after the start of therapy. Several endodontic lesions are present, and bone loss from periodontal disease has continued. Although initially stable, periodontal destruction continued after the patient's compliance decreased and his smoking habit returned.

Reevaluation and End Points in Therapy

Reevaluation is the comparison of current and previous dental and periodontal status. It involves comparing appropriate periodontal and dental parameters and recognizing and evaluating changes that have occurred from the previously established baseline.

Most periodontal diseases are arrestable, not curable. This means that the disease can recur at any time. Therefore, periodic reevaluation plays a key role in controlling these diseases.

The timing of reevaluation varies. It can be performed following initial therapy, following surgical therapy, or during periodontal maintenance. (For more specific information on the maintenance aspect of this process, see chapter 28). Reevaluation is used to judge the efficacy of therapy and to direct future treatment.

Classically, reevaluation of initial therapy occurs 30 to 45 days after active therapy has been completed, and it involves measuring probing depths and assessing inflammatory parameters (such as bleeding on probing) and occlusal factors. The information gathered directs future therapy.

Periodontal diseases occur and recur for many reasons, and acceptable outcomes (end points) vary from patient to patient, within individual patients over time, and from tooth surface to tooth surface within the same patient. Thus, generalizations on specific end points in therapy are difficult to make, at best. Nonetheless, it is still reasonable to have goals for therapy. The end points can be divided into ideal and realistic categories. Ideally, therapy would result in elimination of the disease and regeneration of lost tissues.

Ideal End Points in Therapy

Patient parameters
1. The patient is comfortable.
2. The patient has good oral function.
3. The patient is pleased with the esthetic results.
4. The patient has accepted responsibility for controlling the disease.

Disease (health) parameters
1. There is no inflammation.
2. There are no probing depths greater than 3 mm.
3. There is no tooth mobility.

Unfortunately, in reality ideal end points are often elusive, especially when the patient initially presents with periodontitis. Realistically, the patient and clinician must often accept less-than-ideal outcomes. Not all patients respond as one would wish, comply as they should, or have the time and economic resources to engage in the long-term therapy needed to reach their ideal end points. Given this, what are realistic end points?

Realistic End Points in Therapy

Patient parameters
1. The patient is comfortable.
2. The patient has acceptable oral function.
3. The patient accepts the esthetic results.
4. The patient has accepted as much responsibility as he or she can for disease control.

Disease parameters
1. There is no disease progression.
2. There are minimal clinical signs of inflammation.

Methods of Reconstruction of the Periodontium

If the generalized aggressive periodontitis appears to be stable at reevaluation, ie, there is minimal inflammation and no evidence of disease progression, it is reasonable to consider reconstruction of the periodontium.

Chronic periodontitis with severe attachment loss can be treated successfully with a variety of methods that are often combined in individual patients. These patients are identified by clinical and radiographic evidence of severe destruction of the periodontium. Common findings include severe horizontal or vertical bone loss, probing depths or attachment loss of 7 mm or greater, advanced tooth mobility, class II or III furcation involvement, and pathological migration of teeth. The selection of treatment methods depends on the therapy objective for each patient.

Specific methods include extraction, scaling and root planing, open flap debridement, osseous surgery, root amputation/hemisection, orthodontic therapy, bone and alloplastic grafts, and guided tissue regeneration (GTR) with and without bone grafts. Regeneration is often the objective of therapy in these patients because of the severity of bone loss. When the desired goal is reconstruction of the periodontium, bone grafting and/or GTR are the methods most often used.

Bone Grafts

Periodontal bone grafts have been used for many years to treat chronic periodontitis with severe attachment loss. However, only recently has the biologic basis of this modality become better understood. Advances in bone biology and wound-healing research have enabled clinicians to refine the technique of periodontal bone grafting to make it more predictable. Bone grafting can be very successful with careful patient selection.

Recent advances in bone grafting that have contributed to increased predictability include the following:

1. Improved procurement and availability of bone graft material
2. Improved methods to treat diseased root surfaces
3. Better understanding of the cell biology of wound healing
4. Application of the principles of GTR
5. The use of growth factors to enhance wound healing

The following are the objectives of periodontal bone grafting:

1. Probing-depth reduction
2. Clinical attachment gain
3. Bone fill of the osseous defect
4. Regeneration of new bone, cementum, and periodontal ligament

The first three objectives can be verified clinically, but the last objective requires histologic analysis. Histologic studies of bone grafting supply evidence that regeneration of new cementum, bone, and periodontal ligament (Fig 24-11) is possible on root surfaces previously exposed by periodontal disease.[1]

The two types of grafts most frequently used in periodontal therapy are autogenous grafts (patient's bone) and allografts (bone from another human being). Both types can be obtained either intraorally or extraorally. They may be cancellous bone, cortical bone, or combinations of these. There has been a recent increase in interest in using xenografts (bone from animals). Bone substitutes, usually in the form of hydroxyapatite, have also been used successfully to fill osseous defects, but not for regeneration of periodontal tissues.[2] They are used when autogenous bone is impractical and the patient objects to a bone allograft or xenograft.

Autogenous Bone Grafts

Intraoral autogenous bone grafts are obtained from several sites, including the periodontal surgical site, healing extraction sockets (Fig 24-12), edentulous ridges, tori, exostoses (Fig 24-13), and maxillary tuberosities. None of these sites has been shown superior to the others. The autogenous bone graft decreases cost to the patient, eliminates the possibility of graft rejection, and poses no danger of disease transfer. The amount of bone available from the donor sites is often limited, however. Autogenous

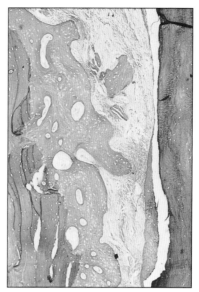

Fig 24-11 Human block section removed 6 months after bone grafting demonstrates regeneration of new bone, cementum, and periodontal ligament.

bone obtained with a bur and mixed with blood is termed *osseous coagulum*.[3] This material is used because its small particles are predictably resorbed and replaced by host bone. The mineralized fragments are also thought to induce bone formation. Intraoral bone obtained with a trephine, chisel, or rongeur is sometimes triturated into a particle size of 100 to 200 μm, called *bone blend* (Fig 24-14).[4] Autogenous bone from healing tooth sockets is usually obtained 8 to 12 weeks after extraction to allow newly forming bone to mature.[5] Bone is obtained from the socket with an instrument like the double-ended Molt curette or trephine, collected in a sterile dappen dish, and then placed in increments into the osseous defect.

Autogenous iliac cancellous bone and marrow is generally agreed to offer the greatest osteogenic potential for regeneration of new bone. All types of periodontal osseous defects have been successfully grafted with this material, including furcations and dehiscence-type lesions.[6] Postoperative root resorption has been reported, but this complication is eliminated by freezing before use.[7] Iliac bone has not received widespread use, however, because of the additional expense, time, and surgical procedure involved. These problems, plus the sometimes-limited quantity of intraoral bone, led to the development of allografts as a source of periodontal bone graft material.

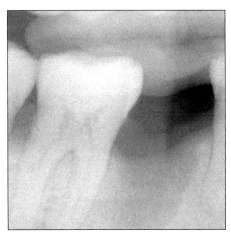

Fig 24-12 Healing extraction site, 3 months after extraction, is a suitable donor site for autogenous bone graft material.

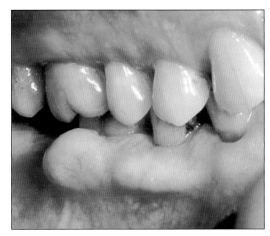

Fig 24-13 Bony exostoses can be used as donor sites for autogenous bone graft material.

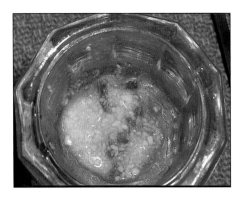

Fig 24-14 Intraoral bone triturated into small particle size is called *bone blend.*

Allografts

When insufficient intraoral autogenous bone is available and iliac grafting is impractical, allografts from tissue banks are often used. The bone is obtained under sterile conditions from fresh cadavers, usually within 24 hours of the death of the donor. Donor bone procurement by a tissue bank includes the following precautionary steps:

1. Elimination of donors from high-risk groups
2. Medical and social screening
3. Human immunodeficiency virus (HIV) antibody and antigen screening
4. Blood culture
5. Serology for hepatitis and syphilis
6. Special lymph node study
7. Histopathological studies of donor tissues
8. Follow-up studies of donor tissues

If these precautions are adhered to and bone is processed according to an established protocol, the risk of disease transfer is 1 in 8 million.[8]

The procedure for processing allografts includes the following:

1. The bone is cut into 0.5- to 5.0-mm particles and immersed in 100% ethanol for 1 hour. Within 1 minute of this treatment, viruses are inactivated.[9]
2. The bone is frozen, further decreasing the risk of disease transfer.
3. Bone is ground to a particle size of 250 to 800 μm. This particle size range was recently shown to be successful in humans.[10]
4. Bone is again immersed in ethanol.
5. The bone may or may not be demineralized.
6. The allograft is freeze-dried to permit long-term storage and reduce antigenicity. It is stored in sterile vacuum-packed bottles.

A study indicates that even if an HIV-infected donor could escape detection by the exclusionary precautions already described, processing the allograft with virucidal agents such as ethanol and hydrochloric acid makes the

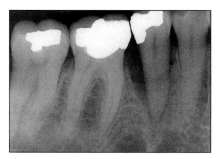

Fig 24-15a An osseous defect with a narrow angle formed between the bone and root surface. This defect has a good prognosis for bone grafting.

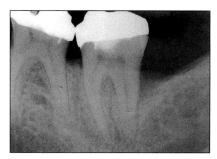

Fig 24-15a Osseous defect distal to the second molar with a wide angle formed between the bone and root surface. The prognosis for bone grafting is not as good as that in Fig 24-15a.

bone safe for human use.[11] An estimated 40,000 periodontal bone allografts are performed annually. From these, there have been no reported cases of disease transfer.

Recent evidence indicates that commercial decalcified freeze-dried bone differs in ability to induce new bone.[12] As the use of allografts in medicine and dentistry increases, the concern about disease transfer will also increase. It is important for practitioners and dental hygienists to understand allograft processing and risks so that patient questions can be answered. Also, the selection of a bone bank that conforms to the standards of the American Association of Tissue Banks[13] is crucial.

Xenografts

A bovine-derived bone xenograft (Bio-Oss, Osteohealth) has recently been used as a bone replacement graft. It is prepared from either cortical or cancellous bovine bone by chemical extraction of all organic material.[14] It is similar to human bone mineral in all physical properties and calcium-phosphorous ratio. In animal models, this xenograft is capable of becoming well vascularized and integrated with new host bone. In humans, Bio-Oss has been shown to be clinically safe, with a risk of disease transmission similar to that of currently available demineralized freeze-dried bone. An immune response does not occur following implantation of this material.[15]

When Bio-Oss was used in the treatment of human vertical osseous defects, a statistically significant gain in clinical attachment and reduction in probing depth were demonstrated when compared with nongraft controls.[16] Results were similar to those of demineralized freeze-

dried bone allograft. Early human histologic evaluations indicate that substantial amounts of new bone, cementum, and periodontal ligament can result from the use of this material.[17] Early findings indicate that Bio-Oss may become a very important graft material.

Success of Bone Grafts

What kind of success can be expected from the use of periodontal bone grafting? A common criterion for the success of bone grafts has been at least 50% fill of the defect.[18] This type of criteria indicates that few grafts are 100% successful. Clinical human studies report a range of 1- to 3-mm mean bone fill following the use of autogenous bone from various sources.[19,20] However, bone fill up to 8.5 mm has been documented.[19] Greater than 50% bone repair is seen on a predictable basis using autogenous bone[18] and allograft.[21]

Generally, two-walled osseous defects respond better than one-walled defects,[19] and deeper lesions respond better than shallow defects.[20] The width of the radiographic defect angle may also be important.[22,23] This angle is formed between the root surface and the defect wall; the wider the angle, the less the potential for repair or regeneration (Figs 24-15a and 24-15b). Optimal plaque control by the patient[24] and appropriate surgical management[25] are also considered critical factors in determining the success of these procedures. From this information, it is obvious that periodontal bone graft success depends a great deal on proper patient and site selection. Not all sites and patients with severe bone loss can be successfully treated with this modality.

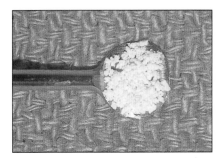

Fig 24-16 Porous hydroxyapatite is used as a graft material when autogenous bone is not available and the patient objects to an allograft. Bone formation has been demonstrated in the pores and on the surface of this material.

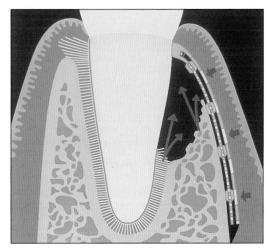

Fig 24-17 Diagram of barrier membrane in place. The purpose of the barrier is to exclude the gingival epithelium and connective tissue, to create a space for migrating and proliferating cells to reconstruct the tissues, and to protect the early clot.

Alloplasts: Bone Substitutes

Alloplasts are biocompatible materials, usually some form of hydroxyapatite, that are used to fill osseous defects. They are not used for regeneration of periodontal tissues. Tricalcium phosphate, nonporous hydroxyapatite, and porous hydroxyapatite are the materials used most often. Healing studies of tricalcium phosphate and nonporous hydroxyapatite indicate that these materials become encapsulated by connective tissue and act only as biocompatible space fillers.[26,27] They do not restore periodontal structures and, therefore, are usually selected when autogenous bone is not available and the patient objects to use of an allograft. The clinical improvement seen at sites treated with nonporous hydroxyapatite was stable in a 5-year longitudinal study.[2]

Porous hydroxyapatite (Fig 24-16) may result in the formation of osseous material in the pores and on the surface of the implants.[28] This cannot be considered regeneration, however, since healing adjacent to the root surface is mainly by a long junctional epithelium. Porous hydroxyapatite has shown favorable clinical results in class II furcation lesions[29] and, therefore, appears to be the best of the alloplastic materials.

Guided Tissue Regeneration

GTR has increased the predictability of regenerating bone destroyed by severe chronic periodontitis. It is not a panacea, however; much research is needed to answer many questions related to this modality. GTR refers to the procedures attempting to regenerate lost periodontal structures through differential tissue response.[30] Cells are manipulated to ensure that cell repopulation of a wound leads to regeneration. GTR alters wound healing by influencing cell proliferation and migration.

Three principles of wound healing form the basis for GTR. The first principle evolved from periodontal wound-healing studies that found that gingival epithelium migrates rapidly into most types of periodontal wounds. This form of healing of the gingival tissues to the tooth, called a *long junctional epithelium*, prevents regeneration. Most periodontal wounds heal in this manner. This form of healing is considered repair and not regeneration, because neither the original architecture nor the function of the periodontium is restored.

If the proliferation of the gingival epithelium and connective tissue, along with their migration into the early wound, can be delayed, reconstruction of the periodontal tissues can progress from pluripotential cells of the periodontal ligament and bone. This delay may be accomplished by placing a physical barrier between the root surface and flap (Fig 24-17). Both nonresorbable and resorbable membranes have been used successfully. Coronally positioned flaps have also been used to delay epithelial migration onto the root surface.[31]

The barrier membrane also creates a space between the mucoperiosteal flap and the periodontal defect, allowing migrating and proliferating cells to reconstruct the defect. This space maintenance is the basis for the second principle of GTR.

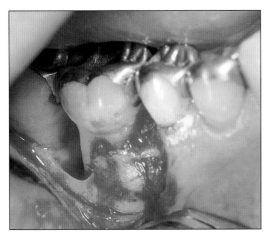

Fig 24-18 Combination of a two- and three-walled defect at the distal aspect of the mandibular first molar is suitable for a guided tissue regeneration procedure.

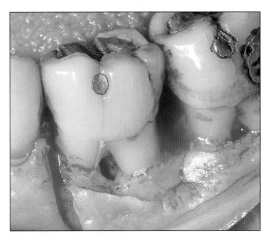

Fig 24-19 Class II furcation involvement of a mandibular first molar is a good indication for guided tissue regeneration.

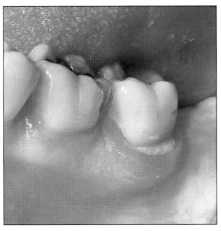

Fig 24-20 Infection of a barrier membrane is seen at the facial aspect of the mandibular second molar at 5 weeks. The membrane was removed immediately.

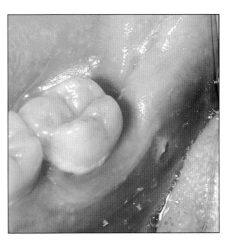

Fig 24-21 Perforation of lingual flap caused by a corner of the barrier membrane is seen in oral mucosa at the distal aspect of the mandibular second molar. Membranes, once trimmed, should have no sharp corners.

Clot stabilization or protection is the third principle of GTR. The barrier membrane protects the newly formed clot in the wound from mechanical and microbiologic injury, as well as stabilizes it. The relative importance of these three factors is not currently understood.

The success of GTR was overestimated during its early use. Periodontal defect features and patient control of dental plaque appear to be major factors influencing the variable results seen with GTR.[24] Success in the treatment of severe periodontitis has been best with two- and three-walled osseous defects (Fig 24-18) and class II furcations (Fig 24-19). Complete regeneration of bone in class III furcations is rare, but many of these lesions can be improved with GTR. Success in treating dehiscence defects has been reported.[32] Some evidence suggests that smoking is a neg-

ative prognosis factor.[33] Combining a membrane barrier with bone graft material has been tested,[32–35] but the findings are not in agreement.

Patients at risk for subacute bacterial endocarditis should not be treated with nonresorbable membranes because when the membrane is exposed to the oral environment, infection is common. Patients with poor oral hygiene should not be considered for GTR. Older age and the presence of nonvital teeth are not considered contraindications.

Complications of GTR include infection of the barrier membrane (Fig 24-20), flap slough and perforation (Fig 24-21), and recession. Infection is the most common complication. Once exposed, the membrane becomes a plaque trap, and infection occurs. Some membranes have to be

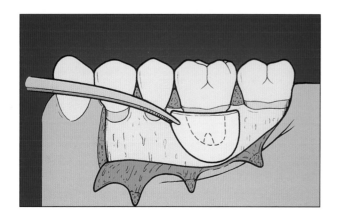

Fig 24-22 Membrane trimmed to extend 2 to 3 mm beyond the borders of the osseous defect. Note that vertical incisions are placed away from the membrane position.

removed because of infection within 2 to 3 weeks of placement. Because the membrane interferes with the blood supply to the overlying mucoperiosteal flap, partial sloughing or perforation of the flap is sometimes seen. Recession of 1 to 2 mm is a predictable outcome of GTR.

Guidelines for clinical application of GTR include the following:

1. Extend membranes only 2 to 3 mm beyond the borders of osseous defects to minimize interference with the blood supply to the flap (Fig 24-22).
2. Keep vertical incisions away from the membrane position. Extend flaps two teeth on each side of the defect (Fig 24-22). Miniflaps that include only one tooth are not recommended.
3. Completeness of root debridement is very important. A combination of curettes, files, ultrasonic instruments, rotating burrs, magnifying lenses, and fiber-optic devices are recommended to increase the thoroughness of root debridement.
4. Antibiotic coverage during the early postoperative period is routine. Antibiotics significantly suppress inflammation at the surgical site.[36]
5. Complete coverage of the membrane with the flap is recommended to minimize the chances of infection of the membrane.
6. Nonresorbable membranes should be left in place at least 6 weeks if there is no evidence of infection.

Postoperative care following GTR procedures should include the following:

1. Avoid mechanical disturbance of the surgical site for 6 weeks after surgery. In place of toothbrushing and flossing at the surgical site, the patient should use chlorhexidine as either a rinse or local topical application. This precaution enhances clot stabilization.[31]
2. Supragingival scaling and gentle probing can be performed at postoperative visits, but no pumice should

be used for the first 6 weeks to avoid a foreign body reaction.
3. Subgingival scaling and probing should be avoided for the first 6 months to allow the newly forming connective tissues to mature.
4. Evidence of infection such as swelling, inflammation, or drainage is an indication to remove the membrane.
5. If there is no evidence of infection, a second surgical procedure with local anesthesia and a mucoperiosteal flap is necessary to remove the nonresorbable membrane at 6 weeks. Resorbable membranes provide the advantage of eliminating a second surgical procedure for removal.
6. Radiographic increases in bone levels or density are usually not seen for at least 6 months (Figs 24-23a and 24-23b).

The following are indications of successful GTR treatment for severe chronic periodontitis:

1. Gain in clinical attachment
2. Reduced pocket depth
3. Minimal recession
4. Radiographic evidence of improved bone levels and density (usually not seen for about 9 months)

Results of controlled GTR studies show a wide variation in success. This variation is related to differences among studies in morphologic features of defects, duration of healing, barrier type, flap position, plaque control, and systemic health of patients. In general, however, the studies show a significant improvement in the parameters previously described, especially in defects with deep initial probing depths. Studies that have extended 5 to 6 years after treatment indicate that the improvements in clinical parameters persist for this time.[37,38]

Emdogain (Biora) is an FDA-approved material used to enhance regeneration of periodontal tissues. It is an enamel matrix derivative (EMD) composed primarily of amelo-

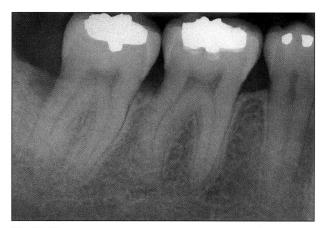

Fig 24-23a Radiograph of an osseous defect at the distal aspect of the mandibular second molar before treatment.

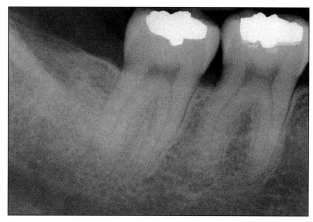

Fig 24-23b Radiograph of the lesion shown in Fig 24-23a taken 9 months after treatment.

genin and related proteins that are derived from porcine tooth buds.[39] These proteins are important for the development of acellular cementum, periodontal ligament, and alveolar bone. The mechanism of action is not well understood, but it has been suggested that the proteins mimic the role of enamel proteins in the cementogenesis that occurs with normal tooth development. The clinical safety of EMD, including its freedom from antigenic problems, has been demonstrated.[40]

In clinical trials, the use of EMD in conjunction with periodontal surgery has been found to reduce inflammation, bleeding on probing, and pocket depth. Its use has also resulted in clinical attachment gains.[41] A human histologic 10-case series indicates that the use of EMD can result in periodontal regeneration on previously diseased root surfaces, but on an inconsistent basis.[42] The reasons for the lack of consistency in results with EMD and all regeneration procedures is related to the many variables that can affect outcome. These variables include patient selection, defect morphology, root preparation, epithelial retardation, wound stabilization, plaque control, periodontal maintenance, graft type, graft placement, occlusal considerations, tooth mobility, flap closure, suturing technique, antibiotic coverage, and endodontic status.

The treatment of aggressive forms of periodontitis, especially severe chronic periodontitis, has been greatly enhanced by periodontal regeneration procedures. The capability of the periodontium to regenerate has been demonstrated. Bone grafting and GTR have contributed to significant advancements in treating severe lesions of periodontal bone destruction. Research and further development of these modalities are constantly improving pre-

dictability. These procedures are not a panacea, however, and their indications, contraindications, and complications are important to understand. At present, regeneration procedures are most successful in two- and three-walled osseous defects and class II furcation lesions. Deep osseous lesions with a narrow angle formed between the bone and root surface respond the best to regeneration procedures. Further research is indicated, but it appears that the goal of predictable periodontal regeneration is attainable.

References

1. Bowers GM, Schallhorn RG, Mellonig JT. Histologic evaluation of new attachment in human intrabony defects. A literature review. J Periodontol 1982;53(8):509–514.
2. Yukna RA, Mayer ET, Amos SM. Five-year evaluation of durapatite ceramic alloplastic implants in periodontal osseous defects. J Periodontol 1989;60:544–551.
3. Robinson RE. Osseous coagulum for bone induction. J Periodontol 1969;40:503–510.
4. Diem CR, Bowers GM, Moffitt WC. Bone blending: A technique for osseous implants. J Periodontol 1972;43:295–297.
5. Amler M. The time sequence of tissue regeneration in human extraction wounds. Oral Surg Oral Med Oral Pathol 1969;27:309–318.
6. Schallhorn RG, Hiatt WH, Boyce W. Iliac transplants in periodontal therapy. J Periodontol 1970;41:566–580.
7. Schallhorn RG. Postoperative problems associated with iliac transplants. J Periodontol 1972;43:3–9.
8. Buck B, Malinin T, Brown M. Bone transplantation and human immunodeficiency virus: An estimate of risk acquired immunodeficiency syndrome (AIDS). Clin Orthop 1989;240:129–133.
9. Resnick L, Veren K, Salahuddin S, et al. Stability and inactivation of HTLV-III/LAV under clinical and laboratory environments. J Am Dent Assoc 1986;255:1987–1993.

10. Fucini S, Quintero G, Gher M, et al. Small versus large particles of demineralized freeze-dried bone allografts in human intrabony periodontal defects. J Periodontol 1993;64:844–847.

11. Mellonig JT, Prewett AB, Moyer MP. HIV inactivation in bone allograft. J Periodontol 1993;63:979–983.

12. Mellonig J, Schwartz Z, Carnes D, et al. Ability of commercial DFDB to induce new bone formation [abstract 687]. J Dent Res 1995;74:97.

13. American Association of Tissue Banks' Standards for Tissue Banking. Arlington, VA: American Association of Tissue Banks, 1984.

14. Spector M. In: Hollinger J, Seyfer AE (eds). Analogs of Bone Mineral as Implants to Facilitate Bone Regeneration. Portland, OR: Leibinger, 1993:386–392.

15. Chen L, Klaes W, Assenmacher S. A comparative morphometric and histologic study of five bone substitute materials. Chin Med J 1996;65:1008–1015.

16. Weisen M, Oringer R, Lynch S, Iacono V. Efficacy of bovine bone mineral in vertical osseous defects [abstract 1165]. J Dent Res 1998;77:777.

17. Mellonig JT. Human histologic evaluation of a bovine-derived bone xenograft in the treatment of periodontal osseous defects. Int J Periodontics Restorative Dent 2000;20:19–29.

18. Rosenberg MM. Free osseous tissue autografts as a predictable procedure. J Periodontol 1971;42:195–209.

19. Carraro J, Sznajder N, Alonso C. Intraoral cancellous bone autografts in the treatment of infrabony pockets. J Clin Periodontol 1976;3:104–109.

20. Renvert S, Garrett S, Schallhorn RG, Egelberg J. Healing after treatment of periodontal intraosseous defects. III. Effect of osseous grafting and citric acid conditioning. J Clin Periodontol 1985;12:441–455.

21. Werbitt M. Decalcified freeze-dried bone allografts: A successful procedure in the reduction of intrabony defects. Int J Periodontics Restorative Dent 1987;7:56–63.

22. Steffensen B, Weber H. Relationship between the radiographic periodontal defect angle and healing after treatment. J Periodontol 1989;60:248–254.

23. Tonetti M, Giovanpaolo P, Cortellini P. Periodontal regeneration of human intrabony defects. IV. Determinants of healing response. J Periodontol 1993;64:934–940.

24. Machtei E, Cho M, Dunford R, et al. Clinical, microbiological, and histological factors which influence the success of regenerative periodontal therapy. J Periodontol 1994;65:154–161.

25. Yukna R. Synthetic bone grafts in periodontics. Periodontol 2000 1993;1:92–99.

26. Baldock WT, Hutchens LH Jr, McFall WT Jr, Simpson D. An evaluation of tricalcium phosphate implants in human periodontal osseous defects of two patients. J Periodontol 1985;56(1):1–7.

27. Froum SJ, Kushner L, Scopp IW, Stahl SS. Human clinical and histologic responses to durapatite implants in intraosseous lesions. Case reports. J Periodontol 1982;53:719–725.

28. Carranza FA Jr, Kenney EB, Lekovic V, et al. Histologic study of healing of human periodontal defects after placement of porous hydroxylapatite implants. J Periodontol 1987;58:682–688.

29. Kenney EB, Lekovic V, Elbaz JJ, et al. The use of a porous hydroxylapatite implant in periodontal defects. II. Treatment of class II furcation lesions in lower molars. J Periodontol 1988;59(2):67–72.

30. American Academy of Periodontology. Glossary of Periodontal Terms, ed 3. Chicago: American Academy of Periodontology, 1992.

31. Garrett S, Bogle G. Periodontal regeneration: A review of flap management. Periodontol 2000 1993;1:100–108.

32. Schallhorn R, McClain P. Periodontal regeneration using combined techniques. Periodontol 2000 1993;1:109–117.

33. Guillemin R, Mellonig J, Brunsvold M. Healing in periodontal defects treated by decalcified freeze-dried bone allografts in combination with ePTFE membranes. I. Clinical and scanning electron microscope analysis. J Clin Periodontol 1993;20:528–536.

34. Wallace S, Gellin R, Miller M, Mishkin D. Guided tissue regeneration with and without decalcified freeze-dried bone in mandibular class II furcation invasions. J Periodontol 1994;65:244–254.

35. Anderegg C, Martin S, Gray J, et al. Clinical evaluation of the use of decalcified freeze-dried bone allograft with guided tissue regeneration in the treatment of molar furcation invasions. J Periodontol 1991;62:264–268.

36. Demolon I, Persson R, Moncla B, et al. Effects of antibiotic treatment on clinical conditions and bacterial growth with guided tissue regeneration. J Periodontol 1993;64:609–616.

37. Gottlow J, Nyman S, Karring T. Maintenance of new attachment gained through guided tissue regeneration. J Clin Periodontol 1992;19:315–317.

38. McClain P, Schallhorn R. Long-term assessment of combined osseous composite grafting, root conditioning, and guided tissue regeneration. Int J Periodontics Restorative Dent 1993;13:9–26.

39. Hammarstrom L, Heijl L, Gestrelius S. Periodontal regeneration in a buccal dehiscence model in monkeys after application of enamel matrix proteins. J Clin Periodontol 1997;24:669–677.

40. Zetterstrom O, Andersson C, Eriksson L, et al. Clinical safety of enamel matrix derivative (Emdogain) in the treatment of periodontal defects. J Clin Periodontol 1997;24:697–704.

41. Heijl L, Heden G, Svardstrom G, Ostgren A. Enamel matrix derivative (Emdogain) in the treatment of intrabony periodontal defects. J Clin Periodontol 1997;24:705–714.

42. Yukna R, Mellonig J. Histologic evaluation of periodontal healing in humans following regenerative therapy with enamel matrix derivative. A 10-case series. J Periodontol 2000;71:752–759.

Host-Modifying Therapeutics

Kenneth S. Kornman and Ray C. Williams
- Biologic Opportunities for Host Modulation of Periodontitis
- Use of Host Modulators in the Clinical Management of Periodontitis Patients

The critical role of bacteria in the initiation and progression of periodontal disease is well documented and discussed in detail in chapter 1. The periodontal pathogens that are implicated in the etiology of periodontitis have enzymes and cell wall components that are able to destroy the extracellular matrix of the gingiva and to activate osteoclastic resorption of bone. However, extensive data indicate that most extracellular matrix and bone destruction in periodontitis is the result of direct action of host-derived enzymes, cytokines, and other mediators. The bacteria, therefore, initiate disease by activating host mechanisms that then destroy the supporting structures of the periodontium (see Fig 1-4).

As evidence accumulated in the 1960s and 1970s to definitively implicate bacteria as the essential "cause" of periodontitis, it was logical to apply systemic and topical antibiotics and antibacterial agents to the proof of the critical role of bacteria and as a means of controlling the disease. An extensive debate arose as to whether periodontitis could and should be treated as a simple bacterial infection.

The authors believe it is reasonable to conclude the following at this stage:

1. Antibiotics alone are not an appropriate means of long-term periodontitis control.
2. Systemic antibiotics, when used as an adjunct to scaling and root planing, may be beneficial in cases with severe generalized periodontitis.
3. Locally applied antibacterial agents, when used as an adjunct to scaling and root planing, may be beneficial in localized sites with probing depths 5 mm or greater in sites with signs of active disease.

At the height of the excitement about the essential role of specific bacteria in periodontitis in the late 1970s and early 1980s, a few diverse research programs made outstanding progress that defined new opportunities for con-

Portions of this chapter are taken from Kornman KS. Host modulation as a therapeutic strategy in the treatment of periodontal disease. Clinical Infectious Diseases 1999;28:520–526. Reprinted with permission from the University of Chicago. Copyright © 1999.

trolling periodontal disease by modulating the host response, instead of directly controlling the bacterial challenge. The following were the major programs at that time:

1. Williams and colleagues,[2] using a beagle dog model of periodontal disease and following up in humans, were able to demonstrate definitively that even in the presence of an excessive bacterial burden, it is possible to block disease progression significantly with a nonsteroidal anti-inflammatory drug. This finding also indirectly suggested that prostaglandins were key players in the bone loss of periodontitis, at least in the beagle dog model. These investigators then examined the role of prostaglandins in human periodontitis by blocking disease progression in subjects with advanced periodontitis with the nonsteroidal anti-inflammatory drug flurbiprofen.[3] This was the first definitive proof that at least one specific host mechanism was in the critical path for periodontitis.
2. Golub and coworkers showed that *(a)* collagenase enzymes were an active component of the destructive process in periodontitis and *(b)* tetracyclines and analogues without antibacterial activity were able to inhibit collagenases.[4-6]
3. Multiple investigators were exploring the ability of bisphosphonates to prevent bone destruction in osteoporosis.[7,8]

The scientific successes of these parallel developments ultimately led to the clinical application of host-modifying agents as a therapeutic approach to the treatment of periodontitis.

Biologic Opportunities for Host Modulation of Periodontitis

The general biologic relationships involved in periodontitis are described in chapter 1 (see Fig 1-4). This biologic map will be used to discuss the biologic opportunities (primary pathogenic mechanisms) that have been considered as targets for therapeutic intervention in periodontal disease. The map depicts the key biologic domains of the disease, including the bacterial challenge that activates the immunoinflammatory mechanisms leading to destruction of connective tissue and bone. It should be noted that many biologic factors interact within each box in the biologic map to regulate the major components described above. The diagram makes it clear that direct bacterial destruction of bone and connective tissue is not a primary

component of disease, thereby emphasizing the critical role of the host response in translating the bacterial challenge into destruction.

Bacterial antigens and lipopolysaccharides appear to explain much of the activation of tissue responses,[1,9] yet many other bacterial products are undoubtedly involved. Similarly, although many mediators are involved in various aspects of the host response, a complex integration of several matrix metalloproteinases (MMPs) and their inhibitors, selected cytokines and their inhibitors, and prostaglandin E_2 (PGE_2) appears to explain much of the tissue destruction.[1,9] The strength of the above host mechanisms will be evident in the following discussion, as disease has been significantly reduced by the use of compounds that specifically inhibit certain mechanisms.

With therapies that control bacteria, "more" is usually better. That may not be the case with host modulators, because the mediators that are being inhibited play complex roles that are intertwined with many other components. Thus, dose-response patterns may be complicated.

Option 1: Block Direct Effectors of Bone and Connective Tissue Destruction

Host modulators with the potential to alter clinical outcomes may be classified based on their targets in the disease process. Figure 25-1 diagrams the current opportunities for host modulation. The destruction of bone and connective tissue produces the clinical signs of disease, so perhaps the most direct opportunity for blocking destructive processes is at the level of osteoclastic bone destruction and destruction of connective tissues by MMPs. This opportunity is seen on the far right of the diagram in Fig 25-1.

Bisphosphonates
Currently used for the treatment of osteoporosis, bisphosphonates are believed to block bone destruction by inhibiting the activation of osteoclasts. Because alveolar bone loss in periodontitis is the result of osteoclastic activity, it is reasonable to consider the use of these agents in chronic periodontitis. Alendronate, a commercially available drug for osteoporosis, significantly reduced periodontal bone loss in two models of periodontitis that involve very high bacterial challenges: *(1)* ligature-induced periodontitis in monkeys[10] and *(2)* progressive periodontitis in beagle dogs.[11]

One study of therapy using bisphosphonates for progressive periodontal disease in humans has been published and showed promising results.[12] Other clinical trials with these agents are in progress.

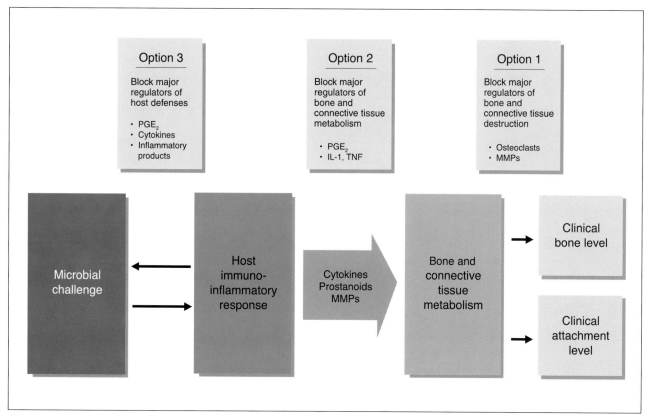

Fig 25-1 Host modulation options are based on different biologic mechanisms. Option 1 involves blocking molecules that are involved in direct destruction of bone and connective tissues. Options 2 and 3 involve blocking molecules that regulate the remodeling of bone and connective tissues and the host protection against bacteria. (IL-1) Interleukin 1; (TNF) tumor necrosis factor.

It should be noted, however, that an unusual dose-response pattern was seen in the monkey study, with the lower dose producing better inhibition of bone loss than the higher dose. This observation was confirmed in a second independent block of the study in which a new series of drug doses was used. This observation points out that attempts to intervene in complex regulatory mechanisms should proceed with caution.

Matrix Metalloproteinase Inhibitors

Because loss of periodontal attachment and bone involves destruction of connective tissues, blocking connective tissue mechanisms is a viable target for prevention of periodontal disease. The chemicals that are responsible for connective tissue remodeling are a group of enzymes, MMPs, and they include the collagenases and gelatinases.

These enzymes play an important role in tissue remodeling, and their activity is tightly regulated by several specific and nonspecific inhibitors.[13] Early studies by Golub and coworkers[4–6] found that tetracyclines directly blocked the action of MMPs. As a result, these agents have been used to prevent connective tissue destruction in multiple

diseases, including periodontitis. The importance of MMPs in periodontal disease has been recently reviewed.[14–21]

Because MMPs are a family of enzymes, the inhibition of specific MMPs by a specific compound will vary. The MMPs that have been studied most extensively in periodontitis are those produced mainly by connective tissue cells: fibroblasts (MMP-1), monocytes (MMP-1), and polymorphonuclear leukocytes (MMP-8). Extracellular matrix changes are involved in so many processes critical to life that it is not surprising to find extensive and redundant regulatory mechanisms. Extracellular matrix remodeling requires multiple cells and a variety of mediators that regulate maturation and phenotypic expression of each cell. These mediators include enzymes, cytokines, prostanoids, and growth factors that regulate the expression of the cells involved.

There appear to be multiple potential opportunities to block MMPs, including blocking production of MMPs, blocking activation of the proenzyme, blocking activity of the enzyme, and activating inhibitors. At least some of the activity of inhibitors involves action in removing Zn^{++} and Ca^{++}, which are essential to the active sites of the MMPs.

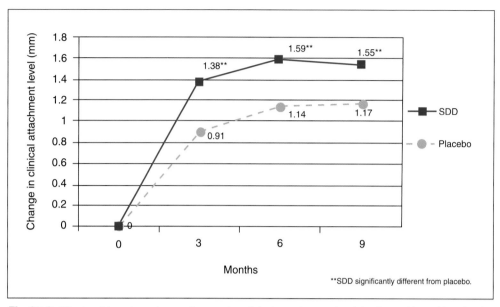

Fig 25-2 Effects of low-dose doxycycline on the clinical attachment level in sites with probing depths greater than or equal to 7 mm. Patients received scaling and root planing at baseline and then either sub-antimicrobial-dose doxycycline (SDD, n = 79) or placebo (n = 78) twice daily for 9 months. (Reprinted from Caton et al,[31] with permission.)

Given the tight regulation in this system, induction of MMPs leads to coordinated activation of specific inhibitors.[22,23] The fact that bacterial products alter the expression and activity of MMPs is important to periodontal disease.[24]

Tetracyclines produce a select MMP inhibition pattern that has some variation by specific compound. In general, the tetracyclines appear to preferentially inhibit the neutrophil collagenase (MMP-8), with a 50% inhibition by doxycycline reported at 15 mmol/L for MMP-8 and at 280 mmol/L for MMP-1.[25–27] An example of that specificity is evident in some clinical applications. For example, the MMP pattern in fluid from failing hip replacements is dominated by MMP-1 and MMP-9, with minimal to no neutrophil MMP (MMP-8).[28] Tetracyclines did not inhibit the MMP activity from loose hip implants, but cephalothin, a member of another class of antibiotics, produced a 49% to 78% inhibition of activity.[29]

A low-dose tetracycline is currently approved by the Food and Drug Administration for treatment of periodontitis. The low-dose tetracycline, when used as an adjunct to scaling and root planing, produced a mean improvement in clinical attachment level that was superior to placebo by approximately 0.4 mm in the deepest sites (Fig 25-2). Perhaps most important, a mean of 3.6% of the deepest sites in the placebo group lost at least 2 mm, compared with a mean of 0.3% in the tetracycline group.[30,31]

Option 2: Block Host Mechanisms That Regulate Direct Effectors

Nonsteroidal Anti-inflammatory Drugs

Prostaglandins, which regulate many aspects of inflammation and extracellular matrix and bone metabolism, have been strongly implicated in the pathogenesis of periodontitis. Several excellent reviews have discussed the evidence supporting a role for prostaglandins in periodontal diseases.[9,32–34]

PGE_2 is produced in the tissues by cyclooxygenase enzymes. In many tissues cyclooxygenase 1 is produced constitutively and appears to be essential to tissue homeostasis. Cyclooxygenase 2, however, appears to be activated in inflammation and contributes primarily to the increase in PGE_2 in periodontitis. In periodontal tissues, monocytes and fibroblasts produce PGE_2 in response to activation by interleukin 1β (IL-1β), tumor necrosis factor α (TNF-α), and lipopolysaccharides.

The relationship of increased levels of PGE_2 to periodontal disease is well established and includes the following, as reviewed recently[9]: (1) PGE_2 levels are associated with disease severity at individual sites and at the patient level; (2) the highest levels of PGE_2 tend to be in actively progressing sites; and (3) the association between levels of PGE_2 and disease is especially strong in patients with systemic conditions that lead to more severe periodontitis, such as diabetes mellitus. Thus, certain systemic conditions that are known to predispose individuals to an increased risk of periodontitis tend to be associated with significantly higher mean gingival crevicular fluid levels of PGE$_2$,[35] independent of the inflammation at the local site.

A variety of nonsteroidal anti-inflammatory drugs have been shown to provide clinical benefit in the treatment of periodontitis. The most well-documented benefit is in reducing bone loss, and the greatest effect in humans has been in patients with progressing disease[36] and in sites with progressing disease.[37] Attachment level results are less clear, although there are positive findings for monkeys.[9]

Although many nonsteroidal anti-inflammatory drugs are currently available in both prescription and nonprescription forms, these agents are not currently used for the treatment of periodontitis. Nonsteroidal anti-inflammatory drugs have not been approved for the treatment of periodontitis in the United States.

Inhibitors of IL-1 and TNF

IL-1 has been strongly associated with the pathogenesis of periodontitis. First, elevated IL-1 levels in the gingival crevicular fluid are associated with more severe periodontal disease.[38] Second, the IL-1β level increases rapidly in experimental gingivitis.[39,40] Third, IL-1β is produced by a variety of cells in the periodontal area, including monocytes, gingival fibroblasts,[41] and polymorphonuclear leukocytes (PMNs).[42] Fourth, IL-1β regulates collagen metabolism and integrity.[43–47] Most important, investigators have shown that specific inhibition of IL-1 and TNF-α locally in the periodontal tissues reduced histologic levels of osteoclasts and bone loss in ligature-induced periodontitis in monkeys.[48]

Multiple TNF-α blocking agents and one IL-1 blocking agent have been approved for the treatment of rheumatoid arthritis in the United States. These agents have not been evaluated in human clinical trials for the treatment of periodontitis.

Option 3: Block Major Regulators of Host Defenses

Compromised antibody and PMN functions have been associated with more severe periodontitis. This suggests that such mechanisms for bacterial control may be reasonable opportunities for therapeutic intervention.[1] The levels and quality of antibody and the localization and function of PMNs are regulated by many factors, including PGE$_2$, IL-1, IL-4, IL-10, TNF-α, and active oxygen species.

Host modulators for periodontal disease have not yet focused specifically on enhancing antibody and PMN function, but agents directed at PGE$_2$, IL-1, and TNF-α

would be expected to favorably influence these protective mechanisms.

Use of Host Modulators in the Clinical Management of Periodontitis Patients

There are considerable data relative to the effectiveness of various therapies for chronic periodontitis. Reasonable bacterial control (at a level that is clinically achievable for many years) and regular professional cleanings to reduce the subgingival bacterial deposits have been shown to predictably control most cases of periodontitis. On the basis of available data, it seems reasonable to conclude that the immunoinflammatory response is sufficiently protective in most individuals such that minimal periodontal destruction will occur with routine oral hygiene measures. Regular bacterial control, therefore, appears to be the most practical approach to periodontal therapy for most patients.

In every periodontal practice there are patients who require more extreme bacterial control to limit their clinical inflammation and loss of attachment. Approximately 8% to 13% appear to be highly susceptible to more severe generalized periodontitis.[49] In addition, increasing data indicate that individuals who exhibit severe generalized periodontitis have an excessive immunoinflammatory response to the bacterial challenge.[9,35,50,51] For such individuals, extreme bacterial control or host modulation plus bacterial control seems to be an appropriate therapeutic strategy.

Most cases of generalized aggressive periodontitis can be explained by a small number of factors that are known to alter the host defense and host destructive mechanisms, including smoking, diabetes mellitus, and genetic predisposition. Such cases appear to be most appropriate for host-modifying therapeutics, because other cases are easily managed with the conventional therapy discussed throughout this book. The role of the above systemic factors that alter pathogenesis is described in detail in chapters 11 to 13.

References

1. Page RC, Kornman KS. The pathogenesis of human periodontitis: An introduction. Periodontol 2000 1997;14:9–11.
2. Williams RC, Jeffcoat MK, Kaplan ML, et al. Flurbiprofen: A potent inhibitor of alveolar bone resorption in beagles. Science 1985;227:640–642.
3. Williams RC, Jeffcoat MK, Howell TH, et al. Altering the progression of human alveolar bone loss with the non-steroidal anti-inflammatory drug flurbiprofen. J Periodontol 1989;60:485–490.

4. Golub LM, Lee HM, Lehrer G, et al. Minocycline reduces gingival collagenolytic activity during diabetes: Preliminary observations and proposed new mechanism of action. J Periodontal Res 1983;18:516–526.

5. Golub LM, McNamara TF, D'Angelo G, et al. A non-antibacterial chemically modified tetracycline inhibits mammalian collagenase activity. J Dent Res 1987;66:1310–1314.

6. Golub LM, Ramamurthy NS, McNamara TF. Tetracyclines inhibit connective tissue breakdown: New therapeutic implications for an old family of drugs. Crit Rev Oral Biol Med 1991;2:297–322.

7. Eastell R, Riggs BL. New approaches to the treatment of osteoporosis. Clin Obstet Gynecol 1987;30:860–870.

8. Fleisch H. Bisphosphonates: A new class of drugs in diseases of bone and calcium metabolism. Recent Results Cancer Res 1989;116:1–28.

9. Offenbacher S. Periodontal diseases: Pathogenesis. Ann Periodontol 1996;1:821–878.

10. Brunsvold MA, Chaves ES, Kornman KS, et al. Effects of a bisphosphonate on experimental periodontitis in monkeys. J Periodontol 1992;63:825–830.

11. Reddy MS, Weatherford TW III, Smith CA, et al. Alendronate treatment of naturally-occurring periodontitis in beagle dogs. J Periodontol 1995;66:211–217.

12. Rocha M, Nava LE, Vazquez de la Torre C, et al. Clinical and radiological improvement of periodontal disease in patients with type 2 diabetes mellitus treated with alendronate: A randomized, placebo-controlled trial. J Periodontol 2001;72:204–209.

13. Jeffcoat MK, Reddy MS. Alveolar bone loss and osteoporosis: Evidence for a common mode of therapy using the bisphosphonate alendronate. In: Davidovitch Z, Norton LA (eds). Biological Mechanisms of Tooth Movement and Craniofacial Adaptation. Boston, MA: Harvard Society for the Advancement of Orthodontics, 1996:365–373.

14. Reynolds JJ, Meikle MC. Mechanisms of connective tissue matrix destruction in periodontitis. Periodontol 2000 1997;14:144–157.

15. Haerian A, Adonogianaki E, Mooney J, et al. Gingival crevicular stromelysin, collagenase and tissue inhibitor of metalloproteinases levels in healthy and diseased sites. J Clin Periodontol 1995;22:505–509.

16. Ingman T, Sorsa T, Michaelis J, Konttinen YT. Immunohistochemical study of neutrophil- and fibroblast-type collagenases and stromelysin-1 in adult periodontitis. Scand J Dent Res 1994;102:342–349.

17. Kubota T, Nomura T, Takahashi T, Hara K. Expression of mRNA for matrix metalloproteinases and tissue inhibitors of metalloproteinases in periodontitis-affected human gingival tissue. Arch Oral Biol 1996;41:253–262.

18. Meikle MC, Hembry RM, Holley J, et al. Immunolocalization of matrix metalloproteinases and TIMP-1 (tissue inhibitor of metalloproteinases) in human gingival tissues from periodontitis patients. J Periodontal Res 1994;29:118–126.

19. Ryan ME, Ramamurthy NS, Golub LM. Matrix metalloproteinases and their inhibition in periodontal treatment. Curr Opin Periodontol 1996;3:85–96.

20. Birkedal-Hansen H, Moore W, Bodden M, et al. Matrix metalloproteinases: A review. Crit Rev Oral Biol Med 1993;4:197–250.

21. Sorsa T, Ding Y, Salo T, et al. Effects of tetracyclines on neutrophil, gingival, and salivary collagenases. A functional and western-blot assessment with special reference to their cellular sources in periodontal diseases. Ann NY Acad Sci 1994;732:112–131.

22. Nomura T, Takahashi T, Hara K. Expression of TIMP-1, TIMP-2 and collagenase mRNA in periodontitis-affected human gingival tissue. J Periodontal Res 1993;28:354–362.

23. Alvares O, Klebe R, Grant G, Cochran DL. Growth factor effects on the expression of collagenase and TIMP-1 in periodontal ligament cells. J Periodontol 1995;66:552–558.

24. Ding Y, Uitto VJ, Firth J, et al. Modulation of host matrix metalloproteinases by bacterial virulence factors relevant in human periodontal diseases. Oral Diseases 1995;1:279–286.

25. Golub LM, Evans RT, McNamara TF, et al. A non-antimicrobial tetracycline inhibits gingival matrix metalloproteinases and bone loss in Porphyromonas gingivalis-induced periodontitis in rats. Ann NY Acad Sci 1994;732:96–111.

26. Golub LM, Sorsa T, Lee HM, et al. Doxycycline inhibits neutrophil (PMN)-type matrix metalloproteinases in human adult periodontitis gingiva. J Clin Periodontol 1995;22:100–109.

27. Suomalainen K, Sorsa T, Golub LM, et al. Specificity of the anticollagenase action of tetracyclines: Relevance to their antiinflammatory potential. Antimicrob Agents Chemother 1992;36:227–229.

28. Takagi M, Konttinen YT, Lindy O, et al. Gelatinase/type IV collagenases in the loosening of total hip replacement endoprostheses. Clin Orthop 1994;306:136–144.

29. Santavirta S, Takagi M, Konttinen YT, et al. Inhibitory effect of cephalothin on matrix metalloproteinase activity around loose hip prostheses. Antimicrob Agents Chemother 1996;40:244–246.

30. Crout RJ, Lee HM, Schroeder K, et al. The "cyclic" regimen of low-dose doxycycline for adult periodontitis: A preliminary study. J Periodontol 1996;67:506–514.

31. Caton JG, Ciancio SG, Blieden TF, et al. Treatment with subantimicrobial dose doxycycline improves the efficacy of scaling and root planing in patients with adult periodontitis. J Periodontol 2000;71:521–532.

32. Williams RC, Beck JD, Offenbacher S. The impact of new technologies to diagnose and treat periodontal disease. A look to the future. J Clin Periodontol 1996;23:299–305.

33. Offenbacher S, Heasman PA, Collins JG. Modulation of host PGE$_2$ secretion as a determinant of periodontal disease expression. J Periodontol 1993;64:432–444.

34. Howell TH, Williams RC. Nonsteroidal antiinflammatory drugs as inhibitors of periodontal disease progression. Crit Rev Oral Biol Med 1993;4:177–196.

35. Salvi GE, Yalda B, Collins JG, et al. Inflammatory mediator response as a potential risk marker for periodontal diseases in insulin-dependent diabetes mellitus patients. J Periodontol 1997;68:127–135.

36. Reddy MS, Palcanis KG, Barnett ML, et al. Efficacy of meclofenamate sodium (Meclomen) in the treatment of rapidly progressive periodontitis. J Clin Periodontol 1993;20:635–640.

37. Jeffcoat MK, Reddy MS, Haigh S, et al. A comparison of topical ketorolac, systemic flurbiprofen, and placebo for the inhibition of bone loss in adult periodontitis. J Periodontol 1995;66:329–338.

38. Yavuzyilmaz E, Yamalik N, Bulut S, et al. The gingival crevicular fluid interleukin-1 beta and tumour necrosis factor-alpha levels in patients with rapidly progressive periodontitis. Aust Dent J 1995;40:46–49.

39. Stashenko P, Fujiyoshi P, Obernesser MS, et al. Levels of interleukin-1β in tissue from sites of active periodontal disease. J Clin Periodontol 1991;18:548–554.

40. Kinane DF, Winstanley FP, Adonogianaki E, Moughal NA. Bioassay of interleukin-1 (IL-1) in human gingival crevicular fluid during experimental gingivitis. Arch Oral Biol 1992;37:153–156.

41. Dongari-Bagtzoglou AI, Ebersole JL. Production of inflammatory mediators and cytokines by human gingival fibroblasts following bacterial challenge. J Periodontal Res 1996;31:90–98.

42. Hendley TM, Steed RB, Galbraith GMP. Interleukin-1β gene expression in human oral polymorphonuclear leukocytes. J Periodontol 1995;66:761–765.

43. DuFour A, Baran C, Langkamp HL, et al. Regulation of differentiation of gingival fibroblasts and periodontal ligament cells by rhIL-1β and rhTNF-α. J Periodontal Res 1993;28:566–568.

44. Ohshima M, Otsuka K, Suzuki K. Interleukin-1β stimulates collagenase production by cultured human periodontal ligament fibroblasts. J Periodontal Res 1994;29:421–429.

45. Okamatsu Y, Kobayashi M, Nishihara T, Hasegawa K. Interleukin-1α produced in human gingival fibroblasts induces several activities related to the progression of periodontitis by direct contact. J Periodontal Res 1996;31:355–364.

46. Irwin CR, Schor SL, Ferguson MWJ. Effects of cytokines on gingival fibroblasts in vitro are modulated by the extracellular matrix. J Periodontal Res 1994;29:309–317.

47. Wahl LM, Corcoran ML. Regulation of monocyte/macrophage metalloproteinase production by cytokines. J Periodontol 1993;64(5 suppl):467–473.

48. Assuma R, Oates T, Cochran D, et al. IL-1/TNF account for most of the inflammatory response in experimental periodontitis [abstract 1298]. J Dent Res 1997;76:176.

49. Papapanou PN. Epidemiology and natural history of periodontal disease. In: Lang NP, Karring T (eds). Proceedings of the 1st European Workshop on Periodontology. London: Quintessence, 1994:23–41.

50. Kornman KS, Crane A, Wang H-Y, et al. The interleukin-1 genotype as a severity factor in adult periodontal disease. J Clin Periodontol 1997;24:72–77.

51. Hernichel-Gorbach E, Kornman KS, Holt SC, et al. Host responses in patients with generalized refractory periodontitis. J Periodontol 1994;65:8–16.

Re-treatment

Thomas G. Wilson, Jr

- When the Tooth Will Be Retained
- Deciding Between Tooth Retention or Extraction
  with Implant Placement

Re-treatment is frequently performed but rarely discussed. The reasons for this lack of discussion include the complexity of the concept, limited knowledge of the disease process, hesitancy to discuss apparent failure with colleagues, and variations in measuring disease activity, to name a few. Still, the subject should be covered, because there is much to learn from the analysis of failure. Everyone agrees that re-treatment is often necessary, but there is great disagreement on how and when to re-treat.

Decisions on when to re-treat are based largely on increases in clinical attachment loss (probing depth). The vast majority of clinicians would say that if probing depths have increased by 3 mm since the last baseline measurement, therapy is indicated. Most would say the same about a 2-mm change. Less change brings less consensus, yet true changes of 1 mm can be clinically significant.

In recent years local and systemic markers of inflammation of the periodontal tissues have received increasing emphasis. No correlation has yet been made between systemic indicators of inflammation (such as C-reactive protein, fibrinogen, and amyloid A) and periodontal infections. Until markers of systemic disease activity are available to the clinician, we must measure the clinical signs of inflammation. The most widely used is bleeding on probing. Most clinicians would agree that the absence of bleeding on probing indicates health, and most would say that they prefer not to see bleeding following probing. However, they disagree on the significance of bleeding on probing and its effect on treatment planning. This parameter will be excluded from the discussion.

When the Tooth Will Be Retained

We assume that the clinician has decided that sufficient attachment loss has occurred to warrant therapy. For patients with a current diagnosis of early periodontitis (4- to 6-mm probing depths with no bone loss in the furcation), therapy usually consists of oral hygiene reinforcement and closed subgingival scaling and root planing. For probing depths of 4 to 6 mm with bone loss in the furcation, advanced ther-

---

The statements and conclusions in this chapter are based on the author's understanding of the current literature and his clinical judgment. The approach described in this chapter should be adapted for each practitioner and each patient.

apy is often needed in the form of the dental endoscope or periodontal surgery. With probing depths greater than 6 mm, the decision often involves whether the tooth should be retained and treated or be removed. In the past, clinicians have decided when to do surgery based on local risk factors (eg, probing depths and degree of compliance) and their clinical experience. However, sufficient data on systemic risk factors now exist to aid the clinician in making this decision.

Bacteria

The deeper the pocket, the more aggressive the bacteria found. Surgical reduction of pockets is often a predictable way to help maintain the dentition. This assumes that closed subgingival scaling and root planing have failed to reduce the pocket depths and that other risk factors are compatible with surgery.

Compliance

Better compliers respond more positively to all forms of therapy. This factor becomes important when deciding between surgery and closed subgingival scaling and root planing. Poor compliers to suggested oral hygiene are usually not candidates for periodontal surgery. Excellent compliers usually respond well to either form of therapy. The problem comes with patients who are partial compliers to suggested oral hygiene and maintenance therapy. For patients who will use a toothbrush daily and return frequently for maintenance, pocket depth reduction often facilitates the use of the interproximal brush, which is more readily accepted by most patients than dental floss.

Diabetes Mellitus

Patients with diabetes mellitus do not handle bacteria as well as those without the disease. Therefore, more aggressive pocket depth reduction procedures, including surgery, are often helpful in good compliers. In general, the less severe the diabetes and the better it is controlled, the more positively the patient will respond to periodontal treatment.

Smoking

Patients who smoke have more tooth loss from periodontitis and do not heal as well following therapy. Suggestions for smoking cessation are appropriate for these patients. Smokers may benefit from either surgical or nonsurgical procedures, but these procedures often need to be performed several times over the life of the patient.

Genetic Factors

According to preliminary information, patients who are positive for the interleukin 1 (IL-1) genotype will not respond as well to regenerative therapy. Because patients with moderate forms of periodontitis are usually not candidates for regenerative therapy anyway, but IL-1–positive patients have been found to harbor more of the pathogens (and greater percentages of those individual pathogens) apparently responsible for inflammatory periodontal diseases, pocket elimination surgery (osseous surgery) is often appropriate for these patients.

Interleukin-1–Positive Smokers

Individuals who smoke and are IL-1 positive will experience more bone and tooth loss than individuals without both risk factors (see chapter 11). This finding would lead the clinician to proceed with any therapy only after informing the patient of the risk and suggesting smoking cessation. Closed subgingival scaling and root planing are often appropriate for individuals in this group until they have stopped smoking.

Deciding Between Tooth Retention or Extraction with Implant Placement

Some teeth with severe periodontitis (probing depths of 7 mm or more) should be removed and replaced with implants. Because several risk factors apply to both teeth and implants, yet teeth and implants may respond differently, these risk factors should be considered during treatment planning. They include the response to bacteria, trauma, compliance, smoking, and genetic factors.

Bacteria

Most agree that bacteria are the primary extrinsic etiologic factors of inflammatory periodontal diseases, but strong disagreement exists about their role in implant loss. Some feel that the influence of bacteria in implant loss is often a primary causal factor, whereas others strongly disagree. This debate has yet to end.

Trauma

Trauma does not cause attachment loss around teeth, but it appears to be an etiologic factor in implant loss. It is also true that some teeth with severe bone loss do not have sufficient support to withstand normal masticatory forces. In general, implants provide greater stability and support than do teeth with severe disease. Patients with parafunctional habits often require splinting of teeth or implants and occlusal therapy, including habit devices (nightguards). Patients with bruxism who receive implants often benefit from additional implants to distribute forces.

Compliance

Patients who clean their teeth and adhere to a schedule of periodontal maintenance visits tend to keep their teeth far longer than individuals who do not follow professional recommendations. There are no studies on the effect of compliance on implant loss, but if trauma or bacteria play a part in this process, then compliance obviously plays a role as well.

Smoking

Smoking has negatively affected the prognosis of both periodontitis and implant therapy. Smoking cessation is optimal, but the author has found that implants have a better prognosis in smokers than do teeth with severe periodontitis.

Genetic Factors

Initial information suggests that patients who are positive for the IL-1 genotype are at greater risk for tooth loss than implant loss. If these data are confirmed, IL-1 patients will fare better with implants than with teeth, all other risk factors being the same.

Interleukin-1–Positive Smokers

Smokers who test positive for the IL-1 gene may be at a greater risk for both implant and tooth loss than individuals with just one of these risk factors. If this proves true,

then smoking cessation is prudent for these patients. Those who refuse to stop smoking should be treated only after the increased risks have been explained.

General Guidelines

How does the practitioner bring all these risk factors together to decide whether to remove or retain teeth affected by severe periodontitis? The author makes clinical decisions using the following generalizations:

1. *Bacteria seem to have a more profound negative effect on teeth than on implants.* Thus, individuals with average levels of oral hygiene (those who brush teeth frequently and clean interproximally occasionally) would tend to fare better with implants than with teeth. This is not meant to suggest that all teeth affected by inflammatory periodontal disease should be replaced by implants. However, the author would suggest implant placement when trying to decide between removing or treating a tooth with severe periodontitis in patients with average oral hygiene.
2. *Smokers are at greater risk for both tooth and implant loss than nonsmokers.* Smokers lose teeth and implants sooner than nonsmokers. Suggestions concerning smoking cessation are therefore prudent. This guideline is not meant to indicate that these patients should not receive therapy, but merely that they should be informed of the consequences.
3. *IL-1–positive patients have more tooth loss than implant loss.* In the author's opinion, patients with severe periodontitis who are IL-1 positive will fare better with implants than with teeth.
4. *IL-1–positive smokers are at special risk.* This small group appears to be at particular risk for tooth loss and perhaps implant loss. The practitioner should make a special effort to inform patients in this group of the potential risks and to encourage smoking cessation.

CHAPTER
27 | Referrals to Specialists

Richard D. Wilson

- Risk Factors
- The Decision to Refer
- Selection of a Periodontist
- The Referral Process

The delivery of periodontal care is shifting in the practice of dentistry as more patients with periodontal conditions are receiving treatment from their family dental practitioners. Patients are primarily referred to periodontists for prerestorative or preprosthetic surgery, for periodontal plastic surgery, for the placement of implants, or for the treatment of conditions that general practitioners view as too complex.

Patients are more likely to seek the care of a general practitioner than in the past. In 1999, approximately three quarters of the US population aged 25 years or older made a dental visit.[1] Complete edentulism in the more mature patient (65 to 74 years) has been reduced by half since the mid-1970s, leaving the profession with the dual legacy of greater numbers of older patients not only having teeth but also desiring to keep them.[2] As more teeth are retained over more years, the risk of periodontal problems increases. From 1980 through 1995, insured patients aged 55 years and older demonstrated an increase in periodontal services in excess of 500%.[1]

The 1985–1986 National Institute of Dental and Craniofacial Research Senior Survey[3] indicated a relatively moderate incidence of periodontal conditions (gingival bleeding, calculus, probing depths greater than 4 mm, and attachment loss greater than 4 mm). In contrast, the more valid New England Elders Dental Study[4] used probing sites that conformed more closely to those normally selected for the diagnosis of periodontal disease. As a consequence, the latter study offered more realistic percent-

ages of periodontal conditions, and they were significantly higher than those of the Senior Survey. Nevertheless, it is apparent to all clinicians that fewer patients have advanced chronic periodontitis. A number of explanations are offered for this decrease, but the most logical is the early diagnosis and therapeutic intervention that takes place in the office of the general practitioner.

In addition, dental patients are increasingly aware of the benefits of oral wellness and are becoming more active participants in preventive oral self-care. Patients are better informed and are influenced by the quantity of available health information (eg, from the Internet, family magazines, and the daily news media). Societal pressures, which stress the symbiosis of oral health and esthetics as a reflection of youth, affect patient preferences. Consequently, patients are receptive to the variety of necessary treatments that general practitioners suggest for periodontal conditions.

The profession is also changing.[5] Ongoing developments in technology, materials, and techniques have improved outcomes. Evolving methods of reconstructing the periodontium, progress in the local delivery of pharmacologic agents,[6,7] microsurgery techniques, and better means of sedation and pain control all have enhanced professional and community confidence in the success of periodontal therapies.

Both general practitioners and periodontists have access to an abundance of educational material, journals, and lectures about periodontal conditions and their treatments. Dental students are taught that the diagnosis and management of periodontal disease is within their purview, provided they have both knowledge and the necessary skills. Consequently, more general practitioners are well informed about the new technologies, as well as educated about, and alert to, the diagnosis of periodontal diseases. They are less reluctant to engage in periodontal therapies and routinely include the treatment of periodontal conditions in their daily office regimens. Their staff members are also better trained and skilled in caring for the periodontal patient. Periodontology involves continual learning as science reveals new layers of knowledge in periodontal diagnosis and treatment.

Risk Factors

Treatment for any dental condition must be preceded by a diagnosis and treatment planning. The new classification[8] of periodontal diseases and conditions now provides the general practitioner and the periodontist with a more orderly, coherent, and clinically useful instrument for planning patient treatment. Although most practitioners inform patients that treatment of chronic periodontitis is punctuated by periodic reevaluation and that the disease is managed and rarely "cured," patients do expect treatment results that are beneficial. Predictable outcomes, however, are occasionally elusive and may cause frustration and disappointment for both the patient and the treating practitioner.

Although pathogenic microbes are responsible for the onset of periodontal disease, other elements influence both the clinical course of the disease and the treatment results. These elements are termed *risk factors*. Included among the risk factors is patient compliance with practitioner-recommended self-care[9] and with regularly scheduled office visits designed to aid in continuing disease management. Correcting poorly shaped restorations that have open, overextended, or rough margins,[10] alleviating recurrent parafunctional occlusal behavior,[11] and educating the patient about the pernicious effects of smoking[12,13] all help to improve success rates. Diabetes mellitus, even when controlled through diet, can hinder therapy and must be monitored both during active treatment and throughout long-term care.[14] Systemic conditions that attack a patient's immune mechanism (eg, human immunodeficiency virus infection,[15] or oncologic and organ implant therapies[16]) also compromise or interfere with treatment success. A careful discussion with the patient of the questions on the history form often reveals domestic, social, or occupational stresses that could contribute to disease progression.[17]

An additional and critically important risk factor has been well documented recently and offers valid research support for clinical opinions about genetic susceptibility long held by practitioners active in periodontology. A specific genotype of the polymorphic interleuken 1 (IL-1) gene cluster has been identified as a genetic marker for adults who, with a bacterial challenge, are much more likely to develop severe periodontitis, especially if they are smokers.[18,19] Genetic testing, therefore, offers clinicians a diagnostic tool for proactively identifying those cases of aggressive periodontitis that may not be as amenable to the nonsurgical treatments frequently employed by a general practitioner.[20–22] See chapter 11 for a more detailed discussion of genetics and periodontal disease.

Ignoring risk factors may lead to disappointing long-term results even after skillfully rendered treatment. The ability to use a curette or scalpel with great dexterity is no longer adequate, of itself, in the treatment of periodontal disease. To be effective, today's oral health care provider must blend clinical abilities with a cognitive application of up-to-date science.

All these considerations confirm the increasing public health role of the general practitioner in dealing with periodontal diseases. Conversely, periodontal diseases may contribute to adverse medical outcomes, such as cardiovascular disease. A number of studies have demonstrated the link of oral health problems (especially periodontal disease) with either coronary heart disease or cerebral vascular accident.[23–28] It is evident that the inclusion of prudently and effectively employed periodontal treatment into the normal routine of a general dental practice is both necessary and appropriate. However, this does not diminish the challenge for general practitioners; it actually compels greater accountability.

By engaging in biologically contemporary periodontal diagnosis and therapy, the general practitioner of the new millennium continues to assume the traditional mantle of the gatekeeper of a patient's periodontal health. In so doing, the general practitioner must also accept the responsibility of deciding who is to deliver the appropriate periodontal treatment.

The Decision to Refer

Although more general practitioners appropriately care for patients with periodontal disease, periodontists have additional formal education in the field. When should this specialist expertise be applied? What guidelines should general practitioners use when referring patients to periodontists, and how should they go about it?

A referral is an awareness of need. If the closed instrumentation (root planing and scaling) implemented in the general practitioner's office does not resolve clinically apparent signs of inflammation or if attachment loss persists, the general practitioner should consider seeking the help of a periodontist. From a patient confidence perspective, the patient should be informed of this possibility before the practitioner initiates periodontal therapy.

Other periodontal conditions that warrant consideration of a referral include the following:

- Non–plaque-induced gingival diseases
- Aggressive periodontitis (especially cases predicted by genotype)
- Combined periodontal-endodontic lesions
- Severe mucogingival deformities
- Multiple sites of surgical crown lengthening
- Edentulous ridge preservation or augmentation
- Complex combination of systemic conditions
- Patients who will not stop smoking
- Esthetic periodontal problems (eg, a "gummy smile")

During the latter two decades of the 20th century, an important new element entered into the relationship of general practitioners and periodontists: implant dentistry. As practitioners and periodontists began learning this rapidly expanding discipline, communication grew and personal and professional alliances strengthened. Reliance on each other's abilities increased as more positive patient results were observed. Improving knowledge about implants was often matched by improving knowledge of the roles of the general practitioner and the periodontist in treating periodontal conditions. Many periodontists now realize that, in addition to their own abilities, their success primarily depends on the periodontal knowledge, restorative skills, and practice success of the general practitioner.

By the same token, general practitioners should confer with periodontists when planning treatment for patients who need sophisticated multidisciplinary care. Often, face-to-face discussions not only develop better treatment but also avoid misunderstandings.

Factors that influence a general practitioner's decision to refer a patient to a periodontist are listed below.

Factors That Influence Referral

The dentist's . . .
- Personal ethical standards
- Preferences
- Knowledge
- Skills
- Business and economic pressures
- Prior experience with periodontists
- Confidence in advanced periodontal therapy (including surgery)
- Conversations with colleagues
- Concern about the patient's condition
- Worries about what a periodontist will say to the patient
- Lack of success in resolving the patient's condition
- Distance from a periodontist
- Desire to transfer a patient requiring difficult treatment
- Uneasiness about the patient's health
- A desire to share responsibility
- A need to increase knowledge
- Restorative requirements
- Desire to learn together

The patient's . . .
- Preferences
- Finances
- Distance from a periodontist
- Prior experience with a periodontist
- Preconceptions or prejudices
- Conversations with other patients
- Confidence in the general practitioner

The periodontist's . . .
- Reputation
- Knowledge
- Skill
- Gentleness
- Staff
- Personality
- Proclivity for gossip
- Tolerance
- Communication abilities
- Fees
- Rapport with general practitioners
- Willingness to be flexible
- Attitude
- Desire to learn

Selection of a Periodontist

The general practitioner usually selects a periodontist the same way a patient selects a general practitioner—based on location and what others say. However, there are different levels of competence in every field, and the referring practitioner should be discriminating. Evaluation of results and patient satisfaction is crucial. If disease recurs in numerous sites or numerous patients, the practitioner must consider a discussion with the periodontist. The periodontist also should be notified if a patient returns to the general practitioner with calculus that is visible during gingival retraction or restorative procedures, if no attached gingiva remains to receive an intracrevicular restoration margin, or if the length of a surgically extended clinical crown is similar to the pretreatment length.

The general practitioner must also make a distinction between legitimate and ethical promotion of a periodontist's skills and other questionable methods of referral inducement. The issues of overtreatment, unnecessary treatment, and treatment beyond one's ability should also be considered in evaluating a referral to any specialist. Clearly, the criterion should be quality of care.

The general practitioner should visit the periodontist's office, be comfortable with the periodontist, and have frequent and informal meetings with the periodontist to discuss treatment philosophy and to review individual cases. Every effort should be made to improve mutual communications and to establish and sustain treatment support, consultative support, and professional support among the general practitioner, the periodontist, and their staffs.

The Referral Process

The general practitioner who decides to refer a patient to a periodontist should employ the same concerns for communication and quality of care that are expected of the periodontist. During the referral consultation, the patient should be informed of the benefits of the treatment to be presented by the specialist. A candid review of risks, options, and disadvantages of treatment should take place to aid the patient in his or her decision.

The general practitioner's open and considerate discussion of the referral with the patient is critical. Spending time on this discussion may appear to be nonremunerative, but it does foster patient confidence and trust and consequently is an important element in building a practice. If this dialogue is hasty, the patient may leave the general practitioner's office confused, uncertain, or even irritated.

The patient should be informed of the reason for the referral. The patient's questions about what the periodontist will do should be answered: "Those are excellent questions, and I encourage you to discuss those openly with the periodontist. As a patient, you have the right to ask questions, and my experience with Dr Periodontist indicates that she always takes time to respond thoughtfully to patient concerns." The referring practitioner should avoid committing the periodontist to a specific treatment or prognosis and should emphasize that the final treatment plan will be developed mutually, with ongoing consultation between the general practitioner and the periodontist.

The patient should be given one periodontist's name. Giving the patient more than one name is confusing and usually results in the patient's trying to evaluate each periodontist by hearsay.

The patient's radiographs should be sent to the periodontist prior to the patient's appointment. They should be recent, clear, and diagnostic. Outdated radiographs, inappropriate bitewing radiographs, or incomplete sets of radiographs usually are not helpful to the periodontist. The patient's learning that the periodontist received inadequate radiographs or no radiographs could lead to loss of confidence. The patient should be informed by the general practitioner that the periodontist may require additional radiographs to aid in periodontal diagnosis.

The periodontist should be informed of the referral and the general practitioner's post–periodontal treatment expectations (eg, crowns or fixed or removable prostheses). This information should be both verbal and written (an electronic form is acceptable). Verbal communication enhances the risk of misunderstanding and litigation.

The periodontist is legally and morally obligated to examine a patient's entire dentition. When a periodontist receives a patient who has been referred for a single procedure (eg, surgical extension of the clinical crown or marginal tissue augmentation via a graft), the periodontist should examine the entire mouth. The general practitioner should inform the referred patient of this during the referral discussion.

The periodontist is responsible for communicating with the referring practitioner. These communications should begin early on and continue during and at the end of active therapy. If the patient is to be under active therapy for an extended time, the general practitioner has a right to be informed of the reasons. If untoward developments occur (eg, unusual postoperative pain or bleeding, unexpected tooth loss, or acute systemic problems such as myocardial infarction or cerebrovascular accident), the periodontist should inform the referring practitioner.

Changes in an established treatment plan should be made mutually and in private. Just as the general practitioner should not commit the periodontist to a specific treatment or prognosis, so too should the periodontist avoid verbally presenting a quick judgment to the patient. It is reassuring to patients to know that both practitioners are taking the time to confer. The patient should be informed that a treatment plan must be flexible and that modifications may be the result of individual response to treatment. Because exceptions always occur, the general practitioner and the periodontist should be thoughtful and prudent in their comments. Criticisms should be confidential between the periodontist and the general practitioner; they should not be made in the presence of patients or staff.

The timing of a referral may be fundamental to treatment success. Delay in a referral could change a treatable situation into a hopeless one; all 7-mm pockets were 4- or 5-mm pockets at one time. Timely inclusion of a specialist in therapy may preserve a patient's confidence, as well as the patient's dentition.

The periodontist and general practitioner must share a continually evolving understanding of each other's treatment philosophies. If the general practitioner has a strong preference for initial root planing and scaling in the office, the periodontist should help shape these skills. If the general practitioner needs guidance in the timing of a referral for surgery, the periodontist should offer such counsel without prejudice. Difficult decisions regarding referral to other specialists, dealing with recurrent periodontal disease or caries, and sharing periodontal maintenance should be addressed early in a referral relationship.[29]

The question of who is to provide periodontal maintenance is controversial. In some cases of periodontal disease that are difficult to manage, the periodontist's office should be primarily responsible for ongoing support of periodontal care. These cases require appropriate communication with the referring practitioner, and the patient should see the general practitioner at least once a year. In most instances, the sharing of patient care is best, but only if the quality of the periodontal maintenance is comparable. Patients who receive an hour of thorough root planing and scaling in one office may not be satisfied with a 20-minute recall visit in another office. Fees may also affect patient preference. Patients may request that periodontal maintenance be performed in one office only. Practitioners should resist these preferences and attempt to keep patients on a mutual-care basis.

Just as the general practitioner should expect quality care from the periodontist, so the periodontist should expect quality care from the general practitioner. There are few components of a general practitioner–periodontist relationship that are as important as the quality of restorative and prosthodontic care. Hasty, overzealous, or poorly designed implementation of these disciplines can irreparably damage an otherwise successful periodontal result. More-over, a clear understanding of the biologic aspects of restorative and prosthodontic treatment is just as important as the traditionally accepted technical aspects of patient care.

Appropriate and complimentary comments about colleagues spoken before patients, staff, and other practitioners are a suitable and ethical extension of professional partnerships. This manifestation of professional support results in an increase of patient confidence in both the referring and the referred therapists, and it often strengthens cross-referrals and practice viability.

The termination of a referral relationship should always be accompanied by an explanation. Frequently, a specialist is bewildered when a general practitioner abruptly stops referring patients. If a correctable problem exists, the specialist should know about it and take steps to correct it.

Finally, both the periodontist and the referring practitioner should be willing to work together to moderate fees and therapy for patients who are highly motivated but cannot afford the proposed treatment plan. In many cases, these patients will eventually be able to complete proper, more sophisticated therapy. As always, these patients must be informed of the risks involved. Professional and personal relationships founded on this basis of respect and care for the patient's well-being create enduring, satisfying, and rewarding intraprofessional rapport for all involved.

References

1. Eklund SA, Pittman JL, Smith RC. Trends in dental care among insured Americans: 1980 to 1995. J Am Dent Assoc 1997;128: 171–178.
2. Marcus SE, Drury TF, Brown LJ, Zion GR. Tooth retention and tooth loss in the permanent dentition of adults: United States, 1988–1991. J Dent Res 1996;75(special issue):684–695.
3. Löe H. Oral Health of United States Adults: Nation Findings. Bethesda, MD: National Institute of Dental and Craniofacial Research, U.S. Department of Health and Human Services, 1987.
4. Douglass CW, Jette AM, Fox CH, et al. Oral health status of the elderly in New England. J Gerontol 1993;48:M39–M46.
5. Brown LJ. Commentary: A proud achievement for American dentistry. J Am Dent Assoc 1997;128:174–181.
6. Jeffcoat MK, Bray KS, Ciancio SG, et al. Adjunctive use of a subgingival controlled-release chlorhexidine chip reduces probing pocket depth and improves attachment level compared with scaling and root planing alone. J Periodontol 1998;69:989–997.
7. Caton JG, Ciancio SG, Crout RJ, et al. Adjunctive use of doxycycline therapy for periodontitis [abstract 2957]. J Dent Res 1998;77:1001.
8. Armitage GC. Development of a classification system for periodontal diseases and conditions. Ann Periodontol 1999;4:1–6.
9. Wilson TG. Compliance: A review of the literature with possible applications to periodontics. J Periodontol 1987;58: 706–714.
10. Wilson RD, Maynard JG. Intracravicular restorative dentistry. Int J Periodontics Restorative Dent 1981;1(4):34–39.

11. Clark GT, Tsukivama Y, Baba K, Watanabe T. Sixty-eight years of experimental occlusal interference studies: What have we learned? J Prosthet Dent 1999;82:704–713.

12. Bergstrom J. Cigarette smoking as a risk factor in chronic periodontal disease. Community Dent Oral Epidemiol 1989;17:245–247.

13. Ah MKB, Johnson GK, Kaldahl WB, et al. The effect of smoking on the response to periodontal therapy. J Clin Periodontol 1994;21:91–97.

14. Emrich L, Shlossman M, Genco R. Periodontal disease in non-insulin dependent diabetes mellitus. J Periodontol 1991;62:123–130.

15. Lucht E, Heimdahl A, Nord CE. Periodontal disease in HIV-infected patients in relation to lymphocyte subsets and specific microorganisms. J Clin Periodontol 1991;18:252–256.

16. Rahman MM, Caglayan F, Rahman B. Periodontal health parameters in patients with chronic renal failure and renal transplants receiving immune-suppressive therapy. J Nihon Univ Sch Dent 1992;34:265–272.

17. Breivik T, Thrane PS, Murison R, Gjermo P. Emotional stress effects on immunity, gingivitis, and periodontitis. Eur J Oral Sci 1996;104:327–334.

18. Kornman K, Crane A, Wang HY, et al. The interleukin-1 genotype as a severity factor in adult periodontal disease. J Clin Periodontol 1997;24:72–77.

19. McGuire MK, Nunn ME. Prognosis versus actual outcome. IV. The effectiveness of clinical parameters and IL-1 genotype in accurately predicting prognosis and tooth survival. J Periodontol 1999;70:49–56.

20. Wilson TG. Using risk assessment to customize periodontal treatment. J Calif Dent Assoc 1999;27:627–632, 634–639.

21. Caffesse RG, Sweney PL, Smith BA. Scaling and root planing with and without periodontal flap surgery. J Clin Periodontol 1986;13:205–210.

22. Lang NP. Indications and rationale for non-surgical periodontal therapy. Int Dent J 1983;33:127–136.

23. Mattila KJ, Nieminen MS, Valtonen VV, et al. Association between dental health and acute myocardial infarction. BMJ 1989;298:779–781.

24. Syrjanen J, Peltola J, Valtonen V, et al. Dental infections in association with cerebral infarction in young and middle-aged men. J Intern Med 1989;225:179–184.

25. Loesche WJ. Periodontal disease as a risk factor for heart disease. Compend Contin Educ Dent 1994;15:976–991.

26. Beck J, Garcia R, Heiss G, et al. Periodontal disease and cardiovascular disease. J Periodontol 1996;67(suppl):1123–1137.

27. Loesche WJ, Schork A, Terpenning MS, et al. Assessing the relationship between dental disease and coronary heart disease in elderly U.S. veterans. J Am Dent Assoc 1998;129:301–311.

28. Loesche WJ. Periodontal disease: Link to cardiovascular disease. Compend Contin Educ Dent 2000;21:463–480.

29. Townsend CH. Guidelines for supportive periodontal therapy intervals and for referral to a periodontist. Periodontal Insights 1994;(4):9–10.

Periodontal Maintenance

Thomas G. Wilson, Jr

- Chart Review and Health History Update
- Clinical Data Collection
- Microbiologic Monitoring
- Review of Oral Hygiene
- Removal of Accretions and Deposits
- Behavior Modification
- Frequency, Efficacy, and Length of Periodontal Maintenance Visits
- Who Should Be Responsible for Periodontal Maintenance?

This chapter covers the specific procedures performed at a typical periodontal maintenance visit for a patient with an inflammatory periodontal disease. Since offices and patients differ widely, these suggestions should be tailored, and improved on, for each specific situation.

Chart Review and Health History Update

The therapist and the patient will benefit from reviewing the patient's health history and the record of the previous periodontal maintenance visit before the patient arrives for treatment. Any medications needed before periodontal maintenance (such as antibiotic prophylaxis to reduce the chance of subacute bacterial endocarditis in a patient with a heart murmur) or any special needs (such as local anesthesia) can be determined in this manner.

Patients can undergo significant medical and dental health changes in the weeks between periodontal maintenance visits. The questions that follow are designed to uncover important new information for the health history, which should be recorded on the patient's chart:

1. Have there been any changes in your health or medications, or have you been hospitalized since your last visit?
2. Is there anything about your mouth or jaws that concerns you?
3. Have you had any dental work since your last visit?
4. What do you routinely do to clean your teeth?

The recent trend has been to deliver dental care rapidly to more and more patients. Professionals sometimes fall into the trap of seeing patients as "mouths to be repaired," not people who have dental problems. Taking a few moments during each visit to get to know each other will have long-term benefits for both the therapist and the patient. Such interchanges can lead to better care and compliance for the patient and more satisfaction for the professional.

Clinical Data Collection

Risk Factors

Compliance to oral hygiene measures, diabetic status, and smoking status can be helpful in determining future therapy. Other risk factors, such as bacterial makeup and genetic factors, can be addressed when appropriate. (See chapters 11 and 19.)

Dental Examination

Tooth Loss

Any teeth lost since the last periodontal maintenance charting should be recorded.

Caries/Prosthetic Examination

The natural teeth are examined for overt signs of dental caries, and any prosthetic replacements of the natural dentition (including implant restorations) are checked.

Fremitus

Movement of the teeth during function (fremitus) is simple to measure and has been associated with advancing disease.[1] Therefore, it may be checked, noted, and eliminated when possible if it is found on a tooth that has clinical signs of active periodontal breakdown.

Periodontal/Implant Examination

Inflammation

It is important to evaluate the soft tissues around implants and teeth for clinical signs of inflammation. In the foreseeable future, a number of more accurate tests for inflammation and prediction of disease activity should be available. At present it is helpful to assess inflammation by checking for bleeding on probing and suppuration. Bleeding on probing can be found by dragging a probe through the sulcus. Suppuration can also be detected by applying coronal finger pressure on the gingival tissues. Because these data may provide information about whether the gingival tissues are inflamed, they should be measured and recorded at each periodontal maintenance visit.

One of the critical issues in periodontal maintenance is how to best use the allotted time. In the past, it was assumed that each surface of each tooth should be thoroughly scaled and root planed. Today, only areas of previous attachment loss, especially those sites with current signs of inflammation, are identified and treated appropriately. Someday it may be possible to predict areas of future attachment loss and provide appropriate local or systemic therapy. In the meantime, emphasis should begin to shift from cleaning teeth to diagnosing and treating disease and the inflammation associated with it.

Probing Depth

The probing depth has been defined as the distance from the gingival margin to the apical depth of periodontal probe tip penetration.[2] These measurements should be taken and recorded at six points around each tooth and in as many areas as the overlying prosthesis will allow around implants. The readings are best obtained by moving a periodontal probe through the sulcus (pocket), with the long axis of the probe parallel to the long axis of the tooth or implant. Records are made of the midfacial and midlingual depths, as well as of the mesiolingual and distolingual and mesiobuccal and distobuccal (facial) aspects. Interproximal readings are best made not at the line angles but by placing the probe tip in the deepest part of the pocket (usually under the contact area) while keeping it as parallel as possible to the tooth's or implant's long axis. This parameter should be checked at each periodontal maintenance visit and any changes from baseline recorded. As discussed in chapter 17, the accuracy and reproducibility of this measurement depend on the diameter of the probe, how forcefully the probe tip is introduced into the pocket, the relative health of the tissue, and the skill and experience of the operator.

Radiographic Examination

Conventional parallel or right-angle radiographs, while limited to showing only gross amounts of bone loss, still provide important information, especially when several sets exposed over a number of years are available for comparison. The number of radiographs should be limited for safety reasons, but in cases of apparently active disease, a full-mouth series every few years with seven vertical bitewing radiographs in intervening years is helpful in making an accurate assessment of bone stability.

Microbiologic Monitoring

For patients whose disease is refractory despite compliance and normally adequate clinical therapy microbiologic monitoring and antibiotic sensitivity testing can be useful. When used in these cases and combined with traditional approaches to therapy, including subgingival scaling and root planing, the appropriate antibiotic and antimicrobial therapy can yield results superior to those of scaling and root planing alone. When possible causal organisms remain after this therapy or if generalized attachment loss or inflammation continues or recurs in spite of the reduction or elimination of other risk factors, periodic microbial monitoring is helpful.

Review of Oral Hygiene

Patients who clean their teeth well tend to keep their teeth longer than those who do not clean optimally. Therefore, personal oral hygiene is of great importance. Unfortunately, a large percentage of patients do not brush well, much less clean between their teeth.[3] Newer mechanical toothbrushes offer improved results when compared with manual brushes and have been well accepted by patients. These mechanical devices should not be suggested for use in individuals with a thin periodontal housing, because of the possible increased risk of recession.

Most disease starts between the teeth, and when no interproximal gingival recession exists, patients must use dental floss. Unfortunately, the average patient does not floss at all or does it incorrectly. For patients with loss of interproximal dental papillae, interproximal brushes are a positive addition to the cleaning regimen.

Most clinicians are looking for a single problem-free method to rid their patients of dental plaque, but this method does not exist. However, in some patients who will not comply otherwise, chlorhexidine rinses have been shown to be useful on a short-term basis, as has the use of oral irrigators.

Removal of Accretions and Deposits

Subgingival

After assessment of attachment loss and inflammation and monitoring and reinforcing of personal oral hygiene, removal of subgingival accretions is the next most important step. This is technically one of the most difficult procedures performed by the dental professional. Inadequate removal of deposits by subgingival scaling and root planing will often produce a positive gingival response that may lead the inexperienced clinician to believe that the disease process has been arrested, when in fact only gingival health has been improved and bone loss continues.

Several studies[4,5] using conventional blind techniques have shown that with diligent effort, the clinician can successfully remove subgingival tooth-borne plaque and calculus from teeth that have 3-mm probing depths using closed subgingival scaling and root planing. These same studies show that as probing depths exceed 5 mm, the probability of removing all subgingival accretions diminishes—this despite as long as three quarters of an hour per tooth spent cleaning. With these greater probing depths, advanced methods for removing subgingival accretions are often warranted. In cases where bone regeneration is a goal, surgery can be useful. This approach also reduces probing depths to facilitate access by the patient and the professional.[6] New devices, such as the dental endoscope, can be considered as another alternative in these situations.

If time for a periodontal maintenance visit is short, then areas that have increased probing depths and clinical signs of inflammation (color changes, bleeding on probing, or suppuration) should be the first to receive closed subgingival scaling and root planing. The patient should then be scheduled for removal of the remaining accretions.

Supragingival

It is unfortunate but true that a great deal of time that could be best spent on more important facets of periodontal maintenance is used for mechanical removal of supragingival accretions. For this reason, the dental professional providing care at the periodontal maintenance visit should complete needed disease assessment, oral hygiene procedures, and subgingival scaling and root planing before removing materials that have accumulated supragingivally. This may require additional visits by the patient.

Behavior Modification

Patient compliance with professional suggestions is critical to long-term success in the treatment of inflammatory periodontal diseases. However, the average patient does not completely comply with recommendations concerning personal health. Most people understand that compliance with suggestions made by health care providers can enrich and lengthen their lives. Still, they find it difficult to adhere to the myriad rules needed for positive change.

One can assume that the average patient will not make sweeping behavioral changes, especially in the long term. This is not to say that one will never be able to turn a non-complier into a complete complier, but only that these victories will be few and far between. Since clinicians deal with chronic diseases for the most part, they must take these facts into consideration during all phases of dental therapy. Expecting a patient with a history of noncompliance to suggested oral hygiene measures and periodontal maintenance to respond well to procedures that require compliance is illogical. Therapy should be based on facilitating compliance, not making it more difficult.

It is possible to improve almost every patient's compliance to some degree using accepted practices for behavior modification. This discussion, while very important, is beyond the scope of this chapter; appropriate techniques are described elsewhere.[3,7,8]

Frequency, Efficacy, and Length of Periodontal Maintenance Visits

In the past, 6 months was the interval most often suggested between periodontal maintenance visits. Some patients with gingivitis and early forms of periodontitis, along with minimal risk factors, do well with this interval, but patients with greater disease severity or more risk factors require more frequent care.

Numerous studies have shown that tooth and attachment loss are found less frequently, and to a lesser degree, in patients on regular periodontal maintenance intervals[9–26] compared with patients seen less often[27–29] or not at all.[30–33] Occasionally, despite the best efforts of therapists and patients, some individuals may lose teeth during periodontal maintenance as a result of continuing disease.[34–36] Patients with this group of diseases may benefit from additional disease analysis and therapy, including more frequent periodontal maintenance visits than necessary for patients with a more typical response.[37,38] A counterpoint to the efficacy of frequent periodontal maintenance visits has been offered in studies that reported no difference in progression of disease in patients seen much less frequently. However, as a rule, the patients who did well with less periodontal maintenance had high levels of personal oral hygiene.[39,40]

For most patients with gingivitis, no previous attachment loss, and few risk factors, periodontal maintenance twice a year will usually suffice.[41] Results from a vast majority of clinical trials suggest that periodontal maintenance intervals of less than 6 months are appropriate for patients with periodontitis, but intervals have varied: 2 weeks,[20,42] 2 to 3 months,[14] 3 months,[12,13,27,43–48] 3 to 4 months,[10,18] 3 to 6 months,[49–51] and 4 to 6 months.[34] While the frequency varies, this body of evidence indicates that patients with a history of periodontitis should be seen at least four times a year, because it decreases the likelihood of advancing disease compared with patients seen less frequently.[11,14,16,21,52] In general, the greater the number of risk factors, the more frequently the patient should be seen.

Specific microorganisms are associated with periodontitis.[53,54] They are usually suppressed following root planing, but they may return to baseline levels days to months later.[55–67] The average time for return to baseline levels is between 9 and 11 weeks, but this may vary dramatically in different patients.[68] If the clinician wishes to maintain a low level of suspected pathogens, periodontal maintenance intervals of 3 months or less appear to be required.

This body of data supports the concept that it is advantageous if periodontal maintenance visits are performed every 3 months for patients with chronic periodontitis; those with aggressive forms of periodontitis often benefit from more frequent periodontal maintenance. This interval should be individualized and, in general, decreased for patients with risk factors as yet uncontrolled. As the prediction of future attachment loss becomes more accurate, periodontal maintenance intervals will vary more among individuals. It should be recognized that periodontal maintenance patients will often need to be returned to active care. Sites that have previous attachment loss are most likely to need active therapy in the future. Active care may involve surgical or nonsurgical therapy and may be required soon after the patient enters periodontal maintenance.

Patients with both dental implants and teeth should be seen as often as needed to maintain periodontal health. Patients with only dental implants should be seen, in general, once a year.

The average periodontal maintenance visit for a patient with inflammatory periodontal disease is about an hour.[24] This is only the average, however; many patients may require a longer time for completion of required periodontal maintenance.

Who Should Be Responsible for Periodontal Maintenance?

The 1989 World Workshop in Clinical Periodontics[28] advised that patients with gingivitis and chronic forms of periodontitis be treated in the general practitioner's office, but that patients with more advanced disease should be the periodontist's responsibility. The following suggestions are made to further clarify the roles of practitioner and periodontist:

1. Patients with a form of dental plaque–induced gingivitis or chronic periodontitis with early attachment loss and few risk factors should be the primary responsibility of the general practitioner.
2. Other forms of gingivitis should be treated and maintained by the periodontist.
3. Patients with chronic periodontitis with moderate attachment loss usually do well by alternating between the general practitioner's and the periodontist's offices.
4. While patients with aggressive forms of periodontitis should be seen by the periodontist for periodontal maintenance, it is important for these patients to have appropriate restorative examinations by their general practitioner.
5. In general, patients with multiple risk factors should be seen more frequently by the periodontist.

References

1. Pihlstrom BL, Anderson KA, Aeppoli D, Schaffer EM. Association between signs of trauma from occlusion and periodontitis. J Periodontol 1986;57(1):1–6.

2. Caton J. Periodontal diagnosis and diagnostic aids. In: Nevins M, Becker W, Kornman K (eds). Proceedings of the World Workshop in Clinical Periodontics, July 23–27, 1989. Chicago: American Academy of Periodontology, 1989:1–22.

3. Wilson TG. Compliance. A review of the literature with possible applications to periodontics. J Periodontol 1987;58:706–714.

4. Waerhaug J. Healing of the dento-epithelial junction following subgingival plaque control. II. As observed on extracted teeth. J Periodontol 1978;49:119–134.

5. Stambaugh RV, Dragoo M, Smith DM, Carasal L. The limits of subgingival scaling. Int J Periodontics Restorative Dent 1981;1:30–41.

6. Caffesse RG, Sweeney PL, Smith BA. Scaling and root planing with and without periodontal flap surgery. J Clin Periodontol 1986;13:205–210.

7. Merchenbaum D, Turk DC. Facilitating Treatment Adherence. New York: Plenum Press, 1987.

8. Haynes RB, Sackett DC. Compliance with Therapeutic Regimens. Baltimore: Johns Hopkins University Press, 1976.

9. Lovdal A, Arno A, Schei O, Waerhaug J. Combined effect of subgingival scaling and controlled oral hygiene on the incidence of gingivitis. Acta Odontol Scand 1961;19:537–555.

10. Suomi JD, Greene JC, Vermillion JR, et al. The effect of controlled oral hygiene procedures on the progression of periodontal disease in adults: Results after third and final year. J Periodontol 1971;42:152–160.

11. Axelsson P, Lindhe J. Effect of controlled oral hygiene procedures on caries and periodontal disease in adults. J Clin Periodontol 1981;8:239–248.

12. Knowles JW, Burgett FG, Nissle RR, et al. Results of periodontal treatment related to pocket depth and attachment level. Eight years. J Periodontol 1979;50:225–233.

13. Ramfjord SP, Morrison EC, Burgett FG, et al. Oral hygiene and maintenance of periodontal support. J Periodontol 1982;53:26–30.

14. Axelsson P, Lindhe J. The significance of maintenance care in the treatment of periodontal disease. J Clin Periodontol 1981;8:281–294.

15. Lindhe J, Westfelt E, Nyman S, et al. Long-term effect of surgical/non-surgical treatment of periodontal disease. J Clin Periodontol 1984;11:448–458.

16. Ramfjord SP, Caffesse RG, Morrison EC, et al. Four modalities of periodontal treatment compared over five years. J Periodontal Res 1987;22:222–223.

17. Westfelt E, Nyman S, Socransky S, Lindhe J. Significance of frequency of professional tooth cleaning for healing following periodontal surgery. J Clin Periodontol 1983;10:148–156.

18. Pihlstrom BL, McHugh RB, Oliphant TH, Ortiz-Campos C. Comparison of surgical and nonsurgical treatment of periodontal disease. A review of current studies and additional results after 6 1/2 years. J Clin Periodontol 1983;10:524–541.

19. Badersten A, Nilvéus R, Egelberg J. Effects of nonsurgical periodontal therapy. II. Severely advanced periodontitis. J Clin Periodontol 1984;11:63–76.

20. Nyman S, Rosling B, Lindhe J. Effect of professional tooth cleaning on healing after periodontal surgery. J Clin Periodontol 1975;2:80–86.

21. Axelsson P, Lindhe J. Effect of controlled oral hygiene procedures on caries and periodontal disease in adults. J Clin Periodontol 1978;5:133–151.

22. Brandzaeg P, Jamison HC. The effect of controlled cleansing of teeth on periodontal health and oral hygiene in Norwegian Army recruits. J Periodontol 1964;35:302.

23. Chawla TN, Nanda RS, Kapoor KK. Dental prophylaxis procedures in control of periodontal disease in Lucknow (rural) India. J Periodontol 1975;46:498–503.

24. Schallhorn RG, Snider LE. Periodontal maintenance therapy. J Am Dent Assoc 1981;103:227–231.

25. Jendresen MD, Hamilton AI, McLean JW, et al. Report of the Committee on Scientific Investigation of the American Academy of Restorative Dentistry. J Prosthet Dent 1984;51:823–846.

26. Kaldahl WB, Kalkwarf KL, Patil KD, et al. Evaluation of four modalities of periodontal therapy. Mean probing depth, probing attachment level and recession changes. J Periodontol 1988;59:783–793.

27. Wilson TG, Glover ME, Malik AK, et al. Tooth loss in maintenance patients in a private periodontal practice. J Periodontol 1987;58:231–235.

28. Nevins M, Becker W, Kornman K (eds). Proceedings of the World Workshop in Clinical Periodontics, July 23–27, 1989. Chicago: American Academy of Periodontology; 1989:II-1–II-20.

29. DeVore CH, Duckworth DM, Beck FM, et al. Bone loss following periodontal therapy in subjects without frequent periodontal maintenance. J Periodontol 1986;57:354–359.

30. Becker W, Berg L, Becker BE. Untreated periodontal disease: A longitudinal study. J Periodontol 1979;50:234–244.

31. Becker W, Becker BE, Berg LE. Periodontal treatment without maintenance. A retrospective study in 44 patients. J Periodontol 1984;55:505–509.

32. Nyman S, Lindhe J, Rosling B. Periodontal surgery in plaque-infected dentitions. J Clin Periodontol 1977;4:240–249.

33. Lindhe J, Haffajee AD, Socransky SS. Progression of periodontal disease in adult subjects in the absence of periodontal therapy. J Clin Periodontol 1983;10:433–442.

34. Hirschfeld L, Wasserman B. A long-term survey of tooth loss in 600 treated periodontal patients. J Periodontol 1978;49:225–237.

35. McFall WT Jr. Tooth loss in 100 treated patients with periodontal disease. A long-term study. J Periodontol 1982;53:539–549.

36. Meador H, Love J, Suddick P. The long-term effectiveness of periodontal therapy in a clinical practice. J Periodontol 1985;56:253–258.

37. Douglass CW, Fox CH. Determining the value of a periodontal diagnostic test. J Periodontol 1991;62:721–730.

38. van Winkelhoff A, Tijhof C, de Graf J. Microbiological and clinical results of metronidazole plus amoxicillin therapy in *Actinobacillus actinomycetemcomitans*–associated periodontitis. J Periodontol 1992;63:52–57.

39. Listgarten MA, Sullivan P, George C, et al. Comparative longitudinal study of 2 methods of scheduling maintenance visits: 4-year data. J Clin Periodontol 1989;16:105–115.

40. Johansson LA, Oster B, Hamp SE. Evaluation of cause-related periodontal therapy and compliance with maintenance care recommendations. J Clin Periodontol 1984;11:689–699.

41. Ramfjord SP. Maintenance care and supportive periodontal therapy. Quintessence Int 1993;24:465–471.

42. Rosling B, Nyman S, Lindhe J, Jern B. The healing potential of the periodontal tissues following different techniques of periodontal surgery in plaque-free dentitions. A 2-year clinical study. J Clin Periodontol 1976;3:233–250.

43. Ramfjord SP, Knowles JW, Nissle RR, et al. Longitudinal study of periodontal therapy. J Periodontol 1973;44:66–77.

44. Ramfjord SP, Knowles JW, Nissle RR, et al. Results following three modalities of periodontal therapy. J Periodontol 1975; 46:522–526.

45. Fleszar TJ, Knowles JW, Morrison EC, et al. Tooth mobility and periodontal therapy. J Clin Periodontol 1980;7:495–505.

46. Hill RW, Ramfjord SP, Morrison EC, et al. Four types of periodontal treatment over two years. J Periodontol 1981;52:655–662.

47. Becker W, Becker BE, Ochsenbein C, et al. A longitudinal study comparing scaling, osseous surgery and modified Widman procedures—Results after one year. J Periodontol 1988;59:351–365.

48. Oliver RC. Tooth loss with and without periodontal therapy. Periodontal Abstr 1969;17:8–17.

49. Lindhe J, Nyman S. The effect of plaque control and surgical pocket elimination on the establishment and maintenance of periodontal health. A longitudinal study of periodontal therapy in cases of advanced disease. J Clin Periodontol 1975;2:67–79.

50. Hamp SE, Rosling B, Lindhe J. Periodontal treatment of multirooted teeth. J Clin Periodontol 1975;2:126–135.

51. Lindhe J, Nyman S. Long-term maintenance of patients treated for advanced periodontal disease. J Clin Periodontol 1984; 11:504–514.

52. Haffajee AD, Socransky SS, Smith C, Dibart S. Relation of baseline microbial parameters to future periodontal attachment loss. J Clin Periodontol 1991;18:744–750.

53. Slots J. The predominant cultivatable microflora of advanced periodontitis. Scand J Dent Res 1977;85:114–122.

54. Slots J. Subgingival microflora in periodontal disease. J Clin Periodontol 1979;6:351–382.

55. Mousques T, Listgarten MA, Phillips RW. Effect of scaling and root planing on the composition of humans' subgingival microbial flora. J Periodontal Res 1980;15:144–151.

56. Listgarten MA, Lindhe J, Helldén L. Effect of tetracycline and/or scaling on human periodontal disease. Clinical, microbiological, and histological observations. J Clin Periodontol 1978;5:246–271.

57. Slots J, Mashimo P, Levine MJ, Genco RJ. Periodontal therapy in humans. I. Microbiological and clinical effects of a single course of periodontal scaling and root planing, and of adjunctive tetracycline therapy. J Periodontol 1979;50:495–509.

58. Magnusson I, Lindhe J, Yoneyama T, Liljenberg B. Recolonization of a subgingival microbiota following scaling in deep pockets. J Clin Periodontol 1984;11:193–207.

59. Lavanchy D, Bickel M, Bachni P. The effect of plaque control after scaling and root planing on the subgingival microflora in human periodontitis. J Clin Periodontol 1987;14:295–299.

60. Greenwell H, Bissada NF. Variations in subgingival microflora from healthy and intervention sites using probing depth and bacteriologic identification criteria. J Periodontol 1984;55:391–397.

61. Van Winkelhoff AJ, Van der Velden U, De Graaf J. Microbial succession in recolonizing deep periodontal pockets after a single course of supra- and subgingival debridement. J Clin Periodontol 1988;15:116–122.

62. Southard SR, Drisko CL, Killoy WJ, et al. The effect of 2% chlorhexidine digluconate irrigation on clinical parameters and the level of Bacteroides gingivalis in periodontal pockets. J Periodontol 1989;60:302–309.

63. Sbordone L, Ramaglia L, Guletta E, Iacono V. Recolonization of the subgingival microflora after scaling and root planing in human periodontitis. J Periodontol 1990;61:579–584.

64. Braatz L, Garet JS, Claffey N, Egelberg JL. Antimicrobial irrigation of deep pockets to supplement nonsurgical periodontal therapy. II. Daily irrigation. J Clin Periodontol 1985; 12:630–638.

65. MacAlpine R, Magnusson I, Kiger R, et al. Antimicrobial irrigation of deep pockets to supplement nonsurgical periodontal therapy. I. Biweekly irrigation. J Clin Periodontol 1985;12: 568–577.

66. Forgas L, Gound S. The effects of antiformin–citric acid chemical curettage on the microbial flora of the periodontal pocket. J Periodontol 1987;58:153–158.

67. Oosterwaal P, Matee M, Mikx F, et al. The effect of subgingival debridement with hand and ultrasonic instruments on the subgingival microflora. J Clin Periodontol 1987;14:528–533.

68. Greenstein G. Periodontal response to mechanical non-surgical therapy: A review. J Periodontol 1992;63:118–130.

Lesions in the Oral Mucous Membranes and Periodontium

Terry D. Rees
• Diseases of the Oral Mucous Membranes

John M. Wright
• Reactive and Neoplastic Lesions of the Periodontium

William F. Ammons, Jr
• Acute Lesions of the Periodontium

Diseases of the Oral Mucous Membranes

A variety of diseases of the oral mucous membranes are of interest to the practitioner who provides periodontal therapy as a part of a general dental practice. The diseases may be localized to the gingiva, or they may involve other intraoral tissues and extraoral sites such as the genitalia, skin, or internal organs. Several mucocutaneous disorders affect the oral cavity, and oral lesions frequently are the earliest manifestations of such disorders. In some instances, the gingiva may be a specific target tissue for autoimmune diseases. A detailed discussion of all diseases of the oral mucous membranes is beyond the scope of this text. Therefore, emphasis will be placed on those diseases most likely to elicit lesions involving the gingiva.

The International Workshop for a Classification of Periodontal Diseases and Conditions recognized that a number of non–plaque-induced conditions may affect the gingiva. These include diseases of specific bacterial, viral, or fungal origin; genetically derived conditions such as hereditary gingival fibromatosis; mucocutaneous or allergic conditions; and traumatic or foreign body reactions.[1] This section will address the more common non–plaque-induced conditions, with emphasis on conditions involving the oral mucosa.

Diagnosis of most mucosal diseases is based on a careful review of clinical, histologic, and immunologic data,

although microbial culturing or specific diagnostic tests are sometimes indicated. In the past, the term *desquamative gingivitis* was used as a pathological diagnosis for an unusual condition of the gingiva characterized by painful, erythematous, erosive, atrophic lesions. On occasion, the involved tissues featured epithelial sloughing or desquamation of the gingiva and the formation of bullae, vesicles, or blebs. The condition was noted to occur frequently in elderly individuals, particularly women, and it was believed to represent an imbalance in sex hormones.[2,3] Today, with improved diagnostic techniques, it is clear that most gingival desquamation is caused by several vesiculobullous mucocutaneous diseases.[4-6] Therefore, in this text, desquamative gingivitis is not considered to be a specific disease diagnosis; rather, it is a clinical feature of several diseases and disorders.

Mucocutaneous Disorders

Lichen Planus
Lichen planus (LP) is a relatively common inflammatory mucocutaneous disease that is immunologically mediated. Its etiology is unknown, although its immunologic makeup suggests that it represents a cell-mediated immune response to intraepithelial antigens in skin or mucous membranes.[7-9] LP may develop spontaneously or in response to a wide variety of drugs, dental hygiene products, or dental restorative materials.[10-12] Drug-related LP appears to be more common among individuals with con-

comitant medical conditions that are associated with granulomatous inflammation. These conditions include rheumatoid arthritis, Crohn disease, hepatitis C, and thyroiditis.[13] A relatively strong association has been suggested between oral LP and chronic hepatitis associated with hepatitis C or its treatment, although the risk appears low in the United States in comparison with the Mediterranean countries, Eastern Europe, and developing countries in Africa and the Middle East.[14–17] Two large studies in Sweden and the United States suggested that LP affects up to 2% of the population, but racial differences may be found.[18,19] The disease may affect the skin, oral mucosa, or genitalia alone or concomitantly. Recent evidence indicates that genital lesions are relatively common in women exhibiting oral LP, and a gynecologic examination may be indicated after diagnosis of oral lesions.[20] However, lesions are confined to the oral cavity in the majority of patients seen in a dental setting. Oral lesions are more common in individuals older than 50 years, and LP is slightly more prevalent in women than in men.[21–23]

Skin lesions usually appear as keratotic, violaceous, pruritic plaques often affecting the flexor surfaces of the extremities, such as the inner aspect of the wrists. The fingers may be involved, which occasionally results in loss of the nails.[22] Oral lesions manifest in more varied forms, and lesions may persist for years.[24] Persistent lesions often change from one oral form to another over time.[24,25]

Oral lesions may appear as papular, reticular, or plaque-like white lesions that are usually asymptomatic. Patients with these types of LP may notice a rough texture to the involved oral tissues. The reticular form occurs most frequently, often affecting the buccal mucosa, although gingival lesions may be present.[26] Painful erosive lesions may occur, either separately or in conjunction with the white lesions. Atrophic, ulcerative, and bullous forms of erosive lichen planus (ELP) have been described, and their presence often causes persistent burning. Atrophic LP appears as diffuse, erythematous lesions that may have lacy, reticular borders. Oral bullous LP is rarely encountered, but a small percentage of patients with LP experience transient small bullae or vesicles on the mucous membranes.[27,28]

Large studies confirm that the buccal mucosa is the most common site of occurrence of LP.[24–26] The gingiva, however, is often affected by ELP, perhaps due to the traumatic stresses imposed on these tissues during mastication and oral hygiene procedures. On occasion, ELP is confined entirely to the gingiva, creating a difficult clinical differential diagnosis because the gingival lesions may appear very similar to those of autoimmune diseases.[27]

The classic histologic features of LP include epithelial hyperkeratosis and acanthosis. In skin, the epithelial rete ridges assume a saw-toothed configuration, although this is not always a feature of mucosal lesions. In the classic histologic manifestation, liquefaction degeneration occurs in the basal cell layer of the epithelium. This degenerative process may account for the tendency for epithelial desquamation in erosive lesions. The final and most distinct histologic feature of LP is a dense band of lymphocytic (T-cell) infiltration in the connective tissue immediately subjacent to the basement membrane. This lymphocytic infiltrate may also occur, however, in other mucocutaneous diseases such as graft-versus-host disease, lupus erythematosus (LE), erythema multiforme (EM), and epithelial dysplasia or malignancy.[29–37]

Immunofluorescence studies of LP do not display distinguishing pathognomonic features, yet direct immunofluorescence (DIF) may be of significant value in confirming the diagnosis and in ruling out other diseases.[38] In skin lesions, the DIF presence of immune reactive cytoid bodies is suggestive of LP. In mucosal lesions, however, several centers have reported that the accumulation of fibrin or fibrinogen in a linear pattern along the basement membrane zone supports the diagnosis.[5,39,40] These immunofluorescence findings are also nonspecific and sometimes may be found in other mucocutaneous diseases, such as lupus erythematosus. Therefore, it is important to stress that DIF studies are supportive of, but not diagnostic for, LP. Ultimately, diagnosis of LP is based on a compilation of clinical, histologic, and immunologic findings. Differential diagnosis of white LP lesions includes leukoplakia, hyperkeratosis, cheek biting, and leukoedema. Differentiation of ELP on the gingiva or other oral sites may be more difficult, since the lesions must be distinguished from conditions such as lupus erythematosus, erythema migrans, secondary syphilis, other vesiculobullous diseases, and dysplasia or even squamous cell carcinoma. A universally accepted diagnostic criteria for LP is needed to better distinguish it from other conditions and to better determine its possible role as a premalignant lesion.[41]

Drug-induced tissue reactions often present features that are indistinguishable from those of LP, based on clinical, histologic, and immunofluorescent evaluation. These lichenoid reactions may occur in response to any drug, but nonsteroidal anti-inflammatory agents, antihypertensive drugs, and antimalarial agents are most often implicated.[42,43] On rare occasions, dental restorative materials have induced allergic lichenoid reactions in soft tissue in close contact with a restoration.[44–48]

The relationship between LP and oral cancer remains contentious.[49,50] Several well-documented case reports and recent prospective studies have suggested that LP—especially the plaque and erosive forms—may be a precancerous condition.[25,26,51–60] Holmstrup et al[25] reported that 1.5% of 611 patients with LP who were observed for 1 to 26 years ultimately developed squamous cell carcinoma. This number was far greater than would have been predicted by chance. The investigators concluded that oral LP met the World Health Organization criteria to be classified as a precancerous condition, which is defined as a generalized state associated with a significantly increased risk of developing malignancy.[61] It is possible that tissue affected by LP is more susceptible to carcinogens, and malignant transformation has been reported among individuals usually not considered at risk for oral cancer.[60,62] Among 675 patients with oral LP being managed at one center, only 7.7% smoked, and only 10.1% used alcohol.[63]

Treatment of LP requires good clinical judgment and the establishment of treatment goals. It is probably inappropriate to administer potent drugs such as systemic corticosteroids to treat asymptomatic reticular LP. On rare occasions, however, malignant transformation has been reported in even these mild conditions.[26] Consequently, proper patient treatment dictates frequent observation of patients to detect any untoward changes at an early stage. The plaque form of LP is more likely to harbor undetected dysplastic changes, and therefore removal of small plaque lesions or frequent biopsy of larger lesions may be indicated. In contrast, painful erosive lesions should be treated vigorously in an effort to eliminate the lesions or to effect a transition to a milder form. Complete resolution of lesions does not predictably occur, but elimination of painful lesions is an appropriate goal.[24,26,27,63,64]

Proper management of oral LP requires the elimination of factors potentially causing lichenoid reactions, the elimination of local irritants such as bacterial plaque, and the effective use of therapeutic agents. The most successful treatment results have been achieved with topical, intralesional, or systemic corticosteroids.[65–69] Success has been reported using topical cyclosporin, retinoids, or tacrolimus; systemic administration of metronidazole or levamisole; and subcutaneous injections of low-molecular-weight heparin.[70–77] However, these therapeutic approaches should be considered experimental at this time. In dental practice, high-potency topical corticosteroids such as fluocinonide, betamethasone dipropionate, or clobetasol have been demonstrated to be effective, but some erosive lesions may prove refractory. In that event, referral to an oral medicine specialist or physician is suggested.

Graft-Versus-Host Disease

Graft-versus-host disease is a common manifestation of bone marrow transplantation in which the engrafted marrow reacts against the tissues of the host. As many as 70% of patients with bone marrow transplants may experience the condition, and the liver, lungs, gastrointestinal tract, skin, and mucosa may be affected. The condition may induce oral lesions that resemble systemic lupus erythematosus (SLE), scleroderma, Sjögren syndrome, or LP. Primary care of affected patients falls within the purview of

the oncologist. However, the dental practitioner may significantly improve oral lesions by initiating meticulous oral hygiene practices and frequent recall visits and by prescribing topical corticosteroid or topical azathioprine and antifungal therapy.[1,78,79]

Chronic Ulcerative Stomatitis

Chronic ulcerative stomatitis is a relatively newly described disease entity that clinically resembles the desquamative gingivitis associated with LP. Although only a few case reports have described the condition, it appears to be more resistant to therapy than LP. Diagnosis is based on immunohistochemistry techniques. Direct immunofluorescence reveals the deposition of antinuclear immunoglobulin G antibody in the basal third of the epithelium, whereas indirect immunofluorescence (IIF) is useful to confirm the presence of stratified epithelium-specific antinuclear antigens. Plaquenil (hydroxychloroquine sulfate) seems to be the drug of choice in treatment, although one case report described successful management using a potent topical corticosteroid.[80,81]

Mucous Membrane Pemphigoid

Mucous membrane pemphigoid, or MMP (cicatricial pemphigoid, benign MMP) is a chronic vesiculobullous autoimmune disease that most often affects the elderly, although the condition has been reported in children and young adults.[82–84] Females are affected twice as often as males. The condition is often extremely debilitating and occasionally life threatening.[85,86] Oral lesions are almost always present, but other mucosa may be involved, including the conjunctivae, nares, larynx, esophagus, upper respiratory tree, rectum, or genitalia.[87–92] On some occasions skin bullae may appear, whereas a related condition, bullous pemphigoid, predominantly affects skin and occasionally involves mucosa. The most common serious complication of MMP occurs when the eyes are affected; loss of vision may follow due to subsequent scarring (symblepharon) and other ocular changes.[93–95]

In MMP, the mouth usually is the first, and often the only, site of involvement. Approximately 90% to 95% of affected patients will have desquamative gingival lesions, although any oral tissue may be involved.[83,96] Affected gingival epithelium may be very fragile, and the epithelial surface is often lost in response to trauma (Nikolsky sign), leaving a shiny, erythematous, painful surface.[96,97] Blistering and ulceration may occur at any oral site, and recurrent lesions in the same site are not uncommon, usually triggered by mild irritation. Untreated lesions may remain constant for many years, although on other occasions they undergo recurrent periods of remission and exacerbation.[98,99]

Mucous membrane pemphigoid is an autoimmune disorder that may be associated with an immune response to one of several antigens found in the basement membrane zone of mucosal tissues.[99,100] The factor that initiates the response is usually unknown, although some internal systemic diseases and disorders may trigger a general autoimmune response, and pemphigoid-like lesions of skin and oral mucosa have been induced by the drugs captopril, carbamazepine, clonidine, furosemide, penicillamine, and practolol,[7,101–104] Some evidence suggests that a paraneoplastic form of pemphigoid may occur in conjunction with a variety of internal malignancies. Therefore, the dental clinician should consider referral to a physician for medical evaluation when oral lesions are diagnosed.[105,106]

Mucous membrane pemphigoid must be differentiated from bullous pemphigoid, pemphigus vulgaris, erosive LP, and a number of less common mucocutaneous conditions.[107] Bullous pemphigoid presents with histologic and DIF features essentially identical to those of MMP, and these conditions are usually differentiated based on clinical features.[102,108,109] Histologically, MMP features subepithelial vesicle formation and vacuolation in the basal lamina immediately below the intact epithelium. Initially, the underlying connective tissue is uninflamed, although a chronic inflammatory infiltrate may appear after the epithelium has separated from the connective tissue.[87,88] Direct immunofluorescence is very helpful in the diagnosis of MMP and in differentiating the condition from other autoimmune diseases. On biopsy, an intact lesion that is still covered by epithelium or even uninvolved mucosa will reveal the presence of immunoglobulins (usually immunoglobulin G) and complement (usually C3) arranged in a linear pattern along the basement membrane zone.[38,102,110] Serum indirect immunofluorescence is of little value, since circulating immunoglobulins are usually not present.[109] Recently, however, IIF techniques have been improved, and smaller quantities of circulating serum antibodies may be detected.[111] It is axiomatic that the diagnosis of oral MMP should be followed by early ophthalmologic evaluation to ensure the detection and treatment of any concomitant ocular lesions. Ocular pemphigoid is often more resistant to treatment than lesions in the oral cavity.[112–114]

Initial treatment of oral MMP is very similar to treatment described for erosive LP. Potent topical or intralesional corticosteroids are useful in managing localized lesions, and control of dental plaque and other local irritants is important.[115] Lesional tissue is often very friable and should be manipulated gently. Systemic intervention by a physician may be required, but the dental practitioner should remain involved in treatment of the patient, especially in helping to control the gingival effects of local irritants. Systemic therapy may include corticosteroids, dapsone, or other immunosuppressive or immunomodulatory agents prescribed by a physician or oral medicine expert.[73,116–119]

Pemphigus

Pemphigus is a life-threatening autoimmune disease that features formation of an intraepithelial blister of skin or mucous membranes. It affects both sexes equally and is more common in older individuals. It occurs in a variety of forms, but pemphigus vulgaris (PV) is the most common and most serious manifestation. If left untreated, the condition can lead to death, although mortality has decreased markedly in recent years due to better diagnostic methods and more effective treatment methods.[98,120,121]

Pemphigus vulgaris is of interest to practitioners because the oral cavity is virtually always involved in the disease, and the mouth is the initial site of involvement in over half of reported cases. The clinical manifestations of PV are very distinct. On skin it manifests as large bullae, often appearing on the trunk. The bullae form and break quickly, leaving painful, eroded surfaces. Death may occur due to loss of fluids and electrolytes from these surface erosions or as the result of secondary infection of the eroded lesions. Oral lesions are very similar in appearance to those described on the trunk. Bullae develop quickly and then rupture, leaving painful, irregular ulcerated lesions. Oral lesions can be very resistant to therapy, and severe oral pain may lead to nutrition deficiency because of poor dietary intake.[111,122,123] Similar lesions may be found on any mucous membranes, but the mouth appears particularly susceptible due to the constant trauma occurring in relation to eating, performance of oral hygiene measures, and exposure to irritants such as smoking or other harmful oral habits. The friability of the epithelium is reflected by the development of bullae under slight traumatic stimulus (Nikolsky sign). The percentage of cases in which the gingiva is involved is not known, although clinical experience suggests that desquamative gingivitis is a common manifestation of the disease. On occasion, the gingiva is the only site involved in early lesions.[124–127]

Other forms of pemphigus have been described, including pemphigus vegetans, pemphigus foliaceus, pemphigus erythematosus (a localized variant of pemphigus foliaceus), and drug-induced pemphigus. Pemphigus foliaceus rarely involves the oral cavity, but pemphigus vegetans may cause the formation of serpiginous, elevated white fungating masses in the mouth. These vegetations develop following the rupture of the initial presenting bullae.[120,127–130]

Differential diagnosis includes the mucocutaneous diseases previously described and other, less common vesiculobullous disorders. Although the irregular eroded oral lesions may be clinically distinct, on occasion LP or MMP may present in a similar fashion, and histologic and immunofluorescence studies are essential. Histologically, a suprabasal separation of the epithelium is evident. It occurs through the process of acantholysis, in which the epithelial intercellular desmosomes are disrupted. The epithelial basal cell layer is usually intact but irregularly arranged, and it forms the base of the histologic lesion.[131,132] Direct immunofluorescence reveals a distinct pattern of immunoglobulins and complement deposited in the intercellular spaces of the epithelium.[133] This occurs in lesional or intact tissue, a feature that may be important in selecting an appropriate biopsy site. Circulating antiepithelial antibodies are often identified in serum of affected patients using IIF, but levels of these antibodies may not be increased in early lesions confined to the oral cavity.[120]

Numerous reports have confirmed a fairly frequent relationship between PV and underlying systemic diseases, and most recently a new manifestation, termed *paraneoplastic pemphigus*, has been identified as an autoimmune response to the presence of certain benign or malignant tumors. The majority of these tumors are malignant and may include lymphoma, leukemia, sarcoma, and squamous cell carcinoma.[98,134,135] Definitive diagnosis of paraneoplastic pemphigus is often difficult, since the condition may induce unusual oral lesions that are similar in appearance to those found in erythema multiforme.[135,136]

Treatment of pemphigus usually involves the use of systemic corticosteroids or other immunosuppressive agents. The practitioner, therefore, primarily serves as diagnostician for oral lesions yet does have a role in control of local irritating factors that may contribute to lesion formation or recurrence.

Lupus Erythematosus

Lupus erythematosus is an autoimmune disease that may occasionally involve the oral cavity along with the skin and internal organs. The condition affects adults of all ages, and it occurs most commonly in women.[137,138] Lupus erythematosus manifests in three forms: systemic, subacute systemic, and discoid.[139,140] The oral cavity is most often affected by the discoid form (DLE), which exclusively involves mucocutaneous tissues. On occasion, the oral cavity is the only site of involvement, and the clinical and histologic features present may make it difficult to distinguish DLE from LP or simple hyperkeratosis.[141,142] The concomitant presence of typical skin lesions may facilitate the diagnosis, but it is important to be aware that mucocutaneous lesions may occur as a component of the systemic (SLE) or subacute systemic forms in up to 40% of affected patients.[143–147]

Classic clinical features of LE include a malar rash and the presence of round, hyperkeratotic plaques on the face and scalp in association with patchy loss of hair (alopecia). Renal involvement is common, and various hematologic and neurologic disorders may occur in SLE.[140,148,149] Lupus erythematosus–associated desquamative gingivitis

may present with the typical shiny, erythematous appearance previously described. More often, however, lesions are located on the palate, the buccal mucosa, or the vermillion border of the lips. Typically, oral lesions feature a central erythematous erosion or ulceration surrounded by radiating keratotic striae on the perimeter of the lesions.[141,142,145,146,150,151]

Diagnosis of DLE in the oral cavity is based on careful compilation of clinical, histologic, and immunologic data. Microscopic features include hyperkeratosis with keratin plugging accompanied by atrophy of rete ridges, liquefaction degeneration of the basal layer of epithelium, and thickening of the basement membrane. A bandlike inflammatory infiltrate is evident in underlying superficial connective tissue.[142,152,153] Because several of these features are similar to those described for oral LP, it is understandable that the diagnosis may occasionally be confused. Direct immunofluorescence usually reveals granular deposits of immunoglobulin, complement, and fibrinogen in the basement membrane and superior lamina propria. This has been described as the *lupus band* and is found in both lesional or normal skin or mucosa. Occasionally, however, this DIF feature may simulate MMP and further confuse the diagnosis.[142,144,154]

As discussed, atypical oral LE may occasionally be indistinguishable from oral LP. The possibility of LE should be considered in any LP lesion that fails to respond to usual therapy. Oral and cutaneous LE may respond favorably to topical or intralesional corticosteroids, but results are unpredictable, and a physician should be involved in the treatment. Antimalarial drugs, systemic corticosteroids, and immunosuppressive or cytotoxic drugs may be necessary to achieve a satisfactory result.[155–157]

Psoriasis

Psoriasis is a genetically determined, chronic mucocutaneous disorder that affects between 1% and 3% of the world population, especially light-skinned individuals who live in colder climates. Skin lesions feature localized or generalized erythematous papules or plaques that are covered with white hyperkeratotic scales (psoriasis vulgaris). On occasion, a pustular form of psoriasis causes serious illness in some patients. Sites of frequent involvement of psoriasis vulgaris include the elbows, knees, sacrum, and scalp. Lesions are believed to occur as a result of an immune stimulus that accelerates epithelial cell mitosis.[27,158]

Not all authorities agree that oral mucous membranes can be affected by psoriasis. Increasing evidence suggests, however, that oral psoriasis does exist and that it may occasionally be confused clinically with desquamative gingivitis.[159–161] Psoriasiform lesions of oral mucosa clearly do occur, manifesting as irregular erythematous areas with raised yellow-white borders. Such lesions have been described in psoriasis, benign migratory glossitis (geographic tongue), stomatitis areata migrans (ectopic geographic tongue), and Reiter syndrome.[162,163] All of these conditions have typical microscopic features of epithelial thickening with elongated rete ridges and lymphocytic infiltration of the submucosa. Intrapapillary microabscesses are common, and polymorphonuclear leukocytes may be found migrating throughout the epithelium.[164] Direct immunofluorescence of psoriatic lesions sometimes reveals the presence of immunoreactants in the stratum corneum of the epithelium, and this feature has been described in an oral biopsy specimen.[158,161,162,165,166]

Differentiation among the various oral psoriasiform lesions is based on clinical appearance and the presence or absence of other lesions or systemic symptoms. Gingival lesions are usually painless, although tongue and palatal lesions are sometimes associated with burning discomfort that may respond to administration of topical corticosteroids.[158]

Allergic Stomatitis

Allergy to a variety of dental hygiene products, soft drinks, candies, mints, and chewing gums has been reported with increasing frequency. The condition is often associated with the development of mucositis and a fiery red, erythematous gingivitis that is clinically consistent with desquamative gingivitis. Granulomatous reactions in the lips and oral mucosa and lichenoid lesions have also been reported. In most instances the causative agent is flavoring used in such products, with cinnamon aldehyde flavoring being the most common. Although allergic stomatitis can present several histologic features, the presence of a dense submucosal lymphocytic infiltrate and perivasculitis deeper in the connective tissue is considered to be highly suggestive of a cinnamon allergic reaction. Treatment involves discontinuance of the allergy-inducing substance, although topical steroid therapy may occasionally accelerate recovery.[167,168]

Other Mucosal Diseases of Interest

Recurrent Aphthous Stomatitis

Recurrent aphthous stomatitis (RAS) is an oral ulcerative condition that affects from 10% to 20% of the general population. Occurrence usually begins in childhood or within the first three decades of life, and outbreaks of lesions tend to be sporadic, with the frequency diminishing with increasing age.[169–171] Three forms of lesions have been described: minor, major, and herpetiform. Minor aphthae are most common. They are small, shallow ulcerations with slightly raised, erythematous borders. Lesions heal without scarring in 10 to 14 days.[172]

Major aphthae (periodontitis mucosa necrotica recurrens) are usually larger than 0.5 cm in diameter. They are indurated and have more irregular borders. The lesions are few in number, but they may persist for months and sometimes heal with scarring. Herpetiform aphthae were so named because they resemble the ulcerations remaining after herpetic vesicles have broken. They are unrelated to the herpes virus, however. They appear as small, discrete crops of multiple ulcerations that heal within 7 to 10 days.[173]

Recurrent aphthous stomatitis affects mobile mucosa that is not firmly bound to bone.[174] The condition is idiopathic, although an antigen-dependent cellularly mediated cytotoxicity has been suggested, and a genetic influence is suspected.[175–177] Precipitating factors have been implicated with outbreak of lesions. These include previous viral or bacterial infection, psychogenic stress, minor traumatic injury, and hypersensitivity to various foods such as nuts, chocolate, cereals, tomatoes, cheese, cow's milk, and citrus fruits. Nutrition deficiencies of iron, folic acid, zinc, vitamin B, vitamin C, or calcium are found in a small number of patients, and replacement therapy may prevent recurrence.[178–196]

A number of hematologic, gastrointestinal, and other disorders, including human immunodeficiency virus (HIV), have been associated with RAS, and the differential diagnosis includes Behçet syndrome, erythema multiforme, ulcerative colitis, Crohn disease, celiac disease, malabsorption syndrome, blood dyscrasias, or the mucocutaneous disorders previously discussed.[197–201]

Treatment for RAS is often empirical. Topical agents are frequently used, and successful results have been reported in controlled studies using antimicrobial mouthrinses, topical corticosteroids, tetracycline rinses, amlexanox, and acemannan hydrogel.[202,203] If lesions persist, a detailed search should be conducted for underlying etiologic factors. On occasion, short-term use of systemic corticosteroids or pentoxifylline may be necessary to manage refractory lesions.[27,204]

Behçet Syndrome

Behçet syndrome is an idiopathic, painful, ulcerative condition involving skin, genitalia, and the mucosa of the eyes and oral cavity. The etiology is unknown, although viral, genetic, and immunologic mechanisms have been suggested.[205] Oral lesions are consistent with recurrent aphthous stomatitis. Symptoms may also include arthralgia/arthritis, central nervous system involvement, intestinal ulcers, and orchitis/epididymitis. The mean age of onset is 30 years, and women may be affected more commonly than men. In some instances the condition appears hereditary, while allergic reactions may occasionally play a role.[206–208]

Oral lesions of Behçet syndrome may be managed as described for RAS.[209,210] Results are not predictable, however, and resistant or disseminated lesions are often best treated using systemic agents such as corticosteroids, cyclosporin, chlorambucil, thalidomide, colchicine, pentoxifylline, or others.[211–218]

Erythema Multiforme

Erythema multiforme is an inflammatory mucocutaneous disease of acute onset that manifests with distinctive skin lesions with or without oral involvement. It primarily affects children and young adults.[219] Erythema multiforme minor causes symmetric erythematous skin wheals surrounded by a circumferential halo (target lesions). The oral cavity may or may not be involved, but on some occasions the oral cavity is the only site of lesions, which appear as bullae that burst rapidly and leave erythematous erosions and ulcerations.[220,221] Oral lesions often develop a grayish pseudomembrane, and a hemorrhagic crust may form on the lips.[222–224] In EM major (Stevens-Johnson syndrome), the oral cavity is usually affected along with the genitalia, conjunctiva, and skin, and multisystem involvement may occur.[225] Both forms tend to recur.

Erythema multiforme lesions may be induced by drugs such as sulfonamides, various antibiotics, anticoagulants, and other miscellaneous agents, or by infectious agents such as *Mycoplasma pneumoniae* or a recent outbreak of herpes simplex. On most occasions, however, no etiologic factor can be identified.[223,226–231]

Clinically, an outbreak of EM may be preceded by prodromal symptoms for 1 to 14 days prior to onset of lesions. Symptoms may include fever, headache, general malaise, nausea, vomiting, and diarrhea. Untreated lesions may continue for 10 days to several months, although spontaneous healing may occur 2 to 3 weeks after onset.[219,223,232] Recurrence is common, and sometimes lesions become chronic.[233]

Histopathologically, EM may feature either intraepithelial or sub-basal bulla formation and a perivascular monocytic inflammatory infiltrate.[234,235] Direct immunofluorescence reveals perivascular and basement membrane zone deposits of immunoglobulins and complement, accompanied by occasional cytoid bodies. Indirect immunofluorescence is negative.[236,237]

Erythema multiforme usually can be differentiated from other bullous diseases by its acute onset and characteristic lesions. Clinical differentiation between oral EM and primary herpetic gingivostomatitis is sometimes difficult, yet most important. Systemic corticosteroids are often used in treatment of EM but are contraindicated in primary herpes. Consequently, on occasion, treatment must be palliative until a clear diagnosis is established. Acyclovir may be useful in management of the recurrent or chronic oral EM that occurs in association with a previous herpes simplex outbreak. Drug-associated EM is managed by withdrawal of the implicated agent.[238,239]

Herpes Simplex Viral Infections

The herpes family of viruses includes the herpes simplex virus types 1 and 2 (HSV-1 and HSV-2), herpes varicella zoster virus, cytomegalovirus, and Epstein-Barr virus. All are capable of causing oral disease. More recently, a number of additional human herpesvirus subtypes have been identified, although the role of these subtypes in disease is generally unknown. However, human herpesvirus 8 has been associated with Kaposi sarcoma in immunocompromised individuals.[240] This discussion is limited to those conditions caused by the HSV.

Most individuals experience a high rate of exposure to the HSV within the first 5 years of life. A second high rate of exposure occurs with the onset of sexual activity. Most oral infections are caused by HSV-1, while genital herpes is caused by HSV-2. HSV-2 can also cause oral lesions, and conversely, some genital HSV infections are caused by HSV-1.[241]

Primary herpetic gingivostomatitis is the most common viral disease that affects the gingiva. It is caused by the first encounter of an individual with HSV, and oral systemic signs and symptoms begin to appear in about 10 to 14 days. Only an estimated 10% of individuals exposed to HSV experience primary gingivostomatitis. The condition features multiple oral vesicles and ulcers, severely inflamed gingiva, cervical and submandibular lymphadenopathy, and increased temperature. Diagnosis is usually made based on the clinical features. In some instances, however, acute necrotizing ulcerative gingivitis (NUG) may be superimposed, making diagnosis difficult, and on occasion, HSV lesions may be suggestive of erythema multiforme, as previously discussed.[239,242]

After the initial infection, the HSV is sequestered in an immunoprivileged site such as the trigeminal ganglion, and it becomes latent. The virus may be reactivated by various stimuli, including trauma, illness, emotional stress, exposure to ultraviolet light, and immunosuppression.[243–245] Reactivation of the virus may occur without symptoms (recurrence), although it often induces coalescing vesicles in the oral cavity (recrudescence) or on the vermilion border of the lip (herpes labialis).[246] An estimated one third to one half of the HSV-infected population experiences recrudescence. Immunocompromised individuals may experience atypical forms of the infection, which tend to be chronic or progressive. In recent years, however, the advent of highly active antiretroviral therapy has resulted in a marked decrease in opportunistic viral, bacterial, or fungal oral infections among individuals infected with HIV.[247]

Differential diagnosis of primary herpetic gingivostomatitis includes severe gingivitis, bacterial stomatitis, acute NUG, erythema multiforme, and vesiculobullous diseases. Viral culturing and viral typing are reliable diagnostic techniques, while cytologic smears and biopsies for the presence of inclusions and multinucleated cells may occasionally be of value. Assay techniques using enzyme-linked immunosorbent assay or immunofluorescence assay are rapid and nearly as sensitive as viral isolation.[248,249]

Palliative and supportive care remain essential in the management of primary or recurrent oral HSV infections. A soft diet, a soothing mouthrinse, analgesics, and antipyretics may be helpful. Systemic administration of acyclovir has not been demonstrated to alter the clinical course of primary herpes, but it may reduce the duration of viral shedding during which the patient is potentially infectious. Systemically administered acyclovir, valacyclovir, or famciclovir may be beneficial for immunocompromised patients, although resistant viral strains have been reported.[250–252] Some patients experience relief from recurrent herpes labialis by application of topical acyclovir, penciclovir, or n-docosanol, provided the therapeutic regimen is initiated in the very early stages of the lesion.[253,254] A recent study indicates that famciclovir combined with a topical corticosteroid gel may be beneficial for herpes labialis with minimal untoward effects.[255] A variety of alternative treatments for herpes labialis have been reported but require further study.[256–259]

Reactive and Neoplastic Lesions of the Periodontium

A variety of reactive and neoplastic lesions arise from the periodontium and as such can simulate the gingival or intrabony manifestations of inflammatory periodontal disease. The soft tissue lesions are characterized by localized tumefaction. Some of these localized overgrowths are not inflammation mediated and can therefore be distinguished from periodontal disease by the lack of the erythema that characterizes inflammatory conditions. It is possible, however, for those overgrowths to result in pseudopockets, with subsequent inflammatory changes superimposed. Many of these tumefactions eventually reach sufficient size that they are incompatible with the minor swelling one sees in chronic gingivitis/periodontitis that results from tissue edema. Many of the reactive gingival lesions are red, and—particularly the early lesions— might be indistinguishable from inflammatory periodontal disease. While practitioners might initially choose to manage these lesions by conventional periodontal therapy, the lack of response to therapy should alert them to the possibility

that the lesions do not represent routine periodontal disease. Biopsy and microscopic examination would then be a prudent course of action.

The intrabony neoplasms and reactive lesions of the periodontium are less commonly mistaken for inflammatory periodontal disease. Radiographically, there is usually a superior margin of bone separating the lesion from the overlying crestal bone, and clinically, there is no communication to the lesion through the sulcus by periodontal probing. Additionally, many of these lesions are characterized radiographically by areas of radiopacity, a feature rarely encountered in chronic periodontitis.

Gingival Lesions

The majority of soft tissue gingival growths are reactive, and most are pyogenic granulomas, peripheral giant cell granulomas, or one of the varieties of fibroma. The most common of the gingival lesions are those of fibrous connective tissue origin, or *fibromas*.[260] Because there is some controversy regarding nomenclature, this lesion has also been called *fibrous epulis, fibrous polyp,* or *fibrous hyperplasia* by those who argue that these lesions represent hyperplastic tissue responses rather than true neoplasms. While it is widely accepted that these fibrous growths are not neoplastic,[261] the author prefers the term *fibroma*, realizing that the suffix comes from the Greek *oma*, which means "tumor," and the term itself does not imply that a growth is neoplastic.

There are two distinct fibrous lesions affecting gingiva— one that arises from gingival connective tissue within the lamina propria and another that arises from superficial periodontal ligament. The latter is referred to as *peripheral odontogenic fibroma* or *peripheral ossifying fibroma* because the lesion arises from an odontogenic tissue and often contains calcification.

Gingival Fibroma
Gingival fibromas are usually sessile swellings of normal color. They often begin within a gingival papilla but can progress to affect both buccal and lingual gingiva and, on occasion, become sufficiently large to move teeth. Surface ulceration with superimposed inflammatory change is seen in some fibromas. Although purely speculative, there is a theory that the fibroma arises from local irritants such as plaque, calculus, poor restorative margins, or denture clasps or margins. These may induce localized inflammation with liberation of growth factors from inflammatory cells.

An interesting variant of the fibroma was first reported in 1974 as giant cell fibroma,[262] which should not be confused with giant cell granuloma. The giant cell fibroma is particularly important when discussing periodontal conditions because approximately 50% of them occur on the

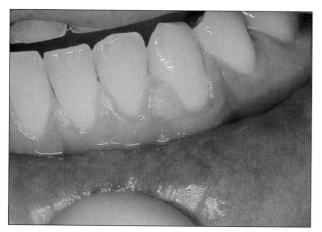

Fig 29-1 Giant cell fibroma between the lateral incisor and canine.

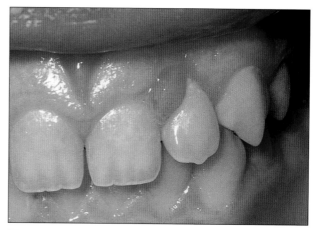

Fig 29-2 Early lesion of peripheral odontogenic fibroma between the left central and lateral incisors.

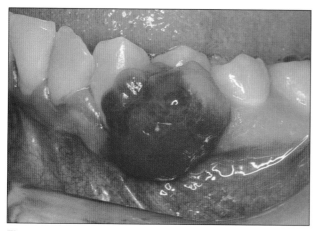

Fig 29-3 Peripheral odontogenic fibroma.

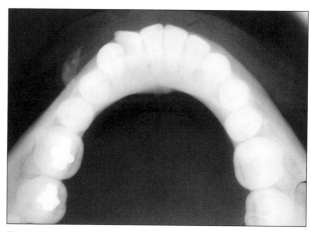

Fig 29-4 Radiograph of peripheral odontogenic fibroma demonstrating calcification.

gingiva.[263] The lesion often has an irregular, almost papillary surface (Fig 29-1); in fact, it is commonly mistaken for a papilloma. The lesion derives its name from the presence microscopically of numerous very plump, stellate, binucleated or trinucleated fibroblasts.

Peripheral Odontogenic (Ossifying) Fibroma

The peripheral odontogenic fibroma is similar clinically to the gingival fibroma except that it presumably arises from cells in the periodontal ligament and occurs only on the gingiva. Early lesions can mimic periodontal disease (Fig 29-2). There are two distinct subtypes of odontogenic fibroma, and they have been reviewed by Gardner.[264] The most common type consists of an exceedingly cellular fibroblastic stroma containing calcifications in the form of bone, cementum, or dystrophic calcification. Occasion-

ally the amount of mineralization is sufficient to be demonstrated radiographically (Figs 29-3 and 29-4). The lesion occurs most often in the second and third decades of life and is commonly ulcerated. Because the lesion presumably arises deep within the gingiva from the periodontal ligament, it is often incompletely removed when "excised," a feature that accounts for its significant recurrence rate of approximately 15%.[265] The second subtype of odontogenic fibroma is that proposed by the World Health Organization[266] and subsequently reviewed by Buchner and colleagues.[267] It is known as *peripheral odontogenic fibroma, WHO type.* This lesion is rare and is characterized histologically by cellular fibrous connective tissue containing odontogenic epithelium and calcification, often in the form of dentinoid.

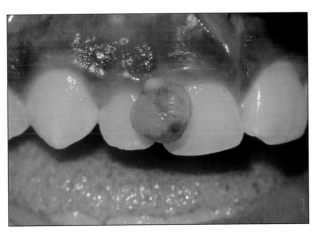

Fig 29-5 Pyogenic granuloma of anterior maxillary gingiva.

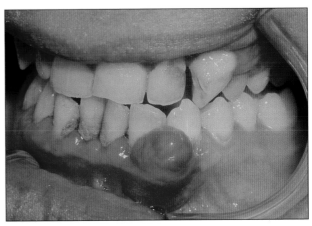

Fig 29-6 Peripheral giant cell granuloma.

Pyogenic Granuloma

One of the most common reactive tumors occurring on skin and oral mucosa is the pyogenic granuloma. Although *pyogenic* means "pus producing," this is a misnomer because the lesion contains no pus and is not caused by bacterial infection. Rather, the pyogenic granuloma is a hyperplastic response of the body's most basic reparative tissue (granulation tissue) to local injury. Although pyogenic granulomas can affect any intraoral site, the preferred site is gingiva. The lesions are usually ulcerated and have a reddish surface because of the prominence and dilation of the blood vessels within the lesions (Fig 29-5). They may bleed spontaneously or following minor trauma. Lesions range from a millimeter to several centimeters, and they may grow rapidly. The pyogenic granuloma occurs over all age ranges but does have a distinct female predilection.[268] This may be due in part to the effect of chorionic gonadotropins on vascular endothelium during pregnancy. In fact, pyogenic granulomas are commonly encountered in pregnant women, where they are also referred to as *pregnancy tumors*.

The pyogenic granuloma is treated by surgical excision. It occasionally recurs, because it is unencapsulated and it is often difficult clinically to determine the margins and extent of the lesion. Recurrence is lessened by removing any irritants or etiologic factors during surgery.

Peripheral Giant Cell Granuloma

The peripheral giant cell granuloma is another reactive soft tissue tumor that occurs exclusively on the gingiva. It is a sessile or pedunculated lesion that is usually red or bluish because of the vascularity and hemorrhage within the lesion and the deposition of hemosiderin (Fig 29-6). The lesion has a predilection for the gingiva anterior to the permanent molars and is more common in women. All ages are affected, but the peak incidence is between 40 and 70 years.[269,270] Lesions do arise on the edentulous alveolar ridge, where they may cause resorption of bone and produce a characteristic "cupping" of the superior aspect of the alveolar ridge seen on radiographs.

The peripheral giant cell granuloma derives its name from the presence microscopically of numerous multinucleated giant cells. The nature and origin of the giant cells have been widely debated, but Bonetti and colleagues[271] recently reported that the giant cells react with a monoclonal antibody for osteoclasts and were negative for typical markers for monocytes or phagocytic cells. It is logical that the cells are related to osteoclasts and arise from bone-related tissues, either periosteum or periodontal ligament. This is supported by the fact that lesions occur only on tissues supported by bone and are not seen in sites such as the tongue, cheek, or lips. The peripheral giant cell granulomas should be removed surgically, and removal of local irritants should reduce recurrence.

Other Gingival Lesions

The majority of gingival tumors are reactive and have been discussed previously. It should be remembered that virtually every soft tissue neoplasm, both benign and malignant, can and does on rare occasion occur gingivally. Most of the odontogenic tumors occur extraosseously in the gingiva.[272] Perhaps one of the most significant other neoplasms that affects gingiva is Kaposi sarcoma, a vascular malignancy of endothelial cells that typically affects immunosuppressed patients. Today, the immunosuppression is invariably secondary to HIV infection, where the presence of Kaposi sarcoma defines acquired immunodeficiency syndrome (AIDS). Oral lesions are common, and almost half of the patients who develop Kaposi sarcoma will have oral or perioral lesions.[273,274] They have a marked predilection intraorally for the palate and gingiva, where they present as single or multiple red to bluish swellings (Fig 29-7).[275]

Finally, the most significant neoplasm to affect the gingiva is squamous cell carcinoma. Although oral cancer does not frequently affect gingiva, it is often more advanced when diagnosed,[276] and it is more lethal in this site.[277] Patients often report pain, swelling, and loosening of teeth. Clinically, the lesions may be papillary, ulcerated, and necrotic, and they may have associated areas of surface redness or whiteness. A distinct type of oral cancer, verrucous carcinoma, is a slow-growing, predominantly exophytic, whitish, papillary carcinoma that has a marked predilection for the gingiva or alveolar ridge[278] and has a strong association with topical tobacco use.[279]

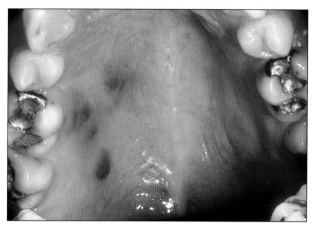

Fig 29-7 Multifocal Kaposi sarcoma of palatal gingiva.

Intrabony Lesions

The entire spectrum of bone pathology affects the jaws, but these conditions are rarely confused with chronic periodontitis. However, there is a group of disorders that presumptively arise from progenitor cells within the periodontal ligament. There is some evidence that individual genes within these progenitor cells can be upregulated or downregulated and that a single cell can differentiate into an osteoblast or cementoblast.[280,281] A proliferation of these cells would be fibrous, and the cells could produce bone, cementum, or both. This has led many investigators to conclude that many of the fibro-osseous or cemento-osseous lesions of the jaws originate in the periodontal ligament (PDL) and make up a spectrum of reactive and neoplastic lesions. The microscopic features of this entire group of disorders are remarkably similar, and most oral and maxillofacial pathologists feel that the most accurate classification is determined only by very careful clinical, radiographic, and histopathological correlation.

Dysplastic Cemento-Osseous Lesions of PDL Origin

The cemento-osseous dysplasias represent a group of related disorders affecting the ability of cells of the periodontal ligament to remodel bone and cementum. These disorders were once thought to be reactive lesions, but there is little scientific evidence to support such speculation. They are more appropriately considered dysplastic conditions, not in the sense that they are considered premalignant but rather because they represent developmental impairment of normal bone and cementum remodeling.[282] These remodeling defects will produce radiographic changes that can be radiolucent, mixed radiolucent/radiopaque, or predominantly radiopaque. Because these lesions are dysplastic rather than neoplastic, they

usually do not move teeth, cause bony expansion, or produce symptoms. The subclassification of these disorders is based on the anatomic site affected and whether lesions are multifocal. When the process is confined to the anterior mandible, it is known as *periapical cemento-osseous dysplasia (PCOD)*. Isolated lesions affecting sites other than the anterior mandible are known as *focal cemento-osseous dysplasia*. When multifocal areas are involved, often all quadrants of the maxilla and mandible, the term *florid cemento-osseous dysplasia (FCOD)* is used.

Periapical cemento-osseous dysplasia. PCOD is also known as *periapical cemental dysplasia* or *cementoma*. Lesions can be single or multiple but characteristically affect the apices of the anterior mandibular teeth. PCOD has a marked predilection for young to middle-aged black females. The female-to-male distribution in the United States is approximately 10:1, and the condition affects blacks in as many as 70% of cases. PCOD is uncommonly seen in patients younger than 20 years old, with most cases being diagnosed in the third to fourth decades of life. Most patients are asymptomatic and experience no bony expansion or, occasionally, minimal expansion.[283,284]

PCOD is usually discovered through the examination of routine radiographs. The radiographic findings are varied and depend on the stage of the condition when discovered. Lesions tend to undergo a maturational sequence in which they begin as completely radiolucent lesions and mature through a mixed radiolucent/radiopaque stage into predominantly radiopaque lesions (Figs 29-8 and 29-9). Maturation, however, may take years.[285] The margins of the lesions are usually noncorticated. The lytic stage of the condition often mimics periapical lesions secondary to devitalized pulps. It is extremely important to perform vitality testing to make this distinction, because teeth affected by PCOD are vital. Failure to determine vitality

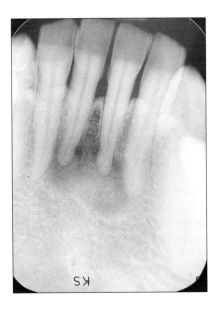

Fig 29-8 Periapical cemento-osseous dysplasia, early radiolucent lesions.

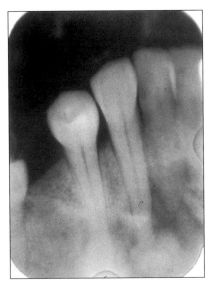 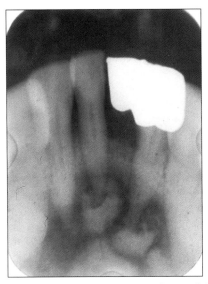 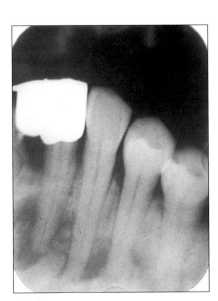

Fig 29-9 Periapical cemento-osseous dysplasia, intermediate radiolucent/radiopaque stage.

often leads to a misdiagnosis of periapical pathology and subsequent mismanagement by extraction or root canal therapy. As lesions become more opaque, the opacities may show ankylosis with the tooth roots.

The diagnosis of PCOD can usually be made from the clinical and radiographic findings; biopsy is usually not necessary. The condition tends to stabilize in the sclerotic stage, and no treatment is necessary. Occasionally, lesions remodel and complete resolution is revealed radiographically,[286] a feature that supports the dysplastic nature of the condition.

Focal cemento-osseous dysplasia. Isolated or focal lesions that are radiographically and histologically similar to PCOD but affect sites other than the anterior mandible have been recognized for years.[287] They have been misdiagnosed as cemento-ossifying fibromas, or COFs (because of the microscopic similarity), and have been treated as neoplasms. In 1994 the condition was first documented, a relationship to POCD was speculated, and the name *focal cemento-osseous dysplasia* was proposed.[288]

Focal cemento-osseous dysplasia is typically discovered during the second to fourth decade of life, the mean age being 29.9 years. The female-to-male ratio is 2:1, and the condition affects the mandible four times more frequently than the maxilla. The most frequently affected site is the posterior mandible. The racial predilection is not nearly as distinct as in PCOD, although approximately a third of

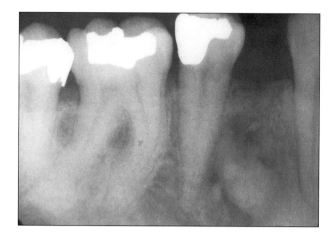

Fig 29-10 Focal cemento-osseous dysplasia, mixed radiolucent/radiopaque lesion.

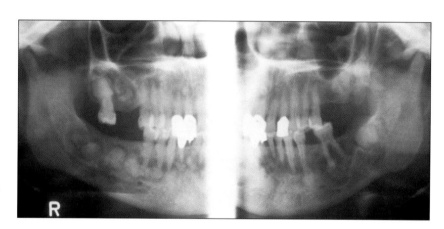

Fig 29-11 Florid cemento-osseous dysplasia, multiquadrant globular opacities with areas of radiolucency.

cases involve African Americans. Most patients are asymptomatic, but some bony expansion is not uncommon.[288]

The radiographic findings are highly variable. Lesions tend to be relatively well demarcated but may or may not show cortication. The average lesion size is approximately 2 cm. Mixed radiolucent/radiopaque lesions are most common (Fig 29-10), but many are completely radiolucent and, as in PCOD, will mimic periapical lesions from devitalized teeth. Teeth affected by focal cemento-osseous dysplasia are vital, however. Predominantly radiopaque lesions are also seen. It is interesting that approximately 21% of cases are found in previous extraction sites.[289] The radiographic maturation of lesions seen in PCOD has not been documented for the focal lesions.

Although the clinical and radiographic features of focal cemento-osseous dysplasia are characteristic, they are not always diagnostic, and biopsy by curettage may be necessary to establish a definitive diagnosis. Once the diagnosis is established, no further treatment is indicated. Occasionally patients develop additional lesions, however, and the pattern of florid cemento-osseous dysplasia evolves.

Florid cemento-osseous dysplasia. Within the spectrum of reactive lesions of periodontal ligament origin are generalized, multiquadrant radiopacities that tend to be globular or rounded and limited to the alveolar processes (Fig 29-11). Historically, the condition has been reported under a bewildering and confusing array of terms, including multiple ossifying fibroma, sclerosing osteitis, multiple enostosis, multiple osteoma, gigantiform cementoma, chronic diffuse sclerosing osteomyelitis, and periapical osteofibroma. The most definitive publication of this condition was in 1976,[290] and today the preferred designation is *florid cemento-osseous dysplasia.*

FCOD has a marked predilection for middle-aged to elderly black females, who in some series account for 90% of cases.[290,291] Most patients are asymptomatic, and lesions tend to be nonexpansible. On radiographic analysis, lesions can be radiolucent, mixed, or radiopaque, but they tend to be rounded and highly sclerotic. Lesions are multiple and affect several sites, often all four quadrants of the maxilla and mandible.

The bone and/or cementum in FCOD is sufficiently dense that it compromises blood flow, and patients are therefore prone to infection. If the bone becomes exposed

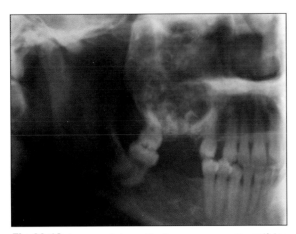

Fig 29-12 Large radiolucent/radiopaque cemento-ossifying fibroma of the right posterior maxilla.

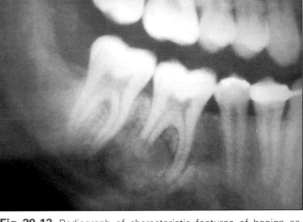

Fig 29-13 Radiograph of characteristic features of benign cementoblastoma. Note the radiopaque tumor fused to the tooth root with a peripheral zone of radiolucency.

through caries, periodontal disease, or extraction, it has little resistance to infection, and acute osteomyelitis ensues, often resulting in sequestration and draining sinuses. Antibiotics are often of little benefit, and the infection may have to be removed surgically. Because patients with FCOD often present with bony infection, the condition has been confused clinically with diffuse sclerosing osteomyelitis. Although infection can induce sclerosing osteomyelitis, the infection in FCOD is caused by the sclerotic bone rather than inducing it.

Gigantiform cementoma. Gigantiform cementoma is a condition that is clinically and radiographically very similar to FCOD. The two conditions are distinguished because gigantiform cementoma is inherited, being transmitted as an autosomal-dominant trait,[292] and FCOD is not inherited.

Neoplasms of PDL Origin

Cemento-ossifying fibroma. One of the more common neoplasms arising from the periodontal ligament is cemento-ossifying fibroma. Although some texts continue to define ossifying fibromas and cementifying fibromas as separate and distinct neoplasms, there is emerging consensus that the two lesions are identical, and whether the neoplastic cells produce bone, cementum, or both has no clinical relevance.[293,294] It was recently suggested that a significant number of lesions that historically would have been classified as COF are in fact dysplastic, and today would be redesignated as FCOD.[288]

COF occurs mostly in middle age, with a marked predilection for the mandible (usually midbody) and a slight predilection for females and blacks. Radiographically, lesions are in association with the roots of teeth, although they do occur in edentulous areas. The neoplasm

is always well circumscribed, and it ranges from completely radiolucent to more radiopaque as the tumor cells produce more bone and cementum (Fig 29-12). COF, however, does not go through a maturational sequence from radiolucent to radiopaque. The condition should be treated by surgical excision, and the lesion classically enucleates when excised.

Benign cementoblastoma. The benign cementoblastoma is a neoplasm of cementoblasts that arises from cementum attached to a tooth root. The neoplasm shows no sex predilection but demonstrates a striking preference for the second and third decades of life. It affects the mandible over the maxilla in a ratio of about 5:1 and most commonly affects the mandibular first molar.[295] The tumor usually affects one tooth, but larger lesions occasionally involve multiple teeth.[296] Most patients present with pain, swelling, or both.

The radiographic features of cementoblastoma are highly characteristic. The neoplasm is usually characterized by radiopacity that shows fusion to the tooth root from which it arose. Because the neoplasm is encapsulated, it also shows a thin radiolucent border that separates it from surrounding normal bone (Fig 29-13).

Treatment of cementoblastoma is surgical excision with removal of the tooth to which it is attached. If the lesion is discovered early, however, the tooth can be treated endodontically and the neoplasm excised from the tooth root.[297]

Langerhans cell histiocytosis. One other condition that occurs in bone deserves mentioning because it classically produces radiographic features that mimic periodontal disease. Originally called histiocytosis X, the condition is often referred to today as *Langerhans cell granulomatosis* or *Langerhans cell histiocytosis*, because it has been doc-

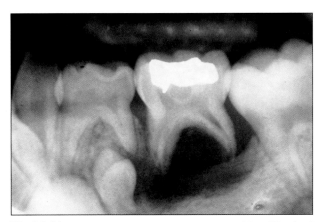

Fig 29-14 Radiograph displaying radiolucency with a "floating" primary molar caused by Langerhans cell histiocytosis.

umented that the lesional cell is a Langerhans cell,[298] a cell of the immune system involved in antigen processing. Langerhans cell histiocytosis is an immune disorder that classically affects children and young adults. Orally, it is primarily a bone condition, and jaw lesions classically affect tooth roots and mimic chronic periodontitis (Fig 29-14).[299]

Acute Lesions of the Periodontium

Acute lesions of the periodontium include a number of pathoses that may affect the periodontium and pose problems for the clinician during diagnosis or treatment planning. Under the new classification of periodontal diseases and conditions proposed at an International Workshop in 1999,[300] the conditions previously referred to as *acute lesions of the periodontium* have been subdivided into a number of categories. This new classification system is used in the following discussion of the lesions and conditions.

Acute lesions have in common an apparent sudden onset and are usually accompanied by pain.[301] Other signs and symptoms may be associated with the lesions to varying degrees. Historically, this category of dental diseases has included periodontal abscess, periapical abscess, pericoronitis, NUG, and necrotizing ulcerative periodontitis (NUP).[302] Occasionally other oral diseases, such as herpetic gingivostomatitis, aphthous stomatitis, and the desquamative lesions, have been included.[29] However, periodontal abscesses, NUG, and NUP are of primary concern to the periodontist.

Oral Abscesses

Abscesses are localized collections of pus that result from infection and suppuration in tissue. While an abscess may occur in any of the oral tissues or structures, the most common oral abscesses are the periodontal abscess and the periapical abscess.

An abscess may affect only the gingival tissues (gingival abscess), or it may affect the deeper structures of the periodontium (periodontal abscess), resulting in the rapid destruction of bone and attachment. An abscess may occur in any of the tissues of the periodontium by traumatic insertion of bacteria or a foreign body into the tissues,[303] but most occur within the wall of a previously existing gingival or periodontal pocket. While an abscess can occur in any pocket, certain configurations and locations of periodontal pockets are more prone to abscess formation than others. Narrow, tortuous pockets are more likely to harbor an abscess than are broad, shallow pockets. The interfurcal area of multirooted teeth is a common site for abscess formation. It is not uncommon for an abscess to occur in a pocket following incomplete instrumentation during scaling and root planing. The resolution of inflammation in the marginal gingiva can result in shrinkage and the development of a purse string–like effect at the pocket orifice (Fig 29-15). This constriction interferes with drainage from the infected area and results in the development of an abscess.[302,304] On rare occasions, abscess formation may occur following periodontal surgery.[304]

Perusal of the periodontal literature indicates that many clinicians believe that the incidence of periodontal abscess formation is higher in patients with diabetes mellitus. The development of multiple abscesses in a patient with periodontitis or the recurrence of abscess formation in a patient with known diabetes mellitus may be an indication for the referral of the patient for appropriate metabolic tests.[304]

Regardless of the inciting event, the result is the development of a localized acute inflammatory response that is characterized by a dense infiltrate of polymorphonuclear neutrophils (PMNs). This acute infiltrate is usually superimposed on the chronic round-cell infiltrate of gingivitis or periodontitis. Indeed, once drainage of the abscess is established via the sulcus or a stoma, in the absence of appropriate therapy, a round-cell infiltrate may become dominant, and a connective tissue capsule may be established around the abscess.[305]

Periapical abscesses are likewise acute inflammatory events that result in pain and swelling of the periodontal tissues; however, the inciting cause is of pulpal origin. The dental pulp can be injured by the extension of caries, chemical irritation from agents placed in proximity to the pulp, thermal damage during injudicious cavity or crown

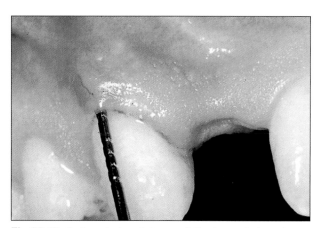

Fig 29-15 Early periodontal abscess following preliminary instrumentation. The facial aspect of a maxillary canine has a deep, narrow pocket associated with a bony dehiscence.

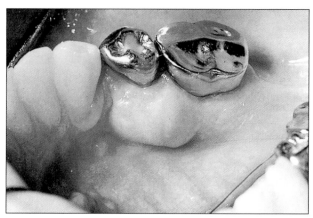

Fig 29-16 Periodontal abscess on the lingual aspect of a mandibular left second premolar. The premolar has been previously treated with endodontics.

preparation, or direct physical trauma. Although rare, it is possible for the pulp to become infected from the extension of a periodontal pocket to involve the apex of the tooth or via a lateral or accessory canal. The result of such injury may be pulpitis and/or necrosis of the dental pulp, with the development of pulpal symptoms; an apical abscess with pain, swelling, and ultimately drainage through the sulcus; a periodontal pocket; or a stoma in the gingiva or mucosa. The challenge to the therapist is to differentiate between the periodontal and the periapical abscess so that appropriate therapy may be provided (Fig 29-16).

Microbiologic Studies

Periodontal abscesses are generally mixed infections of three or more organisms that are residents of the periodontal pocket. A large number of different microorganisms can usually be isolated from an abscess with various culturing methods. The organisms isolated may vary among patients, among sites, and from different locations within the site, but they are predominantly gram-negative anaerobic rods. The common pathogens cultured from apical areas of the abscess are *Bacteroides melaninogenicus* subspecies, *Capnocytophaga* and *Fusobacterium* species, and *Vibrio* corroders. The exudate from the lesion may contain additional organisms, such as facultative streptococci and *Peptococcus* and *Peptostreptococcus* species.[306,307]

Differential Diagnosis: Periodontal Abscess

Patients presenting with periodontal abscesses usually report a sudden onset or recognition of the problem. The most common presenting complaints are pain or discomfort, and/or the appearance of an area of swelling that is

tender to touch, chewing, or toothbrushing. The area of the swelling may be confined to one tooth, or it may involve multiple teeth (Fig 29-17). It may extend along a fascial plane sufficiently to produce an obvious alteration in the facial profile. If the abscess occurs in a site in which periodontitis has resulted in advanced bone loss, a substantial baglike swelling of the soft tissues may result. This sac may contain a large quantity of purulent exudate but result in little or no patient discomfort (Fig 29-18).

Periodontal probing depths are exaggerated in areas of abscess formation. Probing is accompanied by bleeding, and if sufficient exudation has occurred, dilation of the sulcus/pocket with the probe will be followed by a purulent discharge. Because the site of most periodontal abscesses are periodontal pockets, the configuration of the orifice into the abscess is usually broad rather than narrow and tractlike.

The tooth affected by the abscess may display increased mobility if sufficient attachment loss has occurred from the abscess or previously from periodontitis. Rarely is the tooth hypersensitive to percussion unless the interfurcal zone or the apex of the root is involved. Abscesses in the interfurcal area can cause a slight elevation of the tooth in its socket, and thus pain on biting or on percussion of the tooth can result. The degree of discomfort from percussion, however, is usually much less than the discomfort from percussion of a tooth with a periapical abscess.[308]

Periodontal abscesses do not produce pulpal symptoms unless the process is sufficiently advanced to destroy the apical bone and devitalize the tooth via the apex or extension to the pulp through an accessory or lateral canal. The vitality of teeth with periodontal abscesses, as deter-

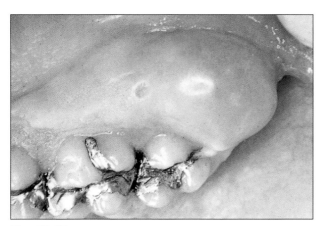

Fig 29-17 Periodontal abscess involving tuberosity and the palatal aspect of the maxillary first and second molars.

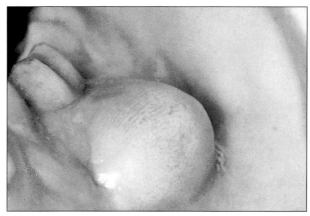

Fig 29-18 Large saclike abscess located on the facial aspect of a mandibular left first molar. Other than the enlargement, the patient was relatively asymptomatic.

mined using either thermal or electrical tests, is normal unless a tooth has been previously treated endodontically or is simultaneously affected by a pulpal lesion (a so-called combined lesion).

Differential Diagnosis: Periapical Abscess

The pain from periapical abscesses, in contrast to the pain from periodontal abscesses, is more diffuse; less well localized; and commonly described as having a sharp, lancinating, intermittent, or throbbing character. Thermal stimuli may either evoke or relieve the pain, depending on the state of pulpal degeneration. Once a sinus tract occurs and drainage is established, the pulp is nonreactive to all forms of pulpal testing. The tooth, however, may remain quite sensitive to percussion.

Therapeutic Management

Appropriate therapy for a periodontal abscess is determined by the stage of the abscess formation, the location and extent of the abscess, the extent and configuration of attachment loss on the affected tooth, and the role of the tooth in the overall periodontal treatment plan.

In any event, the therapy is directed at the resolution of pain and the drainage and debridement of the abscess. Many abscesses occur on teeth with advanced attachment loss or on teeth that are slated for removal for either periodontal or prosthetic reasons. If the abscess is localized and appropriate anesthesia can be obtained by regional nerve block without injecting in the infected area, then extraction and debridement of the socket provide the most expeditious course of therapy.

Many localized periodontal abscesses can be evacuated and thoroughly debrided through the gingival sulcus. Fol-

lowing appropriate anesthesia, the abscess can be explored with the periodontal probe. Then, using appropriate periodontal curettes, hoes, and files, the abscess is evacuated and the root surface and pocket debrided of all debris. If deemed necessary following debridement, the area may be irrigated with sterile saline. Postoperative instructions should be directed at the maintenance of good oral hygiene. Warm oral rinses may be beneficial in the resolution of edema in the site. Most patients require mild or no postoperative medication for discomfort. A large number of over-the-counter or prescription medications are available to patients who require medication. Antibiotic therapy is not indicated for most patients presenting with periodontal abscesses.

Other patients may present with abscesses involving a large area of the dentition or abscesses that are localized at a distance from the periodontal pocket and not amenable to thorough debridement through the sulcus. Such areas are amenable to treatment via two different approaches. One approach is the incision and drainage technique (Fig 29-19), in which a linear incision is placed through the soft tissue wall of the abscess and drainage established through the soft tissues. This is combined with thorough debridement of the root of the affected teeth. For areas that do not drain adequately or for very large abscesses, the insertion of a sterile rubber dam drain in the area is beneficial.

A second approach is seen in Fig 29-20. A patient with a combined periodontal-periapical lesion is treated by an isolated flap procedure. A mucoperiosteal flap of an appropriate dimension is elevated, providing excellent access for visualization and instrumentation of the affected area. Following debridement, the flap is reapproximated

Figs 29-19a to 29-19d Incision and drainage of a periodontal abscess on the palatal aspect of a maxillary right lateral incisor.

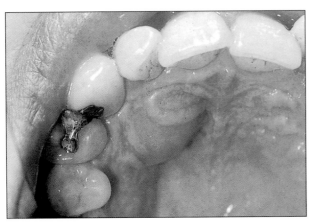

Fig 29-19a Initial appearance of the abscess, 24 hours after first symptoms.

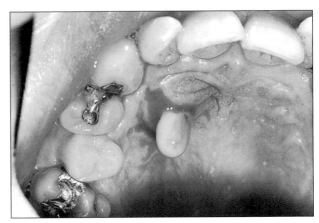

Fig 29-19b Linear incision to provide drainage of exudate.

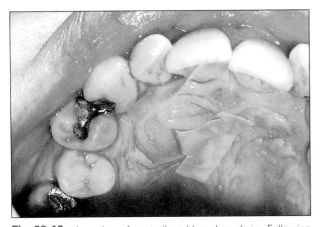

Fig 29-19c Insertion of a sterile rubber dam drain. Following evacuation of the abscess and scaling and root planing of the lateral incisor, an H-shaped drain was inserted through the sulcus and out the palatal incision.

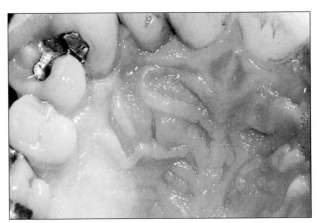

Fig 29-19d Postoperative view at 1 week. The rubber dam was removed after 5 days.

and sutured, and standard postoperative procedures are observed (see chapter 23). The results of both surgical approaches are dramatic in terms of abscess resolution.

Antibiotic therapy is indicated for patients with signs of systemic involvement, for patients requiring antibiotic premedication, or in the presence of diffuse infections that have not localized. Antibiotic administration combined with the application of moist heat is effective in localizing a diffuse infection to a point where it can be effectively drained. Knowledge of the usual oral pathogens associated with abscess formation and of the patient's medication history will allow the selection of an appropriate antibiotic agent.

The treatment of the acute lesion is only the initial step in the therapeutic treatment of the patient. Resolution of the acute incident should be followed by an evaluation of the response to therapy and the institution of appropriate treatment procedures for the management of any residual periodontal lesions and for maintenance of oral health.

Prognosis

The occurrence of a periodontal abscess does not necessarily indicate an unfavorable prognosis for the affected tooth. Indeed, some clinicians believe that chronic lesions that become acute have an increased capacity for repair.[303,309] This is attributed to differences in the chronic

Figs 29-20a to 29-20d Periodontal-periapical abscess on a maxillary left first premolar.

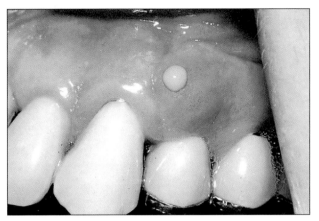

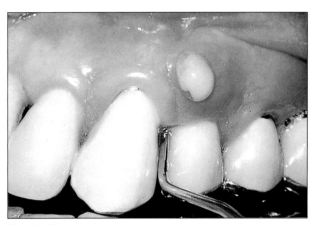

Fig 29-20a Combined lesion: presentation at 6 weeks after endodontic fill; draining stoma.

Fig 29-20b Periodontal probe in mesial periodontal pocket.

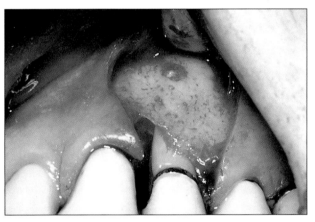

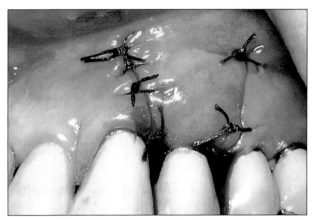

Fig 29-20c Flap reflected to reveal mesial bony periodontal lesion and apical lesion.

Fig 29-20d Flap reapproximated following surgical debridement of the abscess.

versus the acute inflammatory processes and reflects the fact that acute inflammatory sites are sites of intense metabolic activity. The release of the products of inflammation during an acute episode can alter and/or degrade connective tissue elements that are the products of a long-standing chronic inflammatory reaction. Debridement of the site can then establish an environment that is optimal for healing. The clinical response that follows the institution of therapy in acute lesions is often dramatic. It is not uncommon to see bone regrowth sufficient to fill or eliminate intrabony pockets following treatment of an abscess in the intrabony site.[302]

Although dramatic degrees of repair or reattachment may occur in intrabony defects on single-rooted teeth, the

prognosis for an acute abscess in the furcation of a maxillary molar is less favorable. The destruction that occurs may affect each aspect of the furcation. The attachment loss, as well as the complex interfurcal anatomy of the tooth and of the defect that results, can complicate the therapist's ability to successfully instrument the tooth during both active and supportive therapy. A less complex anatomy and greater ease of access to the furcation region of mandibular molars provides for a better prognosis than for maxillary molars. Even though a therapeutic through-and-through (Class III) furcation may occur following an abscess in a mandibular molar, the tooth may be successfully maintained for years if adequate access for home care and professional maintenance can be established.[301]

Necrotizing Ulcerative Gingivitis and Necrotizing Ulcerative Periodontitis

NUG is an acute recurring disease. Although NUG patients are susceptible to recurrences of the disease, the historic terminology of *acute NUG* and *chronic NUG* are misidentifications. The term *acute* as applied to NUG alludes only to the rapidity of its clinical onset, and *chronic* is an allusion to its recurrence in some patients. NUG can occur in patients with chronic periodontitis, and multiple recurrences of NUG can affect the deeper periodontal tissues and result in a loss of periodontal attachment, thus becoming a form of periodontitis. This loss of attachment in patients with recurrent NUG or with HIV infection has been designated as NUP.[310,311]

Historically, various names have been applied to this acute condition to reflect its perceived cause, signs, symptoms, and clinical courses. It has been variously described in the literature as *cheilokake*, ulcerative stomatitis of soldiers, Vincent infection, trench mouth, gangrenous stomatitis,[312] necrotic ulcerative stomatitis,[313] ulceromembranous gingivitis,[314] and acute NUG.[315] More invasive forms described as cancrum oris or noma are described in children in developing countries.[316,317]

The cause of NUG/NUP is not fully understood. The identification of the spirochete and fusiform bacteria, and subsequently a number of different microorganisms, originally contributed to the assumption that NUG was a highly infectious and contagious disease. Indeed, this does not appear to be the case, as efforts to transmit NUG in both animal models and humans have been generally unsuccessful.[318,319] Studies of military populations indicate that NUG is not readily transmissible.[313,314] Likewise, while NUG/NUP appears to have an increased incidence in HIV-infected and AIDS patients, evidence for a sexual transmission of NUG is to date circumstantial.[319–321]

The early observations by Plaut[322] and Vincent[323] implicated spirochetes and the fusiform bacillus as etiologic agents for NUG. Subsequently, other microorganisms have been listed among the possible infecting agents. Loesche et al[324] cultured and identified plaque samples from college students with NUG and identified the dominant bacteria as *Treponema* species, *Fusobacterium* species, *Selenomonas* species, and *Bacteroides intermedius*.

More recently, microscopic analysis of samples from patients with NUG indicated that rods constitute approximately 43% of morphologic forms, followed by 29% cocci and 28% spirochetes. Eight distinct types of spirochetes were seen. Cultural studies have shown that gram-negative rods represent 78% of the total cultivated microorganisms, with *Bacteroides gingivalis (Porphyromonas gingivalis)* and *Fusobacterium nucleatum* being the most commonly identified strict anaerobes.[325] Currently it is believed that *Prevotella intermedia* and an intermediate-sized spirochete (*Treponema* species) are associated with the clinical signs of NUG.[324,326,327]

While microorganisms play a significant role in both the cause and therapy of NUG/NUP, it is unclear whether the infection occurs as a primary response to the presence of specific pathogenic organisms or as a result of bacterial invasion secondary to alterations in host susceptibility.[313,321] Microorganisms are clearly necessary for the development of the oral lesions, but the onset of NUG/NUP likely results from the presence of so-called predisposing or contributing factors that sufficiently alter host tissue resistance to allow bacterial invasion by organisms indigenous to the individual (host). Possible etiologic mechanisms and sequelae are shown in Fig 29-21.

Predisposing/Contributing Factors

In addition to bacteria, a host of other factors have been identified in the periodontal literature as playing a role in the development of NUG. Among these factors are poor oral hygiene and preexisting gingivitis,[321,328,329] emotional and mental stress,[330–334] smoking,[310,325,332,335] socioeconomic status,[315,335,336] and altered host resistance from malnutrition or systemic disease.[317,336,337]

The interruption of normal oral hygiene measures has been observed to lead to an increased incidence of NUG in military and civilian populations.[313,314,320] The prevalence of NUG is higher in patients with poor oral hygiene than in controls. Pindborg[329] reported that 87 of 91 new cases of NUG apparently developed in patients with previous gingivitis. Eighty-seven percent of 218 patients with NUG seen by Barnes et al[338] were deemed to have poor or fair oral hygiene as compared with 40% of 108 age- and sex-matched controls. Heavy deposits of calculus were found in more than 25% of the patients with NUG as compared with only 10% of a control population.[338]

Similar observations in children in developing nations with poor oral hygiene are reported in a number of studies.[317,336,339,340] Taiwo[340] identified a trend for increased prevalence and severity of NUG in Nigerian children with poor oral hygiene. More than 66% of children with very poor oral hygiene had NUG, while only 2 of 83 children (2.4%) with good oral hygiene had the disease. However, the decline in oral hygiene status may be related to the progress of the NUG rather than being the inciting factor.[340]

Factors that alter host resistance or result from lowered host resistance also are identified as contributing to the cause and progress of NUG. Malnutrition is a key factor in the cause of NUG and noma. Noma has been considered a more virulent form of NUG,[316,317,336] and it was once postulated that NUG would progress to noma in the compromised patient. Review of the literature, however, sug-

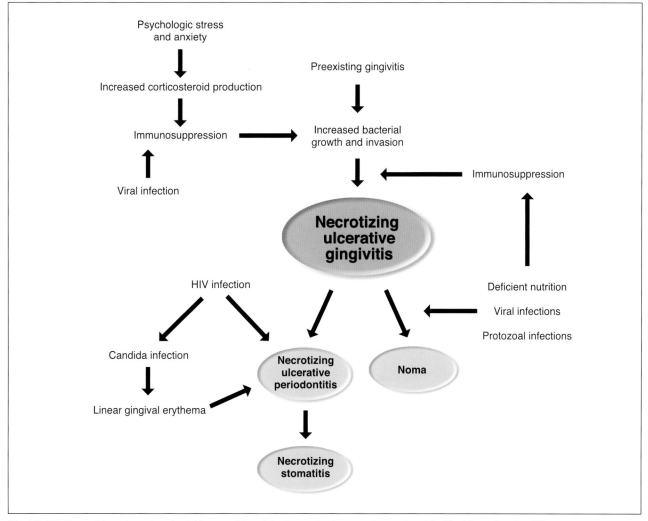

Fig 29-21 Necrotizing ulcerative gingivitis: possible etiologic mechanisms and sequelae. Modified from Rowland[310] with permission.

gests that cases that clearly began as NUG and progressed to noma are uncommon.[341,342] A recent study indicates that noma is associated with elevated cortisol levels and reduced levels of zinc and amino acids in children previously infected with measles or herpesviruses in consort with *Fusobacterium necrophorum* infection.[343] In Nigerian children, measles is the most common predisposing disease to noma.[317]

Stress as measured by psychologic tests or in terms of adrenocortical activity is also suggested to be a predisposing factor. Patients with NUG are reported to be especially nervous,[332] to seek psychologic counseling or care more frequently than control subjects,[330,344] and to be more likely to score as emotionally disordered during psychologic testing than healthy controls.[334] It is also reported that the personality trait of dominance has a positive cor-

relation with the disease, whereas there is a negative correlation between NUG and the trait of abasement.[333]

During periods of stress, there is an increase in adrenocortical activity. Shannon et al[331] measured the mean urinary value of 17-hydroxycorticosteroids in patients with NUG and reported that the mean values were higher than those for patients with gingivitis or periodontitis. However, the differences detected were not at statistically significant levels. Increased levels of steroids during NUG attacks followed by 23% lower levels of 17-hydroxycorticosteroids during periods of disease inactivity were measured by Maupin and Bell.[345]

Smoking is another factor that may predispose individuals to the development of NUG. Patients with NUG are commonly heavy smokers. Although there are few available data that have been adjusted for socioeconomic status, psychological stress, or other possible contributing factors, most reports on large populations, other than children, indicate that patients with NUG are more likely to be smokers and to smoke more heavily than control subjects who smoke.[321,329,346] Melnick et al[321] estimated the prevalence odds ratio between smokers and nonsmokers to be 8.7%. Smoking may influence gingival health both locally and systemically. In addition to its effects on oral hygiene, recent studies have documented a role for smoking in the cause of periodontitis,[347–349] periodontal wound healing,[350] and tooth loss.[351]

Other host resistance factors have been proposed as predisposing factors in the development of NUG. Cogen et al[352] investigated both polymorphonuclear neutrophil and lymphocyte function in patients with NUG. A significant depression in responsiveness of PMNs to both chemotaxis and phagocytosis was detected. The response of NUG lymphocytes to stimulation by nonspecific antigens was less revealing. It suggested that impaired neutrophil chemotaxis and phagocytosis may play a role in NUG. An apparent transient impaired chemotaxis of neutrophils was also reported by Claffey et al[350] in 10 of 11 patients with NUG as compared with 11 healthy control subjects. The impaired chemotaxis was attributed to an intrinsic defect in the leukocytes, because no serum factors were detected that had an effect on chemotaxis. Likewise, the PMNs of NUG patients and control subjects did not differ in their ability to reduce nitroblue tetrazolium or in the intracellular killing of *Candida albicans*. Four of the 11 subjects were reexamined 18 months later when free of NUG symptoms; these four patients demonstrated neither impaired neutrophil chemotaxis nor a phagocytic defect.

Inadequate humoral antibody response to infecting organisms and/or immunosuppression has also been proposed as responsible for the onset of NUG.[325,326,353,354] Using steroid-induced immunosuppression, it has been possible to transmit NUG from animal to animal in a beagle dog model[355,356] and to study the disease. Differences in this dog model and human disease, however, were noted. Thus, the data from the studies to date remain inconclusive and suggest that the relationship between the levels of antibody response and disease onset is poorly correlated and may have little biologic significance.[325,326,354,357]

Recurrent episodes of NUG lead to involvement of the deeper tissues of the periodontium. They can result in the formation of deep craters in the interproximal bone[358] and to a classification as NUP.[310]

Incidence

Necrotizing periodontal disease primarily affects the young. In industrialized nations, the disease is primarily found in young adults,[338] with a mean onset age of 23

years.[321] However, it can occur at any age in the presence of systemic diseases, malnutrition, or blood dyscrasias. In older individuals, it occurs primarily in those with a debilitating disease.[359] Of current concern is the high incidence of NUG/NUP reported in HIV-infected individuals.[360]

The incidence and prevalence of NUG and NUP are low in the general population. In surveyed general populations, NUG is reported to occur at the rate of 0.1 new case per 1,000 person-years.[361] A median period incidence of 0.6% per year with a median point prevalence of 2.0% has been estimated,[321] although occurrence at a higher rate is reported among certain groups of individuals.[317,335,336,362] Recurrence of the disease is relatively common and has been reported in 16% to 33% of patients.[337,363]

Among military service personnel and college-aged students, the incidence rate is estimated by Melnick et al at approximately 30 new cases per 1,000 person-years.[321] Barnes et al identified 218 cases of NUG among 113,000 individuals examined in 1 year at Fort Knox, KY, for an incidence of 0.19%. This is lower than is usually reported for most military installations. NUG was also found to be more prevalent among permanent base personnel than among military trainees.[338]

Epidemiological studies of populations in developing nations report a much higher incidence and prevalence of NUG, particularly in children. Enwonwu found an incidence of 15% in underprivileged Osegere village children and 27% in hospitalized children with protein-calorie malnutrition.[317] A report by Taiwo, also on Nigerian children, found that 117 of 431 children (26.7%) 1 to 11 years old had NUG.[340] This is similar to earlier reports by Emslie[316] and Pindborg et al.[336]

Clinical Features

Classic reports of necrotizing periodontal disease describe an interesting variety of clinical symptoms and signs. However, none of these classic signs and symptoms is present in all cases.[29,338] NUG is characterized by pain, usually of rapid onset; bleeding on manipulation of the gingiva; and the ultimate development of surface necrosis and ulceration. The characteristic areas of necrosis are usually described as craterlike and covered by a whitish gray pseudomembrane that is surrounded by a linear erythematous band. Early in the course of the disease, ulceration may not be obvious, as the lesion commonly begins in the tip of the interdental papilla, and edema and swelling may obscure the area of necrosis (Fig 29-22). As the lesion develops, however, the affected area may assume the punched-out, eroded appearance that is most commonly described in the literature (Fig 29-23). A small, isolated lesion can proceed to the total destruction of the interdental papilla and affect the adjacent marginal gin-

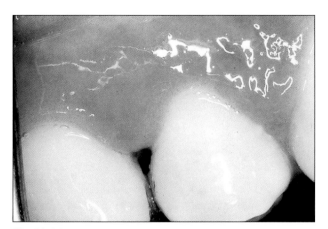

Fig 29-22 Early NUG lesion in the interdental area between the maxillary right first and second premolars. The tip of the papilla is necrotic, but little external involvement of the site is evident.

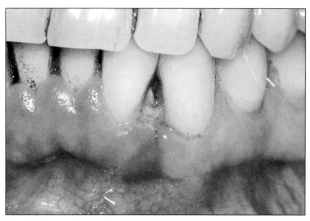

Fig 29-23 More advanced NUG lesion between a mandibular left lateral incisor and canine. Necrosis of the interdental area has extended to destroy the entire papilla. A portion of the pseudomembrane is visible.

giva (Fig 29-24). The extent of involvement may range from an isolated papillary area to multiple interdental sites, although the total involvement of all interdental sites is not reported.[29] Clinical reports indicate that lesions are more common in the anterior than the posterior part of the mouth.[338]

The histopathologic picture of NUG is nonspecific and similar to other inflammatory traumatic ulcers. The inflammatory lesion affects both the epithelium and the underlying connective tissues. The surface of the ulcer may be covered by necrotic debris and an inflammatory exudate. A variety of microorganisms, cellular debris, and inflammatory cells are present. Intracellular edema is present in the adjacent epithelium, and the underlying connective tissue is loose and vascular, with polymorphonuclear cells filling the vascular spaces.

The ultrastructure of the necrotic lesion is described by Listgarten as consisting of four zones.[364] The superficial bacterial zone consists of a layer of microorganisms of many species, including spirochetes. It is separated from the zone of necrosis by a layer of leukocytes consisting primarily of polymorphonuclear neutrophils. The spaces between the neutrophils contain a variety of bacterial cells, including spirochetes of a number of different sizes and shapes. Phagocytosed bacteria are occasionally observed within neutrophils, but the majority of spirochetes, apparently phagocytosed, are seen in mononuclear cells. Within the necrotic zone, spirochetes are the predominant organism. A few microorganisms of a size and shape consistent with fusiform bacteria are also present. Both polymorphonuclear and mononuclear leukocytes are observed, as are histiocytes containing disintegrating PMNs. A plasma cell infiltrate is present in the tissues adjacent to the necrotic zone. At the deepest level of the lesion (250

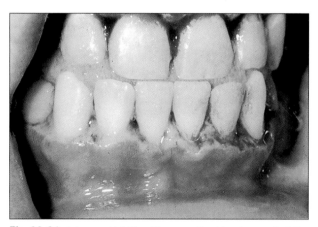

Fig 29-24 Advanced NUG, with generalized involvement of the mandibular incisors and canines. The maxillary incisors, while affected, do not have the same extent of tissue destruction.

μm), the zone of spirochetal infiltration, spirochetes are the only microorganisms observed. Concentrated clumps of predominantly large and intermediate spirochetes are found within the connective tissue. An area of lysis may be present around the clumps of spirochetes. Listgarten's observations, while not indicating a primary role for the spirochete in NUG, demonstrate the capability of these microorganisms to invade non-necrotic tissue in high concentrations.

Therapy

Pain is the most common presenting symptom of patients with necrotizing periodontal disease. Because the perception of pain varies extensively among patients, whether patients view the acute process as an emergency also varies. Some patients report severe pain that interferes

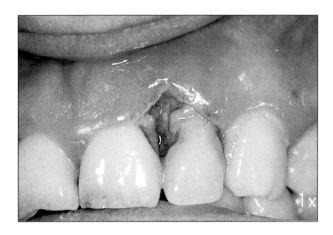

Fig 29-25 Lesion of NUP. Recurrent attacks of NUG have advanced not only to involve the gingival tissues but also to destroy attachment in the interdental area between these maxillary left central and lateral incisors. A permanent gingival deformity may result.

Figs 29-26a and 29-26b Before and after therapy for NUG.

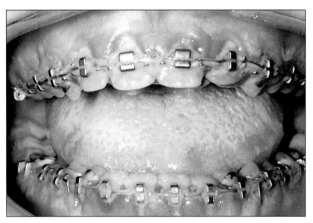

Fig 29-26a Initial presentation, patient aged 14 years. NUG occurred during orthodontic therapy. This patient had multiple episodes of NUG during the 3 years of tooth movement.

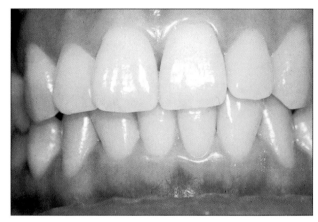

Fig 29-26b Clinical appearance, patient aged 25 years. Following periodontal therapy, including gingival surgery, the patient has been maintained successfully for 7 years with no recurrence.

with eating and oral hygiene practices. Others report little discomfort unless the affected areas are contacted. The discomfort is usually limited to the areas of necrosis, but these areas may be exquisitely sensitive to any form of manipulation, such as periodontal probing. The patient therefore may be reluctant to allow any manipulation of the gingiva.

Unless there are signs of systemic involvement, which is uncommon, the vast majority of NUG cases can be adequately treated by debridement, scaling, and root planing.[29,365] While some discomfort will result from instrumentation, careful curettage with attention to minimal displacement of the tissues can be performed successfully. It is commonly observed that as the debris and pseudomembrane are removed from the area, the discomfort diminishes. If necessary, the use of topical anesthetics can facilitate instrumentation by the operator. Following instrumentation, periodic flushing of the area by the patient with agents such as 3% peroxide diluted 50% with warm

water or one of the commercially available oxygenating agents provides rapid relief. The addition of topical chemotherapeutic agents may be beneficial for immunocompromised patients.[366,367]

The response of patients with necrotizing periodontal disease to measures that reduce the microbial flora in the infected site is dramatic. Both mechanical debridement and antibiotic therapy elicit a rapid reduction in the clinical signs and symptoms associated with the disease. Elimination of the acute signs and symptoms allows a thorough scaling and root planing to be performed. In the presence of systemic signs, systemic disease, or lack of response to local debridement procedures, the addition of antibiotics to the treatment regimen is advisable.

Patients with minimal destruction and mild symptoms may respond to appropriate therapy with resolution of the gingival craters and the reestablishment of a normal gingival form. This outcome is not common for the patient who has enough soft tissue destruction to have resulted in deep gingival craters or who has developed NUP with deep proximal deformities because of recurrent attacks (Fig 29-25).

Following debridement and an initial period of healing, some patients benefit from localized gingivoplasty to alter the gingival form. While not mandatory for successful maintenance therapy, such intervention may facilitate the patient's ability to perform oral hygiene procedures and thereby minimize the potential for recurrence of the disease. In patients with high cosmetic requirements, the improved gingival tone and form may lead to greater patient satisfaction (Fig 29-26).

Patients with advanced periodontal destruction from recurrent necrotizing periodontal disease associated with caries and tooth loss may require more sophisticated therapy. Essential to successful treatment of these patients is the institution of a regimen of personal oral hygiene and professional maintenance that will arrest the disease and prevent recurrence. If an extended period of freedom from the signs of active disease can be achieved, the patient may be a candidate for other periodontal treatment procedures directed at the repair and/or regeneration of the lost periodontal attachment.

References

1. Holmstrup P. Non–plaque-induced gingival lesions. Ann Periodontol 1999;4:20–31.
2. Swenson HM. "D" is for desquamative gingivitis. J Indian Dent Assoc 1984;63:19–21.
3. Karshan M, Ziskin DE, Silvers HF, et al. Studies in the etiology of chronic desquamative and hyperkeratotic lesions of the oral mucous membranes. Oral Surg Oral Med Oral Pathol 1953;6:716–723.
4. Nisengard RJ, Alpert AM, Krestow V. Desquamative gingivitis: Immunologic findings. J Periodontol 1978;49:27–32.
5. Daniels TE, Quadra-White C. Direct immunofluorescence in oral mucosal disease: A diagnostic analysis of 130 cases. Oral Surg Oral Med Oral Pathol 1981;51:38–47.
6. Nisengard RJ, Neiders M. Desquamative lesions of the gingiva. J Periodontol 1981;52:500–510.
7. Williams DM. Dermatology, anti-immune disease and the periodontium. In: Newman HN, Rees TD, Kinane DF (eds). Diseases of the Periodontium. Northwood: Science Reviews, 1993:203–228.
8. Chaiyarit P, Kafrawy AH, Miles DA, et al. Oral lichen planus: An immunohistochemical study of heat shock proteins (HSPs) and cytokeratins (CKs) and a unifying hypothesis of pathogenesis. J Oral Pathol Med 1999;28:210–215.
9. Hakkinen L, Kainulainen T, Salo T, et al. Expression of integrin alpha9 subunit and tenascin in oral leukoplakia, lichen planus, and squamous cell carcinoma. Oral Dis 1999;5:210–217.
10. Katta, R. Lichen planus. Am Fam Physician 2000;61:3319–3324, 3327–3328.
11. Miller RL, Gould AR, Bernstein ML. Cinnamon-induced stomatitis venenata: Clinical and characteristic histopathologic features. Oral Surg Oral Med Oral Pathol 1992;73:708–716.
12. Bratel J, Hakeberg M, Jontell M. Effect of replacement of dental amalgam on oral lichenoid reactions. J Dent 1996;24:41–45.
13. Magro CM, Crowson AN. Lichenoid and granulomatous dermatitis. Int J Dermatol 2000;39:126–133.
14. Lunel F, Cacoub P. Treatment of autoimmune and extra-hepatic manifestations of HCV infection. Ann Med Interne 2000;151:58–64.
15. Varela P, Areias J, Mota F, et al. Oral lichen planus induced by interferon-alpha-N1 in a patient with hepatitis C. Int J Dermatol 2000;39:239–240.
16. Lodi G, Porter SR, Scully C. Hepatitis C virus infection. Review and implications for the dentist. Oral Surg Oral Med Oral Pathol Oral Radiol Endod 1998;86:8–22.
17. Bagan JV, Ramon C, Gonzalez L, et al. Preliminary investigation of the association of oral lichen planus and hepatitis C. Oral Surg Oral Med Oral Pathol Oral Radiol Endod 1998;85:532–536.
18. Bouguot NE, Gorlin RJ. Leukoplakia, lichen planus, and other oral keratoses in 23,616 white Americans over the age of 35 years. Oral Surg Oral Med Oral Pathol 1986;61:373–381.
19. Axell T, Rundquist L. Oral lichen planus—A demographic study. Community Dent Oral Epidemiol 1987;15:52–56.
20. Eisen D. The evaluation of cutaneous, genital, scalp, nail, esophageal, and ocular involvement in patients with oral lichen planus. Oral Surg Oral Med Oral Pathol Oral Radiol Endod 1999;88:431–436.
21. Simpson HE. The age and sex incidence and anatomical distribution of oral leukoplakia and lichen planus. Br J Dermatol 1957;69:178–180.
22. Scully C, El-Kim J. Lichen planus: Review and update on pathogenesis. J Oral Pathol 1985;14:431–458.
23. Mollaoglu N. Oral lichen planus: A review. Br J Oral Maxillofac Surg 2000;38:370–377.
24. Thorn JJ, Holmstrup P, Rindum H, Pindborg JJ. Course of various clinical forms of oral lichen planus: A prospective follow-up study of 611 patients. J Oral Pathol 1988;17:213–218.
25. Holmstrup P, Thorn JJ, Rindum J, Pindborg JJ. Malignant development of lichen planus–affected oral mucosa. J Oral Pathol 1988;17:219–225.
26. Silverman S Jr, Gorsky M, Lozada-Nur F. A prospective follow-up study of 570 patients with oral lichen planus: Persistence, remission and malignant association. Oral Surg Oral Med Oral Pathol 1985;60:30–34.
27. Rees TD. Diseases of the oral mucous membranes. In: Meyerhoff WL, Rice DH (eds). Otolaryngology Head and Neck Surgery. Philadelphia: Saunders, 1992:589–609.
28. Silverman S Jr, Bahl S. Oral lichen planus update: Clinical characteristics, treatment responses and malignant transformation. Am J Dent 1997;10:259–263.
29. Rees TD. Adjunctive therapy. In: Nevins M, Becker W, Kornman K (eds). Proceedings of the World Workshop in Clinical Periodontics. Chicago: American Academy of Periodontology, 1989:X1–31.
30. Heggie AAC, Lacy M, Reade PC. An example of the use of quantitation in histological diagnosis by a comparison of normal human cheek mucosa and cheek mucosa affected by lichen planus. J Oral Pathol 1985;14:483–490.
31. Walker DM. The inflammatory infiltrate in lichen planus lesions: An autoradiographic and ultrastructural study. J Oral Pathol 1976;5:277–286.
32. Dockrell HM, Greenspan JS. Histochemical identification of T cells in oral lichen planus. Oral Surg Oral Med Oral Pathol 1979;48:42–46.

33. Regezi JA, Deegan JK, Hayward JR. Lichen planus: Immunologic and morphologic identification of the submucosal infiltrate. Oral Surg Oral Med Oral Pathol 1978;46:44–52.

34. Peng T, Nisengard RJ, Levine MJ. Gingival basement membrane antigens in desquamative lesions of the gingiva. Oral Surg Oral Med Oral Pathol 1986;61:584–589.

35. Toto PD, Nadimi HT. An immunohistochemical study of oral lichen planus. Oral Surg Oral Med Oral Pathol 1987;63:60–67.

36. Fujii H, Ohashi M, Nagura H. Immunohistochemical analysis of oral lichen planus–like eruption in graft-versus-host disease after allogeneic bone marrow transplantation. Am J Clin Pathol 1988;89:177–186.

37. de Panfilis G. The pathogenesis of lichen planus. Am J Dermatopathol 1987;9:362–363.

38. Yih WY, Maier T, Kratochvil FJ, Zieper MB. Analysis of desquamative gingivitis using direct immunofluorescence in conjunction with histology. J Periodontol 1998;69:678–685.

39. Eversole L. Immunopathology of oral mucosal ulcerative, desquamative and bullous diseases. Oral Surg Oral Med Oral Pathol 1994;77:555–571.

40. Laskaris G, Skalvounou A, Angelopoulos A. Direct immunofluorescence in oral lichen planus. Oral Surg Oral Med Oral Pathol 1982;53:483–487.

41. Van der Meij EH, Schepman KP, Smeele LE, et al. A review of the recent literature regarding malignant transformation of oral lichen planus. Oral Surg Oral Med Oral Pathol Oral Radiol Endod 1999;88:307–310.

42. Daniels TE, Quadra-White C. Direct immunofluorescence in oral mucosal disease: A diagnostic analysis of 130 cases. Oral Surg Oral Med Oral Pathol 1981;51:38–47.

43. Kilpi AM, Rich AM, Radden BG, Reade PC. Direct immunofluorescence in the diagnosis of oral mucosal disease. Int Oral Maxillofac Surg 1988;17:6–10.

44. Potts AJC, Hamburger J, Scully C. The medication of patients with oral lichen planus. Oral Surg Oral Med Oral Pathol 1987;64:541–543.

45. Wright JM. Oral manifestations of drug reactions. Dent Clin North Am 1984;28:529–543.

46. Mobacken H, Hersle K, Sloberg K, Thilander H. Oral lichen planus: Hypersensitivity to dental restoration material. Contact Dermatitis 1984;10:11–15.

47. Eversole LR, Ringer M. The role of dental restorative metals in the pathogenesis of oral lichen planus. Oral Surg Oral Med Oral Pathol 1984;57:383–387.

48. Frykholm KO, Frithiof L, Fernstrom AIB, et al. Allergy to copper derived from dental alloys as a possible cause of oral lesions of lichen planus. Acta Derm Venereol 1969;49:268–281.

49. Lozada-Nur F. Oral lichen planus and oral cancer: Is there enough epidemiologic evidence? Oral Surg Oral Med Oral Pathol Oral Radiol Endod 2000;89:265–266.

50. Silverman S Jr. Oral lichen planus: A potentially premalignant lesion. J Oral Maxillofac Surg 2000;58:1286–1288.

51. Lind PO. Oral lichenoid reactions related to composite restorations. Preliminary report. Acta Odontol Scand 1988;46:63–65.

52. Bolewska J, Hansen HJ, Holmstrup P, et al. Oral mucosal lesions related to silver amalgam restorations. Oral Surg Oral Med Oral Pathol 1990;70:55–58.

53. Pogrel MA, Weldon LL. Carcinoma arising in erosive lichen planus in the midline of the dorsum of the tongue. Oral Surg Oral Med Oral Pathol 1983;55:62–66.

54. Lind PO, Koppang HS, Aas E. Malignant transformation in oral lichen planus. Int J Oral Maxillofac Surg 1985;14:509–516.

55. Fowler CB, Rees TD, Smith BR. Squamous cell carcinoma on the dorsum of the tongue arising in a long-standing lesion of erosive lichen planus. J Am Dent Assoc 1987;115:707–710.

56. Camisa C, Hamaty FG, Gay JD. Squamous cell carcinoma of the tongue arising in lichen planus: A case report and review of the literature. Cutis 1998;62:175–178.

57. Warshaw EM, Templeton SF, Washington CV. Verrucous carcinoma occurring in a lesion of oral lichen planus. Cutis 2000;65:219–222.

58. Lo Muzio L, Mignogna MD, Favia G, et al. The possible association between oral lichen planus and oral squamous cell carcinoma: A clinical evaluation of 14 cases and a review of the literature. Oral Oncol 1998;34:239–246.

59. Hietanen J, Paasonen M-R, Kuhlefelt M, Malmstrom M. A retrospective study of oral lichen planus patients with concurrent or subsequent development of malignancy. Oral Oncol 1999;35:278–282.

60. Rajentheran R, McLean NR, Kelly CG, et al. Malignant transformation of oral lichen planus. Eur J Surg Oncol 1999;25:520–527.

61. McIntyre GT, Oliver RJ. Update on precancerous lesions. Dent Update 1999;26:382–386.

62. Mravak-Stipetic M, Pirkic A, Vidas I. Reduction of epithelial dendritic cells in keratotic lesion of oral lichen planus. Coll Antropol 1998;22(suppl):103–109.

63. Rees TD. Unpublished data. Stomatology Center, Baylor College of Dentistry, March 2001.

64. Murti PR, Daftary DK, Bhonsle RB, et al. Malignant potential of oral lichen planus: Observations in 722 patients from India. J Oral Pathol 1986;15:71–77.

65. Silverman S, Gorsky M, Lozada-Nur F, Giannotti K. A prospective study of findings and management in 214 patients with oral lichen planus. Oral Surg Oral Med Oral Pathol 1991;72:665–670.

66. Lozada-Nur F, Miranda C, Maliksi R. Double-blind clinical trial of 0.05% clobetasol proprionate ointment in orabase and 0.05% fluocinonide ointment in orabase in the treatment of patients with oral vesiculoerosive diseases. Oral Surg Oral Med Oral Pathol 1994;77:598–604.

67. Hurt WC. Pharmacologic management of stomatologic problems. Dent Clin North Am 1984;28:545–554.

68. Cawson RA. Management of oral lichen planus. In: McDonald RE, Hurt WC, Gilmore HW, Middleton RA (eds). Current Therapy in Dentistry, vol 7. St. Louis: Mosby, 1980:63–68.

69. Carrozzo M, Gandolfo S. The management of oral lichen planus. Oral Dis 1999;5:196–205.

70. Pedersen A, Klausen B. Glucocorticosteroids and oral medicine. J Oral Pathol 1984;13:1–15.

71. Eisen D. The therapy of oral lichen planus. Crit Rev Oral Biol Med 1993;4:141–158.

72. Chan ES, Thornhill M, Azkrzewska J. Interventions for treating oral lichen planus. Cochrane Database Syst Rev 2000;(2):CD001168.

73. Lu SY, Chen WJ, Eng HL. Response to levamisole and low-dose prednisolone in 41 patients with chronic oral ulcers: A 3-year open clinical trial and follow-up study. Oral Surg Oral Med Oral Pathol Oral Radiol Endod 1998;86:438–445.

74. Buyuk AY, Kavala M. Oral metronidazole treatment of lichen planus. J Am Acad Dermatol 2000;43:260–262.

75. Hodak E, Yosipovitch G, David M, et al. Low-dose low-molecular-weight heparin (enoxaparin) is beneficial in lichen planus: A preliminary report. J Am Acad Dermatol 1998;38:564–568.

76. Stefanidou MP, Ioannidou DF, Panayiotides JG, Tosca AD. Low-molecular-weight heparin: A novel alternative therapeutic approach for lichen planus. Br J Dermatol 1999;141:1040–1045.

77. Nasr IS. Topical tacrolimus in dermatology. Clin Exp Dermatol 2000;25:250–254.

78. Rees TD. Periodontal considerations in patients with bone marrow or solid organ transplants. In: Rose LF, Genco RJ, Cohen DW, Mealey BL (eds). Periodontal Medicine. Hamilton, Ontario: BC Decker, 2000:205–226.

79. Epstein JB, Gorsky M, Epstein MS, Nantel S. Topical azathiprine in the treatment of immune-mediated chronic oral inflammatory conditions. Oral Surg Oral Med Oral Pathol Oral Radiol Endod 2001;91:56–61.

80. Lorenzana ER, Rees TD, Glass M, Detweiler JG. Chronic ulcerative stomatitis: A case report. J Periodontol 2000;71:104–111.

81. Parodi A, Cozzani E, Cacciapuoti M, Rebora A. Chronic ulcerative stomatitis: Antibodies reacting with the 70-kDa molecule react with epithelial nuclei. Br J Dermatol 2000;143:671–672.

82. Harpenau LA, Plemons JM, Rees TD. Effectiveness of a low dose of cyclosporine in the management of patients with oral erosive lichen planus. Oral Surg Oral Med Oral Pathol Oral Radiol Endod 1995;80:161–167.

83. Francis C, Boisnic S, Etienne S, Szpinglos H. Effect of the local application of cyclosporine A on chronic erosive lichen planus of the oral cavity. Dermatologica 1988;177:194–195.

84. Cheng YS, Rees TD, Wright JM, Plemons JM. Childhood oral pemphigoid: A case report and review of the literature. J Oral Pathol Med 2001;30:372–377.

85. Cole WC, Leicht S, Byrd RP Jr, Roy TM. Cicatricial pemphigoid with an upper airway lesion. Tenn Med 2000;93:99–101.

86. Stallmach A, Weg-Remers S, Moser C, et al. Esophageal involvement in cicatricial pemphigoid. Endoscopy 1998;30:657–661.

87. Laskaris G, Triantafyllou S, Economopoulou P. Gingival manifestations of childhood cicatricial pemphigoid. Oral Surg Oral Med Oral Pathol 1988;66:349–352.

88. Silverman S Jr, Gorsky M, Lozada-Nur F, Liu A. Oral mucous membrane pemphigoid: A study of sixty-five patients. Oral Surg Oral Med Oral Pathol 1986;61:233–237.

89. Farrell AM, Kirtschig G, Dalziel KL, et al. Childhood vulval pemphigoid: A clinical and immunopathologial study of five patients. Br J Dermatol 1999;140:308–312.

90. Foster CS, Ahmed AR. Intravenous immunoglobulin therapy for ocular cicatricial pemphigoid: A preliminary study. Ophthalmology 1999;106:2136–2143.

91. Sallout H, Anhalt GJ, Al-Kawas FH. Mucous membrane pemphigoid presenting with isolated esophageal involvement: A case report. Gastrointest Endosc 2000;52:429–433.

92. Ramlogan D, Coulsom IH, McGeorge A. Cicatricial pemphigoid: A diagnostic problem for the urologist. J R Coll Surg Edinb 2000;45:62–63.

93. Gallagher G, Shklar G. Oral involvement in mucous membrane pemphigoid. Clin Dermatol 1987;5:18–27.

94. Holsclaw DS. Ocular cicatricial pemphigoid. Int Ophthalmol Clin 1998;38:89–106.

95. Messmer EM, Hintschich CR, Partscht K, et al. Ocular cicatricial pemphigoid: Retrospective analysis of risk factors and complications. Ophthalmologe 2000;97:113–120.

96. Shklar G, McCarthy PL. Oral lesions of mucous membrane pemphigoid: A study of 85 cases. Arch Otolaryngol 1971;3:354–364.

97. Leonard JN, Wright P, Haffenden GP, et al. Skin diseases and the dry eye. Trans Ophthalmol Soc UK 1985;104:467–476.

98. Scott JE, Ahmed AR. The blistering diseases. Med Clin North Am 1998;82:1239–1283.

99. Scully C, Carrozzo M, Gandolfo S, et al. Update on mucous membrane pemphigoid. Oral Surg Oral Med Oral Pathol Oral Radiol Endod 1999;88:56–68.

100. Terezhalmy GT, Bergfeld WF. Cicatricial pemphigoid (benign mucous membrane pemphigoid). Quintessence Int 1998;29:429–437.

101. Rogers RS III, Sheridan PJ, Nightingale SH. Desquamative gingivitis: Clinical, histopathologic, immunopathologic and therapeutic observations. J Am Acad Dermatol 1982;7:729–735.

102. Dahl MGC, Cook LJ. Lesions induced by trauma in pemphigoid. Br J Dermatol 1979;101:469–473.

103. Sabet HY, Davis JL, Rogers RS. Mucous membrane pemphigoid, thymoma and myasthenia gravis. Int J Dermatol 2000;39:701–704.

104. Butt Z, Kaufman D, McNab A, McKelvie P. Drug-induced ocular cicatricial pemphigoid: A series of clinico-pathological reports. Eye 1998;12:285–290.

105. Fujimoto W, Ishida-Yamamoto A, Hsu R, et al. Anti-epiligrin cicatricial pemphigoid: A case associated with gastric carcinoma and features resembling epidermolysis bullosa acquisita. Br J Dermatol 1998;139:682–687.

106. Setterfield J, Shirlaw PJ, Lazarova Z, et al. Paraneoplastic cicatricial pemphigoid. Br J Dermatol 1999;141:127–131.

107. Williams DM, Leonard JN, Wright P, et al. Benign mucous membrane (cicatricial) pemphigoid revisited: A clinical and immunological reappraisal. Br Dent J 1984;157:313–316.

108. Ullman S. Immunofluorescence and diseases of the skin. Acta Derm Venereol 1988;140(suppl):1–31.

109. Bean SF, Waisman M, Michel B, et al. Cicatricial pemphigoid: Immunofluorescent studies. Arch Dermatol 1972;106:195–199.

110. Laskaris G, Angelopoulos A. Cicatricial pemphigoid: Direct and indirect immunofluorescent studies. Oral Surg Oral Med Oral Pathol 1981;51:48–54.

111. Korman NJ. New and emerging therapies in the treatment of blistering diseases. Dermatol Clin 2000;18:127–137.

112. Donnenfeld ED, Perry HD, Wallerstein A, et al. Subconjunctival mitomycin C for the treatment of ocular cicatricial pemphigoid. Ophthalmology 1999;106:72–78.

113. Dragan L, Eng AM, Lam S, Persson T. Tetracycline and niacinamide: Treatment alternatives in ocular cicatricial pemphigoid. Cutis 1999;63:181–183.

114. Hashimoto Y, Suga Y, Yoshliike T, et al. A case of antiepiligrin cicatricial pemphigoid successfully treated by plasmapheresis. Dermatology 2000;201:58–60.

115. Damoulis PD, Gagari E. Combined treatment of periodontal disease and benign mucous membrane pemphigoid: Case report with 8 years maintenance. J Periodontol 2000;71: 1620–1629.

116. Laskaris G, Demetriou N, Angelopoulos A. Immunofluorescent studies in desquamative gingivitis. J Oral Pathol 1981;10:398–407.

117. Lamy PJ, Rees TD, Binnie WH, Rankin KV. Mucous membrane pemphigoid: Treatment experience at two institutions. Oral Surg Oral Med Oral Pathol 1992;74:50–53.

118. Aufdemorte TB, de Villez RL, Parel SM. Modified topical steroid therapy for the treatment of oral mucous membrane pemphigoid. Oral Surg Oral Med Oral Pathol 1985;59: 256–260.

119. Ciarrocca KN, Greenberg MS. A retrospective study of the management of oral mucous membrane pemphigoid with dapsone. Oral Surg Oral Med Oral Pathol Oral Radiol Endod 1999; 88:159–163.

120. Rogers RS, Seehafer JR, Perry HO. Treatment of cicatricial (benign mucous membrane) pemphigoid with dapsone. J Am Acad Dermatol 1982;6:215–223.

121. Barth JH, Venning VA. Pemphigus. Br J Hosp Med 1987;37: 326,330–331.

122. Lever WF, Schaumburg-Lever G. Treatment of pemphigus vulgaris. Results obtained in 84 patients between 1961 and 1982. Arch Dermatol 1984;120:44–47.

123. Lynde CW, Ongley RC, Rigg JM. Juvenile pemphigus vulgaris. Arch Dermatol 1984;120:1098–1099.

124. Correll AW, Schott TR. Multiple, painful vesiculoulcerative lesions in the oral mucosa. J Am Dent Assoc 1985;110:765–766.

125. Orlowski WA, Bressman E, Doyle JL, Chasens AI. Chronic pemphigus vulgaris of the gingiva: A case report with a 6-year follow-up. J Periodontol 1983;54:685–689.

126. Markitziu A, Pisanty S. Gingival pemphigus vulgaris. Report of a case. Oral Surg Oral Med Oral Pathol 1983;55:250–252.

127. Barnett ML. Pemphigus vulgaris presenting as a gingival lesion. J Periodontol 1987;59:611–614.

128. Parodi A, Stanley JR, Ciaccio M, Rebora A. Epidermal antigens in pemphigus vegetans. Report of a case. Br J Dermatol 1988;119:799–802.

129. Lamey PJ, Rees TD, Binnie WH, et al. Oral presentation of pemphigus vulgaris and its response to systemic steroid therapy. Oral Surg Oral Med Oral Pathol 1992;74:54–57.

130. Hurt WC. Observations on pemphigus vegetans. Oral Surg Oral Med Oral Pathol 1965;2:481–487.

131. Rice JS, Hurt WC, Rovin S. Pemphigus vegetans. Report of an unusual case. Oral Surg Oral Med Oral Pathol 1963;16: 1383–1394.

132. Coscia-Porrazzi L, Maiello FM, Ruocco V, Pisani M. Cytodiagnosis of oral pemphigus vulgaris. J Acta Cytol 1985;29:746–749.

133. Honma T, Segami N, Hosoda M, Fukuda M. Electron microscopic observation on the epithelial-connective tissue junction of pemphigus vulgaris. A case report. J Submicrosc Cytol 1987; 19:167–174.

134. Stanley JR, Yaar M, Hawley-Nelson P, Katz SI. Pemphigus antibodies identify a cell surface glycoprotein synthesized by human and mouse keratinocytes. J Clin Invest 1982;70:281–288.

135. Kornman N. Pemphigus. J Acad Dermatol 1988;18:1219–1238.

136. Anhalt GJ, Kim SC, Stanley JR, et al. Paraneoplastic pemphigus. An autoimmune mucocutaneous disease associated with neoplasia. N Engl J Med 1990;323:1729–1735.

137. Fullerton SH, Woodley DT, Smoller BR, Anhalt GJ. Paraneoplastic pemphigus with autoantibody deposition in bronchial epithelium after autologous bone marrow transplantation. JAMA 1992;267:1500–1502.

138. Houssiau FA, Lebacq EG. Neonatal lupus erythematosus with maternal systemic lupus erythematosus. Clin Rheumatol 1986; 5:505–508.

139. Stevens MB. Connective tissue disease in the elderly. Clin Rheum Dis 1986;12:11–32.

140. Condemi JJ. The autoimmune diseases. J Am Dent Assoc 1987;258:2920–2929.

141. Standefer JA Jr, Mattox DE. Head and neck manifestations of collagen vascular diseases. Otolaryngol Clin North Am 1986; 19:181–210.

142. Schiodt M, Andersen L, Shear M, Smith CJ. Leukoplakia-like lesions developing in patients with oral discoid lupus erythematosus. Acta Odontol Scand 1981;39:209–216.

143. Jonsson R, Heyden G, Westberg NG, Nyberg G. Oral mucosal lesions in systemic lupus erythematosus. A clinical, histopathological and immunopathological study. J Rheumatol 1984;11: 38–42.

144. Spann CR, Callen JP, Klein JB, Kulick KB. Clinical, serologic and immunogenetic studies in patients with chronic cutaneous (discoid) lupus erythematosus who have verrucous and/or hypertrophic skin lesions. J Rheumatol 1988;15:256–261.

145. Weigand DA. Lupus band test: Anatomic regional variations in discoid lupus erythematosus. J Am Acad Dermatol 1986;14: 426–428.

146. Schiodt M. Oral manifestations of lupus erythematosus. Int J Oral Surg 1984;13:101–147.

147. Schiodt M. Oral discoid lupus erythematosus. II. Skin lesions and systemic lupus erythematosus in sixty-six patients with 6-year follow-up. Oral Surg Oral Med Oral Pathol 1984;57: 177–180.

148. Sontheimer RD. Subacute cutaneous lupus erythematosus. Clin Dermatol 1985;3:58–68.

149. Camisa C. Vesiculobullous systemic lupus erythematosus. A report of four cases. J Am Acad Dermatol 1988;18:93–100.

150. Callen JP. Oral manifestations of collagen vascular disease. Semin Cutan Med Surg 1997;16:323–327.

151. Gonzales TS, Coleman GC. Periodontal manifestations of collagen vascular disorders. Periodontol 2000 1999;21:94–105.

152. Pisetsky DS. Systemic lupus erythematosus. Med Clin North Am 1986;70:337–353.

153. Schiodt M. Oral discoid lupus erythematosus. III. A histopathologic study of sixty-six patients. Oral Surg Oral Med Oral Pathol 1984;57:281–293.

154. Schiodt M, Pindborg JJ. Oral discoid lupus erythematosus. I. The validity of previous histopathologic diagnostic criteria. Oral Surg Oral Med Oral Pathol 1984;57:46–51.

155. Reibel J, Schiodt M. Immunohistochemical studies on colloid bodies (Civatte bodies) in oral lesions of discoid lupus erythematosus. Scand J Dent Res 1986;94:536–544.

156. Newton RC, Jorizzo JL, Solomon AR, et al. Mechanism-oriented assessment of isoretinoin in chronic or subacute cutaneous lupus erythematosus. Arch Dermatol 1986;122:170–176.

157. Clements PJ, Davis J. Cytotoxic drugs: Their clinical application to rheumatic diseases. Semin Arthritis Rheum 1986;15:231–254.

158. Heule F, van Joost T, Beukers R. Cyclosporin in the treatment of lupus erythematosus. Arch Dermatol 1986;122:973–974.

159. Rees TD. Systemic factors in periodontal disease. In: Newman HN, Rees TD, Kinane DF (eds). Diseases of the Periodontium. Northwood: Science Reviews, 1993:55–93.

160. Elliott JR, Bowers GM, Corio RL. The clinical problem of oral psoriasis. Ear Nose Throat J 1985;64:223–227.

161. DeGregori G, Pippen R, Davis E. Psoriasis of the gingiva and tongue. Report of a case. J Periodontol 1971;42:97–100.

162. Pogrel MA, Cram D. Findings in patients with psoriasis with a special reference to ectopic geographic tongue (erythema circinata). Oral Surg Oral Med Oral Pathol 1988;66:184–198.

163. Zhu JF, Kaminski MJ, Pulitzer DR, et al. Psoriasis: Pathophysiology and oral manifestations. Oral Dis 1996;2:135–144.

164. Ulmansky M, Michelle R, Azaz B. Oral psoriasis: Report of six new cases. J Oral Pathol Med 1995;24:42–45.

165. Weathers DR, Baker G, Archard HO, Burkes EJ Jr. Psoriasiform lesions of the oral mucosa (with emphasis on "ectopic geographic tongue"). Oral Pathol 1974;37:872–888.

166. Hietanen J, Salo OP, Kanerva L, Juvakoski T. Study of the oral mucosa in 200 consecutive patients with psoriasis. Scand J Dent Res 1984;92:50–54.

167. Rees TD. Drugs and oral disorders. Periodontol 2000 1998; 18:21–36.

168. Rees TD. Orofacial granulomatosis and related conditions. Periodontol 2000 1999;21:145–157.

169. Fischman SL, Barnett ML, Nisengard RJ. Histopathologic, ultrastructural and immunologic findings in an oral psoriatic lesion. Oral Surg Oral Med Oral Pathol 1977;44:253–260.

170. Axell T, Henricsson V. The occurrence of recurrent aphthous ulcers in an adult Swedish population. Acta Odontol Scand 1985;43:121–125.

171. Crivelli MR, Adler SAI, Quarracino C, Bazerque P. Influence of socioeconomic status on oral mucosa lesion prevalence in school children. Community Dent Oral Epidemiol 1988;16:58–60.

172. Ship II, Morris AL, Durocher RT, Burket LW. Recurrent aphthous ulcerations in a professional school student population. IV. Twelve-month study of natural disease patterns. Oral Surg Oral Med Oral Pathol 1961;4:30–39.

173. Bagen JV, Sanchis JM, Milian MA, et al. Recurrent aphthous stomatitis. A study of the clinical characteristics of 93 cases. J Oral Pathol Med 1991;20:395–397.

174. Cooke BED. Diagnosis of recurrent oral ulceration. Br J Dermatol 1969;81:159–161.

175. Mintz GA, Smidansky ED. Aphthous stomatitis with involvement of attached gingiva. Oral Surg Oral Med Oral Pathol 1985;60:122–124.

176. Shohat-Zabarski R, Kaldeson S, Klein T, et al. Close association of HLA–B51 in persons with recurrent aphthous stomatitis. Oral Surg Oral Med Oral Pathol 1992;74:455–458.

177. Hayrinen-Imminen R. Immune-activation in recurrent oral ulcers (ROV). Scand J Dent Res 1992;100:222–227.

178. Regezi JA, MacPhail LA, Richards DW, Greenspan JS. A study of macrophages, macrophage-related cells and endothelial adhesion molecules in recurrent aphthous ulcers in HIV-positive patients. J Dent Res 1993;72:1549–1553.

179. Kvan E, Gjerdet NR, Bondevik O. Traumatic ulcers and pain during orthodontic treatment. Community Dent Oral Epidemiol 1987;15:104–107.

180. Wright A, Ryan FP, Willingham SE, et al. Food allergy or intolerance in severe recurrent aphthous ulceration of the mouth. Br Med J 1986;292:1237–1238.

181. Hay KD, Reade PC. The use of an elimination diet in the treatment of recurrent aphthous ulceration of the oral cavity. Oral Surg Oral Med Oral Pathol 1984;57:504–507.

182. Wilson CW. Food sensitivities, taste changes, aphthous ulcers and atopic symptoms in allergic disease. Ann Allergy 1980;44:302–307.

183. Field EA, Rotter E, Speechley JA, Tyldesley WR. Clinical and haematological assessment of children with recurrent aphthous ulceration. Br Dent J 1987;163:19–22.

184. Wray D, Ferguson MM, Mason DK, et al. Recurrent aphthae: Treatment with vitamin B12, folic acid and iron. Br Med J 1975;212:490–493.

185. Hutcheon AW, Dagg JH, Mason DK, et al. Clinical and haematological screening in recurrent aphthae. Postgrad Med J 1978;54:779–783.

186. Challacombe SJ, Barkhan P, Lehner T. Haematological features and differentiation of recurrent oral ulceration. Br J Oral Surg 1977;15:37–48.

187. Nelson A, Lamey PJ, Milligan KA, Forsythe A. Recurrent aphthous ulceration and food sensitivity. J Oral Pathol Med 1991;20:473–475.

188. Nelson A, McIntosh WB, Allam BF, Lamey RT. Recurrent aphthous ulceration: Vitamin B, B2 and B6 status and response to replacement therapy. J Oral Pathol 1991;20:389–391.

189. Endre L. Recurrent aphthous ulceration with zinc deficiency and cellular immune deficiency. Oral Surg Oral Med Oral Pathol 1991;72:559–561.

190. Porter SR, Kingsmill V, Scully C. Audit of diagnoses and investigation in patients with recurrent aphthous stomatitis. Oral Surg Oral Med Oral Pathol 1993;76:449–452.

191. Pedersen A, Hornsleth A. Recurrent aphthous ulceration: A possible clinical manifestation of reactivation of varicella zoster or cytomegalovirus infection. J Oral Pathol Med 1993;22:64–68.

192. Scully C, Galloway AR, Main ANH, Russell RI. Effects of dietary gluten elimination in patients with recurrent minor aphthous stomatitis and no detectable gluten enteropathy. Oral Surg Oral Med Oral Pathol 1993;75:595–598.

193. Rees TD, Binnie WH. Recurrent aphthous stomatitis. Dermatol Clin 1996;14:243–256.

194. Ogura M, Yamamoto T, Morita M, Watanabe T. A case-control study on food intake of patients with recurrent aphthous stomatitis. Oral Surg Oral Med Oral Pathol Oral Radiol Endod 2001;91:45–49.

195. Riggio MP, Lennon A, Wray D. Detection of Helicobacter pylori DNA in recurrent aphthous stomatitis tissue by PCR. J Oral Pathol Med 2000;29:507–513.

196. Czerniniski R, Katz J, Schlesinger M. Preliminary evidence for an association of measles virus with recurrent aphthous ulceration. Arch Dermatol 2000;136:801–803.

197. MacPhail LA, Greenspan D, Feigel DW, et al. Recurrent aphthous ulcers in association with HIV infection. Oral Surg Oral Med Oral Pathol 1991;71:678–683.

198. Ferguson MM, Wray D, Carmichael HA, et al. Coeliac disease associated with recurrent aphthae. Gut 1980;21:223–226.

199. Zimmerman HM, Rosenblum G, Bank S. Aphthous ulcers of the esophagus in a patient with ulcerative colitis. Gastrointest Endosc 1984;30:298–299.

200. Coenen C, Borsch G, Muller K-M, Fabry H. Oral inflammatory changes as an initial manifestation of Crohn's disease antedating abdominal diagnosis. Report of a case. Dis Colon Rectum 1988;31:548–552.

201. Charon JA, Mergenhagen SE, Gallin JJ. Gingivitis and oral ulceration in patients with neutrophil dysfunction. J Oral Pathol 1985;14:150–155.

202. Redenos JM, Ortega N, Herranz MT, et al. Cyclic neutropenia: A cause of recurrent aphthous stomatitis not to be missed. Dermatol 1992;184:205–207.

203. Muzyka BC, Glick M. Major aphthous ulcers in patients with HIV disease. Oral Surg Oral Med Oral Pathol 1994;77:116–120.

204. Porter SR, Hegarty A, Kaliakatsou F, et al. Recurrent aphthous stomatitis. Clin Dermatol 2000;18:569–578.

205. Hegab S, Al-Mutawa S. Immunopathogenesis of Behçet's disease. Clin Immunol 2000;96:174–186.

206. Plemons JM, Rees TD, Binnie WH, et al. Evaluation of acemannan in the treatment of recurrent aphthous stomatitis. Wounds 1994;6:40–45.

207. Meiller JF, Kutchen MJ, Overholser CD, et al. Effect of an antimicrobial mouthrinse on recurrent aphthous ulcerations. Oral Surg Oral Med Oral Pathol 1991;72:425–429.

208. Wright VD, Chamberlain MA. Behçet's syndrome with arthritis. Ann Rheumatol Dis 1989;28:95–103.

209. James DG. Behçet's syndrome. N Engl J Med 1979;301:431–432.

210. Marquardt JL, Snyderman R, Oppenheim JJ. Depression of lymphocyte transformation and exacerbation of Behçet's syndrome by ingestion of English walnuts. Cell Immunol 1973;9:263–272.

211. Arbesfeld SJ, Kurban AK. Behçet's disease. New perspectives on an enigmatic syndrome. J Am Acad Dermatol 1988;19:767–779.

212. Wong RC, Ellis CN, Diaz LA. Behçet's disease. Int J Dermatol 1984;23:25–32.

213. Cohen L. Etiology, pathogenesis and classification of aphthous stomatitis and Behçet's syndrome. J Oral Pathol 1978;7:347–352.

214. Mousam ARAM, Marafie AA, Rifai KMA, et al. Behçet's disease in Kuwait, Arabia. A report of 29 cases and a review. Scand J Rheumatol 1986;15:310–332.

215. Benezra D, Cohen E. Treatment and visual prognosis in Behçet's disease. Br J Ophthalmol 1986;70:589–592.

216. Ammann AR, Johnson A, Fyfe GA, et al. Behçet syndrome. J Pediatr 1985;107:41–43.

217. BenEzra D, Cohen E, Chajek T, et al. Evaluation of conventional therapy versus cyclosporine A in Behçet's syndrome. Transplant Proc 1988;20:136–143.

218. Pizarro A, Herranz P, Garcia-Tobaruelaa A, Casado M. Pentoxifylline in the treatment of orogenital aphthosis and Behçet's syndrome. Med Clin (Barc) 2000;115:678–679.

219. Hamza MH. Treatment of Behçet's disease with thalidomide. Clin Rheumatol 1988;5:365–371.

220. Eisenbud L, Horowitz I, Kay B. Recurrent aphthous stomatitis of the Behçet's type: Successful treatment with thalidomide. Oral Surg Oral Med Oral Pathol 1987;64:289–292.

221. Lynch FW. Erythema multiforme: A review. South Med J 1955;48:279.

222. Kalb RE, Grossman ME, Neu HC. Stevens-Johnson syndrome due to mycoplasma pneumoniae in an adult. Am J Med 1985;79:541–543.

223. Ruokonen H, Malmstrom M, Stubb S. Factors influencing the recurrence of erythema multiforme. Proc Finn Dent Soc 1988;84:167–174.

224. Rees TD. Phenothiazine—another possible etiologic agent in erythema multiforme. Report of a case. J Periodontol 1985;56:480–483.

225. Lozada F, Silverman S Jr. Erythema multiforme. Clinical characteristics and natural history in fifty patients. Oral Surg Oral Med Oral Pathol 1978;46:628–636.

226. Lehtinen H, Malmstrom M, Stubb S. Erythema exudativum multiforme and Stevens-Johnson syndrome. A retrospective study. Proc Finn Dent Soc 1986;82:119–126.

227. Welch KJ, Burke WA, Irons TG. Recurrent erythema multiforme due to mycoplasma pneumoniae. J Am Acad Dermatol 1987;17:839–840.

228. Gebel K, Hornstein OP. Drug-induced oral erythema multiforme. Results of a long-term retrospective study. Dermatologica 1984;168:35–40.

229. Kauppinen K, Stubb S. Drug eruptions: Causative agents and clinical types. A series of in-patients during a 10-year period. Acta Derm Venereol 1984;64:320–324.

230. Stutman HR. Stevens-Johnson syndrome and mycoplasma pneumoniae: Evidence for cutaneous infection. J Pediatr 1987;111:845–847.

231. Siegel MA, Balciunas BA. Oral presentation and management of vesiculobullous disorders. Semin Dermatol 1994;13:78–86.

232. McKellar GM, Reade PC. Erythema multiforme and mycoplasma pneumoniae infection. Report and discussion of a case presenting with stomatitis. Int J Oral Maxillofac Surg 1986;15:342–348.

233. Nesbit SP, Gobetti JP. Multiple recurrence of oral erythema multiforme after secondary herpes simplex: Report of a case and review of literature. J Am Dent Assoc 1986;112:348–352.

234. Araujo OE, Flowers FP. Stevens-Johnson syndrome. J Emer Med 1984;2:129–135.

235. Leigh IM, Mowbray JF, Levene GM, Sutherland S. Recurrent and continuous erythema multiforme. A clinical and immunological study. Clin Exp Dermatol 1985;10:58–67.

236. Reed RJ. Erythema multiforme. A clinical syndrome and a histologic complex. Am J Dermatopathol 1985;7:143–152.

237. Caulfield JB, Wilgram GF. An electron microscopic study of blister formation in erythema multiforme. J Invest Dermatol 1962;39:307–316.

238. Orfanos CE, Schamburg-Lever G, Lever WF. Dermal and epidermal types of erythema multiforme. Arch Dermatol 1974;109:682–688.

239. Katz J, Livneh A, Shemer J, et al. Herpes simplex–associated erythema multiforme (HAEM): A clinical therapeutic dilemma. Pediatr Dent 1999;21:359–362.

240. Rivera-Hidalgo F, Stanford TS. Oral mucosal lesions caused by infective microorganisms. I. Viruses and bacteria. Periodontol 2000 1999;21:106–124.

241. Bushkell LL, Mackel SE, Jordon RE. Erythema multiforme: Direct immunofluorescence studies and detection of circulating immune complexes. J Invest Dermatol 1980;74:372–374.

242. Lemak MA, Duvic M, Bean SF. Oral acyclovir for the prevention of herpes-associated erythema multiforme. J Am Acad Dermatol 1986;15:50–54.

243. Lowhagen GB, Jansen E, Mordenfelt D, Lycke E. Epidemiology of genital herpes infections in Sweden. Acta Derm Venereol 1990;70:330–334.

244. Scully C. Orofacial herpes simplex virus infection: Current concepts on the epidemiology, pathogenesis and treatments and disorders in which the virus may be implicated. Oral Surg Oral Med Oral Pathol 1989;68:701–718.

245. Bergstrom T, Lycke E. Neuroinvasion by herpes simplex virus. An in vitro model for characterization of neurovirulent strains. J Gen Virol 1990;71:405–410.

246. Knaup B, Schunemann S, Wolff MH. Subclinical reactivation of herpes simplex virus type 1 in the oral cavity. Oral Microbiol Immunol 2000;15:281–283.

247. Schmidt-Westhausen AM, Priepke F, Bergmann FJ, Reichart PA. Decline in the rate of oral opportunistic infections following introduction of highly active antiretroviral therapy. J Oral Pathol Med 2000;29:336–341.

248. Spruance SL. Pathogenesis of herpes simplex labialis: Experimental induction of lesions with U-V light. J Clin Microbiol 1985;22:366–368.

249. Nahass GT, Goldstein BA, Zhu WY, et al. Comparison of Tzanck smear, viral culture and DNA diagnostic methods in detection of herpes simplex and varicella–zoster infection. JAMA 1992;268:2541–2544.

250. Epstein JB, Scully C. Herpes simplex virus in immunocompromised patients: Growing evidence of drug resistance. Oral Surg Oral Med Oral Pathol 1991;72:47–50.

251. Bayrou O, Gaouar H, Leynadier F. Famciclovir as a possible alternative treatment in some cases of allergy to acyclovir. Contact Dermatitis 2000;42:42.

252. Emmert DH. Treatment of common cutaneous herpes simplex virus infections. Am Fam Physician 2000;15:1697–1706,1708.

253. Habbema L, De Boulle K, Roders GA, Katz DH. n-Docosanol 10% cream in the treatment of recurrent herpes labialis: A randomized, double-blind, placebo-controlled study. Acta Derm Venereol 1996;76:479–481.

254. Boon R, Goodman JJ, Martinez J, et al. Penciclovir cream for the treatment of sunlight-induced herpes simplex labialis: A randomized, double-blind, placebo-controlled trial. Penciclovir Cream Herpes Labialis Study Group. Clin Ther 2000;22:76–90.

255. Spruance SL, McKeough MB. Combination treatment with fam-ciclovir and a topical corticosteroid gel versus famciclovir alone for experimental ultraviolet radiation-induced herpes simplex labialis: A pilot study. J Infect Dis 2000;181:1906–1910.

256. Kaminester LH, Pariser RJ, Weiss JS, et al. A double-blind, placebo-controlled study of topical tetracaine in the treatment of herpes labialis. J Am Acad Dermatol 1999;41:996–1001.

257. Koytchev R, Alken RG, Dundarov S. Balm mint extract (Lo-701) for topical treatment of recurring herpes labialis. Phytomedicine 1999;6:225–230.

258. Willis A, Hyland P, Lamey PJ. Response to replacement iron therapy in sideropenic individuals with recrudescent herpes labialis. Eur J Clin Microbiol Infect Dis 2000;19:355–357.

259. Scalvenzi M, Ceddia C. Research in simple blind with natural interferon alpha at low dosage on subjects affected by labialis and genitalis herpes simplex. Clin Ter 2000;151(suppl 1):13–18.

260. Kfir Y, Buchner A, Hansen LS. Reactive lesions of the gingiva. A clinicopathologic study of 741 cases. J Periodontol 1980;51: 655–661.

261. Barker DA, Lucas RB. Localized fibrous overgrowths of the oral mucosa. Br J Oral Surg 1967;5:86–92.

262. Weathers DR, Calihan D. Giant cell fibroma. Oral Surg Oral Med Oral Pathol 1974;37:374–384.

263. Houston GD. The giant cell fibroma. A review of 464 cases. Oral Surg Oral Med Oral Pathol 1982;53:582–587.

264. Gardner DG. The peripheral odontogenic fibroma: An attempt at clarification. Oral Surg Oral Med Oral Pathol 1982;54:40–48.

265. Buchner A, Hansen LS. The histomorphologic spectrum of pe-ripheral ossifying fibroma. Oral Surg Oral Med Oral Pathol 1987;63:452–461.

266. Kramer IRH, Pindborg JJ, Shear M. World Health Organization Histological Typing of Odontogenic Tumours, ed 2. New York: Springer-Verlag, 1992.

267. Buchner A, Ficarra G, Hansen LS. Peripheral odontogenic fi-broma. Oral Surg Oral Med Oral Pathol 1987;64:432–438.

268. Angelopoulos AP. Pyogenic granuloma of the oral cavity: Statis-tical analysis of its clinical features. J Oral Surg 1971;29: 840–847.

269. Giansanti JS, Waldron CA. Peripheral giant cell granuloma. J Oral Surg 1969;27:788–791.

270. Katsikeris N, Kakarantza-Angelopoulos E, Angelopoulos AP. Pe-ripheral giant cell granuloma. Clinicopathologic study of 224 new cases and review of 956 reported cases. Int J Oral Maxillo-fac Surg 1988;17:94–99.

271. Bonetti F, Pelosi G, Martignoni G, et al. Peripheral giant cell granuloma: Evidence for osteoclastic differentiation. Oral Surg Oral Med Oral Pathol 1990;70:471–475.

272. Buchner A, Sciubba JJ. Peripheral odontogenic tumors: A review. Oral Surg Oral Med Oral Pathol 1987;63:688–697.

273. Abemayor E, Calceterra TC. Kaposi's sarcoma and community-acquired immune deficiency syndrome. Arch Otolaryngol 1983;109:536–542.

274. Lozada F, Silverman S, Migliorati CA, et al. Oral manifestations of tumors and opportunistic infections in the acquired immun-odeficiency syndrome (AIDS): Findings in 53 homosexual men with Kaposi's sarcoma. Oral Surg Oral Med Oral Pathol 1983; 56:491–494.

275. Ficarra G, Berson AM, Silverman S, et al. Kaposi's sarcoma of the oral cavity: A study of 134 patients with a review of the path-ogenesis, epidemiology, clinical aspects, and treatment. Oral Surg Oral Med Oral Pathol 1988;66:543–550.

276. Silverman S, Gorsky M. Epidemiologic and demographic update in oral cancer: California and national data—1973–1985. J Am Dent Assoc 1990;120:495–499.

277. US Dept Health and Human Services, CDC, NIH. Cancers of the oral cavity and pharynx. A statistics review monograph. 1973–1987. Atlanta: Dental Disease Prevention Activity, Na-tional Center for Prevention Services, 1991.

278. McDonald JS, Crissman JD, Gluckman JL. Verrucous carcinoma of the oral cavity. Head Neck Surg 1982;5:22–28.

279. McCoy JM, Waldron CA. Verrucous carcinoma of the oral cav-ity. Oral Surg Oral Med Oral Pathol 1981;52:623–629.

280. Pennypacker JP, Hassel JR, Yamanda KM, Pratt RM. The influ-ence of an adhesive cell surface protein on chondrogenic ex-pression in vitro. Exp Cell Res 1979;121:411–415.

281. Soll DR, Mitchell LH. Differentiation and dedifferentiation can function simultaneously and independently in the same cells in Dictyostelium discoideum. Dev Biol 1982;91:183–190.

282. Wright JM. Reactive, dysplastic and neoplastic conditions of pe-riodontal ligament origin. Periodontol 2000 1999;21:7–15.

283. Neville BW, Albenesius RJ. The prevalence of benign fibro-os-seous lesions of periodontal ligament origin in black women. A radiographic survey. Oral Surg Oral Med Oral Pathol 1986; 62:340–344.

284. Waldron CA, Giansanti JS. Benign fibro-osseous lesions of the jaws. A clinical-radiologic-histologic review of sixty-five cases. Part II. Benign fibro-osseous lesions of periodontal ligament ori-gin. Oral Surg Oral Med Oral Pathol 1973;35:340–350.

285. Waldron CA. Fibro-osseous lesions of the jaws. J Oral Maxillo-fac Surg 1985;43:249–262.

286. Zegarelli EV, Kutscher AH, Napoli N, et al. The cementoma—A study of 230 patients with 435 cementomas. Oral Surg Oral Med Oral Pathol 1964;17:219–224.

287. Waldron CA. Fibro-osseous lesions of the jaws. J Oral Maxillo-fac Surg 1993;51:828–835.

288. Summerlin D, Tomich C. Focal cemento-osseous dysplasia: A clinicopathologic study of 221 cases. Oral Surg Oral Med Oral Pathol 1994;78:611–620.

289. Su L, Weathers DR, Waldron CA. Distinguishing features of focal cemento-osseous dysplasia and cemento-ossifying fibromas. II. A clinical and radiographic spectrum of 316 cases. Oral Surg Oral Med Oral Pathol Oral Radiol Endod 1997;84: 540–549.

290. Melrose FJ, Abrams AA, Mills BG. Florid osseous dysplasia. Oral Surg Oral Med Oral Pathol 1976;41:62–82.

291. Waldron CA, Giansanti JS, Broward BB. Sclerotic cemental masses of the jaws (so called chronic sclerosing osteomyelitis, sclerosing osteitis, multiple enostosis and gigantiform cemen-toma). Oral Surg Oral Med Oral Pathol 1975;39:590–604.

292. Agazzi C, Belloni L. Gli odontomi duri dei mascellari. Arch Ital Otol 1953;LXIV(suppl XVI).

293. Eversole LR, Leider AS, Nelson K. Ossifying fibroma: A clinico-pathologic study of sixty-four cases. Oral Surg Oral Med Oral Pathol 1985;60:505–511.

294. El-Mofty SK. Cemento-ossifying fibroma and benign cemento-blastoma. Semin Diagn Pathol 1999;16:203–207.

295. Farman AG, Kohler WW, Nortje CJY, Van Wyk CW. Cemento-blastoma: Report of case. J Oral Surg 1979;37:198–203.

296. Abrams AM, Kirby JW, Melrose RJ. Cementoblastoma. Oral Surg Oral Med Oral Pathol 1974;38:394–403.

297. Goerig AC, Fay JT, King E. Endodontic treatment of a cemento-blastoma. Report of a case. Oral Surg Oral Med Oral Pathol 1984;58:133–136.

298. Cutler LS, Krutchkoff D. An ultrastructural study of eosinophilic granuloma: The Langerhans' cell—Its role in histogenesis and diagnosis. Oral Surg Oral Med Oral Pathol 1977;44:246–252.

299. Hartman KS. Histiocytosis X: A review of 114 cases with oral involvement. Oral Surg Oral Med Oral Pathol 1980;49:38–54.

300. Armitage GC. Development of a classification system for periodontal diseases and conditions. Ann Periodontol 1999;4(1):1–6.

301. Prichard JF. Management of the periodontal abscess. In: Prichard JF (ed). Advanced Periodontal Disease/Surgical and Prosthetic Management. Philadelphia: Saunders, 1972:602–637.

302. Schluger S, Yuodelis R, Page R, Johnson R. Acute inflammatory periodontal diseases. In: Schluger S, Yuodelis R, Page R, Johnson R (eds). Periodontal Diseases: Basic Phenomena, Clinical Management, and Occlusal and Restorative Interrelationships. Philadelphia: Lea and Febiger, 1990:263–272.

303. Prichard JF. Management of the periodontal abscess. Oral Surg 1953;6:474–482.

304. Goldman HM, Cohen DW. Periodontal Therapy, ed 6. St. Louis: Mosby, 1980.

305. Schluger S, Yuodelis R, Page R, Johnson R. Pathogenic mechanisms. In: Schluger S, Yuodelis R, Page R, Johnson R (eds). Periodontal Diseases: Basic Phenomena, Clinical Management, and Occlusal and Restorative Interrelationships. Philadelphia: Lea and Febiger, 1990:246–254.

306. Labriola JD, Mascaro J, Alpert B. The microbiologic flora of orofacial abscesses. J Oral Maxillofac Surg 1983;41:711–714.

307. Newman MG, Sims T. The predominant cultivable microbiota of the periodontal abscess. J Periodontol 1979;50:350–354.

308. Prichard JF. The periodontal-pulpal quandary. In: Prichard JF (ed). Advanced Periodontal Disease/Surgical and Prosthetic Management. Philadelphia: Saunders, 1972:229–233.

309. Goldman HM, Cohen DW. Special problems in periodontal therapy. In: Goldman HM, Cohen DW (eds). Periodontal Therapy. St. Louis: Mosby, 1980:1021.

310. Rowland RW. Necrotizing ulcerative gingivitis. Ann Periodontol 1999;4(1):65–73.

311. Classification and diagnostic criteria for oral lesions in HIV infection. EC-Clearinghouse on Oral Problems Related to HIV Infections and WHO Collaborating Centre on Oral Manifestations of the Immunodeficiency Virus. J Oral Pathol Med 1993;22:289–291.

312. Hirschfeld I, Beube F, Siegel EH. The history of Vincent's infection. J Periodontol 1940;2:89–98.

313. Schluger S. Necrotic ulcerative gingivitis in the Army: Incidence, communicability and treatment. J Am Dent Assoc 1949;38:174–183.

314. Pindborg JJ. The epidemiology of ulceromembranous gingivitis showing the influence of service in the Armed Forces. Paradontology 1956;10:114–118.

315. Miller SC, Greene HI. A worldwide survey of acute necrotizing ulcerative gingivitis: A preliminary report. J Dent Med 1958;13:66–81.

316. Emslie RD. Cancrum oris. Dent Pract 1963;13:481–495.

317. Enwonwu C. Epidemiological and biochemical studies of necrotizing ulcerative gingivitis and noma (cancrum oris) in Nigerian children. Arch Oral Biol 1972;17:1357–1371.

318. MacDonald JB, Sutton RM, Knoll ML, et al. The pathogenic components of an experimental fusospirochetal infection. J Infect Dis 1956;98:15–20.

319. Schwartzman J, Grossman L. Vincent's ulceromembranous gingivostomatitis. Arch Pediatr 1941;58:515–520.

320. Stammers AF. Vincent's infection: Observations and conclusions regarding the aetiology and treatment of 1,017 civilian cases. Br Dent J 1944;76:147–155,171–177,205–209.

321. Melnick SL, Roseman JM, Engel D, Cogen RB. Epidemiology of acute necrotizing ulcerative gingivitis. Epidemiol Rev 1988;10:191–211.

322. Plaut HC. Studien zur bacteriellen diagnostik der diptherie/und der angien. Deutsche Med Woch 1894;20:920–923.

323. Vincent H. Sur l'etiologie et sur les lesions anatomo-pathologiques de la pourriture d'hopital. Ann Inst Pasteur 1896;10:448.

324. Loesche WJ, Syed SA, Laughon BE, Stoll J. The bacteriology of acute necrotizing ulcerative gingivitis. J Periodontol 1982;53(4):223–230.

325. Falker WJ, Martin S, Vincent J, et al. A clinical, demographic and microbiologic study of ANUG patients in an urban dental school. J Clin Periodontol 1987;14:307–314.

326. Chung CP, Nisengard RJ, Slots J, Genco RJ. Bacterial IgG and IgM antibody titers in acute necrotizing ulcerative gingivitis. J Clin Periodontol 1983;54:557–562.

327. Rowland RW, Mestecky J, Gunsolley JC, Cogen RB. Serum IgG and IgM levels to bacterial antigens in necrotizing ulcerative gingivitis. J Periodontol 1993;64:195–201.

328. Schluger S. The etiology and treatment of Vincent's infection. J Am Dent Assoc 1943;30:524–532.

329. Pindborg JJ. Gingivitis in military personnel with special reference to ulceromembranous gingivitis. Odontol Tidskrift 1951;59:407–499.

330. Moulton R, Ewen S, Thieman W. Emotional factors in periodontal disease. Oral Surg Oral Med Oral Pathol 1952;5:833–860.

331. Shannon I, Kilgoe W, O'Leary T. Stress as a predisposing factor in necrotizing ulcerative gingivitis. J Periodontol 1969;40:240–242.

332. Shields WD. Acute necrotizing ulcerative gingivitis: A study of some of the contributing factors and their validity in an army population. J Periodontol 1977;48:346–349.

333. Formicola A, Witte E, Curran P. A study of personality traits and acute necrotizing ulcerative gingivitis. J Periodontol 1970;41:36–38.

334. Cohen-Cole S, Cogen R, Stevens J, et al. Psychiatric, psychosocial, and endocrine correlates of acute necrotizing ulcerative gingivitis (trench mouth): A preliminary report. Psychiatr Med 1983;1:215–220.

335. Kowolik MJ, Nisbet T. Smoking and acute ulcerative gingivitis. Br Dent J 1983;154:241–242.

336. Pindborg J, Bhat M, Roed-Petersen B. Oral changes in south Indian children with severe protein deficiency. J Periodontol 1967;38:218–221.

337. Jiminez LM, Baer PM. Necrotizing ulcerative gingivitis in children, a nine year clinical study. J Periodontol 1975;46:715–720.

338. Barnes GP, Bowles WF, Carter HG. Acute necrotizing ulcerative gingivitis: A survey of 218 cases. J Periodontol 1973;44:35–42.

339. Sheiham A. An epidemiological survey of acute ulcerative gingivitis in Nigerians. Arch Oral Biol 1966;11:937–942.

340. Taiwo JO. Oral hygiene status and necrotizing ulcerative gingivitis in Nigerian children. J Periodontol 1993;64:1071–1074.

341. Uohara GI, Knapp MJ. Oral fusospirochetosis and associated lesions. Oral Surg Oral Med Oral Pathol 1967;24:113–123.

342. Taiwo JO. Severity of necrotizing ulcerative gingivitis in Nigerian children. Periodontal Clin Investig 1995;17:24–27.

343. Enwonwu CO, Falker WA Jr, Idigbe EO, et al. Pathogenesis of cancrum oris (noma) confounding interactions of malnutrition with infection. Am J Trop Med Hyg 1999;60:223–232.

344. Giddon D, Goldhaber P, Dunning J. Prevalence of reported cases of acute necrotizing ulcerative gingivitis in a university population. J Periodontol 1963;34:366–371.

345. Maupin C, Bell B. Relationship of 17-hydroxycorticosteroid to acute necrotizing ulcerative gingivitis. J Periodontol 1975;46:721–722.

346. Goldhaber P. A study of acute necrotizing ulcerative gingivitis [abstract 18]. Int Agency Dent Res 1957;35.

347. Bergstrom J, Eliasson S. Noxious effect of cigarette smoking on periodontal health. J Periodontal Res 1987;22:513–517.

348. Haber J, Wattles J, Crowlery M, et al. Evidence for cigarette smoking as a major risk factor for periodontitis. J Periodontol 1993;64:16–23.

349. Stoltenberg JL, Osborn JB, Pihlstrom BL, et al. Association between cigarette smoking, bacterial pathogens, and periodontal status. J Periodontol 1993;64:1225–1230.

350. Claffey N, Russell R, Dhanley D. Peripheral blood phagocyte function in acute necrotizing ulcerative gingivits. J Periodontal Res 1986;21:288–297.

351. Holm G. Smoking as an additional risk for tooth loss. J Periodontol 1994;65:996–1001.

352. Cogen R, Stevens JAW, Cohen-Cole S, et al. Leukocyte function in the etiology of acute necrotizing ulcerative gingivitis. J Periodontol 1983;54:402–407.

353. Lehner T, Clarry ED. Acute ulcerative gingivitis. An immunofluorescent investigation. Br Dent J 1966;121:366–370.

354. Wilton J, Ivanyi L, Lehner T. Cell-mediated immunity and humoral antibodies in acute ulcerative gingivitis. J Periodontal Res 1971;6:9–16.

355. Mikx FHM, van Campen GJ. Microscopical evaluation of the microflora in relation to necrotizing ulcerative gingivitis in the beagle dog. J Periodontal Res 1982;17:576–584.

356. Hug HU, Maltha JC, Mikx FHM. Necrotizing ulcerative gingivitis in beagle dogs. II. Histologic characteristics of NUG in relation to interproximal contacts. J Periodontal Res 1984;19:89–99.

357. James K. Immunoserology of infectious diseases. Clin Microbiol Rev 1990;3:132–152.

358. Page RC, Schroeder HE. Periodontitis in Man and Other Animals. A Comparative Review. New York: Karger, 1982.

359. Cogen RB. Acute necrotizing ulcerative gingivitis. In: Genco RJ, Goldman HM, Cohen DW (eds). Contemporary Periodontics. St. Louis: Mosby, 1990:38.

360. Schiodt M, Pindborg J. AIDS and the oral cavity: Epidemiology and clinical oral manifestations of human immune deficiency virus infection. Int J Oral Maxillofac Surg 1987;16:1–14.

361. Skack M, Zabrodsky S, Mrklas L. A study of the effect of age and season on the incidence of ulcerative gingivitis. J Periodontal Res 1970;5:187–190.

362. Smits PAES. Some clinical and epidemiological aspects of Vincent's gingivitis. Dent Pract Dent Rec 1965;15:281–286.

363. Giddon DB, Zackin JS, Goldhabert P. Acute necrotizing ulcerative gingivitis in college students. J Am Dent Assoc 1964;68:381–386.

364. Listgarten MA. Electron microscopic observations of the bacterial flora of acute necrotizing ulcerative gingivitis. J Periodontol 1965;36:328.

365. Buest TB, Albray RA, Hirschfeld I. Oral manifestations and treatment of Vincent's infection. J Dent Res 1930;10:97–108.

366. Ciancio SG. Antibiotics in periodontal therapy. In: Newman M, Gordman A (eds). Guide to Antibiotic Use in Dental Practice. Chicago: Quintessence, 1984:136–147.

367. Lang NP, Brecx MC. Chlorhexidine digluconate—An agent for chemical plaque control and prevention of gingival inflammation. J Periodontal Res 1986;21(suppl 16):74–89.

Part III

Restorative and Esthetic Treatment Aspects of Periodontal Therapy

Periodontal Health and Restorative Procedures

Niklaus P. Lang and William C. Martin
- Preparatory Procedures
- Reconstruction and Periodontal Health
- Esthetic Considerations

The biologic and biophysical aspects of fixed reconstructions have received much attention, starting with the experimental work of the Scandinavian periodontal research community a generation ago.[1–8] The challenge of old dogmas such as the principle of "extension for prevention,"[9] which had dominated reconstructive dentistry for almost a century, paved the way for scientific thinking. However, the practical implications of biologic principles for reconstructive dentistry sometimes conflict with the patient's subjective feelings about esthetics. This chapter documents the biologic basis for acceptable reconstructions and evaluates suggested compromises in light of improved casting techniques, new restorative materials, and additional clinical procedures to improve esthetics.

Preparatory Procedures

Biologic principles must guide both the preparation of the abutment tooth or teeth destined to receive a crown and the choice of dental materials to be used in the procedures. If acceptable periodontal conditions are to be achieved and maintained after cementation of a reconstruction, it is important that gingival inflammation or even periodontitis be successfully treated and eliminated before the pros-

thetic reconstruction is begun. Too often, however, the prognosis of successfully completed periodontal therapy is rendered questionable by the prosthetic treatment that follows it. These negative influences may be attributed to either effects of the prosthetic construction phases (eg, tooth preparation, impression making, and provisional coverage) or functional effects of reconstructions impinging on periodontal health.

Preparation of Abutment Teeth

Rotating instruments used beneath the gingival margin traumatize the gingival tissue, the sulcus epithelium, and possibly even the epithelial attachment and the subjacent connective tissue.[8] The trauma caused by the rotating stone or burr may be reversible (Fig 30-1), but where tooth preparation is carried apical to the base of the attachment level, permanent loss of periodontal attachment may result.[10] Typically, extension into the gingival crevice should not exceed 1 mm, depending on the depth of the sulcus and the level of the osseous crest.[11,12] In areas of esthetic concern, the final crown margin (chamfer or shoulder) should be placed slightly beneath the free gingival margin.[11] Underreduction in this area may lead to overcontouring of the final restoration and chronic irritation.

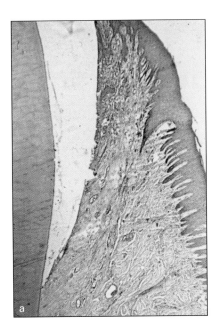

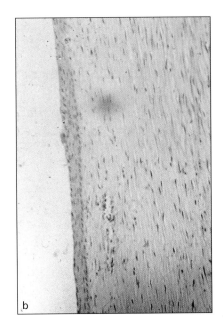

Figs 30-1a and 30-1b *(a)* Treatment of a subgingival environment with a rotating instrument (rubber cup and polishing paste) resulting in removal of most of the junctional epithelium. *(b)* Four weeks following the procedure, an intact epithelial attachment is reestablished. (Courtesy of H. Löe.)

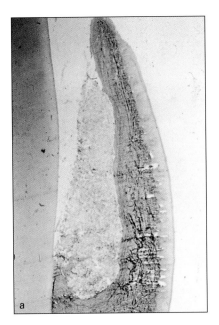

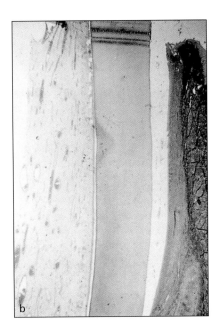

Figs 30-2a and 30-2b *(a)* Retraction cord placed prior to impression taking resulting in damage to the junctional epithelium. *(b)* Four weeks following impression taking, the healing process resulted in the formation of a new junctional epithelium without loss of connective tissue attachment. (Courtesy of H. Löe.)

Impression Making

Damage to the periodontium may occur during impression making, regardless of the impression technique employed. The use of retraction cords to displace the gingiva prior to impression making often damages the subgingival tissues. However, damage is usually reversible[8] (Fig 30-2). A survey of 1,246 members of the American College of Prosthodontists showed that 98% of respondents use retraction cord to displace tissue prior to impression making, and 48% use a double cord technique.[13] Soaking cords in a hemostatic solution prior to placing them in the sulcus is also common. Buffered aluminum chloride is frequently used.[13]

Severe periodontal reactions with subsequent loss of attachment have been reported after the use of elastic impression materials[14] when impression material has accidentally been allowed to remain within the periodontal tissues after the impression was removed. Fortunately, this sort of damage is probably rare in routine dental practice. Impression making is considerably easier if a supragingival tooth preparation is used.

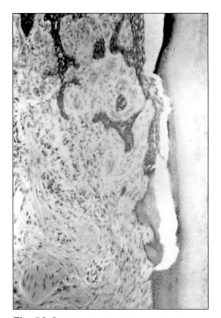

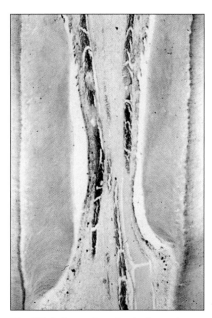

Fig 30-3 Massive burning marks in root cementum and dentin following 1-second application of electrosurgery prior to impression making. (Reprinted from Wilhelmsen et al,[15] with permission.)

Fig 30-4 Secondary dentin formation as a consequence of a electrosurgical needle touching the cementum. (Reprinted from Wilhelmsen et al,[15] with permission.)

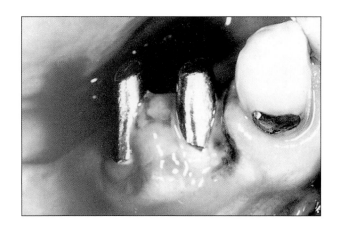

Fig 30-5 Clinical appearance of an electrosurgical wound 6 weeks after therapy. A very prolonged and painful healing period should be expected following the application of electrosurgery prior to impression taking.

Occasionally, local gingivectomies, or opening the gingival sulcus by cutting away the sulcular or pocket lining, using electrosurgery has been advocated. Such "troughing" may result in recession of the gingival margin and loss of attachment. If the electrosurgical needle touches the root surface, hyperemia of the pulp tissues and formation of secondary dentin must be expected (Fig 30-3). Burn marks may easily result from touching cementum or dentin, and as a consequence, attachment loss must be expected[15] (Fig 30-4). From a biologic point of view, electrosurgical therapy in conjunction with the preparation of abutments before making impressions is not recommended

(Fig 30-5). A surgical procedure designed to remove tissues in a controlled mode (crown-lengthening procedure) is preferred prior to finalizing the abutment preparation if the height of the clinical crown is not adequate for retention.

Provisional Restorations

The prepared tooth is usually covered with a provisional restoration made of an autopolymerizing, dual-cured, or light-activated material. Perfect marginal adaptations of provisional restorations are not possible with these materials, and hence a marked gap exists between the prepared

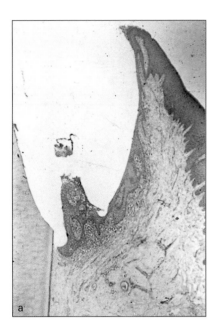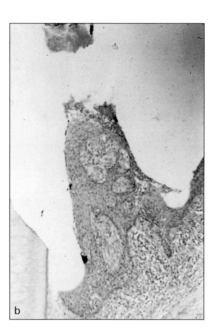

Figs 30-6a and 30-6b Gingival reaction as a result of a subgingivally placed margin of an acrylic (provisional) crown. The marginal gap is 300 μm. (a) Inflammatory infiltrate directly related to the marginal gap. (b) Higher magnification reveals the presence of bacteria in the marginal gap following a wash-out of cementum and adjacent epithelial proliferation. (Reprinted from Waerhaug,[5] with permission.)

tooth and the edge of the provisional crown (Fig 30-6). This gap quickly fills with bacterial plaque, which will provoke a gingival or periodontal lesion. In vitro studies on marginal adaptation of various provisional materials show vertical discrepancies ranging from 0.18 to 0.40 mm.[16] Coupled with the use of provisional cements, clinical provisional restorative margins often induce bacterial plaque accumulation, because resin-based materials are porous and harbor significantly more plaque than do the dental materials used for permanent restorations.[17,18] Provisional restoration contours (emergence, embrasure form, and contact area) greatly influence the ability of the soft tissue to resume its normal architecture. Care must be taken in fabrication of the provisional restoration to allow for sufficient interproximal cleansing with cleaning aids such as interproximal brushes or tufted dental floss.[11]

Reconstruction and Periodontal Health

The term *functional effects* refers to the influences that cemented reconstructions may exert on the periodontium or the gingiva beneath a reconstruction.

Subgingival Preparation Margins

Periodontal Aspects

Follow-up examinations of fixed reconstructions have demonstrated that the position of the crown margin in relation to the gingiva has a significant effect on the Gingi-val Index (GI), as well as the depth of the gingival sulcus (pocket) and the position of the epithelial attachment.[19–25] Crown margins that were positioned subgingivally were associated with the highest GI values, and supragingival crown margins had the lowest GI values[25] (Fig 30-7). Crown margins at the same height as the free gingival margins were associated with intermediate GI values.[24,26,27] Furthermore, the severity of the GI was related to the depth position rather than the crown margin in the gingival sulcus.[25] The Papillary Bleeding Index (PBI) and mean probing depth were also shown to increase when crown margins were placed within 1 mm of the osseous crest.[28] The increased GI and PBI values found with margins placed in the zone of biologic width may impair the long-term periodontal health of the restored teeth. Experimental studies[29,30] have shown that when possible, supragingival margins should be chosen during cavity or crown preparation; furthermore, previously placed subgingival restoration margins should be re-exposed by, for example, surgical lengthening of the clinical crown.

The most significant contribution addressing the long-term periodontal aspects of reconstructions was made by Valderhaug, both independently[26,31] and with colleagues.[27,32] A total of 102 patients with 108 fixed partial dentures were studied for 15 years. Eighty-eight patients with 92 fixed partial dentures were reexamined after 5 years (Fig 30-8), 71 with 77 fixed partial dentures after 10 years, and 55 with 59 fixed partial dentures after 15 years. After 5 years, 282 of the original 343 retainers could be evaluated; after 10 years, 236 retainers; and after 15 years, 187 retainers.[31] Loss of the periodontal supporting apparatus was significantly greater around teeth with subgingival

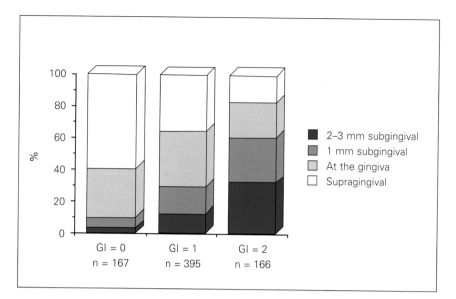

Fig 30-7 Location of the crown margin in relation to the Gingival Index (GI) scores of 0, 1, or 2. A score of 2 occurred significantly more frequently in subgingival locations. (Reprinted from Reichen-Graden and Lang,[25] with permission.)

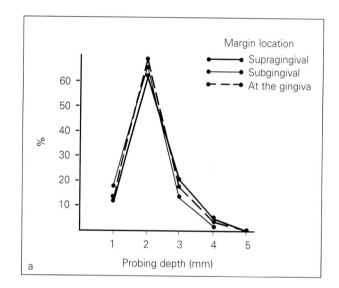

Figs 30-8a to 30-8c Frequency distribution of probing depths: (a) at the time of cementation and (b) 5 years after cementation, for crown margins located supragingivally, subgingivally, or at the gingival margin. (c) Frequency of loss of attachment 5 years after cementation. (Reprinted from Valderhaug and Birkeland,[27] with permission.)

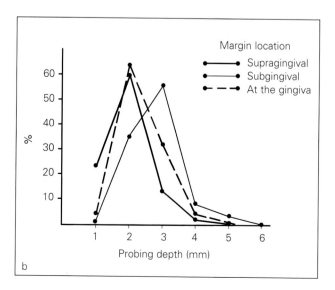

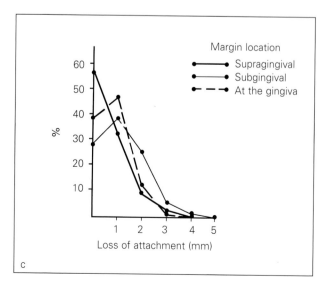

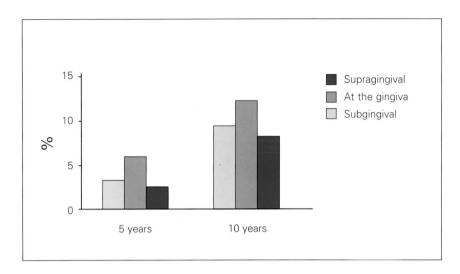

Fig 30-9 Incidence of secondary caries adjacent to crown margins in relation to their location, 5 and 10 years after cementation of the crowns. (Reprinted from Valderhaug,[26] with permission.)

crown margins than around similar teeth with supragingival crown margins. Furthermore, the subgingivally prepared teeth exhibited deeper pockets than teeth that had been prepared either supragingivally or with the margin at the height of the gingiva. The same study showed that 5 years after cementation, 30% of the subgingival crown margins were associated with gingival recession as a result of constant irritation. Most similar clinical trials[25,33–37] agree with the conclusions of the Valderhaug studies. However, a few authors[38–40] claim that no significant differences were found between periodontal conditions of abutment teeth with subgingival crown margins and control teeth without crowns. A significant quantitative relationship exists between intracrevicular marginal discrepancy and GI and crevicular fluid volumes.[41] A precise marginal crown fit was interpreted to be the prerequisite for the stability of periodontal tissues around abutment teeth.

Secondary Dental Caries

Only a very few well-controlled clinical studies are available on the relationship of secondary caries in crowned teeth to the location of the preparation margin.[32] Valderhaug[26] reported a secondary caries incidence of 3.5% in crowned teeth (Fig 30-9). In another study,[42] significantly more secondary caries lesions were found around subgingival preparation margins than around supragingival margins. While 15.4% of supragingival amalgam-restoration margins exhibited secondary caries after 5 years, 30.4% of subgingival amalgam-restoration margins yielded secondary caries. Similar results may be expected for crown retainers.

Plaque Retention on Dental Materials

Even though relatively few studies of the toxicity of dental materials have been performed, available data indicate that dental gold foil, porcelain, and heat-cured acrylic resin irritate the tissues little, if at all.[1,3,43–45] In contrast, according to Waerhaug,[1,5] luting cements have a slight irritating effect on soft tissues. Ørstavik and Ørstavik[46] demonstrated in vitro that luting cements from various manufacturers may have quite different potentials as substrates for bacterial adhesion; these investigators concluded that the choice of a particular type of cement may have prognostic significance for the periodontal condition of crowned abutment teeth.

Rough surfaces can enhance the development of gingivitis because they induce accumulation of plaque.[3,4,18,47,48] A review of the literature suggests a threshold surface roughness (Ra) for bacteria retention of 0.2 μm, below which no further bacteria accumulation can be expected.[49] The range of surface roughness of different intraoral materials is wide, and the impact of polishing procedures on the surface roughness is material dependant. Porosity, therefore, may contribute to the plaque-retentive potential of acrylic resin. However, it must not be forgotten that porcelain and gold also often have surface porosity. For all three materials, the axiom holds that the degree of porosity directly depends on the way the materials were handled and finished.[50] Therefore, it is clear that all three materials must be polished to the highest degree. Dental gold should be polished with an agent that does not increase the risk of subsequent corrosion.

Glantz[44] demonstrated that dental materials possess a greater capacity to accumulate and retain plaque than do either enamel or dentin. It is probable that polymethylmethacrylate accumulates plaque faster than gold and porcelain because of the absorption of fluids. An in vivo study of early dental plaque formation on different dental materials in humans[18] revealed very small differences in colonization of bacteria after 4 and 24 hours. While the plaque composition was qualitatively similar for seven dental materials, dentin, and enamel, surface roughness seemed to influence the amount of plaque development.

Skjörland[51] studied the plaque-retentive capacity of various dental restorative materials in vitro and in vivo. After 6 days plaque that had accumulated on disks inoculated with *Streptococcus mutans* was removed, and its polysaccharide content was measured chemically. In this in vitro experiment, plaque accumulation, which was enhanced by rinsing with sucrose, was studied after 8 hours. In both tests, freshly placed silicate exhibited a plaque-inhibiting effect when compared with the plaque accumulation on amalgam and older silicate restorations. In contrast, the acrylic resin materials exhibited a dramatic tendency for increased plaque accumulation. The findings were confirmed in another study.[17]

Ecological Niche for Periodontopathic Microorganisms

The transition zone, which encompasses the crown margin, the cement, and the prepared tooth, assumes great significance if the crown margin is located subgingivally. A crevice is almost always found in this zone, because no commercially available luting cement provides a perfect closure (seal). The surface of the cement is always rough and porous.[52] It has been demonstrated that the surface area of this "cement line" associated with seated crowns may approach several square millimeters.[34] Histologic investigations by Waerhaug[3] have shown that such subgingival cement roughness enhances plaque accumulation in the gingival sulcus. Thus, this transition zone represents a predilection site for plaque accumulation.[1,3,33,41]

The cement line in the transition zone is all the more significant with regard to periodontal injury in light of the fact that the clinician occasionally observes ill-fitting crowns with obviously open margins. In this respect, Björn et al[6] reported a generally poor marginal fit in retainers for fixed partial dentures. Eighty percent of the radiographically studied reconstructions exhibited marginal defects on the proximal surfaces. Margins that were open by more than 0.2 mm were always associated with alveolar bone loss. In a German survey under private practice conditions,[53] only 18.2% of crown margins were clinically acceptable, and most recent studies yield no better results.

The effects of clinically acceptable and/or overhanging restoration margins on the subgingival microbiota have been studied in a human clinical and microbiologic trial[54] (Fig 30-10). In this study, eight participating students had a healthy dentition but needed a mesio-occlusodistal restoration. Five mesio-occlusodisal cast gold onlays, with 0.5-mm proximal overhanging margins, were placed on mandibular molars for 19 to 27 weeks. They were replaced by five similar onlays with clinically acceptable margins, which served as controls. Another five onlays were placed in reverse order in the remaining patients to fit a crossover experimental design. Prior to placement, and every 2 to 3 weeks afterward, subgingival microbiologic samples were obtained. The predominant cultivable microbiota was determined using continuous anaerobic culturing techniques. Following the placement of restorations with overhanging margins, a subgingival microbiota was detected that closely resembled that of chronic periodontitis. Increased proportions of gram-negative anaerobic bacteria and black-pigmented *Bacteroides* (*Porphyromonas* and *Prevotella* species), as well as an increased anaerobic-to-facultative bacteria ratio, were noted.

Following the placement of the restorations with clinically perfect margins, a microbiota characteristic of gingival health or initial gingivitis was observed. Black-pigmented *Bacteroides* were detected in very low proportions (1.6% to 3.8%). These changes in the subgingival microbiota were obvious both when the restorations with the overhanging margins were placed in the first period of the experiment or during the second period after the crossover (see Fig 30-10). Clinically, increasing GIs were detected at the sites where overhanging margins were placed. Bleeding on gentle probing always preceded the peak level of black-pigmented *Bacteroides*. It was concluded that changes in the subgingival microbiota after the placement of restorations with overhanging margins documented a potential mechanism for the initiation of periodontal disease associated with iatrogenic factors.

Similar changes in the subgingival ecosystem were documented in children receiving orthodontic bands.[55] A more pathogenic microbiota with increased proportions of gram-negative anaerobes (*Prevotella intermedia*) was seen following placement of orthodontic bands. However, these changes in the composition of the microbiota appeared to be of transitional character and limited duration.

Reconstructions and the "Extension for Prevention" Principle

Well-controlled experimental clinical studies have led to the reevaluation of traditional accepted dogmas in reconstructive dentistry. The concept of "extension for preven-

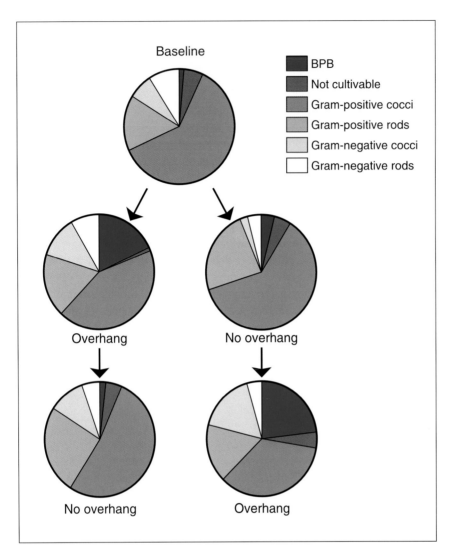

Fig 30-10 Ecological influences of clinically perfect or overhanging margins. Percent colony-forming units (CFU) of bacteria per milliliter sample. Black-pigmenting *Bacteroides* (BPB, or black-pigmenting gram-negative anaerobic bacteria) increase in proportion to the presence of an overhanging margin of the restoration (Adapted from Lang et al,[54] with permission.)

tion," which dates back to Black,[9] demands that the margin of a restoration be placed in a region that is self-cleansing because of the friction of food associated with mastication. Furthermore, it postulates that the cervical margins of all restorations be located subgingivally. The reasoning was that an initial caries lesion could never occur on enamel that was covered by gingiva.[9]

As a result of Black's postulate, extension for prevention was a fundamental principle in the therapy of dental caries and dominated reconstructive dentistry for almost 100 years. However, current knowledge concerning the pathogenesis and etiology of caries and periodontal disease, as well as the accepted principles of preventive dentistry, has made it clear that extension for prevention has become untenable and should be abandoned. The theo-

retical basis for the original concept is now understood to be invalid. It has been demonstrated again and again that without effective oral hygiene, healthy patients will experience massive plaque accumulation.[56] Plaque accumulation, especially on the cervical half of the clinical crown, is hardly ever affected by the self-cleansing effect of chewing, even when very fibrous foods are eaten[7] (Fig 30-11).

For this reason, and because of the eating habits of most people today, self-cleansing can be considered nonexistent. Furthermore, the concept of extension for prevention is based on the assumption that restorations whose margins extend into the gingival sulcus are covered by healthy gingiva. However, as this chapter has shown, all subgingivally placed margins of dental restorations are associated with pathological alterations of the adjacent gingiva (Fig

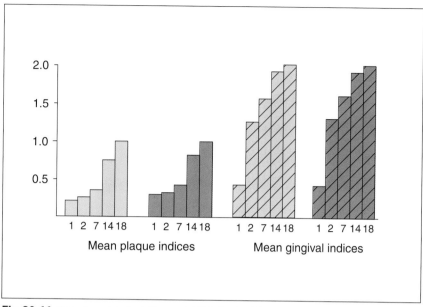

Fig 30-11 Experimental gingivitis model (18 days) with abolishment of oral hygiene practices (control subjects: light bars) or concomitant chewing of fibrous food (test subjects: dark bars). No significant differences for mean plaque indices or gingival indices were found at any time. (Adapted from Lindhe and Wicén,[7] with permission.)

30-12). Thus, all subgingival restoration margins of inlays, crowns, or restorations are, in fact, covered by pathologically altered gingiva.

The greater the marginal inaccuracy of a restoration, the greater the permanent damage to the periodontal tissues[57] (Fig 30-13). This, in turn, means that there is no biologic reason for locating restoration margins in the subgingival area (Fig 30-14). However, if high lip (smile) lines or the patient's demands necessitate such a placement for esthetic reasons, the precision of the marginal fit of the restoration becomes crucial. Optimally, a very precise subgingivally placed margin (narrower than 50 mm) should still be accessible to cleansing devices such as toothbrushes and interdental devices[58,59] (Fig 30-15). The advent of restorations with castable (and pressed) ceramic, in conjunction with porcelain shoulder margins, has diminished the incidence of subgingival margins for esthetic reasons.[41,60] Other nonesthetic reasons, such as retention problems, extensive caries lesions, or previous reconstructions may dictate a preparation extending markedly into the subgingival area. In these instances, surgical lengthening of the clinical crown should be considered. This will be discussed later in this chapter.

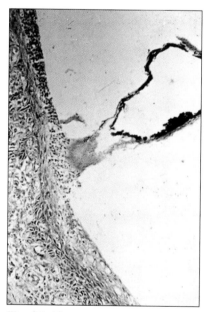

Fig 30-12 Subgingival preparation of restoration with a marginal gap of approximately 60 μm results in cement wash-out, plaque accumulation, and chronic gingivitis. (Reprinted from Waerhaug,[5] with permission.)

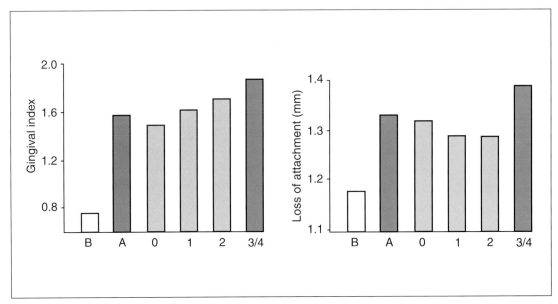

Fig 30-13 Gingival indices and loss of attachment adjacent to subgingival restorative margins of various accuracies. A = all restored teeth; B = control teeth without restorations. 0 = overhang < 0.2 mm; 1 = overhang 0.2–0.4 mm; 2 = overhang 0.4–0.8 mm; 3/4 = overhang > 0.8 mm. (Adapted from Lang et al,[57] with permission.)

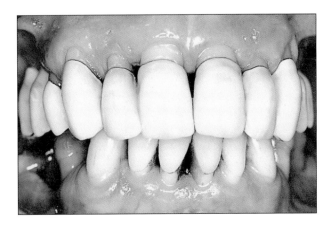

Fig 30-14 Where esthetics do not play a role, crown margins should be located supragingivally.

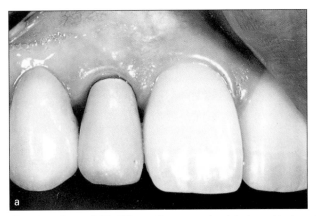
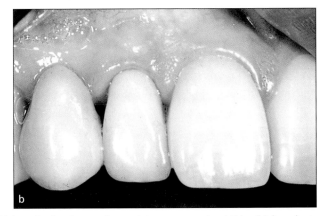

Figs 30-15a and 30-15b (a) Crown on the right lateral incisor. A high smile line leaves the metal crown margin visible. (b) A replacement crown with a porcelain shoulder brings the margin to the level of the gingiva.

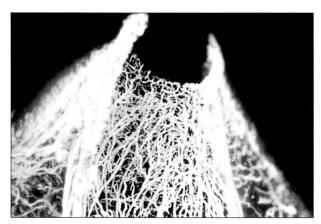

Fig 30-16 A very delicate network of blood vessels subjacent to the junctional epithelium in the interdental col area originating from the periodontal ligament (dog material [beagle], Latex preparation). (Reprinted from Hock[63] with permission.)

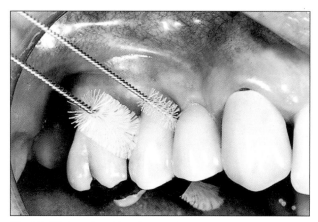

Fig 30-17 Interdental brushes reach into the gingival sulcus approximately 2 to 3 mm. (Reprinted from Waerhaug,[58] with permission.)

Overcontouring of Reconstructions

Interdental Area

Oral hygiene practices may be severely jeopardized by overcontoured reconstructions. The interdental surfaces may impinge on the gingival papillae if inadequate tooth preparation does not provide the necessary space for the prosthetic material. The periodontal significance of correctly formed interdental contacts has been recognized.[61] Food impaction may result in increased plaque accumulation for prolonged periods. Therefore, a tightly fitting, spatially correct relationship of interproximal contact surfaces, along with a correctly designed marginal ridge to avoid the effects of opposing plunger cusps, are prerequisites of biologically acceptable reconstructions. However, clearly open interproximal areas need not affect the periodontal tissues of the adjacent teeth, provided these areas are accessible to cleansing devices. It is important to note that excessively open interproximal areas negatively affect esthetics, impair phonetics, and allow excessive lateral food impaction.[11]

There are no controlled clinical studies on the buccolingual extension of the contact areas in the interproximal space. However, metallurgic in vitro studies suggest that minimal extension of soldering joints must exceed 3 mm, provided that the distance between the two elements to be soldered is 0.1 mm (Métraux Précieux, Neuchâtel). This technical requirement may seriously compromise the health of the interdental area, especially in younger patients with healthy gingival papillae.[62] The very delicate structures (vessel arrangement, supracrestal fibers, and epithelial attachment of the col area) of the interdental papillary region (Fig 30-16) are easily severed by restorative procedures or by plaque accumulation as a result of inad-

equate access by interdental oral hygiene devices. Therefore, dental laboratory technicians must be encouraged to respect the interproximal contact area of reconstructions and provide adequate space for the cleaning devices available today[58] (Fig 30-17).

Furcation Areas

Multirooted reconstructed teeth with beginning furcation involvement often present problems for adequate oral hygiene practices. Special efforts have to be made to accentuate the outline of the root trunk while preparing the tooth to provide adequate access for cleaning devices in the furcation area (Fig 30-18). If roots had to be resected or amputated, and the remaining roots are still used as abutments for fixed reconstructions, the areas of the root concavities must be exaggerated in the reconstruction to avoid overcontouring of regions most susceptible to plaque accumulation (Fig 30-19). Again, proper oral hygiene instructions must be given to patients with such morphologic conditions.

Pontic Design: Edentulous Mucosal Areas

Especially on pontics for fixed partial dentures, the esthetic demands often result in concavities of the pontic body on the apical surface in contact with the mucosa of the edentulous ridge. Such ridge-lap designs inevitably result in mucosal irritation and chronic inflammation and ulceration. An experimental scanning electron microscopic study[64] demonstrated not only that bacterial plaque accumulation is more accentuated on concave fixed partial denture pontics than on convex surfaces but also that the maturation of plaque is much faster. After 48 hours, a filamentous and rod-dominated microbiota may be seen, which contrasts with the predominantly coccoid

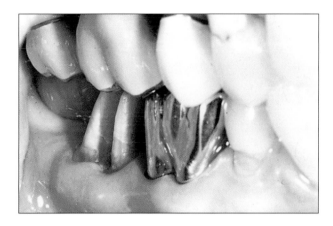

Fig 30-18 Prosthetic reconstruction of the mandibular right first and second molars. Both teeth yielded open furcations following successful periodontal therapy. For easy access with cleaning devices, the furcation is morphologically exaggerated in the reconstruction.

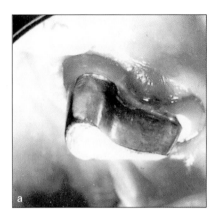

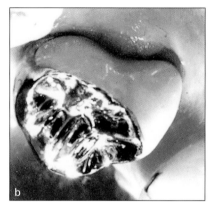

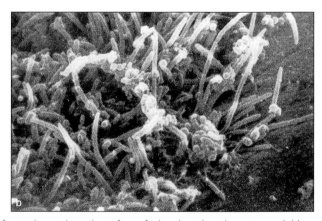

Figs 30-19a to 30-19c Reconstruction of an amputated multirooted tooth. *(a)* Accentuating the concavity during preparation and buildup. *(b)* Correct contouring resulting in healthy gingival tissues. *(c)* Use of appropriate oral hygiene devices (single-tufted brush).

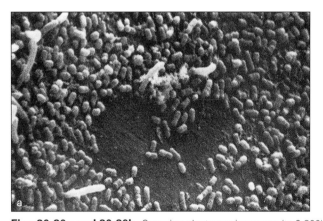

Figs 30-20a and 30-20b Scanning electron microscopy ($\times$ 2,800) of experimental pontic surfaces facing the edentulous mucosal ridge. *(a)* Forty-eight–hour coccoid microbiota on convex surface. *(b)* Forty-eight–hour microbiota on a concave surface characterized by filaments and rods. (Reprinted from Gusberti et al,[64] with permission.)

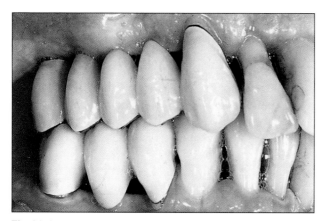

Fig 30-21 Egg-shaped pontics with a convex surface are biologically optimal for plaque control.

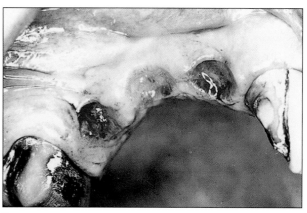

Fig 30-22 Pontics placed into extraction sockets result in permanent irritation and disturbed healing.

microbiota on convex pontic surfaces (Fig 30-20). As a clinical consequence, fixed partial denture pontics should be constructed with only convex (ie, egg-shaped) surfaces (Fig 30-21). However, if esthetic demands dictate a slight ridge-lap design, contact with the mucosal surface should be avoided to provide adequate space for cleaning devices.[65] The shape of the residual ridge, however, will allow the tissue-contacting surface of the prosthesis to be flat or convex, allowing for plaque removal with dental floss.[11]

As the use of ovate pontic designs increases,[66–68] it is important to note that their use is usually at the expense of the underlying soft tissue. If the ovate pontic is to be used, proper site selection is critical, as are a well-keratinized ridge; a convex, highly polished tissue surface of the restoration; and accessibility for oral hygiene procedures. Placement of pontics into extraction sockets has no biologic rationale and must be considered malpractice, since it results in permanent irritation and jeopardizes the healing process of the socket (Fig 30-22).

Esthetic Considerations

Surgical Lengthening of the Clinical Crown

Crown lengthening has been described as a procedure similar to the apical repositioning of the flap with concomitant ostectomy/osteoplasty.[69–73] Some reports describe the importance of a thorough root planing after the ostectomy to avoid reattachment of the surgically separated fibers at a level that would be too coronal, thus positioning the connective tissue attachment deliberately and predictably at a more apical level.[74–76] Few reports

exist on controlled studies of the periodontal changes in the healing phase after surgical procedures designed to lengthen the clinical crown.

One study[77] assessed the changes in the periodontal tissue levels as an immediate result of the surgical crown-lengthening procedure and over a 6-month healing period. Twenty-five patients ranging in age from 20 to 81 years were included. A total of 85 teeth (43 test teeth, and 42 controls not exposed to surgery) were evaluated. After initial periodontal therapy, indications for crown lengthening included the need for increased retention and the lack of accessibility to deep subgingival preparation margins, which hampered impression making. During surgery, the alveolar crest was reduced, thereby creating a distance of 3 mm to the future reconstruction margin.

The study yielded minimal probeable changes in periodontal tissue levels 6 months after surgery when compared with tissue levels obtained immediately after the typical lengthening of the crown. These changes were comparable to changes observed in control teeth not subjected to any surgical procedures. A similar study[78] was designed to assess the alterations of the marginal periodontal tissues both immediately after surgical crown lengthening and over a 12-month healing period. The results showed that over a 12-month period, the tissue exhibited a tendency to grow in a coronal direction from the level defined at surgery. The authors found that the pattern of coronal displacement of the gingival margin was more pronounced ($P < .001$) in patients with "thick" tissue biotypes and was also influenced by individual variations in the healing response ($P < .001$) not related to age or gender.[78]

Frequency analysis of the number of sites with dislocation of the free gingival margin demonstrated that 12% of the sites with crown-lengthening procedures showed 2- to 4-mm recession of the free gingival margin between 6

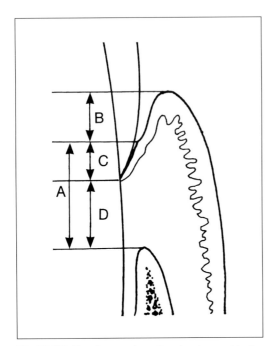

Fig 30-23 The distance from the alveolar crest to the gingival margin (A) is referred to as the *biologic width*[79]: 0.69 mm (B) was identified as the histologic sulcus; 0.97 mm (C) consisted of the epithelial attachment, and 1.07 mm (D) was the area of the supracrestal fiber attachment in human autopsy material. Therefore the biologic width (A = C + D) amounts to slightly more than 2 mm.

- Deep, subgingivally located preparation margins, where impressions can be controlled only with great difficulty
- Deep, subgingivally located caries lesions
- Root fractures in the cervical third
- Root resorptions in the cervical region
- Perforations of parapulpal posts in the cervical third of the root
- Insufficient retention for an artificial crown because of reduced crown height
- Deep subgingivally located, existing margins leading to inflammatory responses that cannot be controlled otherwise
- Odontoplastics, in combination with root sectioning, amputations, and separations of roots in multirooted teeth
- Extremely abraded dentitions prior to reconstruction
- The need for improved esthetic appearance of anterior teeth with short clinical crowns and high lip (smile) lines

Crown lengthening, however, is contraindicated if a comprehensive treatment plan is missing, if the patient's oral hygiene is unsatisfactory, if the respective tooth is of no strategic value, or if the respective tooth reveals a beginning periodontal involvement of the interradicular area.

Tissue Augmentation of Edentulous Ridges

Regenerative surgery, using guided tissue regeneration (GTR), has been successful not only for periodontal tissues lost because of inflammatory periodontal disease[80–84] but also for bone in a variety of jaw defects in animals.[85,86] Furthermore, enlargement of alveolar ridges using GTR has been achieved experimentally prior to the placement of implants[87,88] or at exposed implant threads.[89–91]

The first report of enlargement of reduced alveolar ridge volume in human subjects was published by Nyman et al.[92] Later, a series of case reports also documented successful regeneration of bone in defects of the jaw prior to or after the placement of implants.[90,93] It is therefore obvious that the GTR principle may also be used to enlarge or augment edentulous alveolar bone crests to provide adequate conditions for optimal pontic design and satisfactory esthetics.

A study[94] reported on 19 patients treated with augmentation procedures for alveolar bone volume using the GTR principle. Combined split-thickness/full-thickness mucosal flaps were elevated in the area of missing bone. The size of the defects was assessed by a standardized geometric procedure, and the volume of missing bone under the barrier membrane placed was calculated. At the time of

weeks and 6 months postoperatively. It was therefore concluded that in esthetically critical areas of the dentition, recessions must be closely observed in the healing period after surgical crown lengthening if prosthetic reconstructions are planned.

Also, the creation of a distance of 3 mm from the alveolar crestal bone level to the future reconstruction margin during surgical lengthening of the clinical crown leads to stable periodontal tissue levels. This 3-mm guideline was originally presented by Gargiulo et al,[79] who studied the dimensions of the dentogingival region in human autopsy material (Fig 30-23). On an average, 0.69 mm was attributed to the histologic sulcus depth, 0.97 mm was identified as being occupied by the epithelial attachment, and 1.07 mm was found to constitute a connective tissue attachment, resulting in a total of 2.73 mm, which was defined to represent the *biologic width*.[69] A stable biologic width, without any further uncontrolled attachment loss following the surgical procedure, has been documented in a study by Brägger et al.[77] The surgical lengthening of the clinical crown should always be performed following the successful completion of an initial periodontal or hygienic phase. The following indications may be recommended for crown lengthening:

Figs 30-24a to 30-24f Augmentation of a maxillary anterior region in a 45-year-old woman. *(a)* Bony defect results in a bridge reconstruction with unbiologic contours. *(b)* Following flap elevation, the bony defect (156 mm³) is visible. *(c)* A barrier membrane (Gore-Tex Augmentation Material) is placed and fixed with miniscrews on Memfix supporting devices. *(d)* Healing for 8 months under mucosal coverage using a provisional fixed partial denture reconstruction. *(e)* Regenerated bone after membrane removal. The space volume was 92% filled. *(f)* Final reconstruction following healing of the flap elevated for membrane removal.

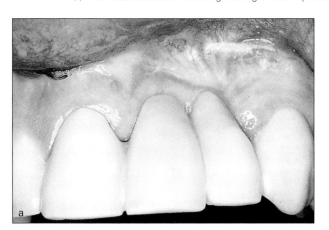

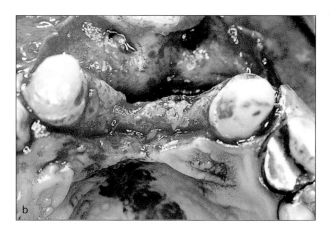

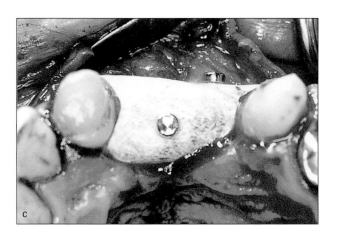

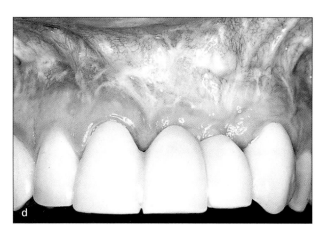

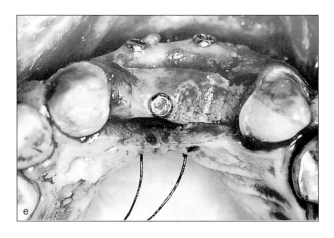

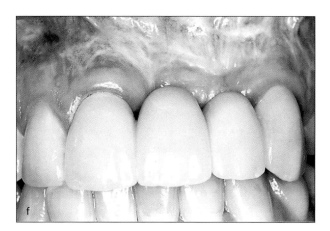

membrane removal, the percentages of regenerated bone in relation to the possible volume for regeneration was determined. In 6 patients in whom the membranes had to be removed early due to infection between 3 and 5 months, bone regeneration varied between 0% and 60%. In 13 patients in whom membranes were left for 6 to 8 months, regenerated bone filled 90% to 100% of the possible volume. It was concluded that successful bone regeneration consistently occurred with an undisturbed healing period of at least 6 months. (Augmentation of a maxillary anterior region prior to the placement of a fixed partial denture reconstruction is depicted in Fig 30-24. See chapters 32 and 39 for more information.)

References

1. Waerhaug J. Tissue reactions around artificial crowns. J Periodontol 1953;24:172–185.
2. Waerhaug J. Observations on replanted teeth plated with gold foil. Reaction to pure gold; mode of epithelial attachment to gold; expulsion of foreign bodies from pockets. Oral Surg Oral Med Oral Pathol 1956;9:780–791.
3. Waerhaug J. Effect of rough surfaces upon gingival tissue. J Dent Res 1956;35:323–325.
4. Waerhaug J. Tissue reaction around acrylic root tips. J Dent Res 1957;36:27–38.
5. Waerhaug J. Histologic considerations which govern where the margins of restorations should be located in relation to the gingiva. Dent Clin North Am 1960;4:161–176.
6. Björn A, Björn H, Grkovic R. Marginal fit of restorations and its relation to periodontal bone level. Part 1: Metal fillings. Odontol Rev 1969;20:311–321.
7. Lindhe J, Wicén P. The effects on the gingivae of chewing fibrous foods. J Periodontal Res 1969;4:193–201.
8. Löe H. Reactions of marginal periodontal tissues to restorative procedures. Int Dent J 1968;18:759–778.
9. Black G. Operative dentistry. Pathology of the hard tissues of the teeth. Oper Dent 1908;1:142–144.
10. Ramfjord S, Costich E. Healing after simple gingivectomy. J Periodontol 1963;34:401–415.
11. Ferencz JL. Maintaining and enhancing gingival architecture in fixed prosthodontics. J Prosthet Dent 1991;65(5):650–657.
12. Goldberg PV, Higginbottom FL, Wilson TG. Periodontal considerations in restorative and implant therapy. Periodontol 2000 2001;25:100–109.
13. Hansen PA, Tira DE, Barlow J. Current methods of finish-line exposure by practicing prosthodontists. J Prosthodont 1999;8(3):163–170.
14. O'Leary T, Standish S, Bloomer R. Severe periodontal destruction following impression procedures. J Periodontol 1973;44:43–108.
15. Wilhelmsen N, Ramfjord S, Blankenship J. Effects of electrosurgery on the gingival attachment in Rhesus monkeys. J Periodontol 1976;47:160–170.
16. Tjan AH, Castelnuovo J, Shiotsu G. Marginal fidelity of crowns fabricated from six proprietary provisional materials. J Prosthet Dent 1997;77(5):482–485.
17. Wise M, Dykema R. The plaque retaining capacity of four dental materials. J Prosthet Dent 1975;33:178–190.
18. Siegrist B, Brecx M, Gusberti F, et al. In vivo early human dental plaque formation on different supporting substances. A scanning electron microscopic and bacteriological study. Clin Oral Implants Res 1991;2:38–46.
19. Silness J. Periodontal conditions in patients treated with dental bridges. J Periodontal Res 1970;5:60–68.
20. Silness J. Periodontal conditions in patients treated with dental bridges. II. The influence of full and partial crowns on plaque accumulation, development of gingivitis and pocket formation. J Periodontal Res 1970;5:219–224.
21. Silness J. Periodontal conditions in patients treated with dental bridges. III. The relationship between the locaton of the crown margin and the periodontal condition. J Periodontal Res 1970;5:225–229.
22. Silness J, Ohm E. Periodontal conditions in patients treated with dental bridges. V. Effects of splinting adjacent abutment teeth. J Periodontal Res 1974;9:121–126.
23. Bergman B, Hugoson H, Olsson C. Periodontal and prosthetic conditions in patients treated with removable partial dentures and artificial crowns. Acta Odontol Scand 1971;29:621–638.
24. Valderhaug J. Prepareringsgrensens beliggenhet-Krone-bro synspunter. Nor Tannlaegeforen Tid 1972;82:386–390.
25. Reichen-Graden S, Lang N. Periodontal and pulpal conditions of abutment teeth. Status after four to eight years following incorporation of fixed reconstructions. Schweiz Monatsschr Zahnmed 1989;99:1381–1385.
26. Valderhaug J. Periodontal conditions and carious lesions following the insertion of fixed prostheses: A 10-year follow-up study. Int Dent J 1980;30:296–304.
27. Valderhaug J, Birkeland JM. Periodontal conditions in patients 5 years following insertion of fixed prostheses. Pocket depth and loss of attachment. J Oral Rehabil 1976;3(3):237–243.
28. Gunay H, Seeger A, Tschernitschek H, Geurtsen W. Placement of the preparation line and periodontal health: A prospective 2-year clinical study. Int J Periodontics Restorative Dent 2000;20(2):171–181.
29. Renggli H. Auswirkungen subgingivaler approximaler Füllungsränder auf den Entzündungsgrad der benachbarten Gingiva. Schweiz Monatsschr Zahnheilkd 1974;84:1–18.
30. Mörmann W, Regolati B, Renggli H. Gingival reactions to well-fitted subgingival proximal gold inlays. J Clin Periodontol 1974;1:120–124.
31. Valderhaug J. A 15-year clinical evaluation of fixed prosthodontics. Acta Odontol Scand 1991;49:35–40.
32. Valderhaug J, Heloe L. Oral hygiene in a group of supervised patients with fixed prosthesis. J Periodontol 1977;48:221–224.
33. Karlsen K. Gingival reactions to dental restorations. Acta Odontol Scand 1970;28:895–901.
34. Silness J, Hegdahl T. Area of the exposed zinc phosphate cement surfaces in fixed restorations. Scand J Dent Res 1970;78:163–177.
35. Landolt A, Lang N. Erfolg und Misserfolg bei Extensionsbrücken. Schweiz Monatsschr Zahnmed 1988;98:239–244.
36. Schatzle M, Lang NP, Anerud A, et al. The influence of margins of restorations of the periodontal tissues over 26 years. J Clin Periodontol 2001;28(1):57–64.
37. Jansson L, Blomster S, Forsgardh A, et al. Interactory effect between marginal plaque and subgingival proximal restorations on periodontal pocket depth. Swed Dent J 1997;21(3):77–83.
38. Koivumaa K, Wennstrom A. A histological investigation of the changes in gingival margins adjacent to gold crowns. Odontol Tidskrift 1960;68:373–385.

39. Kerschbaum T, Meier R. Intraindividuelle Unterschiede am marginalen Parodont überkronter and nicht überkronter, topographisch identischer Zähne. D Zahnärztl Z 1978;33: 499–504.

40. Kancyper SG, Koka S. The influence of intracrevicular crown margins on gingival health: Preliminary findings. J Prosthet Dent 2001;85(5):461–465.

41. Felton DA, Kanoy BE, Bayne SC, Wirthman GP. Effect of in vivo crown margin discrepancies on periodontal health. J Prosthet Dent 1991;65(3):357–364.

42. Hammer B, Hotz P. Nachkontrolle von 1-bis 5-jährigen Amalgam-, Komposit- und Goldgussfüllungen. Schweiz Monatsschr Zahnheilkd 1979;89:301–314.

43. App G. Effect of silicate, amalgam and cast gold on the gingiva. J Prosthet Dent 1961;11:522–532.

44. Glantz P-O. On wettability and adhesiveness: A study of enamel, dentin, some restorative materials, and dental plaque. Odontol Revy 1969;17(suppl):1–132.

45. Leirskar J, Helgeland K. A methodologic study of dental materials on growth and adhesion of animal cells in vitro. Scand J Dent Res 1972;8:120–133.

46. Ørstavik D, Ørstavik J. In vitro attachment of Streptococcus sanguis to dental crown and bridge cements. J Oral Rehabil 1976;3:139–144.

47. Clayton J, Green E. Roughness of pontic materials and dental plaque. J Prosthet Dent 1970;23:407–411.

48. Frank R, Brion M, de Rouffignac M. Ultrastructural gingival reactions to gold foil restorations. J Periodontol 1975;46:614–624.

49. Bollen CM, Lambrechts P, Quirynen M. Comparison of surface roughness of oral hard materials to the threshold surface roughness for bacterial plaque retention: A review of the literature. Dent Mater 1997;13(4):258–269.

50. Craig R, Peyton F. Restorative dental materials, ed 5. St. Louis: Mosby, 1975:37–52.

51. Skjörland K. Plaque accumulation on different dental filling materials. Scand J Dent Res 1973;81:538–542.

52. Silness J. Fixed prosthodontics and periodontal health. Dent Clin North Am 1980;24:317–329.

53. Lange D. Attitudes and behaviour with respect to oral hygiene and periodontal treatment need in a selected group in West Germany. In: Frandsen A (ed). Public Health Aspects of Periodontal Disease. Berlin: Quintessence, 1984:83–97.

54. Lang NP, Kiel RA, Anderhalden K. Clinical and microbiological effects of subgingival restorations with overhanging and clinically perfect margins. J Clin Periodontol 1983;10(6):563–578.

55. Diamanti-Kipioti A, Gusberti F, Lang N. Clinical and microbiological effects of fixed orthodontic appliances. J Clin Periodontol 1987;14:326–333.

56. Löe H, Silness J. Periodontal disease in pregnancy. I. Prevalence and severity. Acta Odontol Scand 1963;21:532–551.

57. Lang NP, Kaarup-Hansen D, Joss A, et al. The significance of overhanging filling margins for the health status of interdental periodontal tissues of young adults. Schweiz Monatsschr Zahnmed 1988;98(7):725–730.

58. Waerhaug J. The interdental brush and its place in operative and crown and bridge dentistry. J Oral Rehabil 1976;3(2): 107–113.

59. Waerhaug J. Plaque control in the treatment of juvenile periodontitis. J Clin Periodontol 1977;4(1):29–40.

60. Magne P, Magne M, Belser U. The esthetic width in fixed prosthodontics. J Prosthodont 1999;8(2):106–118.

61. Hirschfield I. Food impaction. J Am Dent Assoc 1930;17: 1504–1528.

62. Lang NP, Cumming BR, Löe H. Toothbrushing frequency as it relates to plaque development and gingival health. J Periodontol 1973;44:396–405.

63. Hock J. The formation of the vasculature of free gingiva in deciduous teeth of cats and dogs. J Periodontal Res 1974;9:298–304.

64. Gusberti F, Finger M, Lang N. Scanning electron microscopic study of 48 hour plaque on different bridge pontic designs. Helv Odontol Acta 1985;29:1–11.

65. Silness J, Gustavsen F, Mangersnes K. The relationship between pontic hygiene and mucosal inflammation in fixed bridge recipients. J Periodontal Res 1982;17:434–439.

66. Johnson GK, Leary JM. Pontic design and localized ridge augmentation in fixed partial denture design. Dent Clin North Am 1992;36:591–605.

67. Dylina TJ. Contour determination for ovate pontics. J Prosthet Dent 1999;82:136–142.

68. Kois JC, Kan JY. Predictable peri-implant gingival aesthetics: Surgical and prosthodontic rationales. Pract Proced Aesthet Dent 2001;13(9):691–698; quiz 700, 721–722.

69. Ingber JS, Rose LF, Coslet JG. The "biologic width"—A concept in periodontics and restorative dentistry. Alpha Omegan 1977; 70(3):62–65.

70. Palomo F, Kopczyk R. Rationale and methods for crown lengthening. J Am Dent Assoc 1978;96:257–260.

71. Kahldahl W, Becher C, Wentz F. Periodontal surgical preparation for specific problems in restorative dentistry. J Prosthet Dent 1984;51:36–41.

72. Baima R. Extension of clinical crown length. J Prosthet Dent 1986;55:547–551.

73. Davis J, Fry R, Krill D, Rostock M. Periodontal surgery as an adjunct to endodontics, prosthodontics and restorative dentistry. J Am Dent Assoc 1987;115:271–275.

74. Levine H, Stahl S. Repair following periodontal flap surgery with the retention of gingival fibers. J Periodontol 1972;443: 99–103.

75. Tal H, Diaz M. Crown lengthening procedures: An overview. J Dent Med 1985;3:3–7.

76. Brägger U, Lang N. Chirurgische Verlängerung der klinischen Krone. Schweiz Monatsschr Zahnmed 1988;98:644–651.

77. Brägger U, Lauchenauer D, Lang N. Surgical lengthening of the clinical crown. J Clin Periodontol 1992;19:58–63.

78. Pontoriero R, Carnevale G. Surgical crown lengthening: A 12-month clinical wound healing study. J Periodontol 2001;72: 841–848.

79. Gargiulo AW, Wentz FM, Orban B. Dimensions and relations of the dentogingival junction in humans. J Periodontol 1961;32: 261–267.

80. Gottlow J, Nyman S, Karring T. Maintenance of new attachment gained through guided tissue regeneration. J Clin Periodontol 1992;19:315–317.

81. Falk H, Laurell L, Ravald N. Guided tissue regeneration therapy of 203 consecutively treated intrabony defects using a bioabsorbable matrix barrier. Clinical and radiographic findings. J Periodontol 1997;68(6):571–581.

82. Cortellini P, Carnevale G, Sanz M, Tonetti MS. Treatment of deep and shallow intrabony defects. A multicenter randomized controlled clinical trial. J Clin Periodontol 1998;25(12):981–987.

83. Teparat T, Solt CW, Claman LJ, Beck FM. Clinical comparison of bioabsorbable barriers with non-resorbable barriers in guided tissue regeneration in the treatment of human intrabony defects. J Periodontol 1998;69(6):632–641.

84. Tonetti MS, Cortellini P, Suvan JE, et al. Generalizability of the added benefits of guided tissue regeneration in the treatment of deep intrabony defects. Evaluation in a multi-center randomized controlled clinical trial. J Periodontol 1998;69:1183–1192.

85. Dahlin C, Linde A, Gottlow J, Nyman S. Healing of bone defects by guided tissue regeneration. Plast Reconstr Surg 1988;81: 672–676.

86. Dahlin C, Gottlow J, Linde A, Nyman S. Healing of maxillary and mandibular bone defects using a membrane technique. An experimental study in monkeys. Scand J Plast Reconstr Surg Hand Surg 1990;24:13–19.

87. Seibert J, Nyman S. Localized ridge augmentation in dogs. A pilot study using membranes and hydroxyapatite. J Periodontol 1990;61:157–165.

88. Wilson TG Jr, Buser D. Advances in the use of guided tissue regeneration for localized ridge augmentation in combination with dental implants. Tex Dent J 1994;111(7):5,7–10.

89. Dahlin C, Sennerby L, Lekholm U, et al. Generation of new bone around titanium implants using a membrane technique: An experimental study in rabbits. Int J Oral Maxillofac Implants 1989;4(1):19–25.

90. Becker W, Becker BE. Guided tissue regeneration for implants placed into extraction sockets and for implant dehiscences: Surgical techniques and case reports. Int J Periodontics Restorative Dent 1990;10(5):377–391.

91. Jovanovic S, Kenney E, Carranza F, Donath K. The regenerative potential of plaque-induced peri-implant bone defects treated by a submerged membrane technique: An experimental study. Int J Oral Maxillofac Implants 1993;8:13–18.

92. Nyman S, Lang NP, Buser D, Brägger U. Bone regeneration adjacent to titanium dental implants using guided tissue regeneration: A report of two cases. Int J Oral Maxillofac Implants 1990;5(1):9–14.

93. Buser D, Hirt P, Dula K, Berthold H. Gleichzeitige Anwendung von Membranen bei Implantaten mit peri-implantären Knochendefekten. Schweiz Monatsschr Zahnmed 1992;102:1490–1505.

94. Lang NP, Hämmerle C, Brägger U, et al. Guided tissue regeneration in jawbone defects prior to implant placement. Clin Oral Implants Res 1994;5:92–97.

Occlusal Trauma:
Effects and Management

Stephen K. Harrel and William W. Hallmon

- Definitions
- Response of the Periodontium to Occlusal Trauma
- Human Research
- Dental Implants
- Role of Occlusion in the Progression of Periodontal Disease
- Clinical Techniques

The role of occlusion and its interaction with the periodontium has been the subject of extensive investigation and discussion. An injury that results in tissue changes within the attachment apparatus in response to occlusal forces is termed *occlusal trauma*.[1–3] Clinical and radiographic indicators of occlusal trauma may include increased tooth mobility, fremitus, premature occlusal contacts, wear facets, tooth migration, fractured teeth, thermal sensitivity, widened periodontal ligament space, bone loss, and root resorption.[4] Clinician's understanding of the effects of injurious occlusal forces and the adaptive, reparative, and destructive response of the periodontium has largely been based on retrospective observations of human autopsy specimens and studies using laboratory animals.[5–30] Unfortunately, understanding this complex host interaction is complicated by a relative lack of available scientific evidence from well-controlled prospective studies in humans.[2,31,32] This chapter will discuss definitions, the histologic lesion, research findings, clinical and radiographic indicators, and clinical examination and treatment of patients with occlusal trauma.

Definitions

At a recent International Workshop for a Classification of Periodontal Diseases and Conditions, the following working definitions for *occlusal trauma* were developed and listed under section 8, Developmental and Acquired Deformities and Conditions.[1] These definitions will facilitate the reader's orientation and understanding of the relationship between occlusal forces and the periodontium:

- *Primary occlusal trauma*—Injury resulting in tissue changes from excessive occlusal forces applied to a tooth or teeth with normal support. It occurs in the presence of *(1)* normal bone levels, *(2)* normal attachment levels, and *(3)* excessive occlusal force(s)[1] (Fig 31-1).
- *Secondary occlusal trauma*—Injury resulting in tissue changes from normal or excessive occlusal forces applied to a tooth or teeth with reduced support. It occurs in the presence of *(1)* bone loss, *(2)* attachment loss, and *(3)* "normal"/excessive occlusal force(s)[1] (Fig 31-2).

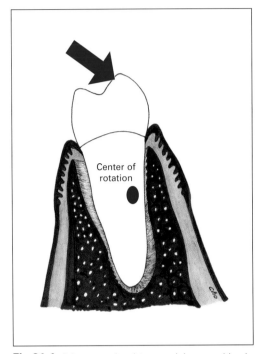

Fig 31-1 Primary occlusal trauma: injury resulting in tissue changes from excessive occlusal forces applied to a tooth or teeth with normal support. The occlusal force applied is too great for the normal supporting structure to withstand, and trauma to the tissue occurs. (Courtesy Dr J. Y. Cho.)

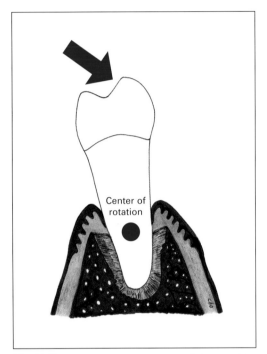

Fig 31-2 Secondary occlusal trauma: injury resulting in tissue changes from normal or excessive occlusal forces applied to a tooth or teeth with reduced support. The supporting structures of the tooth are reduced because of disease and are no longer able to withstand even normal masticatory forces. (Courtesy Dr J. Y. Cho.)

Response of the Periodontium to Occlusal Trauma

The response of the periodontium to occlusal forces depends on the magnitude, direction, location, and duration of the forces, as well as the amount of attachment/support of affected teeth.[6,33] When force is applied, the periodontium sustains areas of tension and pressure. As applied forces increase in magnitude, duration, or both, the ability of the periodontium to adapt to these excess forces may be exceeded, resulting in injury. In such cases, the histologic characteristics of the occlusally injured periodontium may include the following[1,6,33–38]:

- *Pressure zone*—Compression of the periodontal ligament, bone remodeling (frontal/rear resorption), vascular dilation/permeability, hyalinization/necrosis, increased cellularity, thrombosis, and root resorption.
- *Tension zone*—Widening of the periodontal ligament, bone repair, vascular permeability, cemental tears, and thrombosis. These mechanisms are the means by which the periodontium attempts to adapt to the applied injurious external forces. If occlusal trauma is accompa-

nied by a dental plaque–induced inflammatory lesion (preexisting periodontitis), both components should be controlled.[23,39,40]

Earlier investigations of the response of the periodontium to occlusal trauma depended primarily on human autopsy materials for retrospective observations and effects.[5–9] The codestructive theory, which hypothesized that there was a zone of irritation (marginal/interdental gingiva and gingival fibers) and a zone of codestruction (transseptal/alveolar crest fibers, periodontal ligament, cementum, and bone), arose from these investigations. This theory suggested that in the presence of plaque-induced inflammation, occlusal trauma may alter the normal pathway of inflammation and lead to the development of angular bony defects with intrabony pockets. Among the tenets of this theory was that occlusal trauma alone did not cause gingivitis and periodontitis, but that dental plaque was responsible for initiating and sustaining the diseases.[41–43] The role of occlusal trauma in this process has been questioned in other studies, which suggest that the bacterial "plaque front" is the principal determinant of the severity and sites of attachment loss and accompanying bony defects.[44]

Although a great deal has been inferred about the response of the periodontium to occlusal trauma from human autopsy materials, prospective controlled human studies in this area have yet to be conducted. The difficulty and complexity of designing and implementing these types of human studies have resulted in alternative development and dependency on animal models for prospective, clinical, and histologic investigations of this inter-relationship. Among the most widely used animal models for the study of this topic are beagle dogs and squirrel monkeys.[2,16,45] Although such studies provide valuable information about the host tissue response, repair, and adaptive process, findings must be carefully interpreted, because the dynamics of the human masticatory function differ from animal models.

In studies using beagle dogs and in the presence or absence of continuous, excessive jiggling forces (cap splint or bar-spring device) in health and experimentally induced periodontitis, accelerated progression of pocket formation was observed in the presence of ongoing destructive periodontitis. However, no progressive marginal destruction or apical migration of the junctional epithelium was observed in the presence of jiggling trauma in the noninflamed periodontium.[13-21]

The squirrel monkey model was used to study the effects of the presence or absence of jiggling trauma (alternating orthodontic elastic wedging mesial and distal to the septum) in health and induced periodontitis. Associated bone loss and increased tooth mobility accompanied sustained jiggling forces, but little or no loss of attachment occurred. Initiation or progression of periodontal pockets was not observed. Findings from these studies have resulted in decreased emphasis on occlusal factors and increased therapeutic attention to plaque control, and thus periodontal disease.[22-30]

Despite differences between these study approaches and the inherent responses of the animal models employed, there was agreement that in the healthy, noninflamed periodontium, occlusal trauma alone does not result in pocket formation or loss of connective tissue attachment.

Human Research

As previously noted, much of the published literature that has evaluated the effect of occlusal trauma on the human periodontium was based on autopsy material and is descriptive. This means that the patient's occlusal relationships (how the teeth come together in normal function or parafunction) had to be determined after death, and the effects of the occlusion on the periodontium were determined by describing the changes seen in histologic sections. Although the published descriptions of tissue changes are generally accurate and insightful, the correlation of these changes with various occlusal patterns was, at best, conjectural. Some early published works on occlusion described an observed association between advanced periodontal breakdown and the presence of occlusal trauma. However, descriptive studies have limited value in determining the effect of a putative risk factor such as occlusal trauma on the progression of a disease. Studies that follow the progression of a disease over time, with and without treatment (controlled clinical trials), are the best method to evaluate the effect of any risk factor. However, human research in occlusion has been limited because of ethical concerns about withholding treatment over an extended time. Concerns over ethical considerations led the members of the occlusion section of the 1996 World Workshop in Periodontics to conclude that "Prospective studies on the effect of occlusal forces on the progression of periodontitis are not ethically acceptable in humans."[2]

Only a few studies have evaluated the relationship of occlusal trauma to the progression of periodontal disease in humans. It has been reported that patients who have occlusal discrepancies have no more severe periodontal destruction than do patients without occlusal discrepancies.[46,47] However, it was also reported that molars with furcation invasion and mobility have greater pocket depths than molars that are not mobile.[48] The increased mobility noted in this study may have been caused by occlusal factors or to greater loss of bony support due to the furcation involvement. Because it cannot be determined whether occlusal factors or bone loss was first present, from this study it is impossible to establish a clear relationship among occlusion discrepancies, mobility, and probing depths. Another study reported that patients who received occlusal adjustment as part of their periodontal therapy had greater attachment gain than patients who did not receive occlusal adjustment.[49] This study can be viewed as an indication that occlusal adjustment should be performed, where indicated, as a part of periodontal treatment. A series of reports on risk factors for periodontal destruction indicated that mobility and parafunctional habits that are not treated with a bite guard are associated with increased attachment loss, worsening prognosis, and tooth loss.[50,51] This study seems to indicate that untreated (ie, without a bite guard) parafunctional habits may contribute to increased periodontal breakdown

The information found in the noted human studies does not give a clear indication whether excessive occlusal forces cause a more rapid breakdown of the periodontium. Consequently, there has been no agreement as to whether occlusal discrepancies should be treated as part of periodontal therapy. Some educators have interpreted the scant human data as an indication that occlusal trauma plays some role in periodontal destruction and have recommended the use of occlusal adjustment as part of comprehensive periodontal therapy. Others have evaluated the same research material and made the decision not to routinely treat occlusal discrepancies. Based on most published studies, it can be stated that the role of occlusal trauma in human periodontal destruction is not clear, and therefore there is no clear indication for occlusal therapy—with the possible exception of bite guards for parafunctional habits—in the treatment of periodontal disease.

A recent study[52,53] has indicated that occlusal trauma may play a significant role in periodontal destruction. This study looked retrospectively at patients from a private practice who were diagnosed with advanced periodontal disease and had a recommended comprehensive treatment plan that included occlusal adjustment if occlusal discrepancies were detected. Some of these patients self-selected not to have any periodontal treatment (untreated group). Other patients received only nonsurgical periodontal treatment and did not follow through with the surgical portion of the recommended treatment (partially treated group). Others followed through with all the recommended periodontal treatment, including surgery (fully treated group). The effect of occlusal discrepancies was studied in each of these groups, using the tooth as the experimental unit.[52,53] This means that the progression of periodontal destruction or the improvement of the periodontium for each tooth was followed over time. This study design allowed the evaluation of teeth with occlusal discrepancies versus teeth without occlusal discrepancies rather than comparing patients with occlusal discrepancies and patients without occlusal discrepancies.

This experimental approach differs from most past studies, where the patient was the experimental unit and the changes in probing depth or attachment levels were expressed as the patient mean. The patient mean is generated by determining the mean, or average, of all pocket depths/attachment levels around all teeth and using changes in this number to evaluate the effect of occlusal trauma. One of the criticisms of using the patient mean for statistical evaluation is that shallow sites are averaged in with deeper sites that have more periodontal degeneration and, presumably, more active periodontal disease. Using the patient mean may tend to mask changes that are occurring at the more active sites and thereby give results that do not reflect what is actually occurring during localized disease progression.

When individual teeth were used as the experimental unit, teeth that had occlusal discrepancies were noted to have deeper presenting pocket depths and a worse prognosis than teeth that did not have occlusal discrepancies. Furthermore, when teeth with occlusal discrepancies were followed over time, a significant increase in pocket depth and a worsening of prognosis were noted when compared with teeth without occlusal discrepancies. Additionally, teeth in the partially treated group that had received occlusal adjustment showed a slowing of periodontal destruction when compared with teeth with occlusal discrepancies that had not had occlusal adjustment. It was concluded that occlusal discrepancies may contribute to more rapid periodontal destruction and that treatment of occlusal discrepancies seemed to slow periodontal destruction. The authors[52,53] postulated that the reason for the difference in their findings and those of previous studies was the fact that by using the individual tooth as the experimental unit, a more accurate assessment of the effect of occlusal trauma on the periodontium could be obtained.

Dental Implants

The effect of occlusal stress on osseointegrated implants is also controversial. Although practitioners have suggested that excessive occlusal forces on implants may lead to failure, there is little fundamental research or scientific evidence to support this observation.[54] Implant studies in monkeys have reported a significant loss of osseointegration due to occlusal overload; this occurred even in the presence of weekly cleanings. The controls in these studies consisted of implants with heavy plaque and no occlusal overload. No loss of osseointegration was observed in this control group.[55,56] Other studies in the same model using prolonged excessive supraocclusal force (restorations with a "high" contact) in the absence of peri-implant inflammation failed to result in notable peri-implant bone loss. When comparable levels of prolonged excessive supraocclusal force (100-µm cusp height) were combined with experimental inflammation, notable peri-implant bone loss occurred.[57,58] One mechanism suggested for the loss of osseointegration due to occlusal overload has been the formation of microfractures at the coronal aspect of the bone-implant interface.[59] Despite the lack of supporting data, current clinical techniques strongly emphasize the need to avoid overloading the implant-supported prosthesis.[60]

Role of Occlusion in the Progression of Periodontal Disease

The results of animal and human studies do not give a clear picture of the role that occlusal discrepancies and occlusal trauma play in the progression of periodontal disease. Animal studies seem to indicate that occlusal discrepancies and occlusal trauma do not initiate periodontal breakdown. The beagle dog studies may indicate that in the presence of bacterial plaque there will be a more rapid loss of attachment and bone when occlusal discrepancies are present. The role of bacterial plaque as the initiating factor of periodontitis has been well established by a series of studies that showed no significant periodontal breakdown when good oral hygiene was maintained.[61–64] By contrast, none of the human or animal research on occlusion and periodontal disease seems to support the role of occlusal discrepancies/occlusal trauma as a factor in periodontal disease if plaque is not present.

Human research seems to indicate a possible relationship between periodontal breakdown and occlusal discrepancies/occlusal trauma. Human research on occlusion is hampered by the inability to perform a controlled study, however. As noted previously, the gold standard of all human clinical research is the controlled clinical trial, but it is not ethically possible to perform a controlled clinical trial to evaluate the role of occlusion in periodontal disease. The lack of evidence from a controlled clinical trial leaves many unanswered questions about the role of occlusion in the progression of periodontal disease: Are increased probing depths in the presence of mobility due to the presence of occlusal discrepancies or greater loss of bone? Did occlusal discrepancies cause greater periodontal breakdown, or did an area of periodontal breakdown cause the tooth to move and thereby cause an occlusal discrepancy? It is unlikely that clinicians will ever have a satisfactory answer to these questions. However, one retrospective study has shown that when individual teeth with occlusal discrepancies were treated with occlusal adjustment, they showed greater improvement over time than similar teeth that did not have occlusal adjustment.[53] This may indicate that occlusion does in fact serve as a risk factor for periodontal breakdown and that as such, occlusal treatment may need to be considered as part of the comprehensive treatment of periodontal disease.

Clinical Techniques

Clinical Examination

The clinical examination for occlusal discrepancies includes evaluating the patient for signs of current or past occlusal trauma—eg, wear facets, fremitus (movement of the teeth during function), and mobility measured between two instrument handles (see chapter 17). The occlusal relationship of the teeth may also be evaluated by observing the manner in which the teeth make contact. This is usually performed by gently manipulating the pa-

tient's mandible into a retruded position (retruded occlusion/centric relation) and having the patient slowly close until first contact between the teeth is made. The patient is then asked to close to a comfortable intercuspated position (centric occlusion/habitual occlusion). The distance the patient moves from the retruded position to the greatest intercuspation is termed the *centric relation to centric occlusion slide* (or *CR/CO shift*). Both the initial contact point and the approximate amount of slide can be recorded.

Tooth contacts in eccentric jaw positions (ie, lateral and protrusive positions of the jaw) are also recorded. To determine these contacts, the patient is asked to close in the habitual occlusal position (centric occlusion) and then move to the right or left in an unguided movement (ie, the patient is allowed to move the jaw to the side without any manual guidance by the practitioner). The side of the mouth in the direction the patient moves the jaw (eg, the right side of the mouth when the patient moves the jaw to the right) is usually termed the *working side*, and hence the tooth contacts on this side are termed *working contacts*. The side opposite the direction in which the patient moves the jaw (eg, the left side of the mouth when the patient moves the jaw to the right) is usually termed the *balancing side*, and hence the tooth contacts on this side are termed *balancing contacts*. *Protrusive jaw movement* is when the patient moves the jaw to a forward position (ie, protrudes the chin).

For the purpose of recording tooth contact during an examination, contacts are observed visually and may also be marked with a thin inked silk ribbon or Mylar film. The use of paper strips impregnated with ink (occlusal marking paper) is not recommended. Most occlusal marking paper contains wax and may be too thick for accurate recording of occlusal contacts. Ink-impregnated ribbons and Mylar film that is coated with ink do not contain wax and thus are thinner and produce clearer marks on the teeth with less smearing of the ink. However, inked ribbons and Mylar films do not work well in the presence of moisture, and it is necessary to dry the teeth either with air or gauze prior to their use. Figure 31-3 shows a simplified form that can be used to record occlusal findings and tooth contacts during an occlusal evaluation.

Treatment Planning

After occlusal contacts and signs of trauma from occlusion are evaluated, a decision can be made concerning whether occlusal treatment is needed. The decision to treat the patient's occlusion either by adjusting the occlusal surfaces or by the use of an occlusal appliance will be influenced by the patient's symptoms, such as tooth sensitivity to temperature changes or pain on chewing,

Analysis of Occlusion:

Angle classification: R_____   L_____

Presence of fremitus in:

Wear facets on:

Opening deviation and TMJ findings:

Centric prematurities: CR/CO	1	2	3	4	5	6	7	8	9	10	11	12	13	14	15	16
	32	31	30	29	28	27	26	25	24	23	22	21	20	19	18	17
LLE prematurities:	1	2	3	4	5	6	7	8	9	10	11	12	13	14	15	16
	32	31	30	29	28	27	26	25	24	23	22	21	20	19	18	17
RLE prematurities:	1	2	3	4	5	6	7	8	9	10	11	12	13	14	15	16
	32	31	30	29	28	27	26	25	24	23	22	21	20	19	18	17
Protrusive prematurities:	1	2	3	4	5	6	7	8	9	10	11	12	13	14	15	16
	32	31	30	29	28	27	26	25	24	23	22	21	20	19	18	17

Fig 31-3 A simplified form that can be used to record occlusal findings and tooth contacts during an occlusal evaluation. The teeth that are in contact during various movements can be circled to indicate this contact. LLE = left lateral excursion; RLE = right lateral excursion.

mobility, the presence of wear on the occluding tooth surfaces (facets), extent of periodontal destruction, and the patient's ability to adequately function. If the patient is asymptomatic and does not have significant periodontal disease, treatment of the occlusion may not be indicated even if significant occlusal discrepancies are present. If the patient has occlusal discrepancies in addition to periodontal disease, occlusal treatment may be considered.

The preliminary decision to include occlusal treatment in a periodontal treatment plan can often be made at the initial examination appointment. If significant occlusal discrepancies and periodontal destruction are present at the initial appointment, occlusal treatment may be indicated. However, as with all periodontal treatment, the decision to perform occlusal therapy should be made after reevaluation of the patient's response to nonsurgical treatment such as oral hygiene instructions and root planing. Mobility and fremitus will often be greatly reduced by these procedures, and the need for occlusal treatment may be diminished.

Occlusal Treatment

Occlusal treatment is usually performed after periodontal inflammation has been reduced by nonsurgical treatment. When the periodontal supporting structures are inflamed, there is often an increase in the mobility of the teeth. This increased mobility may be due to swelling of the periodontal ligament. When inflammation is controlled, the teeth tend to be less mobile, which allows for a more stable occlusal relationship following occlusal treatment. An exception to this treatment timing would be when the patient has difficulty chewing or has tooth pain when chewing that appears directly related to occlusal trauma. In these cases, occlusal treatment may be indicated as the first step of periodontal therapy to make the patient comfortable. If a decision is made to begin occlusal treatment prior to controlling inflammation, it will probably be necessary to perform further occlusal treatment following control of inflammation. The patient should be informed of this prior to beginning treatment.

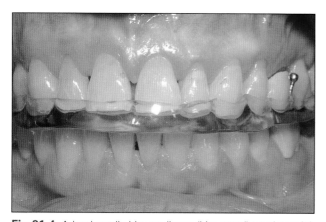

Fig 31-4 A hard acrylic bite appliance (bite guard) used to minimize the forces placed on the teeth during parafunctional movement. A maxillary bite appliance is preferred for most periodontal patients because it will stabilize potentially loose maxillary teeth and prevent anterior flaring.

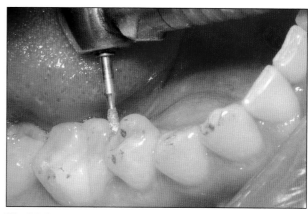

Fig 31-5 Selective grinding of the teeth to permanently change the distribution of the occlusal forces. Selective grinding must be done with care to ensure that the resulting occlusal relationships distribute occlusal forces as evenly and atraumatically as possible.

Occlusal treatment consists of two basic approaches: *(1)* the use of a bite appliance (bite guard) and/or *(2)* adjusting the occlusion by altering the occlusal relationships between the teeth. A bite appliance fits over the patient's teeth and creates an artificial occlusal surface for the opposing dentition to contact. A bite appliance is usually made from hard acrylic, which has the advantage of cushioning contact forces between the teeth. Heat- or cold-cured hard acrylic is usually recommended over a soft acrylic material such as that used for athletic mouth guards. The hard acrylic will offer some cushioning of occlusal forces while allowing the clinician to develop specific occlusal contact relationships between the bite guard and the opposing teeth. When soft acrylic is used, the patient can bite into the material, and if any lateral grinding movements are made, heavy torque forces may be transferred to the teeth. With a hard acrylic bite appliance, the opposing teeth will slide on the acrylic occlusal surfaces, and most torquing forces will be minimized. The use of a maxillary bite appliance (Fig 31-4) is preferred for most periodontal patients because it will stabilize potentially loose maxillary anterior teeth and prevent flaring. If a mandibular bite appliance is used against maxillary teeth with compromised support, flaring of the maxillary teeth is possible.

The relationship between teeth can be permanently altered by orthodontic therapy or by selective grinding of the occlusal surfaces. Altering the occlusal relationship of the teeth, either by selective grinding (Fig 31-5) or orthodontic therapy, has the advantage of creating a permanent change in the distribution of occlusal forces. However, if these therapies are not carried out with care and skill, the possibility exists for creating an occlusal relationship that

is more damaging than the one that previously existed. Creating permanent changes in the occlusion should be approached with great caution and only following adequate instruction in the proper performance of these techniques.[61]

Summary

The role of occlusion in the pathogenesis of periodontal disease and peri-implantitis is controversial. Many clinicians have observed an apparent relationship between occlusal interferences and the progression of periodontal disease and attachment loss. However, animal studies have not consistently borne out this relationship. Most human studies have shown a minimal role for occlusion in periodontal disease. However, one recent human study using the individual tooth as the experimental unit seemed to suggest that occlusal discrepancies are a risk factor in periodontal destruction, so occlusal treatment may need to be considered in the management of periodontal disease. When occlusal discrepancies are present, treatment should be limited to cases where there is evidence of damage to the oral structures, such as tooth wear, mobility, or periodontal destruction. Occlusal treatment can be performed by using removable appliances and/or by altering the contacting surfaces of the teeth. Irreversible changes to the occlusion by adjusting the contacting surfaces should be performed only after adequate instruction in the techniques necessary to obtain acceptable results.

Although there is some evidence that occlusal trauma is a risk factor for periodontal destruction, it should be emphasized that there is no evidence that occlusal trauma will initiate periodontal destruction. All evidence points to bacterial plaque as the initiating factor in periodontal destruction. Effective plaque control and compliance with periodontal maintenance recommendations remain vital to the successful treatment and control of periodontal diseases.

References

1. Hallmon W. Occlusal trauma: Effect and impact on the periodontium. Ann Periodontol 1999;4:102–107.

2. Gher M. Non-surgical pocket therapy: Dental occlusion. Ann Periodontol 1996;1:567–580.

3. Glossary of Periodontal Terms. Chicago: American Academy of Periodontology, 1992:34.

4. Ramfjord SP, Ash MM. Significance of occlusion in the etiology and treatment of early, moderate and advanced periodontitis. J Periodontol 1981;52:511–517.

5. Glickman I, Smulow JB. Effect of excessive occlusal forces on the pathway of gingival inflammation in humans. J Periodontol 1965;36:141–147.

6. Ramfjord SP, Kohler CA. Periodontal reaction to functional occlusal stress. J Periodontol 1959;30:95–112.

7. Stahl SS. The responses of the periodontium to combined inflammation and occluso-functional stresses in four human surgical specimens. Periodontics 1968;6:14–22.

8. Waerhaug J. The infrabony pocket and its relationship to trauma from occlusion and subgingival plaque. J Periodontol 1979;50:355–365.

9. Weinmann JP. The adaptation of the periodontal membrane to physiologic and pathologic changes. Oral Surg Oral Med Oral Pathol 1955;8:977–981.

10. Box HK. Experimental traumatogenic occlusion in sheep. Oral Health 1935;29:9–15.

11. Goldman HM. Gingival vascular supply in induced occlusal traumatism. J Oral Surg 1956;9:939–941.

12. Wentz FW, Jarabak J, Orban B. Experimental occlusal trauma imitating cuspal interferences. J Periodontol 1958;29:117–127.

13. Svanberg G, Lindhe J. Experimental tooth hypermobility in the dog. Odontol Revy 1973;24:269–282.

14. Svanberg G, Lindhe J. Vascular reactions in the periodontal ligament incident to trauma from occlusion. J Clin Periodontol 1974;1:58–69.

15. Svanberg G. Influence of trauma from occlusion on the periodontium of dogs with normal and inflamed gingiva. Odontol Revy 1974;25:165–178.

16. Lindhe J, Svanberg G. Influence of trauma from occlusion on progressive experimental periodontitis in the beagle dog. J Clin Periodontol 1974;1:3–14.

17. Lindhe J, Ericsson I. Influence of trauma from occlusion on reduced but healthy periodontal tissues in dogs. J Clin Periodontol 1976;3:110–122.

18. Ericsson I, Lindhe J. Effect of longstanding jiggling on experimental marginal periodontitis in the beagle dog. J Clin Periodontol 1982;9:497–503.

19. Lindhe J, Ericsson I. The effect of elimination of jiggling forces on periodontally exposed teeth in the dog. J Periodontol 1982;53:562–567.

20. Ericsson I, Lindhe J. Lack of significance of increased tooth mobility in experimental periodontitis. J Periodontol 1983;55:447–452.

21. Nyman S, Lindhe J, Ericsson I. The effect of progressive tooth mobility on destructive periodontitis in the dog. J Clin Periodontol 1978;5:213–225.

22. Polson AM, Meitner SW, Zander HA. Trauma and progression of marginal periodontitis in squirrel monkeys. III. Adaptation of interproximal alveolar bone to repetitive injury. J Periodontal Res 1976;11:276–289.

23. Polson AM. The relative importance of plaque and occlusion in periodontal disease. J Clin Periodontol 1986;13:923–927.

24. Polson AM, Kantor ME, Zander HE. Periodontal repair after reduction in inflammation. J Periodontal Res 1979;14:520–525.

25. Polson AM, Meitner SW, Zander HA. Trauma and progression of marginal periodontitis in squirrel monkeys. IV. Reversibility of bone loss due to trauma alone and trauma superimposed upon periodontitis. J Periodontal Res 1976;11:290–298.

26. Kantor M, Polson AM, Zander HA. Alveolar bone regeneration after the removal of inflammatory traumatic injuries. J Periodontal Res 1976;47:687–695.

27. Perrier M, Polson A. The effect of progressive and increasing tooth hypermobility on reduced but healthy periodontal supporting tissues. J Periodontol 1982;53:152–157.

28. Polson AM, Zander HA. Effect of periodontal trauma upon intrabony pockets. J Periodontol 1983;54:586–592.

29. Polson AM, Adams RA, Zander HA. Osseous repair in the presence of active tooth hypermobility. J Clin Periodontol 1983;10:370–379.

30. Polson AM. Trauma and progression of marginal periodontitis in squirrel monkeys. II. Co-destructive factors of periodontitis and mechanically produced injury. J Periodontal Res 1974;9:146–152.

31. Svanberg GK, King GJ, Gibbs CH. Occlusal considerations in periodontology. Periodontol 2000 1995;9:106–117.

32. Hoag PM. Occlusal trauma. In: Nevins M, Becker W, Kornman W (eds). Proceedings of the World Workshop in Clinical Periodontics, July 23–27, 1989. Chicago: American Academy of Periodontology, 1989:III1–III23.

33. Orban B. Tissue changes in traumatic occlusion. J Am Dent Assoc 1928;15:2091–2106.

34. Bhaskar SN, Orban B. Experimental occlusal trauma. J Periodontol 1955;26:270–284.

35. Oppenheim A. Human tissue response to orthodontic intervention of long and short duration. Am J Orthod Oral Surg 1942;28:263–301.

36. Grant D, Bernick S. The periodontium of aging humans. J Periodontol 1972;43:660–667.

37. Haney J, Leknes K, Lie T, et al. Cemental tear related to rapid periodontal breakdown: A case report. J Periodontol 1992;63:220–224.

38. Ishikawa I, Oda S, Hiyashi J, Arakawa S. Cervical cemental tears in older patients with adult periodontitis. Case reports. J Periodontol 1996;67:15–20.

39. Muhlemann H, Herzog H. Tooth mobility and microscopic tissue changes produced by experimental occlusal trauma. Helv Odontol Acta 1961;5:33–39.

40. Polson AM, Heijl LC. Occlusion and periodontal disease. Dent Clin North Am 1980;24:783–795.

41. Glickman I. Inflammation and trauma from occlusion: Co-destructive factors in chronic periodontal disease. J Periodontol 1963;34:5–10.

42. Glickman I, Smulow JB. Alterations of the pathway of gingival inflammation into the underlying tissues induced by excessive occlusal forces. J Periodontol 1962;33:7–13.

43. Glickman I, Smulow JB. Further observations on the effects of trauma from occlusion in humans. J Periodontol 1967;38:280–293.

44. Waerhaug J. The angular bone defect and its relationship to trauma from occlusion and subgingival plaque. J Clin Periodontol 1979;6:61–82.

45. Polson AM. Interrelationship of inflammation and tooth mobility (trauma) in pathogenesis of periodontal disease. J Clin Periodontol 1980;7:351–360.

46. Pihlstrom BL, Anderson KA, Aeppli D, Schaffer E. Association between signs of trauma from occlusion and periodontitis. J Periodontol 1986;57:1–6.

47. Jin LJ, Cao CF. Clinical diagnosis of trauma from occlusion and its relation with severity of periodontitis. J Clin Periodontol 1992;19:92–97.

48. Wang H, Burgett FG, Shyr Y, Ramfjord S. The influence of molar furcation involvement and mobility on future clinical periodontal attachment loss. J Periodontol 1994;65:25–29.

49. Burgett FG, Ramfjord SP, Nissle RR, et al. A randomized trial of occlusal adjustment in the treatment of periodontal patients. J Clin Periodontol 1992;19:381–387.

50. McGuire MK, Nunn ME. Prognosis versus actual outcome II. The effectiveness of commonly taught clinical parameters in developing an accurate prognosis. J Periodontol 1996;76:658–665.

51. McGuire MK, Nunn ME. Prognosis versus actual outcome III. The effectiveness of commonly taught clinical parameters in accurately predicting tooth survival. J Periodontol 1996;67:666–674.

52. Nunn ME, Harrel SK. The effect of occlusal discrepancies on periodontitis: I. Relationship of initial occlusal discrepancies to initial clinical parameters. J Periodontol 2001;72:485–494.

53. Harrel SK, Nunn ME. The effect of occlusal discrepancies on periodontitis. II. Relationship of occlusal treatment to the progression of periodontal disease. J Periodontol 2001;72:495–505.

54. Quirynen M, Naert I, van Steenberghe D. Fixture design and overload influence marginal bone loss and fixture success in Branemark system. Clin Oral Implants Res 1992;3:104–111.

55. Isidor F. Loss of osseointegration caused by occlusal load of oral implants. A clinical and radiographic study in monkeys. Clin Oral Implants Res 1996;7:143–152.

56. Isidor F. Histological evaluation of peri-implant bone at implants subjected to occlusal overload or plaque accumulation. Clin Oral Implants Res 1997;8:1–9.

57. Miyata T, Kobayashi Y, Araki H, et al. The influence of controlled occlusal overload on peri-implant tissue: A histologic study in monkeys. Int J Oral Maxillofac Implants 1998;13:677–683.

58. Miyata T, Kobayashi Y, Araki H, et al. The influence of controlled occlusal overload on peri-implant tissue: Part 3: A histologic study in monkeys. Int J Oral Maxillofac Implants 2000;15:425–431.

59. Rangert B, Jemt T, Jorneus L. Forces and moments on Branemark implants. Int J Oral Maxillofac Implants 1989;4:241–247.

60. Taylor T, Agar J, Vogiatzi T. Implant prosthodontics: Current perspectives and future directions. Int J Oral Maxillofac Implants 2000;15:66–75.

61. Solberg W, Seligman D. Coronoplasty in periodontal therapy. In: Carranza FA, Newman MG. Clinical Periodontology (ed 8). Philadelphia: W. B. Saunders, 1996:537–558.

62. Axelsson P, Lindhe J. Effect of controlled oral hygiene procedures on caries and periodontal disease in adults. J Clin Periodontol 1978;5:133–151.

63. Axelsson P, Lindhe J. Effect of controlled oral hygiene procedures on caries and periodontal disease in adults: Results after 6 years. J Clin Periodontol 1981;8:239–248.

64. Axelsson P, Lindhe J. The significance of maintenance care in the treatment of periodontal disease. J Clin Periodontol 1981;8:281–294.

Esthetic Periodontics (Periodontal Plastic Surgery)

Richard F. Caudill
• Dentogingival Esthetics

Richard J. Oringer
• Augmentation of Attached Gingiva

Laureen Langer and Burton Langer
• Root Coverage Procedures

Oded Bahat and Mark Handelsman
• Surgical Reconstruction of the Alveolar Ridge

Dentogingival Esthetics

Esthetic Criteria

Gingival Exposure

What constitutes a pleasing dentogingival appearance varies from culture to culture, but usually it depends on the extent of gingival exposure. When a person smiles, the entire crowns of the maxillary central incisors and 1 mm of pink attached gingiva will be evident. Greater amounts of exposed gingiva (eg, 2 or 3 mm) can be cosmetically acceptable as long as the gingiva is not unduly conspicuous, such as a "gummy smile" appearance (Fig 32-1), where more than 3 mm of gingiva is displayed during a relaxed smile.[1] Excessive gingival display is generally not a problem in patients with a moderately long upper lip, unless there has been unusual supraeruption of the maxillary anterior teeth or skeletal hyperplasia.

Anatomic Parallelism

The incisal edges of the maxillary anterior teeth, as well as the posterior maxillary occlusal plane, should be parallel to the interpupillary line. Usually the maxillary incisal

plane parallels this line, along with the border of the lower lip, when a person smiles. It is most pleasing esthetically if the maxillary gingival margins are parallel to these anatomic landmarks.

Tooth Length and Symmetry

Average normal tooth lengths have been determined and reported.[2] The average lengths of the most conspicuous maxillary teeth in the "cosmetic zone" are as follows: central incisor, 11.0 mm; lateral incisor, 10.5 mm; and canine, 11.0 mm.

Where incisal landmarks have been destroyed, once proper incisal edge positions have been phonetically and cosmetically located, recreating average tooth lengths can help locate proper gingival levels. More important than actual tooth lengths are the relationships of the lengths of contralateral teeth. Generally speaking, teeth are equivalent in length in mirror-image fashion on either side of the midline, which is established by the philtrum of the upper lip. The two most important teeth for establishing symmetry in the cosmetic zone are the maxillary central incisors. Many smiles, although not ideal, are acceptable because the central incisors are perfectly symmetric even though there may be unequal lengths of adjacent teeth (Fig 32-2).

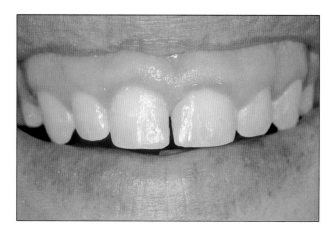

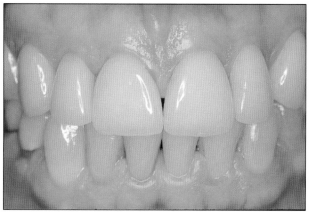

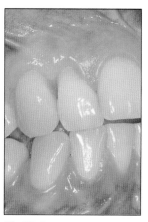

Fig 32-1 In excessive gingival display, more than 3 mm of gingiva is displayed during a relaxed smile.

Fig 32-2 The symmetry of the central incisors masks differing lengths of the adjacent lateral incisors.

Fig 32-3 The maxillary lateral incisor exhibits gingival recession and an altered width-to-length ratio.

Crown Proportions

Normally a maxillary anterior tooth crown exhibits a width-to-length ratio of 8:10.[3,4] Areas of gingival inflammation, gingival overgrowth or enlargement, or altered passive eruption can cause gingival coverage of the clinical crown with a subsequent distortion of normal width-to-length crown ratios. In contrast, excessive tooth wear can shorten the clinical crown and is apparent in that the incisal edge appears wider than normal from an occlusal view. Conversely, crown lengths may appear excessive when there has been gingival recession or supraeruption, which may distort width-to-length ratios as the narrower, more apical portion of the tooth is displaced incisally (Fig 32-3). In such cases, correction of tooth malpositions via orthodontics may be the key treatment factor in proper cosmetic restoration.

Gingival margins can be displaced apically, with tooth intrusion, or coronally, with orthodontic extrusion. In some cases, prosthetic reconstruction may be required, in addition to orthodontics and periodontal surgical interventions, to establish harmonious tooth lengths in proper perspective with the lip and other gingival margins.

Gingival Recession

Indications for Treatment

Gingival recession can be defined as the exposure of the root surface due to an apical shift in the position of the gingiva.[5] Normally, the gingival margin is positioned 1 to 3 mm coronal to the tooth's cementoenamel junction, circumferentially, such that the coronal portion of the root is totally covered with gingival tissue. Prominent teeth with a thin periodontium are subject to gingival recession,[6] especially where there is gingival inflammation.[7] Exposed roots may cause *(1)* hypersensitivity or *(2)* esthetic concerns for the patient and can be covered by a variety of mucogingival surgical procedures described in this chapter.

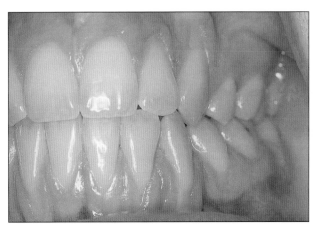

Fig 32-4a This patient exhibits significant gingival recession upon cheek retraction.

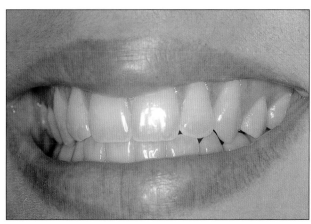

Fig 32-4b The same patient shows little or no gingiva on the maxillary anterior teeth during a relaxed-lip postural position.

Even if a tooth does not exhibit gingival recession at the outset, planned dental therapeutic procedures such as orthodontics, which may cause tooth roots to be more prominent in the dental arch,[8] or the invasive placement of subgingival prosthetic crown margins into areas previously occupied by attached connective tissue fibers[9] or areas of minimal attached keratinized gingiva[10] can promote gingival recession, requiring subsequent surgical correction.

The mere presence of gingival recession may not substantiate treatment in the absence of tooth sensitivity, objectionable visibility in the cosmetic zone, or progressive recession. Patients may be unconcerned about the appearance of clinical crowns lengthened by gingival recession, or they may have long upper lips that cover the gingiva, even during a broad smile. Figures 32-4a and 32-4b show a patient with pronounced gingival recession that is not visible during a relaxed-lip postural position but readily apparent during a broad smile.

If a patient is concerned about the cosmetic effect of "receding gums," correction is appropriate. Teeth that are scheduled for fixed partial dentures may not require surgical techniques for root coverage where the prosthesis will cover the sensitive or unesthetic exposed root. Therefore, where indicated, a complete restorative treatment schedule should be mapped out prior to planning corrective surgical procedures.

Causes

Localized gingival recession may be caused by traumatic tooth-cleaning techniques, especially when teeth are prominent in the dental arch[6] and the overlying soft tissue is thin. Localized gingival recessions such as gingival clefts

have been attributed primarily to local irritants such as plaque and calculus, possibly influenced by excessive occlusal forces,[11] severe orthodontic tipping of teeth,[12] provisional crowns,[13] periodontal surgery,[14–16] mechanical traumatic factors such as fingernail-biting habits,[17] and the extraction of adjacent teeth.[18]

In general, the causal factors implicated in gingival recession include oral hygiene habits,[7,19] high muscle attachments and frenal pull,[20] tooth malpositioning,[21] bone dehiscences,[22] and iatrogenic factors related to various restorative and periodontal procedures.[9,10,14] Surgical correction of gingival recession is often required, together with restorative therapy and/or orthodontics. Total correction, however, may be difficult or impossible, depending on the level of interproximal bone and soft tissues.

Miller[23] classified gingival tissue recessions and predicted the outcome of corrective surgery based on his classification. In Class I defects, where marginal tissue recession does not extend to the mucogingival junction and there is no loss of interproximal periodontium, full coverage of the exposed root can be predicted as a postsurgical outcome (Fig 32-5). Total root coverage can also be anticipated in the correction of Class II recessions, which differ from Class I recessions only in that they extend to or beyond the mucogingival junction with interproximal tissues intact (Fig 32-6). Partial root coverage can be expected in Class III recessions where modest interproximal tissue loss decreases the chance for new attachment gain on the midradicular aspect (Fig 32-7). Due to the pronounced severity of interdental bone and gingival tissue loss and/or tooth malpositioning in the Class IV situation, full root coverage cannot be expected (Fig 32-8).

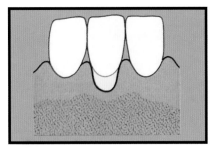
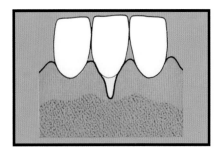

Fig 32-5 Class I Miller defect. The gingival recession does not involve the interproximal papillae or the mucogingival junction. (Reprinted from Miller,[23] with permission.)

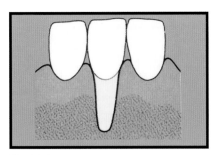
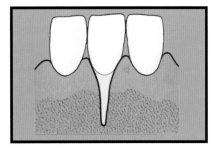

Fig 32-6 The recession in a Class II Miller defect extends past the mucogingival junction but does not involve the interproximal tissues. (Reprinted from Miller,[23] with permission.)

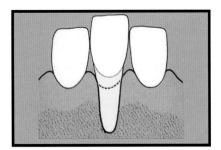
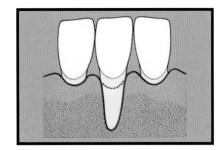

Fig 32-7 The chances for root coverage are decreased when the recession involves the interproximal papillae (Class III Miller defect). (Reprinted from Miller,[23] with permission.)

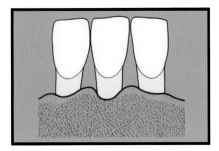
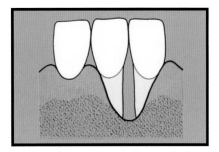

Fig 32-8 Full coverage of exposed root surfaces should not be expected after a soft tissue graft when there is marked loss of the interproximal papillae. (Reprinted from Miller,[23] with permission.)

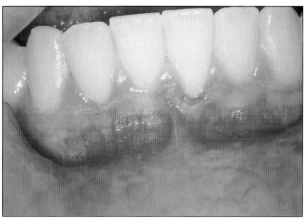
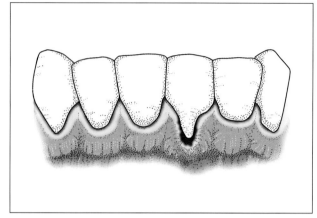

Fig 32-9 The absence of attached gingiva around the mandibular central incisors and the presence of a prominent labial frenum have made it difficult for the patient to maintain this area plaque-free. This situation can lead to gingival recession. Note marginal and papillary erythema around the mandibular central incisors.

Augmentation of Attached Gingiva

Inadequate Attached Gingiva

The term *attached gingiva* refers to gingival tissue that is firmly bound to the tooth and underlying bone. This is differentiated from *keratinized gingiva*, which includes both the attached gingiva and the free gingival margin. It was originally believed that a minimum width of attached gingiva was required to maintain optimal gingival health and prevent recession.[5] However, several longitudinal studies have demonstrated that neither the lack of nor the presence of minimal amounts of attached gingiva necessarily results in the progression of soft tissue recession.[24] Wennstrom found that only 2 of 26 sites with a complete lack, or with only a minimal zone (< 1 mm), of attached gingiva showed further apical displacement of the soft tissue margin during 5 years of observation.[25] Therefore, the concept of adequate attached gingiva is subjective and describes that amount of tissue that is conducive to gingival health in the clinician's opinion.[26] However, there are factors (see box) to help guide the clinician in determining whether a particular site will require a mucogingival procedure to augment the width of attached gingiva (Fig 32-9).

The presence of a minimal or nonexistent zone of attached gingiva is not an absolute indication for a surgical procedure. If the patient exhibits adequate oral hygiene and gingival health, and no restorative dentistry or orthodontic therapy is planned, the site can be monitored periodically at periodontal maintenance visits. Areas that ex-

Indications for Increasing the Width of Attached Gingiva

When there is 1 mm of attached gingiva or less and . . .

1. Recession becomes an esthetic concern for the patient
2. Sites exhibit progressive recession
3. Restorative margins will approach, or be placed apical to, the free gingival margin
4. Teeth will be moved into prominence in the arch during orthodontic therapy

hibit progressive recession or recession disturbing to the patient should be of concern to the practitioner.[27] In these cases a procedure to increase the width of attached gingiva is recommended. If allowed to continue, gingival recession can result in several clinically significant findings: *(1)* exposed roots with increased susceptibility to caries and increased thermal sensitivity; *(2)* difficulty in cleaning, which may lead to further recession and periodontal disease; and *(3)* esthetic concerns.

Other indications for increasing the zone of attached gingiva include restorative procedures that directly involve gingival marginal tissues (eg, full crowns or Class V restorations) or other restorative procedures in which continuous insult to marginal gingival tissues occurs (eg, RPI [rest, proximal plate, and I-bar]–design removable partial dentures and overdentures).[26] In sites where subgingival margins will be placed, it has been suggested that the patient have 5 mm of keratinized gingiva (2 mm of free gin-

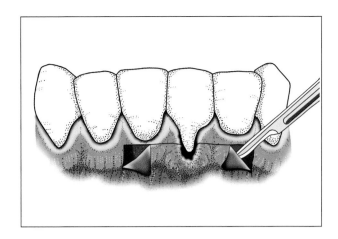

Fig 32-10 After the outline of the recipient site is completed, a No. 15 blade is positioned parallel to the alveolar bone, and a split-thickness flap is elevated and removed. Any remaining frenum attachments are positioned apically by blunt dissection with a periosteal elevator.

giva and 3 mm of attached gingiva).[9] This dimension is based on studies that found a higher incidence of gingival recession following placement of subgingival margins in areas of inadequate attached gingiva.[10]

In addition, patients about to undergo orthodontic therapy who have a site with a minimal or nonexistent band of attached gingiva, and where that tooth will be moved into prominence in the arch, may require a free gingival graft "prophylactically" to avoid future health and esthetic problems. This becomes especially important in patients who demonstrate poor oral hygiene or who have an area with existing gingival recession prior to orthodontic treatment.

Surgical Augmentation

Various techniques have been developed for the augmentation of attached gingiva to prevent further gingival recession. In 1963, the autogenous free gingival graft was introduced.[28] The discussion that follows will focus on this straightforward approach for increasing the band of attached gingiva.

Preparing the Recipient Site
After adequate anesthesia has been achieved, the recipient site is prepared with a trapezoidal-shaped split-thickness flap, which is reflected to expose a firm connective tissue bed to receive the graft. To accomplish this, a No. 15 Bard-Parker scalpel is positioned perpendicular to the tissue, and a horizontal incision is made at the mucogingival junction, preserving the gingival margin. The incision should extend from the mesial line angle of the two teeth adjacent to the site to be augmented. Two vertical incisions extending to the alveolar mucosa are made, again positioning the blade perpendicular to the tissue. This creates an outline of the recipient site, which is trapezoidal and has butt-joint margins.

After the outline is complete, the No. 15 blade is positioned parallel to the alveolar bone, and a split-thickness

flap consisting of epithelium and connective tissue is elevated without disturbing the periosteum (Fig 32-10). The flap will extend apically to the depth of the vertical incisions.

All movable tissues are removed with the tissue scissors so that only an immovable layer of connective tissue remains. If the remaining connective tissue is still mobile, it should be removed, and the graft can be placed directly on bone. Finally, the elevated flap tissue is removed with the scissors or nippers (Fig 32-11). Sterile moistened gauze with pressure is used for hemostasis at the site. A tinfoil template of the recipient bed is fabricated to be used as a pattern for the graft (Fig 32-12).

Harvesting the Donor Tissue
Traditionally, the donor tissue is harvested from the palatal mucosa and should consist of epithelium and a thin layer of connective tissue. To obtain the donor tissue, the tinfoil template is placed against the palatal tissue in the second premolar–first molar area (Fig 32-13). Ideally, the palatal rugae are not included as part of the donor tissue. A shallow incision is traced with the No. 15 Bard-Parker scalpel using the template as a guide. The template is then removed, and the blade is inserted to the desired thickness of 1.0 to 1.5 mm. A corner of the donor tissue is undermined with the blade and held with the tissue forceps. Using the forceps to create tension, the releasing incision is continued until the donor tissue is completely separated from the host (Fig 32-14). To avoid loss of the graft, suction must be used cautiously. Pressure is applied with moistened gauze to the donor site to stop any bleeding (Fig 32-15). Injection of local anesthetic containing a vasoconstrictor can also control hemorrhage at the site. Additionally, the donor site may be sutured to help achieve hemostasis.

The graft may need to be trimmed. Glandular or fatty tissues, as well as irregular surface contours, must be removed while keeping the graft moist. The thickness of the graft should be between 1.0 and 1.5 mm.

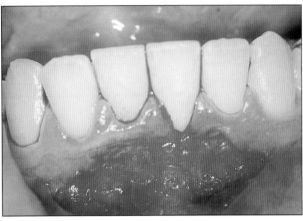

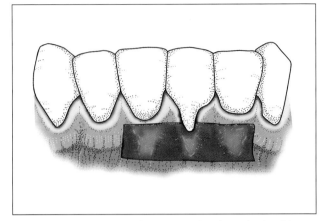

Fig 32-11 After removal of the split-thickness flap and all movable tissues, the site consists of a firm connective tissue bed and is prepared to receive the graft.

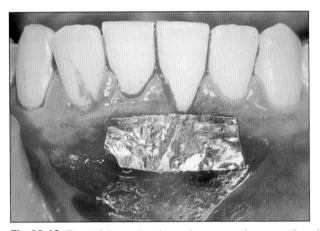

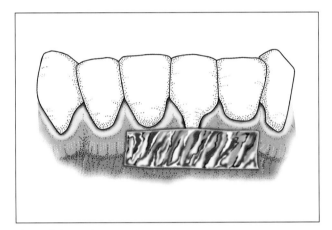

Fig 32-12 The tinfoil template is used to assess the appropriate dimensions of the graft.

Stabilization

The harvested tissue must be positioned and stabilized with the connective tissue side toward the periosteum. Before positioning the tissue, the recipient site should be irrigated to remove any excess clot. A space between the graft and underlying connective tissue will prevent the donor tissue from becoming vascularized, which will result in necrosis and sloughing of the graft.

After the tissue is firmly adapted, sutures are used to secure the graft (Fig 32-16). Initially, the four corners of the graft are sutured to the periosteum. Often a periosteal sling suture in the labial vestibule, wrapped around the lingual surface of the teeth, can help adapt the graft to the underlying tissue. There are many acceptable suturing techniques, which all have the same goal of immobilizing the graft. (Movement of the graft postoperatively can delay healing and result in failure of the procedure.)

Once the graft has been secured, it is covered with periodontal dressing for 1 week. Often the dressing becomes displaced and needs to be reapplied. Pieces of dental floss tied around the teeth may help retain the dressing in position.

Postoperatively, the patient is given an analgesic for discomfort and may be given an antibiotic at the clinician's discretion. The dressing and sutures are removed after 1 week, and the dressing may be repeated for another week if healing is not satisfactory. A palatal stent is fabricated from cold-cure acrylic prior to surgery to alleviate postoperative discomfort caused by mechanical trauma (Fig 32-17). The patient wears the stent continuously for the first 24 hours, and then at meals and during sleep for 8 to 10 days.

In conclusion, the free gingival graft (not for root coverage) has been shown to provide a long-lasting increase in the amount of keratinized and attached gingiva[29] (Figs 32-18 and 32-19). This mucogingival procedure is a predictable treatment option for teeth with restorative or orthodontic needs that have inadequate attached gingiva, as well as for sites with progressive gingival recession.

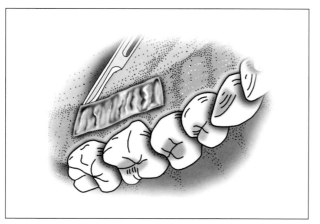

Fig 32-13 The template is placed against the palatal tissue, and an outline is traced with a No. 15 blade.

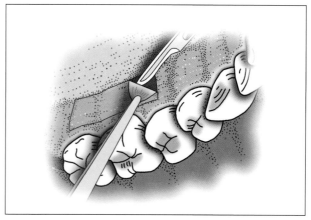

Fig 32-14 A No. 15 blade is used to undermine and reflect the donor tissue, while the tissue forceps are used to create tension. The graft should be 1.0 to 1.5 mm in thickness.

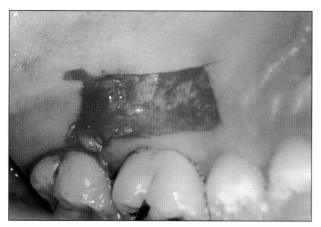

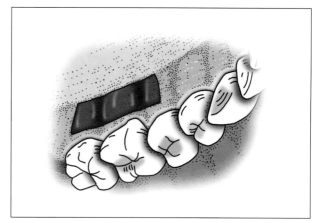

Fig 32-15 Palatal donor site after graft removal. Pressure applied with moistened gauze is usually sufficient for hemorrhage control.

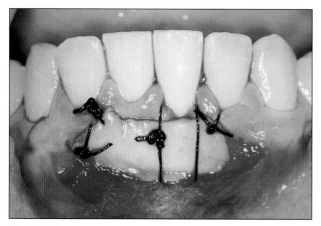

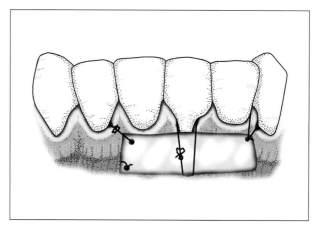

Fig 32-16 Graft positioned and stabilized at the recipient site with a simple interrupted suture and a periosteal sling suture.

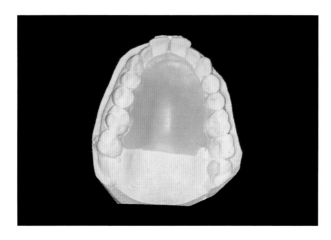

Fig 32-17 Fabrication of an acrylic stent can lessen postoperative discomfort caused by mechanical trauma.

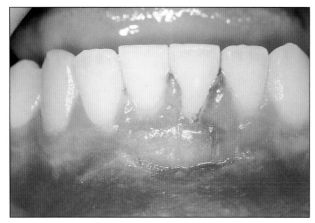
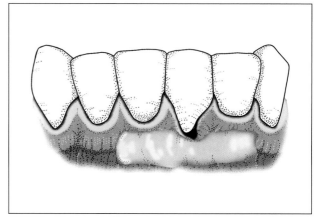

Fig 32-18 Two weeks after surgery. The graft site begins to exhibit a paleness consistent with keratinized palatal mucosa. Note marginal and papillary inflammation as the result of irritation by the sling suture.

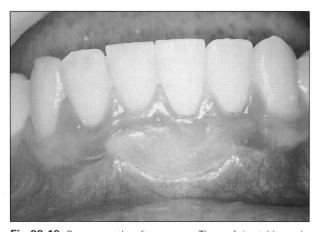
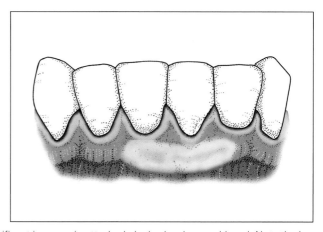

Fig 32-19 Seven months after surgery. The graft is stable, and a significant increase in attached gingiva has been achieved. Note the improvement in gingival health at the graft site.

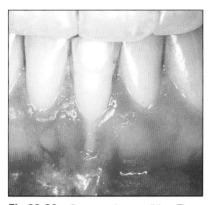

Fig 32-20a Preoperative condition. There is a labial dehiscence and cleft formation on the mandibular left central incisor and an accompanying mucogingival problem and a frenum pull. The adjacent tissue is healthy, and an adequate band of attached keratinized gingiva is present. The vestibular fold is of adequate length to allow the lateral movement of tissue used in a horizontal sliding-flap or pedicle graft.

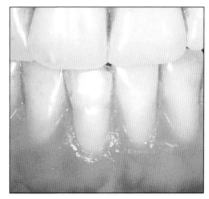

Fig 32-20b Six-year postoperative result. This shows a clinically healthy condition in which the defect over the mandibular left central incisor has been eliminated. There is an adequate band of attached keratinized gingiva, and the frenum pull has been eliminated. The color blend is good, and the root coverage is stable.

Root Coverage Procedures

Historically, indications for treatment of gingival recession included halting progressive recession, enhancing plaque control, preserving a band of keratinized gingiva, decreasing frenum pull,[30–32] and preventing postorthodontic[33,34] and postprosthetic[35] marginal recession. Occasionally, attempts were made to cover denuded roots for cosmetic purposes and to decrease root sensitivity.[36,37] However, total coverage of denuded roots remains a problem for most clinicians because the avascular nature of the root surface hampers the ability of most grafts to survive. Consequently, the wider the area of root exposure, the more difficult a problem for the clinician. The objective of any health professional is not only to arrest and cure a disease process but also, if possible, to regenerate any lost tissue. Such is the goal of root coverage procedures.

In daily clinical practice, decisions must be made to determine which procedures will best resolve an individual patient's recession defect. In general, the anatomy of the area involved dictates the treatment. Following are several graft techniques.

Pedicle Graft

The first major breakthrough in root coverage procedures was the lateral sliding-flap or pedicle graft. Narrow isolated mandibular recessions (Fig 32-20a) with adequate interproximal bone height and adequate keratinized adjacent donor tissue can be successfully treated with a lateral sliding flap, as described by Grupe and Warren.[36] This is a one-stage surgical procedure whereby a pedicle flap is elevated by split-thickness dissection from an adjacent area of keratinized tissue. The blood supply that nourishes the flap over the avascular root surface is supplied by the wide base of the flap and the underlying periosteum surrounding the denuded roots. The color blend and root coverage of an isolated defect in the mandibular anterior region is excellent (Fig 32-20b). However, in cases of wide, isolated recessions or multiple recessions, the horizontal sliding flap has had limited success.

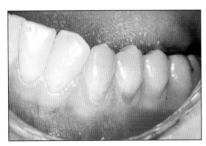

Fig 32-21a Multiple wide shallow recessions. Note minimal keratinized gingiva apical to the mandibular left canine and premolar with wide shallow root denudations, which exhibited hypersensitivity.

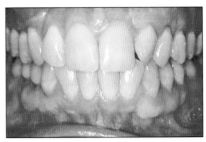

Fig 32-21b Two-year postoperative result. The mandibular left canine and premolar were treated with a thick free gingival graft. The maxillary left lateral incisor, canine, and first premolar were treated with a subepithelial connective tissue graft on the same day. Note thickness and lighter color on the mandible.

Autogenous Free Gingival Graft

The autogenous free gingival graft introduced by Nabers in 1966[30] is designed to increase the width of keratinized gingiva. Unlike the pedicle graft, this procedure takes keratinized palatal connective tissue and epithelium away from its original site, the palate, and relocates it to a remote site. The tissue is placed over a freshly cut bed of connective tissue and sutured in place. Within approximately 4 days, the underlying connective tissue nourishes the graft until it rebuilds its own blood supply and thus survives and functions as keratinized gingiva.

Because this graft retains none of its own blood supply and is totally dependent on the bed of recipient blood vessels, it was originally intended to change alveolar mucosa into keratinized gingiva, not specifically to cover denuded roots.[32] However, several excellent modifications have improved this procedure's root coverage capabilities. Maynard[38] developed two procedures: the initial placement of a free gingival graft to create a band of keratinized gingiva, followed by a second procedure in which the graft is pulled coronally. Holbrook and Ochsenbein[39] used thick, stretched free gingival grafts with intricate suturing to improve the graft's adaptation to the recipient bed and limit the amount of dead space, which could hinder vascularization. Miller[40,41] emphasized root planing and thick butt-jointed free gingival grafts placed over denuded roots that had been treated with saturated citric acid burnished into the root for 5 minutes.

All of these modifications have improved the capability of free gingival grafts to survive over avascular root surfaces. But although coverage of wide deep, wide shallow, and multiple recessions has been improved greatly, the greatest success of the free gingival graft for root coverage remains in the mandible (Figs 32-21a and 32-21b) or on isolated maxillary teeth.

Subepithelial Connective Tissue Graft for Root Coverage

The ridge augmentation procedure as described by Langer and Calagna[42,43] combined the positive features of the pedicle and free gingival grafts to build out edentulous ridges. Its use was expanded by Langer and Langer[44] to gain total root coverage in cases of severe recession on isolated and multiple teeth, especially in the maxilla, where root coverage is most difficult to obtain.

In actuality, the subepithelial connective tissue graft for root coverage is a combination of a pedicle graft and an autogenous free connective tissue graft performed simultaneously (Figs 32-22a to 32-22g).

First, the recipient bed is prepared by carefully elevating a split-thickness flap with a wide base, dissected well beyond the mucogingival junction. This is the pedicle aspect of the procedure. The flap contributes the overlying blood supply that will nourish the graft to be taken from the palate.

Second, a connective tissue graft is dissected from the palate and placed on the recipient bed, which consists of a thin layer of periosteum and connective tissue overlying the bone surrounding the tooth or teeth involved with the recession. This is the autogenous free gingival graft part of the procedure. The recipient bed contributes the second underlying blood supply to the graft and enhances its survival.

Figs 32-22a to 32-22g A 21-year-old woman presented with a chief complaint of extreme sensitivity to cold liquids, air, and toothbrush use bilaterally in the maxilla. The marginal gingiva of the maxillary right first and second premolars is erythematous due to her inability to cleanse the area adequately, as well as to the subsequent plaque accumulation. On the maxillary left lateral incisor, canine, and first premolar, the prominent root position contributed to the pronounced recession.

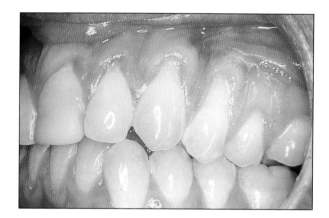

Fig 32-22a Preoperative condition—maxillary left quadrant. The wide deep recessions as seen on the maxillary left canine and first premolar are best treated with a subepithelial connective tissue graft. The visible clinical recession is as follows: lateral incisor, 2 mm × 2 mm; canine, 3 mm × 4 mm; first premolar, 5 mm × 4 mm.

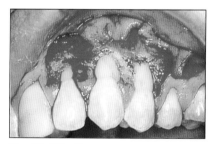

Fig 32-22b Flap elevation. A split-thickness flap is elevated by sharp dissection. The actual or hidden recession is lateral incisor, 5 mm × 3 mm; canine, 5 mm × 5 mm; first premolar, 7 mm × 4 mm. The graft must be large enough to cover the recession and the connective tissue bed in all directions.

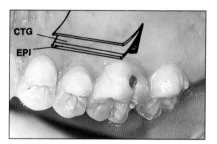

Fig 32-22c Flap design—donor site. Palatally, two horizontal beveled incisions are made. A split-thickness flap is raised. A wedge of connective tissue with its border of epithelium is dissected free, leaving the epithelialized flap to be replaced for primary intention wound closure. (CTG) Connective tissue graft; (EPI) epithelium.

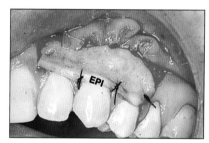

Fig 32-22d Graft stabilization. The subepithelial connective tissue graft measuring 7 mm × 20 mm × 1 mm is positioned over the denuded roots. The thin border of epithelium left on the graft helps with the color blend and suturing and should be placed incisal to the cementoenamel junction. (EPI) Epithelium.

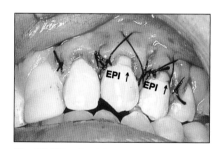

Fig 32-22e Recipient overlying flap. The recipient flap is repositioned coronally to cover as much of the subepithelial connective tissue graft as possible. The epithelial border (EPI) of the connective tissue graft may be visible incisal to the cementoenamel junction.

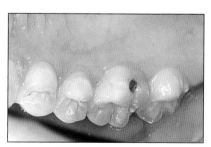

Fig 32-22f Palatal healing. Early wound closure is demonstrated after 10 days.

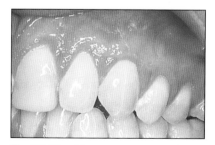

Fig 32-22g Three-year postoperative recipient site healing. The area exhibits a good color blend of the grafted area to the adjacent site and continued total root coverage with minimal probing depth less than 2 mm. (Compare with Fig 32-22a.)

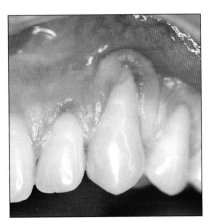

Fig 32-23a Wide deep recession. A 26-year-old man presented with severe hypersensitivity on the maxillary left canine. The tooth had previously been treated by a resin composite restoration that continually chipped away at the most apical margin. The patient was unhappy with his appearance and felt frustrated in his efforts to keep this area plaque-free.

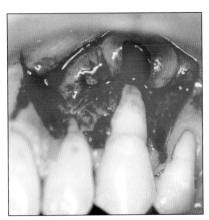

Fig 32-23b Resin composite removal and flap elevation. The resin composite restoration was removed before the initial incision was made. The root surface was planed. A split-thickness flap was elevated beyond the mucogingival junction to expose a thin layer of connective tissue and periosteum.

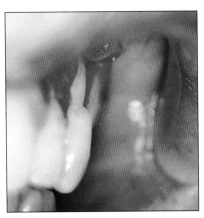

Fig 32-23c Root shaving. A side view reveals the extent to which the tooth had been prepared for the original restoration and shows that it is within the bony housing of the adjacent alveolus.

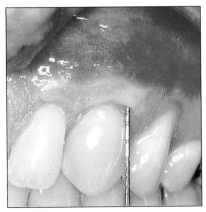

Fig 32-23d Three-year postoperative result. The maxillary left canine shows no loss of original coverage of the denuded root. Probing with pressure reveals minimal sulcus depth and continued root coverage to the cementoenamel junction.

Removal of Restorations

Deep recessions (Fig 32-23a) of maxillary canines are often challenging problems, which can be complicated by previous placement of resin composite restorations. Although the procedure of the subepithelial connective tissue graft is the same as outlined in Fig 32-22, additional consideration must be given to the complete removal of the resin composite material and aggressive root planing prior to grafting to ensure that no foreign material will be left beneath the graft (Figs 32-23b to 32-23d).

Damaged Root Surfaces

Previously damaged root surfaces present a particular challenge to the clinician. In many cases, previous failures can be reversed by employing a subepithelial connective tissue graft (Figs 32-24a and 32-24b).

Multiple Wide Recessions

To cover the multiple recessions in a 32-year-old woman in one session (Fig 32-25a), both sides of the palate were used from the canine to the distal surface of the first molar.

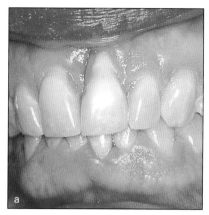
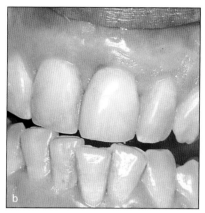

Fig 32-24a Preoperative view. A 29-year-old woman presented with severe recession on the maxillary left central incisor and incipient recession on the maxillary right central incisor, which had been treated previously by a coronally repositioned graft and two pedicle grafts on different occasions. Each procedure increased the recession on the left central incisor and eventually involved the right central incisor. Both teeth were extremely sensitive and increasingly unsightly. Additionally, there was a marked area of hypermineralization from the midlabial to the distal line angle on the left central incisor. Following flap elevation, the root was shaved and treated with citric acid (rubbed with a cotton pellet) for 5 minutes. A subepithelial connective tissue graft was taken from the palate.

Fig 32-24b Postoperative view. One year later there is 90% root coverage on the right central incisor and 100% root coverage on the left central incisor.

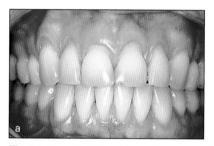
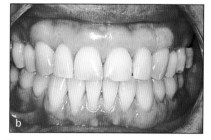

Fig 32-25a Multiple wide maxillary recession. The roots of the maxillary lateral and central incisors and the maxillary left canine are prominent apically. The patient had been using a horizontal-scrub method of toothbrushing that accomplished excellent plaque control but contributed to the increasing recession.

Fig 32-25b Five-year postoperative result. Continued total root coverage of the labial surfaces.

Since the connective tissue graft is taken internally, the rugae in the canine–first premolar areas are not a problem. The overlying flap is composed of the existing labial gingivae, which nourishes the graft and provides a good color blend (Fig 32-25b). Using a free gingival graft in this instance would have denuded an extensive area of the palate.

Coverage of Existing Crown Margins

One of the more exasperating situations in restorative dentistry occurs when a gingival margin pulls away from the margin of a recently placed crown (Figs 32-26a to 32-26d). The patient's attention becomes focused on this one area of the entire reconstruction.

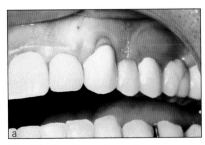
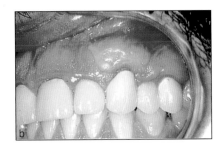

Fig 32-26a Recession adjacent to an existing crown margin. The maxillary right canine shows buccal recession apical to the margin of an existing crown within a maxillary reconstruction.

Fig 32-26b First subepithelial connective tissue graft placed. A portion of the recession has been eliminated after placement of a subepithelial connective tissue graft. Residual recession was still present, and the decision was made to attempt a second procedure.

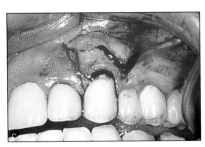
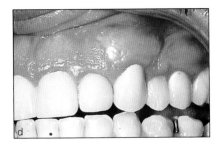

Fig 32-26c Second surgery. The new thickness of the buccal tissue obviates the need for a second surgical site. A split-thickness flap is elevated to expose the underlying connective tissue. The trapezoid-shaped tissue is incised along its lateral and apical borders and then moved coronally.

Fig 32-26d Postoperative view. Thick coverage of the denuded root surface. Some of the gold margin is now obscured by the graft. A gingivoplasty could be performed, if desired.

Surgical Reconstruction of the Alveolar Ridge

The goal of reconstructing an alveolar ridge is to restore function, phonetics, and esthetics. This requires understanding of the bone, oral mucosa, gingiva, and blood supply in relation to the surgical design and strict attention to preserving maximum tissue vascularity. Different surgical designs and techniques will be needed, depending on the site and size of the defect, and the entire reconstruction must be meticulously planned before the first procedure is carried out.

Definition of the Defect

Loss of teeth is followed by resorption of the bone and, often, shrinkage of the soft tissues. Bone loss can occur erratically, producing irregular concavities, and proceeds in different directions in the two jaws (posterosuperiorly in

the maxilla and inferolaterally in the mandible). As bone loss progresses, the anterior ridges come to resemble the edge of a knife, and the occlusal relations of the two jaws deteriorate. The papillae and the scalloped form of the marginal gingiva also disappear. The first step of treatment, therefore, must be a thorough clinical and radiographic definition of the anatomy in three dimensions. The following features must be studied:

1. The type and volume of the deformity that is present or that is expected after tooth extraction. Helpful classifications are those of Seibert and Cohen[45] and Allen et al[46] (Table 32-1).
2. The general contours of the arch and the position and form of the teeth or possible future implants. There are three points to be considered here: the shape of the remaining bone, the relations between the maxillary and mandibular ridges, and the relations of the ridges to the orofacial structures.
3. The thickness of the periodontium.
4. The position of the smile line and lip position.

Table 32-1 Classifications of Ridge Defects

Class	Description of loss
Seibert classification of site[45]	
I	Buccolingual with normal ridge height
II	Apicocoronal with normal ridge width
III	Buccolingual and apicocoronal
Allen classification of extent[46]	
Mild	< 3 mm
Moderate	3–6 mm
Severe	> 6 mm

Once the anatomy has been thoroughly defined, the treatment team determines the appropriate restoration and simulates, in reverse order, the steps needed to reach that goal.

Techniques of Reconstruction

Measures may be required to reconstruct the bone vertically, horizontally, or both. Vertical reconstruction to restore normal ridge height is a particularly complex problem and may necessitate second- and third-stage procedures.[45] Reconstruction may be accomplished with either a soft tissue graft or a bone graft with an exclusion membrane. Four types of grafts are available: autogenous grafts (which necessitate a second surgical site), allografts (eg, freeze-dried bone), alloplastic grafts (synthetic materials), and xenografts (materials from a nonhuman species, such as bovine collagen).

Ridge Preservation
Preserving the ridge at the time of tooth extraction reduces the number of reconstructive procedures needed. However, it also requires preparation of the tooth before the surgical procedure and mandates immediate placement of a restoration. If there is periapical pathosis, the area requires thorough debridement.

Immediate Ridge Augmentation
Like ridge preservation, immediate ridge augmentation at the time of extraction minimizes the number of procedures that will be necessary. It also allows overcontouring of an edentulous area for later gingivoplasty to optimize the relations between the pontics and the soft tissues. However, immediate augmentation has the same disadvantages as ridge preservation, as well as the problems of flap management and maintenance over a large area.

Techniques Relying on Vascular Perfusion
The onlay graft is a full-thickness graft of palatal tissue. Useful when a significant amount of bone height has been lost, it has the advantage of increasing the dimension of the gingiva. However, color matching is unfavorable because of the degree of keratinization of the graft. Stabilization is critical to graft survival, as the graft tissues obtain their blood supply from a single surface during healing. For the same reason, onlay grafts should not be used if the blood supply to the recipient site has been compromised. If onlay grafting is to be used for larger defects, multiple surgeries will be necessary.

The inlay graft provides good color matching. It has better vascularity than the onlay graft and can be stabilized at the desired site. However, it is more difficult to design and manage, especially in the interproximal papillary area.

For two reasons, onlay and inlay grafts are better suited to the repair of smaller defects. First, there is a limit to the amount of soft tissue that can be harvested from a donor site without creating an undesirably large defect. Second, these grafts cannot survive without developing vascular connections with the tissues around their beds, and smaller grafts can do this more easily than large ones.

Both types of graft have the drawback of the unpredictability of postoperative tissue shrinkage. The inlay-onlay graft combines the two, with all of their advantages and disadvantages (Figs 32-27 and 32-28).

Roll Technique
The roll technique maintains the blood supply to the graft as well as the color and texture of the ridge but is limited in available bulk to the relative thickness of the palatal soft tissue adjacent to the target site. It is best suited to the repair of small to medium Seibert Class I defects. A pouch is created on the other side of the ridge; the lingual pedicle, stripped of epithelium, is folded back, inserted into the pouch, and sutured in place.

Although some Class II or Class III defects can be treated with the roll technique, the amount of augmentation available is small. This technique should not be used where the tissue is very thin. Other reconstructive procedures are more useful in augmenting the papilla.

Soft Tissue Management

It must be recognized at the outset that not all patients will have appropriate soft tissues for use in flaps. In some, the tissues in the nondiseased areas of the mouth may be too thin to be reflected and transferred without compromising the blood supply. In other patients, the tissue around the defect may be extensively scarred. In either of these cases, a surgical flap probably will fail.[45]

Figs 32-27a to 32-27g The inlay-onlay graft is a combination of the inlay and onlay graft techniques. It has all the advantages and disadvantages of each individual technique.

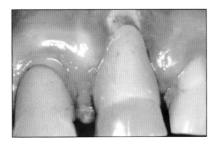

Fig 32-27a Preoperative clinical view, showing advanced attachment loss on the buccal aspect of the left central incisor.

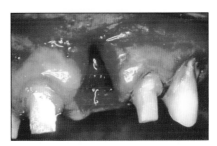

Fig 32-27b Frontal view at the time of extraction of the left central incisor.

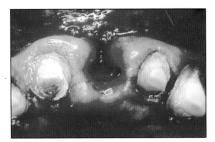

Fig 32-27c Occlusal view after extraction.

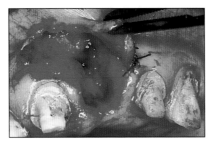

Fig 32-27d Pedicle partial-thickness flap elevated from the buccal surface of the right central incisor and sutured to the mesial aspect of the left lateral incisor to create a buccal wall.

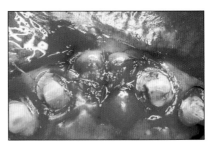

Fig 32-27e Occlusal view of donor material secured in the defect with reconstruction of the buccal ridge contour.

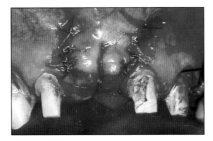

Fig 32-27f Frontal view of final suturing.

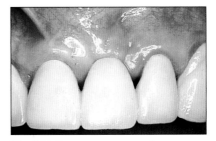

Fig 32-27g Final reconstruction.

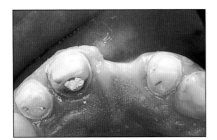

Fig 32-28a Preoperative view. Note the buccal ridge defect (Seibert Class I).

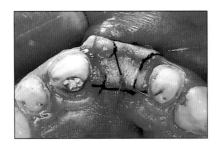

Fig 32-28b Soft tissue graft from the palate is secured with silk sutures.

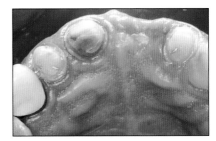

Fig 32-28c View 6 months postoperatively. Note reconstruction of the buccal ridge contour.

Even when the soft tissues appear adequate for reconstruction, careful planning and technique are needed in soft tissue reconstruction. The planning for a flap should start with the recipient site and take into account the possible shortening or shrinkage of the flap during healing, the angle and vectors of movement needed to bring the flap to its new location, and the necessity of avoiding tension and kinking.[47] The tissues must not be stretched excessively, as this would impair their vascularity and make the flap too thin. The final position of the flap, as well as the tissue that will be used to create it, are outlined with methylene blue while the site is under tension.

During flap creation and transfer, all maneuvers must be atraumatic. Crushing of the tissue will compromise vascularity, thereby reducing the likelihood of graft survival and encouraging microbial growth. The same concerns militate against the use of hot sponges or vasoconstrictive drugs to control bleeding. The sutures fixing the flap in its new location should be 2 to 3 mm from the wound or flap edges, and they should not be excessively tight. If these precautions are not observed, there may be damaging vasoconstriction, especially during the inevitable period of postoperative tissue swelling.[47]

Classification of Flaps

All periodontal reconstructive flaps are random-pattern flaps in that they receive their blood supply from various segmental and axial arteries.[48,49] Also, they are all local, in that they are brought from a site adjacent to the defect without detachment from their original blood supply. This proximity is an advantage in that it makes it easier to match the color, texture, and thickness of the graft with those of the new tissue bed.

Most published classifications of periodontal flaps are confusing. Elsewhere,[47] the authors have suggested a system based on the usage in general and plastic surgery, in which a flap is classified according to its mode of transfer and its geometry. This system not only is simpler but also helps the surgeon visualize flap designs.

Mode of transfer. A rotational flap is moved around a pivot point. The line of greatest tension in such a flap is along the radius of the area of rotation. The greater the degree of rotation, the shorter the flap will be.

An advancement flap reaches its target site without rotation or lateral movement. It is created by vertical incisions with or without 100- to 110-degree back cuts, and it may have one or more pedicles.

Anterior advanced flap. The anterior advanced flap[47,50] is an adaptation of the coronally positioned flap (Fig 32-29). With the latter flap, the range was reduced because of the minimal mobilization and dissection of the tissues. However, with modifications of technique, the flap can be used in immediate ridge preservation and augmentation, papilla augmentation, and repair of large ridge deformities, as well as in patients having osseointegrated implants placed. These techniques maintain the vascularity of the tissue even when the flap is extended over a considerable distance. Surgical access and visibility are excellent. However, the method is extremely technique sensitive.

Two vertical incisions are made on either side of the recipient site to allow anterior advancement of the elastic tissue of the rectangular flap. The range of the flap can be extended by back-cut incisions with an angle of approximately 100 degrees on each side of the base. When the flap is advanced, each of these incisions will open into a V.[51,52]

For the advanced flap to be successful, it is necessary that the sharp dissection extend beyond the mucobuccal fold to reduce the tension. The shorter the vestibular depth, the larger the incision into the lip substance must be. The edge of the flap (palatal aspect) should be elevated sufficiently to provide at least 3 mm of effective length.

Customarily, the mesiocoronal and distocoronal edges of the flap are sutured first using 4-0 chromic gut.[47,50] The operator can then confirm the mesiodistal dimensions. The remaining edge is approximated with either continuous or several interrupted sutures, often of 4-0 Prolene. A second procedure occasionally is necessary to release the frenum and muscle pull that has been moved coronally.

Controlled Tissue Expansion

Controlled tissue expansion generates tissue of the proper quantity and color without flap transfer or a residual defect[53] (Fig 32-30). An additional benefit is the greater vascularity of the new tissue. The expander (CUI subperiosteal tissue expander, Cox-Uphoff International) consists of a silicone bag with tubing having a self-sealing valve. An incision wide enough to admit the bag is created on either side of the defect, and the tissue is undermined so that the bag will be in continuous contact with bone. The bag is then sutured in place, taking care not to perforate it with the needle, and inflated until the tissue above it blanches. At intervals, more saline is added through the tubing. After a few weeks, the expander is removed, and the ridge augmentation is completed.

Controlled tissue expansion is bothersome for the patient in that the expander may interfere with the movement of oral soft tissues, and he or she must make several office visits for the addition of saline. There is a risk of infection, and a broad-spectrum antibiotic usually is prescribed. The most common complication is tissue necrosis caused by overly enthusiastic rates of expansion.

Figs 32-29a to 32-29l Anterior advanced flap.

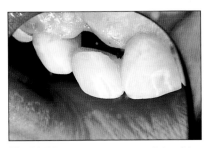

Fig 32-29a Note the extent of the ridge defect, in both horizontal and vertical dimensions.

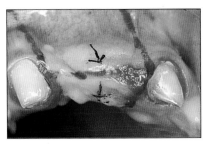

Fig 32-29b Edentulous ridge, with surgical marking pen used to outline the advanced flap design.

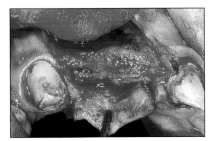

Fig 32-29c Ridge defect; note the reflected palatal edge flap.

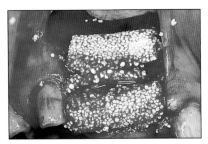

Fig 32-29d Donor material is easily shaped and positioned into the defect.

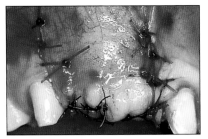

Fig 32-29e Advanced flap is sutured. Note that no tension is created on the flap. Prolene sutures are used on the edge flap margin. Chromic gut is used to secure the buccal margins.

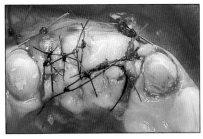

Fig 32-29f Occlusal view showing flap closure and the amount of augmentation achieved in the buccal dimension.

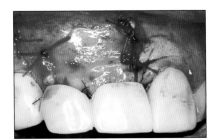

Fig 32-29g Provisional restoration is adapted to allow for swelling during initial healing.

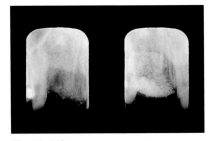

Fig 32-29h Preoperative and postoperative radiographs.

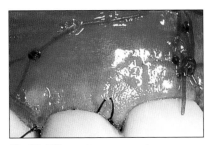

Fig 32-29i Healing at 1 week.

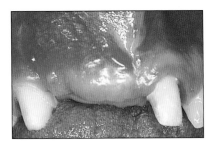

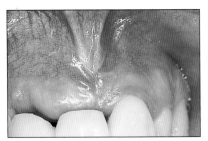

Figs 32-29j and 32-29k Healing at 4 weeks. Provisional restoration can now be adapted to the ideal ridge form.

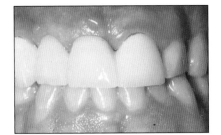

Fig 32-29l Final restorative result. (Courtesy of Dr Bruce Coye.)

Figs 32-30a to 32-30f Controlled tissue expansion.

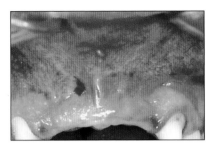

Fig 32-30a Frontal view of alveolar ridge deformity. Structural loss includes vertical and horizontal loss. Observe the adequate tissue thickness and favorable location of the mucogingival junction.

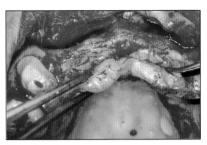

Fig 32-30b Occlusal view shows the extent of the bony ridge deformity.

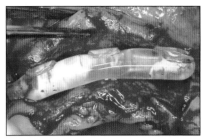

Fig 32-30c The expander is placed into the surgical area that requires tissue expansion. The exit of the inflation tubing through the tissue should be determined to avoid mechanical trauma to mobile tissue and to allow for optimal patient comfort and easy access to the valve for inflation.

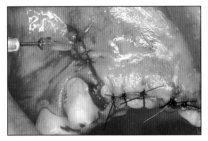

Fig 32-30d Self-sealing valve extends out through the tissue and lies in the vestibule. Note that a 23-gauge needle is inserted and inflated with saline until tissue blanching occurs.

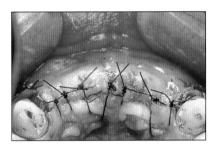

Fig 32-30e Occlusal view of the suturing pattern at the junction of the advanced and edge flaps.

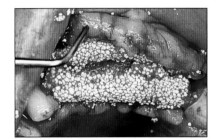

Fig 32-30f Blocks of hydroxyapatite crystals embedded in collagen and placed to reconstruct the edentulous ridge.

Augmentation of the Papilla

The absence of interproximal papillae has adverse esthetic and phonetic effects. Restoration of the papillae tests the limits of surgical precision and soft tissue manipulation, and the potential for catastrophe is considerable.

Because of its small size and its blood supply pattern, the interproximal papilla is, in effect, an end-artery organ. Even a small amount of a vasoconstricting agent may therefore lead to necrosis. This caution against vasoconstrictors applies also to the epinephrine in anesthetics: excessive anesthetic infiltration must be avoided. Clean, sharp dissection and the use of agents other than vasoconstrictors to achieve coagulation are essential.[51]

The advanced flap may be useful in reconstructing the papilla. However, the length-to-base ratio of such a flap is unfavorable, and the need to avoid extending the vertical incisions over adjacent teeth can lead to the creation of an extremely thin flap. It may be appropriate to use minor orthodontic tooth movement to increase the permissible width of the flap.

The suturing technique for the flap is particularly critical in reconstruction of the papilla. Prior to flap apposition, a trial closure should be performed to ensure that there is no tension. Also, the needle should perforate the flap 1 to 2 mm from the cut edge to ensure control of the edge, and it should pass through the flap at an angle greater than 90 degrees so that the edge is everted. To avoid reduction of vascular perfusion, the operator should not perforate the deep edge of the papilla, especially when it is thin. The sutures are removed after 48 to 72 hours.

The goal in reconstructing the alveolar ridge is a functional and esthetic restoration. Different surgical designs and techniques will be needed, depending on the site and size of the defect. The defect must be thoroughly defined and the reconstructive steps necessary to reach the desired goal simulated in reverse order. With careful surgical planning and execution and close teamwork, it is possible to provide most patients with a satisfactory reconstruction of the alveolar ridge.

References

1. Chiche G, Pinault A. Esthetics of Anterior Fixed Prosthodontics. Chicago: Quintessence, 1994:194.

2. Ash M. Wheeler's Dental Anatomy, Physiology, and Occlusion. Philadelphia: Saunders, 1993:129.

3. Shillingburg H, Kaplan M, Grace C. Tooth dimensions—A comparative study. J South Calif Dent Assoc 1972;40:830–839.

4. Bjorndal A, Henderson W, Skidmore A, Kellner F. Anatomic measurements of human teeth extracted from males between the ages of 17 and 21 years. Oral Surg Oral Med Oral Pathol 1974;38:791–803.

5. Carranza FA. Periodontal pathology. In: Carranza FA (ed). Glickman's Periodontology. Philadelphia: Saunders, 1990:118.

6. O'Leary T, Drake R, Crump P, Allen M. The incidence of recession in young males: A further study. J Periodontol 1972;42:264–267.

7. Gorman WJ. Prevalence and etiology of gingival recession. J Periodontol 1967;38:316–322.

8. Maynard J, Wilson R. Diagnostic and management of mucogingival problems in children. Dent Clin North Am 1980;24:683–703.

9. Maynard JG, Wilson R. Physiologic dimensions of the periodontium significant to the restorative dentist. J Periodontol 1979;50:170–174.

10. Stetler K, Bissada N. Significance of the width of keratinized gingiva on the periodontal status of teeth with submarginal restorations. J Periodontol 1987;58:697–700.

11. Novaes A, Ruben M, Kon S, et al. The development of the periodontal cleft. A clinical and histopathologic study. J Periodontol 1975;46:701–709.

12. Batenhorst K, Bowers G, Williams J. Tissue changes resulting from facial tipping and extrusion of incisors in monkeys. J Periodontol 1974;45:660–668.

13. Donaldson D. Gingival recession associated with temporary crowns. J Periodontol 1973;44:691–696.

14. Knowles J, Burgett F, Nissle R, et al. Results of periodontal treatment related to pocket depth and attachment level. Eight years. J Periodontol 1979;50:225–233.

15. Pihlström B, Ortiz-Campos C, McHugh R. A randomized four-year study of periodontal therapy. J Periodontol 1981;52:227–242.

16. Ramfjord S, Caffesse R, Morrison E, et al. Four modalities of periodontal treatment compared over 5 years. J Clin Periodontol 1987;14(8):445–452.

17. Moskow B, Bressman E. Localized gingival recession. Etiology and treatment. Dent Radiogr Photogr 1965;38:3.

18. Lammie G, Posselt V. Progressive changes in the dentition of adults. J Periodontol 1965;36:443–454.

19. Sangnes G. Traumatization of teeth and gingiva related to habitual tooth cleaning procedures. J Clin Periodontol 1976;3:94–103.

20. Trott JR, Love B. An analysis of localized recessions in 766 Winnipeg high school students. Dent Pract 1966;16:209.

21. Parfitt GJ, Mjor IA. A clinical evaluation of localized gingival recession in children. J Dent Child 1964;31:257.

22. Bernimoulin J-P, Curilovic Z. Gingival recession and tooth mobility. J Clin Periodontol 1977;4:107–114.

23. Miller PD. A classification of marginal tissue recession. Int J Periodontics Restorative Dent 1985;5(2):8–13.

24. Kennedy JE, Bird WC, Palcanis KG, Dorfman HS. A longitudinal evaluation of varying widths of attached gingiva. J Clin Periodontol 1985;12:667–675.

25. Wennstrom JL. Lack of association between width of attached gingiva and development of soft tissue recession. J Clin Periodontol 1987;14:181–184.

26. Hall WB. Gingival augmentation/mucogingival surgery. In: Nevins M, Becker W, Kornman K (eds). Proceedings of the World Workshop in Clinical Periodontics, July 23–27, 1989. Chicago: American Academy of Periodontology, 1989:VII-1–VII-21.

27. McFall WT. The laterally repositioned flap-criteria for success. Periodontics 1967;5:89.

28. Bjorn H. Free transplantation of gingiva propia. Sven Tandlak Tidskr 1963;22:684.

29. Egelberg J. Periodontics: The Scientific Way (ed 2). Malmö, Sweden: Odonto Science, 1995:471.

30. Nabers JM. Free gingival grafts. Periodontics 1966;4:243–245.

31. Sullivan HC, Atkins JH. Free autogenous gingival grafts, I. Principles of successful grafting. Periodontics 1968;6:121–129.

32. Sullivan HC, Atkins JH. Free autogenous gingival grafts, 3. Utilization of grafts in the treatment of gingival recession. Periodontics 1968;6:152–160.

33. Alstad S, Zachrisson BV. Longitudinal study of periodontal conditions associated with orthodontic treatment in adolescents. Am J Orthod 1979;76:277–286.

34. Dorfman HS. Mucogingival changes resulting from mandibular incisor tooth movement. Am J Orthod 1978;74:286–297.

35. Silness J. Periodontal conditions in patients treated with dental bridges, 3. The relationship between the location of the crown margin and the periodontal condition. J Periodontal Res 1970;5:225–229.

36. Grupe HE, Warren RF Jr. Repair of gingival defects by a sliding flap operation. J Periodontol 1956;27:92–95.

37. Cohen DW, Ross S. The double papillae repositioned flap in periodontal therapy. J Periodontol 1968;39:65–70.

38. Maynard JG Jr. Coronal positioning of a previously placed autogenous gingival graft. J Periodontol 1977;48:151–155.

39. Holbrook T, Ochsenbein C. Complete coverage of denuded root surface with a one stage gingival graft. Int J Periodontics Restorative Dent 1983;3(3):8–27.

40. Miller PD Jr. Root coverage using a free soft tissue autograft following citric acid application. Part I: Technique. Int J Periodontics Restorative Dent 1982;2(1):65–70.

41. Miller PD Jr. Root coverage using a free soft tissue autograft following citric acid application. Part III. A successful and predictable procedure in areas of deep-wide recession. Int J Periodontics Restorative Dent 1985;5(2):14–37.

42. Langer B, Calagna L. The subepithelial connective tissue graft. J Prosthet Dent 1980;44:363–367.

43. Langer B, Calagna LJ. The subepithelial connective tissue graft. A new approach to the enhancement of anterior cosmetics. Int J Periodontics Restorative Dent 1982;2(2):22–33.

44. Langer B, Langer L. Subepithelial connective tissue graft technique for root coverage. J Periodontol 1985;56:715–720.

45. Seibert JS, Cohen DW. Periodontal considerations in preparation for fixed and removable prosthodontics. Dent Clin North Am 1987;31:529–555.

46. Allen E, Gainza G, Farthing G, et al. Improved technique for localized ridge augmentation: A report of 21 cases. J Periodontol 1985;56:195–199.

47. Bahat O, Handelsman M. Periodontal reconstructive flaps: Classification and surgical considerations. Int J Periodontics Restorative Dent 1991;6:480–487.

48. McGregor IA. The Z plasty. Br J Plast Surg 1966;19:82–87.

49. McGregor IA, Morgan G. Axial and random pattern flaps. Br J Plast Surg 1973;26:202–213.

50. Bahat O, Handelsman M, Gordon J. The transpositional flap in mucogingival surgery. Int J Periodontics Restorative Dent 1990; 10:472–482.

51. Bahat O, Koplin M. Pantographic lip expansion and bone grafting for ridge augmentation. Int J Periodontics Restorative Dent 1989;9:344–353.

52. Stark RB. The pantographic expansion principle as applied to advancement flap. Plast Reconstr Surg 1955;9(15):222–226.

53. Bahat O, Handelsman M. Controlled tissue expansion in reconstructive periodontal surgery. Int J Periodontics Restorative Dent 1991;11:25–30.

Orthodontics and the Periodontium

Terry B. Adams, Thomas G. Wilson, Jr, and Jason B. Cope

- Pretreatment Considerations
- Positive and Negative Effects of Orthodontics
- Orthodontic Therapy and Periodontal Diseases
- Preventing Periodontal Problems
- Case Presentations

Inflammatory periodontal diseases can be exacerbated or improved by orthodontic therapy. This chapter gives an overview of the relationship between these two branches of dentistry.

For patients with periodontal diseases, orthodontic therapy can be used to correct or modify local factors such as malaligned teeth that make oral hygiene difficult, to align the occlusal forces along the long axis of the tooth, to improve gingival and bony form, and to improve tooth position relative to the desired prosthodontic environment.[1] In addition, one can establish a satisfactory occlusion, improve esthetics, and reestablish chewing comfort for the patient.[2]

If used correctly, orthodontic therapy can exert a positive influence on the periodontium.[3] To optimize this outcome, the practitioner must ensure that the periodontal tissues are healthy before orthodontics begins and that they are kept healthy during tooth movement. If left unchecked, inflammation can lead to attachment loss, especially in adults. Therefore, tooth movement should follow resolution of clinical signs of inflammation. In addition, orthodontic therapy should occur only after elimination of active dental caries, placement of dental implants that will serve as anchorage units, or extraction of hopeless teeth that will not be used for anchorage or to support provi-

sional restorations and endodontic therapy. Orthodontic therapy should, however, precede stabilization of mobile teeth, definitive occlusal adjustment, periodontal surgery involving the removal of supporting bone, placement of dental implants that will not be used as anchorage units, and final fixed prosthodontics.[1]

Pretreatment Considerations

The patient must first understand and consent to the needed care. Space must be available or be made available to move the teeth. Adequate anchorage must also be present or be achieved to move the teeth but leave the anchorage units in position. Movement may be accomplished using removable or fixed appliances and can consist of tipping or bodily movement. In most cases, fixed appliances are preferred. Bacterial plaque and other accumulated materials should be removed from the teeth and clinical signs of inflammation eliminated before therapy begins. Plans to control occlusal forces must be made before tooth movement to ensure that occlusal trauma does not interfere with movement. Posttreatment stabilization should also be discussed before tooth movement begins.[4]

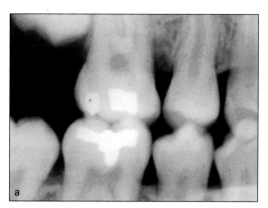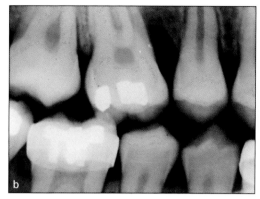

Fig 33-1 *(a)* A radiograph taken at age 12 revealed a radiolucent bony lesion on the mesial aspect of the maxillary first molar. *(b)* At age 14, following orthodontic care without periodontal therapy, the probing depth was 9 mm.

Positive and Negative Effects of Orthodontics

Some professionals say that the long-term health of the periodontium benefits from orthodontic care,[5–7] and some say it does not.[8–11] However, it appears that the type of periodontal disease, the efficacy of the patient's oral hygiene, the presence or absence of systemic risk factors, and the timeliness of maintenance visits dictate the longevity of the dentition to a greater degree than does orthodontic therapy. There are specific ways, however, in which orthodontic therapy can benefit the periodontium:

1. By correcting an overbite that impinges on periodontal tissues[11]
2. By reducing trauma from the teeth in cases of anterior open bite and other severe malocclusions
3. By changing the topography of the periodontium around tipped teeth[12,13]

There are also negative aspects to orthodontic care:

1. Orthodontic therapy results in a small loss of attachment, even in well-maintained cases.[14–16]
2. Orthodontic therapy may contribute to mucogingival problems.[17]

Orthodontic Therapy and Periodontal Diseases

There is a direct relationship between the health of the periodontium and the response of the tissues to orthodontic tooth movement. In the absence of plaque, orthodontic forces alone will not produce gingivitis. However, if bacterial plaque is present when teeth are being moved, attachment loss can occur.[2,17–20]

Most patients who receive fixed orthodontic devices from childhood through puberty develop plaque-induced gingivitis. This usually disappears clinically after removal of appliances.[21] However, during orthodontic therapy, a small number of patients develop periodontitis de novo or exacerbate a previously existing condition (Figs 33-1a and 33-1b); consequently, every patient should be evaluated for periodontal problems before, during, and after orthodontic therapy. Fortunately, in the vast majority of orthodontic cases, irreversible attachment loss does not occur.

Patients with non-plaque–induced forms of gingivitis should not receive orthodontic treatment unless the causal factor can be eliminated or ameliorated to the extent that it will not interfere with orthodontic care. Individuals with chronic periodontitis are not candidates for orthodontics unless the bony destruction can be halted and held in check during tooth movement. Patients with aggressive

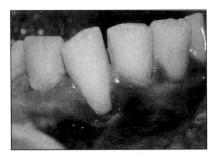

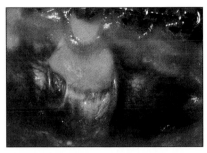

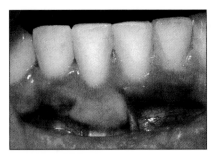

Fig 33-2a This patient will have orthodontic therapy to move the right central incisor into a more prominent position in the arch.

Fig 33-2b Because there was less than 1 mm of attached gingiva and the tooth was being moved into prominence, a free gingival graft was placed prior to tooth movement.

Fig 33-2c The area 5 years after therapy.

forms of periodontitis are not candidates for orthodontic care unless the systemic and local causes of their problems can be successfully controlled. These problems are occasionally discovered during orthodontic care, and if they are successfully treated and closely monitored, then the teeth involved can still be moved orthodontically. Close monitoring is needed, because attachment loss can occur during tooth movement. When it does, tooth movement should be stopped, the periodontal problem treated, and the patient reevaluated to determine whether or not orthodontic therapy should be resumed. Once the disease has been arrested, tooth movement with the gentlest possible orthodontic forces is suggested.

Preventing Periodontal Problems

Before Orthodontic Therapy

Every potential candidate for orthodontic therapy should have a thorough periodontal examination before tooth movement begins. This examination should include an evaluation of oral hygiene, an examination for inflammatory periodontal diseases, a check for the presence of trauma from occlusion, and an evaluation for potential mucogingival problems (see chapter 17).

It is important for the potential orthodontic candidate to have optimal oral hygiene. Absence of proper cleaning can have extremely negative consequences for children and adults who have periodontitis before tooth movement starts. Each individual should be taught to use the most effective means possible for interproximal cleaning. Where space is available, dental floss or interproximal brushes are optimal; where they cannot or will not be used, a mechanical toothbrush is recommended. An oral irrigator is a third choice. Using well-trimmed, bonded brackets and keeping bands as far away from the base of the sulcus as possible leave more room for effective cleaning.[22]

The patient should be screened for the presence of inflammatory periodontal diseases in the usual manner (see chapter 17). If any problems are found, they should be corrected before orthodontic therapy begins. Subgingival deposits should be removed in the most conservative but expeditious manner possible. This usually means closed subgingival scaling and root planing, but in deeper pockets, a flap approach or use of a dental endoscope is often necessary. Supporting bone should not be removed during surgical procedures performed at this stage.

At present there is a question about when, or indeed whether, gaining additional attached gingiva is necessary before orthodontic therapy. Good oral hygiene has been found to reduce the need for soft tissue grafting.[23] However, because perfect oral cleanliness is rare, grafts may be needed before tooth movement begins,[24] because if the teeth are moved through the cortical plate, recession often occurs in a thin periodontium (see Case 2).[25] If oral hygiene is adequate and these same teeth are moved into alveolar bone, little residual damage ensues.[26] However, if oral hygiene is not optimal or if these teeth must be held in a prominent position, permanent and often progressive gingival recession can occur.

Grafts are best placed before orthodontics begins on teeth that have all of the following conditions: there is 1 mm or less of attached gingiva, thin gingival tissues, and less than optimal oral hygiene, and the tooth is to be moved and held in a prominent position (Figs 33-2a to 33-2c) (see chapter 32). This is also an appropriate time to uncover impacted teeth that will not erupt or teeth that will be surrounded by mucosa rather than gingiva if they do erupt. Teeth retain the tissue into which they erupt. If this tissue is mucosa, gingival stripping often occurs. To prevent this problem, these teeth should be uncovered using an apically positioned flap (Figs 33-3 and 33-4).

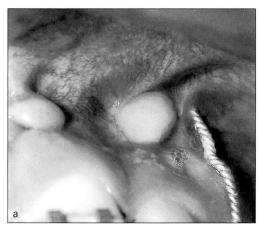
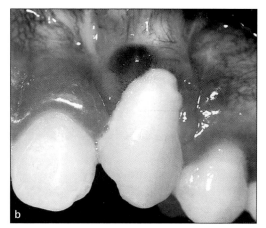

Figs 33-3a and 33-3b This impacted canine was exposed by cutting away the tissue that covered the tooth *(a)*. The tooth was left surrounded by alveolar mucosa as it erupted. This tissue was very tender and quickly became inflamed, and recession started *(b)*. Compare with the case shown in Fig 33-4.

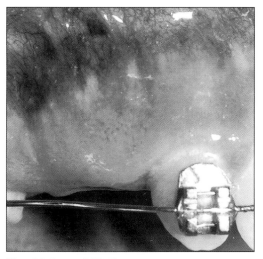
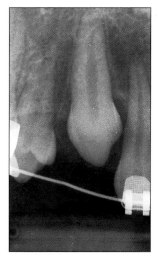

Figs 33-4a and 33-4b This impacted canine would not erupt spontaneously.

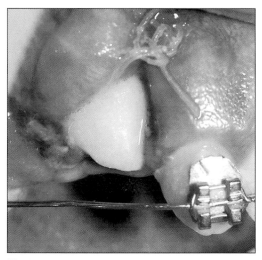
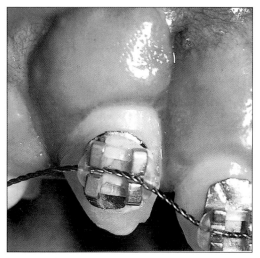

Fig 33-4c An apically positioned flap, which resulted in the tooth being surrounded by keratinized gingiva, was performed.

Fig 33-4d As the tooth actively erupted, the keratinized gingiva migrated with the tooth, preventing gingival recession.

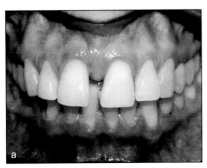
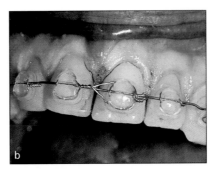
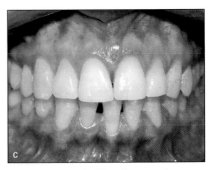

Fig 33-5 This patient's diastema *(a)* was closed and retained for 6 months following active orthodontic care *(b)*. The diastema between the maxillary central incisors recurred as soon as the retainer was removed. A frenectomy was performed, and the diastema remained closed *(c)*.

During Orthodontic Care

Oral hygiene should be monitored, recorded, and reinforced at each periodontal maintenance visit. The patient with less than optimal oral hygiene or with preexisting (or developing) periodontitis should be seen for periodontal maintenance at intervals similar to other patients with these problems. Maintenance intervals can be modified on the basis of probing-depth changes and bleeding on probing (see chapter 28). Fremitus should be monitored and, in patients having clinical signs of inflammatory periodontal diseases, eliminated if appropriate (see chapter 31). In cases of extreme trauma, the fabrication of a disarticulating device may be warranted. Problems are detected by referring to premovement baseline measurements of gingival recession and are treated as previously described.

After Orthodontic Care

Oral hygiene should be monitored as with any other patient. The patient should be kept on appropriate periodontal maintenance and then reevaluated 6 months after tooth movement ends. At this time, any remaining deepened probing depths should be treated in an appropriate manner. Monitoring of fremitus and tooth mobility should continue and an evaluation of these parameters made 6 months after cessation of active orthodontics. Diastemata closed during active tooth movement are evaluated at this time. If spacing occurs when retainers are left off, then interproximal soft tissues, as well as soft tissue and frenum pulls in the area, may need to be modified (Fig 33-5).[27] At that time a final treatment plan to control the occlusion should be developed. For patients with bruxism, a maxillary habit appliance of hard acrylic resin should be worn in place of the typical orthodontic retainer. For a discussion of this aspect of therapy, see chapter 31. It frequently takes time for gingival recession to occur after orthodontic therapy has been completed. Therefore, this parameter should be monitored over time.

Case Presentations

The following cases are presented to demonstrate interdisciplinary cooperation between orthodontists, periodontists, and other specialists in achieving the goal of overall oral health.

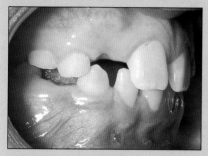
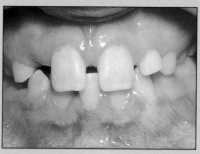
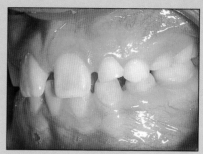

Figs 33-6a to 33-6c Pretreatment records taken at age 11 years, 2 months, for diagnosis, treatment planning, and determination of the timing and sequencing of treatment.

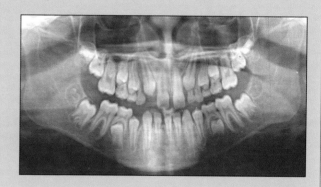

Fig 33-6d Pretreatment panoramic radiograph taken at age 11 years, 2 months, for diagnosis and treatment planning.

An 8-year-old girl was referred to the orthodontist by the general practitioner for an evaluation of congenitally missing teeth. The panoramic radiograph taken at the initial evaluation revealed congenitally missing teeth 7, 10, and 25. Subsequent recall visits to evaluate the eruption of the permanent dentition were at 9-month intervals until age 11 years, 2 months, when complete orthodontic records were made.

Clinical, radiographic, and mounted study cast evaluation revealed a skeletal Class II pattern, mesofacial type, lip competence with no mentalis strain, and pleasing facial esthetics. An end-on Class II relationship was present in the buccal segments when the mandible was manipulated into centric relation. Maxillary and mandibular deciduous second molars, maxillary right and left deciduous first molars, canines, and left deciduous lateral incisor were present.

Teeth 7, 10, and 25 were congenitally missing, and generalized spacing was noted in the maxillary and mandibular anterior areas. Teeth 6 and 11 were erupting into the lateral incisor position, and tooth 20 showed

delayed development. A deep vertical overbite was present. Third molars were developing. Periodontal tissues were inflamed due to poor oral hygiene. No report, history, sign, or symptoms of temporomandibular disorder (TMD) nor myofascial pain dysfunction (MPD) were present.

The patient was referred to a periodontist for control of her inflammatory periodontal disease. Once clinical signs of inflammation were controlled, orthodontic therapy was initiated. Treatment recommended by the orthodontist included full fixed orthodontic appliances, allowing the maxillary canines to erupt into the lateral incisor position and opening space for future dentoalveolar implants at the sites of teeth 7, 10, and 25.

The periodontist evaluated the pros, cons, and timing of implants. The family accepted the recommendation of the orthodontist and periodontist to place implants at the appropriate age.

At age 12 years, 6 months, the patient was referred to an oral and maxillofacial surgeon for extraction of the remaining four deciduous second molars to facili-

(continued)

Case
1 *(continued)*

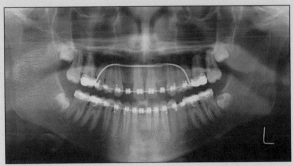

Fig 33-6e Panoramic radiograph showing progress of space and root positions for implants.

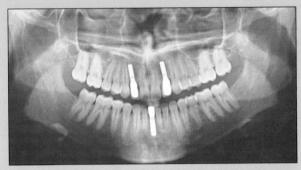

Fig 33-6f Posttreatment panoramic radiograph with implants and restorations placed.

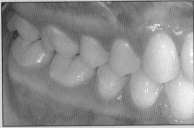
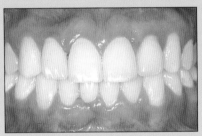
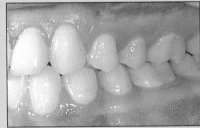

Figs 33-6g to 33-6i Posttreatment photographs reveal good occlusion in the buccal segments; optimum vertical overbite; ideal arch form; restored implants on teeth 7, 10, and 25; and esthetic smile.

tate faster eruption of the mandibular second premolars. At age 12 years, 9 months, full fixed orthodontic appliances were placed, and treatment was initiated to begin optimizing space for future restoration of congenitally missing teeth 7, 10, and 25.

Orthodontic and periodontal treatment proceeded without incident until age 15, when the patient was referred to the periodontist for exposure of tooth 20 to facilitate orthodontic bracket attachment. Cross-sectional tomograms taken at that time revealed inadequate bone in the implant sites.

At age 15 years, 3 months, the patient was referred to the oral and maxillofacial surgeon for third molar extraction and harvesting of corticocancellous bone from the extraction sites to graft in the implant sites of teeth 7, 10, and 25. The grafting procedures were successful, and at age 15 years, 8 months, implants were placed in the sites of teeth 7, 10, and 25. Surgical templates were used for accurate implant placement.

Orthodontic occlusal detailing was accomplished during implant integration, and appliances were removed at age 16. Retainers with pontics were fabricated to maintain ideal space for restoration and esthetics.

The restorative dentist placed provisional restorations for development of papillae and good gingival contour. Final restorations were placed on the implants at age 16 years, 3 months, and new retainers were fabricated by the orthodontist. The patient was placed on recall by the orthodontist and periodontist for implant, periodontal, and retainer maintenance.

The collaborative effort of the orthodontist, periodontist, oral and maxillofacial surgeon, and restorative dentist in diagnosis, treatment planning, and sequencing and execution of treatment was imperative in this case. The patient's goals were attained, and the objectives of ideal dental and facial esthetics and optimum occlusal function with good periodontal health were accomplished.

Connective Tissue Grafts to Treat Tooth Sensitivity and Gingival Recession

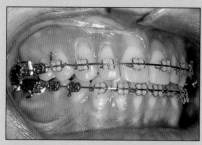 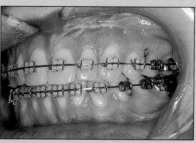 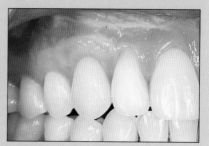

Figs 33-7a and 33-7b Progress photographs following orthognathic surgery and during orthodontic detailing. The patient reported severe sensitivity at the gingival margin on teeth 5, 6, 20, 25, 26, and 29.

Fig 33-7c Posttreatment connective tissue graft on teeth 5 and 6.

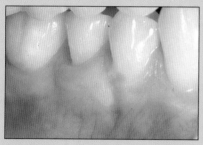 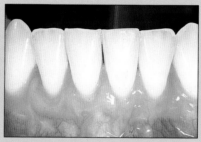 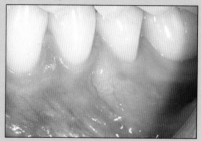

Fig 33-7d Posttreatment connective tissue graft on tooth 29.

Fig 33-7e Posttreatment connective tissue grafts on teeth 25 and 26.

Fig 33-7f Posttreatment connective tissue graft on tooth 20.

This 17-year-old female patient initially presented to the orthodontist with chief complaints of severe anterior open bite, anterior deviate swallow, and a report of TMD and MPD. Treatment included mandibular stabilization using an orthotic, full fixed orthodontic therapy, orthognathic surgery, and myofunctional therapy to reach treatment goals of good dental and facial esthetics, optimal occlusal function, elimination of myofunctional problems, and resolution of the TMD and MPD.

During the finishing and detailing stages of orthodontic therapy, the patient reported severe sensitivity in the areas of teeth 5, 6, 20, 25, 26, and 29. Also, the patient was concerned with the appearance of tooth 6. Gingival recession beyond the cementoenamel junction (CEJ) was noted on these teeth, and the patient was referred to a periodontist for evaluation.

Since the teeth were to move into the alveolar housing, orthodontic treatment was completed. After the inflammation from bracket and band irritation and plaque retention had resolved, the patient returned to the periodontist for placement of subepithelial connective tissue grafts. Connective tissue grafts were placed on the labial and buccal aspects of teeth 5, 6, 20, 25, 26, and 29, with coverage to the CEJ. The patient was pleased with the result and reported minimal discomfort.

The patient was placed in periodontal maintenance. She was given a fixed lingual mandibular canine-to-canine retainer and a maxillary centrically related, mutually protective orthotic for maxillary retention and use as a bruxism guard. The patient was instructed to see the orthodontist on an annual basis for evaluation and any necessary adjustments.

Esthetic Crown Lengthening

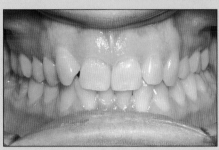

Fig 33-8a The patient exhibits altered passive eruption with excessive gingival display and wide zone of attached tissue beyond the CEJ resulting in short clinical crowns. Asymmetry of gingival contours is also noted.

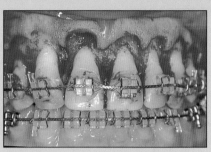

Fig 33-8b Full-thickness flap reflection and osseous surgery completed.

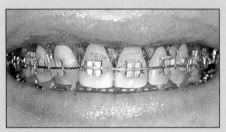

Fig 33-8c Immediate postoperative clinical view. Note the immediate resolution of excessive gingival display.

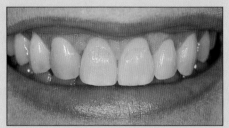

Fig 33-8d Posttreatment. The right canine has been contoured to lateral incisor morphology. Optimum smile line, gingival symmetry, and healthy papilla are noted. The patient is ready for bleaching of the teeth by her restorative dentist.

This 33-year-old woman presented for orthodontic treatment with the chief complaints of a "gummy smile" and malaligned teeth. Clinical and radiographic evaluation, as well as evaluation of mounted study casts, revealed a congenitally missing maxillary right lateral incisor, retroclined maxillary anterior teeth, a deep vertical anterior overbite, generalized malalignment, and a Class II molar and canine in the right buccal segment with the canine in the lateral incisor position.

The patient was referred to the periodontist and restorative dentist for evaluation and consultation. Following appropriate evaluation, the decision was made by the dental team and patient to recontour the maxillary right canine to lateral incisor form in lieu of premolar extraction and distalization of the canine for lateral incisor implant placement. Orthodontic treatment was initiated to align the teeth; to provide for a centrically related, mutually protective occlusal scheme; and to achieve ideal maxillary anterior alignment for peri-odontal plastic surgical procedures to eliminate excessive gingival display, optimize gingival contours, and enhance smile esthetics.

Radiographs and periodontal probing revealed that the level of crestal bone approximated the CEJ with gingival margins extending coronal to it, a condition sometimes referred to as *altered passive eruption*. An apically positioned flap with osseous surgery and re-contouring of the alveolar crestal bone were necessary to meet the treatment objectives. The surgery was performed to reestablish the biologic width at a more apical level, reduce thick bony areas, and elevate the gingival margins.

Collaboration between the orthodontist and periodontist was necessary to achieve an esthetic result with harmonious gingival contours and to satisfy the patient's chief complaints. The patient was referred back to the restorative dentist for tooth bleaching and any necessary restorative procedures.

Forced Extrusion of Tooth, Tissue, and Bone Prior to Extraction and Implant Placement

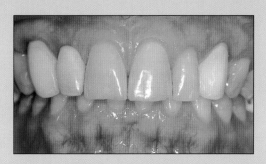

Figs 33-9a Pretreatment. Note the Class II malocclusion, deep vertical overbite, and poor dental esthetics. There is a provisional restoration on tooth 11.

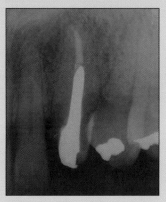

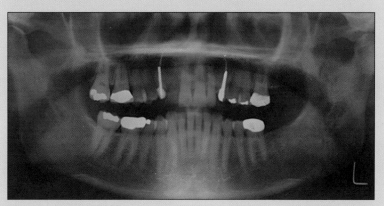

Figs 33-9b and 33-9c Pretreatment periapical and panoramic radiographs.

This 58-year-old woman was referred to the orthodontist by the periodontist for an evaluation and treatment to extrude tooth 11 prior to extraction, dentoalveolar implant placement, and restoration. The restorative dentist had determined that tooth 11 was nonrestorable, with a hopeless prognosis due to internal/external root resorption and root fracture.

Clinical, radiographic, and mounted study cast evaluation revealed a Class II malocclusion, 100% vertical overbite, and undersized maxillary lateral incisors. Teeth 1, 7, 15, 16, 17, 18, and 32 were missing. Significant wear and attrition was noted, especially on the mandibular anterior sextant. There was a history of orthodontic therapy twice in the past, crown-lengthening periodontal surgery on tooth 6, and soft tissue grafting at teeth 6 and 7. Good gingival symmetry was present in the maxillary anterior sextant, with a provisional restoration on tooth 11 and the pontic for tooth 7 cantilevered off tooth 6. Tooth 11 had a 7-mm probing depth on the mesial surface. A brachyfacial pattern, thin competent lips, excessive mentolabial sulcus, and a retrognathic profile were concerns of the patient.

Treatment was initiated following interdisciplinary treatment planning by the periodontist, restorative dentist, and orthodontist. Recommended treatment for tooth 11 included closed subgingival scaling and root planing, followed by slow orthodontic extrusion (5 mm), without concomitant supracrestal fibrotomies, over a period of 8 weeks followed by a stabilization period of 8 weeks. This treatment would improve soft and hard tissue morphology prior to implant placement. Extraction of tooth 11, hard tissue grafting, and pontic placement to the orthodontic archwire as a provisional restoration were performed. Implant placement followed 6 months later, with provisionalization of the implant planned after 3 months of healing. Periodontal and implant maintenance followed the completion of active treatment.

After the initiation of maxillary orthodontic therapy and during forced extrusion of tooth 11, the patient expressed a desire to address the wear and attrition, malocclusion, and facial concerns. Mandibular orthodontic appliances were placed, dental compensations were eliminated, and bilateral mandibular ramus sagittal

(continued)

Case 4 *(continued)*

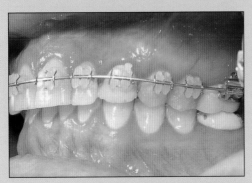

Fig 33-9d Maxillary orthodontic brackets placed; provisional restoration on tooth 11 significantly reduced incisally and lingually to facilitate forced extrusion.

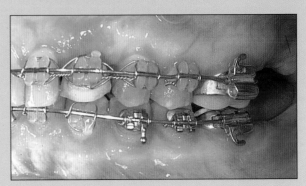

Fig 33-9e Mandibular orthodontic brackets placed to initiate comprehensive interdisciplinary care. Note the level of gingival margin on tooth 11.

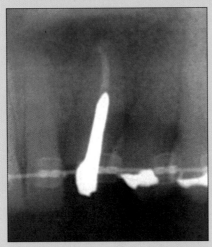

Fig 33-9f Continued forced extrusion of tooth 11 with improved bony architecture.

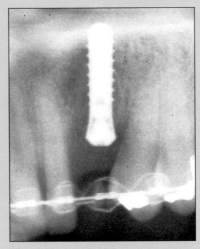

Fig 33-9g Radiograph showing progress after implant placement.

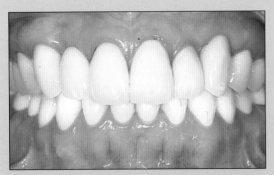

Fig 33-9h Posttreatment occlusion following orthodontics, orthognathic surgery, forced extrusion and implant placement of tooth 11, and complete reconstruction.

split advancement osteotomies were performed to place the mandible in the correct relationship relative to the maxilla, increase anterior facial height, and eliminate the retrognathic facial profile. Following orthodontic therapy, the patient decided to proceed with full-mouth reconstruction by the restorative dentist.

The initial objectives of forced extrusion of tooth 11, extraction of tooth 11, and replacement with an implant were successful. Through the interdisciplinary cooperation of the orthodontist, periodontist, oral surgeon, and restorative dentist, the patient's goals for dental and facial esthetics, stability, function, and improved periodontal health were accomplished.

| Forced Extrusion of Tooth, Tissue, and Bone with Tissue Revision Prior to Tooth Restoration

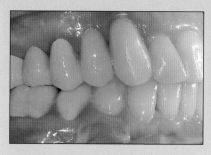

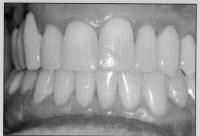

Figs 33-10a and 33-10b Pretreatment. Note excessive clinical crown length on teeth 4, 5, and 6 and asymmetric contour of the gingival margins.

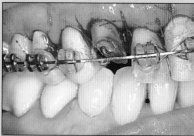

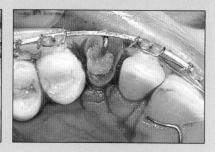

Figs 33-10c and 33-10d Immediate postsurgical repositioned flap. Tooth 6 was orthodontically extruded 5 mm.

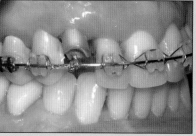

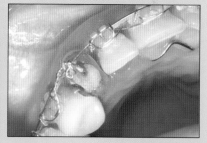

Figs 33-10e and 33-10f Four weeks after periodontal surgery, during orthodontic stabilization.

This 60-year-old woman was referred to the orthodontist by the periodontist and restorative dentist for forced extrusion of tooth 6.

Clinical, radiographic, and study cast evaluation in centric relation revealed a dental Class I occlusion; missing teeth 1, 3, 5, 14, 15, 16, 17, 18, 30, and 31; restoration of the buccal segments; and a fixed partial denture replacing teeth 3 and 5. The fixed restoration margins in the maxillary right buccal segment were restored to the apically receded gingival margins. Excessive and unesthetic clinical crown length on teeth 4 and 6 and the pontic of tooth 5 was noted.

Evaluation by the periodontist revealed an extensive caries lesion 3 mm subgingival, beneath the margin of the full-coverage restoration on abutment 6. A collaborative effort of the periodontist, restorative dentist, endodontist, and orthodontist was necessary to determine the treatment plan. The decision was made to endo-dontically treat tooth 6, disengage tooth 6 from the fixed partial denture, and extrude tooth 6. Orthodontic brackets and a heavy stainless steel archwire were placed on the maxillary teeth to stabilize surrounding teeth during extrusion and to provide for attachment to extrude tooth 6 until tooth structure beyond the caries lesion could be exposed. Orthodontic elastic thread was used from the archwire to the post placed by the endodontist. The tooth, tissue, and bone were extruded, and this procedure was followed by an apically repositioned full-thickness mucoperiosteal flap with bone removal to reposition the gingival tissues on the labial and lingual aspects and to expose tooth structure for restoration margin preparation.

Following healing of the gingival tissues and tooth stabilization, final restoration of the maxillary right buccal segment will be accomplished by the restorative dentist.

Case 6 | Orthopalatal Implant: Maximum Anchorage and Elimination of Headgear

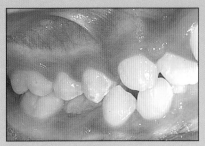

Fig 33-11a Pretreatment. Right Class I molar and end-on Class II canine.

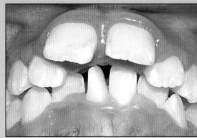

Fig 33-11b Pretreatment. Deep vertical overbite, severe overjet, and gross malalignment.

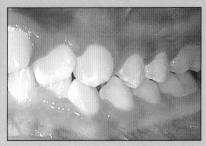

Fig 33-11c Pretreatment. Left Class I molar and end-on Class II canine.

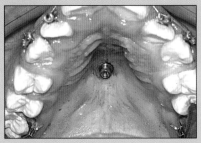

Fig 33-11d Palatal implant is in the predetermined position.

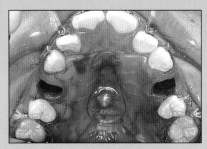

Fig 33-11e The acrylic resin healing stent is placed using acrylic resin in the embrasures of the posterior teeth for temporary anchorage.

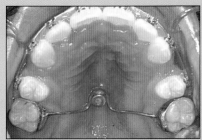

Fig 33-11f Loaded implant. Note good alignment of teeth and ample space remaining for retraction of anterior teeth.

This boy (11 years, 4 months old) presented for orthodontic therapy with chief complaints of severe malalignment, overjet, lip incompetence, and orofacial muscle strain.

Cephalometric evaluation and soft tissue analysis revealed a skeletal Class II pattern, maxillary and mandibular dentoalveolar protrusion, acute nasolabial angle, excessive mentolabial fold, and severe lip incompetence in repose with significant muscle strain where the lips were approximated.

Casts mounted in centric relation revealed Class I molars with end-on Class II canines, severe maxillary and mandibular malalignment, excessive proclination of anterior teeth, 8-mm overjet, and deep vertical anterior overbite. Mouth breathing and generalized gingival inflammation (chronic gingivitis) were present.

There was no report or history of temporomandibular disorder or myofascial pain dysfunction.

The patient's oral hygiene practices were reinforced, and periodontal scaling was performed. The patient was placed in periodontal maintenance.

Orthodontic treatment required extraction of maxillary and mandibular first premolars, anchorage control, and exceptional cooperation from the patient to reach the treatment objectives of ideal dental esthetics, good facial esthetics, lip competence, and a centrically related, mutually protected occlusion. Resolution of the chief complaints would require use of the extraction sites, effective mechanics, and favorable growth.

Traditional anchorage and molar control in this type of case could include transpalatal arch, transpalatal arch with palatal acrylic button, headgear, and sequen-

(continued)

Case 6 *(continued)*

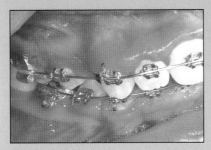

Fig 33-11g Right Class I molar relationship with space available for canine and anterior retraction.

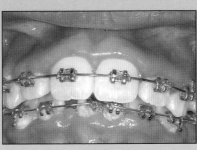

Fig 33-11h Anterior alignment progress.

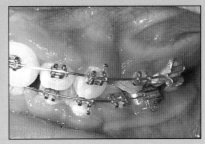

Fig 33-11i Left Class I molar relationship with space available for canine and anterior retraction.

tial retraction of anterior teeth. Reciprocal forces during anterior tooth retraction would result in varying degrees of posterior anchorage loss (the posterior teeth would move forward), depending on the mechanics used and patient cooperation. To eliminate the critical compliance factor and headgear wear, a 6-mm-long, 3.3-mm-diameter sandblasted, acid-attacked palatal implant (2.5-mm neck) was placed. An acrylic resin stent for surgical guidance was used for accurate placement of the implant, and an acrylic resin healing stent was worn to eliminate tongue pressure on the implant and to provide comfort during implant integration. The palatal implant provided 24-hour, stable anchorage control to maximize use of the extraction sites, and it eliminated the need for headgear wear.

Acknowledgment

The authors would like to thank the following practitioners for their work on the cases presented in this chapter: Dr Edward P. Allen, Dr James D. Bates, Dr Farhad E. Boltchi, Dr Michael N. Cohlmia, Dr Arlet R. Dunsworth, Dr Edward Ellis, Dr David McFadden, Dr Ronald S. Stukalin, Dr Keith W. Thornton, and Dr Jeffrey S. Woodson.

References

1. Cooper MB. Minor tooth movement in the management of the periodontal patient. In: Prichard JF (ed). The Diagnosis and Treatment of Periodontal Disease. Philadelphia: Saunders, 1979:462–504.

2. Thilander B. Orthodontic tooth movement in periodontal therapy. In: Lindhe J (ed). Textbook of Clinical Periodontology. Munksgaard: Copenhagen, 1983:480.

3. Roblee RD. Interdisciplinary Dentofacial Therapy. Chicago: Quintessence, 1994:160–167.

4. Marks MH. Tooth movement in periodontal therapy. In: Goldman HM, Cohen DW (eds). Periodontal Therapy. St Louis: Mosby, 1980:564–627.

5. Alexander AG, Tipins AK. The effect of irregularity of teeth and the degree of overbite and overjet on the gingival health. Br Dent J 1970;129:539–544.

6. Kessler M. Interrelationships between orthodontics and periodontics. Am J Orthod 1976;70:154–172.

7. Buckley LA. The relationship between malocclusion and periodontal disease. J Periodontol 1972;43:415–417.

8. Geiger AM, Wasserman BH, Turgeon LR. Relationship of occlusion and periodontal disease. Part VIII. Relationship of crowding and spacing to periodontal destruction and gingival inflammation. J Periodontol 1974;45:43–49.

9. Ingervall B, Jacobsson U, Nyman S. A clinical study of the relationship between crowding of teeth and plaque and gingival condition. J Clin Periodontol 1977;4:214–222.

10. Prichard JF. The effect of bicuspid extraction orthodontics on the periodontium. Findings in 100 consecutive cases. J Periodontol 1975;46:534–542.

11. Gould MSE, Picton DCA. The relation between irregularities of the teeth and periodontal disease. Br Dent J 1966;121:21.

12. Brown J. The effect of orthodontic therapy on certain types of periodontal defects. I. Clinical findings. J Periodontol 1973;44:742–756.

13. Cohen DW. Areas of common concern to orthodontics and periodontics. In: McNamara JA, Ribbens KA (eds). Malocclusion and the Periodontium. Ann Arbor, MI: Center for Human Growth and Development, University of Michigan, 1984:87–105.

14. Zachrisson BU, Alnaes L. Periodontal condition in orthodontically treated and untreated individuals. I. Loss of attachment, gingival pocket depth and clinical crown height. Angle Orthod 1973;43:402–411.

15. Alstad S, Zachrisson BV. Longitudinal study of periodontal condition associated with orthodontic treatment in adolescents. Am J Orthod 1979;76(3):277–296.

16. Richter WA, Ueno H. Relationship of crown margin placement to gingival inflammation. J Prosthet Dent 1973;30:156–161.

17. Ericsson I, Thilander B, Lindhe J, Okamato H. The effect of orthodontic tilting movements on the periodontal tissues of the infected and non-infected dentitions in dogs. J Clin Periodontol 1977;4(4):278–293.

18. Ericsson I, Thilander B. Orthodontic forces and recurrence of periodontal disease. Am J Orthod 1978;74(1):41–50.

19. Ericsson I, Thilander B, Lindhe J. Periodontal conditions after orthodontic tooth movements in the dog. Angle Orthod 1978; 48:210–218.

20. Ericsson I, Thilander B. Orthodontic relapse in dentitions with reduced periodontal support. Eur J Orthod 1980;2:51–57.

21. Zachrisson S, Zachrisson BU. Gingival condition associated with orthodontic treatment. Angle Orthod 1972;42:26–34.

22. Zachrisson BU. Clinical implications of recent ortho-perio research findings. In: Hosl E, Zachrisson BU, Baldaug A (eds). Orthodontics and Periodontics. Chicago: Quintessence, 1985: 169–186.

23. Kennedy JE, Bird WC, Palcanis KG, Dorfman HS. A longitudinal evaluation of varying widths of attached gingiva. J Clin Periodontol 1985;12:667–675.

24. Maynard JG, Ochsenbein C. Mucogingival problems, prevalence and therapy in children. J Periodontol 1975;46:543–552.

25. Engelking G, Zachrisson BU. Effects of incisor repositioning on monkey periodontium after expansion through the cortical plate. Am J Orthod 1982;82:23–32.

26. Steiner GG, Pearson JK, Ainamo J. Changes of the marginal periodontium as a result of labial tooth movement in monkeys. J Periodontol 1981;52(6):314–320.

27. Edwards JG. Soft tissue surgery to alleviate orthodontic relapse. Dent Clin North Am 1993;37:205–226.

Part IV

Dental Implants

The Biology of Implant Dentistry

David L. Cochran and Joachim S. Hermann

- Historic Review
- Structural Biology: Natural Tooth Versus Endosseous Implant
- Submerged Versus Nonsubmerged Implant Placement
- Crestal Bone Loss Around Titanium Implants
- Biologic Width Around Titanium Implants
- Inflammation Around Titanium Implants
- Tissue Implications for Dental Implants

Historic Review

Success in the placement, hard tissue integration, and clinical use of endosseous iron alloy implants has been documented as far back as the first or second century AD.[1] However, in those days, the approach to implant dentistry was purely empirical and carried potential problems such as disease transmission, foreign body reaction, peri-implant inflammation, and fatigue fracture. Implant dentistry did not gain a scientific basis until the first third of the 20th century. Endosseous, root-form implants were introduced in the United States by Greenfield in 1913,[2] and subperiosteal implants were introduced in Sweden by Dahl in 1937.[3–5] However, relatively high numbers of failures were reported using subperiosteal implants, which involved a relatively invasive approach.[6] Removal necessitated by infection caused substantial defects in the residual alveolar bone. Since then, root-form, endosseous implants of varying shapes (cylinder, step cylinder, screw, and combinations thereof) have been used. As a result of an increased need for osteosynthesis after traumatic injury during World Wars I and II, it became evident that titanium, rather than stainless steel or other metals, was the most biocompatible material to use in the attempt to achieve fracture healing by primary intention or hard tissue integration.[7–9]

In the 1940s and 1950s, Bothe et al[8] and Leventhal[9] first described the biocompatibility of titanium for bone surgery. Later, Brånemark and his research group in Sweden defined such hard tissue integration around relatively smooth machined titanium implants as *osseointegration*.[10] Schroeder and his team in Switzerland defined the hard tissue integration adjacent to a rough-surfaced, titanium plasma-sprayed (TPS) surface of implants as *functional ankylosis*.[11–13] Such a functional unit allows only limited movement of the endosseous implant compared with natural teeth, because there is no intervening tissue between the implant surface and the surrounding alveolar bone. The relationship between the endosseous dental implant and the bone tissue dominated the dental implant literature for many years. This was due to the fact that the direct contact of the implant with the bone was completely different from the natural tooth, which has an attachment apparatus between the tooth root and bone consisting of cementum and a periodontal ligament. The endosseous dental implant represented only one part of the dental restoration. It was equivalent to the tooth root, and the final restoration needed an equivalent component to the tooth crown. Consequently, the dental implant restoration, similar to the natural tooth, had to penetrate the oral integument; ie, the restoration also had to pass through the oral soft tissues that were comprised of epithelium and connective tissue. What was unknown was the relationship of the epithelium and connective tissue to the final implant restoration.

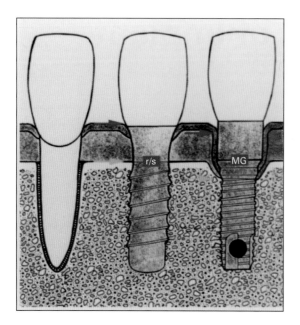

Fig 34-1 Schematic drawing comparing hard and soft tissue reactions around a natural tooth *(left)* with a loaded one-piece, nonsubmerged implant *(middle)* and a loaded two-piece, submerged implant *(right)*. Note that one-piece implants, without a microgap, exhibit a rough/smooth (r/s) implant border at the bone crest level, while two-piece implants have a microgap (MG) at the level of the bone crest between the implant and the abutment. *Red arrows* indicate the level of the gingival margin; *yellow arrows* indicate the level of the first bone-to-implant contact. (Adapted from Cochran and Mahn,[18] with permission.)

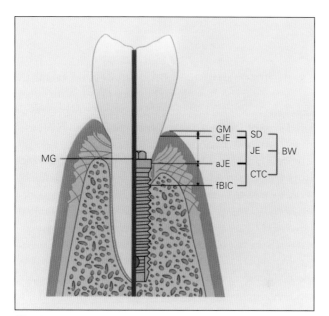

Fig 34-2a Schematic drawing (true to scale) comparing periodontal and peri-implant vertical soft tissue dimensions around a natural tooth[19] and a two-piece, submerged implant,[20] respectively. MG = microgap; GM = gingival margin; cJE = most coronal cell of junctional epithelium; aJE = most apical cell of junctional epithelium; fBIC = first bone-to-implant contact; SD = sulcus depth (distance from GM to cJE); JE = junctional epithelium (distance from cJE to aJE); CTC = connective tissue contact (distance from aJE to fBIC); BW = biologic width (SD + JE + CTC).

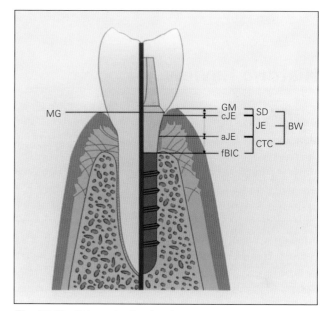

Fig 34-2b Schematic drawing (true to scale) comparing periodontal and peri-implant vertical soft tissue dimensions around a natural tooth[19] and a one-piece, nonsubmerged implant,[21] respectively. Note that both the gingival margin (GM) and the first bone-to-implant contact (fBIC) are located significantly more coronal (*P* < 0.05[20]) as compared with those in Fig 34-2a.

Structural Biology: Natural Tooth Versus Endosseous Implant

In 1921, Gottlieb initially described the epithelial attachment around a natural tooth as epithelial tissue covering distinct areas of the enamel surface or the cementum, not as merely an attachment to the cementoenamel junction (see chapter 3).[14] These findings were confirmed later,[15] and the gingival crevice, or sulcus, was defined. Subsequently, Feneis[16] showed that connective tissue consisted of three-dimensionally oriented fibers firmly connecting tooth structures to the surrounding gingiva. Thus, it became clear that both epithelial and connective tissue attachment contribute to a "protective structure" in an area where the natural tooth penetrates the gingival tissue of the body. Sicher confirmed these findings in 1959 and called this functional unit the *dentogingival junction*.[17]

Both natural teeth and endosseous implants represent a significant challenge for the human body as the only structures piercing the soft tissues of the body (Fig 34-1). However, it has been well documented that few bacteria are found beyond the sulcular area in either healthy periodontal or peri-implant tissues, which fulfill the function of creating a seal around teeth and implants. This "sealing apparatus" between a natural tooth or an endosseous implant and surrounding tissues comprises both hard and soft tissues—namely, hard connective tissue (alveolar bone), soft connective tissue, and junctional epithelium (Fig 34-2). In some cases of long-standing bacterial periodontal or peri-implant colonization of marginal soft tissues, however, soft and hard tissue breakdown can occur, resulting in significant attachment loss.[22–27]

The most coronal connection between tooth surfaces (enamel and cementum) and periodontal soft tissues is provided by the junctional epithelium.[14,28] However, the substance mediating the attachment between the "cuff" of the junctional epithelium and the tooth surface was first described by Schroeder in 1969 as hemidesmosomes attached via the internal basal lamina to the tooth surface.[29] The connective tissue compartment around natural teeth has been shown to consist of intertwined, three-dimensionally and functionally oriented collagen fibers anchored in the cementum, thus firmly connecting tooth structures to the surrounding gingiva.[16] Within the bony housing, natural teeth are anchored via connective tissue fibers inserting into the alveolar bone on one side and into the cementum of the tooth on the other side, forming the periodontal ligament space. Such a functional unit allows movement of the natural tooth within the alveolar socket. In 1961, Gargiulo and coworkers demonstrated that the vertical dimension of the dentogingival junction—composed of sulcus depth, the junctional epithelium, and connective tissue attachment—was stable at about 3.0 mm; they subsequently called it the *biologic width* (see Fig 34-2). In addition, this constant unit was dependent on the location of the crest of the alveolar bone.[19]

Two major clinical procedures have been derived from these findings and are widely used today: surgical crown lengthening[30] and forced eruption.[31] Both procedures are based on the understanding that changing the level of the alveolar bone will predictably move the complete dentogingival junction as a unit in the same direction (apically or coronally). These procedures have a great impact on the location of the gingival margin and the tip of the papilla, and therefore they provide an important tool to achieve stable and esthetic gingival harmony around a healthy natural crown or a tooth-borne restoration (see chapters 23 and 33).

In 1974, James and Kelln realized that a healthy epithelial attachment around endosseous implants made from a cobalt-chromium alloy successfully prevents an apical migration of bacteria along the implant surface.[24] This finding suggested that a functional seal might exist around implants similar to that which was found around the natural tooth. Following this report, this research group and others showed at the electron microscopic level that a hemidesmosomal attachment occurred on cobalt-chromium alloy implants[32,33] and on titanium surfaces,[34,35] as it does on natural teeth. In addition, Buser and coworkers demonstrated an intimate contact between the basal epithelial cell layer and a relatively smooth titanium surface at the light microscopic level.[36] Thus, it can be concluded that the epithelial attachment of a natural tooth and that of an endosseous implant share many similarities.

The connective tissue adjacent to implants has different anatomic structures compared with that adjacent to teeth in the direct vicinity (50 to 100 μm) of a relatively smooth titanium surface. One difference is that the connective tissue fibers run parallel to the implant long axis.[36–39] In addition, almost no neural or vascular structures can be found adjacent to the implant surface; therefore, this tissue compartment resembles a scarlike connective tissue and is different from the periodontal connective tissue attachment apparatus connecting the tooth root to the alveolar bone. Thus, although the epithelium around implants is similar to the epithelium around teeth, the morphology of the connective tissue surrounding teeth and implants is different.

Submerged Versus Nonsubmerged Implant Placement

In the 1960s, as noted above, a Swedish research team led by Brånemark described the concept of osseointegration: the potential of screw-shaped machined titanium endosseous implants to integrate with bone.[10] This research group recommended a submerged approach when placing such endosseous implants, meaning that the screw-shaped implants were placed with their tops at the level of the alveolar bone crest during a first surgical procedure.[40,41] After a submerged healing period under the oral epithelium and connective tissue (3 to 9 months depending on the quality of the bone), a second surgery was carried out, in which the top of the implant was exposed and a secondary implant component (the abutment) was connected to the implant body. This procedure created an implant emerging through the soft tissues, resulting in a two-component transgingival device. This two-piece implant approach results in an interface, or *microgap* (see Fig 34-1), between the implant and abutment within peri-implant soft or hard tissues. The consequences of the interface between the two implant components was originally not known. Subsequent research has indicated that the interface between these implant components has an influence on bacterial accumulation, recruitment of inflammatory cells, and soft and hard tissue dimensions around the implant. For example, some studies have demonstrated that the interface provides space for bacterial colonization.[42,43]

Another approach to placing endosseous dental implants was developed in Switzerland at about the same time. This work, by Schroeder and coworkers,[11-13] was based on extensive research in the field of orthopedic surgery. These implants were either screw-shaped or cylindrical in shape, but rather than having a relatively smooth machined surface, they had a rough surface created by adding titanium by a process using a plasma spray (hence the term *titanium plasma sprayed*). Another major difference with this approach was that the implant extended above the bone level by about 3 mm, which meant that the implant passed through the epithelium and connective tissue. This so-called transgingival top part of the implant had a smooth machined titanium surface and was supracrestal, ie, above the bone crest, at the time of implant placement. This configuration was therefore a one-piece implant that had no interface or microgap and passed from inside the body to outside the body, similar to the natural tooth. More recently, another rough surface has been introduced on the endosseous portion of the implant. This titanium surface is sandblasted with a large grit

and acid attacked (SLA). This SLA surface has been shown to result in a greater amount of bone-to-implant contact and to have a firmer bonding to the bone as determined by higher removal torque values compared with some other implant surfaces, including machined and TPS surfaces.[44,45] Such improvements in surface technology have resulted in earlier loading of the implants with the crown, a large benefit for the patient.[46]

With this one-piece implant, only one surgical procedure is required for implant placement compared to two surgical procedures for the two-piece implant systems. At surgical placement of the one-piece implant, the rough/smooth border at the top portion of the implant is placed level with the bone crest. This results in the top of the implant being immediately exposed to the oral cavity and is called a *nonsubmerged* placement. As is the case with the submerged two-piece implants, the proof of bony integration of the implant (or functional ankylosis) was provided at the light microscopic level. Additionally and importantly, because nonsubmerged implants have only one piece, there is no space between implant components located at the bone level and thus, no potential for bacterial colonization and subsequent inflammatory response within peri-implant soft and hard tissues.

Other implant systems with various surfaces and designs are available, and most companies have a nonsubmerged, one-piece (also known as single-stage) implant design. The biologic consequences of the differences between one-piece and two-piece (nonsubmerged and submerged) implants is not known. Cochran and coworkers have began a series of systematic experimental studies to evaluate the consequences of these two implant designs on the soft and hard (crestal bone) tissues.

Crestal Bone Loss Around Titanium Implants

One consequence of the difference between one-piece (nonsubmerged) and two-piece (submerged) implant designs is the effect on the level of the crestal bone around the implants. In 1981, Adell and coworkers described some crestal bone loss around two-stage implants that had been loaded for approximately 1 year,[40] with minimal crestal bone loss occurring the following years. The initial bone loss averaged 1.5 mm, resulting in a first bone-to-implant contact at approximately the level of the first or second thread of the machined implant (see Fig 34-2a), with a 0.56-mm interthread distance (pitch). Subsequently, such crestal bone changes were defined as one criterion of success when placing two-stage titanium implants.[47] In these studies, radiographic controls were first taken at the time of crown placement (loading), because it was believed that diagnostic radiography might interfere with osseous healing around the implant.[40,48,49] Thus, the protocol did not allow the detection of early crestal bone changes during the initial phases of healing.

In the early 1980s, no similar data existed for one-piece implants. In addition, no data were available to help researchers understand changes in the level of the crest of the bone. Subsequently crestal bone loss for one-stage, nonsubmerged implants was found to be less than 1 mm in a 1-year prospective study.[50,51] This study used a dual-surfaced, one-piece implant[11–13,52,53] with the rough/smooth implant border placed at the bone crest level. In addition, data from an 8-year prospective human radiographic study showed that crestal bone levels, on average, were stable over the entire study period, demonstrating an overall annual crestal bone loss of 0.1 mm.[54]

Based on the early studies and on clinical findings, several experimental studies have been carried out comparing the changes in crestal bone in one- versus two-piece implants placed with submerged and nonsubmerged surgical approaches.[55–58] As time has passed, many clinicians have realized that submerging the dental implant (two-piece) was not required for successful osseointegration. This was due to the success of the one-piece, nonsubmerged implant and the desire to perform only one surgical procedure on the patient. Clinicians then began to surgically place the two-piece implants using a nonsubmerged technique, whereby they connected the abutment to the implant at the time of the so-called first-stage surgery. This essentially resulted in a two-piece implant (with a microgap or interface at the bone crest level) that was nonsubmerged. Alternatively, some clinicians began to place the one-piece implant more apically into the bone and cover (submerge) the implant under the soft tissues. All these possibilities made the nomenclature difficult. For this reason, the authors have chosen to separate the surgical technique from the implant configuration. Thus, *submerged* and *nonsubmerged* are only used to reflect the surgical technique utilized at the time of implant placement. Similarly, *one-piece* and *two-piece* are utilized to reflect only the implant configuration, ie, how many components are required to reach the oral cavity. Thus a one-piece implant reflects the original nonsubmerged or one-stage technique, and a two-piece implant reflects the original submerged or two-stage technique in which the implant stops at the bone crest and a secondary implant component, such as an abutment or crown, is then connected, resulting in an interface at the bone crest. Presently then, the one-piece implant can be placed in a nonsubmerged or a submerged surgical technique, and the two-piece implant can be submerged (still usually without an abutment) or the implant and abutment can be connected and placed in a nonsubmerged surgical approach.

All of these implant configurations and surgical approaches have been examined in relation to crestal bone changes.[55–58] It was found that in one-piece, nonsubmerged implants, crestal bone levels rapidly remodeled to the level of the rough/smooth implant border, originally being located at approximately the alveolar crest (Fig 34-3). In two-piece implant/abutment configurations, approximately 2 mm of crestal bone loss rapidly occurred (Fig 34-4). Importantly, this remodeling was dependent on the location of the microgap in relation to the crest of the bone at the time of implant placement. Furthermore, crestal bone loss around two-piece implant/abutment configurations was independent of whether implants had been placed using a submerged or nonsubmerged surgical technique. These changes occurred relatively rapidly (within 1 month) after implant placement (first-stage surgery) for unloaded one- and two-piece, nonsubmerged implants, whereas crestal bone loss around unloaded two-piece, submerged implants was identified within 1 month after abutment connection (second-stage surgery) when an interface (microgap) was created. Finally, the effect of the microgap was observed to be greater than the effect of the rough/smooth implant border.

Biologic Width Around Titanium Implants

Another difference between one-piece (nonsubmerged) and two-piece (submerged) implant designs is their effects on the linear dimensions (biologic width) of the epithelium and connective tissues around the implant. Initially, the vertical dimension of the soft tissues around dental implants was not well described, because the emphasis was on bone-to-implant contact. In 1991, Berglundh and collaborators[37] presented experimental data on peri-implant soft tissue integration around two-piece, submerged implants. Cochran and collaborators, however, were the first to discuss the biologic width dimensions around endosseous implants.[20,21,59,60] In the case of one-piece, nonsubmerged implants, biologic width was found to be approximately 3.0 mm around both unloaded and loaded implants[20,21,59,60] and therefore was very similar to the dimensions found around natural teeth.[19,61] Hermann et al confirmed that these dimensions are not only physiologically formed but also stable over time.[60] Subsequently, the same research group found that significantly increased amounts of crestal bone loss around two-piece implants also means that the gingival margin is significantly more apical (see Figs 34-6a and 34-6b) around the two-piece

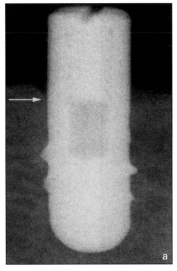
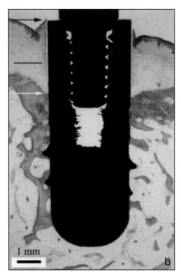
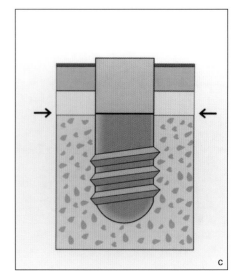

Fig 34-3a A standardized periapical radiograph of a one-piece, nonsubmerged implant after 6 months of unloaded healing and remodeling. The *arrow* indicates the level of the first bone-to-implant contact.

Fig 34-3b A mesiodistal histologic section of a one-piece, nonsubmerged implant. The *white arrow* indicates the level of the first bone-to-implant contact (fBIC), while the *black arrow* indicates the level of the gingival margin (GM). The vertical dimension between the GM and the fBIC is the biologic width. The *black bar* reveals the level of the most apical cell of the junctional epithelium (aJE). The area between the aJE and the fBIC represents the connective tissue contact compartment. Overall, minimal to no signs of peri-implant inflammation (degree of round cell infiltrate) are visible within peri-implant soft tissues. Apical to the fBIC, there is evidence of an intimate hard tissue integration. (Toluidine blue and basic fuchsin stain; original magnification ×2.5).[55–57] (Modified from Hermann et al,[56] with permission.)

Fig 34-3c Schematic drawing of soft and hard tissue dimensions around a one-piece, nonsubmerged implant placed according to standard surgical procedure after 6 months of unloaded healing and remodeling in relation to the rough/smooth implant border *(arrows)*. The red compartment represents the vertical dimension of the sulcus depth, the pink compartment indicates the junctional epithelium, and the yellow compartment represents the connective tissue contact. The sum of these three dimensions equals the biologic width. *Arrows* indicate the level of the crest of the bone at the time of implant placement.

implants compared to one-piece implants. This finding has potentially important implications for final tissue contours in the field of esthetic implant dentistry.[20]

Inflammation Around Titanium Implants

It has been shown that peri-implant inflammatory infiltration is limited around one-piece, nonsubmerged implants having no microgap. This is in contrast to two-piece implants, where moderate to severe degrees of peri-implant inflammation have been observed (compare Figs 34-3b and 34-4b).[62] This inflammation occurred regardless of whether two-piece implants were initially submerged and the abutment attached at a second surgical appointment, or whether an abutment was placed at initial surgery in a two-piece, nonsubmerged implant approach. In addition, the severity of inflammation increased the more apical the

location of the microgap between implant and abutment. This inflammation was likely due to bacterial colonization of the interface, as has been described.[42,43]

Tissue Implications for Dental Implants

Based on findings that a biologic width forms around nonsubmerged, one-piece endosseous implants similar to that around natural dentition,[21] it appears that the oral tissue components are physiologically established with relative dimensions.[60] Results from these and other experimental studies suggest that for tissues around dental implants, *(1)* the level of bone,[55,56] *(2)* the dimensions of the soft tissues,[20,21,60] and *(3)* the degree of inflammation[62] are all important for the final restoration. Pathological changes result in altered tissue relationships, similar to what occurs around teeth, compromising the final restorative outcome.

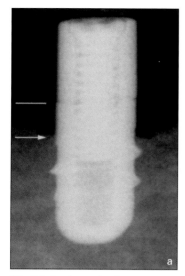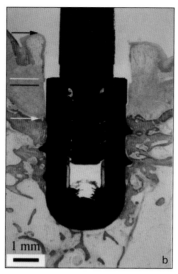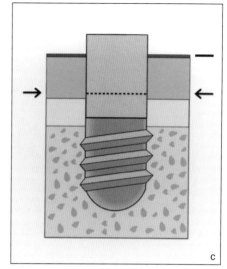

Fig 34-4a A standardized periapical radiograph of a two-piece, submerged implant after 6 months of unloaded healing and remodeling (3 months after abutment connection). The *arrow* indicates the level of the first bone-to-implant contact, while the bar points to the microgap between the implant and abutment.

Fig 34-4b A mesiodistal histologic section of a two-piece, submerged implant. The *white arrow* shows the level of the first bone-to-implant contact (fBIC), the *white bar* delineates the level of the microgap, and the *black arrow* indicates the level of the gingival margin (GM). The vertical dimension between the GM and the fBIC is the biologic width. The *black bar* reveals the level of the most apical cell of the junctional epithelium (aJE). The area between the aJE and the fBIC represents the connective tissue contact compartment. Overall, moderate to severe signs of peri-implant inflammation (degree of round cell infiltrate) are visible within peri-implant soft tissues. Apical to the fBIC, there is evidence of an intimate hard tissue integration. (Toluidine blue and basic fuchsin stain; original magnification ×2.5).[55–57] (Modified from Hermann et al,[56] with permission.)

Fig 34-4c Schematic drawing of soft and hard tissue dimensions around a two-piece, submerged implant placed according to a standard surgical procedure after 6 months of unloaded healing and remodeling and 3 months after abutment connection. Note the relation of the tissues to the microgap *(dashed black line)*. The red compartment exhibits the vertical dimension of the sulcus depth, the pink compartment the junctional epithelium, and the yellow compartment the connective tissue contact. The first bone-to-implant contact and the tip of the gingival margin, indicated by the thick black line, are located significantly more apically ($P <$ .05) compared with the one-piece implant configuration (see Fig 34-3a).[20] *Arrows* indicate the level of the bone crest at the time of implant placement.

Such changes can include necrosis of the junctional epithelium, changes in the connective tissue, and loss of bone. These changes are usually manifested through inflammation and the presence of inflammatory cells and their associated cytokines and inflammatory mediators.[63,64] These altered relationships can be particularly critical in areas of esthetic concern.

The goal for the dental implant restoration, therefore, is to allow for physiologically established, noninflamed tissue relationships. In many cases the clinician can control what tissue changes will occur. This is dictated by the choice of implant design and how the implant is placed relative to the existing hard (Fig 34-5) and soft tissue (Fig 34-6). These choices, in turn, influence the inflammatory infiltrate located around the implant.[62] For example, the clinician must be careful in where the top of the implant is located. Some authors suggest that as the discrepancy increases between an implant shoulder and the diameter of the replaced tooth, the top of the implant should be placed more apically. The rationale is that this placement will improve the emergence profile of the restoration.[65–68]

These recommendations are based on a so-called restoration-driven implant placement technique.[69] Given the scientific data described above, it is clear that such a recommendation is contraindicated, particularly in esthetic areas. Rather, it is proposed that the placement of dental implants be based on a tissue-driven implant placement technique. Such a placement can create physiologically established relationships, minimize altered relationships (often created pathologically), and reduce the degree of inflammation. Furthermore, because such consequences are physiologic, the tissues surrounding the implant will be functional and long lasting. Thus, these recommendations can lead to an esthetically pleasing, tissue-driven implant result.

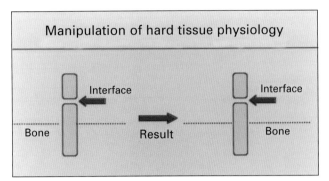

Fig 34-5a Schematic diagram demonstrating the lack of change in alveolar crestal bone when the top of the implant (one piece, nonsubmerged) is located significantly above the original bone crest.

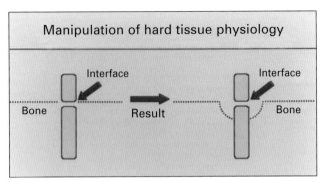

Fig 34-5b Schematic diagram demonstrating the apical movement of alveolar crestal bone when the top of the implant (two piece, submerged) is located at or below the original bone crest. Significant crestal bone loss occurs after abutment placement.

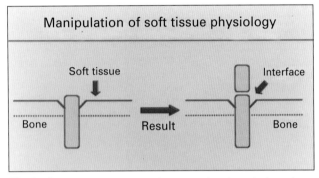

Fig 34-6a Schematic diagram demonstrating the soft tissue location around an implant (one piece, nonsubmerged) placed so the top of the implant is located significantly above the original bone crest. Minimal changes occur in the soft tissues.

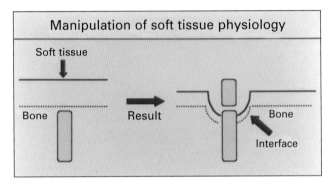

Fig 34-6b Schematic diagram demonstrating the soft tissue changes around an implant and abutment (two piece, submerged and nonsubmerged) when an implant is placed so the top of the implant is located at or below the original bone crest. The peri-implant soft tissues are significantly more apical than when the implant is placed above the soft tissues.

Summary

Replacing missing teeth and roots with artificial devices was first attempted almost 2,000 years ago. Two different surgical approaches and implant configurations have evolved, and both achieve high levels of clinical success. The major difference between these two approaches (the submerged and the nonsubmerged approaches) is the implant configuration, not the surgical technique. The presence of an interface between the implant and abutment, as well as the location of the interface in relation to the alveolar crest, is critical and has significant biologic implications. These implications include the location and dimensions of the soft and hard tissues and the inflammatory response in the adjacent peri-implant soft tissues. A histologic comparison of soft and hard tissue attachment between teeth and implants reveals similar epithelial attachment mechanisms and structures. However, differences are found between teeth and implants in regard to connective tissues and bony integration, because implants do not have cementum or periodontal ligament structures.

The biology associated with implants suggests that they be positioned within the bony housing based on a tissue-driven implant placement technique rather than a restoration-driven technique. With such placement, dental implants can achieve biologically based, physiologic (and therefore natural) tissue relationships.

Acknowledgment

The authors would like to thank Nancy Place and Karen Holt for their artistic help with the figures and Karen Lucas for her excellent help in the preparation of this chapter.

References

1. Crubézy E, Murail P, Girard L, Bernadou JP. False teeth of the Roman world. Nature 1998;391:29.
2. Greenfield EJ. Implantation of artificial crown and bridge abutments. Dent Cosmos 1913;15:364–369.
3. Dahl G. Om Möjligheten för Implantation i Käken av Metallskelett som Bas eller Retention för fasta eller avtagbara Proteser [Possibilities for implantation of subperiosteal implants as a base for retention of fixed or removable prostheses]. Odontol Tidskr 1943;51:440–445.
4. Dahl G. Dental implants and superplants. Rass Trimest Odontoiatr 1956;37:25–36.
5. Dahl G. Subperiosteal implants and "superplants." Dent Abstr 1957;2:685.
6. Obwegeser H. Die chirurgische Vorbereitung der Kiefer für die Prothese [Preprosthetic surgery]. In: Haunfelder D, Hupfauf L, Ketterl W, Schmuth G (eds). Praxis der Zahnheilkunde [Practical Applications in General Dentistry], ed 1. München, Germany: Urban & Schwarzenberg, 1969:1–64.
7. Zierold AA. Reaction of bone to various metals. Arch Surg 1924;9:365–412.
8. Bothe RT, Beaton LE, Davenport HA. Reaction of bone to multiple metallic implants. Surg Gynecol Obstet 1940;71:598–602.
9. Leventhal GS. Titanium, a metal for surgery. J Bone Joint Surg 1951;33-A:473–474.
10. Brånemark P-I, Adell R, Breine U, et al. Intra-osseous anchorage of dental prostheses. I. Experimental studies. Scand J Plast Reconstr Surg 1969;3:81–100.
11. Schroeder A, Pohler O, Sutter F. Gewebsreaktion auf ein Titan-Hohlzylinderimplantat mit Titan-Spritzschichtoberfläche [Tissue response to titanium plasma-sprayed hollow cylinder implants]. Schweiz Monatsschr Zahnheilkd 1976;86:713–727.
12. Schroeder A, Stich H, Straumann F, Sutter F. Über die Anlagerung von Osteozement an einen belasteten Implantatkörper [On hard tissue integration around a loaded endosseous implant]. Schweiz Monatsschr Zahnheilkd 1978;88:1051–1058.
13. Schroeder A, van der Zypen E, Stich H, Sutter F. The reactions of bone, connective tissue, and epithelium to endosteal implants with titanium-sprayed surfaces. J Maxillofac Surg 1981;9:15–25.
14. Gottlieb B. Der Epithelansatz am Zahne [The junctional epithelial attachment around natural teeth]. Dtsch Monatsschr Zahnheilkd 1921;5:142–147.
15. Orban B, Müller E. The gingival crevice. J Am Dent Assoc 1929;16:1206–1242.
16. Feneis H. Gefüge und Funktion des normalen Zahnfleischbindegewebes [Structural and functional aspects of healthy periodontal connective tissue]. Dtsch Zahnärztl Z 1952;2:467–476.
17. Sicher H. Changing concepts of the supporting dental structures. Oral Surg Oral Med Oral Pathol 1959;12:31–35.
18. Cochran DL, Mahn DH. Dental implants and regeneration, Part I. Overview and biological considerations. In: Hardin JF (ed). Clark's Clinical Dentistry (vol 5). Philadelphia: JB Lippincott, 1992:chap 59.
19. Gargiulo AW, Wentz FM, Orban B. Dimensions and relations of the dentogingival junction in humans. J Periodontol 1961;32:261–267.
20. Hermann JS, Buser D, Schenk RK, et al. Biologic width around one- and two-piece titanium implants: A histometric evaluation of unloaded nonsubmerged and submerged implants in the canine mandible. Clin Oral Implants Res 2001;12:559–571.
21. Cochran DL, Hermann JS, Schenk RK, et al. Biologic width around titanium implants: A histometric analysis of the implanto-gingival junction around unloaded and loaded nonsubmerged implants in the canine mandible. J Periodontol 1997;68:186–198.
22. Younger WJ. *Pyorrhea alveolaris* in the times of the pharoahs and the present Egyptians. Am Dent Soc Eur Trans 1905;12:85–89.
23. Younger WJ. *Pyorrhea alveolaris*. Schweiz Vierteljahrsschr Zahnheilkd 1905;15:87–108.
24. James RA, Kelln EE. A histopathological report on the nature of the epithelium and underlying connective tissue which surrounds oral implants. J Biomed Mater Res 1974;8:373–383.
25. Ericsson I, Berglundh T, Marinello C, et al. Long-standing plaque and gingivitis at implants and teeth in the dog. Clin Oral Implants Res 1992;3:99–103.
26. Tillmanns HW, Hermann JS, Cagna DR, et al. Evaluation of three different dental implants in ligature-induced periimplantitis in the beagle dog. Part I. Clinical evaluation. Int J Oral Maxillofac Implants 1997;12:611–620.
27. Tillmanns HW, Hermann JS, Tiffee JC, et al. Evaluation of three different dental implants in ligature-induced periimplantitis in the beagle dog. Part II. Histology and microbiology. Int J Oral Maxillofac Implants 1998;13:59–68.
28. Orban BJ, Bhatia H, Kollar JA, Wentz FM. The epithelial attachment (the attached epithelial cuff). J Periodontol 1956;27:167–180.
29. Schroeder HE. Ultrastructure of the junctional epithelium of the human gingiva. Helv Odontol Acta 1969;13:65–83.
30. Ingber JS, Rose LF, Coslet JG. The "biologic width": A concept in periodontics and restorative dentistry. Alpha Omegan 1977;70:62–65.
31. Ingber JS. Forced eruption: Part II. A method of treating nonrestorable teeth—Periodontal and restorative considerations. J Periodontol 1976;47:203–216.
32. James RA, Schultz RL. Hemidesmosomes and the adhesion of junctional epithelial cells to metal implants—A preliminary report. J Oral Implantol 1974;4:294–302.
33. Swope EM, James RA. A longitudinal study on hemidesmosome formation at the dental implant-tissue interface. J Oral Implantol 1981;9:412–422.
34. Gould TR, Brunette DM, Westbury L. The attachment mechanism of epithelial cells to titanium in vitro. J Periodontal Res 1981;16:611–616.
35. Gould TR, Westbury L, Brunette DM. Ultrastructural study of the attachment of human gingiva to titanium in vivo. J Prosthet Dent 1984;52:418–420.
36. Buser D, Weber HP, Donath K, et al. Soft tissue reactions to non-submerged unloaded titanium implants in beagle dogs. J Periodontol 1992;63:225–235.
37. Berglundh T, Lindhe J, Ericsson I, et al. The soft tissue barrier at implants and teeth. Clin Oral Implants Res 1991;2:81–90.
38. Abrahamsson I, Berglundh T, Wennström J, Lindhe J. The peri-implant hard and soft tissues at different implant systems. A comparative study in the dog. Clin Oral Implants Res 1996;7:212–219.

39. Abrahamsson I, Berglundh T, Moon IS, Lindhe J. Peri-implant tissues at submerged and non-submerged titanium implants. J Clin Periodontol 1999;26:600–607.

40. Adell R, Lekholm U, Rockler B, Brånemark P-I. A 15-year study of osseointegrated implants in the treatment of the edentulous jaw. Int J Oral Surg 1981;10:387–416.

41. Adell R, Lekholm U, Brånemark P-I. Surgical procedures. In: Brånemark P-I, Zarb GA, Albrektsson T (eds). Tissue-Integrated Prostheses: Osseointegration in Clinical Dentistry. London, Chicago: Quintessence, 1985:211–232.

42. Quirynen M, van Steenberghe D. Bacterial colonization of the internal part of two-stage implants. An in vivo study. Clin Oral Implants Res 1993;4:158–161.

43. Persson LG, Lekholm U, Leonhardt Å, et al. Bacterial colonization on internal surfaces of Brånemark system implant components. Clin Oral Implants Res 1996;7:90–95.

44. Buser D, Schenk RK, Steinemann S, et al. Influence of surface characteristics on bone integration of titanium implants. A histomorphometric study in miniature pigs. J Biomed Mater Res 1991;25:889–902.

45. Buser D, Nydegger T, Hirt HP, et al. Removal torque values of titanium implants in the maxilla of miniature pigs. Int J Oral Maxillofac Implants 1998;13:611–619.

46. Cochran DL, Buser D, ten Bruggenkate CM, et al. The use of reduced healing times on ITI implants with a sandblasted and acid-etched (SLA) surface: Early results from clinical trials on ITI SLA implants. Clin Oral Implants Res 2002;13:144-153.

47. Albrektsson T, Zarb G, Worthington P, Eriksson AR. The long-term efficacy of currently used dental implants: A review and proposed criteria of success. Int J Oral Maxillofac Implants 1986;1:11–25.

48. Alm Carlsson G. Dosimetry at interfaces. Acta Radiol Suppl 1973; 332:1–64.

49. Brånemark P-I, Hansson BO, Adell R, et al. Osseointegrated implants in the treatment of the edentulous jaw: Experience from a 10-year period. Scand J Plast Reconstr Surg 1977;16(suppl):1–132.

50. Buser D, Weber HP, Lang NP. Tissue integration of non-submerged implants: 1-year results of a prospective study with 100 ITI hollow-cylinder and hollow-screw implants. Clin Oral Implants Res 1990;1:33–40.

51. Weber HP, Buser D, Fiorellini JP, Williams RC. Radiographic evaluation of crestal bone levels adjacent to nonsubmerged titanium implants. Clin Oral Implants Res 1992;3:181–188.

52. Sutter F, Schroeder A, Buser DA. The new concept of ITI hollow-cylinder and hollow-screw implants: Part 1. Engineering and design. Int J Oral Maxillofac Implants 1988;3:161–172.

53. Buser DA, Schroeder A, Sutter F, Lang NP. The new concept of ITI hollow-cylinder and hollow-screw implants: Part 2. Clinical aspects, indications, and early clinical results. Int J Oral Maxillofac Implants 1988;3:173–181.

54. Buser D, Mericske-Stern R, Dula K, Lang NP. Clinical experience with one-stage, non-submerged dental implants. Adv Dent Res 1999;13:153–161.

55. Hermann JS, Cochran DL, Nummikoski PV, Buser D. Crestal bone changes around titanium implants: A radiographic evaluation of unloaded nonsubmerged and submerged implants in the canine mandible. J Periodontol 1997;68:1117–1130.

56. Hermann JS, Buser D, Schenk RK, Cochran DL. Crestal bone changes around titanium implants: A histometric evaluation of unloaded nonsubmerged and submerged implants in the canine mandible. J Periodontol 2000;71:1412–1424.

57. Hermann JS, Schoolfield JD, Nummikoski PV, et al. Crestal bone changes around titanium implants: A methodologic study comparing linear radiographic with histometric measurements. Int J Oral Maxillofac Implants 2001;16:475–485.

58. Hermann JS, Schoolfield JD, Schenk RK, et al. Influence of the size of the microgap on crestal bone changes around titanium implants: A histometric evaluation of unloaded nonsubmerged implants in the canine mandible. J Periodontol 2001;72:1372–1383.

59. Cochran DL. Implant therapy I. Ann Periodontol 1996;1:707–790.

60. Hermann JS, Buser D, Schenk RK, et al. Biologic width around titanium implants: A physiologically formed and stable dimension over time. Clin Oral Implants Res 2000;11:1–11.

61. Vacek JS, Gher ME, Assad DA, et al. The dimensions of the human dentogingival junction. Int J Periodontics Restorative Dent 1994;14:154–165.

62. Tsai N, McManus LM, Oates TW, et al. An evaluation of inflammation associated with the implant/abutment interface [abstract 197]. J Dent Res 2000;79:168.

63. Assuma R, Oates T, Cochran D, et al. IL-1 and TNF antagonists inhibit the inflammatory response and bone loss in experimental periodontitis. J Immunol 1998;160:403–409.

64. Graves DT, Delima AJ, Assuma R, et al. Interleukin-1 and tumor necrosis factor antagonists inhibit the progression of inflammatory cell infiltration toward alveolar bone in experimental periodontitis. J Periodontol 1998;69:1419–1425.

65. Saadoun AP, Sullivan DY, Krischek M, Le Gall M. Single tooth implant—Management for success. Pract Periodontics Aesthet Dent 1994;6:73–80.

66. Palacci P. Implant placement. In: Palacci P, Ericsson I, Engstrand P, Rangert B (eds). Optimal Implant Positioning and Soft Tissue Management for the Brånemark System. Chicago: Quintessence, 1995:35–39.

67. Spiekermann H. Single-tooth implants. In: Rateitschak KH, Wolf HF (eds). Color Atlas of Dental Medicine—Implantology, vol 1. New York: Thieme, 1995:267–298.

68. Nevins M, Stein JM. The placement of maxillary anterior implants. In: Nevins M, Mellonig JT (eds). Implant Therapy: Clinical Approaches and Evidence of Success, vol. 2. Chicago: Quintessence, 1998:111–127.

69. Garber DA, Belser UC. Restoration-driven implant placement with restoration-generated site development. Compend Contin Educ Dent 1995;16:796,798–802,804.

Treatment Planning for Implant Surgery

Thomas G. Wilson, Jr

- Patient Selection
- Treatment Planning
- Site Selection
- Situations for Initial Implant Experiences
- Choice of Implant System

Until the 1980s, dental implants failed predictably, and failure was often accompanied by extensive bone destruction.[1] These first-generation implants rested either on the bone (subperiosteal implants) or in the bone (blade implants), rather than fusing with the osseous tissue. Most implants failed within 10 years of placement.[1] Failure was often slow and characterized by periods of inflammation and pain. These facts led to less-than-universal acceptance of this mode of therapy,[2] and they still color the thinking of some dental professionals and the lay public.

The discovery of osseointegration[3] began to change the dental profession's attitude toward implants. Osseointegrated implants were found to function for many years,[4] and when failure occurred, the residual damage was usually minimal. Improvements in implant integration with both soft and hard tissues and the development of new methods for stabilizing the implant-prosthesis interface led to even more predictable outcomes.[5]

Implants are now an integral part of dentistry and can enhance almost every dental practice. With new materials and surfaces, as well as the use of new techniques, implant dentistry will continue to benefit patients for the foreseeable future. This chapter is designed to lead the practitioner or student through the issues involved in treatment planning for implant dentistry. Situations that are appropriate for individuals who are beginning their implant experience are emphasized. Advanced scenarios are described in chapter 39. The discussion is confined to osseointegrated dental implants. Both one-stage and two-stage approaches are covered.

Patient Selection

An extensive workup is often needed for the patient who will receive implants. Therefore, a short screening procedure designed to identify individuals most likely to benefit from these devices is suggested. More detailed information can then be gathered for patients who appear to be candidates for implant placement.

Screening Examination

At the first visit, the dental team can perform an abbreviated initial workup that might include the following:

1. *A brief review of the patient's general physical health.* Is the patient's cardiovascular system stable? Does the patient have any bleeding disorders? Does the patient have other major medical concerns (eg, diabetes mellitus)? Is the patient mentally competent to make decisions? Does the patient smoke?
2. *A screening oral examination.* Does the patient appear to have adequate oral hygiene? Do potential surgical sites appear to have sufficient soft and hard tissues? Is there adequate space for implants?
3. *A screening radiographic examination of the implant sites.* Periapical radiographs for individual sites and panoramic radiographs for multiple sites should be obtained.

If the patient is a potential implant candidate, an overview of the implant process and the economics involved, along with any alternative forms of therapy, is then presented. If the patient expresses interest in continuing the process, a comprehensive examination is initiated.

Comprehensive Examination

Gathering information in the following areas should result in a set of treatment plans that include a full range of options from no treatment to the most comprehensive care. The advantages and disadvantages of each plan are then described, and the patient ultimately gives informed consent.

Medical History

The patient usually completes a medical/dental history, which is followed by a dialogue between the practitioner and the patient. Normal considerations for all dental patients should be evaluated, along with these additional factors:

1. *Contraindications to implant placement*—uncontrolled endocrine disorders, such as diabetes mellitus; psychosis; abnormal wound healing that would predictably result in implant failure; uncontrolled bleeding disorders; some immune disorders, including uncontrolled HIV infection; and other diseases or conditions outlined by the patient's physician
2. *Relative medical contraindications to implant placement*—history of head and neck radiation, cigarette smoking, and other areas outlined by the patient's physician

When suitable doubt exists, the practitioner should contact the patient's physician before initiating therapy.

Dental History

The patient's view of his or her dental history is collected on the same written questionnaire as the medical history and is usually followed by a conversation on the topic with the patient. The patient's general dental knowledge, motivation, and understanding of implants should be ascertained.

The relative dental contraindications for osseointegrated dental implants include a lack of ability or willingness on the part of the patient to try to keep the implant clean, especially during the initial stages of healing. This is especially important with single-stage implants, which are exposed to the oral environment from the time of placement. The inability to obtain adequate bone at the implant site also contraindicates placement.

Comprehensive Clinical Examination/Testing

The extraoral clinical examination may detect facial asymmetries, soft and hard tissue pathology, and signs of temporomandibular joint disorders. The intraoral examination includes evaluation of nonperiodontal soft tissues.

The dental examination may reveal dental caries, restorations/prostheses, tooth mobility, cracked or fractured teeth, occlusal habits, interarch distance, maxillomandibular relationships, tooth position, and tooth alignment. The following may also be determined: probing depths (six per tooth and as many as six per implant), gingival recession, bleeding on probing/suppuration, furcation involvement, level of adjacent cementoenamel junctions, amount of keratinized gingiva, and width and height of osseous tissue at the implant site.

Treatment Planning

The treatment planning phase of therapy usually involves the restorative dentist and surgeon, often with input from laboratory technicians and other dental or medical professionals.

Adjunctive Therapy

When the clinical and radiographic examinations, histories, and consultations have been completed and initial consent obtained, treatment planning can begin. While dental implants are an important part of therapy, it must be emphasized that they are only one part and one option. Many other aspects of dentistry affect dental implants and vice versa. Several of these areas of possible interaction are outlined below.

Periodontal Therapy

Microbiota around teeth with healthy gingiva are similar to those found around implants with healthy peri-implant tissues; likewise, teeth with periodontitis and implants with peri-implantitis have similar bacterial ecosystems.[6] While there is discussion on the importance of bacteria in the etiology of implant failure, seeding of bacteria apparently occurs from natural teeth to implants.[6] Thus, a periodontal examination is needed prior to implant therapy, as is appropriate periodontal treatment in conjunction with implant therapy and maintenance following the completion of active implant therapy in dentate patients.

Endodontic Therapy

Endodontic therapy should be started before implant therapy in areas where inflammation from the endodontic lesion could affect the implant site. In addition to reducing the probability of infection around the implant, this approach yields more information on endodontic status before implant therapy begins, thus allowing formulation of a more accurate prognosis for individual teeth in the overall treatment plan.

Orthodontic Therapy

Orthodontic considerations are important in the treatment of implant patients for several reasons (see chapter 33 for more details).

1. Placement of the implants may alter orthodontic treatment planning. For example, when a second molar has tipped into an edentulous first molar site, orthodontics might be used to right the second molar or move it into the site of the missing first molar. With implant therapy, the tooth can be righted and an implant placed in the first molar site, saving time and eliminating the stress of bodily movement of the second molar.
2. Once implants are integrated, they do not move. Therefore, any orthodontic therapy should be planned with the final implant site in mind. In some cases, this can mean delaying implant placement until after completion of orthodontic therapy to ensure proper implant placement.
3. Osseointegrated implants can be used as anchorage units for orthodontic movement.[7,8] These implants are usually placed before orthodontic movement begins.

Implant or Fixed Partial Denture?

In the past, the choice of an implant or fixed partial denture (FPD) was simple, because tooth-supported FPDs lasted longer and were more predictable than their implant counterparts. This paradigm has changed, however. The science of implant dentistry has advanced to the point where an implant is clearly the replacement of choice in most situations. When tooth-supported FPDs fail, the abutment teeth often require repair or removal. This is especially true when endodontic therapy has been previously performed on one of the abutments. On average, implants today clearly have much greater longevity than do FPDs attached to teeth.

The results of two meta-analysis studies summarize the state of the art. One of those studies covered survival rates of FPDs,[9] and the other looked at implant survival.[10] Implants were more successful at all time periods when used to replace a single missing tooth or multiple units. This means that for young patients, implants are preferred, because the average life span of a tooth-supported FPD is less than that of a single implant. The average tooth-supported FPD will need to be replaced several times during the patient's lifetime. In an older patient who has caries on periodontally healthy abutment teeth, a tooth-supported

FPD is often the best choice. Where the abutment teeth are not able to support an FPD, an implant is the clear choice. Between these two extremes, an implant is usually the best choice.

Consider the following scenario: A patient with a single missing tooth is in good health, has an average life expectancy, has acceptable oral hygiene, and his oral environment is conducive to, or can be made conducive to, either implants or an FPD. The primary situations in which an FPD could be justified as the treatment choice would be if the patient is at least 70 years old and has caries on the potential abutment teeth, or if the patient refuses implant therapy. However, implants clearly are superior to FPDs when multiple teeth are to be replaced.

Site Selection

To enhance the probability of success and to make the most of the learning experience, the clinician should be very selective in choosing sites for initial implant experiences. For this reason, it is important to have (1) sufficient bone to surround the implant and provide adequate stability during the healing phase, (2) adequate plaque control during healing (for one-stage implants or two-stage implants placed as one-stage implants), and (3) absence of inappropriate functional loading during the healing phase.

Evaluating Bone Support

Panoramic films and a complete set of periapical and bitewing radiographs (where appropriate) are part of the screening process for most patients. These films will reveal the apicocoronal and mesiodistal dimensions of potential implant sites.

Information on the bony configuration in a buccolingual dimension will help show the amount of bone available for implant placement and indicate the space the implant-supported prosthesis will need to fill. There are two ways to get information on the buccolingual dimension of the bone:

1. *Lateral tomograms.* The information from these films can be enhanced by making a template from a model of the proposed prosthesis, placing a radiopaque marker in the template, and having the patient wear the template while the tomogram is taken. These films are less expensive and deliver less radiation than do computerized tomography scans.
2. *Computerized tomograms.* In some cases, computerized tomograms are preferable to conventional ones. They are more expensive and deliver more radiation, but they can be used with the same radiographic tem-

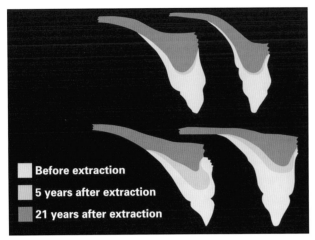

Fig 35-1 Bone resorption seen in representative tracings of cross sections of maxillae on cephalometric radiographs in patients who received immediate dentures. (Modified from Bergman and Carlsson,[11] with permission.)

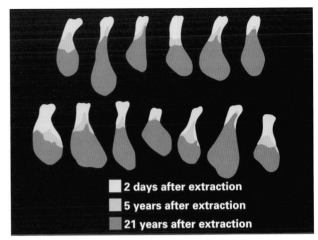

Fig 35-2 Tracings taken from cross sections of the anterior mandible 2 days, 5 years, and 21 years after extraction of teeth in 13 patients. All the patients had maxillary dentures. (Modified from Bergman and Carlsson,[11] with permission.)

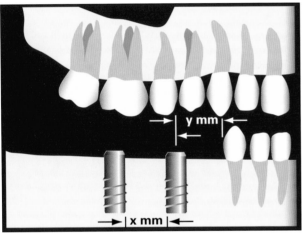

Fig 35-3 Dimensions needed for a partially edentulous site vary depending on implant dimensions. In general, there should be at least 3 mm between tooth root and implant body (y) and at least 3 mm between implant walls (x).

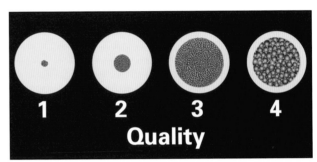

Fig 35-4 In Type 1 bone, most of the osseous tissue is compact. Type 2 bone has a thick layer of compact bone. Type 3 bone has some compact bone that surrounds a core of dense trabecular bone, whereas Type 4 bone has a thin, compact layer and low-density trabecular bone. This classification allows communication on the quality of bone, which is important because there tends to be a higher failure rate in less dense bone. (Modified from Lekholm and Zarb,[12] with permission.)

plates described in chapter 37. These films are useful in cases with multiple potential implant sites. Recent advances in evaluation software for personal computers designed to analyze computerized tomograms make this type of scan more useful.

Buccolingual bone configuration is particularly important in the anterior maxilla, where esthetics is a concern. If a great deal of resorption has occurred and bone augmentation is not an option, a fixed/removable device must be ruled out, because the resulting tooth replacements would be long apico-occlusally and/or very bulky buccolingually (Figs 35-1 and 35-2). To solve this problem, an implant-supported denture may be constructed; proce-dures are also available to enlarge the bone and soft tissue available for implant placement[13] (see chapter 39). In addition, adequate room should be allowed between the implant shoulder and the occlusal surface of the tooth in the opposing arch (Fig 35-3). This requires an evaluation of the apicocoronal height and buccolingual dimension of bone, as well as the interarch distance.

If there is enough bone in the correct location to support implants, the density of the bone should be determined next. A bone density scale has been developed, with the most compact bone termed *Type I* and the least, *Type IV* (Fig 35-4).[12] In general, the densest bone is found in the anterior mandible and the most cancellous, in the posterior maxilla.

Bone quality, width, and height influence the choice of implant diameter and length. When placed in mature bone, an implant should have at least 1 mm of bone on all sides.

Selection of Individual Implants

In general, fewer and shorter implants are needed in denser bone; wider and longer implants are best in patients who grind or clench their teeth; and the greater the percentage of bone-to-implant contact, the fewer implants needed.

Indications for Individual Implant Shapes

At present, there are three general implant shapes: screws, tapered designs, and cylinders. Screws provide the most initial stability, followed by tapered bodies and then cylinders. Proper screw thread angulation can distribute load to the bone in such a way as to increase its density. For these reasons, the screw form is preferable in most situations. Customized shapes and sizes of implant body can be helpful in selected situations.

Situations for Initial Implant Experiences

Single-Tooth Replacement in a Nonesthetic Site

Depending on the site, single-tooth replacement can be one of the simplest or one of the most challenging implant placement procedures. An ideal site for clinicians gaining experience would have the following characteristics:

- At least 1 mm of bone surrounding the implant on all sides and at least 7 mm of interocclusal (interarch) distance measured from the top (shoulder) of the implant to the occlusal surface of the opposing tooth
- At least 3 mm of clearance between the adjacent teeth and the widest portion of the implant
- A posterior site with mature bone
- A buffer zone of approximately 3 mm from the inferior alveolar nerve or the floor of the sinus to the apex of the implant

Completely Edentulous Patients

Some edentulous people do well with conventional full dentures, especially on the maxillary arch. These prostheses can be constructed relatively quickly, and a surgical procedure (with the possible exception of tooth extrac-tion) is usually not needed. Conventional full dentures are also less expensive than their implant-supported counterparts. However, a significant number of people require or prefer an implant-supported prosthesis, some because they cannot tolerate a conventional denture and some because the prosthesis will not function without increased retention. Denture instability may cause tissue irritation, decrease masticatory function, and accelerate its own progressive instability. Implant-supported prostheses are often preferred particularly in the mandibular arch because of the stability they can provide. Three treatment situations are described below, in order of increasing complexity.

Option 1: Denture Retained by Independent Implants

For the patient who is happy with a denture, whose denture is not causing soft tissue irritation, but who needs additional retention, two individual implants with retentive abutments can be used. Normally, the implants are placed in the canine regions. Because the laboratory phase is less complex than for implant-supporting bars, this approach costs less. The disadvantage is that freestanding implants can receive individual forces strong enough to induce failure. Therefore, this approach is most often useful in the mandibular arch, and even then a bar may be appropriate. Retentive anchors that fit into female receptacles placed inside the denture are available (Fig 35-5). If these anchors are used, the implants should be placed as parallel to each other as possible. In most cases, the patient's denture must be remade, because the additional masticatory forces that can be generated with the implants can result in fracture of the original denture. A new denture reinforced with metal is suggested.

Option 2: Denture Supported by a Bar and Clips

Where additional retention and denture stability are desired, implants can be joined with a bar and clips placed inside the denture to provide retention. Generally two implants can support a bar. However, more implants can be added if the patient wants to minimize contact between the denture and the soft tissue (Fig 35-6). The bar is either oval (a round bar) or egg shaped (a Dolder bar) in cross section. The round bar is often preferred because of its additional retention. The clips are processed inside the denture and fit over the bar for retention. The implants should be spaced far enough apart to allow clips to be placed.

Option 3: A Fixed or Fixed/Removable Prosthesis (for Advanced Therapists)

For patients who want a prosthesis that they cannot remove, a fixed/removable prosthesis is often the answer. The term *fixed/removable* refers to a device that is retained

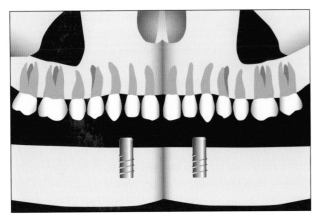

Fig 35-5 For implants with retentive anchors, the implants are usually placed in the canine positions in the mandible.

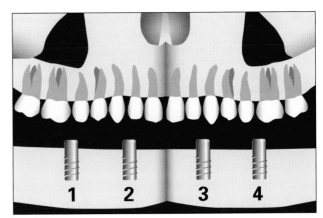

Fig 35-6 For a prosthesis retained by a bar and clip, the 1 and 4 implants are best placed in the first molar/second premolar area unless the distance occlusal to the inferior alveolar nerve precludes an implant. Implants in the 2 and 3 positions are usually in the canine positions or slightly mesial to this position.

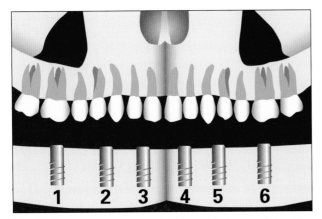

Fig 35-7 Normally, five (or more) long or six (or more) short implants are used to support a fixed/removable restoration. If five implants are to be used, the implant in either the 3 or 4 position is eliminated.

by screws and can be removed by the practitioner but not by the patient. Fixed partial dentures would be retained solely by cement. Both fixed and fixed/removable devices usually require more implants per arch than do other implant-supported full dentures, and the laboratory steps are more complex. Some patients prefer this approach in spite of additional cost and increased difficulty of oral hygiene compared with an implant-supported denture because this prosthesis most closely mimics the natural dentition (Fig 35-7).

When treatment planning is complete, a final consultation is held with the patient. Often several possible treatment plans, ranging from no treatment to comprehensive care, are reviewed. The advantages and disadvantages of each approach should be discussed, and the patient should be given enough information to make an informed decision. Following the patient's informed consent, therapy begins.

Choice of Implant System

There are many different implant systems from which to choose, and the selection of a system may be based on many criteria. It is suggested that the system chosen have well-documented long-term success based on prospective studies, be easy-to-use, have proven strength and accurate fitting, and have strong prosthetic components. It is also convenient if the system has service representatives readily available to answer questions and provide other assistance.

Two basic bone-to-implant interfaces are available: titanium and hydroxyapatite (HA). While HA has been shown to attach more rapidly and more completely to bone initially than does titanium,[14,15] long-term failure is more likely to be seen around HA-coated surfaces.[16–18] In contrast, the bone-titanium interface has been shown to increase over time[4] and can reach levels close to those found with HA.[19] Although new information may lead to the selection of HA-coated implants in the future, titanium is suggested at present.

Several surface modifications of titanium are available. It is suggested that the implant system chosen have a surface modification that allows loading of the implant as rapidly as possible.[19] The more rapidly an implant can be loaded, the less time the patient and the practitioner must spend dealing with the problems (or absence) of provisional restorations.

The relative strength of the implant itself is another important consideration. In general, larger-diameter implants made from stronger grades of titanium fracture less often.

Although the original versions of osseointegrated implants were designed to be covered by soft tissues during initial healing, some implants have been designed specifically for use with a one-stage, transgingival surgical procedure. These implants feature a smooth, polished neck that is designed to move the implant interface coronal to the alveolar bone. Initial concerns that transgingival placement would allow growth of epithelium that would encompass the implant, and therefore lead to failure, have proven to be groundless.[20] In fact, there is more apical migration of the epithelium around implants designed for two-stage placement than one-stage systems. Clinical experience has shown that placement of the implant-abutment interface coronal to the bone decreases inflammation in the peri-implant soft tissues and makes the implant-abutment interface more accessible for cleaning. It should be noted that implant systems originally designed for two-stage approaches (two surgeries) have been suggested for use in a one-stage technique.[21] The advantages of a one-stage approach include reduced trauma to the patient, reduced chair time for the therapist, and decreased expenses (due to fewer visits).

Ease of use and strength of prosthetic components are also important criteria in implant system selection. Because the implants themselves have become less likely to fracture due to larger diameters or stronger grades of titanium, failure is often seen at the prosthetic interface. This argues for a solid, well-fitting prosthetic component. To increase prosthetic options, the implant system chosen should provide multiple prosthetic interfaces, which should include screw-retained and conventional abutments, as well as those designed for use with removable prostheses. In screw-retained prostheses, the occlusal screw is the weakest link in the system, and fracture of these screws causes inconvenience for the patient and significantly increased chair time for the clinician. Selection of a system that has addressed this problem will decrease frustration for all involved.

Selection of an implant system should be based on long-term success as reported by prospective studies, the type of surfaces available, and the prosthetic interfaces available. Customer service and company history are other considerations.

References

1. Bodine RI, Yanase RT. Thirty-year report on 28 implant dentures inserted between 1952 and 1959. [Presented at the International Symposium on Preprosthetic Surgery, Palm Springs, California, May 16–18, 1985.]
2. National Institutes of Health Consensus Development Conference (publication no. NIH-81-1531). Bethesda, MD: National Institutes of Health, 1980.
3. Albrektsson T, Brånemark P-I, Hansson HA, Lindstrom J. Osseointegrated titanium implants: Requirements for ensuring a long-lasting direct bone-to-implant anchorage in man. Acta Orthop Scand 1981;52:155–170.
4. Brånemark P-I, Hansson BO, Adell R, et al. Osseointegrated implants in the treatment of the edentulous jaw. Experience from a 10-year period. Scand J Plast Reconstr Surg Suppl 1977;16:1–132.
5. Schroeder A, et al. Gewebsreaktion auf ein Titan-Hohlzylinder implantat mit Titan-Spritzchichtoberflache. Schweiz Monatsschr Zahnheilk 1976;86:713–727.
6. Mombelli A, van Oosten MA, Schurch E Jr, Lang NP. The microbiota associated with successful or failing osseointegrated titanium implants. Oral Microbiol Immunol 1987;2:145–151.
7. Higuchi KW, Slack JM. The use of titanium fixtures for intraoral anchorage to facilitate orthodontic tooth movement. Int J Oral Maxillofac Implants 1991;6:338–344.
8. Wehrbein H, Merz BR, Diedrich P, Glatzmaier J. The use of palatal implants for orthodontic anchorage. Design and clinical application of the orthosystem. Clin Oral Implants Res 1996;7:410–416.
9. Scurria MS, Bader JD, Shugars DA. Meta-analysis of fixed partial denture survival: Prostheses and abutments. J Prosthet Dent 1998;79:459–464.
10. Lindh T, Gunne J, Tillberg A, Molin M. A meta-analysis of implants in partial edentulism. Clin Oral Implants Res 1998;9(2):80–90.
11. Bergman B, Carlsson GE. Clinical long-term study of complete denture wearers. J Prosthet Dent 1985;53:56–61.
12. Lekholm U, Zarb GA. Patient selection and preparation. In: Brånemark P-I, Zarb G, Albrektsson T (eds). Tissue-Integrated Prosthesis: Osseointegration in Clinical Dentistry. Chicago: Quintessence, 1985:199–209.
13. Buser D, Bragger U, Lang NP, Nyman S. Regeneration and enlargement of jaw bone using guided tissue regeneration. Clin Oral Implants Res 1990;1:22–32.
14. Block MS, Kent JN. Factors associated with soft- and hard-tissue compromise of endosseous implants. J Oral Maxillofac Surg 1990;48:1153–1160.
15. Krauser J. HA-coated root-form implants—Is there cause for concern? Dent Implantol Update 1993;4:37–42.
16. Fugazzotto PA, Gulbransen HJ, Wheeler SL, Lindsay JA. The use of IMZ osseointegrated implants in partially and completely edentulous patients: Success and failure rates of 2,023 implant cylinders up to 60+ months in function. Int J Oral Maxillofac Implants 1993;8:617–621.
17. Wheeler S. Eight-year clinical retrospective study of titanium plasma-sprayed and hydroxyapatite-coated cylinder implants. Int J Oral Maxillofac Implants 1996;11:340–350.
18. Johnson BW. HA-coated dental implants: Long term consequences. J Calif Dent Assoc 1992;20(6):33–41.
19. Buser D, Nydegger T, Hirt HP, et al. Removal torque values of titanium implants in the maxilla of miniature pigs. Int J Oral Maxillofac Implants 1998;13:611–619.
20. Buser D, Weber HP, Donath K, et al. Soft tissue reactions to nonsubmerged unloaded titanium implants in beagle dogs. J Periodontol 1992;63:226–236.
21. Becker W, Becker BE, Israelson H. One-step surgical placement of Branemark implants: A prospective multicenter clinical study. Int J Oral Maxillofac Implants 1997;12:454–462.

Radiography in Dental Implant Assessment

Neil L. Frederiksen
• Intraoral Radiography
• Extraoral Radiography

Osseointegrated dental implants have been found to be a viable treatment alternative for the rehabilitation of the edentulous or partially dentulous patient. Success rates are high for these surgically implanted endosseous implants. This rate of success depends in large part on the careful selection of the patient, the site of implantation, and postsurgical evaluation of the implant over time.

Radiography often provides the only means by which the clinician can evaluate the suitability of the morphologic features of a proposed implantation site.[1] The radiographic technique chosen should provide for a determination of the relationship of anatomic structures, including the relationship of the maxillary sinus and inferior alveolar canal to the site, and for visualization of the inclination of the alveolar process at the site. Radiographic techniques should also provide images on which measurements can be made of bone in the vertical, interdental (mesiodistal or between the teeth), and facial-lingual (cross-sectional) planes. Accurate measurements of available bone at the site are essential prior to implantation.[2] In general, 7.0 mm of interdental bone is required for the placement of a standard-diameter (4.0- to 5.0-mm) implant. For standard implant placement in the mandible, there should be at least 7-mm of bone in the vertical dimension and 7-mm of bone in the facial-lingual dimension. In cases selected for initial implant experiences, additional bone is suggested. These recommendations limit the possibility of contacting the inferior alveolar nerve during the surgical preparation of the implant site. For implant placement in the maxilla, these dimensions should be at least 7 mm in the vertical dimension and 7 mm in the facial-lingual dimension. Smaller dimensions may require bone augmentation procedures prior to the placement of implants and are not suggested for initial implant experiences.

The imaging technique should also allow for evaluation of bone quality. A grading system, from 1 to 4, for the assessment of bone quality has been used by many clinicians.[3] This system is based on the morphology of trabecular bone and the thickness of cortical bone. The greater the thickness of cortical bone and smaller the marrow spaces (grades 1 and 2), the higher the bone quality in terms of the success of osseointegration. The thinner the cortical bone and larger the marrow spaces (grades 3 and 4), the lower the quality of bone.

Several available imaging techniques address these questions, and each has its own usefulness in implant diagnostics.[4–6] It should be noted that no universal imaging technique can answer all concerns relative to the potential site of implantation. The cost and accuracy of the imaging procedure and the radiation dose resulting from the procedure (Table 36-1) should be considered, but they should not be primary determinants of the technique selected. Putting the success of an implantation procedure at risk because of a perceived need to save money or to limit exposure to radiation would be difficult to justify. At present, there is no direct evidence that the magnitude of radiation exposure received as a result of these diagnostic procedures has any adverse biologic effect.[12]

Table 36-1 Effective Dose (E),* Equivalent Natural Exposure,[†] and Probability of Stochastic Effects[‡] by Radiographic Technique

Survey	E (μSv)	Days of equivalent natural exposure	Probability of stochastic effects ($\times 10^{-6}$)
Intraoral			
Round collimation, D-speed film[7]			
Periapical (15 films)	111	13.9	8.1
Interproximal (4 films)	38	4.8	2.8
Complete-mouth survey (19 films)	150	18.8	11.0
Rectangular collimation, E-speed film[8]			
Complete-mouth survey (20 films)	17	2.1	1.2
Extraoral[9]			
Panoramic	26	3.3	1.9
Film tomography[9]			
Anterior			
Round	< 1	<< 1	<<< 1
Rectangular	5.0	0.6	0.4
Premolar			
Round	13	1.6	0.9
Rectangular	30	3.8	2.2
Molar			
Round	11	1.4	0.8
Rectangular	26	3.3	1.9
Computerized tomography			
Maxilla	104[10]–1,202[11]	13.0–150.3	7.6–87.7
Mandible	761[10]–3,324[11]	95.1–415.5	55.6–242.7

*An estimate for the uniform whole body exposure carrying the same probability of radiation effect as a partial body exposure.
[†]The product of the E resulting from the examination and the average daily E (8 μSv) delivered by background radiation.
[‡]An effect whose probability of occurrence increases with radiation dose without a threshold. An example is cancer.

Intraoral Radiography

Periapical Radiography

Analog (X-ray film) or digital (charge-coupled device or storage phosphor) intraoral periapical images may provide evidence for the presence of pathosis, the relative relationship of anatomic structures to the proposed implant site, and an estimate of the quality of trabecular bone. Periapical images allow measurement of available bone in the vertical and mesiodistal planes, assuming image magnification is approximately 6% in films made using the parallel technique. Unfortunately, these images do not always allow a dependable assessment of bone in the vertical plane because the image receptor sometimes cannot be placed parallel to the alveolar ridge in the vertical plane, as directed by the parallel technique (see chapter 18). Information on the interdental dimension is best obtained from clinical examination, but periapical images may confirm these findings and determine that the measurement of bone in this plane is not compromised by the angulation of adjacent tooth roots. Periapical images also provide no information on the quantity of bone in the facial-lingual or cross-sectional plane. The high resolution of analog intraoral images, relative to extraoral images, does allow for the demonstration of pathological changes within bone that may have a negative influence on the success of the implantation procedure.

Digital intraoral images may provide the same information as analog images (Fig 36-1). However, digital imaging has some advantages over analog imaging. Digital images may

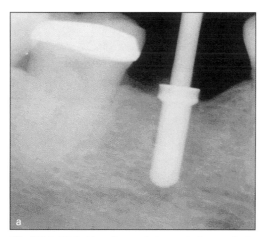
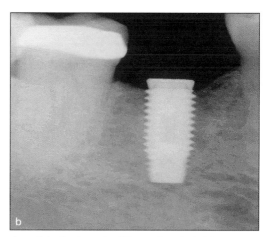

Fig 36-1 Digital imaging techniques during surgical preparation of the implant site (Digora, Soredex). Digital intraoral imaging techniques, while providing the same information as analog imaging techniques, are preferred during surgery because of the speed with which an image may be acquired. (a) An instrument has been inserted into the preparation to assess the pathway of insertion. (b) Image made after implant placement.

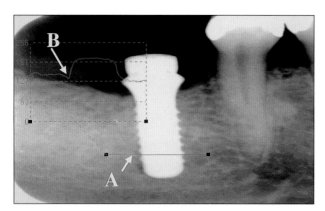

Fig 36-2 Implant evaluation by direct digital imaging (Digora, Soredex). After image acquisition and processing, density values of pixels along a selected line (A) are presented in both numeric and graphic forms. A density profile presents density values along the selected line in graphic form. An area of decreased density (B) adjacent to the implant may indicate a lack of integration.

be electronically processed after acquisition to enhance density and contrast. They may be transmitted electronically to obtain a second opinion, and they require only 10% to 25% of the radiation required to expose a D-speed intraoral radiographic film to diagnostic density. Further, direct digital imaging is almost real-time imaging. This factor makes digital imaging particularly useful for monitoring progress during the surgical placement of implants.

Evaluation of Implants Over Time

The success of an implant can be measured by an absence of mobility, pain, and clinical signs of inflammation; a radiolucency associated with the bone-implant interface;

and a vertical bone loss of 1 to 2 mm or less around machined surface implants in the first year and 0.1 to 0.2 mm in each succeeding year.[2] With the exception of mobility, pain, and inflammation, these factors may be assessed radiographically. The technique of choice for postoperative evaluation is the intraoral parallel technique using either a film or digital image receptor (Fig 36-2).

Intraoral periapical radiography allows the clinician to adjust the central ray of the X-ray beam to each implant individually. Adjustment of the central ray to each implant is necessary because an accurate assessment of the relationship of implant to bone cannot be made if there is a deviation from true parallel technique. Threaded implants have the advantage of making it relatively easy to determine whether or not the central ray has been directed perpendicular to both the plane of the image receptor and the long axis of the implant.[13] When this relationship exists between the implant and the central ray, the implant's threads will be clearly imaged on both sides of the implant. If the threads on the left side are clearly imaged and those on the right are indistinct, the X-ray beam was directed at a more positive vertical angle (inferiorly) than optimal. If the threads on the right side are clearly imaged and those on the left are indistinct, the X-ray beam was directed at a more negative vertical angle (superiorly) than optimal. This finding applies to radiographs of either the maxilla or the mandible. Corrections of approximately 10 degrees are required if the threads are clearly imaged on only one side. If the image of threads on both sides of the implant is obscured, a correction greater than 10 degrees, but in the same direction as noted above, would be required (Fig 36-3).

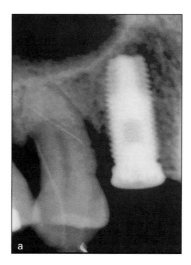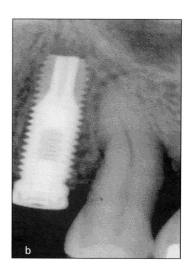

Fig 36-3 Implant evaluation. Parameters of implant success may be assessed radiographically only in images made using the parallel technique. If the central ray of the X-ray beam is not directed perpendicular to the long axis of the implant and/or the film plane is not parallel to the long axis of the implant, an accurate determination of the relationship of implant to bone cannot be made. *(a)* Image acquired using a technique other than the parallel technique. Note the absence of a clear image of the implant's threads. *(b)* Image acquired using the parallel technique. Note the clarity of the threads on both sides of the implant.

After it has been determined that there is no radiolucency associated with the bone-implant interface and the patient is clinically asymptomatic, there may be no reason to include the entire length of the implant in the image. In this case, a smaller film size or a bitewing radiograph can be used and be more easily placed following the principles of the parallel technique.

Occlusal Radiography

Intraoral occlusal radiography may be used to estimate available bone in the facial-lingual plane. However, true cross-sectional imaging in the occlusal plane, unobstructed by superimposition of the images of other structures, is feasible only in the mandibular arch. Occlusal images of the mandible show only the maximum width of the jaw. This characteristic may obscure the image of an anatomic depression such as the submandibular fossa, the presence and location of which may be a significant factor in determining the placement of an implant.

Extraoral Radiography

Cephalometric Radiography

The lateral cephalometric radiograph can provide details of the morphology of both the maxilla and mandible, the relationship of the maxilla to the mandible, and the inclination of the alveolar process and its vertical and facial-lingual dimensions in both the maxilla and mandible. Measurements obtained from these images are relatively accurate, because the technique provides for a determination of image magnification. The lateral cephalometric radiograph is of limited value in implant diagnostics, how-

ever. The observations noted above can be made only in the anterior maxilla and mandible of edentulous patients, and most are redundant because they can be determined by clinical examination.

Panoramic Radiography

The usefulness of the panoramic radiograph in implant diagnostics rests with the film's ability to provide the clinician with a view of the entire maxilla and mandible. The panoramic radiograph is perhaps most useful in the initial diagnostic phase of patient evaluation. This radiograph can be used to evaluate the maxilla and mandible, teeth, maxillary sinus, and temporomandibular joint for gross pathological changes. It indicates the spatial relationships of anatomic structures and their involvement with the alveolar ridge, and it allows the clinician to observe established relationships between maxilla and mandible. However, this film technique has a number of limitations that hinder its contribution to implant diagnostics. An appreciation of these limitations requires an understanding of how the image is made.

The panoramic radiograph is unique in that the focus of projection, or the apparent source of the X-ray beam, is different in the vertical and horizontal planes. In the vertical plane, the effective focus of projection is the focal spot of the X-ray tube, like that of an intraoral periapical or bitewing projection. In the horizontal plane, however, the effective source of X rays is the rotation center of the X-ray beam as it sweeps around the patient. The presence of two foci of projection, at two distinct locations relative to the film, results in the possibility of having a magnification factor in the vertical plane that is different from that in the horizontal plane. In practice, magnification in the vertical plane is relatively constant throughout the image because

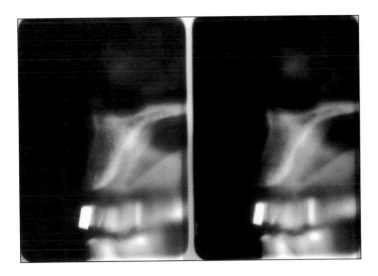

Fig 36-4 Preplacement diagnostics. During the treatment planning phase, an imaging stent with cylindrical markers was made. These markers were placed at the proposed sites using the insertion angles clinically determined to be appropriate for the implants. With the stent in place, octospiral tomograms (Scanora, Soredex) were made of the areas containing the markers. These tomograms of the anterior maxilla show the relationship of the marker to the alveolar ridge and the inferior wall of the nasal fossa. Tomographic slices with a thickness of 4 mm were made to maximize contrast and enhance the perception of detail.

of the relatively constant relationship between focal spot, object, and film. Magnification in the horizontal plane, in contrast, may vary considerably because of the constantly changing distance between the rotational center and the film, as well as the changing rate of movement of the film relative to the X-ray beam. Magnification of the image in the vertical dimension is equal to that in the horizontal dimension only when the dental arches are positioned in the exact center of the curved plane of the focal trough. This means that two factors, patient positioning and the conformity of the patient's dental arches to the focal trough, are important in the production of an image with uniform magnification in both the vertical and horizontal planes. Because of anatomic variability and difficulties encountered in patient positioning, consistently uniform magnification in these two planes is difficult to achieve.

Another principle of panoramic radiography that should be considered is that the X-ray beam is directed upward to the film from below, at a negative vertical angle relative to the occlusal plane. This may misrepresent the amount of available bone in the vertical dimension and the relationship of anatomic structures, such as the maxillary sinus, to the crest of the alveolar ridge. Finally, an assessment of both the quality and quantity of bone at a potential site of implantation cannot be made from the panoramic radiograph, because it is a two-dimensional image of a three-dimensional object.

Film Tomography

Tomography is a technique designed to image more clearly structures lying within a selected layer of the body referred to as the *focal plane*. This goal is accomplished in part by the coordinated movement of the radiographic tube and film, which rotate or pivot around an axis at the focal plane. This movement blurs the images of objects both superficial to and deeper than the layer of interest, leaving the images of objects at the focal plane relatively sharp. There are several types of tomographic motion, ranging from the relatively simple linear, circular, and elliptical to the more complex hypocycloidal and octospiral. As a general rule, the more complex the motion, the more sharply imaged are objects located at the focal plane. Because the tomographic image represents a flat plane rather than a curved plane as produced in panoramic imaging, accurate linear measurements can be made in these images.

The perception of a radiographic image is due in part to image contrast. Image contrast, in turn, is partly related to the thickness of the image layer at the focal plane. Depending on the tomographic equipment used, an image layer thickness of 1 to 8 mm may be achieved. Relatively thin image layers of 1 to 2 mm may not provide sufficient contrast to allow for visualization of the thin cortical border associated with the inferior alveolar canal. Acquisition of image layers of 4 mm appear to represent a compromise between layers too thin to provide adequate contrast and those too thick to provide sufficient detail at the focal plane.

Film tomography can provide the clinician with information that intraoral and panoramic radiography cannot. The technique can accurately assess the alveolar process in the vertical, interdental, and facial-lingual planes. The images can be used to determine the bone quality at the proposed site of implantation. Tomograms can be used to evaluate the inclination of the alveolar process and the relationship of the maxilla to the mandible. Finally, tomograms may demonstrate the spatial relationship of anatomic structures to the proposed site of implantation (Fig 36-4).

Fig 36-5 Multiplanar reformatting of CT data acquired in the axial plane. Following acquisition and reconstruction of all axial images, data pertaining to these images are reformatted to multiplanar images using specially designed software (3-D Dental, Materialise/Columbia Scientific). (A) The relative location of the 38 axial CT scans completed on this patient are shown. The technician then selected a midlevel axial image and electronically drew a curve on the image that was concentric to the anatomic curvature of the dental arch. The software then reformatted three-dimensional and multiple panoramic and cross-sectional images that are concentric with, and perpendicular to, the drawn curve, respectively. Their relative location is noted on the reference axial image (B). (C) Image acquisition technical information. (D) Catalog of the reformatted images.

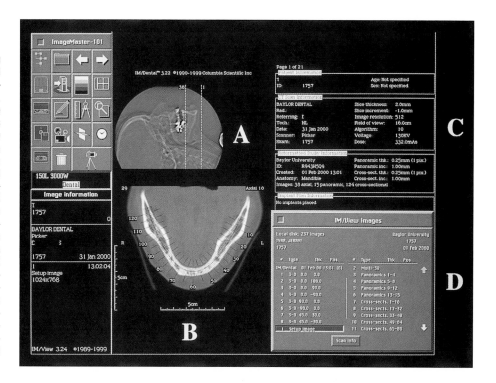

Fig 36-6 Multiplanar reformatting (3-D Dental). Three-dimensional images show the surface of the bony anatomy within the limits of the CT scanning sequence that consisted of 38 axial images.

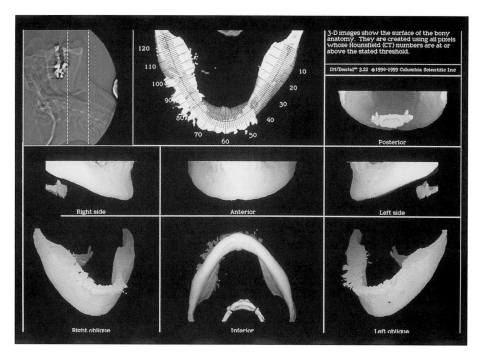

Computerized Tomography

Computerized tomography (CT) is an imaging technique that provides a computer-processed digital image of anatomic structures in a selected plane of the body (Figs 36-5 to 36-9). In conventional or incremental CT, an X-ray tube rigidly connected to an array of radiation detectors revolves around an axis of the patient. This action completes one scan. The remnant radiation exiting the patient is quantified by the detectors, which in turn cause a signal to be transmitted to the computer. Multiple signals acquired during a single scan are analyzed by the computer to produce an image of a layer based on the different thicknesses and densities of objects in the plane traversed by the X-ray beam. In practice, a number of separate scans are necessary to image a specified volume of tissue.

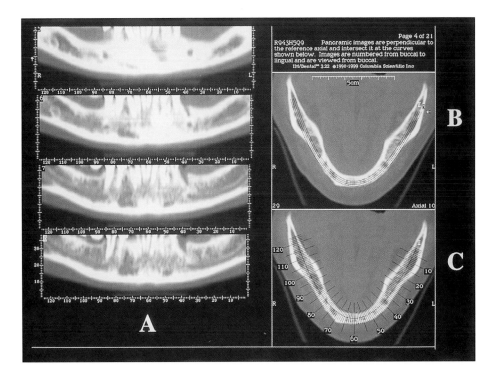

Fig 36-7 Multiplanar reformatting (3-D Dental). (A) Four of the 15 panoramic images that were reformatted in this study are shown. The images are numbered from 5 to 8, top to bottom, and represent the image planes described by the four curves, facial to lingual, in the axial image (B). The thickness of each panoramic image is 0.25 mm, and the images are centered 1.0 mm apart. All images are presented life size. This can be checked by the clinician with the 5.0-cm scale in the image. The patient's left is to the viewer's right. The tick marks along the side of the panoramic images locate the positions of the 38 acquired axial images; the tick marks along the bottom indicate the locations of all reformatted cross-sectional images. The panoramic images represent planes concentric to the electronically drawn curve in the reference axial image (C).

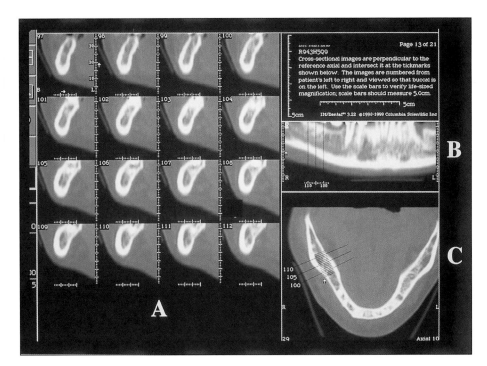

Fig 36-8 Multiplanar reformatting (3-D Dental). (A) Representatives (97 to 112) of the 125 reformatted cross-sectional images in this study are shown. The thickness of each cross-sectional image is 0.25 mm, and they are centered 1.0 mm apart. All images are presented life size. This can be checked by the clinician with the 5.0-cm scale in the image. The facial of each image is to the viewer's left, the lingual to the right. The tick marks along the side of the images locate the positions of the 38 acquired axial images, and those along the bottom show the locations of the 15 reformatted panoramic images. Each cross-sectional image represents a plane perpendicular to the electronically drawn curve in the reference axial image (C). The locations of each cross-sectional image relative to the central panoramic and reference axial images are shown in B and C, respectively.

Images may be acquired in several different planes of the body, but most commonly in the axial or transverse plane. This plane is perpendicular to the body's longitudinal axis. Data representing multiple abutted or overlapped layers acquired in this plane may be reformatted by computer software to produce images in other planes. By multiplanar reformatting or reconstruction, image data of the maxilla or mandible in the axial plane may be processed to produce cross-sectional and panoramic-like images. In contrast to incremental CT, in spiral or helical CT the patient undergoes translation simultaneously with rotation of the X-ray tube and detector array. This allows for a more rapid and continuous stream of image data to be acquired. Following helical scanning, image reformatting is accomplished much like that in conventional CT.

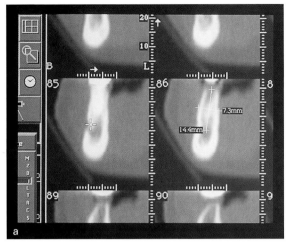 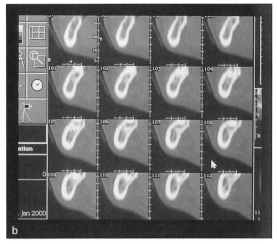

Fig 36-9 Postprocessing of images. The digital images acquired in CT are dynamic. Image density and contrast may be increased or decreased. The image may be magnified, and measurements may be made and recorded directly on the image *(a)*. Note the relative size of the magnified image *(a)* as compared with an image that was not magnified *(b)*. All these manipulations enhance the perception of detail. Additionally, digital images may be transmitted (teleradiology) to remote sites for referral and consultation.

Interactive Computerized Tomography

Images obtained by multiplanar reformatting techniques may be transferred by computer diskette or electronically over the Internet to the referring clinician's personal computer (Figs 36-10 and 36-11). Once these images are acquired by the clinician's computer, the clinician may interact with them.[14] Interactions include manipulating the gray scale to enhance the perception of detail; determining linear and angular measurements; and performing implant, prosthetic, and bone augmentation simulations. The information gained from these interactions assists the clinician in the development of a treatment plan. Once the treatment plan has been established, a permanent record may be made by laser printer. This record would be made available at the time of surgery for consultation by the implant surgeon. This software allows the clinician who ultimately must place the final restorations to direct the placement of implants, which helps ensure a satisfactory outcome.

Magnetic Resonance Imaging

Unlike the techniques previously described, which use X rays for image acquisition, magnetic resonance imaging (MRI) uses nonionizing radiation from the radio frequency band of the electromagnetic spectrum. To produce an image, the patient is placed inside a large magnet, which induces a relatively strong external magnetic field (1.0 T or greater). This magnetic field causes the nuclei of many

atoms in the body, including hydrogen, to align with the magnetic field. Following application of a radio frequency signal, energy absorbed by hydrogen atoms aligned with the magnetic field is released from the body, detected, and used to construct an image by computer. In images from MRI, cortical bone appears dark, because little or no detectable signal is recovered from hydrogen atoms tightly bound in bone. In contrast, cancellous bone appears light because of the relatively high content of mobile hydrogen atoms in the fat of bone marrow. In addition, soft tissue structures such as vessels and nerves are clearly imaged because of the inherently high contrast sensitivity of MRI to tissue differences. Unlike CT, direct multiplanar imaging without repositioning the patient is possible with MRI. This capability of MRI also eliminates the need for additional reformatting software.

The use of MRI for the presurgical evaluation of potential implant sites has been limited, in part because of the relatively high cost of the imaging equipment and in part by the spatial distortion caused by magnetic susceptibility effects at soft tissue–air interfaces. Recently, a low-field-strength (0.2-T) MRI machine, with a capital cost considerably lower than a 1.0-T machine, has shown potential for presurgical assessment. When a magnetic field of this strength is used, all three planes of the body are easily accessible, artifacts are few, and gadolinium markers may be used to accurately locate potential sites of implantation. In addition, vital structures are imaged, cortical and cancellous bone is well delineated, and spatial distortion is not substantial.

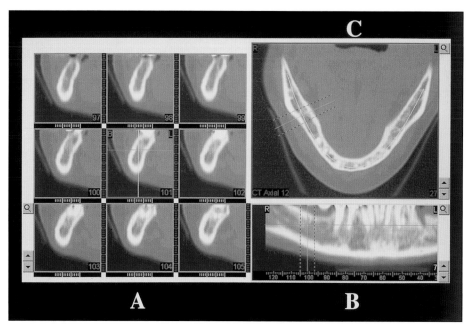

Fig 36-10 Interactive CT. A software program (SIM/Plant, Materialise/Columbia Scientific) allows clinicians planning an implant case to analyze images reformatted by 3-D Dental software on personal computers. The vertical line in cross-sectional image 101 (A) locates the plane of the panoramic image (B). The panoramic image corresponds to the plane described by the curved line in the axial image (C). The horizontal lines in both the cross-sectional and panoramic images locate the position of the axial image displayed. The solid vertical line in the panoramic image locates the position of axial image 101, and the dotted vertical lines include the area described by all cross-sectional images shown. The tick marks along the sides of the images locate the positions of axial, panoramic, and cross-sectional images, as described in Figs 36-7 and 36-8. The clinician may use the up and down arrows associated with each panel to scroll through all images acquired or formatted in that plane.

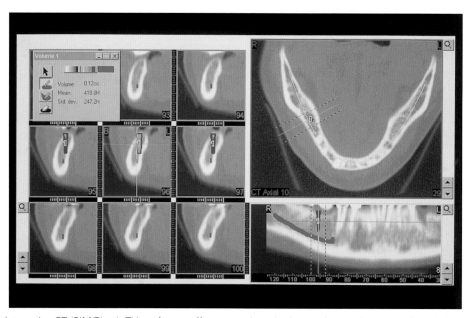

Fig 36-11 Interactive CT (SIM/Plant). This software offers several methods to enhance the perception of detail. In this example, the location of the inferior alveolar canal was not clearly defined in the cross-sectional images. The margins of the canal, however, were evident in one of the panoramic images. This allowed the clinician to "paint" the location of the inferior alveolar canal in the panoramic image. This painted image was automatically transferred to both the cross-sectional and axial images to locate the position of the canal in these views. Seeing the painted location of the canal in the cross-sectional image allowed the clinician to optimize the length, diameter, and insertion angle of the proposed implant. The diameter and length of the simulated implant may be controlled by the clinician and is automatically scaled to the size of the image. In this example, the placement of a tapered implant 11 mm long with a superior diameter of 4 mm and an inferior diameter of 3 mm was simulated.

Conclusion

Today, radiography for dental implant diagnostics shows a large variation in both frequency of use and choice of technique. It is unfortunate that perhaps the most important factors influencing the choice of technique are availability and cost rather than clinical necessity. Although clinicians may prefer to use the radiographic techniques that are readily available, they should keep in mind that optimization of the treatment plan may require referral of the patient to an oral and maxillofacial radiologist for more specialized radiographic examination.

References

1. Tyndall DA, Brooks SL. Selection criteria for dental implant site imaging: A position paper of the American Academy of Oral and Maxillofacial Radiology. Oral Surg Oral Med Oral Pathol Oral Radiol Endod 2000;89:630–637.
2. Jacobs R, van Steenberghe D. Radiographic planning and assessment of endosseous oral implants. Berlin: Springer, 1998.
3. Misch CE. Density of bone: Effect on treatment plans, surgical approach, healing, and progressive bone loading. Int J Oral Implantol 1990;6:23–31.
4. Frederiksen NL. Specialized radiographic techniques. In: White SC, Pharoah MJ. Oral Radiology Principles and Interpretation, ed 4. St. Louis: Mosby, 2000:217–240.
5. Frederiksen NL. Diagnostic imaging in dental implantology. Oral Surg Oral Med Oral Pathol Oral Radiol Endod 1995; 80:540–554.
6. Reiskin AB. Implant imaging. Status, controversies, and new developments. Dent Clin North Am 1998;42:47–56.
7. Avendanio B, Frederiksen NL, Benson BW, Sokolowski TW. Effective dose and risk assessment from detailed narrow beam radiography. Oral Surg Oral Med Oral Pathol Oral Radiol Endod 1996;82:713–719.
8. White SC. 1992 assessment of radiation risks from dental radiography. Dentomaxillofac Radiol 1992;21:118–126.
9. Frederiksen NL, Benson BW, Sokolowski TW. Effective dose and risk assessment from film tomography used for dental implant diagnostics. Dentomaxillofac Radiol 1994;23:123–127.
10. Frederiksen NL, Benson BW, Sokolowski TW. Effective dose and risk assessment from computed tomography of the maxillofacial complex. Dentomaxillofac Radiol 1995;24:55–58.
11. Scaf G, Lurie AG, Mosier KM, et al. Dosimetry and cost of imaging osseointegrated implants with film-based and computed tomography. Oral Surg Oral Med Oral Pathol Oral Radiol Endod 1997;83:41–48.
12. Frederiksen NL. Health physics. In: White SC, Pharoah MJ. Oral Radiology Principles and Interpretation, ed 4. St. Louis: Mosby, 2000:42–65.
13. Gröndahl K, Ekestubbe A, Gröndahl H-G. Radiography in oral endosseous prosthetics. Göteborg: Nobel Biocare, 1996:111–115.
14. Kraut RA. Interactive CT diagnostics, planning and preparation for dental implants. Implant Dent 1998;7:19–25.

Implant Surgery

Frank L. Higginbottom
- Templates

Thomas G. Wilson, Jr
- Surgical Equipment
- Surgical Anatomy
- Practical Aspects of Wound Healing
- Basic Surgical Procedures for Implant Placement
- Postsurgical Care

Templates

When a patient has been determined a candidate for dental implants, additional treatment planning must be done. This planning involves the fabrication of a guide that allows the surgeon to place the implants in the best position possible to ensure a favorable restorative and maintenance phase. Correct placement of an implant is paramount to treatment success. Neither the practitioner nor the technician can make up for bad placement of implants.

The practitioner needs the following information: a medical and dental history of the patient, appropriate clinical information, radiographs of prospective sites, and diagnostic casts (it is important to have three casts of the edentulous area). From this information, the practitioner formulates a treatment plan to present to the patient and to confirm with the surgeon.

The restorative dentist and the laboratory technician should keep the following physical landmarks in mind during planning: inferior alveolar nerve, mental nerve, incisive canal, maxillary sinus, nasal cavity, adjacent teeth, other implants, and floor of the mouth. Additionally, the practitioner needs to know the crestal width of bone available for implant placement. In general, this width should allow at least 1 mm of bone to surround the implant.

The following steps are required to prepare the patient for implant placement:

1. Make a diagnostic waxup of the proposed final restoration.

2. Prepare a clear coping.
3. Prepare a radiographic template.
4. Obtain additional radiographs with the template in place.
5. Fabricate a surgical template to provide to the surgeon prior to the appointment for implant placement.

Fabrication of a Clear Coping

Once the information detailed above has been gathered, the dental laboratory phase begins. First, the practitioner or technician tries to create a vision of the final restoration. Without knowing the proposed position of the final restoration, there is no way to know where to place the implant. The process starts by adding prosthetic teeth or wax to the edentulous sites. This is called the *diagnostic waxup* or *setup* (Fig 37-1a). The diagnostic waxup is duplicated, and a 0.020-inch sheet-resin coping is fabricated over the duplicate waxup via a vacuum-forming process (Fig 37-1b). This coping represents the outline of the final restoration and will be referred to as the *clear coping*.

Fabrication of a Radiographic Template

The clear coping is placed over one of the original casts. Using a 3/32-inch cobalt twist drill in a laboratory handpiece, the practitioner or technician drills through the proposed implant position into the edentulous site. The drill should enter 8 mm into the cast, keeping anatomic landmarks in consideration. Radiographic markers (3/32-inch diameter × 8-mm length) are placed in the cast (Fig 37-1c),

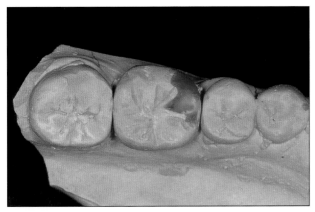

Fig 37-1a A diagnostic waxup represents the clinician's concept of the location for the final restoration (in this case, the first molar).

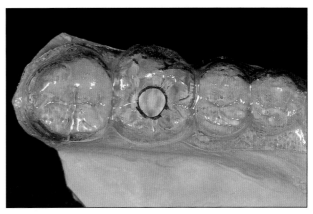

Fig 37-1b A clear sheet-resin coping is adapted to a duplicate of the diagnostic waxup. The cutout in the center of the molar represents the location for the implant.

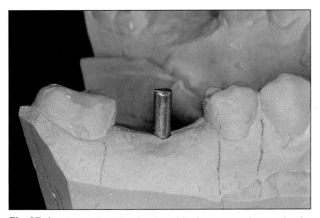

Fig 37-1c A metal marker is placed in the cast at the precise location for the implant.

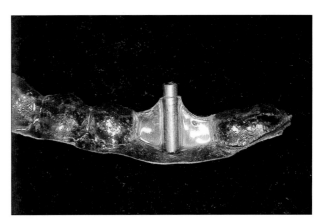

Fig 37-1d The radiographic template will be tried in the mouth and evaluated radiographically for position prior to creating the definitive surgical template.

and a 0.020-inch sheet-resin coping is formed. The coping is recovered from the cast, and 8-mm markers are placed in it. This device is the *radiographic template* (Fig 37-1d).

The radiographic template is placed in the mouth, and radiographs of the proposed site are taken. This procedure will project the proposed implant position in the mesiodistal direction. Tomograms can be used to analyze the faciolingual relationships.

Fabrication of a Surgical Template

Using the radiographic template as a guide, alterations in the proposed implant insertion path can now be made. If needed, a new resin coping is formed. This becomes the surgical template. A surgical template is delivered to the surgeon in ample time for examination and confirmation. The technician or practitioner should provide the surgeon

with all of the diagnostic aids used in the process to generate the surgical template. Surgical templates should be used to dictate proper location of the implant axes, which will allow an optimal restorative outcome.[1] Specific applications are described below.

Partial Edentulism

To ensure a successful restorative phase, the implant must be located accurately. Some clinicians do not use a template for single-tooth gaps. However, visualization is difficult in many parts of the mouth, and use of a template is strongly recommended for all situations. A posterior single-tooth gap is the most common location of a dental implant (Fig 37-2). Anterior single-tooth gaps are more challenging and should be handled by an experienced implant team (Fig 37-3). Use of a surgical template for multiple-tooth anterior gaps and distal extension will help the surgeon to avoid vital structures and interproximal spaces.

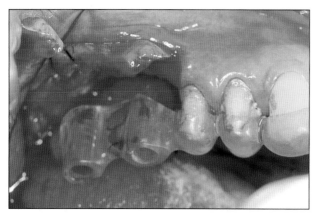

Fig 37-2 Definitive template used for implant placement in a posterior gap.

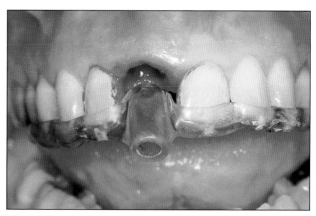

Fig 37-3 Definitive template used for implant placement in an anterior gap.

Complete Edentulism

A different design of surgical template is needed for completely edentulous patients, because the design used for the partially edentulous patient is difficult to position accurately without teeth to serve as an index. The ideal template in this case is a modified version of the patient's existing denture or a duplicate of the denture setup. Use of such a template will help locate the implants in the proper buccolingual dimension, simplifying restorative procedures. Typically, mesiodistal positioning in completely edentulous patients is not as important as in the partially edentulous patient, but adequate spacing between adjacent implants is critical to avoid problems in the restorative phase. Surgeons should attempt to place the shoulders of multiple implants at a similar level to allow passive fit of a tissue bar or a hybrid framework.

Edentulous patients who will receive fixed or fixed/removable metal restorations or fixed ceramic restorations require a more precise template to avoid problems of incorrect mesiodistal placement that tends to position implants in interproximal areas between proposed restorations. This is particularly important in esthetic areas. Implants should be placed under every other tooth in the prosthesis to allow for optimal gingival contours. Anterior sites should be prepared first; depth gauges then can be used to stabilize the template for preparation of the remaining sites. This is probably the most difficult situation for implant placement.

Surgical Equipment

The armamentarium for implant surgery is a variation of that used for periodontal surgery (see box), because the principles of flap elevation, tooth and bone preparation, and flap closure are similar. Slow-speed, high-torque

---

Instruments and Materials Needed for Implant Surgery

Instruments for examination
- Mirror
- Periodontal probe

Instruments for flap preparation and elevation
- Blade handle
- #15 and #12B blades
- Periosteal elevator

Instruments for flap closure
- Needle holders
- Suture material

Instruments for bone modification
- High-speed air rotor handpiece
- High-speed surgical-length round burs (2, 4, 6, and 8)

Instruments for periodontal therapy
- Manual devices for calculus removal (eg, curettes)
- Mechanical devices for calculus removal (sonic, ultrasonic, or piezoelectric devices)

Basic implant equipment
- Slow-speed, high-torgue engine
- Slow-speed, high-torque handpiece
- Implant kit from the manufacturer (including burs, delivery devices, etc)
- Implants

Surgical template specific for the case

---

handpieces and a dental engine are needed, along with an implant surgical kit and an appropriate selection of implants. The engine should be reliable, easy to clean and sterilize; deliver a high torque at a low speed; and have a

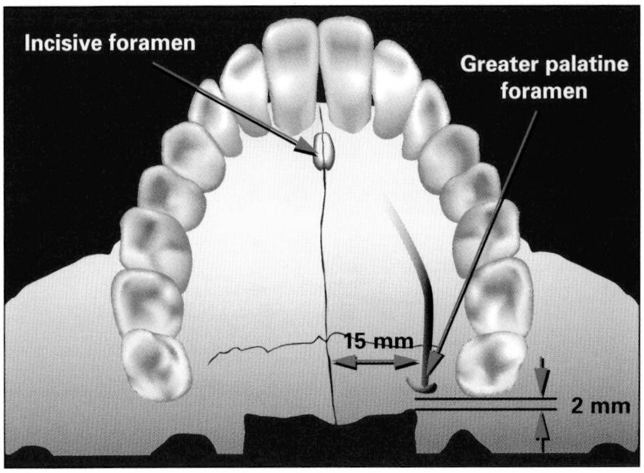

Fig 37-4 The incisive foramen is located dorsal to and between the maxillary central incisors. The greater palatine artery exits the greater palatine foramen and travels anteriorly as its diameter decreases. It usually lies midway between the alveolar crest and the midpalate (curved line).

built-in capacity to deliver sterile coolant.[2] The last feature is important because without it, a second sterile assistant is needed to deliver water to cool the drills.

Surgical Anatomy

Alveolar Ridge

In most cases, when all the teeth are extracted and conventional dentures are placed, bone resorption follows. Although the amount of bone loss varies from patient to patient, significant loss occurs in most[3–5] (see chapter 35) and continues over time.[6,7] This process reduces the amount of bone available for implant placement and often necessitates reconstructive surgical procedures, especially if fixed restorations are to be placed. An implant-supported denture is often the optimal reconstruction in completely edentulous patients whose interarch distance has increased due to ridge atrophy.

Maxillary Arch

The *incisive foramen* is located just dorsal to the nasopalatine papilla and contains nasopalatine vessels and nerves (Fig 37-4). The nerves supply the lingual gingiva and the palatal mucosa from the canines forward. It is rare that patients experience a loss of sensation when the soft tissues in this area are elevated, but cutting the nasopalatine vessels can cause bleeding problems during surgery.[8] Occasionally, the foramen is so large that it precludes implant placement in the maxillary central incisor area, especially when significant bone resorption has occurred.

The *greater palatine foramen* is medial and somewhat anterior to the maxillary third molars. The greater palatine nerve found here supplies the palatal tissues from the foramen to the canines.[9] The greater palatine artery travels approximately midway between the alveolar crest and the

midpalate (Fig 37-4). Incisions (especially vertical ones) should be kept away from this vessel, especially in the molar areas.

Lymph vessels that drain the vestibular gingiva travel to the submandibular nodes in both the maxillary and mandibular arches, as do the vessels from the palatal and lingual gingiva. This is clinically significant only when swelling is seen in these nodes postoperatively, indicating infection.

The general outlines of the floor of the nose and maxillary sinuses can usually be distinguished on radiographs. In practice, if the structures are penetrated, the implant is backed out to rest slightly inferior to, or just at the margin of, these structures. One exception would be if sinus elevation procedures are performed.

Mandibular Arch

The *lingual nerve* arises from the floor of the mouth just medial to the root of the mandibular third molar[10] (Figs 37-5a and 37-5b) and supplies the anterior two thirds of the dorsal surface of the tongue. The practitioner can occasionally feel it just lingual to the mandibular third molar. If possible, vertical incisions distal and lingual to the second molars should be limited to avoid this structure.

An important structure to locate radiographically is the *inferior alveolar nerve*, which supplies the teeth and lingual soft tissue (Figs 37-6a and 37-6b).[11,12] Panoramic radiographs and occasionally tomographic radiographs are useful in determining its position. In some cases, it can loop mesial to the mental foramen.

The *mental nerve* usually exits the facial surface of the mandible in the area of the premolars and travels anteriorly to supply the facial gingiva and mucosa of the lips.[13] It is often helpful to locate the mental foramen during surgery of the mandibular posterior sextant to avoid damaging the nerve. By doing so, the amount of bone coronal to the nerve can be more precisely measured (Fig 37-7).

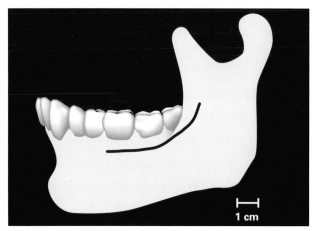

Fig 37-5a Lateral view of the typical course of the lingual nerve.

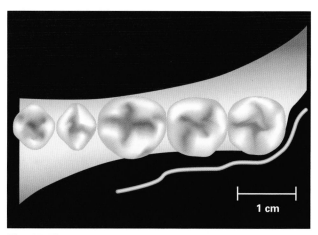

Fig 37-5b Occlusal view of the typical course of the lingual nerve.

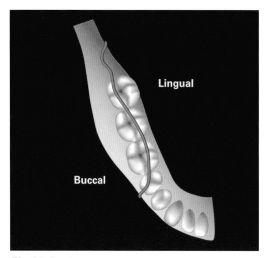

Fig 37-6a Occlusal view of the typical course of the inferior alveolar nerve.

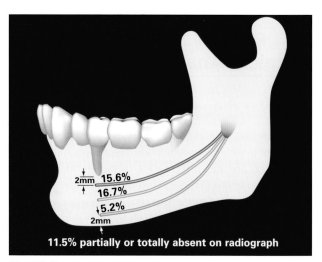

Fig 37-6b The course of the inferior alveolar nerve has been shown to vary considerably.[12] Most often it is located halfway between the root apices and the inferior cortical border, but it can be found within 2 mm of either boundary. Occasionally it can be too indistinct to locate radiographically. (Adapted from Heasman.[12])

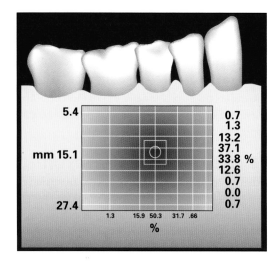

Fig 37-7 Approximately 50% of the time, the mental foramen is located directly apical to the mandibular second premolar, frequently 15 mm apical to the cementoenamel junction. (Adapted from Matheson.[13])

Practical Aspects of Wound Healing

Bone

The likelihood that osseointegration will occur, and occur as rapidly as possible, increases *(1)* the closer the bony wall of the osteotomy is to the implant surface, *(2)* the greater the cell viability, and *(3)* the greater the cellular affinity for the implant surface.[14] The distance from the osteotomy site to the implant wall is governed by many factors, including the accuracy and consistency of drill placement by the operator. Overheating the bone can kill or damage cells important for osseointegration.[15]

Rapid healing is more likely when the following approaches are used during implant placement:

- Apply sterile saline or sterile water either internally (through the drill) or externally to cool cutting instruments.
- Use slow drilling speeds (500 to 800 rpm).
- Use sharp drills, which cut more precisely and with less heat than dull ones.
- Use torque-reduction handpieces.
- Use an intermittent technique when cutting (ie, periodically bring the instrument far enough coronally to flush out any bone chips). If bone fragments are not removed, the risk of overheating bone increases.

To facilitate osseointegration, the implant should first touch the patient's blood (usually in the implant site). Contaminants (eg, glove powder or saliva) should not be allowed to contact the implant surface, because they may interfere with wound healing.[16]

In a clinician's first cases involving edentulous areas, the prosthesis that will cover the implants should not be delivered for 2 weeks after implant placement, if possible. When delivered, the tissue surfaces of these devices should be sufficiently hollowed so no contact with the implants occurs. A soft liner is placed and relieved where it may touch the implant. The patient is told that the denture is meant for esthetic purposes, not function. The soft liner is replaced when it hardens.

Soft Tissue

The healing of soft tissue wounds can affect the ultimate success of the implant. A predictable series of events occurs following surgery, and understanding the process is important. Immediately following suturing, a blood clot forms, and cells that clean the area of damaged tissues and foreign bodies are attracted to the wound. Epithelial cells begin to migrate over the clot from the soft tissue margins. They continue to grow until they meet epithelial cells from the opposite side of the wound or come into contact with the implant surface. At the same time, fibroblasts migrate into the clot, and a new extracellular matrix is formed. This matrix fills in the wound and forms a scaffold for additional cell migration and blood vessel formation. Over the ensuing months, maturation and remodeling occur until wound healing is complete.

Basic Surgical Procedures for Implant Placement

Instrument and Operatory Care

The rules for disinfecting operatories and instruments are constantly being revised. It is strongly recommended that the surgeon and staff be aware of the latest methods for care of the dental facility and dental instruments (see chapter 16). In general, implants are best delivered in a very clean environment. The use of sterile barriers, drapes, and instruments is suggested.[17]

For optimal comfort, the surgical operatory should be large enough to hold needed equipment; be simple to clean; and allow easy access for the patient, surgeon, and other members of the surgical team. As a rule, one chairside and one roving assistant are needed.

Preoperative Procedures and Instructions for the Patient

Broad-spectrum antibiotics administered before surgery (eg, 1 g amoxicillin taken 1 hour before surgery) have been shown to increase implant survival.[18] Assuming no contraindications, nonsteroidal anti-inflammatory medications administered before surgery can help diminish postoperative discomfort. For the anxious patient, an oral sedative (such as a benzodiazepine) taken before the surgical procedure may be helpful. Some patients may require intravenous sedation. The patient's physician should be contacted to answer questions about whether these procedures and medications are appropriate. Just before surgery, rinsing with chlorhexidine digluconate for 30 seconds will greatly reduce oral bacteria.

Standard Surgical Approach

As described in chapter 34, there are two types of implants: submerged and nonsubmerged. One-stage, nonsubmerged implants are placed so that the bone covers the rough surface of the implant. Two-stage, submerged implants

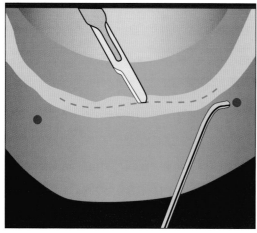

Fig 37-8 In a totally edentulous situation, a midcrestal incision is used. To gain further access, the incision can be carried distally.

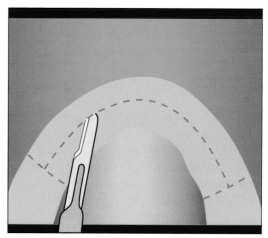

Fig 37-9 An alternative approach in totally edentulous situations involves the use of vertical releasing incisions.

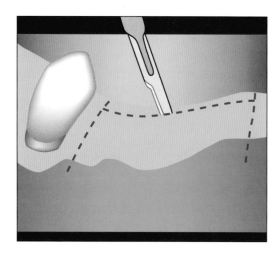

Fig 37-10 Midcrestal incisions can be used in the posterior mandible. The mental foramen should be identified and avoided.

should be placed so that the implant-abutment junction is slightly coronal to the alveolar bone. In one-stage implants and two-stage implants used as one-stage implants, the neck of the implant (or healing screw) is allowed to penetrate the soft tissues. With two-stage implants, the implant is covered with the soft tissues and a second surgery is necessary to uncover it.

In sites with no esthetic concerns, a midcrestal incision is made (or the remaining keratinized gingiva is bisected) (Figs 37-8 to 37-10), and full-thickness flaps are reflected. The incision is often made more lingual in areas of esthetic concern. Bony contours are evaluated, and releasing incisions can be used where additional flap evaluation is needed for the operator to visualize the surgical site. The ridge may be recontoured or augmented as necessary.

The cortical bone is penetrated by a series of burs, beginning at the exact center of the desired implant site. A template should be used to simplify this process (Figs 37-11a to 37-11d).

A hole is drilled to approximately 6 mm deep, using the longest, smallest-diameter pilot drill that will fit in the mouth; a radiopaque point is placed, and a radiograph is exposed and evaluated. Any direction changes can be made and the drill taken to the desired depth. The second pilot drill or a larger-diameter twist drill, if needed, is then taken to the desired depth.

Placement of interim and final restorations is discussed in chapter 38.

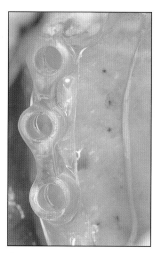

Fig 37-11a The template is placed over the surgical site to help determine where incisions will be made.

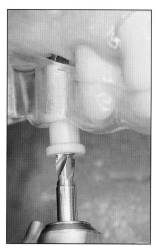

Fig 37-11b Incisions are made and enough soft tissue retracted to evaluate bony anatomy. In sites where the direction or position of the osteotomy site is in question, a radiopaque marker can be placed after the smallest drill is used and a radiograph exposed.

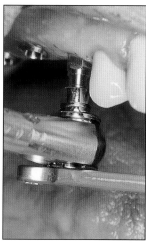

Fig 37-11c The implants are placed and soft tissues sutured.

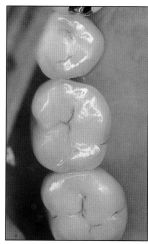

Fig 37-11d Final restorations.

Postsurgical Care

Patient Instructions

The patient is given the following postoperative guidelines:

1. Do not smoke.
2. Keep the head above heart level for least 24 hours.
3. Rest for at least 24 hours.
4. Avoid alcohol.
5. Apply an ice pack to the face for up to 24 hours (10 minutes on, 10 minutes off).
6. Take antibiotics, if prescribed, until all have been used.
7. Take nonsteroidal anti-inflammatory medication (if prescribed) as directed until finished.
8. Rinse with chlorhexidine digluconate twice a day starting 24 hours after surgery, if instructed.

Maintenance by the Surgical Team

First Postoperative Visit (7 to 10 days after surgery)
1. Check soft tissues for signs of infection.
2. Make sure the patient is using chlorhexidine digluconate twice daily or gently cleaning the implant or implant site with a soft-bristle brush. The mouthrinse should be used, on average, for 4 to 6 weeks following surgery.
3. Remove sutures, if necessary. Some are self-dissolving.
4. If the healing is proceeding well, see the patient in 2 to 4 weeks.

Second Postoperative Visit
1. Check soft tissues for signs of infection.
2. Advise the patient to continue with chlorhexidine digluconate or gentle mechanical cleaning.
3. If tissues are healing well, see the patient in 4 to 8 weeks.

Third Postoperative Visit
1. Check tissues for signs of infection.
2. If the tissues are healing normally, tell the patient to discontinue use of chlorhexidine digluconate.
3. Advise the patient to schedule visits at least every 4 to 8 weeks until the implant is sufficiently stable to allow placement of the prosthesis.
4. When implants are stable, the patient is ready for the restorative phase. Implants placed in dense bone are usually loaded sooner than implants placed in less dense (more cancellous) bone.
5. The patient usually continues with postoperative visits until the restoration is finished.

References

1. Higginbottom FL, Wilson TG. Three-dimensional templates for placement of root-form dental implants: A technical note. Int J Oral Maxillofac Implants 1996;11:787–793.

2. Sutter F, Krekeler G, Schwammberger AE, Sutter FJ. Atraumatic surgical technique and implant bed preparation. Quintessence Int 1992;23:811–816.

3. Carlsson GE, Persson G. Morphologic changes of the mandible after extraction and wearing of dentures: A longitudinal, clinical, and x-ray cephalometric study covering 5 years. Odontol Revy 1967;18:27–54.

4. Carlsson GE, Bergman B, Hedegard B. Changes in contour of the maxillary alveolar process under immediate dentures. A longitudinal clinical and x-ray cephalometric study covering 5 years. Acta Odontol Scand 1967;25:45–75.

5. Bergman B, Carlsson GE. Clinical long-term study of complete denture wearers. J Prosthet Dent 1985;53:56–61.

6. Atwood DA. Reduction of residual ridges: A major oral disease entity. J Prosthet Dent 1971;26:266–279.

7. Tallgren A. The continuing reduction of residual alveolar ridges in complete denture wearers: A mixed longitudinal study covering 25 years. J Prosthet Dent 1972;27:120–132.

8. Clarke MA, Bueltmann KW. Anatomical considerations in periodontal surgery. J Periodontol 1971;42:610–625.

9. Westmoreland EE, Blanton PL. An analysis of the variations in positions of the greater palatine foramen in the adult human skull. Anat Rec 1982;204:383–388.

10. Wilson C. Lingual nerve: Anatomic relationship to the mandibular alveolar crest and lingual cortical plate [thesis]. Dallas: Baylor College of Dentistry, 1989.

11. Rajchel J, Ellis E III, Fonseca RJ. The anatomical location of the mandibular canal: Its relationship to the sagittal ramus osteotomy. Int J Adult Orthodon Orthognath Surg 1986;1:37–47.

12. Heasman PA. Variation in the position of the inferior dental canal and its significance to restorative dentistry. J Dent 1988;16:36–39.

13. Matheson BR. Localization of the mental foramen utilizing an intraoral landmark [thesis]. Dallas: Baylor College of Dentistry, 1985.

14. Schroeder A, van der Zypen E, Stich E, Sutter F. The reactions of bone, connective tissue, and epithelium to endosteal implants with titanium-sprayed surfaces. J Maxillofac Surg 1981;9:15–25.

15. Eriksson AR, Albrektsson T. Termperature threshold levels for heat-induced bone tissue injury. A vital microscopic study in the rabbit. J Prosthet Dent 1983;50:101–107.

16. Kasemo B, Lausmaa J. Metal selection and surface characteristics. In: Branemark P-I, Zarb GA, Albrektsson T (eds). Tissue-Integrated Prostheses. Chicago: Quintessence, 1985:99–116.

17. Scharf D, Tarnow D. Success rates of osseointegration for implants placed under sterile versus clean conditions. J Periodontol 1993;64:954–956.

18. Dent CD, Olson JW, Farish SE, et al. The influence of preoperative antibiotics on success of endosseous implants up to and including stage II surgery: A study of 2,641 patients. J Oral Maxillofac Surg 1997;55:19–24.

Restorative Procedures Following Implant Placement

Frank L. Higginbottom and Thomas G. Wilson, Jr
- Interim Restorations
- Final Restorations
- Implant Maintenance
- Case Presentation

Interim Restorations

Interim restorations are very important for both the implant patient and the restorative dentist. The first portion of this chapter addresses both the use of restorations to support function in the edentulous patient during the healing period and the management of the patient at the time of abutment connection.

Management During the Initial Healing Period

Edentulous Patient
The postoperative management of the edentulous patient can proceed in several ways. Ideally, the patient's denture is removed at the time of surgery and not returned to the patient until the soft tissues have healed and the implants have integrated. However, this is not always practical. Most patients do not want to be without teeth. Therefore, at some time after implant placement, patients receive an interim denture. Most patients receive their denture shortly after implant surgery, before soft tissue healing and integration of the implant have occurred. Some patients even receive their removable appliance the day of implant placement. In many cases full dentures are lined with a soft material and delivered 3 to 4 days after implant placement.

Partially Edentulous Patients
Posterior Sites. Early in a clinician's experience with implants, if the patient is missing teeth in the posterior sextants, the best option is not to provide an interim restora-

tion. This will save the patient both unnecessary expense and possible trauma to the healing implant sites. There are few reasons to place a provisional restoration in a posterior single-tooth gap because the surrounding teeth provide enough function, and esthetic considerations do not apply, except on maxillary premolars.

When patients are missing enough posterior teeth to impair function and they desire a removable replacement, they should be informed that the provisional appliance is for appearance only, not for function. The possibility of modifying and relining an existing removable fixed partial denture is limited. Because of the framework design, it is often impossible to use an existing removable partial denture during the healing phase. Other options, for the experienced implant dentist, involve immediate loading of the implants in special circumstances (see chapter 39) or the use of provisional implants (Fig 38-1).

Anterior Sites. Few patients will go without anterior teeth. One form of replacement is a provisional removable partial denture (Fig 38-2). Patients must accept limited function for the luxury of appearance. Additional treatment options include fixed provisional restorations (Fig 38-3); a direct bonded pontic, if adjacent teeth are not to be restored (Fig 38-4); and immediate loading by advanced clinicians, in selected cases (Fig 38-5).

Management at the Loading Appointment

Following osseointegration, the use of provisional restorations on implants allows the patient to return to a functional state and gives the laboratory time to fabricate definitive restorations. Provisional restorations allow the

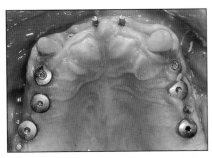

Fig 38-1 Provisional implants used to support an interim prosthesis in the anterior maxilla (seen here between the canines).

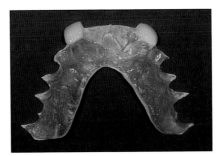

Fig 38-2a An anterior provisional removable partial denture.

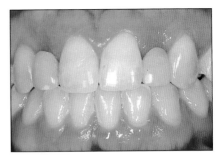

Fig 38-2b Appearance with the interim restoration in place.

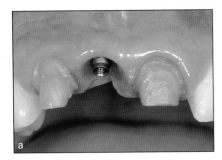

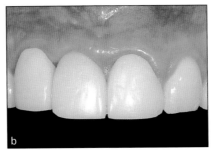

Fig 38-3a Anterior tooth-protected implant site.

Fig 38-3b Interim fixed partial denture in place, covering but not attached to the implant.

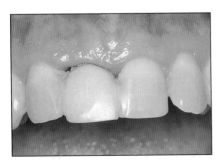

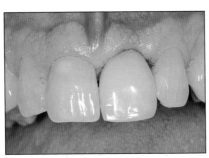

Fig 38-4 *(left)* Direct bonded pontic to replace the maxillary right central incisor (used during healing).

Fig 38-5 *(right)* Anterior implant site loaded immediately with an acrylic interim restoration.

clinician to control loading and to shape the gingival tissues in esthetic sites. They also determine the shape, contour, and occlusal configuration of the final restoration. Impressions for final restorations are made at the loading appointment.

The appliance that was used during the healing period can often be modified for use during the fabrication period, or the implant can be brought into function using a variety of techniques.

Completely Edentulous Patients

Relined dentures. Relining an existing denture and making impressions for the final prosthesis can be performed during a single appointment.

Connect denture to implants. Another way to provide an interim restoration is to connect the patient's existing removable prosthesis to the implants, creating a fixed restoration (Fig 38-6). It provides function for the patient, allows very accurate communication of jaw relations to the laboratory, and can be used to fabricate a verification jig. This prosthesis can also be used as a replacement appliance if the final prosthesis needs future repair.

Fixed provisional restorations. When an edentulous patient will have fixed final restorations, fixed provisional restorations can be placed at the time of abutment connection.

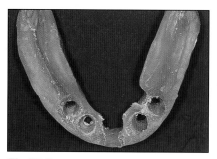

Fig 38-6a Denture modified for pickup of provisional components.

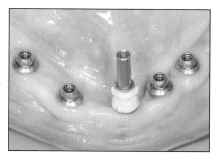

Fig 38-6b Pickup of provisional components with acrylic resin.

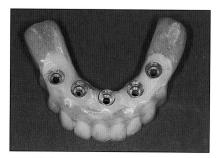

Fig 38-6c Interim hybrid prosthesis, which will be attached to the implants with occlusal screws.

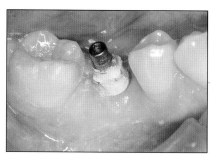

Fig 38-7a Provisional coping reduced, opaqued, and placed with a guide pin in the abutment for a screw-retained provisional restoration.

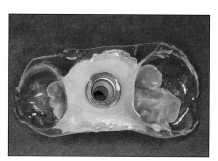

Fig 38-7b Provisional coping picked up in acrylic resin.

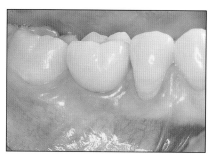

Fig 38-7c Interim restoration screwed into place.

Partially Edentulous Patients

For partially edentulous patients, it is important to fabricate a provisional restoration that will be fixed directly to the implant at the impression or loading appointment.

Screw-retained restorations. For restorations that will be screw retained, the healing abutment is removed and impressions are made. The same abutments used for final restorations can be used for provisional restorations. Provisional copings are customized and fitted to the implant-abutment interface with a guide screw (Fig 38-7a). Provisional resin is adapted to the abutment in the mouth using a vacuum-formed sheet-resin clear coping as a carrier (Fig 38-7b; see also chapter 37). The resin is allowed to polymerize in the mouth and is withdrawn and modified in the laboratory. After the provisional restoration is finished and polished, it is seated in the mouth (Fig 38-7c), and the occlusion is refined. A fixation screw is used to secure the restoration to the implant. The access opening is closed with a small cotton pledget to protect the screw and temporary stopping or resin composite placed 2 mm from the surface of the restoration.

Cemented restorations. When restorations will be cemented, the healing abutment is removed, and an abutment suitable for cementation is placed (Fig 38-8a). The abutment may be modified and impressions made. A vacuum-formed clear coping that resembles the final shape of the restoration is filled with the resin of choice (Fig 38-8b). The material is conditioned in warm water and placed in the mouth to make an impression of the abutment and shoulder of the implant (Fig 38-8c). As the material cures, it is moved on and off. When set, it is returned to the laboratory to refine the marginal area on an analog or implant replica with an actual abutment placed. Resin can be added as needed and cured in warm water. The finished provisional restoration is then polished, adjusted, and seated with provisional cement (Fig 38-8d).

Restorations in the esthetic zone. Provisional restorations in esthetic areas require special consideration. The healing abutment is removed and impressions made at the implant level. An abutment is placed for either cementation or screw retention of a final restoration. Either abutment will allow the fabrication and placement of a provisional

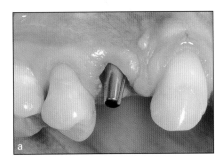

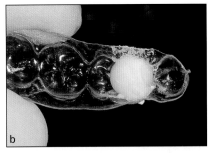

Fig 38-8a Solid abutment seated.

Fig 38-8b Acrylic resin placed in provisional clear coping.

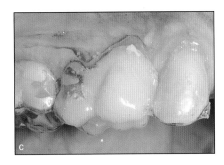

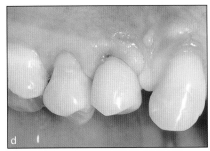

Fig 38-8c Clear coping seated in the mouth to make an impression of the site with the restorative material.

Fig 38-8d Finished provisional in place.

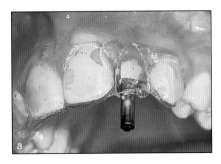

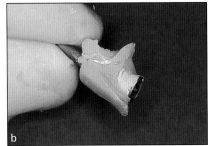

Fig 38-9a Clear coping and guide pin seated over site.

Fig 38-9b A provisional restoration just withdrawn, showing tissue excluding normal crown form. The soft tissues have not allowed formation of a normal emergence profile. The provisional is modified prior to its return to the mouth.

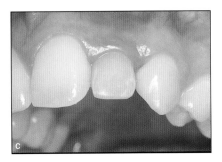

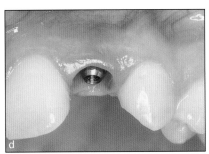

Fig 38-9c The defined provisional restoration in place.

Fig 38-9d Peri-implant sulcus created by the emergence profile provisional (3 months after placement).

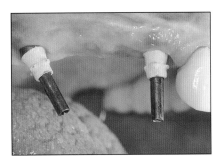

Fig 38-10a Provisional copings seated with guide pins.

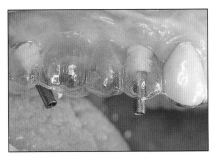

Fig 38-10b Clear coping tried in prior to filling with acrylic resin.

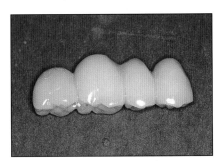

Fig 38-10c Finished multiunit interim restoration.

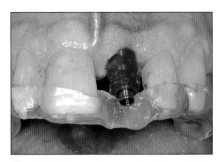

Fig 38-11 Index impression taken at the time of implant surgery.

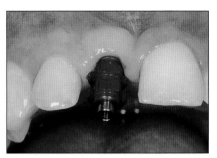

Fig 38-12a Impression coping in place to make an implant-level impression.

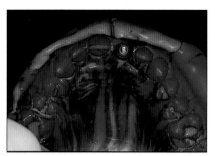

Fig 38-12b Impression recovered and coping picked up.

restoration. It is important to fabricate a provisional restoration that supports and enhances the gingival tissues—an *emergence profile restoration* (Fig 38-9). The process of enhancing the soft tissues is called *guided tissue shaping*. If the clinician does not form the peri-implant tissues during the provisional phase, it will be very difficult to do with the final restoration.

Multiunit restorations. Multiunit provisional restorations are more difficult to fabricate and fit. Care should be taken to ensure the abutment alignment and the fit and strength of the provisional framework (Fig 38-10). Because multiunit restorations involve fixed partial dentures with longer spans and longer treatment times, laboratory-fabricated and reenforced provisionals may be needed.

Final Restorations

Clinical Procedures

Making Impressions
Making impressions marks the start of the final restorative phase. As in any prosthetic procedure, extreme accuracy is needed. Impressions may be made at the time of implant placement or once the implants are stable.

Index at time of surgery. The surgeon or the restorative dentist can make an impression at the time of implant placement. This impression can be sent to the dental laboratory to fabricate a provisional restoration to be used later or to fabricate a final restoration (Fig 38-11).

Implant-level impression. At the beginning of the restorative procedure, the practitioner may elect to make an implant-level impression and forward the impression to the laboratory for abutment selection and restoration construction (Fig 38-12).

Abutment-level impression. At the time the final restorative procedure is started, an abutment can be placed. The abutment type will dictate the impression coping to be used. After the abutment is selected and an impression coping selected, an impression may be made (Figs 38-13 and 38-14).

Making Jaw-Relation Records
After impressions have been made, it is advisable to take records to relate the working casts in the laboratory. A facebow transfer to relate the maxillary cast to the articulator is recommended, as is a centric relation record for the partially edentulous patient to relate the mandibular cast. However, the patient with a distal extension restored with dental implants should have recording material placed between the abutments and the opposing arch. A rigid, fast-setting bite-registration polyvinyl siloxane is the preferred material. Edentulous arches should have reference bases constructed to aid in bite registration. These bases can be stabilized using impression copings.

Laboratory Procedures

Fabrication of Working Casts
The impression is delivered to the dental laboratory. The laboratory technician inspects the impression for accuracy, selects the proper analog, and places it in the impression. The impression is then poured in an accurate die stone material. The impression is recovered and trimmed. The implant working casts are mounted in a semiadjustable articulator with the aid of the diagnostic records gathered. More rudimentary or more advanced instrumentation systems sometimes may be used.

Construction of Screw-Retained Restorations
The technician constructing screw-retained restorations reviews the working casts and selects the components to start the laboratory procedure. The technician selects a

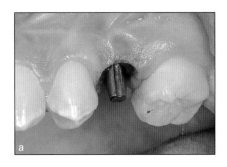

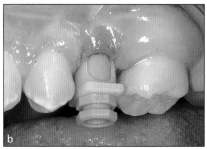

Fig 38-13a Solid abutment for a cemented restoration in place. It has been torqued to the required tightness.

Fig 38-13b Impression coping and positioning cylinder in place.

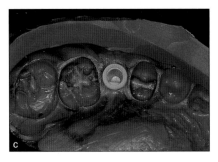

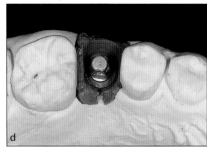

Fig 38-13c Impression recovered and transfers picked up.

Fig 38-13d Working cast for a cemented restoration.

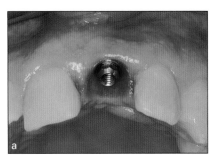

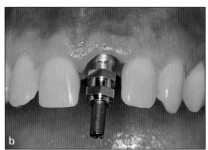

Fig 38-14a Abutment for a screw-retained restoration in place and torqued to the required tightness.

Fig 38-14b Impression transfer coping and guide pin.

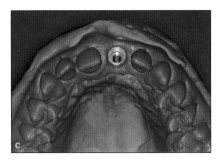

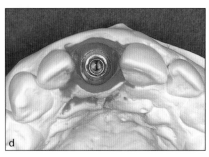

Fig 38-14c Impression recovered with transfer components picked up.

Fig 38-14d Working cast for screw-retained restoration. The cast has been modified with tissue material to provide an accurate soft tissue model, which will be used by the laboratory to develop the subgingival emergence profile.

premachined gold coping—a nonrotating gold coping for single units and round gold copings for multiple units. The gold coping is attached to the analog with a guide pin (Fig 38-15a). The guide pin is shortened to allow for the closure of the articulator. The guide pin is grooved on the top to allow for the use of a screwdriver. The restoration is waxed up to full contour and cut back for porcelain application. The pattern is invested, cast, and refitted to the working cast (Fig 38-15b). Porcelain is applied, and the restoration is finished (Fig 38-15c) and returned to the restorative dentist for placement.

Construction of Cemented Restorations

In constructing cemented restorations, the technician selects the proper burnout coping and shortens it to be flush with the top of the abutment (Fig 38-16a). Wax is then added to full contour and cut back to allow room for porcelain. The pattern is invested and cast, and the casting is refined at the marginal area with a reamer. Porcelain is applied to full contour, adapted to the working cast, and fired to completion. After glazing and final polish, the restoration is returned to the clinician for placement (Fig 38-16b).

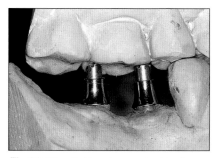

Fig 38-15a Gold copings and guide pins on the working cast.

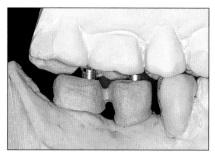

Fig 38-15b Casting fitted and seated on the working cast.

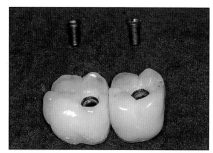

Fig 38-15c Finished restoration after porcelain application.

Fig 38-16a Burnout coping on solid abutment analog on the working cast.

Fig 38-16b Final crown before cementation.

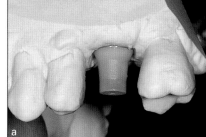

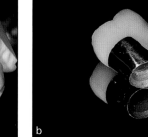

Fig 38-17a Bar components assembled on the working cast with acrylic.

Fig 38-17b Finished bar reconstruction on the working cast.

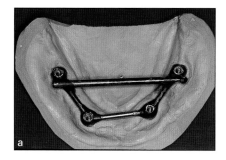

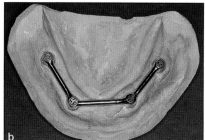

Fabrication of Bar Reconstructions

In fabricating bar reconstructions, the technician selects the appropriate number of round gold copings. They are attached to the analogs on the working cast with guide pins. Bar components can be cut and sized to fit between the gold copings and be connected using resin (Fig 38-17a). The bar assembly can be reinforced at the distal aspect and invested in a quick-setting soldering investment. After soldering, the frame is verified on the working cast and returned to the restorative dentist, along with the tooth setup, to be tried in for accuracy and fit. If the bar fits and the occlusion and fit are verified, the denture setup and bar are returned to the laboratory for processing and the addition of clips. If the bar not does fit, it will be sectioned and indexed with resin and a new impression made, substituting guide pins for the occlusal screws. This will allow the technician to complete the case with an ac-

curate cast (Fig 38-17b). The bar and denture are made in the laboratory and returned to the practitioner for placement.

Fabrication of Hybrid Appliances

For hybrid appliances, the technician selects the appropriate number of round gold copings. They are attached to the analogs on the working cast with guide pins. A boundary of wax or rope caulk can be used to limit the flow of resin. The resin is painted onto the gold copings joining them. The framework is sectioned and replaced on the verification jig. The resin units are reconnected with pattern resin (Fig 38-18a). The pattern is finalized and invested for casting. After casting, the framework is recovered and polished. The framework is returned to the cast, and fit is verified. If the framework does not fit the verification jig, it should be sectioned and soldered. Once the

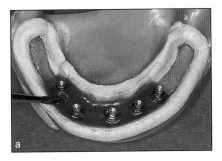

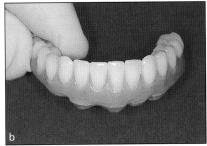

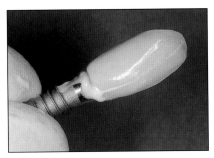

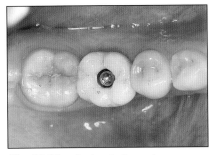

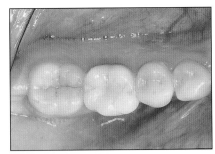

Fig 38-18a Gold copings connected with pattern resin.

Fig 38-18b Final hybrid prosthesis.

Fig 38-19 Crown trial seated on analog. Excess cement will be removed.

Fig 38-20a Occlusal view of screw access channel.

Fig 38-20b Access closed with resin composite.

framework satisfactorily fits the verification jig and the working cast, it is returned to the patient's mouth to see if it fits. If the framework fits, the practitioner can verify the occlusion and the esthetics of the tooth setup and return the framework to the laboratory for completion. If the framework does not seat passively, it should be sectioned and indexed with pattern resin and returned to the laboratory for soldering. A new verification jig should be fabricated from the new index, allowing the technician to have an accurate cast to finish the fabrication. The tooth setup is then finalized, processed, and returned to the practitioner (Fig 38-18b).

Delivery of Final Restorations

Delivery of the final restorations should be simple if previous procedures have been without error. However, if the restorations are not correct and cannot be altered at chairside, they should be returned to the laboratory for correction. Of special concern in esthetic areas is the development of the peri-implant space, which should have been shaped with the provisional restoration.

Cemented Restorations

Restorations to be cemented are fitted, and contacts are evaluated. Tight contacts prevent the complete seating of the restoration. Space should have been captured during the provisional phase to prevent the soft tissues from im-

peding seating of the restoration. Once the seating of the restoration is confirmed either visually or by radiograph, the occlusion may be corrected and the crown polished for cementation. A minimal layer of glass-ionomer cement is used to seat the crown to avoid excess material subgingivally. The crown may first be tried on an analog, and excess cement removed before placement in the mouth (Fig 38-19). Another option is to seat the restoration, remove it to rinse the sulcus of excess cement, then reseat the restoration prior to cement setting. Finally, the occlusion is rechecked.

Screw-Retained Restorations

The restoration is fitted to the abutment, and the fixation screw is tightened. The contacts then are evaluated. Tight contacts or soft tissue may interfere with the seating of the final restoration. The fixation screw seats passively in the first 90 degrees of full metal-to-metal contact. The fixation screw should seat the same way that the crown seats on an analog in the hand. In tightening the screw, keep in mind that it should be tight immediately, without binding. The screw should be tightened to the suggested degree and the access closed with the smallest piece of cotton possible. Warm temporary stopping can be placed up to 2 mm from the top of the screw access channel. Undercuts may be made in the walls of the channel to allow for composite to be placed to occlude the channel (Fig 38-20).

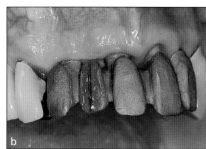

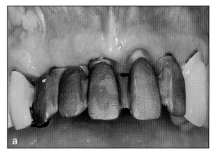

Fig 38-21a Try-in of framework for fit verification. Note that the margins do not close.

Fig 38-21b Framework is sectioned and found to seat passively. The framework is indexed in the mouth using pattern resin and picked up in a new impression.

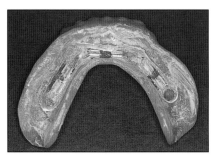

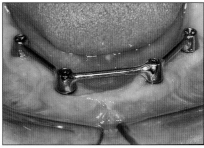

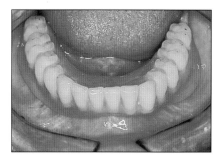

Fig 38-22a Tissue surface of a bar-retained overdenture adjusted with indicator paste.

Fig 38-22b Tissue bar seated.

Fig 38-22c Final denture in place.

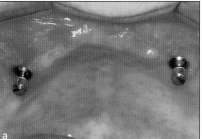

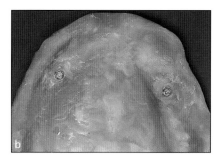

Fig 38-23a Retentive anchor matrices in position.

Fig 38-23b Matrices picked up with acrylic in the patient's existing denture.

Multiunit Fixed Restorations

Multiple units on implants may not fit passively. With natural teeth, the periodontal ligament allows for a slight discrepancy in fit, because the restoration that is close will seat due to repositioning of the teeth. Dental implants, however, do not move. Thus, two or more units must always be tried for fit and verified (Fig 38-21). Castings must fit as passively as possible. With multiunit implant restorations, cement is less likely to stress the framework than are screws.

Bar-Retained Overdentures

The laboratory will deliver the finished prosthesis and tissue bar to the restorative dentist. At the time of placement of the final restoration, provisional appliances are removed. Before the placement of the tissue bar, the denture

is coated with pressure-indicator paste (Fig 38-22a). The denture is adjusted for tissue contacts and occlusion. The tissue bar is placed and verified for fit and accuracy (Fig 38-22b). The denture is placed, occlusion rechecked, and the patient placed in the maintenance phase of therapy (Fig 38-22c).

Anchor-Supported Overdentures

The anchor-supported overdenture is fabricated in the laboratory and delivered to the restorative dentist. The laboratory should allow space to pick up the retentive anchor matrices in the denture (Fig 38-23).

Hybrid Prostheses

With a hybrid prosthesis, the laboratory delivers the final prosthesis to the practitioner for placement. The provisional prosthesis is removed and the implant interface cleansed with water spray and chlorhexidine digluconate. The prosthesis is seated without any occlusal screws and examined for fit. The abutment-implant interface must be closed. If this interface is not visible, radiographs can be used.

Next, and very important, the occlusal screws are seated in the appliance individually. Each screw should seat without binding. The first contact of the screw to its seat should have the same digital feel as a crown seated in the clinician's hand on a laboratory analog. When the screw contacts its seat, it should be tight after 90 degrees of rotation. The way the screw is seated is the best determinant of passive fit. If previous suggestions are followed, this placement will proceed without problems, and one can close the screw access channels. This applies to all screw-retained restorations.

Once the fit is verified, the occlusion is finalized. The appliance is then polished and returned to the mouth. The occlusal screws are torqued to the manufacturer's recommendations, and a small cotton pledget is placed to protect the screw. Temporary stopping is placed to close one half of the remaining channel, and the occlusal portion of the channel is closed with a hybrid composite. The occlusion is checked, and the patient is placed on appropriate maintenance therapy.

Implant Maintenance

A small percentage of implants placed ultimately fail. They appear to fail because of trauma (caused by clenching, bruxism, or an ill-fitting prosthesis), infection, or a combination of these factors. It is not yet known how often failure occurs in the average implant practice, but it has been estimated that as many as 10% of the implants placed will eventually fail. A large number of implants that fail do so early in treatment. Titanium implants that fail after prosthetic restoration fail at highly variable rates; failure appears to be reversible in many cases, so implant maintenance is crucial.

A typical maintenance schedule could include the following:

1. Update the patient's medical and dental history.
2. Review oral hygiene, if necessary. Interproximal brushes are often helpful. For patients who have problems brushing, powered toothbrushes can provide more effective leaning. When other methods prove ineffective, use chlorhexidine short term, and shorten maintenance intervals.
3. Probe (as many as six sites) around each implant, using a standardized plastic probe: record probing depth (from

a fixed position, if possible) and check for bleeding on probing or suppuration.
4. Check for signs of trauma, ie, worn prosthesis; loosened screws; broken abutment screws, abutments, or implants; pain in the implant area; and patient history of bruxism.
5. Check the overlying prosthesis.
6. Remove any implant-borne material, using specially designed nonmetallic curettes. Follow with a rubber cup run at low speed with implant-polishing paste.
7. Take vertical bitewing or periapical radiographs (on average, once a year for the first few years, and more often in cases with active breakdown).
8. Set appropriate maintenance intervals.

The patient should be seen as often as is necessary to keep the periodontium or peri-implant tissues healthy (or usually every 3 months if there is periodontitis present). For completely edentulous patients, at least one visit per year is recommended.

Case Presentation

Collecting the Clinical and Radiographic Evidence

Mrs Pafufnick is a 46-year-old woman in good systemic health. Her chief complaint is that her maxillary full denture is loose and her mandibular removable partial denture is not functioning well. She says that both are a constant bother. In addition, she wants to improve the esthetics of her mandibular anterior teeth.

She wears her maxillary full denture constantly, removing it only for cleaning. Within the last few years, she has had increasing problems with retention; the denture has come loose several times in social situations, causing her extreme embarrassment. The connecting bar of the partial denture, which replaces the mandibular right molars, has been a source of irritation, and she wishes to have it replaced with a fixed prosthesis, if possible.

Interpreting the Evidence

In Mrs Pafufnick's case, there has been a great deal of resorption of the maxillary bony ridge. The clinician knows from her history and the clinical examination that this patient's residual ridge is not sufficient to retain a conventional denture. The bone has resorbed apically and distally, thus increasing the area that must be replaced by the prosthesis and reducing the retentive capacity of the residual ridge. There is, however, adequate bone to support implants. The apicocoronal dimension of the bone in the

THE EVIDENCE

Health History

1. Medical
   - Mrs Pafufnick's health history reveals nothing that would negatively influence her oral health or treatment.
2. Dental
   - All of the patient's maxillary teeth and her mandibular molars on the right side were removed at age 16 because of severe dental caries (Fig 38-24a).
   - The patient is an intelligent person with high dental knowledge.
   - She brushes and uses dental floss twice daily.

Extraoral Examination

1. The head and neck are inspected visually for asymmetries and abnormal features.
   - ➤ None are found.
2. The temporomandibular joints are inspected by palpation during range-of-motion movements; any noise or tenderness is recorded.
   - ➤ The joints move well, and there is no noise or pain on palpation.
3. The lips are examined for any abnormalities (including location and size) noted, since a large percentage of oral neoplasms are found here.
   - ➤ No abnormalities are found.

Intraoral Examination

1. Any discoloration (usually white, red, or black) of the oral mucosal tissues is recorded, including location and size.
   - ➤ No abnormalities are found.
2. The tongue is grasped at the tip with cotton gauze and gently moved anteriorly to inspect the lateral borders, since this is the most frequent site for intraoral neoplasms and changes associated with certain chronic conditions.
   - ➤ No abnormalities are found.

Clinical Examination

1. Dental
   - ➤ All the maxillary teeth are missing, as are the mandibular third molars and mandibular right first and second molars (Figs 38-24b and 38-24c). The re-

maining teeth and dental structures show no clinical signs of pathology except the following.
   - ➤ She has a number of inconsistent margins on the restorations on her remaining teeth.
   - ➤ Resorption of the maxillary edentulous ridge has occurred. The anterior portion of the ridge has resorbed posteriorly and superiorly. This resorption necessitates relining the patient's denture to compensate for loss of hard and soft tissue. The soft tissues are irritated in the vestibular area.

2. Periodontal
   - ➤ The periodontal examination is within normal limits.

Radiographic Examination

Because of the number of potential implant sites, radiographs for this patient should begin with right-angle periapical views of teeth and a panoramic radiograph (Fig 38-24d). Panoramic radiographs provide much information and often help further define significant areas adjacent to the implant site, such as the course of the inferior alveolar nerve, the maxillary sinus, residual roots, and the nasal floor.

Radiographic examination reveals the following:
- Some of the patient's dental restorations show signs of inconsistent margins and recurrent decay.
- Screening radiographs indicate that there is little bone left in the apico-occlusal dimension of the maxilla to receive dental implants. To provide accurate information on the buccolingual dimension of bone available in multiple areas, a computerized tomogram is ordered. In this case, there has been severe resorption of both the maxillary and mandibular ridges, and information on the bone configuration of the site in a buccolingual dimension will be very helpful. In the maxillary arch, this information will show both the amount of bone available for implant placement and the space that the implant-borne prosthesis will need to fill. Filling this space in the anterior maxilla is important, because esthetic results are important to the patient. If a great deal of resorption has occurred, a fixed/removable device is usually ruled out because the resulting tooth replacements would be long (apico-occlusally), very bulky (buccolingually), or both.

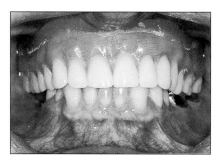

Fig 38-24a This 46-year-old woman has been wearing a maxillary denture since she was 16 years old. She is concerned because her denture no longer stays in place despite numerous relinings and remakes.

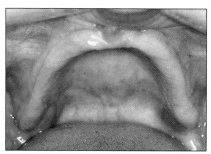

Fig 38-24b The maxillary edentulous ridge has resorbed posteriorly and apically and is no longer capable of retaining a conventional denture.

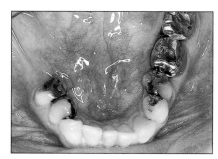

Fig 38-24c The patient reports that her mandibular removable partial denture irritates her tongue.

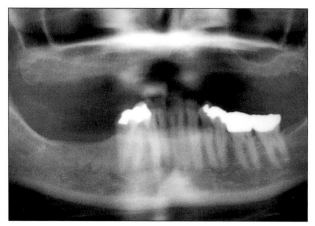

Fig 38-24d Panoramic radiograph.

proposed implant sites ranges from 6 to 10 mm, there is adequate mesiodistal bone, and the buccolingual width of the bone in the proposed sites ranges from 4 to 6 mm. At least 1 mm of bone around the implant is necessary (and preferably more close to important structures such as contiguous teeth and the inferior alveolar nerve). Therefore, an implant system must be chosen that fits within the available bony housing; otherwise, guided bone regeneration must be used to increase the bony housing or the patient should be treated without implants.[1]

The mandible also has adequate bone to surround the appropriate implants.

Patient Goals and Treatment Options

1. What does the patient want?

   To have stable, esthetic tooth replacements and repairs to her existing teeth; she is willing to spend the time and money necessary to achieve her goals.

2. What does the patient need to achieve her goals?
   a. To have stable maxillary and mandibular prostheses.
   b. To eliminate the need for a mandibular removable partial denture, because the connecting bar is a constant bother.
   c. To have the necessary dental repairs made.
   d. To improve the esthetics of the mandibular anterior teeth.

3. What are the maxillary treatment options for this patient?
   a. A new full denture. The existing prosthesis appears well made (and was recently relined). The patient is unable to retain the denture because the residual maxillary ridge is insufficient to hold a traditional denture. Therefore, an implant-borne prosthesis should be considered. Assuming sufficient bone, two types of prostheses are available: a fixed/removable (or fixed) prosthesis or an implant-supported denture.
   b. A fixed or fixed/removable prosthesis. This type of prosthesis in the present environment would, by necessity, be large and not esthetic. If the patient decides on a fixed or fixed/removable device, surgical procedures can change this environment, but an implant-supported denture is a better, less expensive alternative for this patient. She is willing to have a removable prosthesis. There are two possible approaches to an implant-borne denture.
      • A removable denture supported by individual implants. This patient is happy with a denture, but her current prosthesis irritates her soft tissues. Individual implants may not solve this problem, since the denture will still be largely supported by soft tissue. In addition, this approach is more successful in the mandibular arch, where bone is denser. After this option was described in detail, the patient decided that she wanted the stability provided by a bar with additional implants.

- A removable denture supported by a bar. The patient chose implants joined by an interconnective bar and a denture retained with clips inside the denture for the additional retention provided. A round bar is suggested because of its positive lock, which most patients prefer. Inside the denture, a series of clips is processed to fit over the bar (implants should be placed at least 10 mm apart to allow a large enough clip to be made) for retention.

4. What are the mandibular treatment options?

   a. A new removable partial denture. This alternative is recommended for some individuals. However, this patient already has a partial denture that, though well made, is not satisfactory because of constant movement of the prosthesis and trapping of food; so remaking this prosthesis is not an acceptable alternative to her.

   b. An implant-supported fixed partial denture. Because the patient prefers a fixed prosthesis, implants are the treatment of choice. Currently, it is suggested that where small numbers of teeth have been lost, individual teeth should be replaced with individual implants, since this arrangement has all the advantages of single teeth. This requires an implant that achieves a high degree of bone-to-implant contact. The advantages of individual implants include better esthetics, ease of cleaning, and masticatory efficiency. When implants are joined, problems associated with ensuring passive fit of the restoration and oral hygiene emerge. If attachment is deemed necessary, implants should be attached to implants where possible. If this attachment is not possible, tooth-to-implant restorations are the second choice; however, intrusion of teeth can occur when teeth and implants are joined.

Making a Clinical Diagnosis

1. Are there extraoral or intraoral problems that should be dealt with before restorative and implant therapy begins? In Mrs Pafufnick's case, no such problems are evident.

2. Does the disease have a systemic modifier? Since all systemic findings are normal in this case, attention may be focused on dental, periodontal, and implant findings.

3. Signs and symptoms are identified in the periodontal diagnostic process.

   a. Is there inflammation of the periodontal tissues? No.

   b. Is there loss of clinical attachment and/or bone around teeth? No. The pocket probing depths were 3 mm or less, with the soft tissue approximately at the cementoenamel junction. Radiographs indicate no bone loss from periodontal disease.

   c. What is the periodontal diagnosis? Health.

   d. What is the dental diagnosis? All the mandibular premolars and the mandibular left first and second molars have caries.

Formulating a Treatment Plan

1. Periodontal

   a. Restorations will be placed on mandibular teeth, and implant surgery will be performed in both the maxilla and the mandible. These procedures may initially compromise the patient's ability to clean her teeth.

   b. The patient's periodontal condition will be closely monitored during treatment.

   c. She will be placed into periodontal maintenance therapy when active treatment ends. The frequency of the periodontal maintenance depends on the health of the remaining teeth (see the discussion of implant maintenance).

2. Dental

   a. *Arrest caries lesions.* The restorations needed to arrest active dental caries will be placed on the mandibular teeth.

   b. *Provisional restoration.* A provisional maxillary denture will be set up and tried in. This will be painted with barium and worn while a computerized tomogram is taken (Fig 38-25). It may then be used as a surgical stent, or a separate stent may be constructed, following recommendations by Higginbottom[2] (Fig 38-26; see chapter 37). Periapical or panoramic radiographs will then be taken to ensure proper angulation of the drills passing through the surgical stent (Fig 38-27).

   c. *Implant therapy.*

      - Maxilla. The more stability the patient wants, the more implants that should be placed. Because the patient wants a very stable denture, three or more implants should be placed. If three implants are used, they are usually placed in the canine positions (two) and a central incisor position (one). More stability can be gained by placing additional implants in more posterior positions.

      - Mandible. The treatment alternatives for the mandibular right include not replacing the missing teeth, replacing the missing teeth with a removable partial denture, or using dental implants. Following consultation, the patient decides to have dental implants placed. The next decision is whether to splint the implants together or leave them separate. Because keeping the implants separate allows the patient better access for oral hygiene, it is the best choice.

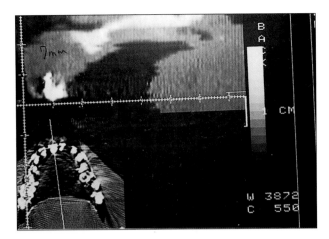

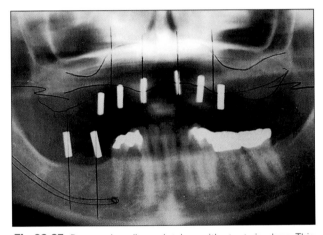

Fig 38-25 A computerized tomogram taken with a barium-coated stent in place shows the amount of resorption that has occurred. The outline of the barium painted around the maxillary central incisors can be seen in the upper left side of the tomogram. The residual ridge is seen in the middle, at the top. The distance between the two will have to be filled in with restorative material. If a fixed/removable device were used, the bulk of the restorative material would interfere with oral hygiene around the implants. An implant-supported denture could be removed for oral hygiene and still support the lip, providing good esthetics and function.

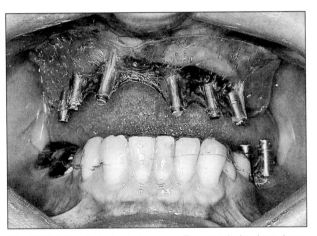

Fig 38-26 Surgical stents in place. The metal pins have been placed using a duplicate of the waxup of the maxillary and mandibular prostheses.

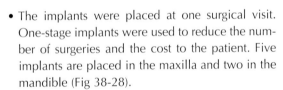

Fig 38-27 Panoramic radiograph taken with stents in place. This film confirms that implant placement through the stent will not interfere with contiguous structures.

- The implants were placed at one surgical visit. One-stage implants were used to reduce the number of surgeries and the cost to the patient. Five implants are placed in the maxilla and two in the mandible (Fig 38-28).

d. *Postoperative care.*
- The patient is placed on systemic antibiotics for 8 days and chlorhexidine mouthrinses twice daily for 4 to 6 weeks. Ten days postoperatively, the original prosthesis is relined with a soft liner. Then the areas immediately surrounding the implants are cut away. The patient is instructed to wear the denture primarily for esthetics and to remove it while sleeping. The denture was relined when the liner hardened.
- The patient is seen on a periodic basis (usually monthly, assuming that healing is progressing normally) until adequate implant stability has been achieved to support the proposed prosthesis. In this case, because no bone augmentation was

necessary, the implant system used allowed the mandibular implants to be restored in 6 weeks, and the maxillary implants in 8 weeks.

e. *Restorative dentistry.* The final denture was fabricated (Fig 38-29a). Provisional restorations were placed on the teeth and implants in the mandible, followed by final restorations a few months later (Fig 38-29b).

g. *Reevaluation of therapy.* At the conclusion of active treatment, a reevaluation of therapy is performed. The final periodontal diagnosis is health. The implants are stable and the surrounding tissues are healthy, so the patient is placed in periodontal maintenance.

h. *Maintenance.* The patient had an exit diagnosis of health. She was seen annually for examination and any needed dental and periodontal maintenance (Fig 38-30). The implants and their overlying prosthesis have been stable for 10 years.

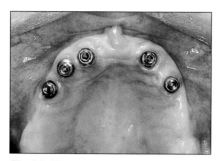

Fig 38-28a A total of five implants were placed in the maxilla. The most posterior implants were placed as far distally as possible without sinus augmentation to provide additional stability for the denture.

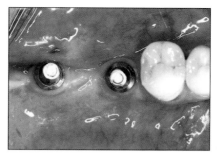

Fig 38-28b Two implants were placed in the right mandible.

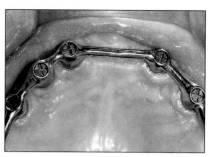

Fig 38-28c A cast bar was constructed over the implants.

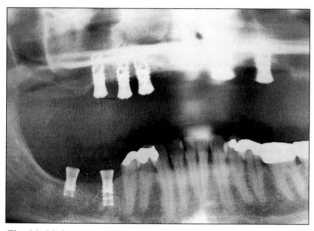

Fig 38-28d Panoramic radiograph taken postoperatively.

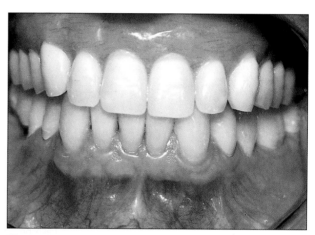

Fig 38-29a Final maxillary prosthesis.

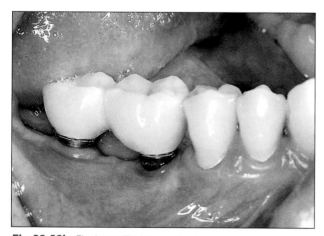

Fig 38-29b Final mandibular prosthesis.

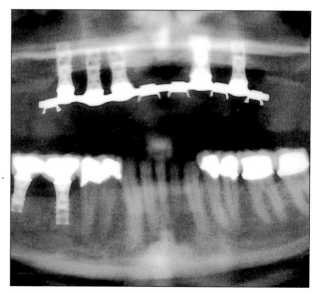

Fig 38-30 Final radiograph.

References

1. Buser D, Brägger U, Lang NP, Nyman S. Regeneration and enlargement of jaw bone using guided tissue regeneration. Clin Oral Implants Res 1990;1:22–32.
2. Higginbottom FL, Wilson TG. Three-dimensional templates for placement of root-form dental implants: A technical note. Int J Oral Maxillofac Implants 1996;11:787–793.

39 | Advanced Implant Therapy

Thomas G. Wilson, Jr
- Multiple-Tooth Replacement in Partially Edentulous Patients
- Implant Placement in Areas of Esthetic Concern
- Implant Placement in Totally Edentulous Patients
- Timing of Implant Placement
- Site Modification
- Immediate Loading

Frank L. Higginbottom and Thomas G. Wilson, Jr
- Case Presentation

Multiple-Tooth Replacement in Partially Edentulous Patients

Multiple-tooth replacement in partially edentulous patients presents special challenges and should be treated by the clinician who has gained experience with single-tooth posterior implants. Proper placement of implants in these cases requires more planning than for cases with single-tooth replacement or for patients who are completely edentulous.

At least 3 mm of space is required between implants to develop a papilla and to allow for ease of cleaning.[1] Therefore, assuming that implants are 5 mm in diameter, at least 8 mm should be allowed between the centers of the implants (10 mm if a retentive clip is to be placed in the space). Additionally, the center of an implant should be at least 5 mm from the adjacent root surface of any contiguous teeth. A larger- or smaller-diameter implant necessitates different separation dimensions. These procedures almost always require templates to properly position the implants.

Implant Placement in Areas of Esthetic Concern

Traditional implant techniques often need to be modified in areas of esthetic concern to the patient, and these areas are not appropriate for initial implant experiences. The clinician should verify the patient's expectations in esthetic areas before undertaking the often extensive (and expensive) procedures needed in these areas. If esthetic results are of concern to the patient, the surgeon will need to preserve or reestablish adequate bone and soft tissue. In areas with minimal loss of supporting structures, implants can be placed simultaneously with soft and hard tissue grafting. In areas with an extensive tissue deficit, it is recommended that lost bone and gingiva be regained before implant placement.

Implant Placement in Totally Edentulous Patients

Cases in which two implants will be used to support a denture are covered in chapter 35. When more than two implants will be used, the implant dentist has two treatment options.

Implant-Supported Complete Denture

The use of three or more implants to support a complete denture should be considered in the following circumstances:

- The patient prefers a denture but wants more stability than that provided by two implants.
- The patient wants to eliminate the palatal portion of the denture. (Doing so usually requires at least six implants, two of which are in the molar regions.)
- The patient with esthetic concerns has a severely resorbed maxilla, but does not want to undergo the surgeries to rebuild lost hard and soft tissues, which would be needed for an esthetic result using a fixed prosthesis.
- The patient's present denture is causing soft tissue trauma, and the patient or therapist wants to eliminate soft tissue impingement of the prosthesis.
- The patient wants or needs the simplified oral hygiene provided by a removable prosthesis (as compared with a fixed/removable or fixed prosthesis).

Implant-Supported Fixed or Fixed/Removable Prosthesis

Four or more implants that support a fixed or fixed/removable prosthesis may be useful in the following situations:

- The patient wants or needs the stability of a fixed prosthesis.
- Available bone and soft tissues approximate (or can be augmented to approximate) the contours found with the natural teeth in areas of esthetic concern. This option is most successful when the patient has good oral hygiene, the implants are properly spaced, and there are enough implants to support the prosthesis.

The position of the implants at surgery should be guided by a template. The longer the implants and the denser the bone, the fewer implants needed. The length of the arch and the force of the occlusion may also dictate the number of implants needed.

When trying to decide between a fixed prosthesis or a removable prosthesis for a totally edentulous arch, consider two points. First, implant-retained removable dentures are easier to clean, often more esthetic, as functional, and less expensive than fixed implant prostheses. Second, it is easier to hide missing bone and soft tissue loss with a removable denture than with a fixed prosthesis.

Timing of Implant Placement

Practitioners in the earlier days of implant dentistry lacked guidelines for the timing of implant placement in relation to tooth extraction. This situation complicated communication between professionals. Four possible relationships between tooth extraction and implant placement have now been classified: immediate sites, recent sites, delayed sites, and mature sites.[2]

Immediate Implant Sites

Immediate implant sites are those in which tooth extraction and implant placement occur during the same surgery, thus preserving the bone of the socket. Under certain circumstances, immediate implants are the preferred approach to implant placement.

To achieve osseointegration in immediate sites, certain guidelines must be followed. The tooth should be extracted in such a manner as to preserve as much alveolar housing as possible. The socket is then cleared of remaining soft tissue. Iodine or chlorhexidine is sometimes needed in selected patients to clean the socket. An important determinate in achieving osseointegration is the distance from the bony socket to the implant surface, termed the *horizontal deficit dimension (HDD)*. Bone has been shown to bridge across HDDs in humans when rough-surface implants (either titanium plasma sprayed or sandblasted and acid etched) are placed in sockets with HDDs of 2 mm or less,[3–5] with or without membranes. Preliminary evidence indicates that to achieve osseointegration with HDDs greater than 2 mm (those often seen at molar sites), the use of sandblasted and acid-etched implants, along with a connective tissue membrane to cover the implant and bony socket, is necessary to allow bone to successfully bridge across these larger HDDs.[6] Immediate implants have become so successful that they should be included routinely in advanced implant practices.

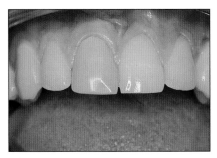

Fig 39-1a This patient had severe external resorption of the maxillary right central incisor. There was insufficient bone to support immediate implant placement.

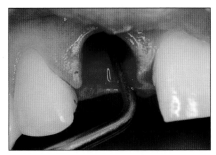

Fig 39-1b Extraction was performed in a manner designed to retain as much bone as possible, and all soft tissues were removed from the socket.

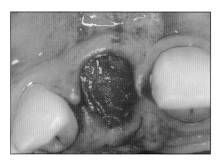

Fig 39-1c A connective tissue membrane has been used to seal the site.

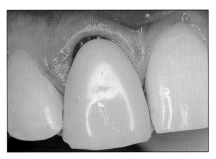

Fig 39-1d Initial support for the soft tissues of the healing site is provided by the pontic on a provisional removable partial denture.

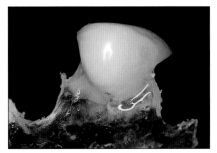

Fig 39-1e The pontic is flat on the facial apical portion and tapers to the palatal portion. The pontic extends 3 mm into the extraction socket. In 1 week the pontic is reduced at the apex by 1 mm to allow the soft tissues to further fill the socket.

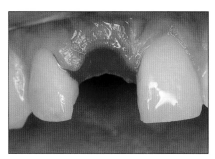

Fig 39-1f Healed site at implant placement 6 months later.

Recent Implant Sites

Recent implant sites are sites where soft tissue healing is allowed prior to implant placement. Implants are usually placed 30 to 60 days later. The rationale for using recent sites is to reduce the probability of infection at implant placement. In practice, however, this concern has not proven valid; therefore, in the author's opinion, this approach is rarely indicated.

Delayed Implant Sites (Extraction Socket Enhancement)

Delayed implant sites are sites where the implant is not placed until dense bone has been generated (usually 6 months or more after tooth extraction). A technique termed *socket enhancement* is frequently used to enhance bony healing in areas where implants will later be placed. It is especially useful in areas of esthetic concern or where contiguous structures (such as the maxillary sinus and the inferior alveolar nerve) will limit the initial stability of the implant. This approach often involves the use of a barrier membrane to seal the socket and to substitute for missing bony walls of the socket. In areas of esthetic concern, it is often combined with soft tissue grafts, autogenous bone grafts, or both (Figs 39-1a to 39-1f).

Mature Implant Sites

By definition, a mature implant site is one in which the surgeon has not been able to guide healing following extraction. Some of these sites will require the generation of additional bone prior to implant placement.[7] The most predictable results of such guided bone regeneration are found in sites with multiple bony walls to provide stability and a source of bone progenitor cells. These sites include areas of previous extraction, fenestration defects, and dehiscence. Sites without lateral walls are less predictable.[7]

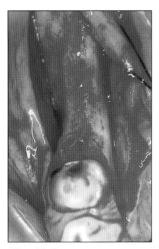

Fig 39-2a This bony ridge was not wide enough to allow implant placement.

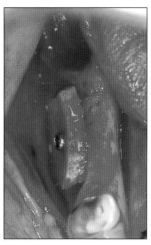

Fig 39-2b A block of autogenous bone was harvested distal to the site and fixed in place with a bone screw.

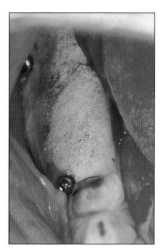

Fig 39-2c The graft was covered with a nonabsorbable membrane, which was stabilized with retaining screws. Absorbable membranes can also be used.

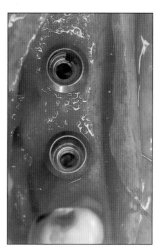

Fig 39-2d Six months later the bony ridge was wide enough to support implants.

The techniques of bone enhancement prior to or at the time of implant placement can provide predictable results. This predictability depends on careful attention to implant selection, proper site selection and enhancement, correct use of guided bone regeneration and socket presentation, and diligent postoperative care on the part of both the surgeon and the patient.

Site Modification

Many potential implant sites cannot be used successfully because they lack adequate bony housing. This predicament has been solved in many cases by the introduction of methods to grow new bone. One of these techniques is *guided bone regeneration*.[8] GBR is the use of materials (usually involving absorbable or nonabsorbable barrier membranes) to selectively exclude gingival tissue from the wound site and to allow the migration of bone-producing cells into the area. This approach was originally introduced for use around teeth and was called *guided tissue regeneration*.[9] Regeneration of bone around implants is more predictable than that around teeth, probably because implants are sterile when first placed and are less likely to cause infection of the hard tissues. Guided bone regeneration has gained rapid acceptance since it was first proposed for use around implants in 1989.[8]

When using GBR, creating space under the membrane is important. This can be accomplished by using a filler material alone (in smaller defects) or in combination with specially designed membrane devices. Autogenous bone is commonly used as a filler (Figs 39-2a to 39-2d), but other materials have proved successful. Autogenous bone can be collected from local or distant sites. Smaller chips, which are packed into place, are preferred. Larger pieces can be held with bone screws. The graft is then covered with a barrier membrane. Healing of graft sites takes at least 6 months, sometimes longer.

The Achilles' heel of barrier membranes is infection, which is most often seen clinically when membranes become exposed to the oral environment. To reduce the chance of exposure, nonabsorbable membranes should be used where possible and covered with soft tissue at the time of placement. Membrane stabilization facilitates correct placement and may enhance bone healing in larger defects. Postoperative care also reduces the chances of infection. Patients are usually administered systemic antibiotics for 8 days, along with twice-daily chlorhexidine rinses for 4 to 6 weeks. With nonabsorbable membranes, the longer they stay in place and the fewer the bacteria allowed to access the surgical site, the greater the production of bone. Primary wound closure also aids in minimizing infection.

While still technique sensitive and prone to occasional infection, in certain circumstances GBR is quite predictable, and the procedure should be part of the advanced implant surgeon's armamentarium.

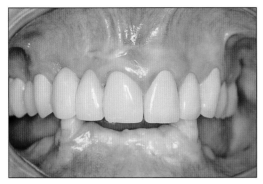

Fig 39-3a This patient has lost all of her mandibular teeth except the canines. She prefers a fixed prosthesis and wants to avoid a provisional full removable denture.

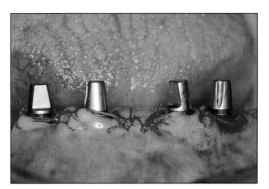

Fig 39-3b The canines are extracted, and four implants are placed.

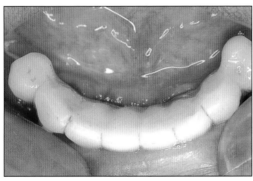

Fig 39-3c Immediately following implant placement, a fixed provisional restoration is relined and cemented into place.

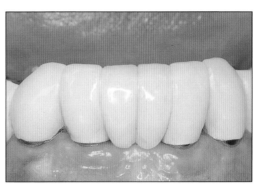

Fig 39-3d The final prosthesis 2 years after placement (restorations courtesy of Dr Douglas Martin).

Immediate Loading

Traditionally, it has been suggested that to achieve optimal osseointegration, excessive functional loading should be avoided for several months.[10] As clinical experience with implants has grown, however, the definition of *excessive functional loading* has changed. When implants were first introduced, it was believed that any load would reduce the possibility of osseointegration. This thinking has evolved to the point where it is now acceptable for implants of a certain size, type, and placement to be put into immediate function (Figs 39-3a to 39-3d).[11] These situations should be handled only by clinicians with advanced experience. The first studies of immediate loading of osseointegration implants used the titanium plasma-sprayed screw[12]; later, this concept was applied to other implant systems and designs.[11]

Case Presentation

Collecting the Clinical and Radiographic Evidence

Ms Buser is a 19-year-old woman in good systemic health. Her chief complaint was congenitally missing maxillary lateral incisors (Fig 39-4).

Interpreting the Evidence

Patient Goals and Options
1. What does the patient want? *To have stable, esthetic tooth replacements.*
2. What does the patient need to achieve her goals? *To have a stable prosthesis to replace the missing incisors.*

THE EVIDENCE

Health History

1. Medical
   - Ms Buser's health history reveals nothing that would influence her oral health or treatment.
2. Dental
   - All the patient's teeth remain except the third molars, which were removed, and congenitally missing maxillary lateral incisors.
   - She is an intelligent person with a high dental IQ.
   - She brushes her teeth and uses dental floss twice daily.

Extraoral Examination

1. The head and neck are inspected visually and palpated for asymmetries and abnormal features. Any deviations from normal are recorded.

   ➤ None are found.

2. The temporomandibular joints are inspected by palpation and sound during range-of-motion movements, and any noise or tenderness is recorded.

   ➤ The joints move freely, and there is no noise or pain on palpation.

3. The lips are examined and any abnormalities (including location and size) noted, since a large percentage of oral neoplasms are found here.

   ➤ No abnormalities are found.

   ➤ The patient's lip line reveals a large amount of tooth and gingival tissue when she smiles. This may require an implant.

Intraoral Examination

1. Any discoloration (usually white, red, or black) of the oral mucosal tissues is recorded, including location and size.

   ➤ No abnormalities are found.

2. The tongue is grasped at the tip with cotton gauze and gently moved anteriorly to inspect the lateral borders, since this is the most frequent site for intraoral neoplasms and changes associated with certain chronic conditions.

   ➤ No abnormalities are found.

Clinical Examination

1. Dental

   ➤ All the teeth are present except the mandibular third molars and maxillary lateral incisors. The remaining teeth and dental structures show no clinical signs of pathology.

2. Periodontal

   ➤ The periodontal examination is within normal limits.

Radiographic Examination

   ➤ The radiographic examination is normal.

---

3. What are the treatment options for this patient?
   a. *Fixed partial dentures.* The contiguous teeth would be suitable abutments, but the potential abutment teeth have no need for restorations.
   b. *A removable partial denture.* The advantages would be good esthetics and an inexpensive prosthesis. The disadvantages would be impingement and pressure on the palatal soft tissues and a possible lack of stability during function.
   c. *Implants.* The advantages would be excellent esthetics and function, as well as greater longevity than a fixed partial denture. The disadvantage would be the need for a surgical procedure.
   d. *No treatment.* The patient is very conscious of esthetics and prefers replacement of the missing teeth.

Formulating a Treatment Plan

The patient chose to have implants placed into the positions of the maxillary lateral incisors. Periapical, panoramic, and tomographic radiographs were taken and evaluated (Fig 39-5). Adequate bone was available for implant placement. Restorative consultations were held, and the patient agreed to proceed with the plan. Radiographic and surgical templates were constructed. Her periodontal condition was normal and will be monitored during implant therapy.

1. *Implant surgery.* In this case, the bone loss was minimal, and implant placement with soft tissue enhancement was performed (Fig 39-6). A subepithelial con-

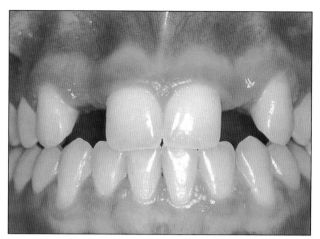

Fig 39-4 Preoperative appearance of a 19-year-old female patient with congenitally missing lateral incisors.

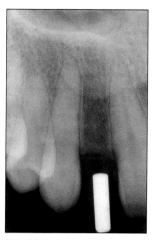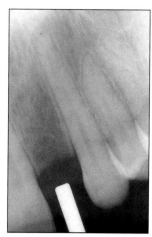

Fig 39-5 Radiographic appearance of the proposed angulation at both lateral incisor sites. Because the facial plate of bone was deficient, the treatment plan called for placement of submerged implants and guided bone regeneration. Subepithelial connective tissue grafts would be done at implant uncovering. A key to esthetic success would be proper angulation of the implants.

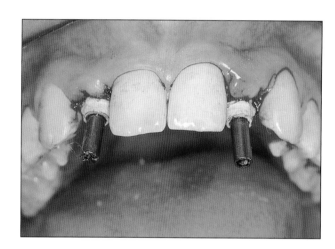

Fig 39-6 Six months after implant placement, the implants were uncovered, membranes removed, and connective tissue grafts placed on the facial bone plate. Abutments for screw retention were placed, impression copings placed, and a final impression made.

nective tissue graft was taken from the palate and placed on the facial aspect of the implants at the same surgery.

2. *Postoperative care.* The patient was given systemic antibiotics for 8 days and asked to use chlorhexidine mouthrinses twice daily for 6 weeks. The patient was seen periodically (visits are usually monthly, assuming that healing is progressing normally) until adequate implant stability to support the proposed prosthesis was achieved. A provisional removable partial denture that did not touch the soft tissue in the implant sites was used during healing.

3. *Restorative dentistry.* Provisional fixed partial dentures were placed to guide soft tissue healing (Figs 39-7a to 39-7c). The final fixed partial dentures were placed a few months later.

4. *Reevaluation of therapy.* Six months after placement of the final restoration, the tissues were normal.

5. *Periodontal maintenance.* The patient exhibited both dental and periodontal health, and she was seen yearly for maintenance (Fig 39-8).

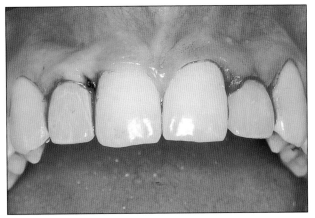

Fig 39-7a Provisional restorations were placed the day of uncovering and abutment connection.

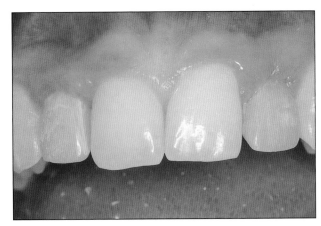

Fig 39-7b Provisionals after 3 months of healing.

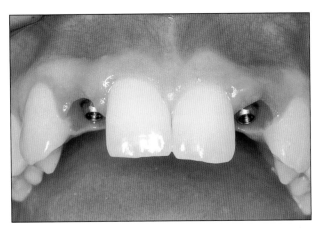

Fig 39-7c Appearance of the peri-implant space created by the emergence profile provisionals on the day the final restorations were delivered.

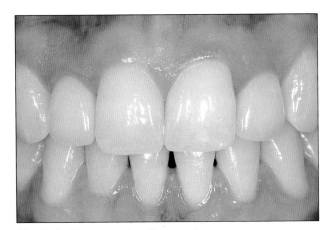

Fig 39-8 Final restorations 7 years after surgery.

References

1. Tarnow DP, Cho SC, Wallace SS. The effect of inter-implant distance on the height of inter-implant bone crest. J Periodontol 2000;71:546–549.

2. Wilson TG, Weber HP. Classification of and therapy for areas of deficient bony housing prior to dental implant placement. Int J Periodontics Restorative Dent 1993;13:451–459.

3. Wilson T Jr, Schenk R, Buser D, Cochran D. Implants placed in immediate extraction sites: A report of histologic and histometric analyses of human biopsies. Int J Oral Maxillofac Implants 1998;13:333–341.

4. Cornelini REA. Immediate one-stage postextraction implant: A human clinical and histologic case report. Int J Oral Maxillofac Implants 2000;15:432–437.

5. Paolantonio M, Dolci M, Scarano A, et al. Immediate implantation in fresh extraction sockets. A controlled clinical and histological study in man. J Periodontol 2001;72:1560–1571.

6. Wilson TG, Carnio J, Schenk R, Cochran D. Immediate implants covered with connective tissue membranes: Human biopsies. J Periodontol 2003 (in press).

7. Buser D, Bragger U, Lang NP, Nyman S. Regeneration and enlargement of jaw bone using guided tissue regeneration. Clin Oral Implants Res 1990;1:22–32.

8. Dahlin C, Sennerby L, Lekholm U, et al. Generation of new bone around titanium implants using a membrane technique: An experimental study in rabbits. Int J Oral Maxillofac Implants 1989;4(1):19–25.

9. Nyman S, Gottlow J, Lindhe J, et al. New attachment formation by guided tissue regeneration. J Periodontal Res 1987;22:252–254.

10. Brunski JB, Moccia AF Jr, Pollack SR, et al. The influence of functional use of endosseous dental implants on the tissue interface. I. Histological aspects. J Dent Res 1979;58:1953–1969.

11. Tarnow D, Emtiaz S. Immediate loading of threaded implants at stage 1 surgery in edentulous arches: Ten consecutive case reports with a 1- to 5-year data. Int J Oral Maxillofac Implants 1997;12:319–324.

12. Ledermann PD. ITI-International Team fur Orale Implantologie. Sechsjahrige Klinische Erfahrungen mit dem Titan-plasma beschichteten ITI-Schrauben implant in der Regio Interforaminalis des Onterkiefers. Separatdruck Aus. Schweiz Monatsschr Zahnmed 1983;93:1070.

Appendix 1: Health History

One essential element in a patient's record is the *health history*. Typically, a form is filled in before the patient is first examined, then updated before any treatment is performed. (A sample form is included in this appendix.)

The form begins by gathering basic *patient information* such as name, age, height, weight, and current address and contact information, as well as the names of the patient's physician and previous dentist. Then the patient is asked about his or her primary dental concern. This is called the *chief complaint* and is important not only as a clue to guide the examination but because addressing patient concerns is one of the primary obligations of the dentist. Identifying these concerns is a precondition of satisfying patient needs, and experience shows that this approach improves patient compliance. Compliance is an essential component of treatment since most periodontal diseases are chronic and require adequate oral hygiene (combined with periodic dental visits) to be controlled.

The health history form should also include information on the patient's *medical history*: past illnesses, medications presently being taken, allergies to medications, the possible need for premedication before dental visits, and other relevant information.

The dentist needs to know about any *illness*, past or present, that could affect a patient's treatment. Examples would include cardiovascular problems (eg, hypertension), pulmonary problems, blood dyscrasias, and other diseases. If there is any question about the effect a problem may have on a patient during therapy, the patient's physician should be contacted.

The dentist should know if the patient takes a *medication* that could directly affect dental and periodontal health. Examples include medications that reduce salivary flow (eg, tranquilizers and antidepressants), those used to treat allergies and asthma, birth control pills, and certain medications for cardiovascular problems.

The dentist should ascertain any patient history of *allergic reaction* to medication. The drugs most commonly used in a practice can be listed and the patient asked to indicate any allergies.

The dentist should know whether a patient needs *antibiotics* before receiving dental treatment. This is often the case before treatments that cause bleeding. The bacteria introduced into the bloodstream during therapy can cause local or distant infections that can be serious or even life threatening. In most cases, specific antibiotic regimens are suggested to reduce the probability of occurrence. Situations requiring premedication include some heart murmurs (such as some mitral valve prolapses), artificial heart valves, and certain other prosthetic devices including joint replacements. (See appendix 2.)

The dentist should know which patients have special conditions affecting treatment. Examples include those who are pregnant or have transmissible diseases. This last category includes patients who are HIV positive and those who are positive carriers for hepatitis.

The health history should cover the patient's *dental history*, including present oral hygiene practices and any history of dental, periodontal, or temporomandibular problems. The patient should be asked about parafunctional habits such as bruxing or clenching, since these problems may contribute to breakdown of the stomatognathic system. Past compliance to suggested oral hygiene and maintenance, and negative experiences in the dental office, are also important elements of dental history, suggesting parameters for potential patient compliance. This is especially important for patients with chronic periodontal problems, since the more they comply with the dental professional's suggestions on proper oral hygiene and frequency of maintenance visits, the more likely they are to keep their teeth.

Family history can be significant and can directly impact the long-term survival of the dentition. Some types of periodontal disease are recurrent within families. In addition, information on cardiovascular problems and parental longevity can give clues to how long the patient will need to maintain the dentition. Family history can also be a predictor of diabetes, which can directly influence the patient's healing capacity as well as the severity of periodontal disease.

PLEASE PRINT AND ANSWER ALL QUESTIONS, INITIAL BOTTOM OF EACH PAGE AND SIGN THE LAST PAGE.
ALL INFORMATION IS CONFIDENTIAL.

Name _____ Age _____ Birthdate _____ Height _____ Weight _____

Single   Married   Separated   Divorced   Widowed   (Please circle)   SS# _____

Residence Address _____ City _____ Zip _____ Phone _____

Fax (Home)_____ Fax (Office) _____

Occupation _____ Position _____ Employer _____

Business Address _____ City _____ Zip _____ Phone _____

Name of Spouse _____

Occupation _____ Position _____ Employer _____

Business Address _____ City _____ Zip _____ Phone _____

Party Responsible for Payment _____ Relation to You _____

Emergency Contact Other Than Spouse _____ Phone_____

Referred by _____ City _____ Phone_____

Current Dentist _____ City _____ How Long? _____ Frequency?_____

Previous Dentist _____ City _____ How Long? _____ Frequency?_____

Your Physician _____ How Long? _____

Physician's Address _____ City _____ Phone _____

Date of Last Complete Physical Examination _____ Purpose of Exam _____

Findings _____

Do You Have Dental Insurance?   Yes _____ No _____ Name of Carrier _____

GENERAL HEALTH (Please circle 'Yes' or 'No'; if in doubt circle 'U', and fill in other information asked for)

Yes   No   U   1. Are you presently under the care of a physician? If so, why? _____

Yes   No   U   2. Do you have any type of health problem? If so, what? _____

Yes   No   U   3. Do you have any type of heart problem? If so, what?_____

Yes   No   U   4. Do you have high or low blood pressure? If so, which? _____

Yes   No   U   5. Do you have shortness of breath after climbing one flight of stairs? _____

Yes   No   U   6. Do you bleed for more than 30 minutes after a minor cut or have any other minor bleeding problems? If so, what? _____

Yes   No   U   7. Are you taking any medications or drugs including aspirin, vitamins, recreational drugs? List each drug, reason for use, and who prescribed the drug. (Use back of page if needed). _____

Yes   No   U   8. Have you been hospitalized in the last 10 years? If so, for what?_____

Yes   No   U   9. Do you faint easily? _____

Yes   No   U   10. Have you taken cortisone or steroids in the last 6 months? _____

Yes   No   U   11. Have you been under the care of a physician in the last 2 years other than for a routine physical? If so, for what? __

Yes   No   U   12. Have you had any major illnesses or serious operations in the last 10 years? If so, please describe. _____

Yes   No   U   13. Do you have any kidney or liver problems? If so, describe._____

Yes   No   U   14. Have you had rheumatic fever? If so, when was it first diagnosed? _____

Yes   No   U   15. Do you have any type of artificial valve, joint pin, prosthetic hip, etc, in place now? _____

Yes   No   U   16. Do you have a heart murmur, mitral valve prolapse, or heart click? If so, which? _____

Yes   No   U   17. Have you ever received psychiatric care or psychotherapy? If so, which? _____

Yes   No   U   18. Have you ever tested positive for tuberculosis? _____

Yes   No   U   19. Do you now or have you ever had hepatitis? If so, when? _____

Yes   No   U   20. Do you have AIDS or AIDS-related complex (ARC) or have you ever tested positive for the AIDS virus?

Please circle each of the following medications to which you are allergic:

Penicillin	Doxycycline	Aspirin	Valium	Phenergan
Erythromycin	Carbocaine	Phenaphen	Demerol	Morphine
Tetracycline	Xylocaine	Codeine	Percodan	List all others:
Keflex/Keflin	Duranest	Novocaine	Stadol	
Halcion	Acetaminophen	Tylenol	Versed	

Date _____ Patient's Initials (Or Parent/Guardian if Under 18 years old)_____

MEDICAL HISTORY: DO YOU NOW HAVE OR HAVE YOU EVER HAD:

Yes No U 1. Anemia?
Yes No U 2. Frequently swollen ankles?
Yes No U 3. Stomach ulcers, diverticulitis, or ulcerative colitis?
Yes No U 4. Excessive thirst or hunger over extended periods of time?
Yes No U 5. The need to get up nightly to urinate?
Yes No U 6. Cuts that tend to heal slowly?
Yes No U 7. Diabetes? If so, how treated? _____
Yes No U 8. Hemophilia?
Yes No U 9. Implant or transplant? If so, describe. _____
Yes No U 10. Thyroid disturbance or taken thyroid tablets?
Yes No U 11. Tuberculosis or emphysema?
Yes No U 12. Kidney or bladder disease?
Yes No U 13. Arthritis or rheumatism?
Yes No U 14. Venereal disease (syphilis, gonorrhea, herpes II)?
Yes No U 15. Epilepsy, convulsions, or seizures?
Yes No U 16. Cancer or radiation therapy?
Yes No U 17. Smoke or use tobacco in any form? If so, frequency? _____
Yes No U 18. Did you know that if you smoke, you have more problems with gum diseases and their treatment and have a higher risk of losing dental implants?
Yes No U 19. Do you wear contact lenses?
Yes No U 20. Are you taking any sort of tranquilizers?
Yes No U 21. Are you taking anticoagulants (blood thinners)?
Yes No U 22. Are you taking antacids regularly? If so, what? _____
Yes No U 23. Are you taking mood elevators such as:

Parnate	Norpramin	Aventyl	Adapin
Marplan	Pertofrane	Sinequan	Nardil
Vivactyl	Elavil	Tofranil	

Yes No U 24. Do you have glaucoma?
Yes No U 25. Do you have asthma, hay fever, or eczema?
Yes No U 26. Do you have liver problems?
Yes No U 27. Do you have prostate problems (males only)?

MEDICAL HISTORY (FEMALES ONLY)

Yes No U 28. Are you pregnant?
Yes No U 29. Have you had a hysterectomy or ovariectomy?
Yes No U 30. Are you taking birth control pills?
Yes No U 31. Have you been through menopause?
Yes No U 32. Have you had a miscarriage?

FAMILY HISTORY

Yes No U 1. Have any of your blood relatives had heart disease or high blood pressure?
Yes No U 2. Have any of your blood relatives had diabetes?
Yes No U 3. Have any of your blood relatives lost teeth as a result of gum disease? If so, why? _____
Yes No U 4. Have we treated any of your relatives? If so, whom? _____

**Do you have any disease, medical condition, or health problem not listed above that you think we should know about or that you believe might affect treatment in any way? _____
_____
_____
_____

**Do you have any questions before the examination? If so, what? (Use back of page if needed) _____
_____
_____
_____
_____

Date _____ Patient's Initials (Or Parent/Guardian if Under 18 years old)_____

DENTAL HISTORY

Yes No U 1. How would you describe your dental health? **Excellent Good Fair Poor**

Yes No U 2. What do you do to clean your teeth at home? Brush_____ How often? _____
Floss _____ How often?_____ Other (bridge cleaners, stimudents, rubber tip, etc) _____
List and describe frequency_____

Yes No U 3. Type of toothbrush used: **Hard Medium Soft**

Yes No U 4. Have you had personal instruction in oral hygiene? By whom and when?_____

Yes No U 5. Do you feel your present oral hygiene is effective in cleaning your mouth?

Yes No U 6. Have you ever had orthodontic treatment (braces)?

Yes No U 7. Are you satisfied with the way your teeth and gums look?

Yes No U 8. If unsatisfied, what would you wish to change? _____

Yes No U 9. Can you chew satisfactorily?

Yes No U 10. Have you noticed spaces developing between your teeth? When did this begin? _____

Yes No U 11. Are your gums receding? If so, where? _____

Yes No U 12. Are your teeth sensitive to hot? If so, which ones? _____

Yes No U 13. Are your teeth sensitive to cold? If so, which ones? _____

Yes No U 14. Are you aware that sensitivity of the teeth to cold can be caused by grinding?

Yes No U 15. Do you clench your teeth? If so, when? _____

Yes No U 16. Do you grind your teeth? If so, when? _____

Yes No U 17. Have you noticed your bite changing? If so, how and when? _____

Yes No U 18. Do you awaken with sore jaws? If so, how often? _____

Yes No U 19. Do you notice popping, clicking, grating, or soreness in the joints just in front of your ears? If so, please describe:
_____

Yes No U 20. Have you ever been treated for TMJ (temporomandibular joint) problems? If so, describe:_____
_____

Yes No U 21. Do you get headaches? If so, where and how often? _____

Yes No U 22. When was your last dental cleaning?_____

Yes No U 23. Date of last FULL MOUTH dental x-rays?_____

Yes No U 24. Have you ever had a frightening experience in the dental office?

Yes No U 25. Have you had previous gum trouble? If so, describe: _____

Yes No U 26. Have you had a previous gum abscess or gum boil? If so, when and in what area? _____

Yes No U 27. If you have had previous gum treatment, who performed the treatment and what type of treatment was performed? _____

Yes No U 28. Would the loss of a tooth (teeth) disturb you?

Yes No U 29. Would wearing a partial denture or false teeth bother you? If so, how much? _____

Yes No U 30. Are any of your teeth loose? If so, which ones?_____

Yes No U 31. What concerns you most about your mouth? _____

Yes No U 32. Do you suck mints, Lifesavers, etc, regularly?

Yes No U 33. Estimate the number of cups, glasses, etc, you consume each day on the average of:
coffee _____ tea_____ soft drinks _____ alcoholic beverages _____

**Do you have any dental problems or questions not covered in the above questions? If so, what? _____
_____
_____
_____

Date_____   Patient's Signature_____
(Or that of parent or guardian if patient is under 18 years of age)

Date first reviewed_____   Periodontist's Signature _____
Thomas G. Wilson, Jr. DDS

MEDICAL HISTORY UPDATE

Date _____   Health History Update: _____
                                 _____
                                 _____
Initialed By: _____ _____

Date _____   Health History Update: _____
                                 _____
                                 _____
Initialed By: _____ _____

Date _____   Health History Update: _____
                                 _____
                                 _____
Initialed By: _____ _____

Date _____   Health History Update: _____
                                 _____
                                 _____
Initialed By: _____ _____

Date _____   Health History Update: _____
                                 _____
                                 _____
Initialed By: _____ _____

Date _____   Health History Update: _____
                                 _____
                                 _____
Initialed By: _____ _____

Date _____   Health History Update: _____
                                 _____
                                 _____
Initialed By: _____ _____

Appendix 2: Premedication*†

For Patients with Specific Heart Defects or Cardiovascular Prostheses

Patients who have had a prosthetic heart valve placed and other patients at risk for developing bacterial endocarditis should have specific antibiotic coverage delivered before and after receiving dental treatment that will induce bleeding. Bleeding is a sign that blood vessels have been opened, allowing the possible inflow of bacteria. When bacteria colonize on prosthetic valves or damaged areas of the heart, the colonies can be locally invasive or can break free, causing serious systemic illness. Problems associated with bacterial endocarditis can be life threatening.

*Readers are referred to the following publication for complete details: Dajani AS, Taubert KA, Wilson W, et al. Prevention of bacterial endocarditis. Recommendations by the American Heart Association. JAMA 1997;277:1794–1801. Also available in J Am Dent Assoc 1997;128:1142–1151.
†Clinicians must use their best clinical judgment in determining the need for antibiotic prophylaxis. They are urged to consult both the patient's physician and related drug information inserts in making this decision.

For Patients with Prosthetic Joints

Bacteria from oral sources can be introduced into the blood during normal daily activities such as chewing or tooth cleaning, but may also be introduced during dental procedures. These bacteria can theoretically come to reside on prosthetic joints, and the fact that some of the organisms cultured from infected joints could have come from oral sources has led some to call for the use of prophylactic antibiotics before dental procedures that could produce these bacteremias. Other groups believe that the need for this coverage has not been documented in the literature. Clinicians are encouraged to consult the patient's physician regarding the need to premedicate.[1]

1. Advisory statement: Antibiotic prophylaxis for dental patients with total joint replacements. J Am Dent Assoc 1997;128:1004–1008.

Cardiac Conditions Associated with Endocarditis

Endocarditis prophylaxis recommended	Endocarditis prophylaxis not recommended
High-risk category • Prosthetic cardiac valves, including bioprosthetic and homograft valves • Previous bacterial endocarditis • Complex cyanotic congenital heart disease (eg, single ventricle states, transposition of the great arteries, tetralogy of Fallot) • Surgically constructed systemic pulmonary shunts or conduits *Moderate-risk category* • Most other congenital cardiac malformations (other than above and below) • Acquired valvular dysfunction (eg, rheumatic heart disease) • Hypertrophic cardiomyopathy • Mitral valve prolapse with valvular regurgitation and/or thickened leaflets	*Negligible-risk category (no greater risk than the general population)* • Isolated secundum atrial septal defect • Surgical repair of atrial septal defect, ventricular septal defect or patent ductus arteriosus (without residua beyond 6 mo) • Previous coronary artery bypass graft surgery • Mitral valve prolapse without valvular regurgitation • Physiologic, functional, or innocent heart murmurs • Previous Kawasaki disease without valvular dysfunction • Previous rheumatic fever without valvular dysfunction • Cardiac pacemakers (intravascular and epicardial) and implanted defibrillators

Adapted, with permission, from Dajani AS, Taubert KA, Wilson W, et al. Prevention of bacterial endocarditis. Recommendations by the American Heart Association. JAMA 1997;277:1794–1801. Copyrighted 1997, American Medical Association.

Dental Procedures and Endocarditis Prophylaxis

Endocarditis prophylaxis recommended*	Endocarditis prophylaxis not recommended
• Dental extractions • Periodontal procedures including surgery, scaling and root planing, probing, and recall maintenance • Dental implant placement and reimplantation of avulsed teeth • Endodontic (root canal) instrumentation or surgery only beyond the apex • Subgingival placement of antibiotic fibers or strips • Initial placement of orthodontic bands but not brackets • Intraligamentary local anesthetic injections • Prophylactic cleaning of teeth or implants where bleeding is anticipated	• Restorative dentistry[†] (operative and prosthodontic) with or without retraction cord[‡] • Local anesthetic injections (nonintraligamentary) • Intracanal endodontic treatment; post placement and buildup • Placement of rubber dams • Postoperative suture removal • Placement of removable prosthodontic or orthodontic appliances • Taking of oral impressions • Fluoride treatments • Taking of oral radiographs • Orthodontic appliance adjustment • Shedding of primary teeth

Adapted, with permission, from Dajani AS, Taubert KA, Wilson W, et al. Prevention of bacterial endocarditis. Recommendations by the American Heart Association. JAMA 1997;277:1794–1801. Copyrighted 1997, American Medical Association.
*Prophylaxis is recommended for patients with high- and moderate-risk cardiac conditions.
†This includes restoration of decayed teeth (filling cavities) and replacement of missing teeth.
‡Clinical judgment may indicate antibiotic use in selected circumstances that may create significant bleeding.

Prophylactic Regimens for Dental, Oral Respiratory Tract, or Esophageal Procedures*

Situation	Agent	Regimen[†]
Standard general prophylaxis	Amoxicillin	Adults: 2.0 g; Children: 50 mg/kg; orally 1 h before procedure
Unable to take oral medication	Ampicillin	Adults: 2.0 g; intramuscularly (IM) or intravenously (IV); Children: 50 mg/kg IM or IV within 30 min before procedure
Allergic to penicillin	Clindamycin	Adults: 600 mg; Children: 20 mg/kg orally 1 h before procedure
	Cephalexin or cefadroxil[‡]	Adults: 2.0 g; Children: 50 mg/kg orally 1 h before procedure
	Azithromycin or clarithromycin	Adults: 500 mg; Children: 15 mg/kg orally 1 h before procedure
Allergic to penicillin and unable to take oral medication	Clindamycin	Adults: 600 mg; Children: 20 mg/kg orally 30 min before procedure
	Cefazolin[‡]	Adults: 1.0 g; Children: 25 mg/kg IM or IV within 30 min before procedure

Adapted, with permission, from Dajani AS, Taubert KA, Wilson W, et al. Prevention of bacterial endocarditis. Recommendations by the American Heart Association. JAMA 1997;277:1794–1801. Copyrighted 1997, American Medical Association.
*Clinicians are advised to consult official product information regarding drugs and their dosages to verify accuracy prior to administering treatment.
†Total children's dose should not exceed adult dose.
‡Cephalosporins should not be used in individuals with immediate-type hypersensitivity reaction (urticaria, anaphylaxis) to penicillins.

Index